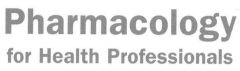

Pharmacology
for Health Professionals

2nd edition

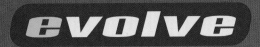

The Latest *Evolution* in Learning

Evolve provides online access to free learning resources and activities designed specifically for the textbook you are using in your class.

The resources will enhance your learning of the material covered in the book and much more.

Visit the website listed below to start your learning evolution today!

LOGIN: http://evolve.elsevier.com/AU/Bryant/pharmacology/

Evolve Online resources for *Pharmacology for Health Professionals 2e* include:

For students and instructors

- Nursing, Midwifery, Paramedic and Complementary Medicines content — discipline-specific resources including learning objectives, additional information, case studies with questions, and crossword puzzles.
- WebLinks — an exciting resource that lets you link to other websites carefully chosen to supplement the content of the textbook.
- Animations — demonstrating important key concepts found in the textbook.
- Student quizzes — includes multiple choice, true/false, fill-in-the-blank and matching questions with instant scoring and feedback at the click of a button.
- Student online drug calculations — an interactive program providing a variety of questions created to help you learn the essential skills of dosage calculations.

For instructors only

- Test Bank with nearly 600 multiple choice questions
- Solutions to end-of-chapter review exercises
- Selected tables from the text including Clinical Interest Boxes and Drugs at a Glance tables
- Image collection

Think **outside** the book...**evolve**.

Pharmacology
for Health Professionals

Bronwen Bryant **Kathleen Knights**

Evelyn Salerno

2nd edition

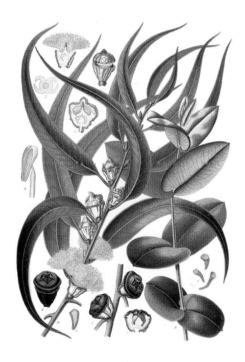

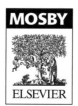

MOSBY

ELSEVIER

Sydney   Edinburgh   London   New York   Philadelphia
St Louis   Toronto

ELSEVIER

Mosby
is an imprint of Elsevier

Elsevier Australia
(a division of Reed International Books Australia Pty Ltd)
30–52 Smidmore Street, Marrickville, NSW 2204
ACN 001 002 357

This edition © 2007 Elsevier Australia

National Library of *Australia Cataloguing-in-Publication Data*

Bryant, Bronwen Jean.
Pharmacology for health professionals.

2nd ed.
Includes index.

ISBN-13: 978-0-7295-3787-2 (pbk.).
ISBN-10: 0-7295-3787-0 (pbk.).

1. Pharmacology. I. Knights, Kathleen M. (Kathleen Mary).
II. Salerno, Evelyn. III. Title.

615.1

Publisher: Debbie Lee
Publishing Editor: Ann Crabb
Developmental Editors: Suzanne Hall & Mae-wha Boadle
Publishing Services Manager: Helena Klijn
Edited and project managed by Kate Ormston-Jeffery & Deborah McRitchie
Proofread by Andy Whyte
Technical checking by Jerry Perkins and Lynne Mackinnon
Cover and internal design by Avril Makula
Index by Jon Jermey and Glenda Browne
Typeset by Egan-Reid Pty Limited
Printed in Hong Kong by China Translation & Printing Services Ltd

Dedications

To my pharmacological mentors, the late Professor Diana Temple, the late Michael
Rand, and David Story, with thanks; and to my daughters Rosemary, Philippa and Alison,
who continually inspire, encourage and amaze me.

Bronwen J Bryant

To my husband, John, who inspires me,
and my family and friends who support me.

Kathleen M Knights

About the Authors

BRONWEN BRYANT

Bronwen originally studied pharmacy at the University of Sydney and became fascinated with pharmacology, so completed an Honours year then a Master of Science degree under the supervision of Associate Professor Diana Temple, with research in areas of biochemical and cardiovascular pharmacology. She also taught pharmacy, science and dentistry students. After two years' research at Riker Laboratories in Sydney, and work in both community and hospital pharmacies to gain registration as a pharmacist, she moved to London and worked as a medical translator and editor.

Returning to Australia, Bronwen accepted a research position at the University of Melbourne in the laboratory of Professor Michael Rand and Dr David Story, where she completed a PhD on negative feedback control of central autonomic transmission. Academic jobs teaching pharmacology followed at various institutions: the Victorian College of Pharmacy, Lincoln Institute, and La Trobe University. Along the way she has managed to do sporadic research in clinical pharmacology (adverse drug reactions and interactions, non-steroidal anti-inflammatory drugs and psychotherapeutics), and has taught students of virtually every health profession.

Eventually greener fields (or bluer seas) beckoned, and Bronwen is currently Associate Professor of Pharmacology at the Fiji School of Medicine in Suva, teaching students of medicine, pharmacy and dentistry from Fiji, the Cook Islands, East Timor, Kiribati, Micronesia, Samoa, the Solomon Islands, Tonga, Vanuatu, and even New Zealand and Australia.

KATHLEEN KNIGHTS

Kathie completed a Bachelor of Science (Honours) degree at North East London Polytechnic (NELP), majoring in pharmacology while working as a research assistant at Guy's Hospital, London. On returning home to Adelaide she accepted a research position in the Department of Anaesthesia and Intensive Care in the School of Medicine at Flinders University. Following receipt of an Australian Commonwealth Postgraduate Research Scholarship, Kathie completed a PhD investigating the hepatotoxicity of the inhalational anaesthetic agent, halothane.

Her academic career has continued to develop throughout her time at Flinders, progressing from her initial appointment as Lecturer to her current position of Reader in Clinical Pharmacology (Associate Professor). She is passionate about the discipline of pharmacology and her teaching crosses discipline boundaries covering medicine, nursing, nutrition and dietetics and paramedic sciences. Recently she steered the development of a pharmacology package delivered on-line to Masters level students in rural and remote areas of Australia.

Kathie's research interests centre on drug metabolism, specifically the metabolism of non-steroidal anti-inflammatory drugs and their mechanisms of renal toxicity. An invited speaker at national and international conferences, she has published over 40 research articles and reviews in peer-reviewed international journals.

Book at a glance

Get the most out of your textbook by familiarising yourself with the key features of this new edition of *Pharmacology for Health Professionals*.

Colours at a glance

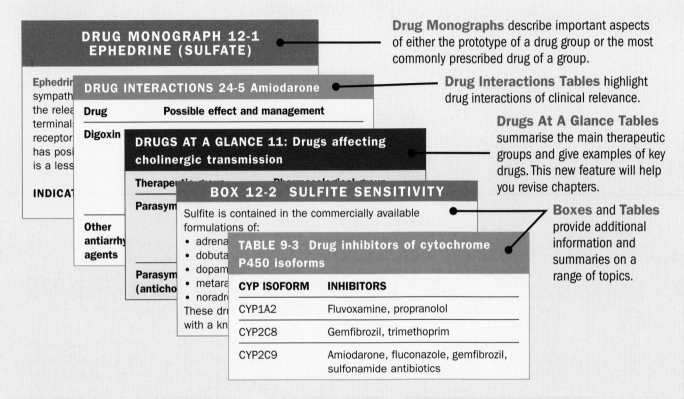

DRUG MONOGRAPH 12-1 EPHEDRINE (SULFATE)

Drug Monographs describe important aspects of either the prototype of a drug group or the most commonly prescribed drug of a group.

DRUG INTERACTIONS 24-5 Amiodarone

Drug	Possible effect and management
Digoxin	

Drug Interactions Tables highlight drug interactions of clinical relevance.

DRUGS AT A GLANCE 11: Drugs affecting cholinergic transmission

Drugs At A Glance Tables summarise the main therapeutic groups and give examples of key drugs. This new feature will help you revise chapters.

BOX 12-2 SULFITE SENSITIVITY

Sulfite is contained in the commercially available formulations of:
- adrena
- dobuta
- dopam
- metara
- noradr

These dr
with a kn

Boxes and **Tables** provide additional information and summaries on a range of topics.

TABLE 9-3 Drug inhibitors of cytochrome P450 isoforms

CYP ISOFORM	INHIBITORS
CYP1A2	Fluvoxamine, propranolol
CYP2C8	Gemfibrozil, trimethoprim
CYP2C9	Amiodarone, fluconazole, gemfibrozil, sulfonamide antibiotics

---

Special interest boxes address items of clinical interest, including drug research, complementary medicines, indigenous issues and lifespan aspects of drug therapy.

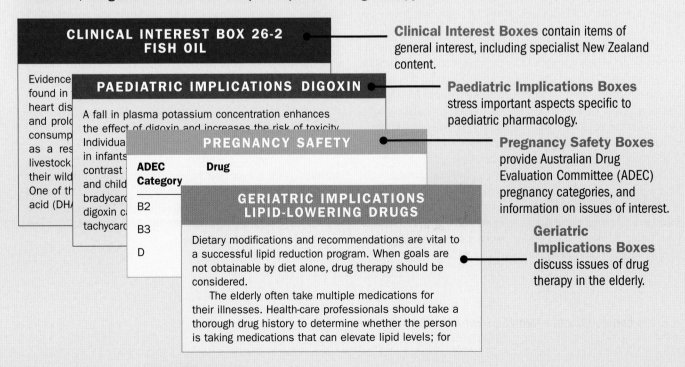

CLINICAL INTEREST BOX 26-2 FISH OIL

Clinical Interest Boxes contain items of general interest, including specialist New Zealand content.

PAEDIATRIC IMPLICATIONS DIGOXIN

A fall in plasma potassium concentration enhances the effect of digoxin and increases the risk of toxicity.

Paediatric Implications Boxes stress important aspects specific to paediatric pharmacology.

PREGNANCY SAFETY

ADEC Category	Drug
B2	
B3	
D	

Pregnancy Safety Boxes provide Australian Drug Evaluation Committee (ADEC) pregnancy categories, and information on issues of interest.

GERIATRIC IMPLICATIONS LIPID-LOWERING DRUGS

Dietary modifications and recommendations are vital to a successful lipid reduction program. When goals are not obtainable by diet alone, drug therapy should be considered.

The elderly often take multiple medications for their illnesses. Health-care professionals should take a thorough drug history to determine whether the person is taking medications that can elevate lipid levels; for

Geriatric Implications Boxes discuss issues of drug therapy in the elderly.

Icons at a glance

 These Clinical Interest Boxes discuss information specific to New Zealand.

Discipline-specific Icons are new to this edition and point to where further Evolve Online resources can be found for:

 Nursing   Midwifery   Paramedic   Complementary medicine

Visit http://evolve.elsevier.com/AU/Bryant/pharmacology/

Text at a glance

Chapters have been carefully structured to aid learning.
Chapter openings are designed to help you focus and mentally organise content.

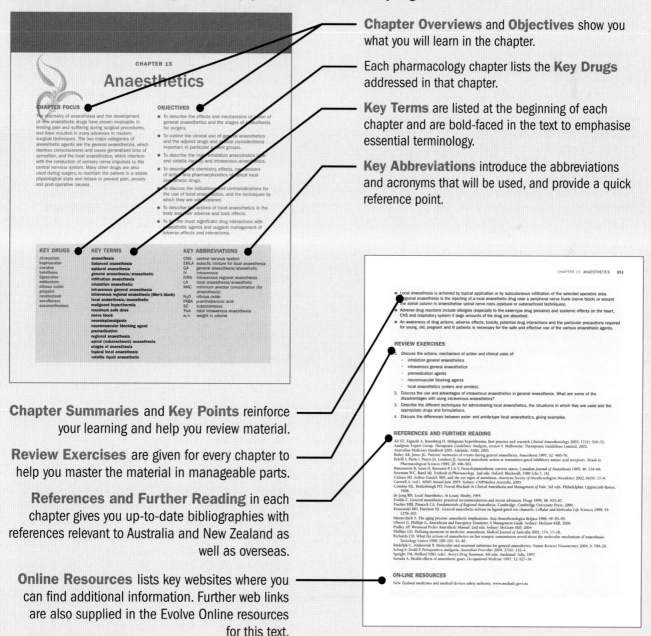

Chapter Overviews and **Objectives** show you what you will learn in the chapter.

Each pharmacology chapter lists the **Key Drugs** addressed in that chapter.

Key Terms are listed at the beginning of each chapter and are bold-faced in the text to emphasise essential terminology.

Key Abbreviations introduce the abbreviations and acronyms that will be used, and provide a quick reference point.

Chapter Summaries and **Key Points** reinforce your learning and help you review material.

Review Exercises are given for every chapter to help you master the material in manageable parts.

References and Further Reading in each chapter gives you up-to-date bibliographies with references relevant to Australia and New Zealand as well as overseas.

Online Resources lists key websites where you can find additional information. Further web links are also supplied in the Evolve Online resources for this text.

CONTENTS

Book at a Glance   vi

Preface   xii

Notes to the User   xv

Figures   xvi

Clinical Interest Boxes   xix

Drug Monographs   xxii

Drug Monographs A–Z   xxiii

UNIT I
Introduction to Pharmacology   1

1   **Drugs, Medicines and Health Professionals   1**
Introduction and definitions   2
A brief history of pharmacology   4
Sources of drugs   7
Drug names and classifications   12
Drug information   16
Dosage measurements and calculations   19

2   **Pharmacotherapy: Clinical Use of Drugs   26**
Quality use of medicines (QUM)   27
Roles of health professionals with respect to drugs   31
Decisions to be made before prescribing drugs   35
Prescriptions   36
Pharmaceutics: formulations of drugs   39
Therapeutic drug monitoring (TDM)   45

3   **Over-the-counter Drugs and Complementary Therapies   50**
Regulation of drugs   51
Complementary and alternative therapies in relation to pharmacology   59

4   **Legal and Ethical Foundations of Pharmacotherapy   73**
Legal aspects of drug use in health care   74
Standardisation of drugs   84
Drug discovery and development   86
Ethical principles related to drug use in health care   96

UNIT II
Principles of Pharmacology   102

5   **Molecular Aspects of Drug Action and Pharmacodynamics   102**
Molecular targets for drug action   103
Pharmacodynamics   106

6   **Drug Absorption, Distribution, Metabolism and Excretion   111**
Pharmaceutical phase   112
Pharmacokinetic phase   113

7   **Pharmacokinetics and Dosing Regimens   128**
Plasma concentration–time profile of a drug   129
Clearance   131
Volume of distribution   133
Half-life   133
Saturable metabolism   134

8   **Individual and Lifespan Aspects of Drug Therapy   137**
Drug use during pregnancy   138
Drug use during lactation   142
Drug metabolism in children   144
Drug use in the elderly   147

9   **Adverse Drug Reactions and Drug Interactions   152**
Definitions   153
History of adverse drug reactions   153
Incidence of adverse drug reactions   153
Classification of adverse drug reactions   154
Risk factors for developing an adverse drug reaction   155
Drug–drug interactions   156
Strategies for limiting adverse drug reactions and drug interactions   159

UNIT III
Drugs Affecting the Peripheral Nervous System   162

10   **Overview of the Autonomic Nervous System   162**
Differences between the parasympathetic and sympathetic nervous systems   164
Action potential generation and neurochemical transmission   165
Transmitters in the peripheral nervous system   169

11   **Drugs Affecting Cholinergic Transmission   177**
Drugs acting at muscarinic receptors   178
Ganglion-blocking drugs   182

12   **Drugs Affecting Noradrenergic Transmission   185**
Adrenergic drugs   186
Adrenoceptor antagonists   193

13   **Overview of the Somatic Nervous System and Drugs Affecting Neuromuscular Transmission   201**
The neuromuscular junction   202
Neuromuscular blocking drugs   204
Anticholinesterase agents   205

UNIT IV
Drugs Affecting the Central Nervous System   212

14 Overview of the Central Nervous System   212

15 Anaesthetics   226
General anaesthesia   227
Local anaesthesia   239

16 Analgesics   251
Physiology of pain   252
Pain management   256
Analgesic drugs and methods   259

17 Antianxiety, Sedative and Hypnotic Drugs   281
Physiology of sleep   282
Sleep disorders   283
Anxiety   284
Drug use in specific groups   285
Benzodiazepines   285
Other antianxiety and sedative/hypnotic agents   289

18 Antiepileptic Drugs   296
Epilepsy   297
Antiepileptic therapy   299

19 Psychotropic Agents   311
Psychotropics and antipsychotics   312
Models used in psychiatry   312
The central nervous system, the mind and emotions   313
Clinical aspects of drug therapy in psychiatry   314
Antipsychotic agents   322
Treatment of affective disorders   325

20 Central Nervous System Stimulants   338
Amphetamines   339
CNS stimulants in treatment of ADHD and narcolepsy   340
CNS stimulants as anorectic agents   342
Methylxanthines caffeine   343

21 Drugs for Neurodegenerative Disorders and Migraine   348
Drug treatment of Parkinson's disease   349
Drugs affecting skeletal muscles   355
Drug treatment of other movement disorders   359
Drug treatment of dementias   360
Drugs used In migraine and other headaches   363

22 Drug Dependence and Social Pharmacology   370
Drug dependence, misuse and abuse   371
Aetiological factors leading to drug abuse and dependence   372
Problems associated with drug abuse   376
Policies related to drug abuse and its management   378
Treating drug dependence   380
Opioids (heroin, morphine and other agonist opioids)   383
Central nervous system depressants   386
CNS stimulants   392
Psychotomimetics   399
Other drugs of abuse   405

UNIT V
Drugs Affecting the Heart and Vascular System   410

23 Overview of the Heart and Vascular System   410
The heart   411
Cardiac function   418
The peripheral vascular system   419

24 Drugs Affecting Cardiac Function   421
Cardiac glycosides   423
Phosphodiesterase inhibitors   428
Antiarrhythmic drugs   428

25 Drugs Affecting Vascular Smooth Muscle   440
Angina   441
Vasodilator drugs—direct-acting   441
Peripheral vascular disease   449
Management of hypertension   450
Vasodilator drugs—indirect-acting   450

26 Lipid-lowering Drugs   461
Dyslipidaemia   462
Management strategies for dyslipidaemia   465

UNIT VI
Drugs Affecting the Kidney and Urinary System   473

27 Overview of the Kidney and Urinary Tract   473
Anatomy and physiology of the kidney   474
Micturition   478

28 Diuretics and Drug Treatment of Urinary Incontinence   480
Diuretics   482
Drugs for urinary incontinence   487

UNIT VII
Drugs Affecting the Blood   491

29 Overview of the Haemopoietic System   491
Blood composition   492
Blood cell formation   492
Red blood cells (erythrocytes)   493
White blood cells (leucocytes)   494
Platelets   494
Coagulation   494
Blood groups and types   497

30 Drugs Affecting Haemostasis, Thrombosis and the Haemopoietic System   499
Anticoagulant drugs   500
Thrombolytic drugs   506
Antiplatelet agents   507
Haemostatic and antifibrinolytic drugs   510
Haemopoietics and haematinics   512

UNIT VIII
Drugs Affecting The Respiratory System   515

31   Overview of the Respiratory System   515
The respiratory system   516
Aerosol therapy   519

32   Drugs Used in Respiratory Disorders   523
Respiratory gases   524
Respiratory stimulants and depressants   528
Drugs affecting secretions and mucociliary
   transport   528
Drug treatment of asthma   531
Drug treatment of chronic obstructive pulmonary disease
   (COPD)   541
Drugs used in respiratory tract infections   542
Drugs affecting the nose   547

UNIT IX
Drugs Affecting the Gastrointestinal System   552

33   Overview of the Gastrointestinal Tract   552
The gastrointestinal tract   553

34   Drugs Affecting the Gastrointestinal Tract   562
Drugs that affect the mouth   563
Drugs that affect the stomach   565
Drugs for nausea and vomiting   567
Drugs used to treat peptic ulcer disease   570
Pancreatic enzyme supplements   573
Drugs that affect the biliary system   574
Drugs that affect the lower gastrointestinal tract   574

UNIT X
Drugs Affecting the Eye, Ear and Special Senses   584

35   Drugs Affecting the Eye   584
Overview of the eye   585
Ocular administration of drugs   586
Autonomic nervous system effects on the eye   588
Antiglaucoma agents   592
Antimicrobial agents   595
Anti-inflammatory and antiallergy agents   597
Ocular local anaesthetics   598
Other ophthalmic preparations   599
Systemic diseases and drugs affecting the eye   602
Ocular adverse drug reactions from systemic drugs   603

36   Drugs Affecting Hearing, Taste and Smell   610
Anatomy and physiology of the ear   611
Common ear disorders   611
Drugs affecting the ear   613

UNIT XI
Drugs Affecting the Endocrine System   620

37   Overview of the Endocrine System   620
Hormones and endocrine glands   621
The major endocrine glands   627

38   Pharmacology of the Pituitary Gland and Hypothalamic–Pituitary Axis   629
The pituitary gland   630

39   The Thyroid Gland and Antithyroid Drugs   639
The thyroid gland   640
Treatment of hypothyroidism   643
Treatment of hyperthyroidism   645

40   Pharmacology of the Adrenal Cortex   652
General aspects of the adrenal glands   653
Glucocorticoids   655
Mineralocorticoids   659
Adrenal steroid synthesis inhibitors   662

41   The Endocrine Pancreas and Management of Diabetes Mellitus   665
The endocrine pancreas   666
Diabetes mellitus   667
Management of diabetes mellitus   671
Hyperglycaemic agents   680

42   The Parathyroid Glands and Calcium Balance   684
The parathyroid glands   685
Calcium balance and mineral homeostasis   687
Bone mineral homeostasis and phosphate levels   690
Bone pathologies   690
Effects of drugs on bone   692

UNIT XII
Drugs Affecting the Reproductive Systems   696

43   Overview of the Female and Male Reproductive Systems   696
Endocrine glands   697
Hypothalamic and pituitary control of reproductive
   functions   698
The female reproductive system   700
The male reproductive system   705

44   Drugs Affecting the Female Reproductive System   708
Female sex hormones   709
Oral contraceptives   712
Menopause and hormone replacement therapy   717
Treatment of gynaecological disorders   720

45   Drugs in Pregnancy, Childbirth and Lactation   724
Drugs in pregnancy   725
Drugs affecting the uterus   726
Drugs in the perinatal period   729
Lactation   730

46   Drugs Affecting the Male Reproductive System   733
The male reproductive system   734
Benign prostatic hyperplasia   736

47   Drugs Affecting Fertility or Sexual Functioning   739
Drugs that affect fertility   740
Drugs that affect sexual functioning   745

UNIT XIII
Drugs Used in Neoplastic Diseases   754

48   Overview of Neoplasia and Cancer Chemotherapy   754
Tumour cell biology   755
Treatment of cancer   760

49   Antineoplastic Agents   769
Cytotoxic agents   770
Hormones   777
Miscellaneous antineoplastic agents   781
Supportive therapy in the treatment of cancer   783
Cancer chemotherapy research   788

UNIT XIV
Drugs Affecting Microorganisms   793

50   Overview of Antimicrobial Chemotherapy and Antibiotic Resistance   793
Infections   794
Antimicrobial therapy   794
Antibiotic resistance   797
Superinfection   798
General guidelines for use of antibiotics   798
Role of host defence mechanisms   800
Dosage and duration of therapy   800

51   Antibacterial drugs   803
Inhibitors of bacterial cell wall synthesis   804
Bacterial protein synthesis inhibitors   812
Miscellaneous antibiotics   819
Urinary tract antimicrobials   820

52   Antifungal and Antiviral Drugs   825
Antifungal drugs   826
Antiviral drugs   831

53   Antiprotozoal, Antimycobacterial and Anthelmintic Drugs   847
Malaria   848
Amoebiasis   854
Toxoplasmosis   855
Trichomoniasis   855
Mycobacterial infections   855
Helminthiasis   862
Anthelmintic drugs   864

UNIT XV
Drugs Affecting Body Defences   869

54   Overview of Mediators of Inflammation, Allergy and the Immune Response   869
The immune system   870
Resistance to disease   871
Natural and acquired immunity   875

55   Anti-inflammatory and Immunomodulating Drugs   878
Non-steroidal anti-inflammatory drugs (NSAIDs)   879
Disease-modifying antirheumatic drugs (DMARDs)   884
Drugs used for the treatment of gout   887

Immunosuppressant drugs   890
Immunostimulant drugs   895
Histamine and histamine-receptor antagonists (antihistamines)   896

56   Drugs Affecting the Skin   903
Structure and functions of the skin   904
Skin disorders   905
Application of drugs to the skin   908
Sunscreen preparations   911
Topical antimicrobial agents   914
Anti-inflammatory and immunomodulating agents   917
Retinoids and treatment of acne   920
Treatment of burns   922
Management of pressure sores   925

UNIT XVI
Special Topics   932

57   Drugs in Sport   932
Drugs and methods banned in sports   934
Drugs restricted in certain sports or competitors   939
Substances and methods permitted in sports   939
Drug testing procedures   941
Ethical aspects of drugs in sport   942

58   Drugs in Obesity   946
Health risks associated with obesity   947
Pathophysiology of obesity   948
Management of obesity   950
Drug therapy   950
The future   953

59   Envenomation and Antivenoms   956
Snakes   957
Spiders   960
Marine envenomation   962

APPENDICES   966

1   Abbreviations   966

2   Antiseptics and Disinfectants   969

3   Herb-, Nutrient- and Food–Drug Interactions   971

4   Glossary   973

5   Australian and New Zealand Schedules for Drugs and Poisons   981
Classification of poisons   981

6   Poisons Information Centres   983
Drug (or Medicines) Information Centres   983

7   The World Health Organization List of Essential Medicines   985

FIGURE AND PICTURE CREDITS   985

INDEX   991

PREFACE

The use of drugs for their curative properties, for their social effects and indeed in many instances for sinister purposes has no cultural, historical or social boundaries. Pharmacy practices during the ancient Egyptian civilisation are recorded in the *Ebers Papyrus* dating back to 1500 BC; the 15th century German physician, Paracelsus, used mercury to treat syphilis; while courtesans of the French court frequently used a preparation of *Atropa belladonna* to dilate their pupils and enhance their mystical qualities. South American native people perfected the preparation of curare and used it as a poison on the tips of their arrows when hunting wild animals and to test the strength of their warriors in trials by ordeal. Australian Aboriginal people used a native tobacco, from *Duboisia* species, for the atropinic alkaloids it contained. In Fiji, kava (yaqona or 'grog') is drunk ritually and socially for its stress-relieving, relaxing and euphoriant properties.

These fascinating aspects of pharmacology are all too often lost when students, faced with an overwhelming wealth of information on a vast array of drugs, see only the need to remember enough facts to pass their next assessment. Drugs in clinical use continue to have a high rate of obsolescence, and the facts learned for a particular drug may be irrelevant when each year brings new drugs with differing modes of action. The challenge for all health professionals is to stay up to date with advances in the field of pharmacology and their impact on the quality use of medicines. We hope the second edition, as with the first, makes the challenge enjoyable, interesting and easy and, as authors, that our continuing fascination with pharmacology is transmitted to you, the readers.

Pharmacology is a universal discipline but the availability of drugs and the patterns of their use differ between countries. Unlike many pharmacology texts, that are biased towards students in the northern hemisphere, this second edition continues to be ideally suited to the needs of all health professionals practising in Australia and New Zealand. The discussion of drugs reflect the names used, the availability and clinical use within the Australasian region, and the material on drug legislation and ethical principles focuses on regional aspects. To complement and enhance this regional flavour, information on traditional medicinal plants and patterns of use of medicines by Australian Aboriginal, New Zealand Māori and Pacific Island people are interspersed in relevant chapters.

Pharmacology texts written especially for medical students continue to emphasise selection, prescription and monitoring of drugs based on diagnosis of a condition in a patient, while those written for pharmacy and science students often give detailed descriptions of the chemistry of the drugs and the biochemistry of the pathways and disease processes in which they act. The needs of other students of health sciences lie somewhere between these approaches: while ambulance paramedics and practitioners of professions such as nursing, podiatry, physiotherapy, dentistry, optometry and orthoptics may not be regularly prescribing or dispensing drugs, they are increasingly finding that their patients and clients are taking many medications, some prescribed and some self-prescribed. Thus it is increasingly important that all health professionals have an appreciation of pharmacology and its important principles, to be able to understand and predict the effects of drugs in people and to consider how drugs may affect a person's health and lifestyle. Throughout this second edition, we have retained both a scientific and a clinical approach, founded on evidence-based medicine, and emphasising always the use and effects of drugs in people. We are confident that this second edition will continue to fulfil the needs of students and academics in all health professions.

In this edition, all material has been updated and revised in the light of recent research findings, introductions of new drugs, withdrawals of old drugs, and changes in recommendations from learned bodies on pharmacological management of disease conditions. Major updates of material have occurred in chapters 9 (Adverse Drug Reactions and Drug Interactions), 16 (Analgesics), 22 (Drug Dependence), 30 (Drugs Affecting Haemostasis, Thrombosis and the Haemopoietic System), 48 and 49 (drugs in cancer), 50–52 (antimicrobials) and 57 (Drugs in Sport, including new listings of banned drugs).

A new chapter, 'Envenomation and Antivenoms', has been included, which contains information on envenomation by spiders, snakes, and marine species and the current recommendations for treatment. Many of the figures and diagrams have been redrawn and new figures included to enhance understanding and interest, e.g. mechanisms of bacterial resistance, platelet activation, sites of action of disease modifying antirheumatic drugs, cellular mechanisms involved in actions of some anticancer drugs, and the step-wise management of pain and of asthma. This new edition also features:

- new and updated Drug Monographs that describe important aspects of either the prototype of a drug group or the most commonly prescribed drug of a group, or, drugs that have gained 'drug of first choice' status; for example, fluoxetine replaces amitriptyline, latanoprost replaces dorzolamide
- more details of drug interactions occurring with major drug groups

- information on recent changes in the pharmacological management of major conditions, including asthma, cardiac failure, dementia, diabetes mellitus, dyslipidaemia, epilepsy, HIV, hypertension, osteoporosis and rheumatoid arthritis
- many interesting new drugs, including verteporfin for ocular macular degeneration, strontium ranelate and teriparatide for osteoporosis, and the antiplatelet drug clopidogrel and the glycoprotein IIb/IIIa receptor inhibitors abciximab, eptifibate and tirofiban
- many new Clinical Interest Boxes that describe items of special interest specific to New Zealand, and references to material from the NZ Medicines and Medical Devices Safety Authority (at www.medsafe.govt.nz)

- enhanced information on the use of complementary and alternative medicine (CAM) modalities, and on interactions between drugs and CAM therapies
- references to new reviews on drugs and management of major diseases, and guidelines for clinical choice and use of drugs (while retaining references to 'classic' scientific papers and reference material)
- a fresh new full-colour treatment to distinguish the text elements and to make navigating the text easy.

Information on the clinical use of drugs is based especially on data in the *Australian Medicines Handbook*, the Therapeutic Guidelines series, and reviews in *Drugs*, the *Medical Journal of Australia* and *Australian Prescriber*.

Acknowledgements

The authors thank all readers (students, academics and colleagues) of the first edition who provided helpful and constructive comments, which we have addressed in this edition.

CONTRIBUTORS
The authors thank and acknowledge the invaluable assistance of the following people, whose time and expertise contributed to the accuracy and clarity of the information:

Rosemary Bryant-Smith, Lawyer, Melbourne

Shaunagh Darroch, Pharmacologist, Melbourne

Gail Easterbrook, Drug Information Pharmacist, Flinders Medical Centre, SA

Dr Paraskevi Gaganis, Postdoctoral Research Officer, Department of Clinical Pharmacology, Flinders University, SA

Dr Thérèse Kairuz, Senior Lecturer, School of Pharmacy, The University of Auckland, New Zealand

Professor Nerida Smith, Head, School of Pharmacy, Griffith University, formerly Department of Pharmacology and Toxicology, University of Otago, New Zealand.

REVIEWERS
The authors and Elsevier Australia are grateful to the following reviewers for their insightful observations and recommendations, which greatly assisted us in developing the second edition:

Robin Fisher, Lecturer in Science, School of Nursing, Australian Catholic University, QLD

Dr Mark S Harvey, Senior Curator, Department of Terrestrial Invertebrates, Western Australian Museum, WA

Anecita Gigi Lim, Senior Lecturer, School of Nursing, University of Auckland, New Zealand

Gayle McKenzie, Lecturer, School of Nursing and Midwifery, La Trobe University, VIC

Gael Mearns, Lecturer, Faculty of Health and Environmental Sciences, Auckland University of Technology, New Zealand

Dr Jennifer Padmanabhan, Lecturer, Faculty of Health Sciences and Technology, Universal College of Learning, Palmerston North, New Zealand

Dr Rachel Page, Director of Sport and Life Science Cluster, Institute of Food, Nutrition and Human Health (IFNHH), College of Sciences, Massey University, New Zealand

Dr Penny Paliadelis, Lecturer, School of Health, University of New England, NSW

Dr Glenn Shea, Senior Lecturer, Faculty of Veterinary Science, University of Sydney, NSW

ANCILLARY AUTHORS
Elsevier Australia would like to thank the following people for developing and updating the content for the Evolve website that accompanies the second edition of *Pharmacology for Health Professionals*:

Helen Aikman, Lecturer, Department of Nursing and Midwifery, La Trobe University, VIC: Student Quizzes and Answers

Shaunagh Darroch, Pharmacologist, Melbourne, VIC: Instructional Designer, Testbank, Solutions to Review Exercises, Weblinks

Patricia Logan-Sinclair, Lecturer, School of Nursing and Health Sciences, Charles Sturt University, NSW: Dosage Calculations program

Lisa McKenna, Senior Lecturer, School of Nursing and Midwifery, Monash University, VIC: Nursing and Midwifery content

Evelin Tiralongo, Lecturer, School of Pharmacy, Griffith University, QLD: Complementary & Alternative Medicines content

Helen Webb, Senior Lecturer, School of Health, Victoria University, VIC: Paramedic content

COLLEAGUES AND EDITORS

We would like to acknowledge the support of our colleagues at Flinders University (KMK), the Fiji School of Medicine and La Trobe University (BJB); and the authors who kindly gave permission to use or adapt their work for our purposes, in particular Professors Bill Bowman, the late Michael Rand, and John Murtagh.

Our role as authors has again been challenging, and we record our thanks to staff and associates of Elsevier Australia, especially Vaughn Curtis, Helena Klijn, Ann Crabb and Mae-wha Boadle for their stimulus, guidance and patience,

editors Kate Ormston-Jeffery and Deb McRitchie for their editorial rigour, and Jerry Perkins and Lynne Mackinnon for their careful technical checking. It is inevitable that recommendations for drug indications and dosage will change—we apologise for any errors and welcome comments and feedback on the second edition of *Pharmacology for Health Professionals*.

Bronwen J Bryant   *Kathleen M Knights*
Fiji School of Medicine   *Flinders University*

October 2006

NOTES TO THE USER

Book structure

In our view, understanding pharmacology is made easier by an appreciation of the relevant underlying physiology, biochemistry and pathology. As with the first edition, this book is divided into Units, each of which begins with an overview of the physiological, and biochemical processes that underpin the subsequent pharmacology chapters. We still believe this enhances understanding of the cellular and molecular aspects of drug action, the rationales for the application of drugs in particular disease processes, and the clinical use of drugs with their therapeutic and adverse effects and drug interactions. As seemed most appropriate, in some chapters information is based on drug groups, with relevant details of the diseases for which they may be indicated, whereas in others the flow of information starts with the disease or condition and leads on to a discussion of the drug groups relevant to treatment.

Units I and II introduce general aspects of the clinical use of drugs and principles of pharmacology. Units III–XII considers drugs acting on the major systems of the body, from the autonomic nervous system through to the reproductive system. Units XIII–XV cover drugs affecting general pathological conditions, including neoplasia, infections and inflammations, and Unit XVI includes discussions of drugs used in sport and in the treatment of obesity, and a chapter on envenomation and antivenoms.

Terms and spelling

With our rich Australasian heritage of language, it is inevitable that there are many spellings and terminologies about which people feel strongly. We have agreed on the following usages, and apologise to those we offend:

- arrhythmia: as the terms arrhythmia and antiarrhythmic drugs are in common usage they have been retained in this book. It is acknowledged that the prefix 'a' means 'without' and in that regard the only arrhythmia is asystole. The correct term is 'dysrhythmia', the prefix dys meaning 'difficulty with'.
- we have now adopted the generally accepted spelling 'fetus' rather than 'foetus' as used in the first edition.
- gonadotrophin, etc: the suffix 'trophic' means bringing nourishment, whereas 'tropic' means turning or moving in response to a stimulus; they appear to have become interchangeable in words like gonadotrophin. There is an understanding that the English term is '-trophin' whereas '-tropin' is American usage. We have standardised on the English form -trophin except where the approved name for a hormone or drug is otherwise, as in somatropin and follitropin.
- receptor: because many drugs interact with molecular targets (e.g. enzymes, ion channels and receptors), we have chosen to standardise the use of the term 'receptor' in accordance with the IUPHAR Committee on Receptor Nomenclature and Drug Classification 1998 (see Chapter 5).
- 5-hydroxytryptamine: in line with accepted terminology, the term '5-hydroxytryptamine', abbreviated as 5-HT, is used throughout this book. Use of the term 'serotonin' is restricted to the first mention of 5-HT in a chapter (as a reminder that this is synonymous with 5-HT) and in reference to specific drug groups, e.g. selective serotonin reuptake inhibitors.
- drug names: throughout the text, Australian approved (generic) drug names are used; when these are markedly different from American and/or Canadian names, this may be noted for clarity; thus ' ... paracetamol, known as acetaminophen in the USA ...'. Since a drug may be marketed under many trade names and subject to frequent changes or deletions, we have not included trade names except in instances where readers may be so familiar with a trade name as to identify most readily with it, e.g. diazepam, marketed as Valium, paracetamol as Panadol, or sildenafil as Viagra.
- although the terms 'adverse effect', 'adverse reaction' and 'adverse event' are often used (mistakenly) interchangeably, we have standardised the use of these terms through out the book. Simply stated, a drug causes an *adverse effect*, a patient suffers an *adverse reaction* to a drug, and an *adverse event* occurs while a person is taking a drug but it is not necessarily due to the drug (see Chapter 9 for full explanations).
- drugs affecting (a system): we have used this term purposely at times, e.g. Drugs Affecting the Skin, to include not only drugs used in treatment of conditions of the organ or system, but also drugs that may have adverse effects particularly in that system, or may be administered to that tissue to have an action elsewhere in the body.

FIGURES

1-1   Chemical structures of some active drugs derived from plant sources
2-1   Typical prescriptions
2-2   Part of a typical medication therapy chart from a patient's hospital record (also known as the patient's drug chart)
2-3   A typical intravenous infusion set-up, showing a secondary 'piggyback' bottle with a reservoir of drug in IV fluid
4-1   Drug Regulation in Australia: from new drug application to the prescription pad
4-2   The 'blue form', on which suspected adverse reactions to drugs and vaccines are reported
5-1   Membrane localisation of a typical G-protein-coupled receptor
5-2   Schematic representation of activation of G-protein-coupled receptors by drugs
5-3   A drug concentration–response curve plotted on an arithmetic scale
5-4   Theoretical concentration–response curves on a logarithmic scale for drugs A, B and C
5-5   Concentration–response curves for three drugs A, B and C, all with the same potency (EC_{50} = 10) but different maximal efficacies
5-6   Competitive antagonism of the response produced by drug A (curve 1) by increasing concentrations (curves 2 and 3) of the competitive antagonist drug B
6-1   Phases affecting drug activity
6-2   The pharmaceutical phase
6-3   Schema of the pharmacokinetic phases, showing absorption, distribution, metabolism and excretion of drugs
6-4   Effect of pH on drug ionisation and transport
6-5   Factors affecting bioavailability
6-6   In this example the volume of the full bucket is 5 L and the amount of drug placed in each bucket is 100 mg. After the drug has distributed a 'blood' sample is removed from each bucket and the concentration of the drug measured
6-7   Relation between drug metabolism and renal excretion
6-8   The drug excretion process
7-1   Plasma concentration–time profile for a theoretical drug administered as a single oral dose
7-2   Plasma concentration–time profiles for a drug administered as (1) a single IV bolus dose followed by an IV infusion, (2) an IV infusion only, and (3) a single IV bolus dose
7-3   Plasma drug concentration versus time curve after an oral dose of a drug
7-4   Concept of total body clearance of a drug from plasma
7-5   In this example, the drug has a half-life of 4 hours and is administered orally every 4 hours
7-6   Effects of volume of distribution and clearance on half-life

7-7   Illustration of the saturable metabolism of the antiepileptic drug phenytoin
8-1   Variation in tetratogenic susceptibility of organ systems during stages of human intrauterine development
8-2   Nomogram for calculating drug doses in children
8-3   How pharmacokinetics change with age
10-1   Divisions of the nervous system
10-2   Schematic diagram of the autonomic nervous system
10-3   Structural components of a neuron
10-4   Electron micrograph of a peripheral myelinated nerve (human skin)
10-5   Primary determinants of the resting membrane potential
10-6   Phases of a nerve action potential
10-7   Chemical neurotransmitters and receptor sites in the autonomic nervous system
10-8   Cholinergic transmission at a neuroeffector junction
10-9   Adrenergic transmission at a neuroeffector junction
12-1   Control of noradrenaline release by presynaptic α_2 receptors
12-2   Nervous system response to high sympathetic drive
12-3   Site of action of drugs affecting noradrenergic transmission
13-1   Diagrammatic representation of motor pathways from the right and left sides of the motor cortex innervating skeletal muscles on the opposite sides of the body
13-2   The neuromuscular junction, showing release of acetylcholine, which acts on both presynaptic and postsynaptic nicotinic receptors
13-3   Summary diagram illustrating the sites of action of various toxins on somatic motor neurons and the motor end-plate
13-4   Sites of action of neuromuscular blocking drugs and anticholinesterase agents
14-1   Organisation of the nervous system, showing the major anatomical subdivisions of the central nervous system
14-2   The human brain, left lateral view
14-3   Components of the limbic system
14-4   Transverse section of the spinal cord
14-5   Major pathways of monoamine-containing fibres
14-6   Neurotransmitter balances in CNS disorders
15-1   Potency and solubility of inhaled general anaesthetics
15-2   Diagrammatic representation of the arrangement and workings of a typical general anaesthetic machine
15-3   Pharmacokinetics of local anaesthetics
15-4   Routes of administration of local anaesthetic drugs
15-5   Technique for Bier's block: IV regional anaesthesia of the upper limb
16-1   Factors affecting pain tolerance
16-2   Scheme illustrating components of pain and suffering
16-3A   Peripheral factors involved in the pain sensation

16-3B Nerve pathways and some neurotransmitters involved in pain sensation

16-4 Pain assessment chart

16-5 Scales for rating the intensity and distress of pain

16-6 Faces Pain Scale

16-7 Flowchart for the 'stepwise' pharmacological management of pain

16-8 Examples of continuous infusion pumps

16-9 Metabolic pathways involving paracetamol

17-1 Stages of sleep

17-2 Sleep–wake cycles across the lifespan

17-3 The reticular activating system

17-4 Chemical structures of some simple sedative drugs

18-1 Electroencephalogram during sleep and in epilepsy

18-2 Non-linear relation between daily dose of phenytoin and steady-state plasma concentration in five individual human subjects

19-1 Proposed mechanisms of action of antidepressant drugs

20-1 Drug interactions between caffeine and alcohol

21-1 Central acetylcholine/dopamine balance

21-2 Levodopa in Parkinson's disease

21-3 Signs, symptoms and implications of myasthenia gravis

22-1 Effects of mind-altering drugs on spiders

22-2 Results of four surveys on the relation between traffic accidents and blood ethanol concentration

22-3 Plasma concentration of nicotine after smoking

22-4 Monoamine neurotransmitters and related hallucinogens

23-1 Schematic diagram of the heart, blood flow and valves

23-2 Structure of heart and cardiac muscle cell fibres

23-3 Coronary blood supply to the heart

23-4 Conduction system of the heart

23-5 **A.** Action potential of a single myocardial cell. **B.** Ion movements across the myocardial cell membrane during an action potential

23-6 Three-phase action potential of a slow-channel fibre, the SA node

23-7 Graphic representation of the normal electrocardiogram

24-1 Signs and symptoms of heart failure

24-2 Schematic representation of cardiac myocyte, indicating sites of action of digoxin, milrinone and β-adrenoceptor agonists

24-3 **A.** Representation of typical effects of digoxin on the electrical activity of the heart as shown on the electrocardiogram (ECG). **B.** Representation of atrial fibrillation as seen on the ECG

24-4 Re-entry phenomenon. Illustration of a branched Purkinje fibre that activates ventricular muscle

24-5 Phases of the cardiac action potential and the effects produced by the various classes of antiarrhythmic drugs

25-1 Mechanism of action of organic nitrates

25-2 Transdermal systems

25-3 Physiological control of blood pressure, and sites of action of currently used oral antihypertensive drugs

25-4 The renin–angiotensin–aldosterone system

25-5 Control of blood pressure

26-1 Schematic diagram of cholesterol transport in the tissues, with sites of action of the main drugs affecting lipoprotein metabolism

27-1 Urinary system and schematic cross-section of a human kidney

27-2 Sagittal sections of the female and male pelvis

27-3 Summary of main transport processes occurring throughout the nephron

28-1 Schematic summary diagram showing the absorption of sodium and chloride in the nephron and the main sites of action of drugs

28-2 Interrelationship of thiazide diuretic therapy and unwanted effects

29-1 Simplified diagram of blood cell production (haemopoiesis) and the involvement of growth factors

29-2 Coagulation mechanisms for intrinsic and extrinsic pathways for blood clotting

30-1 Sites of action of drugs interacting with the coagulation cascade and the fibrinolytic and platelet activation systems

30-2 Platelet activation

31-1 Tracheobronchial tree and bronchial smooth muscle

31-2 Devices for drug administration by inhalation

32-1 Various oxygen delivery systems

32-2 The airways in asthma

32-3 Overview of the mediators of asthma and the effects of various antiasthma medications

32-4 Proposed mechanisms of action of drugs on bronchial smooth muscle

32-5 Stepwise maintenance of asthma in adults

32-6 Sagittal section of head and neck, showing the locations of the respiratory structures

33-1 The gastrointestinal system

33-2 Schematic diagram of stomach, gastric gland and secretory cells

33-3 Schematic diagram of gastric acid secretion and interrelationship of histamine secretion from enterochromaffin-like (ECL) cell and the acid-secreting parietal cells

33-4 The chemoreceptor trigger zone (CTZ) and other sites activating the emetic centre

34-1 Classification of laxatives according to site of action

35-1 Cross-sectional anatomy of the eye (lid not shown)

35-2 Main structures of the eye and enlargements of the canal of Schlemm, showing aqueous humour flow

36-1 Anatomy of the ear

37-1 Locations of the major endocrine glands

37-2 Chemical structures of some naturally occurring steroids

37-3 Levels of endocrine control

37-4 Pituitary hormones

38-1 Levels of control of growth hormone secretion

38-2 Effects of growth hormone treatment in GH deficiency, with catch-up following treatment with human growth hormone (HGH) given over three periods indicated by arrows for a girl with isolated growth-hormone deficiency

39-1 Synthesis of thyroid hormones

39-2   Secretion and control of thyroid hormones

39-3   Effect of thyroxine on growth: response of 6-year-old hypothyroid girl treated with thyroxine

40-1   Biosynthesis of adrenal cortex hormones

40-2   Glucocorticoid secretion

41-1   Control of blood glucose levels

41-2   Insulin pharmacokinetics

41-3   Mechanism of action of oral hypoglycaemic agents (and injected insulin)

42-1   Calcium balance. Flowchart summarising the main factors regulating plasma calcium levels

43-1   The female reproductive system

43-2   The male reproductive system, sagittal section

43-3   Sex hormone secretion and control: the hypothalamic–pituitary–gonadal axis

43-4   Hypothalamic and pituitary regulation of female sex hormones, and gonadotrophin effects on the ovaries

43-5   The menstrual cycle (in the absence of fertilisation and pregnancy)

47-1   Sites of action of various contraceptive methods on the female reproductive tract

48-1   Phases of a cell cycle

48-2   Simplified mechanisms of growth factors in activation of target factors in the cell nucleus

48-3   Synthesis of macromolecules (nucleic acids and proteins)

48-4   Response of cancer cells to therapy

49-1   Chemical structures of representative antineoplastic agents

50-1   Seven mechanisms of antibiotic resistance

51-1   Typical penicillus of *Penicillium notatum*, Fleming's strain

51-2   Sites of action of antimicrobial drugs

51-3   Urticaria, as seen in individuals sensitive to penicillin

52-1   Sites of action of antifungal drugs

52-2   Inhibition sites for HIV replication

53-1   Life cycle of the malarial parasite

53-2   Peripheral blood film (magnification $\times$ 100) showing a normal red cell and a red cell with a trophozoite

of *P. vivax* displaying the typical signet ring form and Schüffners stippling

53-3   Dissemination of tuberculosis

54–1   Location of organs and tissues of the immune system. The inset shows a cross-section of a lymph node

54–2   The complement system

54–3   Schematic of B lymphocyte activation and differentiation into plasma (antibody-secreting) cells and memory B cells

54–4   Primary and secondary immune responses

54–5   The process of acquired immunity

55-1   Simplified diagram of sites of action of NSAIDs and synthesis of thromboxane A_2, prostacyclin, prostaglandin E_2 (PGE_2) and proinflammatory prostaglandins from arachidonic acid, which is released from phospholipid membranes by the action of phospholipase A_2

55-2   Likely sites of action of DMARDs

55-3   Uric acid production and the sites of action of drugs used for the treatment of hyperuricaemia

55-4   Sites of action for immunosuppressive agents

56-1   Structures of the skin

56-2   Different types of skin lesions and some conditions associated with them

56-3   Examples of occlusive dressing to enhance hydration of particular areas of skin

56-4   Extent of body burns: percentage and thickness

56-5   The four stages of pressure sore (decubitus ulcer or bedsore), and recommended treatments

58-1   Energy balance: factors influencing energy intake and energy expenditure

58-2   Schematic representation of food-regulating pathways

58-3   Sites of action for antiobesity drugs in clinical use and drugs under development

59-1   Female redback spider with egg sac and male funnel-web spider

59-2   Box jellyfish

59-3   Stonefish

CLINICAL INTEREST BOXES

1-1 Is alcohol a useful drug?
1-2 History of major drug discoveries and inventions
1-3 Pharmacological properties of some plant drugs
1-4 What's in a (drug) name?
2-1 A drug usage evaluation case study: warfarin prophylaxis in atrial fibrillation
2-2 A new health care strategy
2-3 Clues in the medicine cabinet
3-1 What vitamins should I take?
3-2 Selenium: a little is good, a lot is not!
3-3 Melatonin, the body's timekeeper?
3-4 Facts and figures on complementary and alternative therapies in Australia
3-5 Efficacy of complementary and alternative therapies in clinical medicine
3-6 Indigenous Australian plant remedies
3-7 A herbal remedy case history
3-8 The great Pan Pharmaceuticals recall, 2003
4-1 The thalidomide disaster
4-2 High-throughput screening
4-3 Streptomycin, smoking and statistics
4-4 The Intensive Medicines Monitoring Programme
4-5 An Australian drug discovery: Relenza
4-6 A Hippocratic oath for the 21st century
5-1 Drugs and the theory of receptors
6-1 Named brand and a generic equivalent
6-2 Polymorphism in New Zealand Maori
6-3 Grapefruit juice–drug interactions
7-1 The dilemma of the missed dose
8-1 Fetal alcohol syndrome
8-2 Drug use in pregnancy and breastfeeding
8-3 Grey baby syndrome
9-1 Centre for Adverse Reactions Monitoring (CARM)
10-1 Multiple sclerosis
10-2 Neurotransmitters
11-1 Treatment of Alzheimer's disease
12-1 Phaeochromocytoma
12-2 Withdrawal of a β-blocking agent
13-1 Cosmetic use of botulinum toxin, an inhibitor of acetylcholine release
13-2 Sites of action of toxins on somatic motor neurons and the motor end-plate
13-3 Chemical warfare agents
14-1 Drugs affecting the CNS
14-2 Raised intracranial pressure (ICP)
14-3 Clinical aspects of the blood–brain barrier
15-1 History of anaesthesiology
15-2 Drugs in the anaesthetic drug trolley
15-3 Remifentanil: a rapid-acting opioid for use during general anaesthesia
15-4 Waste anaesthetic gases as an occupational health hazard
15-5 Advantages and disadvantages of intravenous anaesthetics

15-6 Cocaine — the original local anaesthetic
15-7 Calculating the safe dose of a local anaesthetic
16-1 Fears or myths about pain and pain management
16-2 World Health Organization guidelines on analgesic use
16-3 Brompton cocktail
16-4 Opium, opiates, opioids and narcotics
16-5 In praise of opium
16-6 Tips for transdermal administration of fentanyl
16-7 Willow bark, salicylates and *Melaleuca*
16-8 Advantages of paracetamol over aspirin
16-9 A cup of tea, an APC and analgesic nephropathy
16-10 Herbal remedies for pain
17-1 Sleep hygiene
17-2 Falls and fractures in the elderly
17-3 Treatment of panic disorder
17-4 Death by bromide and strychnine
17-5 The 'Mickey Finn'
17-6 Complementary and alternative sedatives
18-1 Triggers of epileptic seizures
18-2 International Classification of Seizures
18-3 Epilepsy support groups
18-4 Eclampsia — toxaemia of pregnancy
18-5 Titrating phenytoin doses
19-1 Historical background to psychiatric drugs
19-2 Neuroleptic extrapyramidal adverse effects
19-3 Thioridazine and arrhythmia; moclobemide and hypertension
19-4 Indigenous mental health
19-5 Principles of psychotherapy
19-6 Signs and symptoms of schizophrenia
19-7 St John's wort and other complementary and alternative therapies in psychiatry
19-8 Tyramine-containing substances
19-9 Prozac beats the blues
19-10 Van Gogh's affect and art
19-11 Therapeutic value of lithium discovered in Melbourne
20-1 Methylphenidate — its (mis)use in New Zealand
20-2 Memory drugs flood the classroom
20-3 Caffeine, anaesthetics and malignant hyperpyrexia
21-1 Parkinsonism induced by drugs
21-2 Levodopa 'on–off' syndrome
21-3 Apomorphine, the archetypal emetic agent
21-4 Myasthenia gravis
21-5 Grievous bodily harm and fantasy
21-6 Bulgarian snowdrops for Alzheimer's disease
21-7 Potentially reversible causes of dementia
21-8 Complementary and alternative therapies in neurological disorders
21-9 Triggering factors in migraines
22-1 Why do people abuse drugs?
22-2 Myths related to drug abuse
22-3 Drug misuse in New Zealand
22-4 'Turning the Tide' on drugs

22-5 Complementary and alternative therapies in management of drug dependence

22-6 The methadone maintenance program

22-7 Alcohols — what's your poison?

22-8 The ecstasy con trick

22-9 Cocaine and Coca-Cola

22-10 Coffee, tea or cocoa?

22-11 Caffeine contents in selected products

22-12 Other hallucinogens

23–1 Coronary heart disease

24-1 Heart failure

25-1 Management of angina

25-2 Hypertension

25-3 New Zealand health information

25-4 ACE inhibitor cough

26-1 Plant sterols

26-2 Fish oil

27-1 Renal disease in indigenous populations

27-2 Urinary incontinence

28-1 Mercurial diuretics

28-2 Use of spironolactone for the treatment of severe heart failure

28-3 Renal damage from drugs, foods and plants

30-1 Coagulation tests

30-2 Aspirin

31-1 Cystic fibrosis and gene therapy

31-2 Puffers and other inhaler devices

32-1 Medical gases

32-2 Oxygen administration in the premature infant

32-3 Asthma in the Australian community

32-4 Asthma in New Zealand

32-5 Not in the script: a case of drug-induced asthma

32-6 Therapeutic tips for asthma

32-7 Smoking

32-8 Complementary and alternative therapies in respiratory disorders

32-9 Flu and the Sydney Olympic Games

33-1 Gastro-oesophageal reflux disease (GORD)

33-2 *Helicobacter pylori*

33-3 Gallstones

33-4 Crohn's disease

34-1 Alcoholic mouth-wash warning

34-2 Fluoridated water

34-3 Milk–alkali syndrome

34-4 Nausea and vomiting in pregnancy

34-5 Activated charcoal

34-6 Australian medicinal plants

34-7 Travellers' diarrhoea

34-8 Peppermint oil

35-1 Sterility of ocular formulations

35-2 Ocular autonomic pathologies

35-3 Trial by anticholinesterases

35-4 The first commandment of eye care

35-5 Winking, blinking and blepharospasm

35-6 Complementary and alternative therapies in ocular medicine

35-7 Beware of those eye-drops!

36-1 Swimmer's ear

36-2 Ménière's disease

36-3 Can't taste the sugar?

37-1 Death from ductless glands — or was it from digitalis?

37-2 Responses to stress

38-1 Creutzfeldt–Jakob disease

38-2 Gigantism, dwarfism and short stature

38-3 Dopamine and lactation

38-4 Diabetes insipidus

39-1 Disorders due to iodine deficiency

39-2 Diagnostic testing for hypothyroidism

39-3 Hyperthyroidism and hypothyroidism: clinical features

39-4 Graves' disease

39-5 Lugol's solution

39-6 Natural antithyroid compounds: cabbages and celery seeds

40-1 Addison's disease and Cushing's syndrome

40-2 Adrenal insufficiency and Conn's syndrome

41-1 Units of insulin activity

41-2 History of diabetes mellitus

41-3 Diabetes in the Australian Aboriginal and Torres Strait Islander population

41-4 Diabetes in New Zealand

41-5 Symptoms of hypoglycaemia and hyperglycaemia

41-6 Effects of commonly abused drugs on diabetes management

41-7 'Sugar-free' oral mixtures

41-8 Complementary and alternative therapies in diabetes mellitus

42-1 Calcium supplements

42-2 Getting enough calcium

42-3 Vitamin D

43-1 Disorders of menstruation

43-2 Should menstruation be optional?

44-1 Clinical uses of oestrogens

44-2 Phased OC hormones

44-3 'The pill'

44-4 HRT — Why? Why not? How? And how long?

44-5 Complementary and alternative therapies in women's conditions

45-1 Ergot, St Anthony, Dale and LSD

46-1 Akhenaton: a pharaoh with Fröhlich's syndrome?

47-1 The 'male pill'

47-2 'Rhythm methods' for natural family planning

47-3 Sex, serendipity, sildenafil and share prices

48-1 Cancers in Australia

48-2 Processes in the typical development of cancers

48-3 A treatment regimen for lung cancer

48-4 What patients want to know

48-5 Safe handling of cytotoxic agents

49-1 History of antineoplastic chemotherapy

49-2 Antineoplastic agents from natural sources

49-3 Complementary and alternative therapies in cancer

49-4 Frequently asked questions about palliative care (relevant to pharmacology)

50-1 Australian medicinal plants

50-2 Antibiotics in animals — the food chain

51-1 Don't take the bite out of antibiotic

51-2 Penicillin rash and anaphylaxis

51-3 More than a lump in the throat

52-1 Australian medicinal plants
52-2 Oral miconazole gel and warfarin
52-3 HIV–AIDS in Australia
52-4 Hepatitis C
52-5 An AIDS vaccine
53-1 East Timor as a new source of malaria infection
53-2 Quinine, gin and tonic, and bitter lemon for malaria
53-3 Global Alliance for Elimination of Leprosy (GAEL)
53-4 Worm treatments
54-1 Meningococcal disease in New Zealand
55-1 COX-2 inhibitors and cardiovascular events
55-2 Update on COX-2 inhibitors in New Zealand
55-3 Complementary medicines
55-4 Colchicine: lower doses for greater safety
56-1 Poisoned through the skin!

56-2 Sunburn, skin cancer and SPF
56-3 Vitamin A, acne and Antarctica
56-4 Spray-on skin, a great Western Australian invention
56-5 Sydney University's *aloe vera*: ancient plants with modern uses
57-1 Some recent doping-in-sport cases
57-2 Anabolic steroid use in Sydney
57-3 Complementary and alternative therapies in sport
57-4 Drug testing at the Sydney Olympic Games
58-1 New Zealand adult obesity rates
58-2 Anorexiants and valvular disorders
58-3 Non-prescription weight loss supplements
59-1 Management of snake bite
59-2 *Latrodectus katipo*
59-3 Irukandji syndrome

DRUG MONOGRAPHS

3-1 Paracetamol
3-2 Ginseng
11-1 Bethanechol
11-2 Atropine
12-1 Ephedrine (sulfate)
12-2 Prazosin
13-1 Pancuronium
13-2 Suxamethonium
13-3 Neostigmine
15-1 Nitrous oxide
15-2 Sevoflurane
15-3 Propofol
15-4 Lignocaine
16-1 Morphine sulfate controlled-release tablets
16-2 Aspirin
17-1 Diazepam
18-1 Topiramate
18-2 Phenytoin
19-1 Chlorpromazine
19-2 Fluoxetine
19-3 Lithium
20-1 Dexamphetamine
20-2 Caffeine
21-1 Levodopa–carbidopa
21-2 Selegiline
21-3 Baclofen
21-4 Dantrolene
21-5 Sumatriptan
22-1 Naltrexone
22-2 Methadone oral syrup
22-3 Alcohol (ethanol)
22-4 Acamprosate
22-5 Nicotine gum
25-1 Glyceryl trinitrate
25-2 Oxpentifylline
25-3 Losartan
26-1 Simvastatin

26-2 Gemfibrozil
28-1 Frusemide
28-2 Hydrochlorothiazide
30-1 Warfarin
32-1 Acetylcysteine
32-2 Salbutamol and terbutaline
32-3 Theophylline
32-4 Beclomethasone inhaled
32-5 Zafirlukast
32-6 Cromoglycate and nedocromil
32-7 Codeine, dextromethorphan and pholcodine
32-8 Pseudoephedrine
32-9 Influenza vaccine
32-10 Zanamivir (Relenza)
34-1 Nystatin
34-2 Metoclopramide
34-3 Ondansetron
34-4 Omeprazole
34-5 Psyllium
34-6 Lactulose
34-7 Diphenoxylate
34-8 Mesalazine
35-1 Latanoprost
35-2 Fluorescein strips
35-3 Botulinum toxin
36-1 Antibiotic–corticosteroid ear-drops and ointments
38-1 Somatropin, recombinant
38-2 Octreotide
38-3 Desmopressin
38-4 Oxytocin
39-1 Thyroxine sodium
39-2 Radioactive iodine
39-3 Carbimazole and propylthiouracil
40-1 Hydrocortisone
40-2 Fludrocortisone
40-3 Aminoglutethimide

41-1 Human insulin
41-2 Glibenclamide
41-3 Glucagon
42-1 Teriparatide
42-2 Salcatonin (salmon calcitonin)
42-3 Calcitriol
42-4 Alendronate, a bisphosphonate
43-1 Human chorionic gonadotrophin (HCG)
44-1 Oestradiol valerate
44-2 Medroxyprogesterone acetate
45-1 Ergometrine
46-1 Testosterone enanthate depot injection
46-2 Finasteride
47-1 Clomiphene citrate
47-2 Intrauterine device with copper
47-3 Sildenafil
49-1 Cyclophosphamide
49-2 Methotrexate
49-3 Tamoxifen
49-4 Calcium folinate (folinic acid, Leucovorin)
52-1 Amphotericin B
52-2 Aciclovir
52-3 Zidovudine
52-4 Indinavir
53-1 Chloroquine
53-2 Isoniazid
53-3 Rifampicin
53-4 Ivermectin
55-1 Allopurinol
55-2 Cyclosporin
56-1 Amorolfine nail varnish
56-2 Tretinoin acne cream
56-3 Silver sulfadiazine
57-1 Epoetin alfa

DRUG MONOGRAPHS A–Z

22-4 Acamprosate
32-1 Acetylcysteine
52-2 Aciclovir
22-3 Alcohol (ethanol)
42-4 Alendronate, a bisphosphonate
55-1 Allopurinol
40-3 Aminoglutethimide
56-1 Amorolfine nail varnish
52-1 Amphotericin B
36-1 Antibiotic–corticosteroid ear-drops and ointments
16-2 Aspirin
11-2 Atropine
21-3 Baclofen
32-4 Beclomethasone inhaled
11-1 Bethanechol
35-3 Botulinum toxin
20-2 Caffeine
42-3 Calcitriol
49-4 Calcium folinate (folinic acid, Leucovorin)
39-3 Carbimazole and propylthiouracil
53-1 Chloroquine
19-1 Chlorpromazine
47-1 Clomiphene citrate
32-7 Codeine, dextromethorphan and pholcodine
32-6 Cromoglycate and nedocromil
49-1 Cyclophosphamide
55-2 Cyclosporin
21-4 Dantrolene
38-3 Desmopressin
20-1 Dexamphetamine
17-1 Diazepam
34-7 Diphenoxylate
12-1 Ephedrine (sulfate)
57-1 Epoetin alfa
45-1 Ergometrine

46-2 Finasteride
40-2 Fludrocortisone
35-2 Fluorescein strips
19-2 Fluoxetine
28-1 Frusemide
26-2 Gemfibrozil
3-2 Ginseng
41-2 Glibenclamide
41-3 Glucagon
25-1 Glyceryl trinitrate
43-1 Human chorionic gonadotrophin (HCG)
41-1 Human insulin
28-2 Hydrochlorothiazide
40-1 Hydrocortisone
52-4 Indinavir
32-9 Influenza vaccine
47-2 Intrauterine device with copper
53-2 Isoniazid
53-4 Ivermectin
34-6 Lactulose
35-1 Latanoprost
21-1 Levodopa–carbidopa
15-4 Lignocaine
19-3 Lithium
25-3 Losartan
44-2 Medroxyprogesterone acetate
34-8 Mesalazine
22-2 Methadone oral syrup
49-2 Methotrexate
34-2 Metoclopramide
16-1 Morphine sulfate controlled-release tablets
22-1 Naltrexone
13-3 Neostigmine
22-5 Nicotine gum
15-1 Nitrous oxide
34-1 Nystatin

38-2 Octreotide
44-1 Oestradiol valerate
34-4 Omeprazole
34-3 Ondansetron
25-2 Oxpentifylline
38-4 Oxytocin
13-1 Pancuronium
3-1 Paracetamol
18-2 Phenytoin
12-2 Prazosin
15-3 Propofol
32-8 Pseudoephedrine
34-5 Psyllium
39-2 Radioactive iodine
53-3 Rifampicin
32-2 Salbutamol and terbutaline
42-2 Salcatonin (salmon calcitonin)
21-2 Selegiline
15-2 Sevoflurane
47-3 Sildenafil
56-3 Silver sulfadiazine
26-1 Simvastatin
38-1 Somatropin, recombinant
21-5 Sumatriptan
13-2 Suxamethonium
49-3 Tamoxifen
42-1 Teriparatide
46-1 Testosterone enanthate depot injection
32-3 Theophylline
39-1 Thyroxine sodium
18-1 Topiramate
56-2 Tretinoin acne cream
30-1 Warfarin
32-5 Zafirlukast
32-10 Zanamivir (Relenza)
52-3 Zidovudine

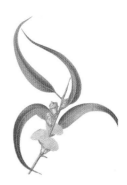

UNIT I
Introduction to Pharmacology

CHAPTER 1

Drugs, Medicines and Health Professionals

CHAPTER FOCUS

Proper selection and clinical use of drugs require a thorough knowledge of pharmacological principles. This chapter focuses on the origin, development and scope of pharmacology, characteristics of drugs, drug nomenclature, classification and sources, dosage measurements and calculations, and selected drug information sources. An understanding of these basic areas of pharmacology is important in the application of pharmacology in many health-care professions.

OBJECTIVES

● To outline the scope of pharmacology and describe the aspects important to health-care professionals.

● To trace and describe the major significant historical events in the development of pharmacology.

● To explain how drugs are named and classified.

● To name the physical characteristics used to describe drugs.

● To name the primary sources of drugs and the types of plant chemicals that are pharmacologically active.

● To explain how drug doses are measured and calculated, with clinical examples.

● To identify authoritative sources for drug information.

KEY TERMS

adverse drug reaction
alkaloid
approved name
chemical name
contraindication
dose calculations
drug
drug information
formulary
generic name
glycoside
history of pharmacology
ideal drug
indication
key, or prototype, drug

'magic bullet'
medicine
organic molecule
over-the-counter drug
pharmacodynamics
pharmacokinetics
pharmacology
pharmacopoeia
potency
prescription drug
proprietary name
selectivity
specificity
steroid
trade name

KEY ABBREVIATIONS

AMH	Australian Medicines Handbook
APF	Australian Pharmaceutical Formulary
BP	British Pharmacopoeia
CPI	consumer product information
CIB	Clinical Interest Box
DM	Drug Monograph
OTC	over the counter
PBS	Pharmaceutical Benefits Scheme
S4	Schedule 4 [Prescription Medicine]
SI	Système International d' Unités scientific units
WHO	World Health Organization

INTRODUCTION AND DEFINITIONS

Pharmacology and drugs

PHARMACOLOGY is the study of drugs, including their actions and effects in living systems. The word **drug** is defined by the World Health Organization as 'any substance or product that is used or intended to be used to modify or explore physiological systems or pathological states for the benefit of the recipient'.* The prefix pharmaco- is derived from the Greek word *pharmakon*, meaning drug or medicine. Hence we have related terms such as pharmacy, **pharmacodynamics**, **pharmacokinetics**, pharmaceutics, pharmacopoeia and pharmacoeconomics (see Table 1-1). The terms medication and **medicine** in this context usually refer to drugs mixed in a formulation with other ingredients to improve the stability, taste or physical form, in order to allow appropriate administration of the active drug.

Pharmacology deals with all drugs used in society today —legal and illegal, prescription and 'over-the-counter' medications, natural and synthetic chemicals, with beneficial or potentially toxic effects. This includes endogenous substances (those produced within the body) such as enzymes, hormones, antibodies, neurotransmitters and ions, and indeed many such chemicals are used therapeutically. Pharmacologists may study the origins, isolation, purification, chemical structure and synthesis, assay (measurement), uses, economics, genetic aspects and toxicity of drugs, as well as their fate in the body, medical uses and effects. The pharmacological agents available today have controlled, prevented, cured, diagnosed and in some instances eradicated disease, and have improved the quality of life.

Medications also have the potential to cause harm, as indicated by the fact that the Greek word for drug was also the word for poison. Health-care professionals should therefore be well informed about each medication before administering it to a patient, or when considering the possible effects of drugs their patients are taking, whether prescribed or self-administered, and whether for medical or social reasons. To administer a drug safely, one must know the usual dose, frequency and route of administration, indications, significant adverse reactions, major drug interactions, dietary implications (if applicable), contraindications, and appropriate monitoring techniques and interventions, and apply this knowledge to the particular patient and situation.

---

*If you asked a random selection of people what the word drug meant to them, you would come up with many very different definitions. Unfortunately, 'drug' has come to have connotations of illicit street drugs, substances more frequently abused than prescribed or administered for therapeutic purposes. However, it has a much simpler and wider meaning: a chemical that affects living tissues.

Characteristics of drugs
Potency, selectivity and specificity

By our broad definition of a drug as a chemical having action on living tissue, virtually every chemical could be classed as a drug; even oxygen, sugar, salt and water affect the body and can be toxic in overdose. To make the definition more descriptive, we can say that useful drugs usually have other important attributes: potency, selectivity and specificity (see Clinical Interest Box 1-1).

CLINICAL INTEREST BOX 1-1
IS ALCOHOL A USEFUL DRUG?

Two commonly taken substances, salbutamol and alcohol, may be compared in terms of their potencies, selectivities and specificities; salbutamol (Ventolin) is used in treatment of asthma (Drug Monograph 32-2), and alcohol (ethanol, Drug Monograph 22-3) is used as a solvent, disinfectant and 'social lubricant'.

	SALBUTAMOL	ETHANOL
Potency: effective at concentrations of:	10^{-8}–10^{-5} M	10^{-2}–10^{-1} M*
Biological selectivity:	β_2-adrenoceptor agonist, bronchodilator, uterine relaxant, plus some cardiac stimulant and vasodilator actions	Increases disorder in lipid membranes, depresses neuronal activity in most excitable cells and tissues
Chemical specificity:	High (closely related to adrenaline and noradrenaline)	Low (depressant actions related to GABA and NMDA receptors and calcium channels)
Specific antagonists	Yes — β-adrenoceptor antagonist (β-blocker)	No — non-specific antagonism by central nervous system stimulation, as with caffeine and amphetamines

As chemicals need to have potency, selectivity and specificity in order to be useful as drugs, by our definition, alcohol is not a useful drug: it requires high doses and has only general effects on most cells of the body.

---

*Note that 0.05% blood alcohol level is approximately equivalent to 1.1×10^{-2} M.
GABA = γ-aminobutyric acid;
NMDA = *N*-methyl-D-aspartate.

TABLE 1-1 Some common pharmacological terms*	
Adverse drug reaction	An unintended and undesirable response to a drug
Clinical pharmacology	Pharmacology applied to the treatment of patients; the study of drugs 'at the bedside'
Dose form	The form in which the drug is administered, e.g. as a tablet, injection, eye-drop or ointment
Indication	An illness or disorder for which a drug has a documented specific usefulness
Medicine	Drug(s) given for therapeutic purposes; possibly a mixture of drug(s) plus other substances to provide stability in the formulation; also, the branch of science devoted to the study, prevention and treatment of disease
Pharmaceutics	The science of preparation and dispensing of drugs
Pharmacokinetics	How the body affects a specific drug after administration; i.e. how a drug is altered as it travels through the body (by absorption, distribution, metabolism and excretion)
Pharmacodynamics	What drugs do to the body and how they do it; refers to the interaction of drug molecules with their target receptors or cells, and their biochemical, physiological and possibly adverse effects
Pharmacoeconomics	The application of health economics to the selection and supply of medical drugs, especially the cost-effectiveness of prescribing
Pharmacopoeia	A reference book listing standards for drugs approved in a particular country; may also include details of standard formulations and prescribing guidelines (a formulary)
Pharmacy	The branch of science dealing with preparing and dispensing drugs; also the place where a pharmacist carries out these roles
Pregnancy safety	A method of classifying drugs according to documented risks in pregnancy
Receptor	A structure on or within a cell or membrane that is capable of binding to a specific substance (such as a transmitter, hormone or drug) and as a result causing a response in the cell
Side-effect	A drug effect that is not necessarily the primary purpose for giving the drug in the particular condition; side-effects may be desirable or undesirable. This term has been virtually superseded by the term adverse drug reaction, which is used throughout this book
Toxicology	The study of the nature, properties, identification, effects and treatment of poisons, including the study of adverse drug reactions

*See the Glossary (Appendix 4) for a more complete list of pharmacological terms.

Potency refers to the amount of chemical required to produce an effect; the more potent the drug, the lower the dose required for a given effect (see Chapter 5 and Figure 5-4). One of the most potent chemicals known is the natural bacterial product botulinum toxin, for which the minimum lethal dose in a mouse is as low as 10^{-12} g (one-millionth of one-millionth of a gram); it has found uses in medicine in treating spasm of eye muscles and spasticity, and in cosmetic surgery (see Drug Monograph 35-3).

Selectivity refers to the narrowness of a drug's range of actions on particular receptors, cellular processes or tissues. The antidepressant drugs known as selective serotonin reuptake inhibitors (SSRIs), such as fluoxetine (Prozac, see Clinical Interest Box 19-9), have fewer adverse effects than older antidepressants because they are more selective in inhibiting the transport of the neurotransmitter serotonin into cells.

The term **specificity** may be used loosely like 'selectivity' to refer to the narrowness of the range of actions of a drug, e.g. cardiospecific or cardioselective β-blocking agents, which are less likely to cause asthma as an adverse effect than are non-specific β-blockers because they are more selective for β_1 receptors, which are found mainly in cardiac tissue. Specificity may also refer to the relation between the chemical structure of a drug and its pharmacological actions; for example, the effects of pseudoephedrine (Drug Monograph 32-9) and related compounds are due to their chemical similarity to the neurotransmitter noradrenaline.

The ideal drug

In designing a new drug, a research pharmacologist might aim for it to be: easily administered (preferably orally) and fully absorbed from the gastrointestinal tract, not highly protein-bound in the blood plasma, potent, highly specific, selective, with rapid onset and useful duration of action, of high therapeutic index (no adverse drug reactions, no interference with body functions), unlikely to interact with any other drugs or foodstuffs, spontaneously eliminated, stable chemically and microbiologically, readily formulated into an easily taken form, and inexpensive. Sadly, not even pharmacologists live in an ideal world, and so we must admit that there is no **ideal drug**, whether natural substance or synthetic. In all cases, the decision to prescribe, administer or take a drug requires a risk–benefit analysis based on the best information available: do the likely therapeutic benefits outweigh the possible harmful effects?

Physical aspects of drugs

In terms of their physical state, drugs may be solids, liquids or gases. Most are solids at room temperature but some are liquids in the pure state, such as nicotine, halothane (a general anaesthetic) and ethanol, and some are gases, especially general anaesthetics such as nitrous oxide and cyclopropane. The solids may be formulated in solid dose forms, such as tablets, capsules, creams, powders or patches, or when dissolved may be formulated in liquid preparations such as cough mixtures, injectable solutions, aerosol sprays, eye-drops or paints. These aspects of the formulation of drugs will be covered in the section on pharmaceutics in Chapter 2.

All drugs, whether found naturally in plants, animals, minerals or microorganisms, or synthesised in a laboratory, are chemicals of one sort or another. They may be inorganic molecules, such as calcium salts used to treat osteoporosis or fluorides used to prevent dental decay. The vast majority of drugs, however, are **organic molecules**, i.e. they contain carbon in their structures. All the major classes of organic compounds, including hydrocarbons, proteins, lipids, carbo-hydrates, nucleic acids and steroids, are represented in pharmacopoeias (see Figure 1-1 later). Many drug molecules are acids or bases, which is important not only for their taste and irritant effects but also for how the drugs move across membranes or are affected by the normal body processes of metabolism and excretion (pharmacokinetics).

The size of drug molecules can also vary enormously, ranging from tiny lithium, the third-lightest element, with an atomic weight of about 7, used as a specific antimanic agent (Drug Monograph 19-3), through to proteins such as insulin (Drug Monograph 41-1), erythropoietin (Drug Monograph 57-1) and influenza vaccine (Drug Monograph 32-9). Most drugs are in a more intermediate size range, with molecular weights (relative molecular masses) between 100 and 1000. For example, gabapentin, an anticonvulsant, has a molecu-lar weight of 171, aspirin 180, caffeine 194, testosterone

(a steroid hormone) 288, penicillin 373, digoxin (a cardiac glycoside) 781, and cyclosporin, an immunosuppressant with a cyclic polypeptide structure, 1203. By comparison, insulin, a relatively small protein, has a molecular weight of about 5700 and erythropoietin, a large glycoprotein, about 30,400. Again, the size and nature of the molecule has important implications for the pharmacokinetic handling of the drug: proteins taken orally would be digested in the gut, so they must be administered by injection; and large molecules will not readily pass through cell membranes and may need to be administered directly into the bloodstream or to their site of action.

A BRIEF HISTORY OF PHARMACOLOGY
Medicines in antiquity

Since the beginning of time, people have searched for substances to prevent, treat and cure disease, so the **history of pharmacology** goes back a long way. Archaeological diggings show that Stone Age people used opium poppies (see Clinical Interest Box 16-5) and Inca civilisations used cocaine (Clinical Interest Box 22-9). The oldest prescriptions found were on a clay tablet written by a Sumerian physician around 3000 BC, i.e. 5000 years ago; these included vegetable and mineral drugs dissolved in milk, beer and wine, showing the longstanding use of alcohol in medicine. Presumably knowledge of pharmacology developed by trial and error, with many fatalities and adverse reactions along the way. Supernatural healing rituals and magical practices involving drugs were—and sometimes still are—carried out by healers and shamans in primitive cultures.

Primitive people through the Egyptian period believed that disease was caused by evil spirits living in the body. Imhotep, the god of medicine, and Isis and Horus, gods of pharmacy, were worshipped. The Ebers Papyrus, dating from about 1500 BC and translated into English in AD 1875, described formulations of over 700 drugs from plant, mineral and animal sources.

Chinese medicine dates back beyond 2000 BC. Methods included the use of herbs, poisons and antidotes, acupunc-ture, diets and moxibustion (burning of herbs for incense and heating the skin). The common practice of using boiling water to make tea probably prevented many intestinal infections and there is documentation of the use of ephedra (ephedrine) for asthma, and seaweeds (iodine) for goitre. Ancient Indian (Ayurvedic) medicine, recorded in sacred writings (the Vedas), described many surgical practices and over 1000 natural drugs, including wine (alcohol) and hemp (marijuana), used for pain relief.

Medicine in the Greek and Roman civilisations

In the Ancient Greek civilisation, the god Asclepias was considered to be the principal god of healing. He combined religion and healing in a temple setting, and his large family represented health or medical ideology. His wife Epione, for example, soothed pain; his daughter Hygeia, the goddess of health, represented the prevention of disease; and Panacea, another daughter, represented treatment. His large temple settings were used to treat both the rich and the poor to cure their illnesses.

Hippocrates (5th century BC) advanced the idea that disease results from natural causes and can be understood only through a study of natural laws and from careful diagnosis. He believed that health was due to a balance of four 'humours' ebbing and flowing in the body (blood, phlegm, black bile and yellow bile); hence we have the terms sanguine, phlegmatic, bilious, choleric and melancholic. He realised that the body has healing powers, and saw the health-care provider's role as assisting the recuperative process. His 'doctrine of opposites', i.e. the concept that opposites cure (cold treats fever, bleeding treats excess humours), was the basis of medicine for many hundreds of years and eventually held up advances in more accurate medical knowledge. Known today as the father of medicine, Hippocrates influenced the principles that control the practice of medicine today, including versions of the Hippocratic Oath that are still read at some medical graduation ceremonies (see Clinical Interest Box 4-6).

Medicine during the Roman Empire (about 100 BC to AD 400) was largely based on Greek traditions of herbal remedies and healing gods. The Romans introduced excellent public health measures, including water supplies and sanitation. Folk remedies included wound dressings of wine, vinegar, eggs, honey, worms and pig dung. Ephedra (ephedrine, a sympathomimetic agent) was used, with good pharmacological rationale, for asthma, cough and haemorrhage. Famous medical men during this era included Dioscorides, a military physician who published a text entitled *De Materia Medica* (on the materials of medicine) on the sources, preparation and uses of hundreds of medically useful natural remedies, including analgesics, antiseptics, emetics and laxatives. Celsus described the four cardinal signs of inflammation, and stressed the importance of moderation, exercise, knowledge of anatomy, and prevention of infection and haemorrhage. Galen of Pergamon wrote voluminously on medical, scientific, philosophical, ethical and religious issues and considered that bleeding (removal of large volumes of blood) was appropriate treatment for virtually all disorders, as they were all due to an excess of a humour in the body. Galen was famous for his knowledge of drugs, both 'simples', i.e. simple herbal or mineral remedies, and complex mixtures that might include exotic herbs, amulets, excrement and antidotes, and which came to be known as 'galenicals'.

The Dark Ages and mediaeval times

The fall of the Roman Empire marked the beginning of the mediaeval period (AD 400–1500). Constantinople (now Istanbul) became the eastern capital of the Byzantine empire, while the West sank into the Dark Ages as barbarians overran Western Europe. The practice of medicine reverted to folklore and tradition similar to that of the Greeks before Hippocrates. During this time, Christian religious orders built monasteries that became sites for learning, including pharmacy and medicine. They aided the sick and needy with food, rest and herbal medicines from their monastery gardens. Learning was carried out in Latin, and libraries held versions of Greek, Roman and Arabic medical texts. Medicine was a combination of both spiritual methods (prayer, exorcism, trust in relics of the saints) and physical methods (diet, drugs, bleeding and surgery).

One of the most famous women of the Middle Ages, Hildegard of Bingen, was a remarkable writer, composer, prophet, healer and abbess. Her books described the causes of many mental and physical diseases, and medical and toxic properties of herbal, animal and mineral preparations. It is thought that her visions were probably due to the migraines from which she suffered. In some countries, women at this period were allowed to practise medicine and midwifery.

Hospitals have been called the greatest medical innovation of the Middle Ages. They were generally hospices attached to monasteries and had multiple purposes, providing religious, nursing and charitable care and also acting as leper houses. Particular saints were attributed the power to heal specific diseases, e.g. St Anthony and ergotism (see Clinical Interest Box 45-3), so a pilgrimage to the appropriate shrine was believed to help cure the condition. Battle wounds always provided a need for surgical and medical care, as victims usually succumbed to infection, haemorrhage and shock. The soporific (sleep-inducing) and analgesic effects of the herbs poppy, henbane and mandrake were known and valued; a 'soporific sponge' containing a mixture of these herbs was prepared for chewing or inhalation by the patient.

During this period, in the Byzantine empire, occurred the Golden Age of Islamic medicine. The Arabs' interest in medicine, pharmacy and chemistry was reflected in the hospitals and schools they built, the many new drugs they contributed and their formulation of the first set of drug standards. Folk medicines included camphor, henna, syrup, aloes, amber and musk. The classic Greek medical works were translated into Arabic and an extensive library was collected in Baghdad. The great contribution of Islamic medicine was the establishment of teaching hospitals such as those in Baghdad, Cairo and Damascus; medical education has depended ever since on this style of training for medical practice.

In AD 1240, the head of the Holy Roman Empire, Frederick II, declared pharmacy to be separate from medicine.

Pharmacy was not, however, truly established separately until the 16th century, when Valerius Cordus compiled the first pharmacopoeia (reference text with standard formulae and recipes) as an authoritative standard.

Medicine in the Renaissance and scientific eras

In the Renaissance (14th to 16th centuries), there was a rebirth of interest in and knowledge of the arts, sciences, politics and economics in Europe. In the medical area, Paracelsus (1493–1541), a professor of physics and surgery at Basel in Switzerland and an alchemist and pharmacologist, denounced 'humoral pathology' and substituted the 'like cures like' theory—that diseases are actual entities to be combatted with specific remedies, especially minerals. He recognised the relationship between cretinism and goitre, and that between gout and the deposition of crystals in tissues, and improved pharmacy and therapeutics for succeeding centuries, introducing new remedies and reducing the overdosing that was so prevalent in that period.

Many important pharmacological discoveries were made in the 16th and 17th centuries, including:

- treating gout with colchicum (colchicine) and restriction of wine intake
- treating malaria with 'Jesuit's bark' (cinchona, containing quinine [see Clinical Interest Box 21-6])
- preventing scurvy (vitamin C deficiency) with oranges and lemons*
- use of willow bark (salicylates) for treatment of fever and foxglove (digitalis) for the treatment of dropsy, a condition we know as oedema
- extracts of opium, mandrake and hemlock in wine to relieve pain and to allow surgical procedures; henbane (hyoscyamus), containing hyoscine and scopolamine, for inducing forgetfulness.

Meanwhile, great progress was being made in pharmacy and chemistry. The first London pharmacopoeia appeared in 1618 and many preparations introduced at that time are still in use today, including opium tincture (Clinical Interest Box 16-5), cocaine and ipecac. Other important national pharmacopoeias were the *French Codex* (1818), followed by the *United States Pharmacopoeia* in 1820, the *British Pharmacopoeia* in 1864, and Germany's in 1872.

In the 18th and 19th centuries, deliberate clinical testing of drugs for their actions was carried out. The gas nitrous oxide and the volatile liquids ether and chloroform were used in surgery, dentistry and obstetrics (see Clinical Interest Box 15-1) and provided the first safe painless surgery. A local anaesthetic, cocaine, had been in use for millennia in extracts of coca bark (Clinical Interest Box 15-6). This was studied, purified and used in eye surgery in the 1870s, and safer synthetic analogues were soon developed. Hypnotics and sedatives such as bromides and chloral hydrate helped relieve insomnia. Antiseptics such as carbolic acid were synthesised and found to be effective in vitro (in test-tubes or Petri dishes) in reducing infection from wounds, but were too toxic in vivo (in the living organism) to be given to patients. The study of dose–response relationships led to the safer use of drugs. Rational medicine had begun to replace empiricism.

Into the 20th and 21st centuries

Early in the 20th century, drugs commonly used in medicine were aspirin and codeine as analgesics, sodium bicarbonate and glycerine for gastrointestinal problems, sodium bromide as a sedative, sodium salicylate as an anti-inflammatory and antipyretic analgesic, strychnine as a 'tonic', and ammonium chloride as an expectorant and urinary acidifier. As knowledge of chemistry, physiology and medicine developed, it was applied to the problem of finding drugs to treat specific conditions. Advances in synthetic organic chemistry led to the establishment of large-scale chemical manufacturing plants to produce drugs, among other chemicals. Structure–activity studies identified series of molecules with agonist or antagonist actions on many types of receptor. The importance of using a control group when testing drugs or other treatments was recognised and the randomised controlled clinical trial became the expected standard (see Clinical Interest Box 4-3).

This was the era of the '**magic bullet**', with the major developments being the production of safe, orally active antimicrobials, both synthetic (sulfonamides) and natural (penicillins). In the 1930s and 1940s penicillin was discovered, isolated and purified (by Fleming, Florey and Chain), which revolutionised the treatment of microbial infections and became the precursor of many other antibiotics, e.g. streptomycin for tuberculosis. These successes led to the expectation that a drug would soon be found to treat every previously life-threatening disease.

During the 20th century, medicine made enormous advances, leading to therapeutic revolutions in all areas of medicine (see Clinical Interest Box 1-2). Of 36 major events identified as the most significant in modern medicine from 1935 to 1999 (Le Fanu 1999), at least half have been directly due to the development of effective drugs that either treated diseases that were previously life-threatening, or permitted safe surgery or diagnosis.

*The actual antiscorbutic factor, vitamin C or ascorbic acid, was eventually isolated in 1927 by Albert Szent-Gyorgyi, who was awarded the Nobel Prize for Medicine in 1937 for this discovery. Previously, while puzzling over the identification of the factor, which was known to be related to glucose, he had suggested that it be named 'ignose' or 'godnose'.

It is interesting to note at the beginning of the 21st century that, as major acute conditions are generally now treatable with drugs, most of the top 10 drugs (Table 1-3) are said to be for lifestyle diseases, including calcium channel blockers and angiotensin-converting enzyme inhibitors for cardiovascular diseases, proton pump inhibitors for peptic ulcers, selective serotonin reuptake inhibitors for depression, statins for high cholesterol levels, inhaled corticosteroids for asthma, and the fluoroquinolone antibiotics for infections resistant to safer antibiotics.

The scientific revolution brought about by molecular biology techniques has enabled the cloning and expressing of genes that code for therapeutically useful proteins, including monoclonal antibodies. In addition, many receptors have been purified, identified and cloned, and the biochemical pathways important in cell division are being elucidated, leading to new anticancer agents (see Clinical Interest Box 49-1). The recognition that many treatments used in medicine have never been subjected to scientific scrutiny has encouraged the development of meta-analysis techniques to analyse the results of all the clinical trials and medical research, and to evaluate scientific data to encourage implementation of evidence-based medicine.

In many countries, increasing numbers of older people and escalating costs of medical treatments have required dramatic changes to reform health-care systems, with an emphasis on providing quality health care in a more cost-effective manner, leading to a redefinition of professional roles and decision-making responsibilities among health professionals. An integrated interdisciplinary health-care delivery team approach centred on high-quality patient-focused care includes assessment, planning, monitoring, counselling, accountability for therapeutic outcomes, and patient advocacy. Because drugs are usually the primary therapies used in treatment and rehabilitative care, today many different health-care professionals—not only the apothecaries and doctors, as in previous centuries—need to have a solid basic understanding of pharmacology.

SOURCES OF DRUGS

Drugs and biological products have been identified or derived from several main sources:
- microorganisms, e.g. fungi used as sources of antibiotics, and bacteria and yeasts genetically engineered to produce drugs such as human insulin
- plants, e.g. *Atropa belladonna* (atropine), *Cannabis sativa* (marijuana), *Castanospermum australe* (castanospermine), *Coffea arabica* (coffee, caffeine), *Digitalis purpurea* (digitalis), *Duboisia* species (hyoscine, nornicotine), *Eucalyptus* spp. (eucalyptus oil), *Papaver somniferum* (opium, morphine)

- humans and other animals, from which drugs such as adrenaline, insulin (Drug Monograph 41-1), human chorionic gonadotrophin (hCG; Drug Monograph 43-1) and erythropoietin (Drug Monograph 57-1) were or are obtained, sometimes by recombinant techniques
- minerals or mineral products, e.g. iron, iodine (Drug Monograph 39-2) and Epsom Salts
- substances synthesised in laboratories, such as sulfonamides, β-blockers and antidepressants. Drugs may also be classed as semisynthetic, when the starting material is a natural product such as a plant steroid or microbial metabolite, which is then chemically altered to produce the desired drug molecule.

The processes and stages of drug discovery and development are discussed in more detail in Chapter 4.

Safety of natural products

There is a widely held belief that 'natural' products are safer than synthetic, man-made drugs. This belief is encouraged by many in the health-food industry and by alternative therapy practitioners. However, a quick scan through a list of naturally occurring substances such as arsenic, botulinum toxin, cantharidin, cocaine, cyanide, deadly nightshade, ipecacuanha, mercury, methanol, physostigmine, strychnine, thallium, tobacco and uranium will prove the belief false. Equally, it would be foolish to expect all substances extracted from microorganisms, plants, animals or minerals to be automatically safer than those synthesised in laboratories. In all cases, whether natural or synthetic, a drug's safety and efficacy must be tested and proved before it is approved for clinical use (see Smith 2002).

Active constituents of plant drugs

The leaves, roots, seeds and other parts of plants may be dried, crushed, boiled and extracted, or otherwise processed for use as a medicine and, as such, are known as crude drugs or herbal remedies; these are discussed in Chapter 3. Although they may appear more 'natural' than tablets, ointments or injections, their therapeutic effects are produced by the chemical substances they contain (see Clinical Interest Box 1-3).

When the pharmacologically active constituents are separated from the crude preparation and purified and quantified, the resulting substances have similar pharmacological actions to the crude drugs but are more potent, usually produce effects more reliably, and are less likely to be affected by other constituents in the crude preparations. Some of the types of pharmacologically active compounds found in plants, grouped according to their physical and chemical properties, are alkaloids, glycosides, steroids, hydrocarbons, alcohols, proteins, gums and oils. Note that the groups are not mutually exclusive—there can be glycoproteins and phenolic glycosides etc. Figure 1-1 shows the chemical formulae of some drugs that are extracted from plant sources.

Alkaloids

Alkaloids are organic nitrogen-containing compounds that are alkaline and usually bitter-tasting; the nitrogen atom is usually in a heterocyclic ring of carbon atoms (Figure 1-1A) and, as many alkaloids are amines, their names often end in

---

CLINICAL INTEREST BOX 1-2
HISTORY OF MAJOR DRUG DISCOVERIES AND INVENTIONS

TIME PERIOD	COMMENTS
1500 BC	Ebers papyrus, with details of Egyptian pharmacy and surgical practices; disease considered due to wrath of the gods
400 BC	Hippocrates, Greek physician: emphasis on humours and doctrine of opposites
1st century AD	Dioscorides' *De Materia Medica*: information on use of >600 medicinal plants; translated into Latin, Arabic and Persian. Celsus' medical textbook
2nd century	Galen, Greek physician/surgeon/druggist: pharmacy based on 'simples', and complex mixtures now called galenicals
5th–11th centuries	Dark Ages in Europe: herbal medicine, magic and cosmology interwoven in monasteries. Meanwhile in Arabia, China and India, medicine and herbal pharmacy developed, with teaching hospitals and medical libraries
12th–14th centuries	In Europe, medical schools developed in Salerno, Bologna and Montpellier; apothecaries documented use of herbs and spices
16th–17th centuries	More scientific: Vesalius (anatomist), Gerard and Culpepper (herbalists) and Paracelsus (alchemist, botanist); opium tincture, coca (cocaine), ipecac and antiscorbutic agents (antiscurvy) — important drugs, still used today
18th century	Digitalis: source of cardiac glycosides (digoxin, digitoxin); smallpox vaccine developed
19th century	Important alkaloids isolated: morphine, quinine, atropine and codeine, all still available for use today; ether and chloroform, first general anaesthetics available (rare or obsolete now)
1860s	Important advances in chemistry, especially coal-tar (organic) chemistry
20th century	Application of organic and synthetic chemistry to drug discovery
1922	Insulin isolated, the most important discovery for treatment of diabetes mellitus
1930s–1940s	The first safe oral antimicrobials: sulfonamides and penicillins developed. Use of muscle relaxants with general anaesthetics making major surgery safer
1949	Cortisone, an important hormone from the adrenal cortex, identified and synthetically prepared
1940s–1950s	Autonomic pharmacology studies, structure–activity relationships on α- and β-receptors; tuberculosis cured with combination antimicrobial therapy
1952	Chlorpromazine, the first effective antipsychotic drug, revolutionised treatment of schizophrenia (see Clinical Interest Box 19-1)
1950s	Oral contraceptives developed — chemicals similar to natural oestrogen and progesterone hormones, and which have been used by millions of women worldwide
1955, 1961	Poliovirus vaccines (inactivated and live oral, respectively) eliminating deaths and paralysis from polio epidemics
1960s	Levodopa used to treat Parkinson's disease; immunosuppressants make organ transplantation feasible; effective treatment of hypertension with thiazide diuretics and β-blockers helps prevent strokes; cytotoxic agents (alkylating agents, antimetabolites and antibiotics) developed to treat cancers. The thalidomide disaster, when thousands of infants are born with severe malformations, leads to tightening of regulations for testing the safety and efficacy of drugs
1970s	Antivirals developed for prophylaxis and treatment of viral diseases. Childhood leukaemia treated successfully with cytotoxics and steroids. Ovulatory stimulants used in in-vitro fertilisation
1980s–1990s	New drugs for thrombolysis, reduction of cholesterol levels, combination therapy of AIDS and treatment of impotence, and new antineoplastic agents for chemotherapy of cancers; refinement of treatment protocols
2000 on	Examples of some recent innovations include chiral versions of optically active drugs (levobupivacaine, escitalopram), genetically engineered molecules (insulin glargine), prostaglandin analogues for glaucoma (latanoprost, travoprost), and monoclonal antibodies in cancer chemotherapy (trastuzumab)

CLINICAL INTEREST BOX 1-3
PHARMACOLOGICAL PROPERTIES OF SOME PLANT DRUGS

The pharmacological actions of drugs from plants are determined by their active chemicals. Useful plant drugs with actions affecting virtually every body system have been found, as shown in the table below.

DRUG	SOURCE	MAIN PHARMACOLOGICAL ACTIONS
Caffeine	*Coffea arabica* (coffee)	CNS stimulant, diuretic
Cocaine	*Erythroxylum coca*	CNS stimulant, local anaesthetic
Strychnine	*Strychnos nux vomica*	CNS stimulant, convulsant
Morphine	*Papaver somniferum* (opium poppy)	Analgesic, sedative, constipating, cough suppressant
Pilocarpine	*Pilocarpus microphyllus*	Muscarinic agonist, Rx glaucoma
Atropine	*Atropa belladonna* (belladonna lily)	Antimuscarinic, premedication, Rx asthma
Ephedrine	*Ephedra sinica*	Sympathomimetic, Rx asthma
Digoxin	*Digitalis lanata* (foxglove)	Cardiac glycoside, Rx heart failure
Quinine, quinidine	*Cinchona* bark	Antimalarial, Rx cardiac arrhythmias
Nicotine	*Nicotiana tabacum* (tobacco)	Vasoconstrictor, CNS stimulant, addictive
Coumarins	Sweet clover	Anticoagulants, prevent thrombosis
Ipecacuanha	*Cephaelis* root	Expectorant, emetic, Rx poisoning
Bran	Indigestible vegetable fibre	Laxative, Rx constipation
Aromatic oils	E.g. from eucalyptus, pine, mint	Decongestant, Rx common cold, mild antiseptics
Benzoin	Resin from *Styrax* spp.	Inhalant, decongestant, antiseptic, astringent
Phyto-oestrogens	Clover, soybeans	Oestrogenic, Rx menopausal symptoms
Ergot alkaloids, e.g. ergometrine	Mould on *Claviceps* spp.	Oxytocic, Rx postpartum bleeding
Salicylates	*Salix* spp. (willow)	Anti-inflammatory, analgesic, antipyretic
Colchicine	*Colchicum autumnale* (crocus)	Anti-inflammatory, Rx gout
Emetine	Ipecacuanha (*Cephaelis*) root	Antiamoebic, Rx dysentery
Vincristine	*Vinca rosea* (periwinkle plant)	Antineoplastic, Rx cancer
Paclitaxel	Yew tree bark	Antineoplastic, Rx cancer

Source: Evans (2002), *Trease & Evans' Pharmacognosy*. 15th edn. ch. 6.
CNS = central nervous system; Rx = treatment of.

the suffix '-ine'. They are combined as salts to make them more soluble, e.g. morphine sulphate. It is thought that plants may have evolved the ability to synthesise bitter alkaloids as a defence mechanism against herbivorous animals. Examples of pharmacologically useful plant alkaloids are listed below, with cross-references to interesting relevant Drug Monographs (DM) and Clinical Interest Boxes (CIB):
* the analgesic agents morphine (CIB 16-4 and 16-5, DM 16-1), cocaine (CIB 15-6 and 22-9) and codeine (DM 32-7)
* the antiasthma drugs ephedrine (DM 32-8), theophylline (DM 32-3) and atropine
* anticancer agents, such as the vinca alkaloids (CIB 49-2), and antiretroviral agents, e.g. castanospermine

* alkaloids used in gout (colchicine), malaria (quinine [CIB 21-6]), obstetrics (the ergot alkaloids [DM 45-1]), and glaucoma (pilocarpine; Table 35-4)
* 'social' drugs: nicotine (DM 22-5), caffeine (CIB 22-10 and 22-11, DM 20-2) and mescaline
* poisons such as strychnine, muscarine, antithyroid compounds (CIB 39-6) and the ergot alkaloids from mouldy grains (CIB 45-1).

Formerly, the drug company Drug Houses of Australia (earlier known as Felton, Grimwade and Duerdins Pty Ltd) manufactured hyoscine and atropine from Australian *Duboisia* species; this was important during World War II, when supplies of the antinauseant drug hyoscine from European

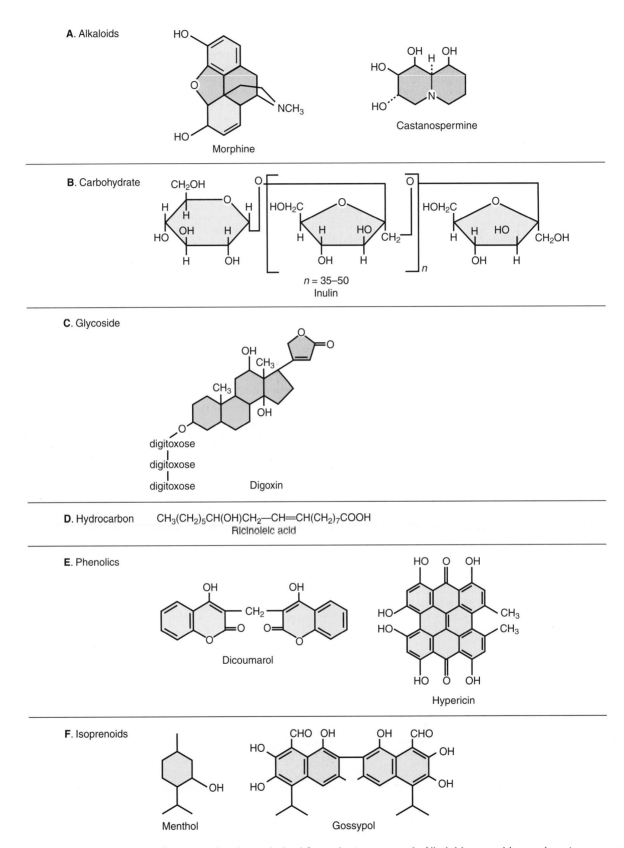

FIGURE 1-1 Chemical structures of some active drugs derived from plant sources. **A.** Alkaloids: morphine and castanospermine. **B.** A carbohydrate: inulin. **C.** A glycoside: digoxin. **D.** A hydrocarbon: ricinoleic acid. **E.** Phenolics: dicoumarol and hypericin. **F.** Isoprenoids: menthol and gossypol.

sources ran out.* In Tasmania, the opium poppy *Papaver somniferum* is grown and harvested for production of opium alkaloids. *Castanospermum australe* is a source of the effective antiretroviral alkaloid castanospermine.

Carbohydrates

Carbohydrates are organic compounds of carbon, hydrogen and oxygen. Carbohydrates used in medicine include sugars such as glucose; starches and fibres such as cellulose and inulin (a fructose–furanose polysaccharide used in kidney function tests [Figure 1-1B]); gelling agents such as agar; and gums such as tragacanth and *Aloe vera* products.

Gums and mucilages are plant exudates. When water is added, some of them will swell and form gelatinous masses. When taken orally, they tend to remain unchanged in the gastrointestinal tract, where they act as hydrophilic (water-attracting) colloids, forming watery bulk and exerting a laxative effect. Agar and psyllium seeds are examples of natural laxative gums, whereas methylcellulose and sodium carboxymethylcellulose are synthetic colloids. Gums are also used to soothe irritated skin and mucous membranes, and may be a rich source of starch.

Glycosides

Glycosides are a particular type of carbohydrate, which, on hydrolysis, yields a sugar plus one or more additional active substances. The sugar moiety (part) is combined chemically via ester-type glycosidic linkages to another sugar molecule or to a hydroxyl group on another chemical entity. The sugar is believed to increase the solubility, absorption, permeability and cellular distribution of the glycoside. An important plant glycoside used in medicine is digoxin (Figure 1-1C), found in *Digitalis* (foxglove) plants and known as a cardiac glycoside because of its stimulant actions on the heart. Glycosides present in other Australian plants, including the oleanders *Cerbera* and *Carissa*, are responsible for the poisonous nature of these plants. Cane toads also contain cardioactive glycosides.

The nucleotide subunits of RNA and DNA contain ribose in a glycosidic link. Glycosides are also produced during the processes of drug metabolism in the human body, particularly in the liver; many drug molecules and their metabolites are combined in a glycosidic link with glucuronic acid. Such large compound metabolites are known as glucuronides and are more soluble and hence more excretable than the parent drug molecules; they are also less pharmacologically active, as the large drug–glucuronide molecule cannot activate receptors, as can the parent drug.

---

*FG & D were able to supply enough hyoscine for prophylaxis of motion sickness for all of the troops crossing the English Channel in the D-Day landings of June 1944.

Hydrocarbons

Plants contain many hydrocarbon components, including fats and waxes; oils such as castor, olive and coconut oil; and fatty acids, prostaglandins and balsams. Derivatives such as organic alcohols and esters contribute the fragrances to many plants and perfumes. Castor oil is mainly composed of ricinoleic acid (Figure 1-1D).

Phenols

Many pharmacologically active plant constituents are **phenolic**, i.e. they contain a benzene ring with a hydroxyl substituent. Examples are the salicylates, including aspirin-like compounds and flavouring agents (e.g. vanillin); iso-flavones, including phyto-oestrogens (Clinical Interest Box 44-5); coumarins, including the anticoagulant dicoumarol (Figure 1-1E); cannabinols from marijuana; hypericin (from St John's wort, used in depression, Clinical Interest Box 19-7 and Figure 1-1E); and poisonous aflatoxins from mouldy peanuts. (Ethanol from fermented plants and grains is not phenolic but is the prototype alcohol.)

Tannins are astringent plant phenolics that have the ability to tan hides (animal skins) by precipitating proteins. Tannins are common plant constituents, especially in bark, and account for some of the brown colour in swamps and rivers, also indeed in cups of tea. In Australian native medicine, kino, the gum exuded from eucalyptus trees, was an important source of tannins, which were used to treat diarrhoea, haemorrhages and throat infections.

Terpenes and steroids

Many plant chemicals, including **steroids**, are synthesised naturally from terpenes, 10-carbon molecules built up from small 5-carbon building blocks called isoprenes. Plant steroids, with their characteristic 4-ring structures (Figure 37-2), are used as the starting material for the production of many hormones. For example, the production of oestrogenic hormones for use as contraceptives was very difficult and expensive until methods were devised to use the plant sterol diosgenin, from *Dioscorea* species, in the synthesis of oestrogenic compounds. Other isoprenoid compounds are gossypol, a Chinese male contraceptive agent (Figure 1-1F); the active ingredients of the herbs gentian, valerian, feverfew and ginkgo; carotenoids such as β-carotene (Clinical Interest Box 56-3, Drug Monograph 56-2); and the poison picrotoxin.

Salicylates, a group of phenolic terpenoid compounds, are important analgesic drugs based on saligenin from willow tree bark; the chemical name for aspirin is acetylsalicylic acid (Clinical Interest Box 16-7, Drug Monograph 16-2). Pyrethrins, terpene-type compounds with effective insecticidal actions, have been used for centuries: it is reported that Napoleon ordered that the dried flowers of the chrysanthemum plant be used to delouse the French army! Australian research in the pyrethrin industry has discovered semisynthetic derivatives that have longer half-lives than the natural compounds and are therefore more useful in the plant production industries and as insecticides for animals.

Oils

Oils are highly viscous liquids that are high in hydrocarbon content, often flammable, and immiscible with water and aqueous solvents. They may be terpene-type compounds, and contain many types of chemicals including ketones, phenols, alcohols, esters and aldehydes. Oils are classified as being of two kinds, volatile or fixed: a fixed oil dropped onto filter paper will leave a greasy stain, whereas a volatile oil will not, as it evaporates. Volatile oils may impart aromas to a plant.

Oils are frequently used as flavouring agents, in perfumery, in chemical industries, and for therapeutic actions as antiseptics, carminatives (soothing to the stomach) and antispasm agents. Eucalyptus, peppermint and clove oils are examples of volatile oils used in medicine. Castor oil is an example of a fixed oil used in medicine, while olive oil is a fixed oil used in cooking. Camphor, menthol (Figure 1-1F) and thymol are related aromatic agents used in respiratory medicine. The Australian species myrtaceae and melaleucas contain many fragrant and useful oils, including eucalyptus and tea-tree oils.

DRUG NAMES AND CLASSIFICATIONS

Drug names

As a drug passes through the investigational stages before it is approved and marketed, it collects three different types of name—the chemical name; the approved (or generic or non-proprietary) name; and the proprietary (or brand or trade) name or names. For example, the chemical name of amoxycillin, a commonly prescribed antibacterial antibiotic, is D(-)-α-amino-p-hydroxybenzylpenicillin. Its approved (generic) name, amoxycillin, is derived from parts of its chemical name, and it is marketed under dozens of proprietary names, including Alphamox, Amohexal, Amoxil, Bgramin, Cilamox and Moxacin, in various formulations such as injections, capsules, tablets, syrups, suspensions and paediatric drops, and in combinations with other anti-bacterials.

Chemical names

The **chemical name** is a precise description of the drug's chemical composition and molecular structure. It is particularly meaningful to medicinal chemists, who should be able to draw

the chemical structure if given the chemical name, but may be virtually unintelligible to others. As chemical names are too complicated to remember easily, or fit on a prescription pad or pharmacy bottle label, drugs likely to reach the market and be used medically are given a name that is simpler, more euphonious and easier to spell.

Approved (generic) names

The **approved name** is usually assigned by the manufacturer with the approval of the local drug regulating authority; it becomes the official drug name, e.g. the Australian Approved Name (AAN) or European Approved Name (EAN). It is a shorter name usually derived from the chemical name, and is the name listed in official compendia such as the *Australian Medicines Handbook* or the *British Pharmacopoeia*. The approved name needs to be distinct in sound and spelling so that it is not easily confused with other drugs, and preferably related to the names of pharmacologically similar drugs (see Table 1-2).*

---

* A musical spoof on drug names, and on the drug industry generally, was written and recorded by two British comedians, Adam Kay and Suman Biswas; the lyrics of 'Paracetamoxyfrusebendroneomycin', to be sung to the tune of 'Supercalifragilisticexpialidocious' from 'Mary Poppins', can be found via the Google search engine.

TABLE 1-2 Families of drugs

PREFIX OR SUFFIX	DRUG GROUP	EXAMPLE GENERIC NAME
-caine	Local anaesthetics	Lignocaine, bupivacaine
-cillin	Penicillins	Ampicillin
-olol	β-blockers	Propranolol
-tidine	Histamine H_2-receptor antagonists	Cimetidine
cefa/o-	Cefalosporins	Cefotaxime
-oxacin	Quinolone antibiotics	Norfloxacin
-statin	HMG-CoA reductase inhibitors	Simvastatin
-pril	ACE inhibitors	Captopril
-azepam	Benzodiazepines	Diazepam
-artan	Angiotensin-II-receptor antagonists	Candesartan
-a/oquine	Quinine antimalarials	Chloroquine
-a/ovir	Antivirals	Aciclovir
-azole	Azole antifungal agents	Ketoconazole
-coxib	Cyclo-oxygenase-2 inhibitors	Celecoxib
-cycline	Tetracycline antibiotics	Doxycycline
-dipine	Calcium channel blockers	Nifedipine
-dronate	Bisphosphonates	Alendronate
-eplase	Fibrinolytic agents	Alteplase
-floxacin	Quinolone antibiotics	Ciprofloxacin
gli-	Sulfonylureas	Glibenclamide
-glitazone	Thiazolidinediones (glitazones)	Rosiglitazone
-i/ythromycin	Macrolide antibiotics	Erythromycin
-lutamide	Antiandrogens	Flutamide
-mab	Monoclonal antibodies	Trastuzumab
-onidine	$α_2$-adrenoceptor agonist	Clonidine
-oprost	Prostaglandin analogues	Latanoprost
-prazole	Proton pump inhibitors	Omeprazole
-setron	$5\text{-}HT_3$ antagonists	Ondansetron
-stim	Colony-stimulating factors	Filgrastim
-tinib	Tyrosine kinase inhibitors	Imatinib
-triptan	$5HT_1$ agonists	Sumatriptan
-zolamide	Carbonic anhydrase inhibitor	Acetazolamide

Note: It would be useful if all drugs had names related to other similar drugs; however, this tends to be true only of more recent drug groups. Names can be deceiving: names of most β-blockers end in '-olol'; however, stanozolol is not a β-blocker but an anabolic steroid, so it is not safe to assume that drugs whose names sound similar always have similar effects and uses. Similarly, while drugs ending in '-mycin' all come from fungi (Eumycetes) or are related to fungal metabolites, they may be antibacterial antibiotics or anticancer drugs. And the table cannot be read backwards, i.e. while the suffix -vir implies the drug is probably an antiviral, not all antiviral drugs end in -vir (think zidovudine and ribavirin).

ACE = angiotensin-converting enzyme (converts angiotensin I to angiotensin II, which acts to decrease the diameter of arteries and arterioles [vasoconstriction] and hence to raise blood pressure); HMG-CoA = 3-hydroxy-3-methylglutaryl coenzyme A (a coenzyme involved in the early stages of cholesterol synthesis).

Strictly speaking, the term **generic name** refers to a group name, e.g. the penicillins, the salicylates, the β-blockers; however, it has come to be used interchangeably with the approved name. For example, we speak of generic prescribing, meaning doctors prescribing using the approved name of a drug (amoxycillin) rather than one proprietary or brand name (e.g. Amoxil). In this text we will always use generic (approved) names for drugs but may sometimes add a trade name if it is well known enough (e.g. Valium, Prozac or Viagra) to help students identify a particular drug. Note that approved names use lower-case letters, whereas a trade name always begins with an upper-case letter.

Proprietary (trade or brand) names

When a drug company markets a particular drug product, it selects and copyrights a **proprietary** or **trade name** for its drug (see Clinical Interest Box 1-4). This copyright restricts the use of the name to that individual drug company and refers only to that formulation of the drug. To encourage doctors to prescribe particular versions of the drug and to promote sales of trade name drugs, extensive advertising is usually necessary; this expense is eventually borne by the consumer.

Generic prescribing and bioequivalence

As numerous brand names may exist for the same drug, such as those shown above for amoxycillin, prescribers are encouraged to use the generic name. The use of generic names is also widely advocated to avoid confusion between drugs with similar trade names. With some exceptions, most generic drug products sold (assuming same dose and type of formulation) are considered therapeutically equivalent (bioequivalent); and some generic products are often much less expensive than a particular brand name drug. For this reason, and because pharmacists cannot possibly carry and store every brand of every marketed drug, in some defined situations pharmacists are allowed to substitute between brand names if the named products are considered to be identical in terms of bioequivalence (dose, availability to sites of action, pharmacokinetic parameters etc.). Thus the Australian Pharmaceutical Benefits Scheme (PBS; see Chapters 2 and 4) allows brand substitution between the six brands of amoxycillin listed earlier, for formulations of the same strength (dose), unless the prescriber checks a box on the prescription form to indicate 'Brand substitution not permitted' (see Figure 2-1B). The substitution can be confusing to patients if, for example, the colour, shape, name, taste and packaging of the tablet change but the pharmacist insists that the medicine is the same; this situation requires sensitive counselling.

International Non-Proprietary Names (INN) and European Approved Names

Since the United Kingdom's entry into the European Community (EC) in 1973, and the recent adoption of European Approved Names for drugs, the British medical and pharmaceutical establishments have had to accept the use of INN in the EC as the European Approved Names for drugs. Examples of INN are norepinephrine (formerly noradrenaline), sulfonamides (sulphonamides), furosemide (frusemide), diethylstilbestrol (stilboestrol) and ciclosporin (cyclosporin) (see Longmore et al 2004). These changes have not yet been adopted in Australia or New Zealand. We suspect and hope that the old terminology will stay on; for example, although the INN for the sympathomimetic neurotransmitter is 'norepinephrine' in the EC, USA and Canada, the type of neurotransmission is still called 'noradrenergic' and the receptors 'adrenoceptors'.

American names

It would be ideal for safety and convenience if the approved name for a drug molecule could be the same worldwide: indeed, the World Health Organization (WHO) is encouraging the use of International Non-proprietary Names (INN). Approved names in Australia generally follow the British names, as Australian pharmacy has long been legally dependent on the *British Pharmacopoeia* as the standard for drugs. Sometimes, however, other approved names are used in the USA (USAN, the US Approved Name), Canada and countries that follow their lead, so Australian and New Zealand students can become confused if they do not realise, for example, that adrenaline (UK, Australia, New Zealand) = epinephrine (USA).

Major reference texts such as *Martindale: The Complete Drug Reference* (Sweetman 2005) usually list alternative approved and many trade names, which helps clarify the issue.

Drug classifications
Classification systems

Drug classification can be approached from many perspectives. Using the example of amoxycillin again, this could be classified by:

- source, i.e. where the drug comes from (semisynthetic antibiotic from *Penicillium* spp.)
- chemical formula, type of chemical structure of the drug (β-lactam, penicillanic acid derivative)
- pharmacokinetic parameters, e.g. relating to how the drug is absorbed or metabolised in the body (acid-resistant, β-lactamase-sensitive, intermediate half-life)
- activity, relating to the effects of the drug in the body (wide-spectrum antibacterial agent)

- mechanism of action, explaining how the drug works (inhibitor of bacterial cell wall synthesis)
- clinical use, conditions for which the drug is prescribed (indicated for treatment of infections by sensitive Gram-positive and Gram-negative organisms)
- body system affected by the drug (for infections of respiratory system; ear, nose and throat; genitourinary tract etc)
- drug schedule, i.e. the group into which the drug is classified for legal purposes (e.g. S4 [PRESCRIPTION-ONLY] medicine—see Chapter 4 and Appendix 5)
- pregnancy safety schedule, grouping drugs depending on their safety for use in pregnancy (A: considered safe) (see Clinical Interest Box 45-1)
- popularity (most commonly prescribed drug in the world)
- whether its use is allowed in sporting competitions (yes—approved by the World Anti-Doping Agency).

Not surprisingly, students are often confused by drug classification, particularly as sometimes the same drug may be classified into various groups depending on the clinical use, e.g. aspirin-like drugs may be classified as analgesics, antipyretics, anti-inflammatory agents or antithrombotics. Probably the most useful methods involve classification by clinical indication, by body system or by mechanism of action. This book uses these approaches where appropriate; examples include Chapter 26: Lipid-lowering Drugs, and Chapter 52: Antifungal and Antiviral Drugs. An example of drugs classified by body system can be found in Unit IV: Drugs Affecting the Central Nervous System, whereas in Chapter 19: Psychotropic Agents, antidepressants are grouped together under 'Tricyclic antidepressants' (a chemical class), 'Monoamine oxidase inhibitors' or 'Selective serotonin reuptake inhibitors'. Such drug classifications can help the health-care professional understand and learn about the individual agents available for drug therapy.

Prototype drugs

Pharmacology is easier to understand and learn when **key**, or **prototype**, **drugs** are studied. A prototype drug is usually the most important drug in a particular drug class, to which other drugs in the class can be compared. In this text, many prototype drugs are described in detail in a consistent format called a Drug Monograph; thus, diazepam can be viewed as the prototype benzodiazepine antianxiety agent (Drug Monograph 17-1). When a new similar drug becomes available, the practitioner can associate it with its drug group and prototype, and make inferences about many of its basic qualities before focusing on specific properties to differentiate it from the prototype and other drugs in the same group.

Prescription only or OTC drugs

A drug may be classified as a **prescription only drug**, which means that it requires a legal prescription to be dispensed, or it may be a non-prescription, or **over-the-counter (OTC) drug**, which means that it may be purchased without a prescription, possibly in a pharmacy, supermarket or general store. Some prescription drugs may be purchased OTC, usually in lower drug dosages that are considered to be relatively safe for sale, for conditions that may not warrant a person visiting a doctor, or for which important drugs need to be readily available. An example is the non-steroidal anti-inflammatory drug naproxen, which is available as an OTC drug (S2, Pharmacy Only) in a 220 mg to 275 mg strength for treatment of dysmenorrhoea, but requires a prescription (S4) for the 250, 500, 550, 750 or 1000 mg tablets, 500 mg suppositories or 25 mg/mL suspension for arthritis and bone pain.* Drug schedules are considered in more detail in Chapters 2 and 4, and OTC medicines in Chapter 3.

WHO essential drugs list

It is recognised that with the enormous range of drugs available, few countries or health services can subsidise or provide the whole range of drugs, and no pharmacies could stock them all. To assist in decision making with respect to which drugs are the most important, the World Health Organization, WHO, through its Department of Essential Drugs and Medicines (EDM), has derived a model list of about 300 individual drugs from some 27 categories (see Appendix 7), which are considered essential to provide 'safe and effective treatment for the majority of communicable and non-communicable diseases'. This is useful for all countries attempting to curtail rapidly increasing expenditure on drugs, and is particularly useful for developing countries, allowing them to concentrate on providing the most important drugs. A statement by WHO defines essential drugs as 'those that satisfy the health-care needs of the majority of the population . . . they should therefore be available at all times in adequate amounts and in the appropriate dosage forms, and at a price that individuals and community can afford'.

The selection of drugs is determined by a committee of scientists and clinicians and is updated at regular intervals. These drugs first require market approval on the basis of efficacy, safety and quality as well as value for money. Listing 'essential' drugs inevitably raises concerns, particularly from

---

*There is some logic here — the cost of many drugs is subsidised by the government, so low-income earners with health-care cards may be able to obtain drugs more cheaply if they have been prescribed, than they could by buying the same drugs OTC.

the manufacturers of drugs not on the list, which may be seen as 'non-essential'. A table adapted from the WHO model list of drugs is included as Appendix 7, showing categories of essential drugs and, where possible, an example of therapeutic groups.

Australian top 10 drugs

The Commonwealth Department of Health regularly audits the usage of prescription drugs in Australia and publishes lists of the top 10 drugs, scored by numbers of daily doses, by prescription counts, and by cost to the government (i.e. to taxpayers). The lists for drug use in the year 2004/05 are summarised in Table 1-3; note that only subsidised drugs are audited here, not those bought OTC or provided under private prescriptions.

Understandably, the government is concerned about the widespread use of the 'statin' drugs, used to lower blood cholesterol levels. As can be seen, in each of the lists statins occupy the top two places. When these drugs were listed on the PBS there was a massive blow-out in their use, partly by people wishing to reduce their cardiovascular risk without the inconvenience of raising their exercise levels or decreasing their food intake. The two statins together accounted for A\$266 million greater expenditure in the 2004/05 health budget than they had in 2000/01. There are now strict guidelines that must be met before these drugs can be prescribed on the PBS, including documentation of blood lipid levels and risk category (cardiovascular, diabetes, family history, age), and at least 6 weeks of dietary therapy attempted. There is concern, however, that patients who are denied a prescription by one doctor may simply 'shop around' until they find a doctor who will decide that they meet the criteria.

DRUG INFORMATION
Important drug information

The basic **information** important for a major drug includes its:
- approved/generic name
- drug group or category
- pharmacodynamic effects
- mechanisms of action
- particular pharmacokinetic parameters
- **indications** for clinical use
- common adverse effects (**adverse drug reactions**)
- **contraindications** and precautions
- significant drug interactions
- monitoring techniques.

Contraindications are the medical conditions in which a drug should not be prescribed, e.g. a particular drug may be contraindicated in patients with kidney failure, or during pregnancy. Information as to potential toxic effects

and treatment of poisoning may also be relevant, as well as safety of use in particular cohorts of patients, such as premature infants or the elderly. The Australian Drug Evaluation Committee's Pregnancy Safety category indicates the likely safety or risks with the use of a drug during pregnancy (see Chapter 8 and Table 8-1).

Drug information sources

Publication of new information on old drugs and the release of new drugs are ongoing processes. Research papers in scientific journals, news releases, articles, patient information brochures, reference books and textbooks are written in an attempt to keep up with the new discoveries. Because no one reference is a complete source of drug data to meet the varied and specialised needs of clinical practice today, students need to be familiar with the primary drug reference sources available. It is always important to read critically and consider what credibility can be given to the author and the publication, particularly with information found on the worldwide web.

Official sources, pharmacopoeias and formularies

Official sources of drug information are published by governments and government bodies such as departments of health and hospitals, and by pharmaceutical societies and medical colleges, and contain legally accepted standards for drugs. **Pharmacopoeias** are reference texts containing a compendium or collected body of drug information relevant to a particular country. The pharmacopoeia usually contains information on all of the authorised drugs available within the country, including their descriptions, formulae, strengths, standards of purity and dosage forms.

Formularies are similar but may also include information on drug actions, adverse effects, general medical information, guidelines for pharmacists dispensing medicines, and the 'recipes' for formulation or production of different medicines, such as tablets, injections, ointments and eye-drops. A national formulary may also be used by the government to limit the drugs available or subsidised to encourage rational, cost-efficient prescribing and enhance the quality use of medicine (QUM; see Chapter 2).

Examples of official drug information sources are:
- the *Australian Pharmaceutical Formulary* (APF) and *Australian Pharmaceutical Handbook* (Pharmaceutical Society of Australia)
- the *Paediatric Pharmacopoeia* (Pharmacy Department, Melbourne Royal Children's Hospital)
- the *British Pharmacopoeia* (BP; British Pharmacopoeia Commission)
- the *British National Formulary* (BNF; Royal Pharmaceutical Society of Great Britain and British Medical Association)

TABLE 1-3 Australia's top 10 drugs, 2004-05*

Top 10 drugs counted by number of people taking the standard daily dose every day per thousand population

ORDER	DRUG (INDICATION)	DAILY DOSES PER THOUSAND PEOPLE
1	Atorvastatin (lipid-lowering)	98.2
2	Simvastatin (lipid-lowering)	56.0
3	Ramipril (hypertension)	33.7
4	Diltiazem (angina)	30.1
5	Omeprazole (oesophageal reflux)	20.6
6	Irbesartan (hypertension)	20.1
7	Salbutamol (bronchodilator)	18.9
8	Frusemide (diuretic)	18.8
9	Aspirin (antiplatelet, anti-inflammatory)	18.2
10	Sertraline (antidepressant)	17.6

Top 10 drugs by prescription counts (in millions)

ORDER	DRUG (INDICATION)	MILLIONS OF PRESCRIPTIONS
1	Atorvastatin (lipid-lowering)	8.07
2	Simvastatin (lipid-lowering)	6.28
3	Paracetamol (analgesic)	4.77
4	Omeprazole (oesophageal reflux)	4.41
5	Irbesartan (hypertension)	3.37
6	Atenolol (hypertension, angina, arrhythmias)	3.25
7	Salbutamol (bronchodilator)	3.06
8	Esomeprazole (oesophageal reflux)	2.98
9	Irbesartan with hydrochlorothiazide	2.94
10	Ramipril (hypertension)	2.90

Top 10 drugs by cost to government (in A$ millions)

ORDER	DRUG (INDICATION)	COST TO GOVERNMENT (A$ MILLIONS)
1	Atorvastatin (lipid-lowering)	461
2	Simvastatin (lipid-lowering)	370
3	Omeprazole (oesophageal reflux)	177
4	Fluticasone with salmeterol (asthma)	166
5	Clopidogrel (thromboembolism)	151
6	Olanzapine (schizophrenia, mania)	149
7	Esomeprazole (oesophageal reflux)	143
8	Pravastatin (lipid-lowering)	120
9	Alendronic acid (osteoporosis)	109
10	Pantoprazole (peptic ulcer)	104

*Note that the audit does not score drugs prescribed by private prescription or bought OTC.
Source: Australian Prescriber 2006; 29(1): 5.

- the *European Pharmacopoeia and European Pharmacopoeia Supplement* (Council of Europe, Strasbourg)
- *Martindale: The Complete Drug Reference* (Pharmaceutical Press, London)
- the *United States Pharmacopeia* (USP) and *United States National Formulary* (US Pharmacopeial Convention)
- *Handbook of Nonprescription Drugs* (American Pharmaceutical Association).

In New Zealand, there is no national formulary, but the BNF and APF are legal standards and are used for teaching. The Pharmaceutical Schedule from PHARMAC lists subsidised medicines and is updated every few months (see www.pharmac.govt.nz).

Semiofficial sources

Semiofficial sources of drug information may be published by government bodies or other groups, such as medical and pharmacology societies or independent publishers, and may include drug bulletins, reference books and updates, but no drug advertisements. While not official standards, they attempt to provide up-to-date, independent and unbiased information on drugs. Depending on the publication, information such as lists of food additives, patient support organisations, poisons information centres and prescribing guidelines may be included. Examples include the Therapeutic Guidelines series, Adverse Drug Reactions Advisory Committee (ADRAC) bulletins and *MediScene* newsletters, reference books such as *Australian Drug Information for the Health Care Professional* (AusDI), the *Australian Prescription Products Guide* (known as the PP Guide), the *Merck Index*, *Drug Interactions: Facts*, and *Drug Interactions Analysis and Management*, and journals such as *Current Therapeutics* and *Drugs*.

Handing out consumer medical information (CMI) pamphlets to patients is encouraged as an important way to improve people's involvement with and understanding of the drugs they are prescribed. In Australia, all products have had CMI handouts since the end of 2002. They are particularly important when a drug is first provided, the dose or formulation changed, or the information revised. In particular, patients want answers to three questions:
- what is this medicine for?
- what will it do to me?
- how do I take it? (also: what will it cost?).

Some reference texts, e.g. the *MIMS Annual*, *Mosby's GenRx* and the United States Pharmacopeial Convention's *Drug Information for the Health Care Professional* (USP DI), provide actual photographs of drug formulations to assist in identifying an unknown tablet or capsule. In addition, manufacturers often place numbers with letters on their solid-dose formulations to aid in identification.

The Cochrane Collaboration is an international organisation that prepares systematic reviews of the effects of health-care interventions, such as clinical trials of drugs or other therapeutic techniques, with the aim of helping all people make well-informed decisions about health care. It aims to avoid duplication of studies, minimise bias and provide relevant, up-to-date easily accessible information. There are Cochrane databases of reviews, clinical trials, methodologies and economic evaluations, among others.

Drug or poisons information centres and pharmacists

Drug information centres, usually located in the pharmacy departments of major teaching hospitals, are set up to disseminate information about drugs and treatment of drug overdoses, and other related information, to maximise safety, efficacy and economy in drug use (see Appendix 6, and *Australian Medicines Handbook*, Appendix F.) Their advice is based on medical and scientific literature and expertise in the areas of identification of drugs, adverse reactions, drug interactions and poisoning. They are excellent sources of information for both the public and health professionals and for answering difficult pharmacological questions. In addition, pharmacists in hospitals and retail chemist shops are usually available and willing to provide drug information.

A new arm of the Community Quality Use of Medicines program was launched in Australia in January 2004, with pocket-sized 'Medimate' booklets distributed to doctors and pharmacists for patients. The program was supported by advertisements on national TV and in magazines. Each booklet contained general information about medicines, other therapies, CMI leaflets, use of OTC medicines, side-effects and information sources, and questions that consumers should ask about their medicines, and provided a tear-off slip that could be filled in to summarise the person's drug therapy.

Other drug information sources

An up-to-date pharmacology textbook is a valuable source of drug information for inclusion in the health-care professional's library. Various 'drug guides' also exist, acting as quick reference sources of summarised information on drugs. Most of these have grown rather too large to fit in the pocket of a doctor's, nurse's or pharmacist's uniform, but are useful on the desk or ward station. Examples are *Havard's Nursing Guide to Drugs*, *Mosby's Medication Guide*, and the *MIMS* bi-monthly drug reference guide.

Drug companies applying for registration of their products must supply to health authorities an enormous amount of information on all aspects of the drug, to prove safety, efficacy and cost-effectiveness. A summary of this information is available in publications such as the *MIMS Annual*, the PP Guide and in CMI sheets, advertisements and promotions. (Ethical aspects of drug advertising are discussed in Chapter 4.) It is important to consider the source of such information and beware of bias or selectivity of information.

With the proliferation of medical sites on the Internet, many search engines and directories are available to provide both general and specialised drug information for everyone—health-care professionals and consumers/patients. Some professional journals (medical, pharmacy and nursing), databases, indexes and abstracting services also provide current drug information on the Internet. It is essential to read Internet sites critically when seeking drug information because there is no screening system to determine the accuracy of Internet information, and erroneous or biased information may be posted. Therefore the best approach may be to consider the credibility and reputation of the provider of the information. For example, does it come from reputable drug information centres; pharmacy, medical or nursing schools; professional journals; medical societies or colleges; government bodies; drug companies; or even individuals wanting to publicise or sell their own favourite remedies or products?

Many other sources of drug information are available. The criteria for using any particular source should be based on the information desired and the currency and accuracy of the source.

DOSAGE MEASUREMENTS AND CALCULATIONS

The main system of measurement in use for administering drugs is the metric system, based on **SI units** (Système International d' Unités)—this is the most widely used and the most convenient, as units change in multiples of 10. The 'household system', utilising measures readily available in the home setting, such as the teaspoon (about 5 mL), the tablespoon (15–20 mL) and cup (250 mL), is a less accurate system. The apothecary system, dating back hundreds of years and based on the English system of measures, was phased out in Australia in the 1960s, to the relief of all who had been required to learn its tables of measures.* Useful conversion tables to convert between metric measures and imperial ones such as inches or pints are included in some reference books, e.g. the introductory general section of the *MIMS Annual* (Caswell 2005).

---

*Basic units of weight were the grain (equivalent to about 65 mg), the apothecary's ounce (31 g) and the pound (454 g). One scruple was equal to 20 grains, and one drachm 60 grains. The basic unit of fluid volume was the minim, equal to the volume of water that would weigh a grain — a very small amount (about 0.06 mL). Other volume measures were the fluid dram (1 teaspoonful, i.e. about 5 mL), the fluid ounce (28.4 mL), and the pint (about 568 mL).

Metric system

The metric system has several basic units of measure, including:
- length, the metre (m)
- time, the second (s)
- mass, the kilogram (kg)
- amount of substance, the mole (mol).

Other useful units are: for volume, the cubic metre (m^3) and the litre (L, about 4 cups); for area, the square metre (m^2); and for mass, the gram (g, a little more than the weight of a small paper clip).

The mole is the amount of any substance that contains Avogadro's number (about 6.022×10^{23}) of atoms or molecules of the substance, and is equivalent to the molecular weight expressed in grams. The mole is therefore a different weight depending on the substance; for example one mole of sodium chloride (molecular weight 58.5) is present in 58.5 g pure NaCl, and one mole of water in 18 g pure H_2O. This unit is used mainly in laboratories and research situations, not for dosing drugs. A one molar solution (1M = 1 mol/L) contains one mole of the particular solute dissolved in 1 litre of the solvent.

The metric system is a decimal system in which the basic units can be divided or multiplied by 10, 100 or 1000 to form a secondary unit. The names of the secondary units are formed by joining a Greek or Latin prefix to the name of the primary unit (Table 1-4); for example, the gram is the metric unit of weight commonly used in weighing chemicals and various pharmaceutical preparations. A gram is 1/1000 of a kilogram, and 1000 times greater than a milligram. Hence to change milligrams to grams, divide by 1000, and to change metres to centimetres, multiply by 100.

The following is the recommended style of notation as proposed for the International System of Units:
- units are not capitalised (gram, not Gram)
- no full stop should be used with unit abbreviations (mL, not m.L. or mL.)
- only decimal notation should be used, not fractions (0.25 kg, not 1/4 kg)
- quantities less than 1 should have a zero placed to the left of the decimal point (0.75 mg, not .75 mg) to avoid mistakes
- abbreviations should not be made plural (kg, not kgs).

There are some situations in medicine in which SI units are not used. These include:
- measurement of blood pressure. The sphygmomanometer used to measure blood pressure is calibrated in millimetres of mercury (mmHg) rather than in units of pressure (pascals, Pa)
- percentage solutions, where the strength of a solution may be expressed as a percentage (e.g. 2% solution) rather than in mol/L or g/L. By convention, in this context '%' means grams of solute per 100 mL solution. Thus a 2% lignocaine solution contains 2 g lignocaine per 100 mL

solution, and a 0.1% solution contains 0.1 g/100 mL, i.e. 1 mg/mL
- drip rates for infusion sets. Note that the drip rate may vary, as may the volume of a drop, so each unit should be checked according to the manufacturer's advice. Commonly, a standard set delivers 20 drops of aqueous liquid per mL (15 drops for blood), whereas a microdrip set delivers 60 drops per mL
- the strengths of solutions of electrolytes, which may be expressed in milliequivalents (mEq), best explained by the following example: 1 L of a 1 mM solution of calcium chloride ($CaCl_2$) contains 1 mEq calcium ions and 2 mEq chloride ions.

Dosage calculations

A thorough understanding of arithmetic (fractions and ratios) is necessary for safe drug administration in the health-care setting. When in doubt, it is advisable to double-check all calculations with another health-care professional, especially with a pharmacist who will be highly trained in medication calculations. The following examples of **dose calculations** are the types of problems that may be encountered by health professionals. Each problem is solved in a stepwise manner and, where appropriate, a helpful hints section is included.

Sample calculation for oral administration of tablets or capsules

Example 1. The prescriber orders paracetamol 1 g orally every 6 hours for a patient with a high temperature. The label on the package states that each tablet contains 500 mg paracetamol. How many tablets do you administer to the patient every 6 hours?

Step 1.   Convert both weights to the same unit of weight, in this case milligrams.
Prescribed dose = 1 g × 1000 mg/g
= 1000 mg 6-hourly.

Step 2.   To calculate the number of tablets required, apply the formula:

$$\text{Tablets required} = \frac{\text{prescribed dose}}{\text{tablet strength}}$$

$$= \frac{1000 \text{ mg}}{500 \text{ mg}}$$

$$= 2 \text{ tablets.}$$

The patient should take 2 tablets every 6 hours.

Example 2. An elderly patient is prescribed 0.125 mg digoxin once daily, which is available in your care facility

pharmacy only as a 250 mcg tablet. How many tablets do you administer daily?

Step 1.   Convert both weights to the same unit of weight, in this case micrograms.
Prescribed dose = 0.125 mg × 1000 mcg/mg
= 125 mcg daily.

Step 2.   To calculate the number of tablets required, apply the formula:

$$\text{Tablets required} = \frac{\text{prescribed dose}}{\text{tablet strength}}$$

$$= \frac{125 \text{ mcg}}{250 \text{ mcg}}$$

$$= 0.5 \text{ tablet.}$$

The patient should take half a tablet once a day.

Helpful hints:
- Never use less than half a tablet, and preferably use a smaller-dose tablet if one is available; here, 2 × 62.5 mcg tablets would be preferable.
- Exercise care, as some tablets or capsules should never be broken, especially enteric-coated or sustained-release preparations, unless otherwise indicated as safe to break.
- Take care when converting from milligrams to micrograms. Always use the abbreviation 'mcg' and not the Greek symbol μ.

Calculation for oral administration of liquids

Example 3. A child has been prescribed the antibiotic erythromycin 250 mg orally every 12 hours as prophylaxis for rheumatic fever. The stock liquid suspension contains 200 mg/5 mL. What volume of the mixture should be given every 12 hours?

Step 1.   Conversion is not required because in this example both prescribed dose and stock suspension strength involve the same unit of weight, mg. The strength of the stock suspension is 200/5 mg/mL = 40 mg/mL.

Step 2.   To calculate the volume of suspension required apply the formula:

$$\text{Volume required} = \frac{\text{prescribed dose}}{\text{strength of stock suspension}}$$

$$= \frac{250 \text{ mg} \times 5 \text{ mL}}{500 \text{ mg}}$$

$$= 6.25 \text{ mL.}$$

The child should be given 6.25 mL twice daily.

TABLE 1-4 Metric prefixes, meanings, and relations

PREFIX	MEANING	POWER OF 10
tera (T)	million millions	10^{12}
giga (G)	billions	10^{9}, 1 000 000 000
mega (M)	millions	10^{6}, 1 000 000
kilo (k)	thousands	10^{3}, 1 000
hecto (h)	hundreds	10^{2}, 100
deca (da)	tens	10^{1}, 10
deci (d)	tenths	10^{-1}, 1/10, 0.1
centi (c)	hundredths	10^{-2}, 1/100, 0.01
milli (m)	thousandths	10^{-3}, 1/1000, 0.001
micro (μ or mc)	millionths	10^{-6}, 0.000001
nano (n)	billionths	10^{-9}
pico (p		10^{-12}
femto (f)		10^{-15}

Note that the units hecto-, deca-, and centi- are not commonly used; that micro (μ) should be written out or mc used if there is possibility of confusion with 'm' (a mistake, e.g. dosing a patient with 250 mg digoxin instead of 250 μg, could be fatal); that the term billion may mean 10^{9} or 10^{12} depending on local custom; and that a zero should be used before the decimal point if the number is <1, e.g. 0.5, not .5.

Calculation of dosage based on body weight

Example 4. A child has been prescribed the antibiotic ampicillin and the recommended dosage is 10 mg/kg every 6 hours. What will be the size of a single dose for a child weighing 30 kg?

Step 1.   Conversion is not required because in this example the body weight of the child and that in the recommended dosage are in the same units, kg.

Step 2.   To calculate the size of a single dose, apply the formula:

Prescribed dose = recommended dose (mg/kg)
$\times$ body weight (kg)
= 10 mg/kg $\times$ 30 kg
= 300 mg.

The child should be given 300 mg every 6 hours.

Example 5. A child is to be given the antiprotozoal drug metronidazole to treat giardiasis. The recommended dosage is 30 mg/kg/day in three divided doses (i.e. 8-hourly). What is the size of a single dose if the child's weight is 18 kg?

Step 1.   Conversion is not required because in this example the body weight of the child and that in the recommended dosage are in the same units, kg.

Step 2.   To calculate the total daily dose apply the formula:

Prescribed dosage = recommended dosage
(mg/kg/day)
$\times$ body weight (kg)
= 30 mg/kg/day $\times$ 18 kg
= 540 mg/day total dose.

Step 3.   To calculate the size of a single dose, apply the formula:

$$\text{Single dose (mg)} = \frac{\text{total dose (mg)}}{\text{number of doses}}$$

$$= \frac{540 \text{ mg}}{3}$$

$$= 180 \text{ mg.}$$

The child should be administered 180 mg every 8 hours.

Calculation of dosage based on surface area

In some circumstances (e.g. critical-care situations, cancer chemotherapy), dosages of some drugs are calculated in terms of body surface area (see Chapter 8). These calculations usually involve a nomogram that relates height (or length), weight and surface area (Figure 8-2).

Example 6. A woman is to be administered epirubicin for treatment of cancer. The prescribed dosage is 100 mg/m^2 and her body surface area has been determined as 1.5 m^2. The stock solution of epirubicin is 2 mg/mL. What volume should be drawn up for injection?

Step 1.   Conversion is not required because in this example the body surface area of the patient and that in the prescribed dosage are in the same units, m^2

Step 2.   To calculate the total dosage, apply the formula:

Prescribed dosage = recommended dosage (mg/m^2)
        × body surface area (m^2)
        = 100 mg/m^2 × 1.5 m^2
        = 150 mg.

Step 3.   To calculate the volume to be drawn up for injection, apply the formula:

$$\text{Volume required} = \frac{\text{prescribed dosage}}{\text{strength of stock suspension}}$$

$$= \frac{150 \text{ mg}}{2 \text{ mg}} \times 1 \text{ mL}$$

$$= 75 \text{ mL}.$$

The volume to be drawn up for injection is 75 mL. Note that this drug is available for injection in several pack sizes, ranging from 10 mg/5 mL to 50 mg/25 mL.

Calculation of drug dosage for injection

Example 7. A patient has been ordered 75 mg pethidine for pain relief. The ampoules available to you contain 100 mg in 2 mL. What volume is required for injection?

Step 1.   Conversion is not required because in this example the units of weight are the same, mg. The strength of the solution in the ampoules is 100/2 mg/mL
        = 50 mg/mL.

Step 2.   To calculate the volume to be drawn up for injection, apply the formula:

$$\text{Volume required} = \frac{\text{prescribed dosage}}{\text{strength of stock suspension}}$$

$$= \frac{75 \text{ mg}}{50 \text{ mg/mL}}$$

$$= 1.5 \text{ mL}.$$

The volume to be drawn up for injection is 1.5 mL from the 2 mL ampoule.

Helpful hints:
- Measuring drug dosages for injection is important, as too high a dose may be dangerous and too low a dose may be ineffective. Always check your calculation with another qualified health professional if you have any doubts at all.
- For drugs administered by injection, the number of decimal places in an answer should match the graduations on the syringe. For less than 1 mL, calculate to two decimal places (e.g. 0.75 mL, 0.25 mL, 0.64 mL), as syringes are often graduated in hundredths of a mL, i.e. 0.01 mL graduations. For more than 1 mL, calculate to one decimal place (e.g. 1.8 mL, 8.7 mL, 12.5 mL), as syringes may be graduated in either fifths (0.2 mL graduations) or tenths (0.1 mL graduations).

Calculation of drug dosage for intravenous infusion (by drip rate)

Example 8. A patient has been ordered an infusion of sodium chloride and glucose, 500 mL over 24 hours. The IV infusion (giving) set delivers 20 drops/mL. At what rate (in drops/minute) should the giving set drip?

Step 1.   Convert time to the same units, minutes:
        = 24 hours x 60
        = 1440 minutes.

Step 2.   To calculate the drip rate, apply the formula:

$$\text{Rate (drops/minute)} = \frac{\text{volume to be delivered} \times \text{drops/mL}}{\text{time (minutes)}}$$

$$= \frac{500 \text{ mL} \times 20 \text{ drops/mL}}{1440 \text{ minutes}}$$

$$= 6.9 \text{ drops/minute}$$

$$= 7 \text{ drops/minute (using next whole number).}$$

The giving set should be adjusted to a drip rate of 7 drops/minute.

Calculation of drug dosage for intravenous infusion (by infusion pump)

Example 9(a). For the same patient as in Example 8, an infusion pump becomes available. At what rate should the pump be set to deliver the sodium chloride/glucose solution?

Step 1.   The calculation here is much simpler, and can be done by simple proportions, as we know that 500 mL need to be delivered over 24 hours.

Thus: in 24 hours, deliver 500 mL

so   in 1 hour, deliver $\dfrac{500 \text{ mL} \times 1 \text{ h}}{24 \text{ h}}$

= 20.8 mL.

The infusion pump should be set to deliver approximately 21 mL/hour.

Example 9(b). The patient (a man weighing 80 kg) is then prescribed gentamicin 3 mg/kg/day in 3 doses/day by IV infusion, given every 8 hours over a 2-hour period. Each dose is to be diluted in 100 mL sterile normal saline. How should the infusion pump be set?

Method (1): Calculation by first principles:

Total daily dosage = 3 mg/kg/day × 80 kg
                             = 240 mg/day

divided into 3 equal doses = 240/3 mg/dose
                                            = 80 mg/dose.

Dose is to be diluted in 100 mL saline. Gentamicin Injection BP is provided as vials containing 80 mg/2 mL, so 1 vial contains 1 dose.
For each dose, contents of 1 vial are diluted to 100 mL in normal saline, giving 80 mg/100 mL, i.e. 0.8 mg/mL. Solution is to be run in IV over 2 hours, i.e. 100 mL/2 h, so pump is set at an infusion rate of 50 mL/h.

Method (2): Calculation by formula:

Infusion rate (mL/h) $= \dfrac{\text{Drug required (mg/h)} \times \text{volume (mL)}}{\text{Total amount (mg)}}$

From Method (1), each dose = 80 mg over 2 h = 40 mg/h, in a volume of 100 mL for a dose of 80 mg.

Hence infusion rate $= \dfrac{40 \text{ mg/h} \times 100 \text{ mL}}{80 \text{ mg}}$

$= \dfrac{4000 \text{ mg.mL}}{80 \text{ mg.h}}$

= 50 mL/h.

Calculation using strength of a solution

Example 10. An ophthalmologist has prescribed timolol eye-drops 5 mg/mL, one drop in the affected eye twice daily. You have available timolol 0.25% solution drops. How many drops are needed for the required dose?

Step 1.   Convert the concentration of the stock solution to mg/mL:

0.25% solution means 0.25 g/100 mL.

Step 2.   To calculate mg/mL, apply the formula:

$\text{mg/mL} = \dfrac{\text{g} \times 1000}{\text{volume (mL)}}$

$= \dfrac{0.25 \text{ g} \times 1000}{100 \text{ mL}}$

= 2.5 mg/mL.

Step 3.   To calculate the number of drops required, apply the formula:

$\dfrac{\text{number}}{\text{of drops}} = \dfrac{\text{prescribed dose}}{\text{strength of stock solution}} \times \dfrac{\text{number}}{\text{of drops}}_{\text{prescribed}}$

$= \dfrac{5 \text{ mg/mL}}{2.5 \text{ mg/mL}} \times 1 \text{ drop}$

= 2 drops.

You should instil two drops in the affected eye twice daily; however, note that two drops do not usually fit in the conjunctival sac, as discussed in Chapter 36, so a 0.5% solution will have to be obtained.

Calculation for safe maximum dose of a local anaesthetic

Example 11. The safe maximum dose (SMD) of lignocaine as a local anaesthetic in adults is set at 3 mg/kg body weight. You are provided with 5 mL ampoules of Lignocaine Hydrochloride Injection BP 2%. What is the maximum number of ampoules you would expect to require for an average-sized adult?

Assuming a mean adult body weight of 70 kg,
SMD = 70 × 3 mg/kg
        = 210 mg
2% solution means 2 g lignocaine hydrochloride per 100 mL solution,
i.e. 2000 mg are present in 100 mL
so 210 mg are present in (210/2000) × 100 mL
        = 10.5 mL.
So the safe maximum dose will be present in 10.5 mL solution and, as the ampoules provided contain 5 mL, two ampoules (10 mL) will probably be adequate.

KEY POINTS

- Pharmacology is the study of drugs, which are substances used for their effects on living systems. Useful drugs have the characteristics of potency, selectivity and specificity.

- Drugs may be solids (most commonly), liquids or gases. Most are organic (carbon-containing) chemicals. They may come from natural sources or be synthesised in laboratories. Pharmacologically active compounds derived from plants include alkaloids, glycosides, steroids, phenols and oils.

- People have searched for, been fascinated by, and used and abused drugs throughout recorded history. Initially, natural compounds were discovered by trial and error, then were studied for their medical actions and adverse effects. Now drugs and even receptors may be synthesised or genetically engineered and their mechanisms of action determined.

- Each drug is identified by three names: a chemical, generic (or approved), and proprietary (or trade) name. Generic prescribing is encouraged and substitution of products considered bioequivalent is sometimes permitted.

- Drugs may be classified by many systems, including by chemical formula, by body system affected, by mechanism of action, by clinical use or by legal schedule. Drug classifications help facilitate the student's understanding of pharmacology by comparing the common characteristics of an example of a drug group or classification (the key, or prototype, drug) with those of any new drugs released in the same classification or category.

- Maintaining a current source of credible drug information is a necessity in clinical practice today. Types of drug information range from official legal standards through prescribing guidelines to drug advertisements.

- To ensure correct drug dosage calculations and safe administration of medications, health-care professionals must have a working knowledge of the SI units of measurement and the methods of performing dosage calculations.

REVIEW EXERCISES

1. Name the three measuring systems used for administering medications and outline the advantages of the SI system.

2. The physician prescribes for a patient an investigational drug that is new to you. Which drug information source would you select to find information on this drug? What credibility could you give the information?

3. What are the differences between an alkaloid, a glycoside, a steroid and an oil? Name one drug from each category.

4. Work through the dosage calculations sample questions again without looking at the suggested method.

5. Compare the advantages and disadvantages of doctors prescribing using approved (generic) names rather than trade names.

6. Define the pharmacological terms in Table 1-1, giving examples where possible.

REFERENCES AND FURTHER READING

Adverse Drug Reactions Advisory Committee (ADRAC). *Australian Adverse Drug Reactions Bulletin*. Canberra: ADRAC.

American Pharmaceutical Association. *Handbook of Nonprescription Drugs*. Washington, DC: American Pharmaceutical Association, 2000.

Anonymous. Top 10 drugs. *Australian Prescriber* 2006; 29(1): 5.

Australian Medicines Handbook 2005. Adelaide: AMH, 2005.

Bennett PN, Brown MJ. *Clinical Pharmacology*. 9th edn. Edinburgh: Churchill Livingstone, 2003.

Birkett D. Generics—equal or not? *Australian Prescriber* 2003; 26(4): 85–7.

Blainey G. *Pharmacy 40,000 Years Ago*. Melbourne: Pharmaceutical Society of Victoria, 1977.

Bowman WC, Rand MJ. *Textbook of Pharmacology*. 2nd edn. Oxford: Blackwell, 1980 [chs 7, 16].

British Medical Association, Royal Pharmaceutical Society of Great Britain. *British National Formulary 41*. London: BMJ Books, 2001.

British Pharmacopoeia Commission. *British Pharmacopoeia 2000*. London: Her Majesty's Stationery Office, 2000.

Brown M, Mulholland JL. *Drug Calculations: Process and Problems for Clinical Practice*. 5th edn. St Louis: Mosby, 1996.

Budavari S, O'Neil MJ, Smith A, Heckelman PE (eds). *The Merck Index: An Encyclopedia of Chemicals, Drugs and Biologicals*. Whitehouse Station, NJ: Merck, 2001.

Caswell A (ed.). *MIMS Annual June 2005*. Sydney: CMPMedica Australia, 2005.

Collins DJ, Culvenor CCJ, Lamberton JA et al. *Plants for Medicines: A Chemical and Pharmacological Survey of Plants in the Australian Region*. Australia: CSIRO, 1990.

Commonwealth Department of Health and Family Services. *MediScene* newsletters. Canberra: CDHFS.

Council of Europe. *European Pharmacopoeia*. 3rd edn & Supplement 2000. Strasbourg: Council of Europe, 1996 & 2000.

Cribb JW. Australia's medicinal plants. *Medical Journal of Australia* 1985; 143: 574–7.

Davis R, Rees N, Lovitt H, Bebee R. *Mosby's Medication Guide 1999/2000*. Sydney: Mosby, 1999.

Downie G, Mackenzie J, Williams A. *Calculating Drug Doses Safely: A Handbook for Nurses and Midwives*. Edinburgh: Churchill Livingstone, 2006.

Duffin J. *History of Medicine: A Scandalously Short Introduction*. Toronto: University of Toronto Press, 2000.

Evans WC. *Trease and Evans' Pharmacognosy*. 15th edn. Edinburgh: Saunders, 2002.

Fogg S. Informing the consumer. *Australian Prescriber* 2003; 26(1): 2–3.

Gatford JD, Anderson RE. *Nursing Calculations*. 5th edn. Edinburgh: Churchill Livingstone, 1998.

Gaut B. Defining moments in medicine: a golden age defined, fifty years of medical advances. *Medical Journal of Australia* 2001; 174(1): 8.

Hanson BA. *Understanding Medicinal Plants: Their Chemistry and Therapeutic Action*. New York: Haworth Herbal Press, 2005.

Hassali A, Stewart K, Kong D. Quality use of generic medicines. *Australian Prescriber* 2004; 27(4): 80–1.

Herxheimer A. The importance of independent drug bulletins. *Australian Prescriber* 2002; 25(1): 3–4.

Le Fanu, J. *The Rise and Fall of Modern Medicine*. London: Little Brown, 1999.

Longmore M, Wilkinson IB, Rajagopalan SR. *Oxford Handbook of Clinical Medicine*. 6th edn. Oxford: Oxford University Press, 2004.

Magner LN. *A History of Medicine*. New York: Marcel Dekker, 1992.

Mann J. *Murder, Magic and Medicine*. Oxford: Oxford University Press, 1992.

Parker GB. Would the pharmaceutical companies please mind their Ps and Qs, and their Xs, Ys and Zs. *Medical Journal of Australia* 2000; 173: 662–3.

Pharmaceutical Care Information Services. *AusDI: Australian Drug Information for the Health Care Professional*. 1st edn. Curtin, ACT: Pharmaceutical Care Information Services, 1999.

Pharmaceutical Society of Australia. *Australian Pharmaceutical Formulary and Handbook*. 17th edn. Curtin, ACT: PSA, 2000.

Pharmacy Department, Royal Children's Hospital Melbourne. *Paediatric Pharmacopoeia*. 12th edn. Melbourne: Royal Children's Hospital, 1997.

Radford DJ, Gillies AD, Hinds JA, Duffy P. Naturally occurring cardiac glycosides. *Medical Journal of Australia* 1986; 144: 540–4.

Rang HP, Dale MM, Ritter JM. *Pharmacology*. 4th edn. Edinburgh: Churchill Livingstone, 1999 [ch. 32].

Rang HP, Dale MM, Ritter JM, Moore PK. *Pharmacology*. 5th edn. Edinburgh: Churchill Livingstone, 2003 [chs 5, 50]

Shargel L, Mutnick AH, Souney PF et al. *Comprehensive Pharmacy Review*. 3rd edn. Baltimore: Williams & Wilkins, 1997.

Smith A. It's natural so it must be safe. *Australian Prescriber* 2002; 25(3): 50–1.

Speight TM, Holford NHG (eds). *Avery's Drug Treatment*. 4th edn. Auckland: Adis International, 1997.

Sweetman SC (ed.). *Martindale: The Complete Drug Reference*. London: Pharmaceutical Press, 2005.

Tatro DS (ed.) *Drug Interactions: Facts*. St Louis, MO: Facts and Comparisons, 2001.

Thomas J (ed.). *Australian Prescription Products Guide*. 30th edn. Melbourne: Australian Pharmaceutical Publishing, 2001.

Thorp RH, Watson TR. A survey of the occurrence of cardio-active constituents in plants growing wild in Australia. *Australian Journal of Experimental Biology* 1953; 31: 529–32.

Tiziani, A. *Havard's Nursing Guide to Drugs*. 7th edn. Sydney: Mosby-Elsevier, 2006.

United States Pharmacopeial Convention. *USP DI: Drug Information for the Health Care Professional*. 18th edn. Rockville, MD: USP Convention, 1998.

United States Pharmacopeial Convention. *United States Pharmacopeia* (USP). 29th edn. Rockville, MD: USP Convention, 2005.

United States Pharmacopeial Convention. *United States National Formulary*. 24th edn. Rockville, MD: USP Convention, 2005.

Various authors. Articles on Australian industries in alkaloids, pyrethrums and marine-derived drugs. *Chemistry in Australia* 1989; 56(10): 348–61.

ON-LINE RESOURCES

Adverse Drug Reactions Advisory Committee (ADRAC), *Australian Adverse Drug Reactions Bulletin*. Canberra: ADRAC: www.tga.gov.au/adr/aadrb.htm

Cochrane Library: www.cochrane.org

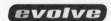 More weblinks at http://evolve.elsevier.com/AU/Bryant/pharmacology/

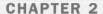

CHAPTER 2

Pharmacotherapy: Clinical Use of Drugs

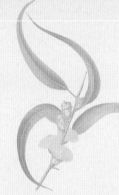

CHAPTER FOCUS

Pharmacotherapy refers to the use of drugs in people for treating or preventing disease, and is sometimes referred to as clinical pharmacology, as distinct from theoretical or experimental pharmacology, in which drugs may be studied to understand their mechanisms of action and effects. In this chapter, we focus on the medical use of drugs, from government policies on drug use, through prescribing, dispensing and formulations for medicines, to altering and monitoring the person's responses to drugs.

OBJECTIVES

● To outline ways in which the quality use of medicines (QUM) can be maximised.

● To describe the roles of health professionals with respect to drugs.

● To give a brief outline of pharmaceutics, the science of producing drugs in forms suitable for administration.

● To suggest decisions that need to be made before prescribing or administering drugs.

● To explain how prescriptions are written.

● To list some of the many factors that modify people's responses to drugs.

● To describe how drug therapy is monitored: therapeutic drug monitoring (TDM).

KEY TERMS

adverse drug reactions
compliance
drug interactions
drug usage evaluation
enteric coating
evidence-based medicine
five rights
formulations
health professionals
parenteral administration
pharmaceutics
pharmacoeconomics
placebo
polypharmacy
prescription
quality use of medicines
randomised controlled clinical trial
sustained release
tablets
therapeutic drug monitoring

KEY ABBREVIATIONS

ADR   adverse drug reaction
ASCEPT Australasian Society of Clinical and Experimental
            Pharmacologists and Toxicologists
DUE   drug usage evaluation
EBM   evidence-based medicine
EC   enteric-coated
NMP   National Medicines Policy
OTC   over the counter
PBS   Pharmaceutical Benefits Scheme
PHARM Pharmaceutical Health and Rational Use of
            Medicines
QUM   quality use of medicines
RCCT   randomised controlled clinical trial
script   prescription
TDM   therapeutic drug monitoring

QUALITY USE OF MEDICINES (QUM)

IN a review of pharmacotherapeutics in Australia in the 20th century (Day & Mashford 2001), two eminent clinical pharmacologists described the progress in pharmacology up to the 1950s as "an impressive story of rapid progress from empiricism towards a rational, biologically based approach to disease", and since the 1950s, as "an explosion in the numbers and variety of drugs available and illnesses that are treatable . . . (and) a marked improvement in general levels of efficacy and tolerability of medicines". To optimise the use of these new drugs in a rational, clinically and cost-effective manner, it is important that health professionals understand the information required before drugs are prescribed or advised, how prescriptions are written by doctors (or dentists or nurse practitioners) and dispensed by pharmacists, the types of formulations in which drugs are administered, the factors that can affect how people respond to drugs, and how drug therapy is monitored to assess the person's progress—in fact, basically the whole of clinical pharmacology!

Some professional groups have incorporated a QUM policy within their own charter; for example, the Royal College of Nursing Australia has produced a position statement around registered nurses and QUM (see On-line resources at the end of this chapter).

Evidence-based health care

Health professionals generally are encouraged to practise evidence-based health care, commonly referred to as **evidence-based medicine** (EBM)—the conscientious, explicit and judicious use of current best evidence in making decisions about the medical care of individual patients.* The practice of EBM requires the integration of individual clinical expertise with the best available external clinical evidence from systematic research. This should apply whatever the style of treatment, whether with drugs, physiotherapy techniques, orthoptic eye exercises or optometric lens prescriptions, podiatric or dental surgery, nursing care, ambulance and paramedic emergency aid, or complementary and alternative remedies. In the context of drug therapy, the **randomised controlled clinical trial** (RCCT) has long been accepted as the 'gold standard' of evidence; many other types of therapy, which may have been in traditional use for decades

---

*While the term 'medicine' is sometimes used to imply health care provided by doctors, in the wider sense the term is defined as 'the branch of science devoted to the prevention of disease and the restoration of the sick to health' (Youngson, 1998); thus medicine is a discipline studied and practised by a wide range of health-care professionals.

or centuries without any evidence of efficacy, are now being subjected to clinical trials (see Chapter 4).

Four levels of evidence

The Australian National Health and Medical Research Council (NHMRC) has classified the strength of evidence on which EBM is based into four levels:

- meta-analyses: evidence from a systematic review of all relevant RCCTs, such as Cochrane reviews (see Chapter 1)
- evidence from at least one properly designed RCCT
- evidence from well-designed non-randomised trials, or cohort or case-controlled studies
- evidence from case series.

Evidence based on clinical experience and descriptive studies, from committees or colleagues, is considered a low form of evidence on which to base clinical decision making. An electronic search of databases such as the Cochrane Collaboration, AustHealth or Medline usually quickly reveals available evidence about a particular treatment. Drug information and prescribing advice in semiofficial sources such as the *Australian Medicines Handbook* or *Therapeutic Guidelines* is based on the highest-level evidence available.

The evidence–relevance gap

Even with the optimal amount and level of evidence available, the gap between scientific evidence at the population level and what is relevant to a particular patient remains challenging to health professionals. For example, many women bombarded with an overload of information in the lay press about hormone replacement therapy (HRT) in menopause from large-scale clinical trials found it impossible to decide its relevance to their particular situation (suffering symptoms? predisposed to breast cancer? colorectal cancer? cardiovascular disease?), and to weigh the short-term benefits of relief of menopausal symptoms and long-term protection against osteoporosis against the possible long-term higher risk of cancers. In fact, the changes in long-term outcome are so small as to be irrelevant for many women (see Neeskens 2002).

Drug availability in Australia
Approval by the Therapeutic Goods Administration (TGA)

The TGA is a division of the Australian Commonwealth Department of Health and Ageing, in Canberra. It has evolved from the Australian Drug Evaluation Committee, set up in 1963 after the thalidomide disaster of the late 1950s, which caused many countries to act rapidly to control the safety of medicines. The TGA has the responsibility to register all drugs for which therapeutic claims are made, on the basis of quality, safety and efficacy; cost-effectiveness is also an important consideration.

The Pharmaceutical Benefits Scheme (PBS)

The PBS is a scheme whereby the Australian Commonwealth Department of Health and Ageing subsidises a large number of drugs considered essential to optimal heath care in the population. Originally (1948) about 140 drugs were available free of charge; a nominal co-payment was soon introduced, from which pensioners were exempt. The cost and number of drugs is continually rising, the population (especially the elderly) and its demands for drugs increasing, advances in health care are calling for greater access to new drugs, and costs involved in drug discovery and development always escalating. Hence pressure is put on doctors to prescribe, and governments to subsidise, an increasing number of drugs, leading to a relentless escalation in costs of the PBS to taxpayers.* Attempts are made to rationalise the subsidies while maintaining the appropriate level of availability of drugs at reasonable costs; for example, the 'minimum pricing policy', whereby the basic cost of a drug is based on the cheapest available brand, and campaigns for rational prescribing, e.g. limiting the overuse of antibiotics. The government attempts to maintain a balance between competing interests in terms of quality of drugs, equity of access, quality use of medicines, and a viable drug industry.

Availability under other schemes

There are several other ways whereby drugs can be accessed:
- a 'private' prescription, for which the patient pays the full cost of the drug, not subsidised by the government
- the Special Access Scheme of the TGA, which provides for the importation and/or supply of an unapproved therapeutic good (e.g. drug) for single patients on a case-by-case basis. The categories of patients for whom drugs may be made available are: (a) those terminally or seriously ill; (b) those with a life-threatening medical condition; and (c) those with a serious medical condition
- on application, potential importation of drugs for personal use
- investigational drugs sometimes made available for testing in clinical trials.

And, of course, many drugs are available over the counter (OTC) in pharmacies, general stores, health shops or supermarkets.

Targeting QUM
A National Medicines Policy

During the 1980s, many consumer organisations and medical activists campaigned for rationalisation of government policies with respect to medicines, leading to the establishment

---

*The cost is currently increasing at about 6% per annum, with the total annual cost in the year ending June 2005 over A$5.3 billion.

---

under the auspices of the PBS of a National Medicines Policy (NMP) to achieve **QUM**. The stated aims of the NMP are:
- timely cost-effective access to medicines that Australians need
- medicines meeting high standards of quality, safety and efficacy
- quality use of medicines
- maintenance of a responsible and viable medicines industry.

Several effective arms to this policy have been implemented. The Pharmaceutical Health and Rational Use of Medicines (PHARM) Committee has placed QUM high in priority on the national health agenda. QUM is considered to mean: (1) selecting management options wisely; (2) choosing suitable medicines if considered necessary; and (3) using medicines safely and effectively. Information sources supported include the journal *Australian Prescriber*, the Therapeutics Resource and Educational Network for Doctors (TREND), *Therapeutic Guidelines* and the *Australian Medicines Handbook*, and Consumer Medicine Information (CMI) handouts, which are usually included inside packs of medicines or are available from pharmacists. Barriers to QUM were identified, such as waste or hoarding of medicines, inappropriate demand and poor compliance. Many campaigns on using medicines wisely have been supported at national, state and local levels.

The Australian National Prescribing Service (NPS) was set up (1998) with representation from doctors and pharmacists to improve health outcomes for all Australians, enhance continuity of QUM programs and coordinate activities influencing prescribing. The NPS has the mission to improve health outcomes for all Australians through QUM. Through its educational activities targeted to doctors, pharmacists, nurses, other health practitioners, consumers and the pharmaceutical industry, the NPS has achieved some significant savings in drug costs. In New Zealand, the Preferred Medicines List provides guidelines aimed at achieving QUM in the health system in that country (see also Clinical Interest Box 2-2 later).

Some examples of recent studies and programs in QUM include alerting people to the possibility of interactions between prescription medicines and alternative therapies, education about the development of antibiotic-resistant microorganisms and the need to rationalise prescribing of antibiotics, advice that paracetamol is often overused in treating childhood fevers, and information about the use in arthritis of the new cyclo-oxygenase-2 (COX-2) inhibitors, and their adverse effects.

Drug usage evaluation (DUE)

The process of maximising QUM, particularly in the hospital context, requires regular monitoring and evaluation of the use of drugs in the institution in order to define patient groups that will best benefit from drugs, to optimise hospital prescribing and to face the implications of spiralling costs and capped budgets. **Drug usage evaluation** (DUE) teams include clinicians, pharmacologists, pharmacists and nurses interested in QUM in their institution.

Many members of the Clinical Interest Group of the Australasian Society of Clinical and Experimental Pharmacologists and Toxicologists (ASCEPT) have established a DUE network to encourage, review and discuss DUE activities in hospitals; an interesting study on prophylaxis of stroke is reviewed in Clinical Interest Box 2-1. Other recent DUE studies have been in the areas of:

- determining the list of drugs for acute care use in remote Aboriginal community health centres
- understanding and reporting of adverse drug reactions (ADRs)
- the relative merits of flucloxacillin and dicloxacillin with respect to ADRs
- complementary medicines in public hospitals
- continuity of pharmacological care as patients are moved from hospital to the community
- reducing the prescribing of benzodiazepines in the community
- appropriate drug therapy of chronic obstructive pulmonary disease (Dartnell et al 2000).

Such studies have been shown to save not only lives and time but also money. A recent survey (Dooley et al 2003) in eight major teaching hospitals across six Australian states looked at changes initiated by clinical pharmacists to drug therapy regimens and patient management. Altogether, 1399 interventions were documented, evaluated by independent panels and costed. The commonest reasons for intervention were to decrease potential adverse events or morbidity or mortality, and to increase efficacy and symptom control. The most frequent outcomes were avoidance of admissions and procedures, and changes to laboratory monitoring of drug plasma concentrations. Annualised savings at the eight sites totalled over A$4.44 million; for every dollar spent on pharmacist time, $23 were saved. This study demonstrated that routine clinical pharmacist review of inpatient drug therapy is an essential component of QUM programs, and significantly reduces length of hospital stay and potential for readmission.

It is hoped that as research is implemented, flow-on will occur to maximise QUM in general practice as well.

Changes in drug use with time

Pharmacopoeias and formularies are in a constant state of change, and health professionals need to keep up to date with current drug information. Some of the influences on evolving drug use are described below, with examples of drugs affected.

New technologies

Until the early 20th century, most drugs were from natural sources such as plants (morphine, cocaine), minerals (iodine,

---

**CLINICAL INTEREST BOX 2-1
A DRUG USAGE EVALUATION CASE STUDY: WARFARIN PROPHYLAXIS IN ATRIAL FIBRILLATION**

Despite evidence that warfarin prophylaxis can significantly reduce the risk of stroke in patients at risk of thromboembolism secondary to atrial fibrillation (AF), many patients do not receive warfarin. A recent study in the Royal Adelaide Hospital assessed the impact of various interventions (audit of anticoagulation procedures for AF, development and dissemination of local guidelines and a sticker placed by a clinical pharmacist in the patient's casenotes) on prophylactic prescribing of warfarin in medical units.

An audit carried out 6 months after the intervention showed that appropriate use of warfarin increased significantly—by 41% (Clark et al 2005).

---

iron) and animals (vaccines, tissue extracts). As chemical industries developed, synthetic and semisynthetic drugs such as antibacterial sulfonamides, thiazide diuretics, volatile general anaesthetics, corticosteroids and oral contraceptives, safe antihypertensives and effective antipsychotic agents became available. Genetic engineering has produced human insulin and other hormones and proteins. Older, less effective and less safe drugs have become obsolete.

New uses for old drugs

Drugs are sometimes found to have additional uses to those for which they were initially developed. Minoxidil, an antihypertensive agent, was found to cause increased growth of hair and found a new use as a hair restorer. Methylphenidate, originally an appetite suppressant, found new application in treating attention deficit hyperactivity disorder.

Better understanding of mechanisms

The discovery of the mechanism of action of aspirin (inhibiting synthesis of prostaglandins) led to further evaluation of its actions. Results of clinical trials showed that subjects receiving aspirin suffered fewer adverse cardiovascular events, demonstrating the antithrombotic actions of aspirin, hence its use prophylactically against heart attacks and strokes.

Better understanding of aetiology of disease

The evolution of better drugs to treat peptic ulcers followed studies of the causes of peptic ulcers. First, sedatives were prescribed to reduce stress, then antacids to neutralise gastric acid, then histamine H_2-receptor antagonists and proton pump inhibitors to reduce production of acid, and finally antibacterials to reduce infection with *Helicobacter pylori* were added to the gastroenterologist's armamentarium.

Old 'remedies' proven useless

For centuries syphilis was treated with mercury-containing compounds, perhaps because no effective treatment was available. These very toxic medicines were used for hundreds of years despite total lack of efficacy. Only when safe oral antibacterials became available (and the concept of clinical trials developed) did mercury compounds drop out of pharmacopoeias.

Drug combinations shown to be unjustified

Complex combinations of drugs (galenicals) date back to the time of the ancient Greek physician Galen. Even in the mid-20th century, doctors often wrote prescriptions for complex mixtures 'for nerves' or as 'tonics'. Frequently, combinations of antimicrobials or of antihypertensives were formulated together. It is now recognised that it is usually better to prescribe drugs individually, as doses can then be adjusted individually and the drug with the longer half-life does not accumulate and cause toxicity.

Changes in popularity of drugs

There is a recognised cycle in popularity of many new drugs: as a drug is developed and marketed (often aggressively to both prescribers and consumers), it rapidly surges in popularity. As adverse reactions inevitably become apparent and its expense is noted, its use wanes. Then, as rational evidence of the benefits and risks are evaluated, the drug regains a medium but more stable position in the drug usage charts.

Changes in availability of drugs

There may be a major change in the use of a drug as it is moved between drug schedules (see Chapter 4) and becomes either more or less readily available or expensive. When the histamine H_2-receptor antagonists were introduced, they rapidly became very popular and hospital drug budgets blew out. Restrictions were placed on the frequency of their prescribing to rationalise their use and costs. Similarly, when new COX-2 inhibitors (celecoxib, rofecoxib) were introduced in Australia, they were very expensive. Public (and drug company) pressure led to their being subsidised and listed on the PBS (2001), when their use sky-rocketed.

Withdrawal of useful drugs

Drug companies may decide to discontinue production and marketing of a useful drug for various reasons: an old drug may have become redundant or unprofitable, an old manufacturing process obsolete, rare unexpected adverse reactions may become apparent, a disease may become much less prevalent, or company mergers may bring competitor products into the same 'house'. However, there can be important implications for patients who may have been stabilised on a particular drug for many years and are intolerant or unresponsive to other drugs. Change to a new drug may cause withdrawal reactions, recurrence of illness, or new adverse drug reactions or interactions. A coordinated approach between drug companies, government and health professional organisations is required to minimise these problems.

When to use a new drug

The safety and efficacy of new drugs are now determined in RCCTs and the information soon becomes readily available to add to the evidence base for treating certain conditions. Knowledge about the drug, however, is still quite limited, and post-marketing use of the drug may bring evidence of unusual adverse reactions and efficacy in subgroups of the population, e.g. pregnant women, children and the elderly. Prescribers then need to consider carefully when they prescribe new drugs. The cautious approach suggests that doctors limit their prescribing of new drugs until post-marketing surveillance provides accumulated data on clinical and cost-effectiveness in large populations.*

A good example of the caution necessary in rapidly prescribing new drugs is the case of the COX-2 inhibitor rofecoxib (Vioxx). This anti-inflammatory agent was introduced in Australia in 1999 after trials in over 5000 patients who had received it for less than 6 months; there was a low overall incidence of thromboembolic events. Rofecoxib rapidly became very popular (as was celecoxib) for treatment of painful and inflammatory conditions in patients who might be at risk of gastrointestinal side-effects from the older NSAIDs. Meanwhile, analyses of cardiovascular events occurring during larger-scale longer trials and post-marketing use showed that people taking 25 mg rofecoxib daily had about double the risk of heart attacks and strokes compared to placebo. The drug was withdrawn in Australia in 2004; since that time, related COX-2 inhibitors have been closely monitored for similar effects. Hundreds of patients in Australia have joined legal class actions against the manufacturer of rofecoxib, claiming that the manufacturer knew about the increased risk of cardiovascular events long before the drug was withdrawn.

---

*However, this requires many doctors to prescribe and many patients to take the new drugs. Someone somewhere has to start the ball rolling . . .

Pharmacoeconomics

Because of the blow-out in demands for and costs of drugs, no country can provide all the drugs that might be desirable; hence, economic rationalism is essential and decisions must be made to ration drugs and contain costs, if possible without compromising good health care (**pharmacoeconomics**). Such decisions have both clinical and ethical implications (the latter will be discussed in Chapter 4).

While detailed study of health economics is beyond the scope of this text, some of the issues involved have already been mentioned, such as the costs of developing and providing drugs, the increasing need for drugs by the growing elderly proportion of the population, and the increasing demands for 'lifestyle' drugs. Health economists need to evaluate many aspects of drug use, including indirect aspects such as savings from shorter hospital admissions, improved quality of life, and surgery avoided. Overall, policies such as generic substitution (dispensing the cheaper alternative among medicines considered bioequivalent) and rational-isation of drug policies and QUM help optimise access to essential drugs.

Cost-effectiveness of new drugs

To be listed by the Australian Pharmaceutical Benefits Scheme (PBS) as a subsidised drug, a drug must be proved to be not only safe and effective but also cost-effective, which requires an economic evaluation of the additional cost of any extra benefit over the current standard therapy. Listing as a 'restricted benefit' or as 'authority required to prescribe' helps limit the PBS use of a drug to those in whom it will be most effective.

For example, a cost-effectiveness analysis of the platelet aggregation inhibitor clopidogrel compared to aspirin showed that on average it would require 115 people to be treated for 2 years each to prevent one additional stroke, heart attack or cardiovascular death; this would cost approximately $252,000 (2003 $). The approved indications for authority to prescribe clopidogrel list only six very specific situations in which the drug can be subsidised by the PBS.

ROLES OF HEALTH PROFESSIONALS WITH RESPECT TO DRUGS

Traditionally, the **health professionals** involved with drugs were doctors (and dentists and veterinary surgeons), who prescribed them; pharmacists, who dispensed them; and nurses, who administered them. Medicine as a profession in England developed with physicians allowed to prescribe 'physic' (medicine) compounded by apothecaries

(pharmacists). Apothecaries had developed along with grocers, as they both used scales for weighing. Apothecaries became specialist medicine sellers and used leeches, herbal remedies, pills and potions. Surgeons and barbers were also originally associated because they used the same tools of trade (razors and knives, basins and towels). During the Great Plague (1660s), however, many physicians fled London, leaving apothecaries to care for the sick and dying. After that time, apothecaries gained in popularity and became the general practitioners of the day, even delivering babies. It was not until the 19th century that these roles diverged into those we are familiar with today.

Now, however, the roles of health professionals are changing, the boundaries between them are breaking down and many more health professionals are involved with drugs or with people who are taking them; hence the need to know, if not the same depth of pharmacology, at least some of the language and principles of pharmacology. The roles of many of these professionals will be described briefly.[†] Specialised aspects, such as details of nursing roles in drug administration and nursing implications of drug therapy, are beyond the scope of this text. Information in Clinical Interest Box 2-2 describes the integration of many health professionals in Primary Health Organisations in New Zealand.

Ambulance and 'MICA' paramedics

These specialists in first aid and emergency care are often the first health professionals to respond to situations such as accidents, acute myocardial infarctions (heart attacks), cerebrovascular accidents (strokes) and severe asthma attacks. The roles of standard ambulance paramedics include rapid assessment of the person after medical or trauma emergencies in the pre-hospital setting—especially for central nervous system, cardiovascular and respiratory functions—to provide life-saving support and stabilise the condition until the patient is received at a medical facility. Under written standing orders in medical protocols, paramedics can administer drugs, including chewable aspirin and sublingual glyceryl trinitrate for chest pain, IM midazolam for seizures, inhaled methoxyflurane as an analgesic, glucose buccal gel for hypoglycaemic attacks and IM naloxone for opioid overdoses. Paramedics with extra training for the Mobile Intensive Care Ambulance (MICA) service also need to be able to administer more powerful drugs, including antiarrhythmic agents, cardiac stimulants, bronchodilators, corticosteroids, muscle relaxants and potent analgesics, and to set up intravenous fluid administration drips.

[†]In alphabetical order, to avoid implying some hierarchy in position or knowledge.

**CLINICAL INTEREST BOX 2-2
A NEW HEALTH CARE STRATEGY**

The Government in New Zealand introduced a new Health Strategy in 2005. The Primary Health Care Strategy places emphasis on prevention of illness by improving access to, and funding of, primary health care services. The aim is to improve the health of all New Zealanders and promote community involvement in the maintenance of health.

The Primary Health Care Strategy included the formation of Primary Health Organisations (PHOs); these organisations include doctors, nurses and other trained, skilled health professionals working together to provide primary health services. Patients need to enrol as members of the PHO, and their visits to the GP are then subsidized by the government. This makes the visit cheaper for the patient, and health services more accessible to the public. Children and students at school receive subsidised visits and medicines, and within the PHO structure this has been extended to include 18 to 24 year olds.

PHOs receive their funding from the local District Health Board (DHB) and are not-for-profit organisations. Not all New Zealanders are members of a PHO, and not all GP practices are PHOs.

Adapted from: www/moh.govt.nz, accessed 16 January 2006.

Complementary and alternative medicine practitioners

Complementary and alternative medicine (CAM) practitioners use techniques including provision of herbal products, massage, acupuncture, naturopathy, homeopathy and iridology. (These areas are covered in Chapter 3.) It is being increasingly recognised that there can be interactions between practices in Western medicine and CAM, e.g. drug interactions between prescribed drugs and CAM preparations that patients may be taking concurrently, so it is important that such practitioners have some understanding of pharmacology and the potential for problems to occur.

Dentists

Dentists are allowed to prescribe drugs related to their treatment—in particular, antibiotics and analgesics. They frequently administer local anaesthetics during dental procedures to prevent and relieve pain.

Dietitians

Dietitians are particularly involved with the principles of nutrition and food as they relate to health. There is overlap with pharmacology in areas such as parenteral nutrition, supplementation of nutrition and food–drug interactions.

Doctors

Doctors (medical practitioners) are responsible for diagnosing disease and initiating and monitoring therapy, including prescribing drugs that are not available OTC. Doctors therefore require extensive knowledge of pharmacology in all aspects: actions and mechanisms of drugs (pharmacodynamics), drug handling by the body (pharmacokinetics) and, in particular, clinical aspects, including adverse drug reactions, drug interactions, dosages, indications and contraindications for drug use, in all situations and patients, whether children, adults, the elderly or those with concurrent diseases and being administered other therapies. Doctors may specialise in many fields of medicine, such as obstetrics and gynaecology (women's conditions, pregnancy and childbirth), paediatrics (children), oncology (cancers), anaesthetics etc. Specialists will obviously require particular knowledge of the drugs used in that area. It is said that anaesthetists are the world's best clinical pharmacologists because, during a surgical operation, they are continually administering many drugs, monitoring the patient's responses, checking for adverse reactions and drug interactions, altering doses, and responding to the clinical situation minute by minute (see Clinical Interest Box 15-2).

Traditionally, doctors visiting patients in the community carried a black bag, holding various drugs that the doctor could supply as needed, particularly in emergencies. These 'doctor's bag' supplies may also be important for emergencies that occur in the surgery or office or when on calls. The PBS still allows doctors to carry such drugs, most of them in parenteral (injectable) form. Examples are adrenaline (for cardiac arrest and severe allergic reactions), atropine (for cardiac arrhythmias or poisoning with insecticides), benzylpenicillin (for bacterial infections), chlorpromazine and haloperidol (for psychiatric emergencies), frusemide (a potent diuretic drug used in hypertension), hydrocortisone (an anti-inflammatory and immunosuppressant agent), lignocaine (a local anaesthetic), morphine and tramadol (to treat severe pain) and naloxone (an opioid antagonist used to treat overdose with opioids such as heroin). Other non-injectable drugs include soluble aspirin tablets (first-line treatment for anyone suspected of having had a heart attack), diazepam (sedative, antianxiety and anticonvulsant), glyceryl trinitrate spray or patch (for angina), salbutamol aerosol (for asthma), and possibly antiemetics (to prevent vomiting), antibiotics and analgesics.

Health information managers

Health professionals trained in health information management specialise in managing databases in epidemiology and clinical trials data, coding data from patient hospital records, evaluating reports on accreditation and standards, and analysing 'casemix' information (that related to hospital admissions, patient diagnoses and records, and funding). These health workers need to understand basic concepts in pharmacology and to know the major groups of drugs in order to understand the patient and the medical record and, for example, to be able to code accurately whether a condition is a primary one or an adverse drug reaction, or to understand why treatment of some conditions requires lengthy hospital stays.

Indigenous health workers

Indigenous Australians (Aboriginal and Torres Strait Islanders) make up approximately 2.4% of the population; about 25% live in areas classified as remote or very remote. These people are disadvantaged across a range of socioeconomic factors, and continue to suffer a greater burden of ill-health than the rest of the population. In the indigenous Aboriginal community-controlled health services in some remote areas of Australia, indigenous health workers, in collaboration with visiting nurses and pharmacists, provide essential knowledge about health, society and culture. For example, in the Kimberley region of Western Australia, health workers who recognise problems and are familiar with a range of common medicines and their effects play important roles in home medicine reviews, improvement of compliance, help with interviews and communication and information about social circumstances (Larkin & Murray 2005).

Midwives

Midwifery is the area of health care specialising in antenatal care, labour and childbirth; most midwives are trained nurses. Midwifery is generally concerned with normal pregnancy and labour, whereas in difficult or abnormal situations or where medical conditions complicate pregnancy, obstetricians are called in. Midwives involved in antenatal care may recommend drugs such as iron and folic acid to treat anaemias. During childbirth, nitrous oxide or oxygen may be administered and, in the absence of a doctor, midwives in some jurisdictions are allowed on phone order to administer one or two doses of pethidine, oxytocin and/or ergometrine for a woman in labour, and metoclopramide as an antiemetic. Such doses must be followed up with a written doctor's prescription within 24 hours. A midwife may top up an epidural anaesthetic if a cannula is in place. The neonate may require oxygen, naloxone for reversal of opiate-induced respiratory depression, and vitamin K administered IM.

Nurses

Traditionally, nurses have worked in hospitals, community health centres, specialist medical clinics and private practice, and in many other areas such as industry and rural and district nursing services. Nurses are involved, among other

roles, in ensuring safe and reliable administration of drugs and in monitoring adverse reactions. In the hospital situation this could include:

- taking a drug history
- assessing the patient
- noting the prescription, checking dosage and calculations, and ensuring correct administration (the **'five rights'**—right patient, drug/form, dose, route, frequency)
- signing the patient record after administering a dose
- identifying problems relating to drug therapy
- ensuring compliance with therapy
- ensuring safe storage of drugs
- following institutional procedures and maintaining documentation and records, advocacy with respect to patients' rights and responsibilities, and education about important drug information, missed doses and continuation of therapy after discharge from hospital.

Nurses may be the first to recognise adverse reactions such as hypotension, constipation or nausea and vomiting, and have the responsibility to ensure appropriate treatment is instituted. Nurses may refuse to administer a drug if they feel that the situation has changed and it is not in the best interests of the patient, and have the responsibility to prevent medication errors. Nurses are not allowed to initiate or change drug therapy or alter labels on drug packs. In an emergency, nurses may implement verbal directions from a doctor to administer a drug, but this must be followed by a written prescription as soon as practicable or, usually, within 24 hours.

In several countries, laws have been changed recently to allow nurses with special expertise and training (including pharmacology) to apply for endorsement as nurse practitioners. The scope of the role is not yet fully established and many models are being trialled and evaluated in consultation with doctors and pharmacists. It is envisaged that the scheme might include permission to:

- manage therapeutic medication, including the right to prescribe a limited number of Schedule 4 drugs (see Chapter 4) formerly limited to doctors and dentists
- refer patients to specialists
- order diagnostic tests and procedures
- admit patients to health-care agencies
- complete and issue 'leave of absence' certificates.

In part, this is in response to the problems in country areas where there are insufficient doctors. In Australia, there is at present no published formulary of drugs that nurse practitioners may prescribe, but the process of diagnosis, drug choice, prescribing, counselling and monitoring therapy would be within the guidelines of the QUM program. Examples of areas in which nurse practitioners may specialise are rural health, diabetes management, palliative care, and drug dependence and withdrawal.

Occupational therapists

Occupational therapists work particularly with people who have physical, emotional, psychological or social disorders that affect how they carry out activities of daily living, such as looking after themselves, cooking, driving and job skills. Occupational therapists try to facilitate and rehabilitate the person through the use of activities, group therapy, and adaptation of equipment and of the environment. While they do not themselves prescribe or administer drugs, they may need to know the language of pharmacology in order to understand information about the drugs that their patients/clients are taking and how these may affect functioning or cause adverse reactions.

Optometrists and orthoptists

Optometrists specialise in examining the eyes, testing vision and prescribing spectacles (glasses) and contact lenses. Recently, in some Australian states, optometrists have been given the opportunity, after undertaking accredited extra training in pharmacology, to have their registration endorsed so that they can prescribe a limited range of Schedule 4 drugs for optometric use. The list of drugs includes ocular preparations of antimicrobials (antivirals, antibacterials), local anaesthetics, anti-inflammatory drugs, antiallergy drugs, drugs to dilate the pupil (mydriatics), and many drugs for treating glaucoma.

Orthoptists generally work with ophthalmologists (doctors specialising in eye disorders) and are involved in the treatment of eye movement disorders such as strabismus (squint), and of people with low vision. Recently the training of orthoptists has been extended to equip them to prescribe spectacles and lenses.

Pharmacists

Pharmacists are specialists in drugs and are involved with their storage, supply and distribution. They generally work in hospital or retail pharmacies and in nursing homes. Some of the many roles of pharmacists are:

• dispensing medications according to the prescriber's intentions, with correct labelling, recording and checking
• counselling patients to ensure safe and effective administration of drugs
• detecting potential inappropriate doses, adverse drug reactions or drug interactions, or drug misuse
• monitoring sales of S2 and S3 medicines
• supervising staff, students and dispensary assistants
• ensuring that the pharmacy is conducted according to the law and to standards of good pharmaceutical practice
• ordering and safe storage of drug supplies
• maintaining all required equipment and reference materials.

In hospitals, pharmacists also carry out many specialist roles, such as filling and maintaining ward stocks of drugs (imprest cabinets and drug trolleys); preparing sterile parenteral solutions, parenteral nutrition solutions and oncology drugs; and participating in ward rounds, medication history reviews, therapeutic drug monitoring, advice on drug therapy and provision of drug information as specialists in drug therapy. Pharmacists in retail practice often take on responsibilities for medication management services, i.e. overview of the drug therapy of people in nursing homes, and domiciliary medication reviews for patients in their own homes.

Physiotherapists

Physiotherapists (also known as physical therapists) deal with problems of movement, muscle coordination and posture, and with impairments caused by physical injury. Many of their patients have neurological, cardiovascular, respiratory or orthopaedic conditions (fractures, soft tissue injuries, vertebral syndromes), have been through surgery or childbirth, have major pain control problems, or require rehabilitation after surgery, accidents or neurological damage. Physiotherapists use physical methods of therapy, such as heat, cold, electrical stimulation, exercise, massage and manipulation, electromagnetic radiation and biofeedback, rather than chemical methods (drugs).

Because virtually all their patients are likely to be taking some drugs for their underlying medical conditions or for the problems for which they present for therapy, physiotherapists need to have a good general understanding of the language and principles of pharmacology and, in particular, a thorough knowledge of drugs used in obstetrics, neurological and cardiovascular conditions, asthma and inflammatory conditions, and for pain control.

Podiatrists

Podiatrists specialise in disorders of the lower limb, especially of the ankle and foot, and deal with biomechanical, medical, surgical and sports-related problems, especially in diabetes and rheumatology. The drug groups that their patients are likely to be using include cardiovascular drugs, hypoglycaemic agents, anti-inflammatory drugs, analgesics and antimicrobials. Podiatrists are allowed to administer local anaesthetics for pain relief in procedures and surgery involving the foot. Those with extra training in pharmacology are allowed in some Australian states to prescribe a limited range of Schedule 4 drugs, such as antimicrobials, anti-inflammatory drugs, antianxiety agents and long-acting local anaesthetics.

Prosthetists and orthotists

These health professionals specialise in provision of prostheses (artificial limbs) and orthoses (devices to support limbs). Many of their patients have problems with poor circulation, especially diabetes, so they need to know about drugs used to improve circulation and treat diabetes.

Speech pathologists (speech therapists)

Speech pathologists deal with people who have difficulties with verbal communication, language development and speech, hearing and swallowing. As such, they are not themselves likely to be advising on drug therapy but they may well be dealing with clients who are taking drugs for an underlying clinical problem, such as strokes or other neurological impairments, or for psychiatric or behavioural disorders. Speech pathologists may therefore find it useful to understand the language of pharmacology and be able to read drug information sources.

DECISIONS TO BE MADE BEFORE PRESCRIBING DRUGS

Any therapeutic intervention—whether administering a drug, implementing a physiotherapeutic electrotherapy program, carrying out a dental or podiatrical surgical procedure, altering a person's diet or administering a CAM therapy such as acupuncture, herbal remedy or massage—may interfere with the person's body systems, either physically or chemically. The first priority before carrying out any intervention must be based on the advice of Hippocrates: FIRST DO NO HARM. Then there are many questions that need to be answered, consciously or intuitively, before intervening, and, in the context of drug therapy, the rest of this book attempts to provide useful answers to these questions.

What is the problem?

The question is 'What is going wrong here?'. A full health history may take at least 30 minutes to complete and should list all the patient's current problems, medications, past drug history, allergies, adverse drug reactions and interactions, relevant family history, use of social drugs such as alcohol and tobacco and CAM therapies, and all treatment modalities being used. For effective treatment the starting point is the problems specified in terms of pathophysiology or altered anatomy or psychology, not necessarily a diagnosis.

Is there a drug-based solution? What other sorts of therapy could help?

There may not be a drug-based solution to the problem—not all medical problems are currently treatable with pharmacotherapy. It is important to attempt to identify what

changes need to be brought about in the person's functioning and whether drug treatment can cure the condition or improve symptoms. Practitioners should keep an open mind here and consider all modalities—surgery, physiotherapy, lifestyle changes (e.g. diet, exercise, stress levels), psychotherapy, CAM methods, and combinations of therapies, as well as drug treatment. Assuming that there are safe, effective drugs available to treat the problem, then there are many decisions to be made:

• What class of drugs is appropriate?
• Which particular drug from the class should be selected? Are they all bioequivalent?
• What do QUM guidelines recommend about this drug? What experience do we have with it?
• Is more than one drug required?
• Are there pharmacoeconomic factors (costs) to consider?

What does the drug do and how does it act?

What is known about the drug's pharmacodynamics? What actions does it have and what is the mechanism—does it affect receptors, enzymes, ion channels, transport processes? How will this affect the person's problems? What do we not know that could be important? What are the common adverse reactions (side-effects) and potential drug interactions? Checking a drug monograph for the drug is helpful here.

How long will the patient be treated?

This requires knowing the usual course of the condition and prognosis. Will the patient get better after a few days of treatment (e.g. after an acute infection), might there be ongoing relapses and remissions (as with multiple sclerosis) or will the condition progress relentlessly (as do diabetes and cancer)?

How will you monitor therapy?

The patient's progress must be monitored to evaluate effects of the therapy. It is possible to monitor several parameters (see later section on therapeutic drug monitoring):
• improvement in the problem (e.g. reduction in blood pressure after an antihypertensive agent)
• adverse reactions to the drug (e.g. fall in white cell count after a cytotoxic drug used in cancer)
• plasma levels of the drug (e.g. of drugs with a low therapeutic index [safety margin], such as cyclosporin and lithium).

How much drug should be given?

What dose is being prescribed, for what effect, and is it appropriate? Doses need to be individualised so do not feel you have to rely on memory—look it up! Pharmacokinetic principles will determine the frequency of dosing and possibly the appropriate route. The drug's therapeutic index will determine how critical the exact dose is. The route may determine the formulation or there may be choices: if oral, will it be tablets, capsules, a mixture, a sustained-release form?

What is special about this patient?

If the patient is not the standard 70-kg fully functioning adult, what is the patient's age and weight? Might a woman patient be pregnant or breastfeeding? How effective are the liver and kidney functions likely to be? (These affect pharmacokinetic parameters such as protein binding and drug elimination, and are discussed in Chapters 6–8.) Are there other concurrent medical conditions? Is the drug contraindicated in any of these situations? Are there relevant sociocultural aspects relating to values, beliefs, cultural differences or restricted income that might affect compliance or responses to therapy? Is the person taking any other medications, whether prescribed, OTC or CAM? If so, what drug interactions are possible or clinically significant?

Can you write (or fill or administer) the prescription?

Are the 'five rights' right (patient, drug, dose, route, time)? Does the prescription seem appropriate? Does it conform with PBS and institutional requirements and QUM guidelines? Are the instructions to the patient adequate and correct? (See later under Prescriptions.)

Are there any warnings for the patient or staff?

Patients have the right to get as much medical information as they want. In particular, they need to know about their condition, why a drug is being prescribed and for how long, whether it is to treat the disease or to relieve symptoms, and how and when to take the medicine. Patients need to be warned about possible significant adverse reactions, how to recognise them and what to do if they occur, drug and food (and alcohol) interactions and what to do if they miss a dose.

Printed consumer product information should be included in the drug package with all relevant details. Patients' carers, both family and nursing staff, may also need warnings about some adverse reactions to help them in their roles.

PRESCRIPTIONS
Prescription orders

A **prescription** (script) is a written direction for the preparation and administration of a drug, containing the names and quantities of the active ingredients. It is written by a licensed prescriber (medical practitioner, dentist or veterinary surgeon)* and may present in two formats: on a prescription form or an institutional order sheet (Figures 2-1 and 2-2). Prescriptions must comply with legal formats, e.g. as laid down in the Australian *Drugs, Poisons and Controlled Substances Act, and Regulations 1981*. Prescriptions are then dispensed (filled) by a registered pharmacist.

Doctors' prescriptions

A **prescription** must be clear, concise and correct. It has elements that can be correlated with the **five** nursing **rights** of medication administration: the patient's name and address (right patient); date written, generic or proprietary drug name (right drug); drug strength and dosage (right dose); route of administration (right route); dosage instructions or frequency of administration (right time); and bears the signature, name and address of the prescriber. The number of times the prescription can be repeated should also be specified. All the elements should be clearly written to avoid any chance of error; for example, if there is any chance that 'μg' might be read as 'mg', then the word 'microgram' should be written in full or abbreviated to mcg. Formerly, it was required that prescriptions be written indelibly in the prescriber's own handwriting, but now they can be computer-generated and printed. All efforts must be made to prevent forgery of details or of entire prescriptions. If any confusion or doubt exists, the prescriber is contacted for clarification.

It is suggested that for good prescribing practice, doctors should have a finite list of 'personal preferred drugs' with which they are very familiar, and feel confident in their ability to evaluate new information and prescribe wisely. In practice, most doctors regularly prescribe only 40–60 different drugs.

---

*In some Australian states, other appropriately qualified health professionals such as nurse practitioners, optometrists and podiatrists are licensed to prescribe a limited range of Prescription Only drugs.

A.

FOR PNEUMONIA	
Iodide of Potassium	ℨ ╪
Creosoti	ℨ SS
Rectified Spirits of Wine	ℨ ╫
Ext. Glycyrrhizae Liq.	ℨ ╫╪
Water	ℨ V╪
Dose: One tablespoonful to be taken every four hours till temperature becomes normal.	

Adapted from: Disabled Men's Association of Australia. *Medical Prescriptions (for all diseases and ailments)*. Melbourne: Disabled Men's Association, c. 1929. Note that potassium iodide (1 drachm) is still included in some cough mixtures as an expectorant; creosote (1/2 fluid drachm), a mixture of phenols obtained from distillation of wood tar, has disinfectant and expectorant properties; Rectified Spirits of Wine (2 fluid drachms), aka Spiritus Vini Rectificatus (SVR) is Alcohol 95%; and Ext. Glycyrrhizae Liq. (3 fluid drachms) is a chloroform–water extract of unpeeled liquorice (the dried root of the plant *Glycyrrhiza glabra*), used as a demulcent (soothing agent), flavouring agent and expectorant. The mixture is made up with water (6 fluid ounces).

B.

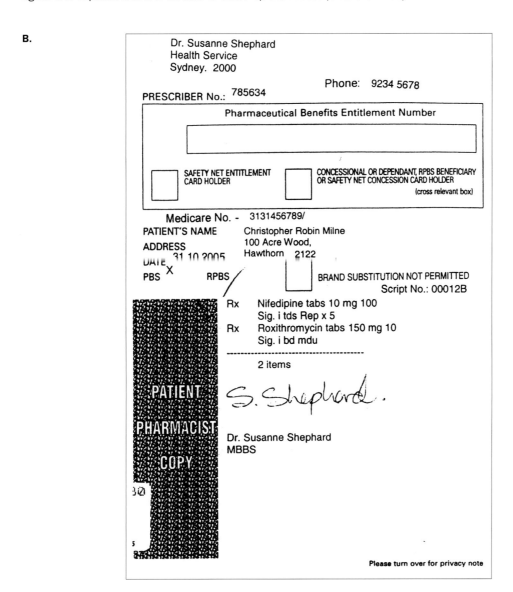

FIGURE 2-1 Typical prescriptions. **A.** An example of a prescription from the early 20th century. **B.** A typical current Pharmaceutical Benefits Scheme prescription; names and details have been changed.

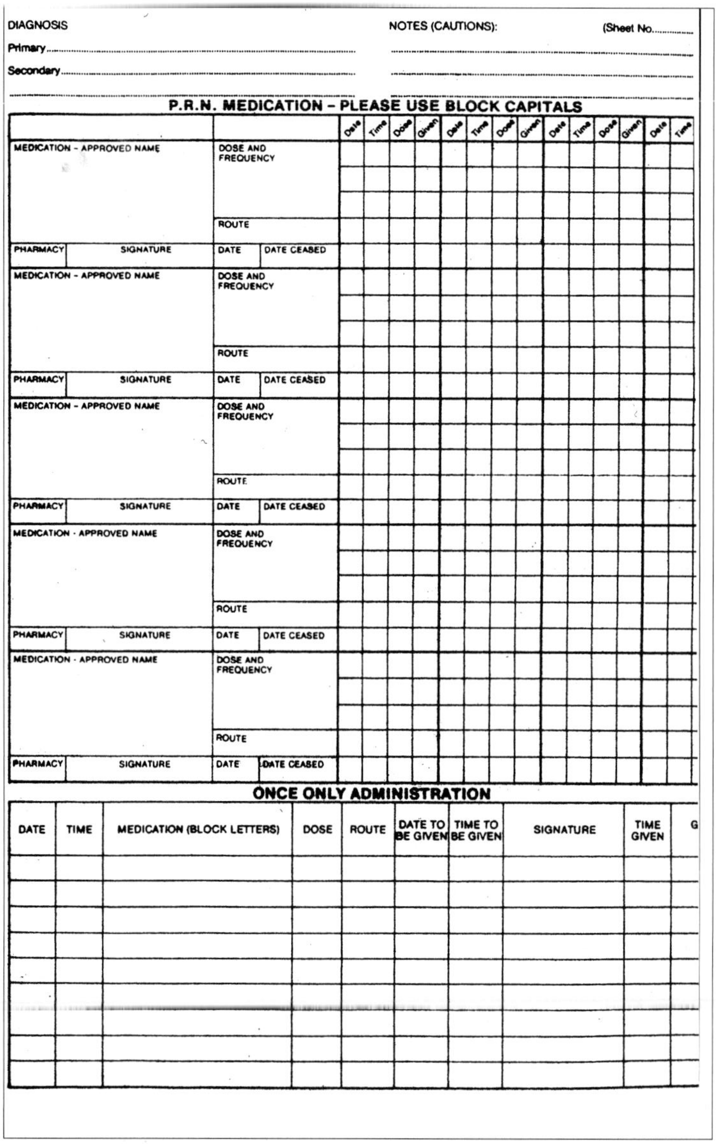
DIAGNOSIS
Primary
Secondary
NOTES (CAUTIONS):
(Sheet No.

P.R.N. MEDICATION - PLEASE USE BLOCK CAPITALS

MEDICATION - APPROVED NAME	DOSE AND FREQUENCY	Date	Time	Dose	Given	Date	Time	Dose	Given	Date	Time	Dose	Given	Date	Time
	ROUTE														
PHARMACY SIGNATURE	DATE / DATE CEASED														
MEDICATION - APPROVED NAME	DOSE AND FREQUENCY														
	ROUTE														
PHARMACY SIGNATURE	DATE / DATE CEASED														
MEDICATION - APPROVED NAME	DOSE AND FREQUENCY														
	ROUTE														
PHARMACY SIGNATURE	DATE / DATE CEASED														
MEDICATION - APPROVED NAME	DOSE AND FREQUENCY														
	ROUTE														
PHARMACY SIGNATURE	DATE / DATE CEASED														
MEDICATION - APPROVED NAME	DOSE AND FREQUENCY														
	ROUTE														
PHARMACY SIGNATURE	DATE / DATE CEASED														

ONCE ONLY ADMINISTRATION

DATE	TIME	MEDICATION (BLOCK LETTERS)	DOSE	ROUTE	DATE TO BE GIVEN	TIME TO BE GIVEN	SIGNATURE	TIME GIVEN	G

FIGURE 2-2 Part of a typical medication therapy chart from a patient's hospital record (also known as the patient's drug chart). (Designed and printed by Rolls Printing P/L; reproduced with permission.)

Telephone orders and standing orders

Drugs are also sometimes prescribed by doctors as 'telephone orders' or standing orders if the doctor cannot be present at the time. A doctor may telephone a drug prescription through to a pharmacist, who is legally entitled to dispense the prescription, and to a nurse entitled to administer it on the oral instructions. The doctor must then, as soon as is practicable, write out the drug order on a prescription pad, sign it and post or deliver it to the pharmacy, or use the hospital drug chart. A faxed prescription copy can confirm an oral order but is not legally acceptable, as the signature has to be original, i.e. in the doctor's handwriting; the pharmacist must see the original prescription before releasing the drug to the client.

'Standing orders' are sometimes left by doctors as ongoing prescriptions in a hospital, nursing home or residential care setting. These have no legal validity unless properly written, dated and signed as for any normal prescription.

Hospital drug charts

Prescriptions in hospitals are usually written on a drug chart, or medication therapy chart (Figure 2-2). These can become quite complicated and may run to many pages in a patient's medical record, as patients in hospital are frequently prescribed 10–15 drugs during one stay. In the sample chart, only one page of which is shown, the users are instructed:

- to use approved names for drugs

- not to alter existing orders
- to record all instances when drugs are administered, or when the drug was not administered, giving reason
- that IV fluid orders are to be recorded on a separate IV orders chart
- that nurse-initiated therapy (e.g. mild analgesics, laxatives, antacids) is to be countersigned by a doctor.

This form also has sections for general medications, and for admission and discharge drugs (those the patient was using when admitted, and those prescribed when discharged).

Specialised medication charts are also available to record phone orders, comments on administration discrepancies and errors, IV orders (covering fluids administered, drip rates and additives), diabetes management and fluid balance. There are also forms designed for recording other aspects of health care, such as for physiotherapy and podiatry progress notes, nursing admission data, neurological observations, patient's consent to treatment, delivery and neonatal records, and residential care information.

Instructions and abbreviations in prescriptions

A clearly written drug order specifies the conditions for drug administration; for example, a routine order means that the drug is administered until discontinued by the prescriber; a prn (pro re nata = when necessary) order is administered only when needed by the patient, while a stat (statim = immediately) order is for immediate administration of one dose of medication.

Many abbreviations and symbols are used in drug ordering (see Table 2-1 for a list of common accepted forms). Drug names should not be abbreviated; if there is any possibility of confusion, all words should be written in full: 'If in doubt, write it out!'.

Electronic prescribing

General practitioners (GPs) in Australia have been encouraged to adopt the use of computers in their practices. A study in 2000 showed that about 65% of GPs used electronic prescribing packages. While there are some disadvantages (initial cost, information overload, invasion of patient's privacy, intrusiveness of advertising), the advantages are many:

- improved legibility
- improved access to patient's past history
- access to prescribing guidelines and drug information
- warnings as to potential adverse reactions, allergies and drug interactions
- possibility of accumulating epidemiological and prescribing patterns data
- improved efficiency in the health-care system.

PHARMACEUTICS: FORMULATIONS OF DRUGS

Depending on the route by which a drug is administered (e.g. whether by mouth, topically onto the skin, by injection, into the eye or ear), different drug dosage forms are possible or appropriate (see Box 2-1). **Pharmaceutics** is the science of formulating drugs into different types of preparation, e.g. tablets, ointments, injectable solutions or eye-drops. It also includes study of the ways in which various drug forms influence pharmacokinetic and pharmacodynamic activities of the active drug.

Many drugs are available in different **formulations**. This variety assists the prescriber in choosing a formulation that is best suited to the individual patient and route of administration, and according to whether it is intended that the drug act locally or be absorbed into the systemic circulation. Box 2-1 shows a comprehensive listing of various forms of drug preparations, with a brief description of each form. More details of formulations specific to particular drug groups are given in the relevant chapters, as follows:

- drugs administered by inhalation: Chapter 32
- drugs administered to the eye: Chapter 35
- drugs administered to the ear: Chapter 36
- drugs applied to the skin: Chapter 56.

The routes of drug administration and the ways in which the route affects absorption of drugs are discussed in Chapter 7.

Formulations for oral administration

An oral drug may appear in solid form (e.g. tablet, capsule or powder) or in liquid form (solution, elixir or suspension). Disintegration of the solid dose form must occur before dissolution, a process by which a drug goes into solution and becomes available for absorption. The form of the drug dose is important because the more rapid the rate of dissolution, the more readily the compound crosses the cell membrane and is absorbed into the systemic circulation to be circulated to the site where it acts. Oral drugs in liquid form are therefore more rapidly available for gastrointestinal absorption than those in solid form.

Tablets

The oral route of administration is by far the most common: about three-quarters of all drugs prescribed are administered orally and, of these, about 60% are in tablet form. **Tablets** are compressed mixtures of active drug with various other chemicals, called excipients, which assist in the formulation.

TABLE 2-1 Common abbreviations and symbols in prescriptions*

ABBREVIATION	UNABBREVIATED FORM	MEANING
*ac	Ante cibum	Before meals
ad lib	Ad libitum	Freely
am	Ante meridiem	Morning
*aq	Aqua	Water, aqueous
*bd, bid	Bis die, bis in die	Twice each day
c	Cum	With
*cap	Capsule	Capsule
cc, cm³	Cubic centimetre	Cubic centimetre (= 1 mL)
D5W	Dextrose 5% water	5% Dextrose in water
D/C or DC	Discontinue	Terminate
DW	Distilled water	Water purified by condensation from steam
EC	Enteric-coated	Tablet or capsule formulation whose coating prevents dissolution until reaching the small intestine
elix	Elixir	Elixir
*g, gm	Gram	1000 milligrams
gtt	Gutta	Drop
h, hr	Hora	Hour
hs	Hora somni	At bedtime
IA	Intra-arterial	Into an artery or arteriole
IC	Intracardiac	Into the heart
ID	Intradermal	Into the skin
*IM	Intramuscular	Into muscle
inj	Injection	Injection
IT	Intrathecal	Into the subarachnoid space
IU	International Unit	Unit of pharmacological activity for a particular drug, as defined by an international convention
*IV	Intravenous	Into a vein
IVPB	IV piggyback	Secondary IV line
kg	Kilogram	1000 grams
KVO	Keep vein open	Very slow infusion rate
L	Litre	Litre (1000 cm³)
M	Mitte	Send, supply
*mane	Morning	In the morning
µg, mcg	Microgram	One millionth of a gram
*mg	Milligram	One thousandth of a gram
mEq	Milliequivalent	One thousandth of the gram equivalent weight of a solute in an electrolyte solution
mist	Mistura	Mixture
*ml, mL	Millilitre	One thousandth of a litre, 1 cm³

TABLE 2-1 Common abbreviations and symbols in prescriptions*—cont'd

ABBREVIATION	UNABBREVIATED FORM	MEANING
NG	Nasogastric	Into the stomach via the nose
*nocte	At night	At night
NS	Normal saline	0.9% Sodium chloride solution
oc	Oculorum	Eye
os	Os	Mouth
OTC	Over the counter	Non-prescription drug
otic	Otikos	The ear
*pc	Post cibum	After meals
*pm	Post meridiem	After noon
PO	Per os	By mouth, orally
PR	Per rectum	Into the rectum
prn	Pro re nata	According to necessity (lit. for the thing [i.e. need] having arisen)
PV	Per vagina	Into the vagina
q	Quaque	Every
*qd, qid	Quater in die	Four times a day
qh	Quaque hora	Every hour
q4h, qqh	Quaque quarta hora	Every 4 hours
qs	Quantum satis	Sufficient quantity
Rx	Receipt, recipe	Take (or dispense, provide)
s	Sine	Without
SC	Subcutaneous	Into subcutaneous tissue
Sig.	Signature	Label, instructions
SL	Sub linguam	Under the tongue
SOS	Si opus sit	If necessary
ss	Semis	A half
*stat	Statim	At once
*tab	Tablet	Tablet
tbsp	Tablespoon	Tablespoon (15 mL)
*tid or TDS	Ter in die	Three times a day
TO	Telephone order	Order received over the telephone
top	Topically	Applied to the skin
tsp	Teaspoon	Teaspoon (4 or 5 mL)
U	Unit	A dose measure for insulin, heparin
ung	Unguentum	Ointment
VO	Verbal order	Order received verbally
×	Times	As in two times a week

*Only the abbreviations marked with an asterisk are approved by the *Australian Medicines Handbook*.

BOX 2-1 VARIOUS FORMS OF DRUG PREPARATIONS

Preparations for oral use
Liquid
- Aqueous solution (substances dissolved in water)
- Aqueous suspension (solid particles suspended in water; must be shaken well before measuring out)
- Draught (oral liquid in single-dose volume, e.g. 50 mL)
- Elixir (aromatic, sweetened alcohol and water solution)
- Emulsion (two-phase system of two immiscible liquids, with fine droplets of one phase dispersed in the other by action of an emulsifying agent)
- Extract (syrup or dried form of pharmacologically active drug, usually prepared by evaporating solution)
- Fluid extract (concentrated alcoholic liquid extract of plant or vegetable)
- Mixture (liquid preparation of drugs in aqueous vehicle for oral administration)
- Spirit or essence (alcoholic solution of volatile substances)
- Syrup and linctus (aqueous solution containing high concentration of sugars)
- Tincture (alcohol extract of plant or vegetable substance)

Solid
- Capsule (soluble case [usually gelatin] that contains liquid, powdered, or beaded drug particles; convenient for drugs with an unpleasant taste)
- Lozenge (flavoured, medicated tablet that dissolves slowly in the mouth)
- Pill (spherical or ovoid mass containing a single dose of drug mixed with excipients)
- Powder/granule (loose fine/moulded drug substance in dry form for drug administration)
- Tablet (compressed, powdered drug(s) in a small disc for single dose administration)

Preparations for parenteral use (injections)
- Ampoule (sealed glass container for sterile liquid injectable medication for single use)
- Cartridge (single-dose unit of parenteral medication to be used with a specific injecting device)
- Injection (sterile solution or suspension for parenteral administration)
- Vial (glass container with rubber stopper for liquid or powdered medication)

Intravenous infusions (container suspended on hanger at bedside)
- Glass bottles, flexible collapsible plastic bags, or semirigid plastic containers in sizes from 100 to 1000 mL used for continuous infusion of fluid replacement with or without drug
- Heparin lock or angiocath (a port site for direct administration of intermittent IV medications without the need for a primary IV solution)
- Intermittent intravenous infusions (usually a small secondary IV set to which drug is added; it runs as a 'piggyback' to the primary IV infusion)

Preparations for topical use
- Aerosol (fine mist of powder or solution, may contain a propellant)
- Cream (semisolid emulsion that contains a drug incorporated into both an aqueous and an oily base)
- Dusting powder (dry substances in fine powder form for application to skin or mucous membranes)
- Gel or jelly (semisolid preparation in a non-fatty base)
- Liniment (liquid preparation for lubricating or soothing, applied by rubbing)
- Lotion (liquid preparation that can be protective, emollient, cooling, astringent, antipruritic, cleansing etc)
- Ointment (semisolid preparation in an aqueous or oily base for local protective, soothing or astringent effects, or for transdermal application for systemic effects
- Paste (thick ointment primarily used for skin protection)
- Plaster (solid preparation spread on fabric; may be adhesive, protective or soothing)
- Transdermal patch (adhesive patch impregnated with drug, which is absorbed continuously through the skin and acts systemically)

Preparations for use on mucous membranes
- Aqueous solutions of medications, usually for topical action but occasionally used for systemic effects, including enemas, douches, mouth-washes, nasal and throat sprays, and gargles
- Aerosol sprays, nebulisers and inhalers (deliver aqueous solutions of drug in fine droplet form, or very finely dispersed powders, to the target membrane, e.g. bronchodilators to the bronchial tree)
- Drops (aqueous solutions, with or without gelling agent to prolong retention time; used for eyes, ears or nose)
- Foam (powders or solutions of medication in volatile liquids with a propellant, such as vaginal foams for contraception)
- Lamella (small gelatine disc impregnated with drug for use in the eye, e.g. to treat glaucoma)
- Pessary (a vaginal suppository)
- Suppository (a small bullet-shaped solid form containing drug mixed in a firm but malleable base [e.g. cocoa butter] to facilitate insertion into the rectum; may be for local or systemic effect)

Miscellaneous drug delivery systems
- Intradermal implant (sterile pellet or rod containing a small deposit of drug for insertion into a dermal pocket. Designed to allow drug to leach slowly into tissue; usually for administration of hormones such as testosterone or oestradiol)
- Micropump system (a small external pump, attached by belt or implanted, that delivers medication via a needle in a continuous steady dose; e.g. for insulin, anticancer chemotherapy or opioid analgesic)
- Targeted drug-carrier system, e.g. liposomes, protein drug carriers (designed to deliver a specific drug to a particular capillary bed, cell or receptor)

For example, pharmacologically inert chemicals may be present as diluents (fillers), binders, adhesives, disintegrants, lubricants, flavours, colours, sweeteners or absorbents. Thus the active drug may make up only a very small fraction of the total tablet weight.

Tablets may appear as simple white discs or may be multilayered or coated with a film* to mask an unpleasant taste. Some tablets are prepared for sublingual administration (dissolved under the tongue) or as effervescent tablets that fizz and dissolve in water so that they are easier to take.

Tablets may also be available for use by a pharmacist or scientist in preparing solutions of particular strengths.

The rate of release of active drug from a tablet—and thus the drug concentration in the circulation and at the active site — can be manipulated by pharmaceutical processing. It is possible to combine an active drug with a resin or other substance from which it is slowly released, to delay absorption (**sustained-release** [SR], or controlled-release [CR] preparations). In addition, it is possible to prepare a tablet with a coating that offers relative resistance to the digestive action of stomach contents (enteric coating, EC). **Enteric coatings** on drugs are used:

- to prevent decomposition of chemically sensitive drugs by gastric secretions (e.g. penicillin G and erythromycin are unstable in an acid pH)
- to prevent dilution of the drug before it reaches the intestine
- to prevent nausea and vomiting induced by the drug's effect in the stomach
- to provide delayed action of the drug.

Other oral dose forms

Other formulations for oral administration include capsules, solutions, elixirs, powders, syrups and lozenges; further pharmaceutical detail about these dose forms is beyond the scope of this text.

Parenteral dose forms
Parenteral solutions

Parenteral administration of drugs is the administration of drugs by injection and is the most rapid form of systemic therapy. The intravenous (IV) route, in which the drug is injected directly into the circulation, avoids any delay during absorption. Because any injection is an invasive procedure with the potential for infection being introduced, drugs formulated as solutions for parenteral administration must be sterile, filtered, particle-free and preferably isotonic with body solutions (i.e. with normal saline, 0.9% sodium chloride

solution) and buffered to body pH. Solutions that are acidic or alkaline, hypertonic or contain irritant drugs can damage tissues into which they are injected. If solid particles are injected, they can cause granulomas, ischaemia or phlebitis.

Usually, parenteral solutions consist of the drug dissolved in an aqueous solution, but in some cases a drug that is very insoluble in water and which must be administered parenterally, such as the general anaesthetic propofol (Drug Monograph 15-3), can be formulated in an oily emulsion suitable for injecting.

Equipment and solutions for parenteral administration

Solutions for injection are usually presented in glass ampoules or bottles or plastic bags. The equipment for delivery of a drug by an IV infusion is complicated (Figure 2-3) and may include sterile tubing, an in-line filter and drip chamber, clamps to adjust the flow rate, and a cannula for insertion into the vein. Most institutions will have guidelines as to the use of such IV sets, with lists of appropriate infusion solutions and possible admixtures (agents added to IV fluids). The general rule is

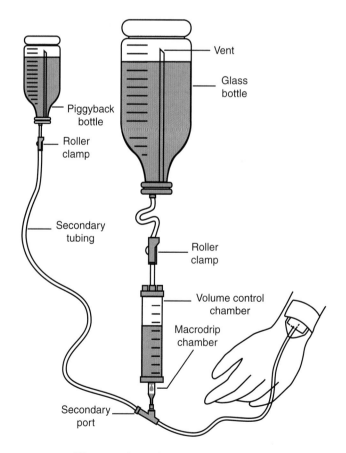

FIGURE 2-3 Diagram of a typical intravenous infusion set-up, showing a secondary 'piggyback' bottle with a reservoir of drug in IV fluid.

---

*Brightly coloured film-coated tablets look remarkably like sweets such as 'Smarties', and account for many cases of childhood poisoning annually.

that unless an admixture is specifically allowed, it should not be made, unless a hospital pharmacist or drug information centre has approved the addition.

Factors modifying responses to drugs

If the same dose of drug (on a mg drug per kg body weight basis) is given to similar people—or indeed to the same person on different occasions—their responses are likely to be different. Many factors can modify drug responses and these need to be anticipated by the health professional before prescribing and administering a drug, and also afterwards, when observing responses and monitoring drug therapy. Pharmaceutical factors affecting response, such as the form in which the drug is administered (whether liquid or oral, simple tablet or sustained-release form, patch or ointment etc), were discussed in the previous section.

Pharmacokinetic factors

Factors that affect how the body handles drugs, i.e. how the drug is absorbed from its site of administration, distributed around the body in the bloodstream and eliminated by metabolism and excretion, will obviously help determine how much drug is available at any time to act. Pharmacokinetic principles are studied in Chapter 6, and applied in Chapters 7 and 8 to dosage regimens and individual and lifespan aspects of drug therapy.

Pharmacokinetic factors affecting drug responses may be influenced by:
• body composition (proportion of fat)
• diet and presence of food in the stomach
• smoking (may alter clearance of a drug from the body)
• age and gender (may affect cardiac, liver and kidney functions)
• pregnancy (alters distribution)
• genetic factors (may determine enzyme levels)
• liver disease and kidney disease (impair metabolism and excretion of drugs, potentially leading to accumulation and toxicity)
• hypermotility of the gastrointestinal tract (may rush drugs through before adequate absorption occurs).

Pharmacodynamic factors

Pharmacodynamics refers to what the drug does in the body —its actions and effects, including useful therapeutic effects and adverse reactions (side-effects), as well as studies of the mechanism of action of the drug at the molecular level. These aspects of pharmacology are discussed in Chapters 5 and 9, and in sub-sequent chapters under drug groups and in Drug Monographs.

While the mechanism of action of a drug is generally similar in all individuals—unless they happen to have unusual amounts or types of the receptor or other cell component on which the drug acts—there are still factors that can affect pharmacodynamic aspects of an administered drug and hence affect responses. Such factors include tachyphylaxis and desensitisation (rapid decreased effect of a drug) and tolerance (slowly acquired reduction in responsiveness, e.g. in opioid-dependent persons).

Individual and clinical factors
COMPLIANCE

Obviously the primary determinant of drug response is whether or not the person takes the drug.* **Compliance** means following all aspects of a treatment plan. In the context of drug therapy, it implies administering the drug according to the five rights (see Doctors' prescriptions, earlier). All the other advice given related to therapy must also be followed, including lifestyle aspects such as weight reduction, cessation of smoking, and moderation in alcohol intake. This can be demanding and, when many drugs are prescribed, may become a formidable exercise.

There are many causes of poor compliance:
• confusion over complicated drug regimens
• bad taste or pain on administration
• adverse effects occurring
• not wanting to disturb or wake the patient for night-time doses
• poor communication and lack of information about the treatment
• lack of support and monitoring of therapy
• cost or difficulty in obtaining medicines.

The consequences of poor compliance are more than just wasted drugs and time. Drug levels in the body may fall below the therapeutic range, leading to inadequate responses and lack of effect. The doctor cannot properly monitor and adjust therapy if lack of response is due to poor compliance, and may waste effort in revising the diagnosis, increasing doses, adding more drugs or sending the patient for more tests. In particular situations, poor compliance with therapy may result in pregnancy (oral contraceptives), convulsions (antiepileptic drugs), strokes or heart attacks (anticoagulant or antithrombotic drugs).

Studies have shown that good compliance is the exception rather than the rule, and despite Hippocrates' warning, doctors

*This has been recognised for thousands of years. The ancient Greek physician Hippocrates, writing about compliance, advised his medical students to: 'Keep a watch also on the faults of patients, which often make them lie about the taking of things prescribed. For through not taking disagreeable drinks, purgative or other, they sometimes die. What they have done never results in a confession, but the blame is thrown upon the physician.'

are not good at predicting which patients are likely to be good or poor compliers. Ways of assessing compliance include careful counts of tablets or other dose forms remaining after a specified period, and assays (measurements) of drug levels in blood samples.

It must be recognised that people have a right to autonomy in their own medical care and may justifiably refuse to take drugs for good reasons; however, it is important that the prescribers be made aware if drugs are not being taken as directed, so that allowances can be made and, possibly, different drugs substituted.

DRUG INTERACTIONS

After a person has been stabilised on repeated doses of a drug, the responses to the drug may be affected by interactions with any other drug taken, including non-prescribed OTC drugs and CAM therapies, as well as other ingested compounds such as food and drinks. As a person takes, or a patient is prescribed, more and more drugs, the possibility of **drug interactions** rises exponentially. The topic of drug interactions is discussed in Chapter 9, and in individual drug monographs where clinically relevant. There are exhaustive lists of common drug interactions in reference texts such as the *Australian Medicines Handbook* (Appendix A), *MIMS Annual* (Index to Drug Interactions Table) and *Avery's Drug Treatment* (Appendix B: Guide to Clinically More Important Drug Interactions).

Drug interactions may affect either the pharmacokinetics of the drugs involved (e.g. monoamine oxidase inhibitors inhibiting the metabolism of many other drugs) or pharmacodynamic aspects (e.g. antihistamines and alcohol having additive CNS-depressant effects).

POLYPHARMACY

Polypharmacy is defined as 'the concurrent use of multiple medications'. In the clinical context, it has the connotation of implying prescription and use of too many or unnecessary drugs, or use at frequencies greater than therapeutically essential. Polypharmacy is thus a situation in which multiple drug interactions can occur, and is potentially harmful to the patient.

An Australian National Health Survey (1995, reviewed in *NPS Newsletter 13*, 2000) found that 10.7 million Australians—almost 60% of the population—were taking prescribed or OTC medications (excluding CAM therapies) at any one time. If CAM had been included, the proportion may well have been much higher. Of those using at least one medication, 14.5% were taking four or more drugs, and 4.6% were taking six or more. In persons over 75 years, the proportions were about 40% and 17% respectively. This very high reliance on drugs (Australia has been called 'the overmedicated society') means that many people are at high risk of adverse drug reactions and drug interactions.

Polypharmacy is not the sole responsibility of prescribing doctors; various health professionals can initiate the steps recommended for managing and avoiding polypharmacy:

- prevention: avoid prescribing or administering drugs for minor complaints
- regular medication review: assess appropriateness and need for therapy, dosage and formulation, ADRs and drug interactions, and compliance
- non-pharmacological approaches: use lifestyle measures whenever possible
- communication: with the patient, about concerns, expectations and difficulties with compliance, and with other health carers about changes in drug regimens
- simplification: reduce regimens to essential drugs, at the lowest effective doses and frequencies; limit use of optional, trivial and placebo medications.

A case involving polypharmacy, and a successful resolution of the problems, is described in Clinical Interest Box 2-3.

PLACEBO EFFECT

The Latin word *placebo* literally means 'I will please'. In the pharmacological context, it refers to a harmless inactive preparation prescribed to satisfy a patient who does not require an active drug. In a clinical trial, it is formulated to look identical to the active drug under trial, to maintain 'double blinding', so that neither subject nor clinician knows which treatment group the subject is in. Patients and subjects in trials frequently appear to respond to placebos, with therapeutic or adverse effects. This '**placebo response**' may be a significant but temporary alteration in the person's condition, due to the person's expectations or other unexplained psychological effect. Factors possibly inducing the response include the relationship between the patient and the health professional, the wish to be seen to respond, response to the increased care and attention, and aspects such as the colour and taste of the dose form or pain on injection (no gain without pain).

THERAPEUTIC DRUG MONITORING (TDM)

Therapy can be monitored in various ways, including simply observing the patient's progress and changes in signs and symptoms. In the specific case of checking on results of drug therapy, there are three main ways of carrying out TDM—observing and/or measuring therapeutic effects, **adverse drug reactions**, or levels of the drug in the body. The purpose of **TDM** is to provide evidence on which to base rational adjustment of dosage.

Drugs commonly monitored are:
- those in which there is a good relation between plasma concentration and clinical effect (e.g. theophylline)

CLINICAL INTEREST BOX 2-3   CLUES IN THE MEDICINE CABINET

Doctor D was called with a request that a home visit be made to an elderly woman living at home: 'Mother is going downhill . . . someone has to come around and sort things out.' The doctor visited the woman, armed with the files on her medical history, which revealed many years of hypertension, angina, heart failure, a heart attack, osteoarthritis, depression, obesity and surgical repair of a hiatus (oesophageal) hernia. Most recently she had been diagnosed with heart failure and peripheral vascular disease, and doses of digoxin and frusemide had been increased.

Mrs X's current complaints were of worsening dyspnoea (difficulty in breathing) and ankle swelling, poor circulation in the legs and cold feet, cramps, anorexia and nausea, and postural hypotension (dizziness when standing up). On examination she was unwell, pale, with pitting oedema, irregular pulse with atrial fibrillation, high blood pressure (180/95), and bilateral pulmonary crepitations (crackling noises indicating abnormal fluid in the lungs). Possible causes of her problems were myocardial infarction (heart attack), renal failure, digitalis toxicity, hypokalaemia, anaemia and drug interactions.

A tactful request to view the medicine cabinet was greeted with relief, and proved 'a revelation almost beyond belief'. The hoarded contents included:
- verapamil, a calcium channel blocker and antiarrhythmic agent
- two β-blockers, atenolol and propranolol, as antihypertensive drugs
- digoxin, a cardiac glycoside for heart failure, at the usual adult dose
- two diuretics: frusemide, a loop diuretic; and chlorothiazide, a thiazide diuretic
- a potassium supplement
- two tricyclic antidepressants, amitriptyline and doxepin
- glyceryl trinitrate tablets for angina, many months beyond their use-by date
- prochlorperazine, a phenothiazine antiemetic drug

- atropine plus diphenoxylate tablets, for diarrhoea
- a fibre supplement, to treat constipation
- several anti-inflammatory agents: indomethacin, dextropropoxyphene plus paracetamol, paracetamol, aspirin, and sustained-release aspirin
- pheniramine, an antihistamine
- sodium citrotartrate, for urinary alkalinisation or gastric hyperacidity
- eight assorted ointments and creams.

Mrs X was confused about her medicines (not surprisingly, as several had no instructions for administration) but thought she took most of them. Review of the many potential drug interactions and ADRs revealed that several of the drugs are contraindicated in heart failure, the anti-inflammatory agents could be exacerbating fluid retention, potassium supplementation was probably inadequate for two potassium-depleting diuretics, and digitalis toxicity could be contributing to arrhythmias and gastrointestinal upsets.

Most of the medicine cabinet was cleared out and several tests ordered to monitor digoxin levels (high), potassium (low), renal function and haemoglobin (normal). With fluid restriction and weight reduction after stabilisation on therapy, Mrs X was maintained on digoxin (1/4 the previous dose), amiloride plus hydrochlorothiazide (one potassium-conserving and one potassium-depleting diuretic), and paracetamol as necessary for pain. Her blood pressure was monitored carefully but required no medication.

The case highlights many problems of polypharmacy, including:
- overuse of drugs by those with ready access to them
- requirement for well-maintained medical records and drug charts
- the importance of good labelling of medicines and provision of drug information for patient and carers
- regular review of drug therapy regimen and medicine cabinet.

Source: Murtagh 1992; used with permission.

- drugs with well-defined therapeutic and toxic levels (e.g. digoxin, phenytoin, antidepressants)
- drugs with a low therapeutic index (e.g. digoxin)
- those with no easily measured response (e.g. anticonvulsants, antiarrhythmics and immunosuppressants)
- in overdose, when the plasma level determines the treatment of overdose (e.g. paracetamol overdose).

Monitoring of therapeutic effects

The effects of drugs can be monitored by measuring various physiological parameters. Examples include measuring blood pressure in a patient receiving an antihypertensive agent,

measuring various clotting times with anticoagulant drug therapy, and gauging the effects of hypoglycaemic agents by measuring the patient's blood glucose levels.

Monitoring of adverse reactions

Particularly in the case of drugs with a low therapeutic index, the **adverse reactions** may limit the level to which the dose can be increased. Cytotoxic therapy is frequently monitored by checking the patient's white blood cell count; if this falls too low, the patient is at risk of overwhelming infections. The white cell count is monitored after a course of chemotherapy; only when it has recovered sufficiently is another course of chemotherapy instituted. A common adverse reaction to the non-steroidal anti-inflammatory drugs is dyspepsia and exacerbation of peptic ulcers. A way to monitor this effect might be for the prescriber to advise the patient 'Stop taking the drug if you start to feel sick, and let me know'. The aminoglycoside antibiotics can cause severe damage to the kidneys and to hearing, so patients who require these drugs may have their hearing function monitored.

Indications for monitoring

The main indications for TDM, i.e. the situations in which it is considered useful, include:
• to check compliance or the progress of therapy
• to obtain baseline data before changing drug (or other) therapy
• to check for drug abuse, overdose or underdosing
• if there is unstable renal, liver or cardiovascular function
• monitoring of clinical trials.

Monitoring plasma concentration of drug

TDM probably refers most commonly to monitoring of the concentration of the drug in a sample of the patient's blood plasma. For drugs that require frequent monitoring, automated drug screens are available: a blood sample will be taken and sent to the clinical pharmacology or biochemistry laboratory for the drug levels to be assayed.

Monitoring plasma concentration is most useful for drugs with a low therapeutic index, for which a well-defined therapeutic range has been established. Drugs commonly monitored this way include digoxin, lithium, theophylline, anticonvulsants, antiarrhythmics, anticoagulants, toxic antibiotics, and paracetamol if an overdose is suspected.

Procedures for monitoring by plasma concentration

The drug concentration measured will be compared to the **therapeutic range** (published values of the concentration of the drug in plasma at steady state during effective therapy

$[C_{ss}]$). This is reached after about five half-lives during regular dosing. Therapeutic ranges are valid for about 80% of the population and are a good guide to expected plasma concentration of the drug. Trough levels (the lowest level likely to be in blood, measured by taking a blood sample immediately before the next dose) are usually measured. In some situations, e.g. to avoid toxic levels, peak levels are measured at the time of maximum plasma concentration.

Drug concentration is measured by highly accurate and specific techniques such as immunoassay, high-performance liquid chromatography (HPLC), gas chromatography, or flame photometry.

Typical procedure

The usual procedure for TDM is:
• collect 2–5 mL blood in a heparinised tube, just before the next dose, in a patient stabilised on a regular dose
• record all relevant information: dose schedule (amount, route, frequency), time of last dose, time of sampling, other drugs being taken
• send the sample to a laboratory for chemical assay
• evaluate the results in terms of published therapeutic levels and clinical data and problems.

If the therapy appears well controlled, further measurements may be taken 6–8 weeks later and again at 6–12-monthly intervals.

Drug screens

Drug screens are a particular example of TDM by drug blood levels, in which samples taken from patients are screened for presence of a range of drugs, usually for medicolegal reasons. They may be carried out to detect drugs of abuse, drugs possibly taken in overdoses or, in the forensic context, to detect poisons. Almost any body fluid can be screened, as well as solid tissues such as hair, bone or nails. False-positive results may arise from interference from other drugs that have been appropriately taken, and false-negatives because of levels below the detection limit, owing to inappropriate sampling time or insufficiently sensitive methods. Some toxic substances, including insulin, succinylcholine and potassium, may not be detected by any method after a delay.

KEY POINTS

● With the enormous range of drugs available and the increasing costs of new drugs, it is essential that quality use of medicines be encouraged; government policies on prescribing, schemes limiting availability of drugs, educational bodies disseminating objective information, and studies of drug usage in hospitals all contribute to cost-effective clinical pharmacology.

● Effective use of drugs in the clinical situation requires thorough knowledge of all aspects of the drugs and understanding of the patient's condition as it relates to how the drug is affected by the body and how the body responds to the drug.

- Before a drug is prescribed or administered, the health professional needs to: identify the patient's problem and its likely course; attempt to find a solution to the problem, considering possibly useful drug groups; choose a suitable drug about which pharmacokinetic and pharmacodynamic details are known; relate the drug to this patient in terms of relevant conditions that may affect therapeutic or adverse effects; determine how drug response will be monitored; and decide what warnings need to be given to patient and carers.

- Prescriptions are legally regulated documents, with specific requirements for format; abbreviations in prescriptions should be used only cautiously to avoid confusion.

- Drugs may be formulated in many dose forms to maximise effective administration and clinical effect; formulations for oral and parenteral administration are common in general practice and hospital use, respectively.

- Many factors may affect how a person responds to drugs, including pharmacodynamic and pharmacokinetic aspects; in the clinical situation, compliance, drug interactions, polypharmacy and placebo effects are particularly important.

- Responsible prescribing and use of drugs require that therapy be monitored, and altered if ineffective or potentially toxic; drug therapy may be monitored by measuring the therapeutic effects, adverse reactions and/or plasma concentration of drug.

REVIEW EXERCISES

1. Discuss the basis for campaigns for the quality use of medicines and describe some attempts being made to rationalise drug use.

2. Describe the role of your health profession with respect to drug usage and compare it to three or four other professions.

3. List at least 10 decisions that need to be made before a drug is prescribed or administered, explaining what information is important.

4. Describe the 'rights' that must be checked before a drug is administered to a patient.

5. Explain why it is important for drugs to be available in various dose forms and describe typical formulations for oral and parenteral administration.

6. Discuss how variations in compliance, polypharmacy and placebo effects can determine how a person responds to a drug.

7. List the reasons why drug therapy is monitored, the clinical situations in which it is important, and drugs that are commonly monitored.

8. Describe the three main methods by which therapeutic drug monitoring is carried out, giving examples.

9. Set up a class debate on the topic: 'If a drug to treat a condition exists, the government should provide it for all patients who need it'.

REFERENCES AND FURTHER READING

Anderson DM (ed.). *Dorland's Illustrated Medical Dictionary*. 30th edn. Philadelphia: Saunders-Elsevier, 2003.
Australian Medicines Handbook 2005. Adelaide: AMH, 2005.
Australasian Society of Clinical and Experimental Pharmacologists and Toxicologists. *Development of Drug Usage Evaluation in Hospital Practice in Australia and New Zealand* [Position paper]. Melbourne: ASCEPT, 1998.
Braun L, Cohen M. *Herbs and Natural Supplements: An Evidence-Based Guide*. Sydney: Mosby-Elsevier; 2005.
Buckley N. Drug screens. *Australian Prescriber* 2001; 24(4): 90–1.
Burridge N (ed.). *Australian Injectable Drugs Handbook*. 3rd edn. Melbourne: Society of Hospital Pharmacists of Australia, 2005.
Butler CC, Rollnick S. *Compliance*. London: Mosby, 2003.
Caswell A (ed.). *MIMS Annual June 2005*. Sydney: CMPMedica Australia, 2005.
Clark EA, Shakib S, Nigro O, Puri R, Psaltis P, Ryan R, Bochner F. An intervention to increase the rates of warfarin prophylaxis in general medical inpatients with atrial fibrillation. *Proceedings of the joint meeting of ASCEPT and APSA* 2005; 11: O157.
Dartnell J. Activities to improve hospital prescribing. *Australian Prescriber* 2001; 24(2): 29–31.
Dartnell J. *Understanding, influencing and evaluating drug use*. Melbourne: Therapeutic Guidelines, 2001.
Dartnell JG, Campbell DA, Nosworthy JC et al. Combining disease management and DUE improves acute management of COPD. *Proceedings of the Australian Society of Clinical and Experimental Pharmacology and Toxicology* 2000; 8: 29.
Darzins P, Pugh M. Are we there yet? Travel along the information highway seeking evidence-based medicine. *Australian Prescriber* 2001; 24(5): 116–19.
Dawes M, Davies P, Gray A, Mant J, Seers K, Snowball R. *Evidence-Based Practice: A Primer for Health Care Professionals*. 2nd edn. Edinburgh: Elsevier Churchill Livingstone, 2005.
Day RO, Mashford ML Pharmacotherapeutics: what a difference five decades make! *Medical Journal of Australia* 2001; 174(1): 48–51.
Disabled Men's Association of Australia. *Medical Prescriptions (for all diseases and ailments)*. Melbourne: Disabled Men's Association, c. 1929.

Dooley MJ, Allen KM, Doecke CJ, Galbraith KJ, Taylor GR, Bright J, Carey DL. A prospective multicentre study of pharmacist initiated changes to drug therapy and patient management in acute care government funded hospitals. *British Journal of Clinical Pharmacology* 2003; 57(4): 513–21.

Gilbert A, Roughead L, Sansom L. I've missed a dose; what should I do? *Australian Prescriber* 2002; 25(1): 16–18.

Hopkins H, Wade T, Weir D. 'Take as directed', whatever that means. *Australian Prescriber* 2000; 23(5): 103–4.

Humphries JL, Green J (eds). *Nurse Prescribing*. 2nd edn. Basingstoke: Palgrove, 2002.

Larkin C, Murray R. Assisting Aboriginal patients with medication management. *Australian Prescriber* 2005; 28(5): 123–5.

Lexchin J. Are new drugs as good as they claim to be? *Australian Prescriber* 2004; 27(1): 2–3.

Lyndon B. Withdrawal of useful drugs from the market. *Australian Prescriber* 2003; 26(3): 50–1.

Mant A. Quality use of medicines: ten years down the track. *Australian Prescriber* 2001; 24(5): 106–7.

Moulds R. Combination products—love them or loathe them? *Australian Prescriber* 2001; 24(5): 127–9.

Murtagh J. *Cautionary Tales: Authentic Case Histories from Medical Practice*. Sydney: McGraw-Hill, 1992.

National Prescribing Service. To prescribe or not to prescribe: issues surrounding our approach to new drugs. *NPS Newsletter 19,* 2001.

Neeskens P. The evidence–relevance gap: the example of hormone replacement therapy. *Australian Prescriber* 2002; 25(3): 60–2.

Pharmacy Board of Victoria. *Guidelines for Good Pharmaceutical Practice 2002*. Melbourne: Pharmacy Board of Victoria, 2002.

Phillips S. The National Prescribing Service and *Australian Prescriber*. *Australian Prescriber* 2002; 25(2): 26–7.

Rang HP, Dale MM, Ritter JM, Moore PK. *Pharmacology*. 5th edn. Edinburgh: Churchill Livingstone, 2003 [chs 5, 50].

Roller, L. *Pharmaceutics and Pharmacy Practice I, Practical Manual*. Melbourne: Victorian College of Pharmacy, Monash University, 1994.

Shargel L, Mutnick AH, Souney PF et al. *Comprehensive Pharmacy Review*. 3rd edn. Baltimore: Williams & Wilkins, 1997.

Shenfield GM. Therapeutic drug monitoring beyond 2000. *British Journal of Clinical Pharmacology* 1998; 46(2): 93–4.

Speight TM, Holford NHG (eds). *Avery's Drug Treatment*. 4th edn. Auckland: Adis International, 1997.

Stephenson H. Electronic prescribing in hospitals: the road ahead. *Australian Prescriber* 2001; 24(1): 2–3.

Sweeney G. *Clinical Pharmacology: A Conceptual Approach*. New York: Churchill Livingstone, 1990.

Therapeutic Guidelines Groups. *Therapeutic Guidelines: Antibiotic*. Version 12 [and other titles in the Therapeutic Guidelines series]. Melbourne: Therapeutic Guidelines, 2003.

Various authors. Adopting best evidence in practice. *Medical Journal of Australia* 2004; 180(6) Suppl: S43 and following 11 articles.

Walker R, Edwards C (eds). *Clinical Pharmacy and Therapeutics*. Edinburgh: Churchill Livingstone, 2003.

Youngson RM. *Collins Dictionary: Medicine*. 2nd edn. Glasgow: HarperCollins, 1998.

ON-LINE RESOURCES

Australasian Society of Clinical and Experimental Pharmacologists and Toxicologists (ASCEPT): www.ascept.org/

Cochrane Library: www.cochrane.org

National Medicines Policy (NMP): www.health.gov.au/internet/wcms/publishing.nsf/Content/National+Medicines+Policy-2

New Zealand Medicines and Medical Devices Safety Authority: www.medsafe.govt.nz

Royal College of Nursing Australia. Position Statement: Registered Nurses and Quality Use of Medicines: www.rcna.org.au/pages/welcome.php

Therapeutic Goods Administration (TGA): www.tga.gov.au

evolve   More weblinks at http://evolve.elsevier.com/AU/Bryant/pharmacology/

CHAPTER 3

Over-the-counter Drugs and Complementary Therapies

CHAPTER FOCUS

With proper use, over-the-counter (OTC), or non-prescription, drugs are considered safe for the treatment of minor illnesses without the regular supervision of a licensed health-care professional. Problems relating to the use of these products can occur, such as adverse effects, drug interactions, drug toxicity, and drug overuse or misuse. Complementary and alternative medicines (CAM) such as herbal therapies are also commonly employed today. Because some of these products are not assessed for safety and effectiveness, health-care professionals need to be informed about the use of and potential problems associated with such products. This chapter reviews the regulatory differences between prescription-only and OTC drugs, herbal remedies and nutritional supplements, and discusses general considerations on drug marketing and consumer education for safe administration of OTC drugs, herbal remedies and various complementary and alternative therapy modalities.

OBJECTIVES

- To describe the basis on which drugs are regulated and classified as listed, registered, OTC and/or prescription-only.

- To discuss the advantages and possible disadvantages of people self-medicating in treating minor illnesses.

- To explain the basic information necessary for proper selection of an OTC drug in the following categories: analgesics, antacids, laxatives, cough/cold preparations and antidiarrhoeal agents.

- To describe the prevalence and reasons for use of complementary and alternative therapies, and some of the issues involved.

- To discuss the differences between Eastern and Western approaches to illness, the laws governing herbal remedies in Australia, and the health-care professional's role regarding safe use of OTC drugs and complementary and alternative therapies.

KEY DRUGS

ginseng
paracetamol

KEY TERMS

complementary and alternative
  therapies
contamination
drug schedule
evidence-based medicine
herbal remedies
homeopathy
over-the-counter medicines
self-medication
Therapeutic Goods Administration
traditional Chinese medicine

KEY ABBREVIATIONS

CAM	complementary and alternative medicine
EBM	evidence-based medicine
NSAIDs	non-steroidal anti-inflammatory drugs
OTC	over the counter
SUSDP	Standards for the Uniform Scheduling of Drugs and Poisons
TCM	traditional Chinese medicine
TGA	Therapeutic Goods Administration

REGULATION OF DRUGS

THE Australian **Therapeutic Goods Administration** (TGA), a section of the Commonwealth Department of Health and Ageing, provides a framework for the regulation of therapeutic goods to ensure their safety, efficacy, quality and timely availability. The National Drugs and Poisons Scheduling Committee imposes controls on drugs by setting the Standards for the Uniform Scheduling of Drugs and Poisons (SUSDP) and deciding which **Schedule** a drug, poison or other chemical should be placed into. The Schedules related to drugs are numbered 2, 3, 4, 8 and 9. (Schedules are discussed in further detail in Chapter 4, and outlined in Appendix 5).

Self-medication

Over-the-counter (OTC) medicines are bought and used by the general public to self-treat minor illnesses. Such preparations may be readily available in pharmacies, supermarkets or other non-pharmacy outlets for selection by people who wish to be involved in their own health care, feel competent in undertaking **self-medication**, and wish to avoid the time and expense involved in going to a prescriber. It has been estimated that most people visit their physicians for only 10% of their illnesses and injuries, and that six out of every 10 medications purchased are OTC medications; thus OTC drugs represent a huge market.

Background and benefits of OTC availability of drugs

Factors that have led to the increase in self-medication include:

- growing media emphasis on health and health promotion
- reduced times of hospital stays
- rising costs of prescription drugs
- increased accessibility of information about health care and drugs
- higher marketing pressure and advertising of OTC products.

When used wisely, OTC drugs result in time and money savings, reduced workload for health professionals and, ultimately, reduced overall health-care costs. Other benefits include reduced chance of abuse or misuse of drugs than if they are not controlled at all, and fewer adverse effects or fatalities than might occur if OTC drugs were unscheduled and available without professional oversight or counselling.

Characteristics of OTC drugs

Differences between prescription-only and over-the-counter drugs

PRESCRIPTION-ONLY DRUGS

Drugs not considered safe enough for use by the general public without medical supervision are restricted to prescription-only status (Schedule 4 or 8 in the Australian system [see Chapter 4 and Appendix 5]). These products require the intervention of an authorised prescriber (usually a doctor) to consider the patient's problems, diagnose pathological medical conditions, choose the most effective treatment for the patient and provide appropriate information about how to use the medicine safely and effectively. Examples might be antibiotics to treat infections, or drugs for heart disease or depression. Schedule 8 includes drugs liable to cause addiction, such as narcotic analgesics and amphetamines, which require tighter controls. Once prescribed in a legally valid prescription, these drugs are available only when dispensed by a pharmacist.

OTC DRUGS

It is recognised that some conditions are sufficiently mild and/or self-limiting that people should be able to access drugs to treat themselves. Some chronic conditions require regular medication with drugs, such as analgesics for pain, or bronchodilators for asthma, and to require a patient to visit a doctor's surgery to renew a prescription could be life-threatening or cause undue pain. These types of drugs are therefore made more available than prescription-only constraints would allow. The stated aim of the Australian TGA in scheduling some drugs for OTC access is that "consumers have adequate information and understanding to enable them to select the most appropriate medications for their condition and to use them safely and effectively, taking into account their health status" (Galbally 2000).

Commonly, **OTC drugs** are those considered relatively safe and effective for self-treatment by the public, assuming good manufacturing practices are followed by the manufacturer and the label directions are followed by the consumer. They are drugs with a high therapeutic index (safety margin) and/or are available in low doses or in limited supplies.

SAFETY. The drug product has a low incidence of severe adverse reactions and a low potential for harm, assuming that proper instructions and adequate warnings are given on the label.

EFFECTIVENESS. When used properly, the drug ingredient will provide relief of the minor symptom or illness in a significant proportion of the population.

Some drugs are **unscheduled** in the SUSDP and may be sold through any retail outlet, including supermarkets, health-food stores and general merchants. Such drugs include most vitamins and minerals and small packs of simple pain-relievers (analgesics) such as paracetamol. These may also be included under the umbrella of OTC drugs, depending on the definition.

Schedule 2 (PHARMACY-ONLY) drugs are non-prescription drugs that can be bought off the shelf from a pharmacy where professional advice is available; the safe use of these drugs may require advice from a pharmacist. Schedule 3 (PHARMACIST-ONLY) products are considered to require a pharmacist's advice in their supply, to ensure they are used safely and effectively. Indeed the pharmacist has a responsibility to counsel the person on safe administration of the drug.

OTC drugs should not be considered completely harmless —as with all drugs, the possibility always exists for adverse reactions, depending on the dose and the patient. Also, a drug should not be considered to be either OTC or prescription-only—many drugs fall into various **drug schedules** depending on the dose to be administered, the route by which it is given or the condition for which it is indicated. In certain situations, costs of drugs may be subsidised when prescribed but not when bought OTC. Examples of some drugs that may appear in Schedules 2, 3 and/or 4 are shown in Table 3-1.

CHANGE OF A DRUG BETWEEN PRESCRIPTION-ONLY AND OTC STATUS

The TGA may from time to time suggest that prescription-only drugs be changed to OTC status (or vice versa). This is based on expert findings that the drug in a particular formulation is safe and effective for use by the general public, that drug information is available and that compliance is appropriate. Certain formulations of salbutamol, hydrocortisone and ranitidine, for example, have been moved down to S2 or S3 Schedules, as shown in Table 3-1.

On the other hand, experience sometimes shows that particular drugs do need the extra safeguards of being classified S4 (PRESCRIPTION-ONLY), which encourages doctors and pharmacists to exercise professional judgement as to the prescribing of this drug and advice that may help the patient. For example, in Australia recently, all insulin formulations were moved back to Schedule 4 from Schedule 3, where they had been placed for a few years.

TABLE 3-1 Examples of prescription drugs also available OTC

DRUG	OTC SCHEDULE, DOSE AND INDICATION	PRESCRIPTION-ONLY SCHEDULE, DOSE AND INDICATION
Ranitidine tablets (H_2-receptor antagonist)	S2: 150 mg; relief of gastro-oesophageal reflux in adults >18 years	S4: 150 mg, 300 mg tablets, injections; e.g. treatment of peptic ulcer, duodenal ulcer, Zollinger–Ellison syndrome
Glyceryl trinitrate (vasodilator)	S2: 0.4 mg sublingual spray; S3: 0.6 mg tablets; prevention or treatment of angina pectoris	S4: 5–15 mg patches, injection; perioperative hypertension, unresponsive angina, acute myocardial infarction
Codeine phosphate (opioid analgesic)	S2 or S3: 8–9.6 mg (with aspirin or paracetamol); moderate to severe pain, relief of symptoms of colds and flu, dry cough	S4: 30 mg with aspirin or paracetamol; S8: codeine alone, codeine injections; moderate to severe pain
Nystatin oral, topical, vaginal (antifungal)	S2 or S3: 100,000 IU; oral, vaginal or cutaneous candidiasis	S4: combination ointment or ear-drops with other antibiotics and corticosteroid; inflammatory and infected dermatoses
Salbutamol inhaler (bronchodilator)	S3: 100–200 mcg/dose; asthma reliever and prophylaxis against exercise-induced asthma	S4: nebulising solution; asthma when inhaler administration is inappropriate; S4: obstetric injection; to delay premature labour
Beclomethasone (corticosteroid)	S3: nasal spray/pump 50 mcg/dose; prophylaxis and treatment of hay fever	S4: 50 mcg/dose inhaler; bronchial asthma
Hydrocortisone (corticosteroid)	S2: 0.5% cream and ointment, S3: 1% cream and ointment; minor skin irritations, inflammations and itching	S4: cream and ointment, 50 g pack, 1%; S4: injections, eye-drops, rectal foam, tablets; inflammatory conditions and as corticosteroid replacement therapy

IU = international units of activity.

TABLE 3-2 Examples of drugs available OTC

SYSTEM OR INDICATION	CONDITION TREATED	DRUG GROUP (EXAMPLE)
Gastrointestinal tract	Peptic ulcers	H_2-receptor antagonists (ranitidine); antacids (magnesium trisilicate)
	Constipation	Laxatives (lactulose, sennosides)
	Diarrhoea	Antidiarrhoeals (loperamide, atropine)
	Nutritional supplements	Vitamins (folic acid, vitamin C); minerals (iron, calcium); amino acids (creatine, amino acid chelates)
Cardiovascular system	Angina	Vasodilators (glyceryl trinitrate)
	Thrombosis, myocardial infarction	Antithrombotics (aspirin)
Central nervous system	Insomnia	Sedatives (diphenhydramine)
	Nausea/vomiting	Antihistamines (promethazine); antimuscarinics (hyoscine)
Nervous system	Pain	Simple analgesics (aspirin, **paracetamol**); plus low-dose codeine
Musculoskeletal system	Pain, inflammation	NSAIDs (naproxen); salicylates (aspirin, methyl salicylate)
Genitourinary system	Urinary tract infections	Antiseptics (hexamine), urinary alkalinisers (sodium citrotartrate)
	Vaginal infections	Antifungals (miconazole, nystatin)
Infections and infestations	Worm infestations	Anthelmintics (mebendazole)
	Mild infections	Antiseptics (chlorhexidine)
Respiratory system	Coughs and colds	Decongestants (pseudoephedrine); antitussives (pholcodine); antihistamines (pheniramine); various (menthol, camphor, vitamin C)
	Asthma	Bronchodilators (salbutamol inhaler)
Allergic disorders	Allergy, inflammation	Antihistamines (pheniramine, loratidine)
Ear/nose/throat conditions	Swimmer's ear	Solvents (isopropyl alcohol)
	Nasal congestion	Decongestants (oxymetazoline)
	Dental caries (prophylaxis)	Fluoride (drops, toothpastes)
	Sore throat	Antiseptics (cetylpyridinium); local anaesthetics (benzocaine)
Eyes	Infections	Antimicrobials (sulfacetamide)
	Allergies, red eyes	Decongestants (phenylephrine)
	Dry eyes	Lubricants (hypromellose)
Skin	Acne	Antiseptics (cetrimide, peroxides)
	Dandruff	Medicated shampoos (selenium sulfide, coal tar)
	Warts	Keratolytics (salicylic acid)
	Fungal infections	Antifungals (miconazole, terbinafine)
	Leg ulcers	Gels (propylene glycol); dressings (calcium alginate fibres)
	Perspiration	Antiperspirants (aluminium salts)
	Alopecia	Hair restorers (minoxidil)
Surgical preparations	Pain	Anaesthetics (lignocaine nasal spray, cream)
	Infections	Antiseptic sprays, gels, dressings, irrigations etc
Diagnostic agents	Diabetes	Test kits for urinary glucose
	Pregnancy	Pregnancy test kits; ovulation time test kits; spermicidal contraceptive gels

NSAIDs = non-steroidal anti-inflammatory drugs.

The range of OTC drug categories

Thousands of drugs are available OTC. Many of these are discussed in detail in the systematic pharmacology chapters of this text, where their actions, mechanisms of action, clinical uses, adverse reactions and interactions and doses are described. Some of the most common groups are mentioned briefly here and the types of drugs available OTC are summarised in Table 3-2. This information should assist the health-care professional in identifying and evaluating the multitude of OTC medications on the market. By understanding basic information and checking package ingredients and consumer product information, a safer and more logical approach to product selection can be taken. As an example of the Drug Monographs found throughout this book that summarise all the information about clinically important drugs, in Drug Monograph 3-1 we consider the analgesic paracetamol, one of the most commonly taken OTC drugs, available in both supermarkets and general stores (unscheduled) as well as in pharmacies (Schedule 2, 3 or 4, depending on formulation and dose of other active ingredients).

ANALGESICS

Pain is one of the most common and feared symptoms. For minor pain such as headache, toothache, muscle and joint aches, swelling (inflammation) and fever, many people obtain relief inexpensively with OTC analgesics. Examples are paracetamol (Drug Monograph 3-1), aspirin, and other non-steroidal anti-inflammatory drugs (NSAIDs). Analgesic agents

---

DRUG MONOGRAPH 3-1 PARACETAMOL

Paracetamol, having little anti-inflammatory action, is rather different from the other non-steroidal anti-inflammatory drugs (NSAIDs), but is safer than aspirin as an analgesic (see Clinical Interest Box 16-8 and Figure 16-12, showing metabolic pathways of paracetamol and explaining why the drug is toxic when taken in massive overdose). Its analgesic and antipyretic (antifever) actions are thought to be due to inhibition of prostaglandin synthesis in central nervous system tissues via cyclo-oxygenase inhibition.

INDICATIONS Paracetamol is indicated for relief of fever and of mild to moderate pain associated with headaches, muscular aches, period pain, arthritis and migraine.

PHARMACOKINETICS After oral administration, paracetamol is rapidly and completely absorbed from the gastrointestinal tract; peak plasma concentration of the drug is reached 10–60 minutes later. Absorption is delayed by food in the gastrointestinal tract. Distribution via the bloodstream is uniform to most body fluids and tissues, with an apparent volume of distribution (V) of about 1–1.2 L/kg, implying some sequestration (binding) of paracetamol in tissues. There is negligible plasma protein binding, hence little risk of interactions with other protein-bound drugs. Paracetamol does cross the placenta in small amounts and so can affect the fetus. It is excreted in only small amounts in the milk of lactating women; hence it is the analgesic of choice in breastfeeding mothers.

   The metabolism of paracetamol occurs in the liver by hepatic microsomal enzymes. In adults the main metabolites (65%–85%) are the glucuronide and sulfate conjugates (see Figure 16-12), whereas in children it is the sulfate derivative. (When it is taken in great overdose, the normal metabolic pathways are saturated and toxic metabolites are formed that can irreversibly damage the liver and kidneys.) Excretion is via the urine as paracetamol metabolites (95%) within 24 hours. The elimination half-life is 1–3 hours, hence doses must be given regularly every 3–4 hours to maintain therapeutic blood levels.

ADVERSE DRUG REACTIONS In normal doses, paracetamol rarely causes adverse effects; dyspepsia (stomach upsets), allergy and blood reactions have been suggested. Because of the high therapeutic index (safety margin), accidental overdose is rare. If taken in overdose, e.g. 20 tablets instead of one or two, it is potentially fatal, with acute liver failure occurring 2–3 days later. As there may be few or only mild symptoms in the early stages after overdose (vomiting, abdominal pain, hypotension, sweating and CNS effects), any suggestion of paracetamol overdose is taken seriously. Treatment is instituted as soon as overdose is suspected, with attempts to remove the drug by gastric lavage or activated charcoal, and administration of the specific antidote acetylcysteine (see Box 16-2).

DRUG INTERACTIONS There are few clinically significant drug interactions. Paracetamol may prolong bleeding times in patients previously stabilised on warfarin.

WARNINGS AND CONTRAINDICATIONS Caution should be used before administering paracetamol to persons with renal or hepatic dysfunction, as the drug or its metabolites may accumulate. Paracetamol is considered safe in pregnancy (Category A) and in breastfeeding. In children it should be used strictly as directed and the stated doses not exceeded except on the advice of a doctor. Packets of paracetamol tablets or capsules, and liquid formulations, should be kept out of reach of children (as should all medicines).

DOSAGE AND ADMINISTRATION Paracetamol is available in a multitude of formulations and dosages, and mixed with other active ingredients. The standard adult dose form is 1–2 tablets, capsules or suppositories, each containing 500 mg paracetamol, with the dose administered every 3–4 hours, not exceeding a maximum of eight per day (four for suppositories). Formulations suitable for children include infant drops, elixirs, suspensions and suppositories; dose recommendations on the basis of the child's age or weight should not be exceeded.

are discussed in detail in Chapter 16, where morphine and aspirin are considered as the prototype analgesics.

ANTACIDS

Various medical conditions, overeating or eating certain foods may result in dyspepsia (stomach upset), heartburn and indigestion. Antacids—drugs that buffer, neutralise or absorb hydrochloric acid in the stomach, and thus raise gastric pH—are commonly used for these conditions. The major ingredients in antacids are alkalis such as bicarbonate, sulfate, trisilicate and hydroxide, as aluminium, magnesium or calcium salts. Simethicone may be added to these preparations as a defoaming or antigas agent.

LAXATIVES

Laxatives—drugs given to induce defecation—may be classified according to their site of action, degree of action or mechanism of action (see Chapter 34). Many older people are overly concerned about their bowel habits, and laxatives are often misused or abused.

ANTIDIARRHOEAL AGENTS

The term diarrhoea describes the abnormal passage of stools with increased frequency, fluidity or weight, and an increase in stool water excretion. Diarrhoea is acute when it is of sudden onset in a previously healthy individual, lasts about 3 days to 1–2 weeks, is self-limiting, and resolves without sequelae. Excess fluid and electrolytes can be lost and severe morbidity and even death can occur in malnourished populations, the elderly, infants and debilitated people.

COUGH/COLD PREPARATIONS

Every year, especially in winter, millions of dollars are spent on cough, cold and influenza (flu) preparations such as antitussives, antihistamines, expectorants and decongestants (see Chapter 32). Many cough/cold products contain a combination of ingredients, some of which are subtherapeutic dose combinations or are unnecessary for the particular symptoms they purport to treat. Such preparations are not considered rational and may not be safe and effective.

ANTIHISTAMINES

Antihistamines are drugs that compete with histamine for its H_1-receptor sites. They are commonly used to treat allergic symptoms, itching, motion sickness, and as sedatives. Part of their usefulness in 'cough and cold cures' is due to their antimuscarinic actions, which help dry up nasal and airways secretions.

NUTRITIONAL SUPPLEMENTS

Many people feel constrained (or convinced by advertising) to supplement their diets with extra ingredients, especially vitamins, minerals and amino acids as 'ergogenic aids'. Most medical authorities agree that, provided a person regularly eats

---

CLINICAL INTEREST BOX 3-1
WHAT VITAMINS SHOULD I TAKE?

A healthy 54-year-old woman presented to the surgery requesting advice as to what vitamins she should take. She was a non-smoker, not on any special diets, who was confused by media reports that 30% of the population use vitamin supplements.

Her physician considered several approaches:
- the medical-school teaching that vitamin supplements are a waste of money for people on a good diet
- that vitamin supplements (e.g. folic acid in pregnancy) can prevent serious clinical conditions
- that vitamins are pushed by the health-food industry for profit
- that few good randomised controlled clinical trials have been carried out to provide evidence-based proof of efficacy
- that results from many trials conflict, especially in terms of evidence for reduced risks of cancer or heart disease.

Based on a wide review of medical literature on folic acid, vitamins A, B_6, B_{12}, C, D, E and multivitamin preparations, and considering advice from some professional societies and government panels, the physician's advice was that "a daily multivitamin that does not exceed the RDA (recommended daily allowance) of its component vitamins makes sense for most adults . . . however, a vitamin pill is no substitute for a healthy lifestyle or diet . . . and cannot begin to compensate for the massive risks associated with smoking, obesity or inactivity".
Adapted from: Willett & Stampfer 2001.

---

a varied diet with appropriate amounts of the different food types on the food pyramid, there is no need for nutritional supplements. Many supplements are available as OTC drugs or in products sold in health-food stores. There are, however, some groups in the community who may benefit from dietary supplements, particularly those with special needs, such as pregnant women or elite athletes, and those who do not have a good varied diet, such as elderly people living alone, strict vegetarians, alcoholics and food faddists (see Clinical Interest Box 3-1).

Vitamins are organic compounds essential in small amounts for the body to maintain normal function and development. They were so named as a contraction of the term 'vital amine', as the first such essential compounds identified were amines. Many of the vitamins are considered in detail in later chapters, especially:
- vitamin A (retinol), essential to normal growth, bone formation, epithelial tissues formulation, retinal function and reproduction (see Drug Monograph 56-2 and Clinical Interest Box 56-3)
- vitamin B_{12} (cyanocobalamin), essential for blood (Chapter 30) and nervous system functions

- vitamin D (calciferol derivatives), essential for calcium and phosphate balance (see Drug Monograph 42-3 and Clinical Interest Box 42-3)
- vitamin K (phytomenadione derivatives), essential to blood coagulation (Chapter 30)
- folic acid, essential in many one-carbon transfer reactions in biochemistry, in blood functions and in fetal development.

Minerals are inorganic substances (not containing carbon); some are required in the diet to maintain health. Deficiency is comparatively rare, except for calcium and iron. Essential minerals are:

- calcium, necessary for structure of bones and teeth, clotting of blood, functions of cell membranes, excitation–contraction coupling in muscle, and in many enzyme reactions (see Clinical Interest Box 42-1)
- iron, essential in the formation of haemoglobin and the carrying of oxygen in the blood (Chapter 30)
- iodine, essential for synthesis of thyroid hormones (see Drug Monograph 39-2 and Clinical Interest Box 39-5)
- sodium, important in excitable properties of nerves, muscle and gland cell membranes (the 'sodium pump'), for regulation of pH and osmotic pressure, and in bone salts
- magnesium: enzyme reactions, transmitter release

- chloride: extracellular ion in membrane potentials, osmotic pressure
- phosphorus: important constituent of bone, interacts with calcium in calcium balance
- potassium: transmembrane potential, pH, osmotic pressure
- zinc: DNA synthesis and cell division, enzyme reactions, insulin binding, wound healing and tissue repair
- copper, fluorine and selenium as trace elements in minute amounts (see Clinical Interest Box 3-2)
- lithium, not recognised as an essential mineral, but interesting in pharmacology as being the smallest drug. As the third-lightest element, it has an atomic number of 3 and is a key drug in psychiatry, being the most effective antimanic agent available (see Drug Monograph 19-3).

Other **dietary supplements** are of a wide range and number and are more the focus of nutrition than of pharmacology.

CLINICAL INTEREST BOX 3-2
SELENIUM: A LITTLE IS GOOD, A LOT IS NOT!

Selenium is an essential trace element, chemically related to sulfur. It is not normally present in the body in detectable amounts but deficiency has been known to cause fatty infiltration of the liver, whereas excess can cause alopecia (hair loss) and is teratogenic in animals (causes congenital malformations). It is used as the selenium disulfide form in antidandruff shampoos.

Although concentrations of selenium in New Zealand soils are low, there is no indication that this has resulted in any detrimental effects on the health of New Zealanders. Supplementation of animal and poultry feeds and consumption of imported plants seem to ensure that the selenium intake of most New Zealanders is at recommended levels.

Some New Zealanders take selenium supplements with the intention of reducing the oxidative damage caused by free radicals, in the hope that this will prevent cancer and cardiovascular disease, but its value in these respects has not been established.

The NZ National Poisons Centre receives reports from time to time that some people have consumed animal selenium supplements, well exceeding the safe daily human intake of 0.4 mg. There is no antidote for selenium overdosing, and management lies in stopping the selenium and providing symptomatic care.
Adapted from: New Zealand Prescriber Update No. 20: 39–42, Feb 2001. (www.medsafe.govt.nz/)

CLINICAL INTEREST BOX 3-3
MELATONIN, THE BODY'S TIMEKEEPER?

Melatonin is a hormone secreted by the pineal gland. Chemically, it is an indole derivative synthesised from tryptophan via serotonin (5-hydroxytryptamine, 5-HT), to which it is closely related. The metabolic activity of the pineal gland is sensitive to light and darkness, melatonin being secreted during periods of darkness and serotonin during exposure to light. Melatonin has been called 'the endocrine messenger of darkness' and many wonderful claims are made for its actions and uses, most largely unsubstantiated. It is not currently available for medical use in Australia but is readily available in many other countries and is often imported by travellers.

By virtue of its actions in entraining the body's circadian rhythms, melatonin can be useful in sleep management, e.g. for treating jet-lag, sleep disorders in blind people and neurologically impaired children, and insomnia in the elderly.

Reductions in melatonin secretion occur in many disorders, including cardiovascular diseases, Alzheimer's disease, diabetes, migraine and in ageing, but the role of melatonin in their aetiology or pathophysiology has not been established. Secretion is reduced by alcohol, caffeine and some other common drugs.

Other roles proposed for melatonin include:
- as a potent scavenger of oxygen free radicals: it may be useful in delaying ageing, tissue damage or cancer
- reducing the severity of lesions in the gastric mucosa induced by NSAIDs
- as an immunomodulator: melatonin enhances the immune response, and is proinflammatory.

Melatonin is not without adverse effects, causing tolerance and fatigue, so it is recommended that only the lowest effective hypnotic dose should be taken, and use on consecutive nights should be avoided.
Adapted from: Kendler 1997.

Many have been used in sport in attempts to enhance performance, e.g. pyruvate, creatine (see Clinical Interest Box 57-3); however, the fact that they are allowed by bodies such as the International Olympic Committee shows that they have never been proven to enhance performance! Others are used to enhance formation of neurotransmitters, as prophylaxis against heart disease (vitamin E, folic acid) or cancer (selenium, vitamin E), or to assist in other physiological functions deemed inadequate (see Clinical Interest Box 3-3).

The terms 'nutraceuticals' and 'functional foods' have been coined to cover a wide range of (usually) natural supplements that may confer health benefits. Examples are: soy protein and phyto-oestrogens (sources of oestrogens, for menopausal symptoms and bone health), citrus flavonoids (antioxidants, anticancer and cholesterol-lowering), red wine and tea tannins (cardiovascular disease), dietary fibre (coronary heart disease and gastrointestinal tract regularity), probiotics, active microorganisms in yoghurt (balance gut microflora), and omega-3 fish oils (cardiac arrhythmias, insulin resistance and arthritis); see Table 3-3.

Potential problems with use of OTC drugs

Although OTC medications are generally considered to be safe and effective for consumer use, it is apparent that problems can result from their use.

Self-diagnosis

Self-medication follows self-diagnosis of the signs and symptoms of a clinical condition. Generally, the public may consider most illnesses to be minor, however self-treating a potentially serious condition with OTC medications may mask the condition and delay the seeking of professional help for appropriate treatment.

Adverse effects and drug interactions

OTC medicines may contain potent drugs, many of which were previously prescription-only. There has been a trend recently to transfer more drugs to OTC status. The TGA uses a risk management approach, considering whether a product contains scheduled drugs, whether significant adverse reactions are likely, if it is used to treat very serious conditions and if there may be adverse effects from prolonged or inappropriate use. Health-care professionals should therefore be aware that many OTC products (new and old) are capable of producing both desired and undesirable effects, drug interactions and drug toxicity. Post-marketing surveillance is carried out to monitor for adverse effects or drug interactions of both OTC and prescription-only drugs, and other therapeutic goods.

Labelling

The TGA regulates the appearance and content of OTC package labelling so that important information is provided in terms that are likely to be read and understood by the average consumer. Many consumers may nevertheless find that some labels are confusing and that often the print is too small to read, especially by elderly people. OTC labelling that is difficult to understand and apply may result in unsafe and possibly improper use of the medication. Restrictions on labelling, packaging and storing of OTC drugs are useful but also have the potential for adding to costs and reducing competition in the marketplace.

Drug marketing

In Australia, all therapeutic goods must be registered by the TGA before they can be supplied. Therapeutic goods include anything represented to be or likely to be taken or used for a therapeutic purpose, including for disease prevention or treatment; modifying a physiological process; testing, controlling or preventing conception; or replacing or modifying body parts. (There are a few specific exclusions of well-known ingredients with a long history of safe use, such as vitamins, sunscreens and soaps.) Therapeutic goods must be assessed and monitored to ensure safety, efficacy and quality. Manufacturers must be licensed and manufacturing processes must comply with the principles of 'Good Manufacturing Practice'. Advertising is also regulated by the TGA. This compares favourably with the situation in the USA, where many goods are allowed onto the market as OTC products with little regulation, provided that they are identified as 'Generally recognized as safe and effective'.

While such regulations are essential to protect the public, it can be argued that the scheduling of substances reduces individual freedoms by placing restrictions on who may supply or administer substances to whom and in what circumstances. This could be seen as an impediment to competition and a limit on consumer access to and choice of drugs.

Potency and efficacy

Another important concept to understand is the difference between drug potency and drug efficacy (effectiveness). Drug potency relates inversely to the amount of drug required to produce a desired effect: the more potent the drug, the lower the dose required. Potency determines dose but is rarely an important aspect to consider when selecting a drug—actions, adverse effects and pharmacokinetic aspects are more relevant clinically. When drug manufacturers claim that their product is more potent than another product, this usually means that less of the drug is necessary to produce the same effect, but does not mean that the more potent drug is also the more effective drug. This terminology is often used and may be misleading if the difference between potency and effectiveness is not understood by health-care providers or consumers.

Combination products

Combination products may contain substances that are not necessary for the person's symptoms. If the individual has an adverse reaction to the combination drug, it will be difficult to determine the ingredient responsible. Change in dosage will alter the dose of all active ingredients, which may not be appropriate. Raising the dose may cause accumulation of the drug with the longest half-life, leading to toxicity.

Consumer education for over-the-counter drugs

OTC drugs are often misconceived as being very safe and thus not requiring the special precautions used to take a prescription drug safely; however, these products also have the potential for being misused or abused and inducing adverse effects. They also may be dangerous if taken in certain disease states or if taken concurrently with other drugs, food or alcohol. Health-care professionals need to be aware of these risks before administering or advising use of an OTC preparation, and need to be able to access and understand information about OTC drugs. All the potential problems with OTC drugs listed above should be considered and, if relevant, discussed with the consumer.

Selection of drug

Product ingredients have either proven or questionable effectiveness; therefore a careful check of active ingredients is necessary to select the appropriate product in a specific drug category for treatment of the specific symptom the consumer is experiencing.

Multiple dosing with similar drugs

Many different products may have the same or very similar active ingredients that may or may not differ in strength, dosage form (liquid, tablet, capsule) or in other ingredients in combination, contributing to the problem of polypharmacy (considered in Chapter 2 [see Clinical Interest Box 2-3]). If the ingredients are not carefully checked, accidental overdosing is possible by taking the same or similar drugs in many different products.

Another aspect of different products having the same ingredients is that it may allow for product substitution. For example, hundreds of antacid products are available that primarily contain only four or five recognised active ingredients. Many OTC antacids are thus virtually duplicate preparations. The generic product is often as effective as the 'upmarket' brand name product, so there is usually little, if any, advantage in buying the more expensive item.

Tampering with packages

Consumers should check the selected package for tampering. There have been recent instances of commercial sabotage, in which, for example, disgruntled former employees tampered with products to insert dangerous ingredients. Most products are now contained in tamper-resistant packaging or tampering-evident packaging, which allows the consumer to detect signs of tampering. If the package is suspect, it should be taken to the pharmacist or store manager. The expiry date should also be checked to ensure that it has not passed.

Sensitivity to ingredients

Consumers should read labels very carefully if they have ever had an allergic or unusual response to any medication, food or other substance, such as food dyes or preservatives, to ensure that such an ingredient is not included. Caution should be used if the individual is on a special diet, such as low-sugar, low-sodium or phenylalanine-free, because many OTC drugs contain more than just their active ingredients, and liquid preparations may contain high concentrations of sugar or alcohol. Women who are pregnant or breastfeeding should not take OTC medications without first consulting the health-care provider. People with underlying medical conditions, such as hypertension or diabetes, should read labels carefully to assess whether the medication may be contraindicated in their condition.

OTC medicines are drugs

OTC drugs are still drugs and should be reported to any health-care provider when a drug history is being taken. A question phrased in neutral terms like 'Do you ever take any medicines?' is likely to elicit a more positive and instructive response than 'What drugs are you on?'. Instructions and warnings on the label need to be followed carefully. If the instructions seem unclear, it may be helpful to ask the pharmacist for clarification. If the symptoms for which the OTC drug is being taken are not relieved in an appropriate time as indicated on the label, a health-care provider should be consulted.

STORAGE

Unless instructions state otherwise, both prescription and OTC medicines should be stored in closed containers in a cool dry place, out of the reach of children. Do not store in the bathroom, near windows or in damp places because heat, moisture and strong light may cause deterioration or loss of drug potency. 'Use-by' dates should be carefully observed.

"TAKE AS DIRECTED"

The old Latin abbreviation 'mdu', meaning 'take as directed', is now considered unhelpful. Patients are often anxious and inattentive when prescribers or pharmacists give advice about conditions and drugs, and forget what has been said. It is much more effective for the instructions to be written on the package label in specific terms such as 'Take one tablet with a full glass of water three times a day after meals'.

All solid-dose medications (tablets and capsules) should be taken with a full glass of water, and the person advised to remain sitting or standing up for about 15–30 minutes afterwards, to reduce the potential for oesophageal irritation or injury. If the person has a problem with dry mouth or minor problems in swallowing, drinking a small amount of water before taking a tablet or capsule is helpful. If the drug is a sustained-release or enteric-coated form, it should be swallowed whole. If the medication is in a liquid form, a specially marked measuring spoon or glass should be used to measure each dose accurately.

COMPLEMENTARY AND ALTERNATIVE THERAPIES IN RELATION TO PHARMACOLOGY

What is complementary and alternative medicine?

The term **complementary and alternative medicine** (CAM) implies some treatment modality not usually taught or practised in mainstream scientific (Western) medicine. Although the terms alternative and complementary are generally used interchangeably, there may be a distinction between them. *Complementary* indicates that some scientific documentation exists, the practice is accepted, and it may be integrated in mainstream health-care practice, whereas *alternative* generally refers to practices that are either scientifically unfounded or lacking in support data. Usually, complementary therapies include diet, exercise, counselling, biofeedback, massage therapy, relaxation, herbal therapy, acupuncture and hypnosis. Other therapies, such as homeopathy, macrobiotics and many others, are classified under the alternative label.

The primary pharmacological modality in complementary and alternative therapies is the use of herbal or other natural products. Use of such products dates back to the earliest records of mankind, when it was believed that herbal extracts, home remedies or folk medicines could treat or cure many illnesses. Table 3-3 lists some common home or folk remedies still in use today, available from the kitchen.

Prevalence of use of complementary and alternative therapies

In the past 20 years, there has been a vast increase reported in the interest in and use of alternative medical approaches in many Western countries. Recent data on usage in Australia are given in Clinical Interest Box 3-4. It is estimated that about 50% of the population use complementary and alternative therapies (not including minerals such as calcium or iron, or prescribed vitamins).

In New Zealand, it has been shown that a substantial proportion of children hospitalised with acute medical illness had received complementary and alternative therapies before hospitalisation, as an adjunct rather than as an alternative to conventional medical care. Receiving such treatment had no effect on the severity of the illness, investigations performed, treatment administered or length of hospital stay.

In the USA, the number of visits to complementary health-care practitioners in 1990 exceeded the number of visits to primary care physicians, with the cost of alternative therapies estimated at US$14 billion annually.

CLINICAL INTEREST BOX 3-4
FACTS AND FIGURES ON COMPLEMENTARY AND ALTERNATIVE THERAPIES IN AUSTRALIA

- More than 60% of Australians use at least one complementary health-care product each year, including vitamins, minerals and herbal products.
- About A$2 billion per year are spent in this sector of the health market, two-thirds on complementary medicines and one-third on other complementary therapies.
- There are at least 2.8 million consultations with traditional Chinese medicine practitioners yearly, with a turnover of $84 million.
- The person most likely to use complementary and alternative therapies (in both Australia and the USA) is female, 30–50 years old, with tertiary qualifications, earning over $50,000 annually and employed in a professional or managerial position.
- Over 50% of children attending a major children's hospital had used CAM in the preceding year; most of these had not discussed this with their treating doctor.

Adapted from: the website of the Office of Complementary Medicines, TGA, Canberra 2002; McCabe 2005; Lim et al 2005.

TABLE 3-3 Common home or folk remedies

REMEDY	POTENTIAL USES OR INDICATIONS	COMMENTS
Celery	Anti-inflammatory; to lower serum cholesterol, chemoprotection against cancers	High in sodium; contains coumarins and flavonoids; potential interactions with warfarin
Cranberry	Bacteriostatic, antioxidant	Prevention and treatment of urinary tract infections
Fish oils	Antiarrhythmic, lower cholesterol levels and high blood pressure, antithrombotic, anti-inflammatory, neuroprotective, chemoprotective against cancers	Contain two polyunsaturated fatty acids, also various vitamins (Bs, E) and minerals
Garlic (*Allium sativum*)	Antimicrobial, antiplatelet, coronary artery disease, lowers high blood cholesterol, hypertension, antitumour, antioxidant	Garlic contains alliin, which is converted to allicin and is responsible for both the garlic odour and the potential antibacterial effects. Other ingredients such as ajoene are considered to be at least as potent as aspirin and may be responsible for its antithrombotic and antiplatelet effects
Green tea	Antioxidant, antimicrobial, anticancer; protection against cardiovascular disease	Contains flavonoid polyphenols, caffeine and other methylxanthines; green tea is made from leaves that have not been oxidised
Honey	Antibacterial, antiseptic; used in burns and to enhance wound healing	Constituents depend largely on nectar from which it is derived; may include many acids, esters, flavonoids, enzymes and beeswax
Horseradish	Irritant to mucous membranes; circulatory and digestive stimulant	Roots contain peroxidase enzymes, volatile oils, glycosides, coumarins, acids
Licorice (liquorice)	Has mineralocorticoid and expectorant actions; extract is used as a flavouring agent and in cough mixtures	The root of the plant *Glycyrrhiza glabra*; as a sweet it is compounded with sugars. Main saponin is glycyrrhizin; many other ingredients, including flavonoids, sterols, coumarins, amines, sugars and oils
Mussels, NZ green-lipped	Anti-inflammatory, especially in rheumatoid and osteoarthritis	Bivalve molluscs; contain many proteins (especially pernin) and lipids
Oats and oatmeal	Lipid-lowering actions, also antihypertensive and hypoglycaemic	Contain soluble fibre, saponins, alkaloids, starch, protein, coumarins, flavonoids, plus minerals and vitamins

Note that 'kitchen remedies' also include various herbs and spices (see Table 3-4). *Source*: Braun & Cohen 2005.

In the UK, about 20% of people surveyed had used complementary and alternative therapies in the preceding year, with the most popular therapies being herbalism, aromatherapy, homeopathy, acupuncture/acupressure, massage and reflexology. The annual expenditure for the country was estimated at £1.6 billion for the whole nation in 1999. In other European countries, 20%–50% of residents reported using complementary and alternative therapies; herbal remedies and homeopathy are particularly popular in German-speaking countries.

Unfortunately, scientific evidence concerning the safety and efficacy of alternative medicine is often lacking. The prevalence of use and enormous expenditure on complementary and alternative therapies makes it imperative that scientific studies be carried out to validate through its commitment of time and money. The Australian TGA, through its Expert Committee on Complementary Medicines in the Health System, is reviewing many aspects of complementary and alternative therapies, including definitions of terms, advertising, fees and charges, post-marketing surveillance, and administrative arrangements. (The US National Institutes of Health, which includes the Office of Alternative Medicine, is devoting millions of dollars annually to research into complementary and alternative therapies.)

**CLINICAL INTEREST BOX 3-5
EFFICACY OF COMPLEMENTARY AND
ALTERNATIVE THERAPIES IN
CLINICAL MEDICINE**

The use of complementary and alternative therapies in clinical medicine has been shown to be effective in many situations, using EBM levels of proof. Some of the data are summarised in the following Clinical Interest Boxes (CIB):

- CIB 16-7: Willow bark, salicylates and *Melaleuca*
- CIB 17-6: Complementary and alternative sedatives
- CIB 19-6: St John's wort and other complementary and alternative therapies in psychiatry
- CIB 21-8: Complementary and alternative therapies in neurological disorders
- CIB 22-5: Complementary and alternative therapies in management of drug dependence
- CIB 32-8: Complementary and alternative therapies in respiratory disorders
- CIB 35-6: Complementary and alternative therapies in ocular medicine
- CIB 39-6: Natural antithyroid compounds: cabbages and celery seeds
- CIB 41-8: Complementary and alternative therapies in diabetes mellitus
- CIB 44-5: Complementary and alternative therapies in women's conditions
- CIB 49-3: Complementary and alternative therapies in cancer
- CIB 57-3: Complementary and alternative therapies in sport

Reasons for use of complementary and alternative therapies

This interest in what is part of the 'back to nature movement' may have been encouraged by numerous warnings that were issued on food additives, preservatives and synthetic products that were said to be cancer-producing substances. Other reasons given by users and practitioners of complementary and alternative therapies include:

- the perception that only complementary and alternative therapies treat the whole person (holistic medicine)
- dissatisfaction with conventional medicine if found to be hard to access or too technologically oriented; 'post-modern' philosophies
- the belief that natural methods are better and safer than scientific methods and products
- to prevent illness such as colds, whereas conventional medicine is seen as useful only for treating symptoms
- the allure of promised efficacy without adverse effects
- perceived lower cost if scientific medicine is unaffordable
- offer of comfort for those with a poor prognosis in a

severe condition, or a disorder with a major psychological component
- desire to participate in therapy, leading to self-empowerment.

Whatever the reason, the general public appears to be more interested than ever in taking personal responsibility for their health and wellbeing, and for trying alternative methods to self-treat their health problems. The result is a vast proliferation of alternative healers, health-food stores, natural products, organic fruits and vegetables, and the use of herbal remedies. This movement has evolved into a multimillion-dollar enterprise that is not limited to any specific cultural or ethnic groups.

Complementary and alternative therapies are used in a wide variety of disorders, in both prevention and treatment. In later chapters, we have included in Clinical Interest Boxes relevant information, based on evidence-based medicine (EBM) levels of proof, as to clinical situations in which CAM has been shown to be effective. These are summarised in Clinical Interest Box 3-5.

Regulation of complementary and alternative therapies

In Australia, products used in complementary and alternative therapies, including vitamins, herbal remedies, aromatherapy and homeopathic preparations, are regulated by the TGA, as are OTC and prescription-only drugs. The system is seen as an excellent one and other countries have looked to it as a model. All products for which therapeutic claims are made must be assessed by the TGA for risk category. They may then be banned, exempt, listed or registered, depending on the ingredients and the claims made. The TGA has committees with particular responsibilities for complementary medicines and for complementary health care.

Listed products

Products considered of low risk are allowed to be self-assessed by the proposer, who must have documentation to back up any claims of efficacy such as 'may help in the condition . . .'.
The TGA evaluates the product for quality of manufacture and safety. Most complementary and alternative medicines are listed rather than registered.

Registered products

Products considered of higher risk and those containing ingredients listed in SUSDP Schedules are subjected to rigorous assessment, regulation and monitoring by the TGA for quality, safety and efficacy. They are then classified into the various drugs and poisons schedules, which determines their availability, labelling, storage etc, or become 'unscheduled'.

TABLE 3-4 Some commonly used herbal remedies

HERB (SCIENTIFIC NAME)	PART USED	CLAIMED ACTIONS AND USES	COMMENTS
Aloes (*Aloe vera*)	Leaves produce resin and gel	Orally, for constipation; topically, heals external wounds and burns; also promoted as a hypoglycaemic agent, anti-inflammatory and for dozens of other uses	Use of aloes to treat burns dates back to ancient Egypt (Cleopatra). A preparation of fresh aloes is effective topically for burns (sunburn, radiation burns) and wound healing; orally, it is a potent laxative
Damiana (*Turnera aphrodisiaca*)	Leaves	Aphrodisiac	There is little scientific evidence to support this claim
Dandelion (*Taraxacum officinale*)	Leaves, root	Tonic, gastrointestinal distress, mild diuretic, mild laxative	Old native American remedy and food; good source of vitamin A; used to make wine and coffee substitute (roasted roots)
Echinacea (*Echinacea* spp.)	Root and leaf	Antiseptic, stimulates immune system, used in respiratory tract infections; anti-inflammatory	Commonly used in respiratory tract infections
Evening primrose (*Oenothera* spp.)	Whole plant, oil from seeds	Anti-inflammatory, antithrombotic, speeds wound healing; for cough, sedation, atopic eczema, mastalgia; premenstrual syndrome	Also used in hypertension and diabetes
Feverfew (*Tanacetum parthenium*)	Leaves	Relaxes smooth muscle; anti-inflammatory, analgesic; prophylaxis of migraine	Inhibits 5-HT release and blocks receptors
Ginger (*Zingiber officinale*)	Rhizome	Soothes the gastrointestinal tract; prevention of motion sickness	Antiemetic, commonly used in nausea of pregnancy
Ginseng, Chinese or Korean (*Panax ginseng*) (see Drug Monograph 3-2)	Root	Immunostimulant, tonic, panacea for many illnesses, including adrenal disorders, debility, stress; claimed to provide chemoprotection against cancers	All ginsengs are adaptogens, i.e. they help the person adapt to physical and mental stress, fatigue and cold. There are claims that ginseng is abused in the West where it is taken as a tonic instead of a medicine (i.e. it should not be taken for more than 6 weeks)
Hawthorn (*Crataegus* species)	Flowers, leaves and berries	Heart remedy, lipid-lowering, for hypertension	Prescribed in Europe as a substitute for digitalis, as hawthorn has flavonoids with cardiotonic effects, but may take months to produce effects; self-treatment for cardiac problems is not recommended
Maidenhair tree (*Ginkgo biloba*)	Mucilage from leaves, seeds	Has antioxidant, vasodilator and antiplatelet actions; alters many CNS transmitters; as a tea, for asthma and bronchitis; for circulatory insufficiencies and cognitive impairment	Used for many varied indications
Saw palmetto (*Serenoa serrulata* [or *repens*])	Fruit	Diuretic, urinary antiseptic, endocrine and anabolic effects; treatment of prostatic enlargement	Inhibits 5-alpha-reductase and binding of androgens to receptors
Slippery elm (*Ulmus fulva*)	Bark	Gastrointestinal distress, cough, sore throat; topically as a lubricant and poultice for boils and splinters	Has demulcent properties, soothes irritated surfaces such as the gastrointestinal tract and throat
St John's wort (*Hypericum perforatum*)	Herb, flowers	Sedative, astringent for wound healing; neuroses, depression	Many pharmacological actions; enhances many CNS neurotransmitters
Valerian (*Valeriana officinalis*)	Dried root	Tranquilliser, antispasmodic	Used in insomnia and anxiety

Adapted from lists in: Bellamy & Pfister 1992; Geng et al 1991; Caswell 2000; Braun & Cohen 2005.

Other regulation

CAM professions are gradually coming under regulation and registration requirements; the state of Victoria established the first Chinese Medicine Registration Board in the Western world, and chiropractic and osteopathy are registered. (However, some people consider that granting of registration status to less mainline professions would confer legitimacy on dubious practices.) Some universities in Australia now grant bachelor's degrees in Chinese medicine, naturopathy, Western herbal medicine, homeopathy, chiropractic and osteopathy. The Australian Taxation Office recognises some professional CAM associations, and Medicare, the universal health-care system, subsidises claims for treatment by some CAM practitioners after referral by a general practitioner (GP). Almost all private health funds offer rebates for consultations by major CAM therapists. These social and regulatory forces are moving CAM closer to mainstream health care.

Types of complementary and alternative therapies

There is a very wide range of modalities, outside the scope of conventional scientific medicine, for which therapeutic claims are made. The range includes:
- psychological methods (including counselling, hypnotherapy, music therapy, cognitive behavioural therapy, prayer, homeopathy, relaxation, humour and laughter therapy, and twelve-step programs such as that of Alcoholics Anonymous)
- dietary changes (megavitamins, vegetarianism, other specialised diets)
- physical methods (Alexander technique, massage, chiropractic, dance therapy, osteopathy, yoga, acupuncture, biofeedback, Pilates, Qi Gong, t'ai chi, reflexology and electromagnetic applications)
- pharmacological means (herbal medicines, traditional ethnic medicines, essential oils, chelation therapy and some aromatherapy, Bach flower remedies and homeopathic preparations).

Some of these are grouped under the umbrella of 'naturopathy', which focuses on self-healing and disease prevention through changes in lifestyle, and there are other eclectic practitioners who apply various methods in holistic therapy, e.g. mind–body medicine. To discuss all these is beyond the scope of a pharmacology textbook, so we will concentrate on the pharmacological group, particularly herbal remedies.

HERBAL REMEDIES

Herbal remedies, i.e. using parts or extracts of plants for treatment of illness, have been used for millennia. As described in Chapter 1 in the section on the history of medicine, ancient civilisations including the Chinese, Egyptian, Greek and Byzantine peoples used natural remedies and have left documentation of recipes and clinical uses. Today, herbal remedies are used with the main purposes of increasing the body's natural resistance and restoring the balance of health. (Some plants from which active drugs are extracted, and the chemicals present in these drugs, are discussed in Chapter 1; the formulae of typical structures are shown in Figure 1-1.)

HERBAL PRODUCTS IN AUSTRALIA. The principal outlets for sale of herbal products in Australia are health-food stores, dispensaries of complementary and alternative practitioners, traditional herbal dispensaries operated by ethnic Australians, and the Internet; pharmacies and supermarkets may also carry these products. A wide range of plants is used; a list summarising commonly used herbal remedies is given in Table 3-4. The *MIMS OTC* (2000) includes 12 monographs on commonly taken herbal products. The definitive textbook in this field is *Herbs and Natural Supplements: An Evidence-Based Guide* (Braun & Cohen 2005). Relevant information on ginseng is summarised in Drug Monograph 3-2, in the same format used for all other drugs, as an example of a herbal remedy; however, it will be noted that information is often unavailable for herbal products.

HERBAL PRODUCTS IN THE UNITED KINGDOM. The British have a long history of interest in and clinical use of herbal remedies. There is an official *British Herbal Pharmacopoeia 1996*, produced by the British Herbal Medicine Association. This gives detailed monographs for about 170 standard herbal remedies, with information on their characteristics, identification, quantitative standards and claimed actions. Appendices give methods of analysis to determine the strength and purity of the preparations.

OTHER PHARMACOLOGICAL COMPLEMENTARY AND ALTERNATIVE THERAPIES

ESSENTIAL OILS AND AROMATHERAPY. Other pharmacological natural products include essential oils and the extracts used in aromatherapy, in which the volatile oils, esters, alcohols and many other chemicals from the plants may contribute to the aromas and their effects on the senses and body functions. Aromatherapy with wildflower essences is used in some hospitals for stress and pain management. Tea-tree oil has become one of the most commonly used natural remedies in Australia, and its popularity has spread internationally. The essential oil from *Melaleuca alternifolia*, it contains many active constituents, including terpenes such as cineole. Its main proven actions are antifungal, antibacterial and antiviral (Herpes simplex); it is used particularly in skin infections and in podiatry.

HOMEOPATHY. Homeopathy is a form of treatment in which substances (minerals, plant extracts, chemicals or microorganisms) that in sufficient amounts would produce

DRUG MONOGRAPH 3-2 GINSENG

Ginseng is a herbal product, the dried root of plants of the **Panax** species; Oriental (or Chinese or Korean) ginseng is from **Panax ginseng**. The active constituents are mainly a group of saponin glycosides known as ginsenosides or panaxosides from the roots.

PHARMACODYNAMICS The pharmacological actions of ginseng are complex, as the product contains a wide variety of ingredients, some of which have opposing actions to others; this is said to contribute to its 'adaptogenic' effects (helping the body respond to stresses). It inhibits the reuptake of many neurotransmitters and is said to improve physical performance, psychomotor performance, mental ability and wellbeing, and inhibit the development of morphine tolerance. Ginseng has anti-inflammatory and gonadotrophin-like activities, including oestrogenic effects. It has some actions similar to those of corticosteroids but it has antidiabetic rather than hyperglycaemic effects. In the cardiovascular system, it has antiarrhythmic actions and may either increase or decrease cardiac performance. Low doses lower blood pressure but higher doses may raise blood pressure. The blood lipid profile is improved. It is claimed to be hepatoprotective; in some situations it is cytotoxic and in others it has antitumour activity owing to its immunostimulating actions.

In traditional Chinese medicine (TCM), it is considered a stimulant, diuretic and tonic for the spleen and lungs.

INDICATIONS The herbal preparation is used as a demulcent (soother), stomachic (to relieve dyspepsia), thymoleptic (modulator of the immune system) and, possibly, an aphrodisiac. It is indicated for nervous disorders, insomnia and depression, and menopausal symptoms. In TCM, it is indicated for leucopenia, shock, diabetes and mental fatigue.

PHARMACOKINETICS Ginseng extracts have a sweet, slightly bitter taste. Little other information on absorption, distribution, metabolism or excretion is available.

ADVERSE REACTIONS Ginseng is considered to have low toxicity but adverse effects are difficult to assess objectively because of differences between preparations as to the type of ginseng, dose and purity of preparations. Adverse reactions noted include insomnia, hypertension, diarrhoea, mastalgia, vaginal bleeding and skin eruptions. In TCM, it is noted that 'allergies' can lead to palpitations, insomnia and pruritus (itching).

DRUG INTERACTIONS Because of its widespread effects in many body systems, ginseng has the potential to interact with a wide range of drugs, either enhancing or inhibiting their actions, especially warfarin, digoxin, and all drugs metabolised by CYP1A. All of these potential interactions emphasise the importance of people who are using ginseng discussing this with health-care professionals, especially any considering prescribing other drugs.

WARNINGS AND CONTRAINDICATIONS Guidelines suggest that ginseng is contraindicated in acute illness and haemorrhage, and should be avoided by people with nervousness or schizophrenia, by healthy people aged under 40 years and by pregnant or lactating women. Long-term use should be avoided. Ginseng should be used with caution by patients with cardiovascular disease or hypertension.

DOSAGE AND ADMINISTRATION Ginseng is usually formulated as an alcoholic tincture, extract, injection or tablets; the dose is quoted as equivalent to 1–3 g of root, usually combined with other herbs.

---

a set of symptoms in healthy persons, are given in minute amounts to produce a 'cure' of similar symptoms. It is based on the teachings of a German physician–pharmacist Samuel Hahnemann (1755–1843). Homeopathic 'remedies' based on extracts of plant drugs such as atropine, quinine and arnica, and copper, zinc, calcium and mercury are used.

The homeopath is said to encourage the body's own healing by stimulating a 'vital force' by administration of an extract of fresh natural product, a process known as 'proving' the drug. The mother tincture is then diluted thousands of times,* with vigorous shaking and tapping (succussion), which is said to release the power to heal. Each serial dilution is said to increase the power of the medicine. Care must be taken not to contaminate the preparation with anything that could affect its 'potency'. Formulations include tablets, drops, tinctures and powders.

The lack of scientific rationale for homeopathic principles, in particular the total negation of accepted dose–response relationships, and lack of scientifically acceptable and repeatable evidence for clinical efficacy in randomised controlled double-blind trials, make this modality anathema to most pharmacologists. It is nonetheless widely practised in Europe and followed by many influential people, including royalty. In Australia, homeopathic preparations are exempt from regulation by the TGA unless they contain ingredients of human or animal origin, but labels must state that they are not approved by the TGA.

---

*In fact, so many times that the dilution goes well below Avogadro's number, i.e. less than 1 in 10^{26}. As a chemist asked at a seminar on homeopathy: 'By my calculations, you have a solution with a concentration equivalent to one molecule in the whole Pacific Ocean. How do you know that you've captured it in your bottle?'.

CLINICAL INTEREST BOX 3-6 INDIGENOUS AUSTRALIAN PLANT REMEDIES

Active constituents of plants are known to vary in strength, both seasonally and geographically. Traditionally, plants may be prepared in a range of ways:

- for inhalation: leafy branches may be placed over a fire with the patient inhaling the aromatic oil vapour; sprigs of aromatic leaves may be crushed and inhaled or inserted into the nasal septum
- for infusion: the leaves or bark of the plants are soaked in hot water and the resultant liquid is drunk or used as a wash
- for topical administration as poultices: the leaves or roots are ground up and mixed with ash, or the crushed seed paste, fruit pulp, animal oil or milky plant sap is applied
- for ointments: crushed leaves are mixed with animal fat.

Effective antibacterial activity has been proven for extracts of leaves from many Australian plants used in traditional indigenous ways, including:

- *Eremophila duttonii*, *E. maculata* and *E. alternifolia*
- *Acacia auriculoformis* and *A. bivenosa*.

Adapted from: Collins et al 1990; Cribb 1985; Cribb & Cribb 1988; Lassak & McCarthy 2001; Low 1990; Zola & Gott 1992; Palombo & Semple 2001.

TRADITIONAL MEDICINE PRACTICES

AUSTRALIAN INDIGENOUS MEDICINE. The traditional Australian Aboriginal beliefs about causation of illness emphasise social and spiritual dysfunction as the main causes, with supernatural intervention causing serious illness. Some quite sophisticated 'bush medicine' methods were developed (see Clinical Interest Box 3-6). The medicinal properties of many Australian native plants may have been used by indigenous people for over 60,000 years. The diversity of plant species throughout Australia enabled the many distinct Aboriginal tribes and clans to develop a great range of traditional remedies, which were administered by various routes. Plants commonly included *Eucalyptus* (gum tree) and *Melaleuca* (tea-tree) species for coughs and colds, *Barringtonia* as a fish poison, *Leichhardtia* as an oral contraceptive, and *Euphorbia* topically for skin lesions.

The knowledge of preparation and use of medicinal plants has largely been inherited through oral tradition. Unfortunately, as these practices become more infrequent and the number of tribal elders with such knowledge diminishes, there is concern that much of this invaluable information may be lost, so it is important that the information be documented. There are many scientific journals, reference books, interest group newsletters and government reports in which the identification of useful species, their active ingredients and medicinal uses are noted. This information is fragmentary, however, often focusing on only one species or one region; for example, the central and northern Australian remedies have been more widely documented than those of eastern states.

Comparatively few native plants have been tested for their chemical or pharmacological properties. It is promising to note, however, that studies on the active ingredients of indigenous plants are being conducted in both Australian and overseas laboratories. Aromatic leaves, tannin-rich inner barks and 'kinos' (resins and gums) of several species have well-documented therapeutic effects. Other plants undoubtedly contain alkaloids or other compounds with pronounced clinical effects. As yet, no comprehensive database has been constructed to make this information easily accessible to the general public, although a chemical and pharmacological survey of Australian plants was carried out by the Commonwealth Scientific and Industrial Research Organisation (CSIRO) some years ago (Collins et al 1990).

TRADITIONAL EASTERN COMPARED WITH WESTERN MEDICINE. There is a major difference between the Eastern (Asian) and Western philosophical approaches to health care. In Eastern or Asian medicine, the emphasis is on health promotion or stabilisation, as opposed to Western concepts of illness intervention and treatment. In the West, the concentration is on treating symptoms or treating the area where the symptoms originated, both pharmacologically and non-pharmacologically. For example, bronchitis symptoms may include excessive mucus secretion in the bronchi, cough, frequent chest infections, and cyanosis. Treatment may include a systemic antibiotic for the infection, an expectorant and postural drainage for the mucus, and advising the patient not to smoke. If necessary, a bronchodilator and oxygen may be ordered. Eastern treatment might use some of these therapies but would also include approaches to help the individual regain energy balance to reduce further episodes. Depending on the practitioner, the approaches can vary considerably. Meta-analyses of some TCM remedies are beginning to appear in medical literature, to attempt to bring TCM into the era of evidence-based medicine (see Li et al 2003).

TRADITIONAL CHINESE MEDICINE. In traditional Chinese medicine (TCM), maintaining an energy balance in the body is considered most important; a balance between yin (negative) and yang (positive) forces is necessary to maintain good health. The Chinese physician may thus prescribe a variety of interventions such as herbal therapy, acupuncture, diet changes, exercise, meditation, or the services of a spiritual healer. Herbal remedies have been studied for thousands of years, so this knowledge is used with other therapies to achieve a balance within the body to help regain and maintain good health.

In Chinese herbal medicine, herbs are either taken orally or applied externally to correct the physical disorder.

Herbs are described by their properties, e.g. heat-clearing herbs, Qi-regulating herbs, or Yin-tonifying herbs. Texts such as the *Chinese Materia Medica* (Zhu, 1998) describe the philosophy and techniques of TCM materia medica (pharmacology), with guidelines for the harvesting, production and application of the materials. Monographs on products may describe the chemistry, pharmacology, adverse effects and toxicity, the traditional description, indications for use and applications of the remedy, and the dose and how it is administered.

In TCM it is believed that herbal preparations are much more effective when used in a balanced formula (see Clinical Interest Box 3-7), and that ingredients have synergistic effects, i.e. actions are magnified when taken as mixtures (however, there is little scientific evidence for this). **Ginseng**, for example, may energise the body (especially the lungs, spleen and pancreas) but it can also cause strong adverse effects if used alone. The ginsenosides in ginseng can constrict arteries but if ginseng is combined with other herbs such as kudzu or astragalus, the adverse effects are believed to be balanced. Another example is the combination of bitter orange, ginseng and ginger; the bitter orange stimulates the body's vital energy (Qi), ginseng energises the body, and ginger is included as an assisting herbal (i.e. it helps to relax muscle tissue). This combination is chosen for the individual effects and the effects in combination. In this formula the key herbal may be the bitter orange for the person who needs to strengthen his or her body Qi energy (cold). The balancing herbal is ginseng because it energises the body by providing a warmer energy, and ginger serves as an assistant herbal. This combination may be used to treat muscle aches (muscle relaxant) and digestive tract problems, and in people who need to strengthen their Qi energy.

AFRICAN TRADITIONAL MEDICINE. Traditional medicine practitioners in many African countries include herbalists, midwives, bone setters, faith healers and spiritualists. Disease is considered to arise not only from physical and psychological causes but also from astral, spiritual and other esoteric causes. African traditional medicine provides holistic treatment, and may include herbal, mineral and animal remedies, administered orally as liquids, topically as powders, ointments or balsams, or by inhalation. Parenteral routes are rarely used. Other types of African traditional medicine include diets and fasting, hydrotherapy or dry heat therapy, surgical operations, blood letting, spinal manipulation, faith healing and occultism.

Several important drugs have come into Western medicine from traditional African remedies, including physostigmine (an anticholinesterase), yohimbine (an α-receptor antagonist resembling the ergot alkaloids), reserpine (an alkaloid from *Rauwolfia* and a former antihypertensive and neuroleptic agent that caused severe depression), and ouabain (from *Strophanthus* species, a cardiac glycoside).

**CLINICAL INTEREST BOX 3-7
A HERBAL REMEDY CASE HISTORY**

A woman patient was brought into the medical ward with possible atypical pneumonia, plus postviral fatigue after severe glandular fever and Epstein–Barr virus infections. Recently she had been taking herbal tablets prescribed by the local TCM practitioner, 30 (yes, thirty) tablets per day. Each tablet allegedly contained:

- *Prunella vulgaris* spine 40 mg
- *Scrophularia nodosa* root 25 mg
- *Angelica polymorpha* root 9 mg
- *Mentha haplocalxy* herb 9 mg
- *Citrus aurantium* fruit 9 mg
- *Rheum palmatum* root 9 mg
- *Fritillaria thunbergii* bulb 9 mg
- plus various other natural products.

The concerned emergency department doctors did a quick search through reference sources to determine whether any of the ingredients might be potentially either effective or toxic in this situation. In summary:

- *Prunella vulgaris* spine is used in traditional medicine at a dose of 10–15 g to clear liver fire and phlegm fire.
- *Scrophularia nodosa* root (10–15 g) is used for sore throat, boils, goitre and fevers.
- *Angelica polymorpha* root, 'angelica', is a stimulating expectorant, used in confectionery and to raise blood sugar levels.
- *Mentha haplocalxy* herb, 'mint' (2–10 g), is used to clear the head and liver, and as a mild antiseptic and anticolic agent.
- *Citrus aurantium* fruit, sweet orange fruit (3–10 g), is used for liver, spleen, cough, and as a flavouring agent.
- *Rheum palmatum* root, rhubarb, is a laxative and astringent.
- *Fritillaria thunbergii* bulb is distasteful and poisonous.

It was quickly realised that while some of the herbs were possibly useful in respiratory infections, the 'doses' in the tablets were far too low to be effective, even if 30 tablets were taken daily. On the other hand, *Fritillaria thunbergii* is potentially poisonous.

The patient was advised to cease taking the herbal tablets and, after treatment with appropriate antibiotics, made a full recovery.

Source: Personal communication from Dr Philippa Smith, Geelong, 2005.

Issues related to complementary and alternative therapies
Evidence-based medicine?

One major difference between modern Western medicine and complementary and alternative therapies is that the former is required to be based on sound scientific principles of safety

TABLE 3-5 Some herbal preparations with a potential for toxicity

BOTANICAL NAME	COMMON NAMES	TOXICITY AND COMMENTS
Aconitum spp.	Monkshood	Contains various alkaloids that may be cardiotoxic and cause convulsions
Aesculus spp.	Buckeyes, horse chestnut, aesculus	Contains coumarin glycosides that may interfere with normal blood clotting
Amanita spp.	Mushrooms	Contains alkaloids, including muscarine and muscimol; powerful cholinergic effects in the autonomic nervous system
Areca catechu	Betel nut and leaf	Chewed in many cultures as a euphoriant and intoxicant; contains arecoline; users have a high incidence of mouth cancers; also used in veterinary medicine to expel worms
Arnica montana	Arnica flowers, wolfsbane, mountain tobacco, Flores Arnicae	Extracts affect the heart and vascular systems. Arnica is extremely irritating and can induce a toxic gastroenteritis, nervous system disturbances, extreme muscle weakness, collapse and even death
Aristolochia spp.	Birthwort, serpentary	Aristolochic acid is carcinogenic and causes renal damage
Artemisia absinthium	Wormwood, absinthe, madderwort, absinthium, mugwort	Contains a narcotic poison (oil of wormwood); can cause nervous system damage and mental impairment
Atropa belladonna	Belladonna, deadly nightshade	Contains the toxic alkaloids atropine, hyoscyamine and hyoscine. Anticholinergic symptoms range from blurred vision, dry mouth and inability to urinate, to unusual behaviours and hallucinations
Conium maculatum	Hemlock, conium, spotted hemlock, spotted parsley, St Bennet's herb, spotted cowbane, fool's parsley	Contains the toxic alkaloid coniine and other related alkaloids; the poison that killed Socrates
Datura stramonium	Thornapple	Formerly used in witches' brews and initiatory rites; source of hyoscyamine and atropine (see *Atropa*)
Digitalis purpurea	Foxglove	Contains digitalis and related cardiac glycosides; can cause arrhythmias and hypotension
Glycyrrhiza spp.	Liquorice	Has mineralocorticoid actions; may cause hypertension
Lobelia inflata	Lobelia, Indian tobacco, wild tobacco, asthma weed, emetic weed	Contains lobeline plus other alkaloids; excessive use can result in severe vomiting, pain, sweating, paralysis, low temperature, collapse, coma and death
Ephedra sinica	Ma huang, Ephedra	Contains ephedrine (30%–90%, depending on species) and possibly pseudoephedrine, sympathomimetics producing effects similar to noradrenaline. Can raise blood pressure and heart rate; also has been used to make methamphetamine ('speed') and as an alternative drug to 'ecstasy', an illegal street drug
Panax **ginseng** (and others)	**Ginseng**	Oestrogenic effects, hypoglycaemia, hypertension (see Drug Monograph 3-2)
Symphytum spp.	Comfrey	Pyrrolizidine alkaloids, which are hepatotoxic
Vinca major, Vinca minor	Periwinkle, vinca	Contain toxic alkaloids (vinblastine, vincristine) that are cytotoxic (and are used to treat cancer) and may cause liver, kidney and neurological damage

and efficacy, for which a high standard of objective reproducible evidence must be published in peer-reviewed scientific journals (**evidence-based medicine**). Complementary and alternative therapies, on the other hand, are often based on anecdotal evidence and personal experiences, and few remedies have been submitted to randomised controlled clinical trials. Practitioners of complementary and alternative therapies often argue that their types of treatments are not conducive to scientific testing but are individualised to each patient. If, however, complementary and alternative therapies are to be accepted as part of mainstream therapy and subsidised by governments, their practitioners will need to agree to the same high standards of proof and evidence and not evade objective examination. Some treatments that have been shown to be effective have been discussed in later chapters where relevant (see Clinical Interest Box 3-4). Herbal remedies for which good supporting evidence at the EBM standard exists include St John's wort, *Ginkgo biloba*, echinacea, ginger and valerian.

The potential risks of CAM have been neatly summarised as follows:

- economic harm, e.g. people wasting money and governments committing funds to regulation and investigation of ineffective 'treatments', and money spent by companies on marketing and advertising
- direct harm, such as adverse drug reactions and interactions, e.g. liver impairment from black cohosh and chaparral
- indirect harm, from delay in obtaining effective treatment due to misinformation about effectiveness of a CAM method, e.g. laetrile touted as a cancer cure.

Adverse drug reactions

Just as prescribed and synthetic drugs can cause adverse reactions, so many natural products can cause harm,* depending on the herb itself, the quantity consumed, whether the correct plant or part of the plant is present in the product, the presence of contaminants, and other factors. Although not many herbal toxicities are reported in the consumer literature, some very serious problems have been reported in the medical literature (see Table 3-5). Chaparral, for example, was promoted in the USA as a blood purifier and cancer cure (not on the label, which would then involve the FDA, as this is a medicinal use promotion), but its use has caused

---

*There is a widespread belief that 'if it's natural, it can't harm you', whereas drugs made into tablets, ointments, injections etc must be viewed as dangerous. A cursory consideration of a few natural substances such as arsenic, strychnine, uranium, thallium, atropine, digoxin, opium, deadly nightshade and tobacco will soon show this belief to be naive and unfounded (see Smith 2002).

CLINICAL INTEREST BOX 3-8 THE GREAT PAN PHARMACEUTICALS RECALL, 2003

Prior to mid-2003, Pan Pharmaceuticals was the largest Australian manufacturer of CAM products, a multimillion-dollar industry that produced 40%–50% of all vitamin and mineral tablets and capsules. Pan's Managing Director was considered the 'grandfather of the CAM industry' in Australia. However, he had previously been found guilty of professional misconduct, in which lactose had been substituted for paracetamol, manufacturing records falsified and ingredients from a banned manufacturer used.

Early in 2003, problems surfaced when 60 people became ill and 19 were hospitalised after taking the product Travacalm (formulated by Pan) for prevention or treatment of motion sickness; these tablets nominally contained dimenhydrinate 50 mg (an antihistamine), hyoscine hydrobromide 0.2 mg (an atropine-like antimuscarinic) and caffeine 20 mg. However, some tablets were found to contain no or very little active ingredient and others many times more than the specified amounts. The product was recalled, and the company's analyst was blamed and sacked. After TGA inspections of the company's premises and manufacturing processes, the manufacturing licence of Pan Pharmaceuticals was suspended for 6 months for serious breaches of quality control and widely varying content, inadequate cleaning, and substitution of beef cartilage for shark cartilage. Initially more than 200 Pan products were recalled, then eventually over 1600 products, including cold and flu capsules, children's medicines, folic acid, evening primrose oil and calcium supplements in a 'class 1' recall (where the recalled product may cause serious illness), the world's biggest ever recall of health products.

Following the scandal, many other CAM companies that had relied on Pan for their supplies were facing losses and/or closure, and Pan customers and creditors were seeking legal redress. The TGA was accused by Pan of being heavy-handed, acting as 'judge and jury', using scare tactics and being out to destroy Pan. As Pan did not have sufficient assets to meet potential claims for compensation, it went into voluntary administration.

Since this episode, the Australian government has established an Expert Committee on Complementary Medicines in the Health System, which has produced a report containing 49 recommendations covering the regulation of complementary medicines and complementary health-care practitioners, research, information, education and other aspects of the CAM industry. The already established two-tier system of registration and listing of all medicines is still considered to lead the world in the regulation of complementary medicines (see TGA 2005).

serious liver damage in some patients. In at least one case the need for a liver transplant was reported after 10 months of chaparral use.

The Australian TGA issues alerts about complementary medicines on its website; alerts have included warnings of interactions between St John's wort and many prescription medicines, that preparations containing kava are linked to hepatotoxicity, and that Chinese herbal medicines in Australia have been found to contain samples of *Aristolochia*, a herb considered so toxic that it is banned.

Contaminants (adulterants) are frequently found in natural products. They may be natural, such as the heavy metals lead, arsenic, mercury and thallium found in some imported preparations. In other cases, synthetic drugs have been found in supposed natural products, including NSAIDs in supposed 'herbal' preparations for the treatment of inflammation, and synthetic oral hypoglycaemic agents in herbs used to treat diabetes. Such **contamination** is potentially very dangerous if the patient is taking the 'natural' products in addition to prescribed drugs or is allergic to any of the unexpected ingredients.

Complementary and alternative therapies other than herbal remedies have also caused serious adverse effects. Examples are:
- cervical manipulations causing cerebrovascular accidents (strokes)
- acupuncture leading to infections, trauma and pneumothorax
- homeopathic preparations containing toxic concentrations of heavy metals.

Drug interactions

The mushroom Kombucha has been associated with illnesses and death. A tea made from Kombucha is said to be a tonic, but several people have been hospitalised and one woman died after taking this product. The cause could not be directly attributed to the Kombucha, but several theories were offered, e.g. the tea might have reacted with other medications that the woman was taking, or bacteria might grow in the Kombucha liquid and, in patients with suppressed immunity, might prove to be fatal.

The toxicity of Kombucha indicates potential problems that may not have been considered before taking the product; that is, what effect would the active ingredients in the herb have on other medications that the individual may be consuming? Many active medications in current use were originally discovered from plants, such as digitalis glycosides from foxglove, vinca alkaloids from periwinkle, or ephedra (ephedrine) from MaHuang. Natural or herbal products may therefore contain active ingredients that have or have not been identified and that, in combination with other medications or other herbal products, may cause serious drug interactions or may interfere with the results of laboratory tests.

The risk of interactions rises exponentially with the number of medicines a person takes. Many clinically significant interactions with herbal remedies are being documented and published as lists in journals and as posters and brochures for health professionals to consult (see Braun & Cohen 2005; Fugh-Berman 2000; Faulding Healthcare 2000). Virtually all commonly used herbal remedies have some serious drug interactions related to their use, so such lists should be consulted before advising their use and particularly if adverse effects or interactions are suspected.

A full drug (including complementary and alternative therapies) history

As many herbal remedies may be harmful to some individuals, health-care professionals taking a medication history should inquire about the use of OTC, health-food-store and herbal products. Such products are often not considered to be drugs or medications by the consumer and therefore are not generally reported. Caution with respect to complementary and alternative therapies should particularly be exercised by women who are pregnant or breastfeeding, and by people with medical conditions.

There are also ethical and legal issues relating to the interface between CAM and conventional medicine. Doctors should recognise that most patients do take CAM products or use CAM methods, and should be prepared to discuss the risks and benefits of all relevant treatments, and become familiar with qualified and competent CAM practitioners in their area to whom referrals can confidently be made.

Other issues

The main issues with respect to the use of complementary and alternative therapies relate to: the level of scientific evidence available to prove safety and efficacy; purity, strength and the variability between different preparations of the same herb; and the belief that natural methods and substances are harmless. Other aspects of the use of complementary and alternative therapies that may result in problems include:
- practitioner qualifications possibly not being subject to regulation and substantiation
- a wide range of treatments often being recommended, with little agreement between practitioners as to the remedy of first choice in a particular condition
- the fact that CAM treatments shown by clinical trials to be effective are often ignored by practitioners
- patients being unlikely to admit to using complementary and alternative therapies
- unsubstantiated claims for safety and efficacy, with 'statistics' being perpetuated despite absence of proof
- complementary and alternative therapies being used for conditions in which they are contraindicated or dangerous

- issues related to costs: people and governments may waste money on useless 'remedies'
- health policy makers being subjected to pressure from proponents of complementary and alternative therapies and neglecting the need for clinical trials
- labelling of remedies being often inadequate, with insufficient information as to dose, storage, contraindications, likely adverse effects and interactions, antidotes or instructions for use
- people rarely being warned to use the remedies only for short periods.

Many of these issues were exemplified in the Pan Pharmaceuticals debacle in Australia in 2003 (see Clinical Interest Box 3-8).

KEY POINTS

- With proper use, over-the-counter (OTC) drugs are considered safe for use in the self-medication of minor illnesses without the regular supervision of a health-care professional.
- Wise selection and use of OTC drug products can be very cost-effective.
- Because of the widespread use of OTC drugs, problems relating to the products can occur, such as prescription drug–OTC drug interactions and drug overuse or overdose.
- The most commonly used OTCs are analgesics, antacids, laxatives, cough/cold preparations, antidiarrhoeals and nutritional supplements.
- Consumers should be informed on how to review the label on OTC medications before purchase (e.g. ingredients, precautions and contraindications, as related to their documented health problems).
- A wide range of complementary and alternative therapies is available for use, including psychological, physical, dietary and pharmacological types. Herbal remedies contain potentially active drugs and need to be used with care.
- With the increased interest in and use of herbal, home and natural remedies today, the health-care professional needs to be informed on such products. A thorough medication history and close patient monitoring are recommended.
- The consumer and the health-care professional are responsible for detecting any unusual or adverse reactions with listed products because the TGA does not assess some herbal products for quality, safety or effectiveness before these are marketed.
- Traditional medical practices in indigenous Australian, Asian and African countries may differ in philosophies and ranges of treatments from Western scientific medicine; combinations of types of medical treatments are commonly used now.
- The main issues related to the increasing use of complementary and alternative therapies are the frequent absence of proof of safety and efficacy; the potential for adverse effects and drug interactions; inadequate information as to strength, purity and administration; cost; and delay in effective treatment of serious conditions.

REVIEW EXERCISES

1. Describe the differences between, and regulations governing, OTC medicines and prescription-only drugs in Australia; for OTC drugs, explain why drugs are unscheduled or in Schedules 2 and/or 3.
2. Describe the range of OTC products available, giving examples of drugs acting in 10 body systems.
3. What potential problems are there if people self-medicate with OTC drugs?
4. What advice and counselling could you give a person who had a basket of OTC products in the family medicine cabinet?
5. Discuss the prevalence of and rationales for use of complementary and alternative therapies.
6. Define the term 'complementary and alternative medicine', giving examples of different types of therapeutic modalities.
7. List and discuss briefly potential problems with the widespread use of complementary and alternative therapies in your community.
8. Set up a class debate on the topic 'That in the context of safety and efficacy of medical treatments, anecdotes can never be evidence'.

REFERENCES

Balinski AA. Use of Western Australian wildflower essences in the management of pain and stress in the hospital setting. *Complementary Therapies in Nursing and Midwifery* 1998; 4(4): 111–17.

Barrett B, Kiefer D, Rabago D. Assessing the risks and benefits of herbal medicine: an overview of scientific evidence. *Alternative Therapies* 1999; 5(4): 40–9.

Bellamy D, Pfister A. *World Medicine: Plants, Patients and People*. Oxford: Blackwell, 1992.

Bowman WC, Rand MJ. *Textbook of Pharmacology*. 2nd edn. Oxford: Blackwell, 1980 [chs 42, 43].

Braun L, Cohen M. *Herbs and Natural Supplements: An Evidence-Based Guide*. Sydney: Elsevier Mosby, 2005.

British Herbal Medicine Association. *British Herbal Pharmacopoeia 1996*. 4th edn. Guildford: Biddles, 1996.

Caswell A. *MIMS OTC*. 3rd edn. Sydney: MIMS Australia, 2000.

Caswell A (ed.). *MIMS Annual June 2005*. Sydney: CMPMedica Australia, 2005.

Chang K, Cheung L. *Interactions Between Chinese Herbal Medicine Products and Orthodox Drugs*. Amsterdam: Harwood Academic, 2000.

Clark MJ, Robson T. *What's the Alternative? Orthodox and Complementary Remedies for Common Complaints*. Melbourne: Melbourne University Publishing, 2005.

Coates P, Blackman MR, Cragg G, Levine M, Moss J, White J (eds). *Encyclopedia of Dietary Supplements*. New York: Marcel Dekker, 2005.

Collins DJ, Culvenor CCJ, Lamberton JA et al. *Plants for Medicines: A Chemical and Pharmacological Survey of Plants in the Australian Region*. Canberra: CSIRO, c. 1990.

Cribb AB, Cribb JW. *Wild Medicine in Australia*. Sydney: Collins, 1988.

Cribb JW. Australia's medicinal plants. *Medical Journal of Australia* 1985; 143: 574–7.

Ernst E, ed. *The Desktop Guide to Complementary and Alternative Medicine: An Evidence-Based Approach*. Edinburgh: Mosby, 2001.

Ernst E, White A. The BBC survey of complementary medicine use in the UK. *Complementary Therapies in Medicine* 2000; 8(1): 32–6.

Evans WC. *Trease and Evans' Pharmacognosy*. 15th edn. Edinburgh: Saunders, 2002.

Faulding Healthcare. *Herb Drug Interaction Guide*. Australia: FH Faulding, 2000.

Fugh-Berman A. Herb–drug interactions. *Lancet* 2000; 355(9198): 134–8.

Galbally R. *Final Report of the National Competition Review of Drugs, Poisons and Controlled Substances Legislation*. Canberra: Therapeutic Goods Administration, Commonwealth of Australia, 2000.

Geng J, Huang W, Ren T, Ma X. *Practical Traditional Chinese Medicine and Pharmacology: Medicinal Herbs*. Beijing: New World Press, 1991.

Green D, Halat K. Are your patients taking herbal meds? *Podiatry Today* 2003; 16(12): 28–34.

Hathcock J. Dietary supplements: how they are used and regulated. *Journal of Nutrition* 2001; 131(3s): 1114S–17S.

Kendler BS. Melatonin: media hype or therapeutic breakthrough? *Nurse Practitioner* 1997; 22(2): 66–77.

Kerridge IH, McPhee JR. Ethical and legal issues at the interface of complementary and conventional medicine. *Medical Journal of Australia* 2004; 181(3): 164–6.

Kotsirilos, V. Complementary and alternative medicine: Part 2—evidence and implications for GPs. *Australian Family Physician* 2005; 34(8): 689–91.

Lassak EV, McCarthy T. *Australian Medicinal Plants*. Kew: Reed-New Holland, 2001.

Latz P. *Bushfires & Bushtucker: Aboriginal Plant Use in Central Australia*. Alice Springs: IAD Press, 1995.

Li GQ, Duke CC, Roufogalis BD. The quality and safety of traditional Chinese medicines. *Australian Prescriber* 2003: 26(6): 128–30.

Lim A, Cranswick N, Skull S, South M. Survey of complementary and alternative medicine use at a tertiary children's hospital. *Journal of Paediatric and Child Health* 2005; 41(8): 424–7.

Liu C, Douglas RM. Chinese herbal medicines in the treatment of acute respiratory infections: a review of randomised and controlled clinical trials. *Medical Journal of Australia* 1998; 169(11–12): 579–82.

Low T. *Bush Medicine. A Pharmacopoeia of Natural Remedies*. Sydney: Angus & Robertson, 1990.

MacLennan AH, Wilson DH, Taylor AW. Prevalence and cost of alternative medicine in Australia. *Lancet* 1996; 347: 569–73.

McCabe, P. Complementary and alternative medicine in Australia: a contemporary overview. *Complementary Therapies in Clinical Practice* 2005; 11: 28–31.

Maher P. A review of 'traditional' Aboriginal health beliefs. *Australian Journal of Rural Health* 1999; 7(4): 229–36.

Mann J. *Murder, Magic and Medicine*. Oxford: Oxford University Press, 1992.

Murcott T. *The Whole Story: Alternative Medicine on Trial?* New York: Macmillan, 2005.

Ong YC, Yong EL. Panax (ginseng)–panacea or placebo? Molecular and cellular basis of its pharmacological activity. *Annals of the Academy of Medicine Singapore* 2000; 29(1): 42–6.

Palombo EA, Semple SJ. Antibacterial activity of traditional Australian medicinal plants. *Journal of Ethnopharmacology* 2001; 77(2–3): 151–7.

Pengelly A. *The Constituents of Medicinal Plants: An Introduction to the Chemistry and Therapeutics of Herbal Medicine*. 2nd edn. Sydney: Allen & Unwin, 2004.

Pinn G. Herbal medicine: an overview. *Australian Family Physician* 2000; 29(11): 1059–62.

Schraub S. Unproven methods in cancer: a worldwide problem. *Supportive Care in Cancer* 2000; 8(1): 10–15.

Shang A, Huwiler-Muntener K, Nartey L, Juni P, Dorig S, Sterne JA, Pewsner D, Egger M. Are the effects of homoeopathy placebo effects? Comparative study of placebo-controlled trials of homoeopathy and allopathy. *Lancet* 2005; 366(9487): 726–32.

Smith A. It's natural so it must be safe. *Australian Prescriber* 2002; 25(3): 50–1.

Sofowora A. Plants in African traditional medicine—an overview. Ch. 39 in: Evans WC. *Trease and Evans' Pharmacognosy*. 14th edn. London: Saunders, 1996.

Spencer JW, Jacobs JJ. *Complementary/Alternative Medicine: An Evidence-Based Approach*. St Louis: Mosby, 1999.

Therapeutic Goods Administration. *Australian Regulatory Guidelines for Complementary Medicines (ARGCM): Part 1: Registration of Complementary Medicines*. Canberra: Australian Department of Health and Ageing; June 2005.

Thomas KJ, Nicholl JP, Coleman P. Use and expenditure on complementary medicine in England: a population based survey. *Complementary Therapies in Medicine* 2001; 9(1): 2–11.

Trounce J, Gould D. *Clinical Pharmacology for Nurses.* 16th edn. Edinburgh: Churchill Livingstone, 2000 [ch. 29].

Vaughn GN. Australian medicinal plants. Ch. 6 in: Steiner RP (ed.). *Folk Medicine: The Art and the Science.* Washington: American Chemical Society, 1986.

Webb LJ. The use of plant medicines and poisons by Australian Aborigines. *Mankind* 1959; 7: 137–46.

Weir M. *Complementary Medicine: Ethics and Law.* Brisbane: Prometheus, 2000.

Wildman REC (ed.). *Handbook of Nutraceuticals and Functional Foods.* Boca Raton: CRC Press, 2001.

Willett WC, Stampfer MJ. What vitamins should I be taking, Doctor? *New England Journal of Medicine* 2001; 345: 1819–24.

Zhu Y-P. *Chinese Materia Medica: Chemistry, Pharmacology and Applications.* Amsterdam: Harwood Academic, 1998.

Zola N, Gott B. *Koorie Plants, Koorie People: Traditional Aboriginal Food, Fibre and Healing Plants of Victoria.* Melbourne: Koorie Heritage Trust, 1992.

ON-LINE RESOURCES

New Zealand Medicines and Medical Devices Safery Authority: www.medsafe.govt.nz
Therapeutic Goods Administration: www.tga.gov.au

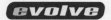 More weblinks at http://evolve.elsevier.com/AU/Bryant/pharmacology/

CHAPTER 4

Legal and Ethical Foundations of Pharmacotherapy

CHAPTER FOCUS

Health-care professionals who prescribe, dispense or administer drugs are legally accountable for their actions, especially as they relate to drug therapy. This chapter reviews the laws relating to the regulation of prescription and over-the-counter drugs, poisons, controlled substances, proscribed substances and investigational drugs, particularly those of Australia and New Zealand. Many ethical principles also apply to drug use, based on human rights and ethics; these can give rise to controversy as to how ethical principles are applied in clinical situations. To practise safely and professionally, health-care professionals must have a working knowledge of the relevant drug Acts and Regulations, and principles of bioethics.

OBJECTIVES

- To outline the various pieces of Commonwealth and state legislation relating to the regulation, use and testing of drugs in Australia, especially the Therapeutic Goods Act, and Drugs, Poisons and Controlled Substances Acts and Regulations.

- To describe the roles of the Commonwealth and states with respect to proscribed drugs, and the implications of the relevant Customs, Crimes and Narcotic Drugs Acts.

- To compare the scheduling of drugs and controlled substances in Australia and New Zealand.

- To describe how drugs are assayed and standardised.

- To outline the routes and stages of drug discovery and development.

- To identify and explain the phases and important elements in clinical trials of investigational drugs.

- To explain the human rights principles on which bioethics are based and discuss some relevant current issues.

KEY DRUGS	KEY TERMS		KEY ABBREVIATIONS	
thalidomide	animal rights	International	ADEC	Australian Drug Evaluation Committee
zanamivir	assay	Narcotics Control	ADRAC	Adverse Drug Reactions Advisory
	Australia Pharmaceutical	Board		Committee
	Formulary	International Units	APF	*Australian Pharmaceutical Formulary*
	bioassay	of Activity	BP	*British Pharmacopoeia*
	bioethics	meta-analysis	CSIRO	Commonwealth Scientific and Industrial
	biological variability	null hypothesis		Research Organization
	British Pharmacopoeia	orphan drug	CSL	Commonwealth Serum Laboratories
	clinical trial	proscribed drug	CTN	Clinical Trial Notification
	controlled drugs	regulation of drugs	CTX	Clinical Trial Exemption
	drug development	scheduling of drugs	FDA	Food and Drugs Administration
	drug regulation	screening	HREC	Human Research Ethics Commitee
	gene therapy	Single Convention	HTS	high-throughput screening
	high-throughput	on Narcotic Drugs	IEC	institutional ethics committee
	screening	standardisation of	IMMP	Intensive Medicines Monitoring Programme
	Hippocratic Oath	drugs	IU	International Units
	human rights	statistical methods	PBS	Pharmaceutical Benefits Scheme
	institutional ethics	the new genetics	RCCT	randomised controlled clinical trial
	committee		SUSDP	Standard for the Uniform Scheduling of
				Drugs and Poisons
			TGA	Therapeutic Goods Administration
			USP	*United States Pharmacopeia*

LEGAL ASPECTS OF DRUG USE IN HEALTH CARE

BEFORE the 20th century, there were few controls on the use of drugs, most of which were natural products, many with low efficacy. There was little information available about drugs compared with what we expect today, such as research studies proving the safety and effectiveness of the preparation, content analysis and strength, drug consistency from one pack to another of the same preparation, and information on administration and adverse reactions. As chemical industries developed, more potent and efficacious drugs were synthesised, and trade in drugs of dependence (addictive drugs) increased, it was recognised that controls on drugs were required. The early 1900s marked the beginning of national and international legislation relating to drugs.

International drug controls
Controls on narcotic drugs

Control of drugs in international law began in 1912 when the first Opium Conference was held at The Hague, Netherlands. International treaties were drawn up, calling on governments to:

- limit to medical and scientific needs the manufacturing of and trade in medicinal opium
- control the production and distribution of raw opium
- establish a system of governmental licensing to control the manufacture of and trade in drugs covered by the treaties.

In 1961, government representatives formulated the United Nations **Single Convention on Narcotic Drugs**, which became effective in 1964. The convention needs to be ratified and signed by a country before it binds that country. The country then has to enact appropriate legislation. This convention consolidated all existing treaties into one document for the control of all narcotic substances* by:

- outlawing the production, manufacture, trade and use of narcotic substances for non-medicinal purposes

---

*The term 'narcotic' literally means 'causing numbness, sleep or unconsciousness', and so could apply to all central nervous system depressants. It was originally used to refer to the 'narcotic analgesics', such as opium and opiate derivatives like morphine and codeine, to distinguish them from the 'non-narcotic analgesics', like aspirin. The term came to be extended to all drugs likely to cause addiction, and thus came to include drugs such as cocaine, and even LSD and marijuana. It is now used more or less interchangeably with the term 'illicit', to refer to all drugs for which there are international controls on trade and importation.

- limiting possession of all narcotic substances to authorised persons for medical and scientific purposes
- providing for international control of all opium transactions by the national monopolies (countries designated to produce opium, such as Australia and Turkey) and authorising production only by licensed farmers in areas and on plots designated by these monopolies
- requiring import certificates and export authorisations.

The **International Narcotics Control Board** was established to enforce the Single Convention on Narcotic Drugs. This board is an international organisation of representatives from governments and the World Health Organization, established to monitor compliance with the Single Convention on Narcotic Drugs and with other United Nations conventions regarding the manufacture and traffic of drugs, international trade in drugs, and government control over chemicals used in the illicit manufacture of drugs.

Because enforcement is an immense task, it is impossible to prevent illicit trafficking in drugs. For example, during a 1-year period it was estimated that 1200 tons of opium were circulated in the illicit market, while 800 tons were considered sufficient for world medical needs. Laws need to be frequently updated and strictly enforced, but the unfortunate fact is that the available financial support for regulation and enforcement is sometimes not equal to the task, and is less than the money to be made by illicit trafficking and pushing of narcotics. New means of distribution, such as 'Internet pharmacies', most commonly used by consumers in Europe and the United States, pose new problems. Also, international treaties are not automatically binding, even on countries that have signed the treaty, unless those countries introduce local laws and enforce them. For this reason, treaties and international attempts to control illicit drugs are only as strong as the determination of their member countries.

Controls on drugs for use in health care

It is recognised that drugs used therapeutically also need to be controlled, as people cannot assess the safety and efficacy of all drugs. The public want access to drugs but also expect to be protected from harm. Governments generally take a risk assessment role and require that drugs to be made available in their country are assessed for safety, efficacy, quality of manufacture (aspects such as purity, stability and strength), availability and marketing. This provides protection not only for the public but also for drug manufacturers. The principles generally adopted are that most people are not sufficiently knowledgeable about health care and drugs to self-medicate safely in all conditions, that all drugs are inherently potentially dangerous and should be assessed for risks and benefits, that a licence to market a drug is granted for a specified period subject to review, that licences can be revoked, and that government guidelines with respect to Good Laboratory

Practice (GLP), Good Manufacturing Practice (GMP) and Good Clinical Practice (GCP) should be observed.

As world trade and health practices become ever more based on a global economy, it is increasingly important that requirements for drug registration and licensing be uniform in all developed countries. If, for example, the regulations were different in the major markets of Europe, Asia and the USA–Canada, it would add enormously to the costs of developing and introducing new drugs. Most developed countries require similar standards of preclinical testing, clinical trials and post-marketing surveillance, as described in the later section on drug discovery and development. A tragic situation that developed in the early 1960s, after widespread use of the seemingly safe sedative **thalidomide**, led to much more rigorous testing and strict controls on the approval and supply of drugs (see Clinical Interest Box 4-1).

Regulation of drugs in Australia

Australian laws related to **drug regulation** can be broadly divided into two types: laws that regulate drugs used for medicinal purposes in humans (discussed in this section under Drug Regulation), and laws that prohibit the possession, production and supply of **proscribed** (i.e. prohibited) **drugs** (discussed in this section under Drug Offences). Legal non-medicinal drugs such as alcohol and tobacco are also subject to much regulation, which is primarily related to their sale, advertising and packaging (not considered in this chapter).

In Australia, drugs are controlled by Commonwealth, state and territory laws (see Table 4-1). There is no uniform Australian scheme for drug regulation or drug offences, partly because the Commonwealth legislation cannot apply in all situations for Constitutional reasons. Broadly, state and territory laws control 'poisons', and Commonwealth legislation controls 'therapeutic goods'. Offences related to international drug trafficking are set out in Commonwealth legislation, while the state and territory criminal laws cover the production, possession, use and distribution of proscribed drugs within those jurisdictions. Additional legislation in most states covers drug use related to road safety.

In addition to specific Acts and Regulations relating to drug development and use, there are relevant aspects of Common Law (developed by judicial precedence and interpretation). For example, health professionals are considered to have a

CLINICAL INTEREST BOX 4-1 THE THALIDOMIDE DISASTER

In the years 1959–1962, it appeared that a new 'epidemic' was sweeping England, Europe and other countries, including Australia. Dozens, then hundreds, and eventually thousands of babies were born with congenital malformations, commonly with absent or rudimentary limbs and deformities of other organs and systems. The condition was termed phocomelia, meaning 'seal-like limbs', and had up until that time been an incredibly rare congenital malformation. Causes were sought, including viral infections, radiation damage or environmental contaminants.

Dr W Lenz, of Hamburg in Germany, asked mothers of affected babies to list all the drugs they had taken during pregnancy; Contergan, an apparently safe sedative, appeared in about 29% of the lists. At a meeting of paediatric physicians, Dr Lenz suggested that a drug might have been responsible.

Meanwhile in Sydney, Dr William McBride had been consulted about several babies with phocomelia; all the mothers had taken Distaval, a mild sedative, during pregnancy. McBride wrote to the journal *Lancet*, asking if similar cases had been reported in the UK. Lenz replied with his findings and it became apparent that the same drug, **thalidomide**, was implicated in all the cases. More case reports flooded in and the drug was withdrawn; however, cases kept appearing, partly because the drug was marketed under many trade names and warnings were unheeded, so bottles of tablets lay around for some time.

Other reasons why it took so long for the link between the drug and the adverse effect to be established were that the critical period was so short—between the 37th and 54th days of pregnancy—and the effects were not observed until many months later.

The drug had not been released in the USA, as the Food and Drug Administration was concerned, not about its teratogenicity (ability to cause birth defects) but that it appeared to have adverse effects on the nervous system. Overall, it is estimated that in Germany alone about 10,000 babies were affected, of whom half survived, most with severe malformations. Law suits against the drug companies concerned, relating to damages claims, were still being pursued in the courts decades later.

Thalidomide had appeared to meet a public need for a safe and effective drug to treat a mild condition—insomnia—and had been submitted to the testing required at the time, yet had set in train a disaster for all affected. A positive benefit was that, after public outcry as to how it could have occurred, regulations regarding the testing, approval and availability of drugs were severely tightened, to the extent that for some years it became very difficult for new drugs to be approved.

For many years thalidomide was totally banned in most countries; however, it became apparent that it does have some useful immunosuppressant and anti-inflammatory actions. In Australia it is now an 'orphan drug', available for use in very strictly controlled situations, for treatment of some skin conditions in leprosy, and for multiple myeloma. In some countries it is less tightly controlled and the warnings on the packs are in English rather than the native language so, tragically, cases of phocomelia still occur.

Adapted from: Cartwright & Biddiss 1972.

TABLE 4-1 Principal Australian legislation involved in the regulation of drugs

JURISDICTION	DRUG REGULATION LEGISLATION	ADDITIONAL DRUG OFFENCES ACTS
Commonwealth (Cth)	*Therapeutic Goods Act 1989* (Cth) *Therapeutic Goods Regulations 1990* (Cth) *National Health Act 1953* (Cth)	*Customs Act 1901* (Cth) *Crimes (Traffic in Narcotic Drugs and Psychotropic Substances) Act 1990* (Cth) *Narcotic Drugs Act 1967* (Cth) *Criminal Code Act 1995* (Cth) *Criminal Code (Serious Drug Offences) Amendment Act 2004* **(Cth)**
Australian Capital Territory (ACT)	*Poisons and Drugs Act 1978* (ACT) *Poisons Act 1933* (ACT) *Poisons Regulations* (ACT) *Drugs of Dependence Act 1989* (ACT) *Drugs In Sport Act 1989* (ACT) *Drugs of Dependence Regulations 2005* (ACT)	
New South Wales (NSW)	*Poisons and Therapeutic Goods Act 1966* (NSW) *Poisons and Therapeutic Goods Regulations 1994* (NSW)	*Drug Misuse and Trafficking Act 1985* (NSW)
Northern Territory (NT)	*Poisons and Dangerous Drugs Act 1983* (NT) *Therapeutic Goods and Cosmetics Act 1986* (NT) *Poisons and Dangerous Drugs Regulations 2004* (NT)	*Misuse of Drugs Act 1990* (NT)
Queensland (Qld)	*Health Act 1937* (Qld) *Health (Drugs and Poisons) Regulations 1996* (Qld)	*Drugs Misuse Act 1986* (Qld)
South Australia (SA)	*Controlled Substances Act 1984* (SA) *Controlled Substances (Poisons) Regulations 1996* (SA) *Drugs of Dependence (General) Regulations 1985* (SA)	*Drugs Act 1908* (SA)
Tasmania (Tas)	*Poisons Act 1971* (Tas) *Poisons Regulations 1975* (Tas) *Alcohol and Drug Dependency Act 1968* (Tas) *Therapeutic Goods Act 2001* (Tas) *Therapeutic Goods Regulations 2002* (Tas)	*Misuse of Drugs Act 2001* (Tas)
Victoria (Vic)	*Therapeutic Goods (Victoria) Act 1994* (Vic) *Drugs, Poisons and Controlled Substances Act 1981* (Vic) *Drugs, Poisons and Controlled Substances Regulations 1995* (Vic)	
Western Australia (WA)	*Poisons Act 1964* (WA) *Poisons Regulations 1965* (WA)	*Misuse of Drugs Act 1981* (WA)

'duty of care' to the people with whom they deal, and so are expected to carry out their roles with the best interests of their clients/patients as a priority. Underpinning all health-care-related law are fundamental principles of human rights and ethics (see later section on Ethical principles related to drug use in health care). Drug availability can also be controlled at the local level, for example by a hospital's drug committee.

Drug regulation

Dwyer and Newgreen (1998) point to three primary aims of the **regulation of** medicinal **drugs**: to control the supply of drugs prone to abuse; to regulate the availability of substances for therapeutic use (to ensure safety and quality); and to include certain products on government-sponsored assistance schemes. The criteria of quality, safety and efficacy are mentioned as objects of the *Therapeutic Goods Act 1989* (Cth).

In Australia, there exist extensive, complex and overlapping pieces of Commonwealth, state and territory legislation regulating drugs. Although the regulation of drugs has traditionally been the domain of the states, the role of the Commonwealth has increased steadily, with the introduction of the Therapeutic Goods Act. Because a substance may be either a poison or a therapeutic good or both, it may be subject to both Commonwealth and state regulation. Note that the term 'poison' is used broadly to cover drugs used clinically as well as veterinary, agricultural and domestic chemicals.

Classification of poisons in the Standard for the Uniform Scheduling of Drugs and Poisons (SUSDP)

To restrict the availability of drugs of certain types, drugs are classified with others requiring the same level of regulation, into Schedules. Historically, scheduling in Australia was a state responsibility, which led to anomalies such as a drug being available over the counter (OTC) in one state, e.g. in Albury, NSW, whereas in its sister town, Wodonga, on the other bank of the Murray river in Victoria, a prescription might be required.

The need for reform of the **controlled substances** system was recognised and a National Competition Review of Drugs, Poisons and Controlled Substances legislation was set in train; an Options Paper and Final Report were published (Galbally 2000, 2001). The Review considered all aspects of the legislation relating to drugs, including how **scheduling of drugs** determines access, supply and provision of drugs, their labelling, packaging and storage, records and advertising. The controls and restrictions imposed, their effects, costs and benefits were all discussed, and options and alternatives were suggested. The Review strongly supported a uniform regulatory scheme across states and territories, more closely integrated with related legislation, and noted the benefits in terms of quality use of medicines flowing from effective counselling by pharmacists. A uniform system of control also ensures a balance between the many vested interests involved in drug scheduling. For example, drug companies want drugs to be as widely bought and used as possible, governments want to contain costs and protect the public, while health professionals may wish to maintain their powers and protect their unique roles in the supply of drugs. The Review recommended that funds be provided for further research in the area and that administrative arrangements be amended to streamline functions of the relevant committees. The Review, and the Australian Health Ministers Advisory Council Working Party response, were unanimously approved by the Council of Australian Governments in June 2005.

The SUSDP has attempted to implement the Review's recommendations by setting uniform schedules and expecting all states to move towards adhering to them. The SUSDP classifies drugs in relation to their possible therapeutic uses. It is published annually and comprises the recommendations of the National Drugs and Poisons Schedule Committee (NDPSC). The decisions of the NDPSC in relation to the Standard have no force in Commonwealth law but are recommended for incorporation into state and territory drugs and poisons legislation. Most states and territories have adopted the Standard, in whole or in part, to designate which substances are subject to regulation. The SUSDP also attempts to unify scheduling and control of drugs and poisons between Australia and New Zealand. This is referred to as Trans-Tasman Scheduling Harmonisation and has been largely effective, with a few minor discrepancies still existing.

The Australia New Zealand Therapeutic Products Authority, the new trans-Tasman regulatory agency for therapeutic products, is expected to commence during 2007. This agency will replace the Australian TGA and New Zealand's Medicines and Medical Devices Safety Authority (MedSafe).

DRUG SCHEDULES

The SUSDP contains nine Schedules of chemicals (drugs and poisons) that are subject to varying levels of control. Schedule 9 includes some drugs of abuse (such as heroin), and drugs that may be required for research or investigational purposes but are considered too toxic for therapeutic use. Schedules 2, 3, 4 and 8 include drugs used medically; Schedules 5, 6 and 7 include mainly non-drug chemicals used domestically or in agriculture. Schedules 2 and 3 include OTC drugs, and have been discussed in Chapter 3 (see Tables 3-1 and 3-2). Drugs are now labelled with the name of the classification rather than the 'S' number (e.g. 'Prescription Only' rather than 'Schedule 4'). This change was made to counteract the false perception in the community that higher S numbers necessarily meant higher toxicity. Definitions and important aspects of the Schedules are listed in Appendix 5.

The decision to classify a substance into a particular schedule depends not only on the drug's potential toxicity but also on the purposes for which it is used, the dose in the particular preparation, its potential for abuse, other ingredients present and the need for the drug to be readily available in the community. A drug may appear in more than one schedule, e.g. codeine phosphate is scheduled as follows:

- small quantities (20) of compound analgesic tablets containing low-dose codeine (8 mg) are S2 (PHARMACY ONLY)
- larger quantities (50, 100) of these tablets are S3 (PHARMACIST ONLY) (except in NSW [S2])
- some codeine cough-suppressant preparations are available as S2 in higher doses, e.g. syrups with 19.2 mg/10 mL dose
- higher doses (15 or 30 mg) in compound analgesics, with aspirin or paracetamol, are S4 (PRESCRIPTION ONLY)
- codeine alone (30 mg) in tablets is in S8 (CONTROLLED DRUGS).

If a substance does not appear in a Schedule of the SUSDP, it is not a poison by definition and can be supplied freely to the public (unless it is subject to other legislative controls). Where a preparation contains two or more poisons included in a schedule, the preparation takes the Schedule that is the most restrictive.

In some Australian states, the SUSDP has been adopted as the basis for determining whether or not a drug is a proscribed drug, so that production or supply of a Schedule 8 or Schedule 9 drug constitutes an indictable offence. In other states there are separate lists in the legislation related to the relevant offences, but these lists correlate closely with the SUSDP Schedules.

Regulation of poisons

Poisons are subject to strict regulation in all Australian states and territories from the moment of their manufacture until their administration. Usually only registered doctors and dentists are allowed to prescribe drugs, and pharmacists to dispense them. There are exceptions; for example, in some states of Australia, specially qualified nurse practitioners, optometrists and podiatrists have the right to prescribe a limited number of relevant S4 (Prescription Only) drugs. The roles of various health professionals with respect to drugs have been described in Chapter 2.

MANUFACTURE AND WHOLESALING OF POISONS (DRUGS)

All states and territories require manufacturers and whole-salers of Schedule 2, 3, 4 and 8 poisons (and Schedule 9 for wholesaling) to be licensed. The licence may relate exclusively to a poison of a particular Schedule, or it may be a licence to manufacture poisons in a particular poisons Schedule or Schedules, classes of substances or specific substances. The security and record-keeping obligations are less rigorous for Schedule 2, 3 and 4 poisons than for S8 or S9. Licences are generally issued by the relevant state or territory Minister or department, for a fee.

The Therapeutic Goods Act also contains provisions covering counterfeiting, recall procedures, reporting of adverse effects, and record keeping by manufacturers.

RETAILING

In all jurisdictions except Western Australia, poisons legislation authorises pharmacists to possess, manufacture and supply poisons without a licence in the practice of their profession. The circumstances and manner in which the supply can be made, e.g. whether or not a prescription is required, and record-keeping requirements, depend on the Schedule of the substance in question.

SAMPLING

State and territory legislation usually permits representatives of licensed manufacturers and wholesalers to possess and supply samples of certain poisons.

PACKAGING AND LABELLING

The labelling and packaging of drugs for use in humans are governed by orders and regulations made under the *Therapeutic Goods Act* and by the SUSDP, as transcribed or adopted by state and territory legislation. It is an offence in

Commonwealth and state laws to fail to comply with labelling and packaging standards for therapeutic goods.

Part of the pharmacist's role is to ensure that medicines are labelled correctly to ensure safe storage and administration. Some labels are advisory, e.g:
• THIS MEDICINE MAY CAUSE DROWSINESS
• DISCARD CONTENTS AFTER dd/mm/yyyy.
• RINSE MOUTH WITH WATER AFTER EACH USE
• REFRIGERATE: DO NOT FREEZE
Other labels are explanatory or reminders, such as:
• CERTAIN FOODS AND DRUGS SHOULD NOT BE TAKEN WITH THIS MEDICINE
• SHAKE THE BOTTLE
• THIS PRESCRIPTION MAY BE REPEATED . . . TIMES
• KEEP OUT OF REACH OF CHILDREN
• TAKE IMMEDIATELY BEFORE FOOD
Many of the requirements for labelling are determined by the Schedule into which a drug or poison is classified (see *Australian Medicines Handbook* Appendix D).

POSSESSION

Certain persons are authorised to possess Schedule 4 and 8 poisons for legitimate commercial, professional, academic, research or emergency purposes. In all states and territories the unauthorised or unlicensed possession of Schedule 8 or 9 poisons is a criminal offence (see Drug Offences, below).

PRESCRIPTION

Generally, Schedule 4 or 8 poisons can be prescribed by medical practitioners, dentists and veterinary surgeons in the lawful practice of their respective professions for the treatment of persons (or animals) under their care. The circumstances in which these poisons can be prescribed differ across the states. There are also special prescribing requirements for patients whom medical practitioners believe are drug-dependent. (The requirements for prescription writing, and sample prescriptions, are discussed in Chapter 2.)

DISPENSING

Legally valid prescriptions for Schedule 4 and 8 poisons can be filled by pharmacists or by the prescriber for his or her own patients. For certain poisons in these Schedules, e.g. dextromoramide, hydromorphone and methadone, there are extra controls on dispensing (see Drug Monograph 22-2). In all states and territories except the ACT, pharmacists can prescribe Schedule 4 drugs without a prescription in an emergency; however, a valid written prescription must be provided by the prescriber as soon as is practicable.

ADMINISTRATION

As a general rule, the administration of Schedule 4 and 8 poisons to a person requires the written or verbal authorisation of a medical practitioner or dentist. There are significant exceptions to this rule, such as administration in emergency situations and by certain professionals such as podiatrists and nurses. (Regulations with respect to telephone orders and standing orders are described in Chapter 2.)

STORAGE AND DESTRUCTION

There are strict security requirements concerning the storage and destruction of Schedule 4 and 8 poisons by manufacturers, wholesalers and pharmacists, and in hospitals.

It is usually essential for some drugs to be stored on hospital wards, to provide ready and out-of-hours access. An 'imprest' system of lockable cupboards, trolleys and bedside drawers is used. Strict procedures must be maintained with respect to security of drugs, accuracy of records, 'loaning' of drugs between wards, monitoring access by staff, control of keys to drug stores, and disposal of unused or expired drugs. The hospital's director of pharmacy or chief pharmacist should have ultimate responsibility and control.

The storage requirements imposed on doctors, dentists and veterinary surgeons are less stringent, in recognition of the fact that these practitioners are less likely to store large quantities of Schedule 4, 8 or 9 poisons.

RECORD KEEPING

People involved in the manufacture, supply, dispensing or administration of Schedule 4 and 8 poisons (except the patient who actually receives the drug) are required to account in writing for every instance that the poison is dealt with.

Therapeutic goods

The Commonwealth *Therapeutic Goods Act* regulates 'therapeutic goods', defined as medicines, blood products and medical devices. As mentioned above, a substance may be a poison and a therapeutic good, in which case both the state poisons legislation and the Commonwealth therapeutic goods legislation may apply.

Because of Constitutional restrictions, the *Therapeutic Goods Act* can regulate therapeutic goods only in certain circumstances. Much of the regulation of therapeutic goods exists in the state poisons legislation, discussed above.

Before a drug (or other therapeutic good) can be marketed in Australia, it must be evaluated by the Therapeutic Goods Administration (TGA), a division of the Commonwealth Department of Health and Ageing, which assesses the product for quality, safety, efficacy and cost-effectiveness, and considers the extent to which the drug should be made available to the public (see Figure 4-1). Sponsors, usually drug companies, are required to submit to the TGA an enormous amount of material relevant to the application for approval, including chemical and manufacturing data and results from pharmacological testing in vitro, in vivo and in clinical trials. This material is examined closely by experienced evaluators, a process that may take some months, and may be referred to an expert committee (the Australian Drug Evaluation Committee, ADEC) for its comments. The TGA makes the final decision on whether or not to register the drug for therapeutic use in Australia and decides into which Schedule it should be put.

The process also applies to non-prescription drugs (OTC and 'listed' drugs [see Chapter 3]), complementary and alternative remedies (as discussed in Chapter 3) and to medical devices such as breast implants, diagnostic test kits, dental materials, contact lenses and tampons. There is a 'Special Access Scheme' covering approval for supply of unapproved therapeutic goods for a specified purpose.

MANUFACTURE

Irrespective of whether the goods are or are not in a poisons Schedule, manufacturers of therapeutic goods for supply in Australia for use in humans must hold a licence under the *Therapeutic Goods Act*. Some types of drug and certain persons are exempt from the licensing requirements.

Examples of drugs that are exempt goods are homeopathic remedies, antiperspirants and acne cleansers. Examples of exempt persons are most registered health professionals, such as doctors and pharmacists in the usual practice of their professions, and a wide range of practitioners of alternative health-care modalities.

SUPPLY AND WHOLESALING

It is an offence to supply by wholesale therapeutic goods that are not on the Australian Register of Therapeutic Goods. Because the Therapeutic Goods Act cannot always apply for Constitutional reasons, New South Wales, Victoria and the Northern Territory have created similar offences under state law.

ADVERTISING

Various state Acts, based on the *Therapeutic Goods Regulations (Cth)* and the SUSDP, have prohibited the advertising of Schedules 4, 8 and 9 poisons to the general public. Such advertisements are allowed to be included in bona fide professional publications. Unscheduled substances and poisons in Schedules 2 and 3 can be advertised directly to the public in certain circumstances.

CLINICAL TRIALS

Complicated provisions in the *Therapeutic Goods Act* and its Regulations govern the use of experimental drugs and testing in animals and humans. These are discussed in subsequent sections of this chapter.

ORPHAN DRUGS

Orphan drugs are highly specialised drugs used to treat, prevent or diagnose rare diseases. It is recognised that, while such drugs might not be commercially viable, patients with rare conditions have as much right as all others to access drugs that are safe and effective for their treatment.

In 1983 in the USA, the Food and Drug Administration (FDA) established the *Orphan Drug Act*, which provided grants to encourage research to find drugs for treatment of rare chronic diseases. Because such research was unprofitable, it was very limited before this Act. Among the disorders that benefit from this research are cystic fibrosis, von Willebrand's disease, leprosy (Hansen's disease), AIDS and rare cancers.

Australia's TGA has based its Orphan Drug Program (formerly known as Section 100 Items) on that of the FDA. The program encourages sponsors (drug companies) by reducing the costs associated with drug research, approval and marketing. Fees for application and evaluation processes are waived, exclusive approval of a drug may be given and approval times are shortened. The drugs are usually supplied only through hospitals with appropriate specialist facilities, and funding is subsidised by the government only for the listed indications.

The criteria under which a drug may be considered for 'orphan status' are that there are fewer than 2000 affected individuals in Australia, or, for vaccines, the vaccine would be given fewer than 2000 times per year; or the costs involved in developing the drug are prohibitive. Most of the conditions involved are serious diseases. The drug does not need to be the only drug for treatment for the condition, but if it is a new drug, it must be clinically superior. Drugs already rejected on safety grounds, or already registered or considered essential drugs, are not considered for the program. If approved and registered, the drug may be considered for listing on the Pharmaceutical Benefits Scheme (PBS), and will be required to be subjected to post-marketing surveillance for safety and efficacy. Examples of orphan drugs are listed in Table 4-2.

The Pharmaceutical Benefits Scheme (PBS)

Set up under the *National Health Act 1953* (Cth), the PBS is a program in which already registered drugs deemed to be essential to the community but too expensive for individual purchase are subsidised by the government to some extent. Over 100 million prescriptions are subsidised each year and the numbers and costs are increasing, currently 0.7% of GDP. The overall process is shown diagrammatically in Figure 4-1.

On the advice of an expert committee, the Pharmaceutical Benefits Advisory Committee (PBAC), the government lists recommended drugs for subsidy and negotiates a price. This of course encourages wider use of the drugs, as they are more affordable, and so members of the committee, government and doctors are under considerable pressure from drug companies to ensure that their drugs are PBS-listed. There has been great concern recently as to the composition of the committee and the blow-out in costs when new drugs have been subsidised and used to a far greater extent than anticipated (e.g. celecoxib, a newer anti-inflammatory agent, and bupropion, for quitting smoking).

SUBSTITUTION OF DRUGS (GENERIC PRESCRIBING)

In an attempt to keep down the escalating costs of drugs to the community, doctors are encouraged to prescribe generic rather than name brand drugs considered equivalent; this allows the pharmacist to supply (and the government to subsidise) the cheapest alternative. This is allowed only if the doctor agrees, and if the alternatives are considered 'bioequivalent' (see mock prescription, Figure 2-1B, and

TABLE 4-2 Examples of orphan drugs (S100 Items)

ORPHAN DRUG	RARE CONDITION TREATED
Aldesleukin (interleukin-2)	Metastatic renal cell carcinoma, metastatic malignant melanoma
Nandrolone decanoate	Debilitated patients with HIV infection
Specified antifungals and antivirals	Patients with AIDS-related infections
Recombinant blood factors VIII and IX	Haemophilia A and B
Enzymes for replacement	Congenital metabolic diseases, e.g. lipid storage diseases, Fabry's disease, Gaucher's disease
Peritoneal dialysis solutions	End-stage renal disease
Rabies vaccine	Contacts with rabid animals
Recombinant human growth hormone	Specific conditions involving short stature, e.g. Prader–Willi syndrome
Some antineoplastic agents	Cancers unresponsive to usual therapy: multiple myeloma, ovarian cancer, metastatic melanoma
Thalidomide	Leprous skin reactions, multiple myeloma
Tobramycin inhalation solution	Cystic fibrosis patients with respiratory tract infections
Tumour necrosis factor α 1-a	Soft tissue sarcoma

Drug regulation: from new drug application to the prescription pad

Below is a brief representation of the main processes of drug regulation in Australia.

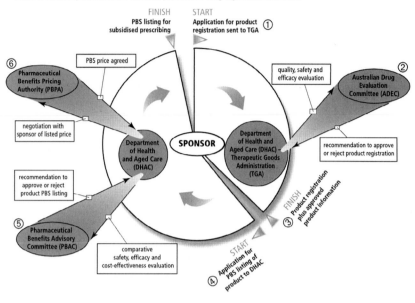

Diagram is a simplified schematic representation of the process.
The time taken for individual applications to move through the system does differ.

How it works

1. A sponsor (usually a pharmaceutical company) applies to the Therapeutic Goods Administration (TGA) to register a new drug, a new presentation of an existing drug, or a new indication for an existing drug, for use in Australia.

2. The Australian Drug Evaluation Committee (ADEC) advises the TGA on the quality, safety and efficacy of the new drug application.

3. Once approved by the TGA, the pharmaceutical company can market the new drug for its approved indications. At this stage, the drug can be prescribed by GPs on private prescriptions only.

4. The pharmaceutical company may decide to apply to the Department of Health and Aged Care for listing on the Pharmaceutical Benefits Scheme (PBS).

5. The Pharmaceutical Benefits Advisory Committee (PBAC) advises the Minister for Health and Aged Care on the comparative safety, efficacy, cost-effectiveness, and clinical role of the new drug relative to existing therapies on the PBS.

6. If PBS listing of the drug is recommended, the pharmaceutical company negotiates the PBS-listed price with the Pharmaceutical Benefits Pricing Authority (PBPA).

   The PBS listing of a new drug allows Commonwealth-subsidised prescribing of the new drug for those indications listed in the Schedule of Pharmaceutical Benefits (yellow book) only. PBS-listed indications may be a subset of the approved indications for the drug; there is no subsidy for drugs used for indications which are not listed on the PBS.

FIGURE 4-1 Drug Regulation in Australia: from new drug application to the prescription pad.
Source: National Prescribing Service Newsletter 2001: 19; used with permission.

related discussion). Drugs for which bioavailability can vary markedly between different formulations, and which therefore are not allowed to be substituted, are those with a low therapeutic index (safety margin) and low lipid solubility. Such drugs include digoxin (a cardiac glycoside used in heart failure), theophylline (a smooth muscle relaxant used for relief of bronchospasm in certain respiratory conditions) and phenytoin (an antiepileptic drug).

Legal aspects of concern to pharmacists

As the supplier of many OTC and all prescription-only drugs, the final responsibility for safe supply rests with the pharmacist; hence there are many regulations as to the pharmacist's professional roles and conduct. State and territory Acts, Regulations and Pharmacy Board guidelines cover aspects such as:

- training, examination and registration of pharmacists
- the practice of pharmacy, including control of the dispensary, dispensing, labelling, counselling and record keeping
- possession, storage and supply of drugs
- good pharmaceutical practice
- services to residential care facilities.
  Typical day-to-day issues for pharmacists involve:
- requests for excessive supplies
- clients who appear to be 'doctor shopping' for excessive numbers of prescriptions

- prescriptions for Schedule 8 (CONTROLLED DRUGS) for which the pharmacist is concerned about possible forgery
- loss or theft of drugs
- suspected self-prescribing by doctors
- ensuring that requests for Schedule 3 (PHARMACIST ONLY) drugs are warranted by an appropriate condition being diagnosed
- administration of the methadone maintenance program, if they are involved (see Drug Monograph 22-2).

Medicines in pregnancy

The Australian Drug Evaluation Committee has set up an 'Australian categorisation of risk of drug use in pregnancy' (see Table 8-1). The categories are described in detail in Chapter 8. In order of increasing potential risk, they are:

- A: drugs that have been taken by a large number of pregnant women without harmful effects on the fetus (e.g. most penicillins, salbutamol, iron, folic acid)
- B1 (e.g. anthelmintics, H₂-antagonists), B2 (e.g. antihistamines, some vaccines), B3 (e.g. oestrogens, trimethoprim)
- C (e.g. morphine, β-blockers, some NSAIDs)
- D: drugs that have caused or may cause fetal malformations or damage (e.g. cytotoxic agents, ACE inhibitors)
- X: drugs that have such a high risk of permanent fetal damage that they should not be used in pregnancy or when there is a possibility of pregnancy (e.g. isotretinoin, misoprostol).

The classification is a warning to users and prescribers of the dangers of drug use in pregnancy, and a reminder that there are two individuals being administered the drug (the woman and the fetus), and it also offers the opportunity for the user or prescriber to select the safest drug that will have the desired effects.

Drugs in sport

The use of drugs by athletes and during sporting competition is regulated not so much by the government (although there is some state legislation, e.g. *Drugs in Sport Act 1999* [ACT]) as by the International Olympic Movement and its Anti-Doping Rules, and the World Anti-Doping Agency (see Chapter 57). In Australia this is implemented by the Australian Sports Anti-Doping Authority, set up in March 2006 in Canberra. Drugs are classified into groups depending on whether they are allowed, allowed under certain circumstances, prohibited, or prohibited in some sports.

Drug offences

Laws relating to drugs are relatively recent, dating from the 1890s in relation to opium, and the early 1900s in relation to other drugs. The enactment of drug legislation in Australia has followed the social trends and scientific knowledge of the time. In his book *From Mr Sin to Mr Big*, Desmond Manderson argues that historically in Australia the selective enactment of drug laws has also been influenced by racism, powerful international pressures and the vested interests of the medical profession, bureaucrats and politicians. He uses the example of opium:

> In nineteenth-century Australia, opium was the preserve of neither the creative few nor the urban poor. It was freely available and freely used. Furthermore, perhaps partly as a consequence of the weakness of the medical profession, the line which is now seen to divide medical 'use' from non-medical 'abuse' was not yet apparent.

By the late 1880s, however, opium was seen as a 'pollutant, moral as well as physical' and was associated with Chinese 'opium dens'. Soon after, its use was criminalised.

Foreign trends and international law have also influenced Australian drug policy. Two pieces of Commonwealth legislation that relate to certain dealings in drugs, both within and outside Australia, the *Crimes (Traffic in Narcotic Drugs and Psychotropic Substances) Act 1990* (Cth) and the *Narcotic Goods Act 1967* (Cth), were introduced pursuant to United Nations Conventions.

There is much debate about whether the criminalisation of certain drugs reduces or increases the harm associated with drug use. The negative consequences of criminalisation are said to include social problems, related criminal offences and the high cost of enforcement. Proponents of decriminalisation argue that without the adverse reactions associated with their illegal character, drug offences are 'victimless': consumers, producers and suppliers share an interest in continued production and supply of drugs. In this way, drug offences are unlike other serious crimes. Some commentators believe that certain drugs should be decriminalised (e.g. marijuana) or have their regulation modified (e.g. heroin) to reduce the associated harm.

Legislation

Like the laws regulating poisons and therapeutic goods in Australia, drug offences are set out in Commonwealth, state and territory legislation. Dealings with drugs can be an offence under both Commonwealth and state and territory laws. Responsibility for the policing of drug laws is shared by the Commonwealth, states and territories.

Commonwealth legislation proscribes the importation and exportation of narcotic drugs, the possession of drugs that have been illegally imported, and certain dealings in drugs within and outside Australia. Commonwealth laws also regulate the manufacture of certain **proscribed drugs**.

State legislation proscribes the possession, production and distribution of certain drugs. Because of the historical origins of these offences, they appear in the same legislation that governs poisons and, in some states and territories, also appear in the state or territory's Crimes Act or Criminal Code.

Generally, for offences for which possession of the drug is a necessary part, it will be a defence to show that the possession was authorised (for example, the defendant holds a licence or is authorised under the relevant state law to deal with the drug as part of his or her profession).

Which drugs are proscribed (illegal)?

The drugs that are proscribed in the states, territories and the Commonwealth are very similar, although the means of definition and classification of proscribed drugs varies across the jurisdictions. Drugs that are proscribed are usually set out in an authoritative list, which is often based on the SUSDP.

Commonwealth offences

The principal piece of Commonwealth legislation containing drug offences is the *Criminal Code Act 1995* (Cth). The Criminal Code is supplemented by the *Customs Act 1901* (Cth) and the *Narcotic Goods Act*. Part 9.1 of the Criminal Code addresses the trafficking, illegal manufacture, supply and possession of controlled drugs and plants. Prohibited conduct under the Criminal Code includes: the cultivation of certain plants (e.g. opium poppy) to produce narcotic drugs; making narcotic drugs or psychotropic substances; and the sale, supply or possession of a narcotic drug or psychotropic substance. Offences under the Criminal Code relate to conduct wholly or partly in Australia, dealing in drugs on board an Australian aircraft in flight or an Australian ship at sea, and dealings outside Australia in various circumstances.

The *Customs Act* also details offences relating to importing or exporting narcotic goods. The *Narcotic Goods Act* forbids the manufacture of a drug unless the manufacturer holds a licence to do so. It contains other restrictions on the manufacture of drugs, including constraints on the premises, conditions of licence, labelling requirements and permission to destroy drugs, narcotic preparations or byproducts.

State and territory offences

In all Australian states and territories it is an offence to possess, produce, use, sell, distribute or supply drugs that are proscribed, unless the Act in question was otherwise authorised. In some jurisdictions there exist related offences, such as the possession of equipment for use in relation to proscribed drugs. In most jurisdictions it is an offence, unless authorised, to:

- use or have within one's possession a proscribed drug or plant
- consume, use or self-administer a proscribed drug or allow someone else to administer a drug to oneself
- produce or manufacture a proscribed drug or cultivate a proscribed plant

- take part in a step in the process of production of a proscribed drug or plant
- deal in, distribute, traffic in, sell, supply or offer to sell or supply a proscribed drug
- possess more than a prescribed quantity of a proscribed drug (prescribed quantities are set out for particular drugs).

A range of related offences exists in certain states and territories, such as the theft of proscribed drugs, the possession of property derived from drug dealing, possessing instructions or equipment for producing proscribed drugs, and various offences related to prescriptions for proscribed drugs. The practices of health professionals are usually governed by relevant Acts of Parliament (such as the *Nurses Act*) and by regulations of the appropriate professional board (e.g. the Podiatrists Registration Board of Victoria). These are specific to the profession concerned, and details of their functions are beyond the scope of this book.

While drug offences are dealt with in state and territory criminal justice systems, some states have set up 'drug courts' and diversion programs to divert illicit drug users from prisons into treatment programs.

New Zealand drug regulations
Scheduling and subsidisation of drugs

In New Zealand, legislation relevant to drugs is contained in the *Medicines Act* 1981 and Regulations (1984). Drugs are scheduled, more simply than in Australia, into three main categories:

- prescription-only
- restricted (pharmacist-only)
- pharmacy-only, or licensed shops where they are more than 10 km from the nearest pharmacy.

All other products are for general sales. There are no registration numbers assigned to products to show that they have been approved for sale, as there are in the Australian system.

Despite efforts at Trans-Tasman Harmonisation and simplification, there are still some differences in the scheduling of drugs. Single-agent sedating (old) antihistamines, for example, are S3 (pharmacist-only) in Australia, except when used as antiemetics against travel sickness (S2), but pharmacy-only in New Zealand, except in small packs as 'sleeping aids', when they are pharmacist-only. Nicotine replacement gums are pharmacy-only in Australia but general sales in New Zealand, whereas salbutamol metered-dose inhalers are pharmacist-only in Australia but require a prescription in New Zealand, possibly reflecting the concern over some decades about higher than expected mortality rates due to asthma there.

Some nurses in New Zealand also have limited prescribing rights, as do midwives, and New Zealand allows direct-to-consumer advertising of drugs, which is usually prohibited in Australia. With respect to categories of safety of drugs in pregnancy, New Zealand follows the Australian guidelines and categories.

PHARMAC is a New Zealand Crown body with the responsibility for managing the pharmaceutical budget. It tenders for the subsidised drugs and its committees set the access criteria applying to expensive items. In the year 2000/01, it negotiated subsidy reductions worth about NZ$50 million. The top six expenditure groups of drugs in New Zealand recently were lipid-modifying agents, antiulcerants, antipsychotics, agents affecting the renin–angiotensin system, antidepressants and inhaled corticosteroids. This list can be compared with the lists of the top 10 drugs in Australia (Table 1-3); despite the differences in how the lists are compiled, the similarities are striking.

Controlled drugs (drugs of dependence)

The *New Zealand Dangerous Drugs Act 1927* dealt with the controls required for opium and non-opiate drugs for which regulation was required by the League of Nations. Before this, opium was readily available in many pharmaceutical preparations; however, the main drugs causing problems (then as now) were alcohol and tobacco.

After World War II, cannabis and amphetamines began to appear as problem drugs and in the 'hippy' days of the 1960s and 1970s people experimented with *Datura* (containing the plant alkaloids atropine and hyoscine), amphetamines, hallucinogens and solvent sniffing. The *Narcotics Act 1965* included controls on mescaline, cocaine and LSD as well as opiates. The *Misuse of Drugs Act 1975* and subsequent Regulations (1977) classified **controlled drugs** into different schedules to allow different penalties depending on the severity of the abuse. Alcohol and tobacco are excluded from the Acts; alcohol is subject to the *Sale of Liquor Act 1989* and amendments.

The United Nations Single Convention on Narcotic Drugs (1961, 1972) imposed wider controls on possession and use as well as production and trafficking in drugs, including marijuana. Countries signatory to this Convention are constrained to abide by its international agreements. There is some debate in New Zealand as to the wisdom of including marijuana along with drugs such as heroin and cocaine; drug trafficking and abuse of the latter two cause much more devastating consequences (Fastier 1998).

STANDARDISATION OF DRUGS

Medicines (formulations of drugs) may vary considerably in strength and activity depending on the amounts of active drug(s) they contain. Drugs obtained from plants such as

opium and digitalis may fluctuate in strength depending on where the plants are grown, the season during which they are harvested and how they are preserved or extracted. Because accurate dosage and reliability of a drug's effect depend on uniformity of strength and purity, **standardisation** and publication of standards are necessary. (Drug information resources, pharmacopoeias and formularies are reviewed in Chapter 1.)

Standards for drug quality and actions
Drug standards in Australia

The main standards for drugs in Australia are those published in the **British Pharmacopoeia*** by the British Pharmacopoeia Commission, and those in the **Australian Pharmaceutical Formulary** (APF). The BP gives detailed, legally accepted standards for hundreds of drugs, with chemical information and the approved formulations that contain the substance, and lists criteria for purity, chemical methods for identification and **assay**, tests for likely contaminants, and maximum levels allowed for impurities. Preparations shown to meet these standards are then referred to as the BP preparation; for example, 'Morphine Sulphate BP' must contain 98%–102% of the stated amount; methods for identification and assay are given and limits set for the levels of iron, codeine, pseudomorphine and hydroxymorphine.

The BP also has monographs for natural substances. For Opium BP it notes that "Raw opium is the air-dried latex obtained by incision from the unripe capsules of *Papaver somniferum* . . . it contains not less than 10.0% of morphine and not less than 2% of codeine . . . Raw opium has a characteristic odour and a blackish-brown colour." Test methods are given for its identification (under microscope and by thin-layer chromatography) and assay by liquid chromatography. The maximum limit for the contaminant thebaine is 3%.

The **APF** by contrast, is more a reference and 'recipe book' for pharmacists. As well as much useful medical information and dispensing practice guidelines, it gives the standard formulae for many formulations. For Calamine Lotion APF, for example, it lists the six ingredients and their amounts, gives the method for preparation of the lotion, and describes its uses.

Assays

The technique, either chemical or biological, by which the strength and purity of a drug are measured is known as an **assay**. Chemical assay is a chemical analysis to determine the ingredients present and their amounts. Opium, for example,

---

*The 'BP', as it is fondly known by generations of pharmacy students and pharmacists.

is known to contain certain alkaloids and these may vary greatly in different preparations; the BP's official standard gives details of assay methods for these alkaloids.

Bioassays

For some drugs, either the active ingredients are not completely identified or there are no available chemical methods of analysing and standardising them. These drugs may be standardised by biological methods, or **bioassay**. A bioassay is a biological test method for measuring the amount of a pharmacologically active substance in a preparation (tissue extract or pharmaceutical formulation). **Bioassays** are typically performed by determining the amount of a preparation required to produce a defined effect on a suitable laboratory animal or tissue under certain standard conditions, and then comparing the response to that produced by a standard preparation in the same bioassay. Examples of early bioassays were for the potency of a sample of insulin measured by its ability to lower the blood glucose levels of rabbits, or the strength of digoxin preparations by their effects on human electrocardiogram tracings.

    Bioassays are especially applicable to:
- substances that are poorly defined chemically
- mixtures containing chemically very similar substances (e.g. optical isomers, of which only one is active)
- highly active substances, especially endogenous mediators, present in very small amounts
- testing drugs in animals to predict effects in humans.

    Bioassays require setting up a model system on which pharmacological activities can be measured. The classic is the isolated guinea-pig ileum smooth muscle preparation, which responds to stimulation by several neurotransmitters and other endogenous mediators. The test method may be *in vitro* (in glass), e.g. using a suspension of an enzyme, a cell or tissue culture, a microbiological culture, a standard preparation of an antibody, or an isolated organ or tissue,* or *in vivo* (in the living organism), e.g. testing the effect of a drug on blood pressure or behaviour.** Some drug actions are virtually impossible to test either *in vitro* or *in vivo*, particularly effects of centrally acting agents on mood, perception and thought processes.

    Because of **biological variability** there may be variations in results and lack of precision in quoting the absolute amount of biologically active material. Bioassays are no longer used as frequently as previously because techniques such as radioimmunoassay (RIA, itself a type of bioassay) and high-performance liquid chromatography (HPLC) have allowed very low levels of chemicals to be measured accurately without using animals. The BP 2000 gave methods for bioassay of several drugs, including:
- depressor substances (tested for activity in lowering cat blood pressure, against a histamine standard)
- histamine activity (on isolated guinea-pig intestinal smooth muscle, against a histamine standard)
- corticotrophin (activity increasing the function of adrenal glands in hypophysectomised rats)
- tests for acute toxicity (24 hours, in five mice).

    There are also BP biological tests for biological products such as blood-clotting factors, cytokines (e.g. interferons), vaccines, antibiotics and pyrogens (substances that cause fever), and tests for microbiological sterility or contamination.

    The design of bioassays usually involves comparison of two preparations, a standard and an unknown, by testing many concentrations of each on the same model and constructing log dose–response curves. If the substances act by similar mechanisms, the curves will be roughly parallel in their mid-sections and so the potency ratio can be determined, allowing the strength of the unknown to be calculated compared to the known standard (see Figure 5-4).

    Clinical trials (see later section) are essentially bioassays in humans: the new drug (unknown) is tested against the best currently available therapy (standard), and compared for safety and efficacy.

International Units of Activity

The strength of extracts of natural substances for which the purity is not 100% cannot be expressed in absolute terms such as grams or milligrams, as it cannot be assumed that the whole weight is due to the active ingredient. For such preparations that are assayed biologically, a unit of pharmacological activity must be defined to compare the unknown with the standard. In the past a particular standard, e.g. of an animal hormone,

---

*The use of isolated tissues to assay responses reached an extraordinarily sophisticated level in the classic experiments of Sir John Vane at the Royal College of Surgeons in London in the 1960s. A set of five organ-baths was set up in vertical series such that the physiological saline solution from the top bath flowed down over (superfused) the next bath, and so on down the cascade. Small samples of GIT smooth muscle from four different species were set up in the baths, and the pattern of responses to seven endogenous mediators, including noradrenaline, bradykinin, prostaglandins, and antidiuretic hormone, was studied. Using this technique, Vane discovered the mechanism of action of aspirin and other non-steroidal anti-inflammatory drugs, viz. inhibition of the synthesis of prostaglandins, for which he was subsequently awarded the 1982 Nobel Prize for Medicine (Vane 1971).

**There is currently a worldwide dearth of pharmacologists with the skills necessary to carry out in-vivo studies in medical research or to train new generations of students in these techniques. This has come about largely because of the decrease in the number of practical classes held in pharmacology courses and the replacement of animal experiments with computer-modelled 'practicals'. In-vivo work, however, is vital for the analysis of drug actions and development of new drugs.

enzyme preparation or plant alkaloid, was designated the International Standard preparation, against which other national standard preparations were assayed, and then these latter were used to standardise all preparations. In Australia, for example, the Commonwealth Serum Laboratories (CSL) in Melbourne maintained the national standards for insulins, and all CSL insulin preparations were compared to them. The strengths of preparations were expressed in terms of **International Units of Activity** (IU), for whatever activity was measured in the particular bioassay (see Clinical Interest Box 41-1).

Statistical methods in bioassays

Variability in responses to drugs may be due to many causes, including errors in measurement and inherent biological variability both within and between individuals. In bioassays the same dose repeated may therefore give differing responses and the dose required to give the same response varies. Consequently, biological experiments need to be repeated many times to get an average or mean result, which is taken to represent the true value. Variability in responses can be partly reduced by refining methods and using a very homogeneous population of animals or very similar subjects, but this reduces the wide applicability of the results.

Statistical methods are then applied to deal with random variations and to extrapolate from the sample mean to the population. (Such techniques are the province of a text on biostatistics rather than pharmacology—see Clinical Interest Box 4-3.) In the pharmacological context, statistical methods are typically applied to bioassays studying dose–response relationships, cause–effect correlations, differences between groups of subjects treated in different ways, and clinical trials. Usually a '**null hypothesis**' is defined (i.e. that there is no statistically significant difference between the groups being studied), and when results are analysed the null hypothesis is either accepted or rejected. The probability level at which the results are accepted as being due to a real difference rather than occurring by chance is usually set at 0.05, i.e. there is only 5% chance (1 in 20) that the results could have occurred by chance. Typical statistical tests employed are either parametric (assuming a normal distribution of results) such as Student's *t*-test, analysis of variance, or variance ratio; or non-parametric (when normality cannot be assumed), e.g. the sign test, or Wilcoxon rank-sum test.

DRUG DISCOVERY AND DEVELOPMENT

Drug discovery

There are several main ways in which drugs are 'discovered', i.e. ways in which the potential therapeutic uses of chemicals are determined. The routes to drug discovery are not mutually exclusive and an eclectic approach is often the most successful. This has been summarised as "three steps: understand the science, unravel the story, and . . . apply the technology" (Handen 2005).

Development from herbal or traditional remedies

For thousands of years people have been trying natural products—plants, minerals and parts of animals—to see if they were useful as foods or in treating disease (these sources of drugs have been discussed in detail in Chapters 1 and 3). Examples of drugs developed from natural sources include morphine and codeine from the opium poppy *Papaver somniferum*, atropine from the belladonna lily *Atropa belladonna*, growth hormone from extracts of pituitary gland, insulin from beef and pig pancreas, and iron and iodine from mineral resources. The natural products may be used as crude extracts, such as raw opium or herbal teas, or purified and/or synthesised and then formulated as pharmaceutical preparations, such as tablets and injections.

This route to new drugs is sometimes called the 'reefs and rainforests' approach, as it is recognised that there are millions of natural chemicals out there needing to be identified and tested before exploitation and despoilation of the world's resources permanently terminate our chances of finding novel anticancer or antibiotic agents (for example).

Serendipity (sheer good luck)

While luck plays a part in some drug discoveries, such as Fleming's bacterial culture plate becoming contaminated with a growth of the fungus *Penicillium notatum*, it usually takes lateral thinking (e.g. questioning why growth of the bacterial culture was inhibited near the fungus), intelligence and years of hard work (extracting the natural antibacterial agent or antibiotic, determining its structure and developing methods of mass production) to exploit the lucky find (producing enough penicillin to treat people with bacterial infections).

Other examples of serendipity in pharmacological discovery are the finding that patients treated with the first safe oral antibacterial agents, sulfonamides, had a lowering in their blood glucose levels, which had a 'spin-off' to the development of the sulfonylurea oral hypoglycaemic agents; the finding that hypertensive patients treated with the vasodilator minoxidil tended to grow more hair (the drug is now mainly used as a hair restorer); and the finding that sildenafil, undergoing clinical trial as a vasodilator in cardiovascular disease, was unexpectedly popular with the male subjects in the trial, leading to its exploitation as a treatment for impotence (see Drug Monograph 47-3 and Clinical Interest Box 47-3).

Empirical chemistry plus pharmacological studies

As chemical techniques developed in the 20th century, the chemical structures of pharmacologically active substances

---

CLINICAL INTEREST BOX 4-2
HIGH-THROUGHPUT SCREENING

High-throughput screening (HTS) refers to the process whereby millions of chemicals can be put through automated biochemical tests, in minute amounts, in very rapid times. The aim is to discover 'lead compounds'—those that lead to potentially useful drugs. Such screens have been described as 'fishing trips', trawling through millions of compounds in the hope of catching something interesting.

The tests are carried out in an array of tiny 'cells' (minute test-tubes) or on silicon chips, leading to the term 'in silico' for this type of assay, as distinct from in vitro and in vivo. Most tests involve a particular protein (e.g. receptor, enzyme, ion channel or antibody), gene or RNA fragment in the cell or on the chip, and the amount of binding of the new compounds to the protein or gene is determined. Tests may be based on enzyme-linked immunosorbent assays (ELISA) and commonly use high-performance liquid chromatography–mass spectrometry technologies (HPLC–MS) and/or fluorescence methods.

Binding is picked up electrically by a voltage-sensing detector and registers as a 'blip' signal. Positive binding can be followed up in laboratory assays to determine the nature and strength of the binding, e.g. whether the compound is an agonist or antagonist at a receptor or whether a particular enzyme activity is enhanced or inhibited

Gene fragments and RNA molecules from the huge databases of the Human Genome Project can be checked in different disease states, to test for under- or overexpression of encoded proteins, identify genes implicated in disease or diagnose inherited diseases or predisposition to cancers. HTS methods can also be applied to pharmacokinetic aspects of new compounds, checking for enzymes responsible for metabolism, rapidity of metabolism and inhibition or induction of drug-metabolising enzymes.

Pharmaceutical characteristics of the compounds can be tested, such as solubility and permeability, and potential for crossing the blood–brain barrier. HTS procedures are also applied to toxicological analysis, e.g. detection simultaneously of several different compounds in forensic samples in criminal cases, or doping control in sport.

The procedures are highly automated, using robot technology, and are computer-controlled. In an HTS facility, millions of compounds can be screened per month. Using HTS, drug companies hope not only to discover new drugs but also to reduce the drop-out rate of compounds in the later, more expensive stages of animal and human testing.

---

could be determined and similar substances synthesised and then tested for activities. These structure–activity relations led to the development of many drug groups; for example, all the sympathomimetic amines were initially noradrenaline 'look-alikes', and the second- and third-generation penicillins were adapted from the first penicillin.

Active metabolites of existing drugs

Sometimes drugs have been found to be more active after metabolism in the body and so the metabolites are tested as drugs. Paracetamol is one of the metabolites of phenacetin, an early antipyretic analgesic agent, and is much safer. Many of the benzodiazepine antianxiety agents have pharmacologically active metabolites, some of which are marketed as distinct drugs in their own rights.

Rational molecular design

Structure–activity studies can lead to speculation as to the shape of the active site of a receptor and to the design and synthesis of drugs that may be agonists or antagonists at that receptor. Studies of *Ephedra sinica*, long known in traditional Chinese medicine to be useful in respiratory conditions (asthma), led to the purification of the active ingredient, ephedrine, then synthesis of the related compounds isoprenaline (a useful antiasthmatic drug), salbutamol (a β_2-adrenoceptor agonist with fewer cardiovascular adverse reactions), and the β-blockers such as metoprolol (a selective β_1-receptor antagonist useful in cardiovascular diseases and with less likelihood of causing asthma than non-selective forms). The early antihistamines were modelled on the histamine molecule, and subsequent brilliant pharmacology by Sir James Black led to the discovery of histamine H_2-receptors and development of specific H_2-antagonists that revolutionised the treatment of peptic ulcer.

Computer-aided design

Drug receptors, enzymes, ion channels and transporters are no longer simply 'black boxes' referred to by pharmacologists wishing to explain drug mechanisms, but are proteins with known amino acid sequences and tertiary structures (three-dimensional shapes), able to be cloned and genetically engineered. Computer modelling of the active sites of such proteins assists drug design, as chemical structures can be modelled and tested for virtual affinity for binding to the active sites. Using such techniques, inhibitors of the angiotensin-converting enzyme (ACE) inhibitors were designed for use in hypertension, dopa-decarboxylase inhibitors were designed for administration with levodopa in Parkinson's disease, and potential anticancer drugs are designed to inhibit various stages in the pathways of macromolecular synthesis.

Monitoring the activity of the scientific community

Research carried out by pharmacologists, biochemists and chemists in universities and research institutes may lead to the discovery of new drugs in unexpected ways. The pharmaceutical industry monitors such research via the scientific literature, patent applications and scientific conferences.

Drug development

Development of new drugs is regulated by government legislation and administered by government authorities—the TGA in Australia. Regulation is necessary because consumers need protection so that only safe and effective drugs are approved, and the sponsoring drug companies need protection for their investment in terms of intellectual property, patents and copyright. The main processes of drug regulation in Australia are summarised in Figure 4-1.

The stages of drug development

Drug development has traditionally been described as occurring in several clearly defined phases:

- the new idea or hypothesis: the routes to drug discovery (see above) include ideas for new molecules, purification of new natural products, new hypotheses for disease causation, and research with new technologies such as molecular biology and genetic engineering techniques
- design, purification or synthesis of the new molecule: combinatorial chemistry techniques make it possible for millions of new molecules to be synthesised, either actually or virtually
- **screening** for useful pharmacological activities or possible toxicological effects: screening may be broad, to detect all actions, or specific, for affinity for a particular receptor or enzyme; **high-throughput screening** allows millions of compounds to be run through automated initial screens (see Clinical Interest Box 4-2)
- preclinical pharmacology: this includes in-vitro and in-vivo studies (see earlier section on bioassays); pharmacodynamic actions, pharmacokinetic aspects (the fate of the chemical in the body) and possibly drug interactions are studied on at least three mammalian species, including only one rodent species
- toxicology studies (adverse effects): these include acute toxicity, long-term toxicity (chronic effects and effects on reproduction) and tests for mutagenicity and carcinogenicity; requirements depend on anticipated exposure and clinical use, whether acute or chronic
- pharmaceutical formulation and manufacturing scale-up, including stability tests and assay methods
- an application to drug-regulating authorities for approval to test on humans: this requires that all results,

manufacturing information, proposed clinical protocols, names of personnel in the clinical trial team, approval from an ethics committee etc be submitted
- if the drug appears to be safe, effective and worth testing, it will go to clinical trial while being closely monitored by authorities
- depending on the results of the clinical trial, the sponsors may apply for registration of the drug, i.e. for approval to market it; this requires rigorous scientific evaluation of all the data available on the drug
- ongoing post-marketing studies then follow up the drug, monitoring its effects in the wider community for longer periods.

The costs in time, money and effort

The development of a drug takes a prodigious amount of time, money and effort. It has been estimated that drug development from idea to market takes 12–24 years and that from active compound to clinical trials takes 7–9 years. Once the idea, chemical or process is patented (to protect the developers from other companies stealing their ideas) the clock starts ticking! In most countries, the duration of a patent is usually 15–17 years, with a possible short extension. When the patent expires, other companies can manufacture and market the drug as a 'generic' product under their own trade names. Consequently, companies need to minimise the time taken to get their drug onto the market.

The financial costs involved in bringing a drug to market are so great now that very few companies can afford to carry out the research and development. It is estimated that every new drug costs around A$1.2 billion and that a drug company needs 1–2 new drugs every 3–4 years to remain financially viable. While the spin-offs from research into the human genome have been incredibly exciting in terms of potential targets for drug actions and disease treatment, this research is very expensive to exploit and there are estimated to be 3000–10,000 protein targets to be explored, of which the G-protein receptors are likely to be especially important to pharmacology (see later section on Future drug development and the new genetics).

The costs in terms of effort involved are also immense and may eventually be wasted. It was formerly estimated that only one out of every 10,000 chemicals synthesised made it to the marketplace; the proportion would be far smaller now in the era of combinatorial chemistry and high-throughput screening. This is because drug development may be abandoned at any stage if the drug is 'thrown out' because of problems with safety, efficacy, changes in fashion or a better competitor drug. Drug companies are trying to streamline testing procedures and get early information on toxicity or pharmacokinetic problems so as to waste as little time and money as possible.

CLINICAL INTEREST BOX 4-3 STREPTOMYCIN, SMOKING AND STATISTICS

Before the 1950s, medical practice was based on accumulated wisdom acquired through everyday experience, passed down to succeeding generations of doctors. In 1950, however, two events occurred that caused a paradigm shift in medicine, such that statistical proof became the criterion for scientific evidence on which practice should be based (evidence-based health care).

Both events were due to Professor Austin Bradford Hill, of the Medical Statistics department of the London School of Hygiene and Tropical Medicine. Bradford Hill had intended to follow his father into medical practice but contracted tuberculosis (TB) during World War II, and so could not enter clinical medicine. He studied economics and **statistical methods**, and then applied these studies to epidemiology.

Bradford Hill's first major contribution to medicine was the demonstration that two drugs together, streptomycin and para-aminosalicylic acid (PAS), given over a period of several months, resulted in a marked improvement in patients with TB and reduced the development of resistance to the antibiotic. When invited to join the Tuberculosis Trial Committee, Bradford Hill realised that streptomycin, an antibiotic discovered in 1943, had to be given for several months before any improvement became obvious; that the British supplies of the drug were very limited; and that patients with TB sometimes underwent spontaneous remission, making proof of drug efficacy difficult. He argued persuasively that investigation of the two drugs in a

clinical trial could be conclusive only if a control group were used and if the patients were randomly allocated into the control group, 'treated' with bed-rest and collapse of the lung, or the treatment group on streptomycin (and in later trials, PAS as well). The trials demonstrated conclusively that the drug combination considerably reduced deaths from TB and the risk of development of streptomycin-resistant TB.

The second achievement was the convincing proof that smoking causes lung cancer. Because a very large proportion of the population smoked cigarettes during and after World War II, and pollution levels in cities were very high, the association of tobacco smoking with respiratory disease was not obvious. By applying **statistical methods** to this epidemiological issue and separating subjects into groups based on their smoking habits, Bradford Hill was able to demonstrate convincingly that the more cigarettes people smoked, the greater their risk of lung cancer.

Bradford Hill is credited with showing that 'the detached objectivity of statisticians inherent in the notion of randomisation is more likely to get at the truth than the subjective impressions generated from clinical experience'. The gold standard of the randomised controlled **clinical trial** was to prove indispensable in evaluating the enormous number of new drugs that were produced in the 1950s and 1960s, and medical statistics proved invaluable in demonstrating associations between lifestyle factors and conditions such as cancers and cardiovascular disease.
Adapted from: Le Fanu 1999.

Clinical trials of drugs

A **clinical trial** is a prospective study carried out in humans to determine whether a treatment that is believed to benefit a patient actually does benefit; thus it is a type of human experiment. The treatment being tested may be investigational (new) or a new version of an established treatment; it may be a drug, diet, medical device, surgical or physical procedure* or other modality. In the context of testing a new drug, the trial provides scientific data on safety (by rate or severity of adverse drug reactions) and efficacy (by statistically significant evidence of difference between treated and control groups). The 'gold standard' of clinical trials is the **randomised controlled clinical trial** (RCCT).

Typically, each subject enrolled in the trial is randomly allocated into a treatment group, to be administered the new drug under test, or to a control group, usually given the current best therapy or a placebo if there is no available treatment. It must be noted that the treatments are considered

equivalently beneficial before the trial, otherwise it is unethical to deny one group the better treatment, and that the results are applicable only to this treatment regimen and cannot be widely extrapolated to other similar drugs or patient groups. All tests in humans must be approved by a local **institutional ethics committee** (IEC).

Clinical trials are generally required for all new drugs and for new uses or formulations of old drugs; however, there are exceptions:

- toxic drugs (e.g. anticancer drugs) may go straight to phase II studies (see below) in a small number of patients with the disease, so that volunteers without cancer are not subjected to the likely adverse effects
- the rules are bent for orphan drugs (non-patentable, or for very rare diseases; see earlier discussion)
- there is public pressure for fast-tracking drugs potentially useful in otherwise fatal diseases such as AIDS.

The objectives of RCCTs need to be realistic, efficient, compatible, valid and specific, yet allow for generalisation. The criteria for efficiency and validity require that statisticians become involved in planning, to ensure that enough subjects are involved for the results to be statistically acceptable (see Clinical Interest Box 4-3). Clinical trials are a staged process with distinct phases, which allows for lower risk (few patients

---

*Many therapeutic techniques used unquestioningly by therapists for decades in professions such as physiotherapy, podiatry, orthoptics and speech pathology are now being subjected to clinical trials (often by Honours and postgraduate students), as part of the move to evidence-based medicine.

in early phases) and stepwise decisions (trials can be stopped if clear differences or toxicities become apparent); but are slow, expensive, and put pressure on the participants involved.

PHASE I: THE FIRST TESTS IN HUMANS

After extensive testing in vitro and in animals, the drug is administered initially in very low doses to a small number of healthy volunteers, e.g. in a research centre or institution, under close medical and scientific supervision. The objectives are to determine pharmacological activities in humans, pharmacokinetic parameters, a safe dosage range and any acute toxicity. Few Phase I trials are done in Australia, mainly because relatively little drug discovery and development work is done here (however, see Table 4-3).

PHASE II: THE FIRST ADMINISTRATION TO PATIENTS

These are the initial efficacy studies to test if the drug is indeed effective in treating the condition of interest, in a small number of closely supervised patients (10–200) in tertiary hospitals (usually major metropolitan teaching hospitals). The tests are 'single-blind', which means that the patients do not know which treatment they are getting but the investigators do. The investigators are specialists in the appropriate field of medicine, such as endocrinologists, psychiatrists, anaesthetists or rheumatologists. Phase II studies give an indication of the therapeutic range of doses, maximum tolerated dose and common adverse reactions in patients with the disease; again, few are carried out in Australia.

After the Phase II trial the drug company may apply for approval to conduct a RCCT. In Australia, data are sent to the Australian Drug Evaluation Committee and its specialist subcommittees, which assess formulation, production, efficacy, adverse reactions, protocols in the proposed trials and ethical aspects. If the drug appears to be safe and efficacious, with likely benefits outweighing risks, it progresses to the next phase.

PHASE III: THE FULL-SCALE RANDOMISED CONTROLLED CLINICAL TRIAL

This is 'the **Clinical Trial**', in which the drug is administered to numerous patients under experienced clinical investigators.

TABLE 4-3 Some drugs developed and/or trialled in Australia

DRUGS OR COMPOUNDS	RESEARCH INSTITUTE OR DRUG COMPANY
PI-88, a potential anticancer drug targeting the enzyme heparanase, important in the growth and spread of cancers	Progen Industries and John Curtin School of Medical Research at the Australian National University
Compounds that inhibit hepatitis-C-virus-directed protein expression in cell cultures	Virus Research Centre at the Royal Children's Hospital, Brisbane, and AMRAD Corporation, Melbourne
Novel crystalline carbohydrates, with applications in preventing adverse gut reactions with antibiotics, and graft rejection after transplant surgery	Alchemia P/L and the University of Queensland's Centre for Drug Design and Development
Pravastatin, subjected to RCCTs for prevention of death from heart disease and strokes	NHMRC Clinical Trials Centre, the University of Sydney, and Bristol-Myers Squibb Pharmaceuticals
Blood products: vaccines, sera, factors for bleeding disorders, antibodies for preventing severe infections; interferon beta-1a for treating multiple sclerosis	CSL Ltd, Melbourne
Plant products (isoflavones and phyto-oestrogens) to prevent degenerative changes in reproductive, cardiovascular and musculoskeletal systems	Novogen
Thebaine, used to synthesise the opioids oxycodone and buprenorphine, produced in high yields from new strains of opium poppy	Tasmanian Alkaloids P/L
Zanamivir (Relenza): treats influenza by stopping production of neuraminidase protein in flu virus (see Clinical Interest Box 4-5)	Victorian College of Pharmacy, CSIRO, Australian National University and Biota Holdings Ltd
Specialised drug delivery methods, especially for delivery of drugs and nucleic acids into cells, and viral vectors carrying material into chromosomes; topical and aerosol formulations technology	F.H. Fauldings Co. Ltd

Adapted from: Harrison 2000.

The aim is to ascertain whether, under the defined conditions, the drug shows clinical benefit for the disease state, with acceptably low rate and severity of adverse drug reactions. The trial is usually 'multicentre', i.e. carried out simultaneously in several medical centres in different countries, to increase the number of subjects and investigators, achieve quicker results, and enrol different ethnic groups; many are carried out in Australia. Statistically significant results able to be extrapolated to a wide range of populations are desirable. An RCCT may cost up to US$5 million, so it is important that it be designed carefully to ensure valid results. Other aspects that may be included in the study are the drug's pharmacokinetics, effects of other concurrent diseases or drugs, and costs of therapy.

Important elements of the RCCT are as follows:

- the design, which must minimise bias between groups
- the investigators must initially believe that the new treatment is at least as good as the old
- comparison between groups: various designs are possible (paired, crossover, parallel)
- whether the control group is to be administered the current established therapy or placebo
- criteria for inclusion and persons to be excluded from participation
- randomisation of subjects to ensure groups are initially similar in characteristics such as gender, age range, weight range, severity of disease
- blinding, i.e. who knows which treatment each group is getting; double-blinding is usual, with coded packs of drugs so that neither investigators nor subjects know who received the new drug until the trial has concluded and results are analysed
- any participant in an investigational drug study should be an informed volunteer; the 'informed consent' form should contain detailed information about the study, and potential benefits and adverse reactions
- a pretrial pilot study may be run, to detect problems with the protocol or non-compliance among the subjects.

It is essential that the trial be planned well to determine in advance parameters such as the maximum length, end-points, justification (who benefits?), information to be given to patients, consent forms, protocols, inclusion criteria, withdrawal procedures and follow-up schedules. Ethical aspects must be considered (discussed later) and an application made to the institutional ethics committee for approval to run the trial.

During the execution of the trial, subjects are monitored closely and the trial is regularly audited for safety, ethics and quality control. If it becomes apparent that one group is benefiting far more (statistically significantly) than the other,* or suffering more adverse reactions, the trial must be halted. Usually the statistical basis for the trial is the null hypothesis—that there is in fact no difference between the two treatments (i.e. the new drug is as good as the current therapy); results are analysed for statistical equivalence and the null hypothesis is accepted or rejected.

PHASE IV: POST-MARKETING STUDIES

Assuming that the clinical trial process is concluded and the new drug is shown to be safe, efficacious and cost-effective, it may be approved for marketing. It is recognised, however, that there are several limitations in the testing and trialling processes. The number of people studied and the time allotted to the study are limited. Also, certain types of individuals are excluded from the study, such as children, pregnant women, persons with multiple disease states or taking other drugs, and the elderly. If a drug is considered safe and effective during the time of study, with the previously mentioned limitations, it is marketed when approval has been granted. Once marketed, the drug is used in much greater numbers of patients and probably for longer periods. It is therefore inevitable that the drug will be reported to produce additional effects (possibly therapeutic but often adverse) that were not noted during the trial studies, such as rare adverse reactions, effects in subgroups of the population, and effects in patients taking other drugs with which the new drug may interact.

Post-marketing surveillance by the TGA also involves laboratory investigations of products on the market, and ongoing monitoring of products to ensure compliance with legislation. Later, **meta-analysis** (or overview analysis) may be carried out to combine and analyse data from several similar clinical trials. This has the advantage of increasing the statistical power of analysis by increasing the numbers of subjects, making significant results more likely; however, meta-analysis suffers inevitably from 'publication bias', as negative results are less likely to be published than positive results. Sometimes, different trials will produce conflicting results; the choice of which drug to prescribe then becomes one based on the clinical judgement of the prescriber.

THE 'BLUE FORM'

Through its Adverse Drug Reactions Advisory Committee (ADRAC), the TGA has instituted a voluntary program to

---

*A study carried out in 1990–92 on more than 9000 Australians and New Zealanders was halted 6 months early because results showed that one group of subjects was suffering a significantly greater risk of dying from heart attack than the other. The independent coordinator realised that the death rate in the control (placebo) group was higher than in the test group of subjects receiving the cholesterol-lowering drug pravastatin. The success of this and two similar major trials of the drug had a substantial impact on clinical practice and led to widespread prescribing of the drug and a massive blow-out in expenditure on the drug when subsidised (*The Age*, Melbourne, 5 May 1997).

CLINICAL INTEREST BOX 4-4 THE INTENSIVE MEDICINES MONITORING PROGRAMME

The Intensive Medicines Monitoring Programme (IMMP) was initiated in New Zealand in 1977 as part of post-marketing surveillance of new drugs, to identify adverse reactions early, see who is particularly at risk and ensure appropriate actions for safe use of medicines.

IMMP intensively monitors new medicines using a method known as 'prescription event monitoring'. New Zealand has made valuable contributions to this world-wide programme by identifying previously unrecognised adverse effects. For example, New Zealand took the lead in taking regulatory action over agranulocytosis caused by mianserin, and the liver toxicity that resulted from nefazodone. It is the only drug monitoring system that can help to protect groups of people (such as Maori and Pacific Islanders) in whom the metabolic pathways of drugs are genetically affected, by collating post-marketing data.

In 2004 there were reports that the NZ government was withdrawing its funding of the IMMP. This raised concerns worldwide, some of which were published in the British Medical Journal. However, the Ministry of Health responded by stating that the NZ Government was committed to strengthening its pharmacovigilance services, but felt that the labour-intensive manner in which IMMP had operated in the past required reviewing. The Ministry is using an innovative approach to monitor the use of a new vaccine which had been developed to deal with the meningococcal epidemic in New Zealand.

Source: Matheson D. *British Medical Journal* 2004; 329:460.

enhance the reporting by health-care professionals of adverse reactions they suspect are related to medications and medical devices. The verification of an adverse reaction is not necessary. It is important to inform the agency of medication- or medical-device-related events suspected to have resulted in adverse reaction. Confidentiality is maintained in the reporting. The paperwork is a one-page form (the 'blue form', see Figure 4-2) that is readily available and is regularly sent to prescribers of drugs, along with copies of the *Adverse Drug Reactions Bulletin*. Reports of adverse reactions are reviewed, coded, entered into a database and analysed for patterns. Some are forwarded to ADRAC, which updates and informs health professionals about adverse reactions, and can recommend actions ranging from no action required, change of aspects of prescribing or dispensing, through to withdrawal of a drug from the market. (New Zealand has a similar Intensive Medicines Monitoring Programme; see Clinical Interest Box 4-4.)

In Australia, adverse reactions can now be reported on-line, via the TGA's website, following links to the Online Services. Consumers can also report their own adverse reactions, via

Report of Suspected Adverse Reaction to Drugs and Vaccines
(See reverse for statement about use of personal information)

Patient *(Initials or Record No. only)* Date of Birth: / /
Sex: M / F Weight: ___kg

Adverse Reaction Description: Date of Onset of Reaction: / /

All Drug Therapy /Vaccines Prior to Reaction *(please use trade names and asterisk suspected drug)*	Daily Dosage *(Dose No for vaccines, e.g. 1st DTP etc)*	Date Begun	Date Stopped	Reason for Use

Treatment *(of reaction)*:
Outcome: Recovered ☐ Date of Recovery: / / Not Yet Recovered ☐
Unknown ☐ Fatal ☐ Date of Death: / /
Sequelae: No ☐ Yes ☐ *(describe)*
Severity: Life threatening ☐ Hospitalised ☐ Required a visit to Doctor ☐
Comments *(eg. relevant history, allergies, previous exposure to this drug)*:

Reporting Doctor, Pharmacist, etc:
Name: Postcode ____
Address:

Signature ______________ / /

FIGURE 4-2 The 'blue form', on which suspected adverse reactions to drugs and vaccines are reported (published by the Australian Adverse Drug Reactions Advisory Committee, Woden, ACT; reproduced with permission).

a 1300 telephone number designated the Adverse Medicine Events (AME) Line: 1300 134 237.

The pharmaceutical industry

The pharmaceutical industry is constantly screening substances with potential to market as new drugs; worldwide the industry is estimated to be worth about US$250 billion/year.

Prospective drugs take years and large amounts of capital for basic and clinical studies and for the costs of application and promotion. The increasing emphasis on 'lifestyle drugs', which may be taken for decades and hence require studies of long-term safety; the prevalence of polypharmacy, with its inherent risks of drug interactions and, the insistence of governments on proof of cost-effectiveness, all contribute to the enormous costs of testing drugs. In addition, drug companies carry out research aimed at new drug discovery. Because of the huge commitment and

CLINICAL INTEREST BOX 4-5 AN AUSTRALIAN DRUG DISCOVERY: RELENZA

More than 40 million people have died from influenza in the past 100 years. Although vaccines are effective, they need to be continually updated, as the virus has the ability to mutate frequently to new strains that are not inactivated by old vaccines. Research carried out by Dr Peter Colman, a scientist with the CSIRO, has led to the development of a novel anti-flu drug, **zanamivir** (Relenza). The history of the discovery and development of the drug is as follows.

1978   Dr Peter Colman and Dr Jose Varghese, at CSIRO's Division of Protein Chemistry in Parkville, Melbourne, recognised that the only invariant (unchanging) part of the flu virus when it mutates is part of the neuraminidase protein on the viral cell surface. (Neuraminidase is an enzyme that hydrolyses sialic acid residues in sugar groups in biological membranes.) Working with Dr Graeme Laver at the Australian National University, they set out to determine the three-dimensional structure of the protein.

1983   The structure of the protein was elucidated, and the next step was to find funds to set up a team to synthesise chemicals that might inhibit the functions of the protein and thus inactivate the virus.

1985   A local entrepreneur, Mark Crosling, formed Biota Holdings Ltd to back the development, and a licensing agreement was signed. Biota subsequently funded research at both CSIRO and the Victorian College of Pharmacy (VCP), Parkville.

1986   A synthetic chemistry program was started in the Pharmaceutical Chemistry department at the VCP,

led by Dr Mark von Itztein, to custom-design an organic molecule that would inactivate the viral neuraminidase enzyme.

1989   The first potent inhibitor was synthesised. As much more funding was required to develop the drug and submit it to clinical trials, the drug company GlaxoWellcome, which had earlier shown interest, was contacted and a collaboration initiated.

1990   A formal agreement was signed between Biota and Glaxo, allowing Glaxo access to Biota's intellectual property and the marketing rights to the drug.

1992–93 Glaxo took the lead compound into exploratory development, and the efficacy of the most active compound in animal trials (code-named GG167) was established.

1994–97 Phase I, II and III clinical trials.

1998   Registration applications in Australia, Europe, Canada and USA for zanamivir (Relenza, GG167).

1999   Market release of zanamivir in Australia, Europe and USA; shares in Biota Holdings soar!

It is estimated that the Australian investment in the research and development that led to the development of zanamivir totalled A$26.3 million in 1994/95 dollars. This included funding by CSIRO and Biota and extra government top-up grants. The costs of clinical trials, manufacturing scale-up and marketing were funded by the sponsoring company, GlaxoWellcome.

Based on information from: Warrick Glynn, CSIRO Parkville, and CSIRO 1998.

risks involved, drug companies have been merging over the past few years, for economies of scale and to combine their research and development efforts and achievements, with the result that there are only a few major drug companies left worldwide.*

It is interesting to note that, on average, drug companies allocate 1% of their expenditure to research and 20% to marketing. The major markets are of course the USA, Europe and Japan; Australia takes only 1%–2% of world sales of pharmaceuticals.

Drug development in Australia

There is little basic research carried out in drug companies in Australia; most companies are offshoots of multinational companies based overseas. Scientific work carried out in

---

*With complicated triple-barrelled merged names, including Pfizer/Warner-Lambert; GlaxoWellcome/SmithKline Beecham; Bristol-Myers-Squibb; and Pharmacia-Upjohn/Monsanto.

Australia is mainly pharmaceutical work on formulations suitable for Australian conditions, and preparation of submissions for the marketing in Australia of drugs that have been developed and trialled overseas. Australian companies such as Fauldings, GlaxoWellcome Australia and AMRAD try to carve out niches for themselves in areas such as parenteral formulations or developing products of local biotechnology companies like Biota Holdings.

CLINICAL TRIALS IN AUSTRALIA AND NEW ZEALAND

In Australia the TGA has overall control of therapeutic goods via pre-market evaluation and approval of products, licensing of manufacturers, and post-market surveillance. Therapeutic goods not yet registered may be accessed for clinical trials by application to the TGA, which thus regulates **clinical trials** in Australia. Details of the relevant regulations and guidelines are covered in the TGA booklet *Access to Unapproved Therapeutic Goods: Clinical Trials in Australia* (Therapeutic Goods Administration 2001).

There are two main schemes under which drugs (and medical devices) may be trialled. The first is application under the Clinical Trial Exemption (CTX) scheme. An application to conduct a trial is submitted to the TGA, whose delegate reviews the data and may object to the trial or comment on the proposal. When any objections have been satisfactorily met and the local Human Research Ethics Committee (HREC) has approved it, the trial may go ahead without further assessment from the TGA. Early Phase I and II studies and trials of medical devices most commonly come under the CTX scheme. The scheme is complex, and few trials now come under these rules.

The second approach is notification under the Clinical Trial Notification (CTN) scheme, under which data are submitted to the local HREC of the institution where the trial will be conducted. The HREC reviews the data and the trial design and advises the institution if it approves the trial. A CTN form must be submitted to notify the TGA of the trial. Phase III and IV trials and bioequivalence studies are best suited to the CTN scheme. The HREC can refer the application to the CTX scheme if it is uncomfortable with making its decision based on the data available.

The TGA has strict regulations relating to the roles of HRECs, trials involving gene therapy and related therapies, preventing or stopping a trial, and indemnity and compensation. The Code of Good Clinical Practice must be followed. This covers aspects such as the responsibilities of the chief investigator and of the drug company; drug product handling, storage and accounting; reporting of adverse effects; and keeping and archiving of records. There are potential problems relating to delaying or withholding of negative results, applying 'spin' to make drugs look better than they really are, participating doctors accepting funding or gifts from sponsoring drug companies, and lack of transparency about procedures.

In New Zealand, approval to trial a new drug not yet registered is submitted to the Standing Committee on Therapeutic Trials (SCOTT). Quite a few clinical trials are carried out in NZ, as it is a small, closed, not too mixed population. The *New Zealand Regulatory Guidelines for Medicines,* Volume 3, contains the Interim Good Clinical Research Practice Guidelines, which aim to make those involved in the design, performance and analysis of clinical studies aware of the minimum requirements for high-quality research. The guidelines are based on the European Union, UK, Nordic, Australian, World Health Organization and Committee for Proprietary Medicinal Products (CPMP) guidelines and codes for Good Clinical Research Practice.

The New Zealand guidelines outline the need to evaluate the risks and benefits, requirements for obtaining informed consent, quality control, audit, data recording, analysis, interpretation of the results and reporting of adverse events for studies conducted in New Zealand. Pharmaceutical companies conducting clinical research have to comply with the principles contained in the guidelines. It is essential that doctors are familiar with Good Clinical Research Practice requirements and assess the proposed research for compliance before participating.

DRUGS DEVELOPED IN AUSTRALIA

Australian medical schools and medical research institutes have had an enviable reputation worldwide for health-care research; however, commercial exploitation and 'value-adding' of the research usually happens overseas. Some drugs that have recently been developed and/or trialled in Australia are summarised in Table 4-3, and a case study of the discovery and development of **zanamivir** is given in Clinical Interest Box 4-5 (clinical aspects of this drug are described in Drug Monograph 32-10).

Future drug development and the new genetics

Drugs are still being discovered by the old methods, including structure–activity studies on drugs binding to receptors, and 'fishing' for interesting leads in reefs and rainforests (and other natural sources). There has been great interest and excitement in the hope for new drugs from **'the new genetics'**—the application of molecular biology and its techniques to health care. This has led to reports of genes to combat cancer, ageing and arthritis, and hope for cures after discovery of the genes for cystic fibrosis, breast cancer, type 1 diabetes and various anaemias. While there have been some successes, as yet the promises of the new genetics have not been extensively fulfilled.

Genetic engineering

Genetic engineering, commonly referred to as biotechnology, is basically another route for the synthesis of proteins and other complex molecules using recombinant DNA techniques. Once the gene that codes for a particular protein is discovered, it can be inserted into a micoorganism such as a strain of bacteria, so that the bacteria will now synthesise the protein. The first drug to be made this way was human insulin (in 1978), which previously had been synthesised by changing the amino acid sequence of pig insulin. Now, human insulin is readily produced by the bacterium *Escherichia coli* and the yeast *Saccharomyces cerevisiae* (see Drug Monograph 41-1).

Other 'biotech' products in therapeutic use by 1995 included interferon-alpha, human growth hormone, erythropoietin, interleukin-2, factor VIII (antihaemophilic factor), and many other growth-stimulating factors and monoclonal antibodies.

Genetic screening

There are about 4000 diseases resulting from the mutation of single genes; most of them are very rare except for conditions such as cystic fibrosis, Huntington's chorea and some congenital blood disorders. New genetic techniques in the 1980s allowed the identification of many of these genes, so that some of these disorders can now be diagnosed prenatally by genetic testing of an 'at-risk' fetus in the uterus. (However, this does not help people in whom the disorder arises spontaneously by mutation.) Genes, or fragments of them, involved in at least 42 conditions have been identified, including cystic fibrosis, Huntington's chorea, sickle-cell anaemia, thalassaemia, haemophilia and muscular dystrophy. These conditions can therefore now be diagnosed in utero, making it possible for parents to decide whether to terminate the pregnancy or allow it to continue. Genes that predispose to cancers are also being hunted; however, cancers closely linked to a particular gene are very much in the minority, e.g. only about 5% of breast cancers are related to the two main breast cancer genes.

Gene therapy

This refers to the concept that if a normal copy of a gene can be inserted into a cell carrying a genetic error, the error can be corrected and the genetic disease cured by physically changing the gene itself. This leads to the dream that humans might no longer be constrained by their genetic make-up. For **gene therapy** to be feasible, first the gene for a condition must be identified, then a copy of the normal gene must be inserted via a 'vector' into certain cells, which use the gene to make the missing proteins. The vector is usually a virus that has been inactivated so as to be no longer pathogenic. Gene therapy has been carried out in several situations, including inserting the gene for the enzyme adenosine deaminase into T lymphocytes of patients with a deficiency in this enzyme; in cystic fibrosis, administering the normal gene via a nasal solution into the airways of children with the disease; and in muscular dystrophy, injecting primitive muscle cells containing the normal gene into the muscles of boys with muscular dystrophy.

Unfortunately, none of these methods has worked for long; the main problems appear to be that the vectors are not sufficiently effective in taking the gene into the appropriate cells, that the genes require many other helper genes to regulate their actions, and that there may be immunological reactions to the inserted genes and their proteins. So dreams for gene therapy on a wide scale have not yet been realised.

Human genome targets: pharmacogenomics

The exciting work that led to the publication in 2001 of the genetic code for the whole human body—the human genome—has provided a huge amount of information that can potentially be exploited for the benefit of the human race. Even just in the field of pharmacology it is estimated that there are 3000–10,000 protein targets that may be important in terms of drug actions. This field is now known as 'pharmacogenomics', and can be considered a branch of pharmacogenetics (see Chapter 6).

Likely to be of particular interest are proteins related to G-protein receptors, and genes with sequences similar to those coding for receptors. It is conceivable that researchers may study a protein similar to a receptor, find a ligand (a chemical that binds to the protein) and study the binding or substances that inhibit binding, all without knowing whether the receptor look-alike is implicated in any biological function or disease. The possibilities are endless and the costs enormous, which is why drug companies are merging to pool their research efforts and resources in this exciting new field of pharmacology.

Some examples of recent research and drug development in pharmacogenomics are:

* the neuropeptide nociceptin/orphanin FQ, a novel bioactive substance identified as the natural ligand of the opioid-receptor-like 1 receptor; it has a wide spectrum of activities including either facilitation or inhibition of pain perception
* the SPARC gene and protein (Secreted Protein Acidic and Rich in Cysteine; also known as osteonectin), implicated in cell adhesion, growth and cell–matrix interactions; its role is being studied in pathologies as diverse as human breast cancers, astrocytomas and gliomas, melanoma, ovarian carcinoma, scleroderma, cataracts and retinal scarring, and kidney transplant rejection
* studies of the gene expression profiles for drug resistance markers in subtypes of acute lymphoblastic leukaemia (ALL), providing insight into the genetic pathways of drug resistance, and facilitating the targeting of drug therapy to children with ALL
* expression profiling of cancer-specific proteins is helping identify early cancer markers, which will improve treatment of patients in early stages of cancers
* paraoxonase-1, and its associated gene; this enzyme is involved in protecting low-density lipoproteins from oxidation, metabolising some drugs, and metabolising some organophosphorus insecticides; genomic studies of variants of the enzyme have been applied to protection against bioterrorism threats with sarin poison.

ETHICAL PRINCIPLES RELATED TO DRUG USE IN HEALTH CARE

Human rights, the basis for bioethics

The basic **human rights**, acknowledged by the United Nations and accepted by most countries, are the rights for life, security, health, dignity, privacy, autonomy, marriage and procreation, and freedom of thought and religion. Codes of **bioethics** are based on these human rights and date back as far as the **Hippocratic Oath** (5th century BC). More recently, bioethics are based on the Declaration of Geneva (1948) and the International Code of Ethics (1949), agreed to by the United Nations after World War II; modern versions of the **Hippocratic Oath** have been devised (see Clinical Interest Box 4-6).

Medical ethics are the principles that define the manners, modes and morals of medical practitioners, and by extension apply to all health practitioners. They are usually listed as:

- non-maleficence (not doing harm)
- beneficence (doing good); together these first two principles are part of the duty of care owed to patients and clients, and imply the importance of risk–benefit analysis and the potential for failure in duty of care being seen as (and sued for) negligence
- justice, whereby all persons should have equal access to health and health care; while lip-service is paid to this principle, in practice access often depends on factors such as funds (both public and private) available for health services, and geographical situation (closeness to doctors and major hospitals)
- veracity, i.e. that the truth will be told to all persons about their condition and treatment; this may sometimes be waived if it is truly in the patients' best interests that they not be given certain information
- confidentiality of personal and health records: health privacy principles relate to collection of information, use and disclosure of information, data quality, data security and retention, openness of policies, access to and correction of information, assignment of identifiers to individuals, possibility of anonymity, data flow across borders and transfer of information between providers and to other health services
- autonomy of the patient: the patient always retains the right to refuse treatment and has the right to have sufficient information to make informed decisions about choosing ('informed consent') or refusing treatment or participation in a trial.

The principles of **bioethics** put responsibilities on health practitioners to practise ethically. This implies that they will

remain competent and up-to-date in their practice, that they will use all appropriate resources in the best interests of their patients and will accord their patients all basic human rights, including observing confidentiality of information. What constitutes unethical conduct may be hard to determine; in the health-care context, it has at times been taken to mean serious misconduct compared with what would reasonably be expected by a general body of colleagues.

Bioethics issues arise frequently. Typically these involve professional secrecy, consent to treatment (must be valid, informed and specific), and procedures with legal problems (sterilisation, abortion, assisted pregnancies, maiming and experimentation). This section cannot attempt to cover all

---

CLINICAL INTEREST BOX 4-6 A HIPPOCRATIC OATH FOR THE 21ST CENTURY

Hippocratic oaths, or modernised versions, are still proclaimed at graduation or medical registration ceremonies at approximately half of Australia's medical schools (McNeill & Dowton 2002). This is not just for sentimental reasons (although there is hardly a dry eye among parents), but for the purposes of imparting a professional bond, stating high aims and a moral commitment, for continuity in the medical tradition, as a reminder of professional standards and to affirm core values publicly. As an example, below is the 'Declaration of Ethical Intention' written and proclaimed by the graduating class of 2003 from Monash University in Melbourne:

- In acknowledging the privilege of practising medicine, I make this declaration freely and sincerely in front of my family, friends, colleagues and teachers.
- In the practice of medicine, the care of patients is my first concern. I will use my knowledge and skills to the best of my ability in striving to prevent and treat disease, improve quality of life and provide support in times of suffering, for the individual and the community.
- I will endeavour to earn my patients' respect and confidence and to treat all equally and without prejudice. I will honour their freedom and dignity, both in living and in dying.
- I recognize the unique role I fulfil in their lives and accept the importance of taking responsibility for my actions and acting with integrity.
- I will seek to gain in knowledge and understanding, and to freely share this with others.
- I acknowledge that to honour these commitments I should seek to maintain my personal well-being and that of my family, friends and colleagues.
- May these affirmations guide and inspire me in practising the art and science of medicine.

(With thanks to the Faculty of Medicine, Nursing and Health Sciences, Monash University; and Dr Philippa Smith, Geelong.)

aspects of medical ethics relevant to pharmacology, but some aspects of selected current issues are summarised below.

Current issues in bioethics
Animal rights

It is now generally recognised that animals should be used in testing of drugs and medical devices or procedures only when absolutely necessary. While results from animal tests cannot automatically be extrapolated to humans, such tests do protect humans. When it comes to the decision, few people would be prepared to take drugs in a life-threatening condition or allow drugs to be administered to their children if the drugs had not previously been tested in some animal or human. The Australian and New Zealand Council for the Care of Animals in Research and Teaching (ANZCCART) works diligently to protect **animal rights**, minimise the use of animals in testing, and promote 'the three Rs': replacement of animals wherever possible, reduction in the numbers of animals used, and refinement of techniques to minimise harm and use.

Information technology/ 'telemedicine'

The advent of the Internet and availability of instantaneous communication and information have raised new issues. Should medical information and consultations be available to all people, e.g. on the worldwide web, should doctors be allowed to prescribe on-line and pharmacists supply drugs by mail? Does this erode the doctor's role or the clinical relationship between health professional and patient, or is it the patient's right to know about and obtain drugs? Does it disperse responsibilities from the doctor to the patient or to whoever publishes information on the web?

Warnings and consent forms

Patients need enough information on which to base their consent to, or choice of, treatment or participation in a trial; however, if every possible adverse effect or drug interaction is explained in detail, they may never take any drug, thus putting their health further at risk. In realistic practice, it is usual for doctors and pharmacists to discuss with the person all real risks, considering how much information the person wishes to be told; however, the fear that extensive information will put the person off treatment altogether does not justify withholding information. Equally, health professionals have an ethical obligation *not* to recommend inappropriately risky treatments. The High Court of Australia has said that the patient must be informed about 'material' (i.e. significant) risks. Equally, health-care professionals have an ethical obligation *not* to recommend inappropriately risky treatments.

Population studies, especially of particular groups

During the normal procedures for clinical trials or epidemiological studies, many groups may be excluded from participation, e.g. children, pregnant women or people of particular indigenous or ethnic groups. On the other hand, trials that would not be approved in countries with strong regulations regarding clinical trials may be carried out in underdeveloped countries.* Some of the ethical issues are those of informed consent, the ownership of intellectual property of the data, access of all people to equally high standards of health care, and the exploitation and/or stereotyping of people.

In particular, children have been described as 'therapeutic orphans' (see Gazarian 2003). Children are rarely included as subjects in clinical trials, so if the drug is subsequently approved for use, this will usually be only in adults, so children will be denied access to many new medications. Also, drugs commonly used in children may never be tested for safety and efficacy. Extrapolating results from adult studies to children poses many risks, and new drugs are unlikely to be formulated into forms suitable for children. 'Off-label' prescribing is risky for the doctor and costly to the patient (or parents), as it is not subsidised. Some drug studies are now being carried out in children overseas, but only in potentially profitable drugs.

Institutional ethics committees (IECs)

The TGA requires that all institutions in which human or animal testing is carried out, including universities, research institutions and hospitals, have properly constituted **institutional ethics committees** to respond to and judge ethical questions in the specific environment. One IEC may approve a trial protocol that another rejects. There are many potential problems, including:
- the possibility that proposed, worthwhile innovative research may never be approved
- that multicentre trials may require simultaneous approval from several IECs
- that unless there is communication and integration between IECs, there can be great wasting of time and overlap in work, as well as 'reinvention of the wheel'
- that the autonomy of individual IECs is limited by guidelines and protocols.

Pharmacoeconomics and rationing of drugs or medical care

The increasing costs of medical technologies and new drugs, the demands of an ageing population, patients' expectations,

*As described graphically in the book and movie version 'The Constant Gardener' by John LeCarre.

doctors' fear of litigation, and governments' need for tight budget controls all make the rationing of health care a difficult ethical issue. The agenda on public health is often set by the commercial demands of the pharmaceutical industry. (Some of these aspects of pharmacoeconomics have been discussed in Chapter 2.) Principles of equity and fairness need to be applied or high-quality care will only be available to the wealthy. Hospital drug and therapeutics committees may need to draw up guidelines in advance to prioritise needs and allocation of resources.

Promotion or advertising of medicines

The World Health Organization has a code of 'ethical criteria for medical drug promotion', both to health professionals and to the public. Drug companies obviously consider promotion of drugs to doctors as being effective in increasing the prescribing and use of particular products, otherwise it would not be carried out. Advertising adds to the already heavy cost of new drugs.* In Australia, 'detailing' of drugs to doctors is regulated by TGA legislation, guidelines and the Code of Conduct of Medicines Australia (formerly the Australian Pharmaceutical Manufacturers Association), and by complaints from consumers and 'watchdogs'. Breaches of the code can require withdrawal of promotional material and heavy fines, plus exposure in professional journals. Advertising needs to be monitored to check that it is objective and not biased; it can often be noted that the benefits of a drug are emphasised rather than the risks and that adverse reactions are mentioned only in the finest print.

Advertising of prescription medicines to the public is not permitted in Australia but advertising of OTC drugs is allowed. 'Direct-to-consumer' drug advertising is legal in NZ and the USA, and is very effective in increasing demand for prescription medicines. Drug companies can also boost the demand for their products by defining common, mild problems as diseases requiring drug treatment, e.g. mild dyspepsia, headache, baldness or anxiety, and by running 'disease-awareness' campaigns. This adds to the heavy costs of drugs to governments.

Advertisements generally, whether in medical journals, glossy magazines or on television or the Internet, should be monitored for superficial or misleading information, shock tactics, insidious comparisons, and stereotyping. It is instructive, for example, to check for advertisements aimed at the middle-aged male doctor, with subtle references to the anxious housewife, children who may 'need' antibiotics for a cold, confused elderly women or stressed hypertensive male business executives. Advertisements should emphasise the

information supplied, rather than aiming to catch the eye or shock with sexist or racist images.

Relationships between health practitioners and the pharmaceutical industry

Doctors and other health professionals in a position to prescribe or encourage drug use are often 'wooed' by representatives from drug companies to increase their prescribing of a particular drug. Incentives may range from equipment for the desk to subsidisation of trips to overseas conferences or funding for research. While doctors generally maintain that they can resist such pressures, studies have shown that even subconsciously their prescribing patterns are affected by pressure from drug company 'reps'. As more health professionals (nurse practitioners, optometrists, podiatrists) gain the right to prescribe drugs, they will be subject to similar pressures. There is a range of positions that prescribers can adopt, from refusing all gifts so as to avoid all compromise, through to acceptance of lavish gifts while hoping to maintain independence.

The chief concerns about these practices are that commercial objectives override properly prioritised health care, education and research; that advertising inevitably increases prescribing of the company's drugs; and that there may be distortions in scientific evidence, evaluations and publications. Most biomedical journals now require that authors declare all conflicts of interest. Institutions and learned colleges expect there will be minimal acceptance of gifts or support, and that research and publication will be guided by scientific and ethical values.

Ethical aspects of clinical trials

The Declaration of Helsinki, recognised internationally, outlines ethical considerations related to clinical trials:

> Every biomedical research project involving human subjects should be preceded by careful assessment of predictable risks in comparison with foreseeable benefits to the subject or to others. Concern for the interests of the subject must always prevail over the interests of science and society.

Many of the general issues in medical ethics discussed above also apply to the situation of a clinical trial. Some ethical issues particularly relevant to clinical trials are:

- personal autonomy and the subject's right to withdraw at any stage
- every treatment is experimental in each patient unless the person has taken it before
- can ethics be applied or adequately monitored by a committee?
- the doctor is in a position of potential conflict: the healer versus the investigator
- clinical trials by their design manipulate subjects and use controls

---

*Drug companies are estimated to spend A$1–1.5 billion per year promoting their drugs in Australia (Lexchin 2000).

- randomisation into groups denies the control group access to the test drug, and the test group access to the current best treatment
- use of placebo is usually considered unethical, as it denies the placebo group access to treatment
- should subjects or patients have the right to refuse to participate in the advancement of medical knowledge? (welfare rights versus individual rights)

- to what extent should subjects be paid, or be compensated for expenses?
- what is the appropriate make-up of ethics committees?
- what are the rights and responsibilities of the investigators?
- what special arrangements or guidelines need to be made for testing of reproductive technology, or for patients who cannot give consent (e.g. minors, or those who have dementia, are aggressive or unconscious)?

KEY POINTS

- Drugs are controlled at many levels: international, national and state. Laws apply to the classification and control of chemicals, poisons, drugs and other therapeutic goods. Some chemicals are proscribed and criminal law relates to offences under these Acts.
- The road to market of a new drug product requires an initial drug discovery or design, drug development, animal and human testing, and approval before a new drug is marketed and reaches the consumer.
- During this process, legal requirements for drug regulation remove or eliminate unsafe or ineffective drugs from reaching the marketplace; drugs are classified into various schedules to protect the consumer.
- Special arrangements exist for 'orphan drugs' to treat very rare diseases, for classifying drugs for safe use in pregnancy and with respect to drug use in sport.
- Post-marketing surveillance is important in identifying adverse reactions or serious problems not previously identified. This voluntary program requires the cooperation of health-care professionals.
- During the process of testing drugs, assays are carried out to determine their strength and purity; these can be chemical or biological assays. Bioassays may be of various types: in vitro, in vivo, or in silico; drugs need to be tested in animals and humans before being approved as safe and effective.
- Drug testing in humans, both preclinical testing in volunteers and testing in patients in clinical trials, is closely controlled and monitored. Randomised controlled clinical trials are the best method of objectively gathering information as to the safety and efficacy of proposed treatments.
- Application of new technologies, including those of combinatorial chemistry, high-throughput screening and genetic engineering, provides hope for the discovery of new drugs and diagnostic methods.
- The ethical principles on which clinical practice is based are underpinned by protection of basic human rights. Application of these principles can be controversial in many current situations but it is important for health professionals to consider and discuss ethical issues.

REVIEW EXERCISES

1. Outline the laws relating to the regulation and use of drugs in your country or state and describe how these may affect your practice as a health professional.
2. Describe the Schedules into which drugs and poisons are classified, naming two substances that fall under each Schedule.
3. Explain why drugs need to be assayed and standardised, and give examples of in-vitro, in-vivo and in-silico tests.
4. Describe the advantages and disadvantages of investigational animal and human studies of drugs.
5. Trace the main phases of clinical trials of drugs from preclinical testing to post-marketing surveillance.
6. Discuss drug discovery and development, giving examples of drugs discovered by each of several different methods.
7. List the internationally accepted basic human rights and explain their role as the basis of bioethics.
8. Give examples of how principles of bioethics may be compromised during the process of clinical trials of new drugs.
9. Choose one of the topics currently of interest and concern in the area of bioethics and either set up a class debate on the issue or list several arguments that could be used to support each side of a debate on the topic.

REFERENCES AND FURTHER READING

Australian Medicines Handbook 2005. Adelaide: AMH, 2005.

Australian Pharmaceutical Manufacturers Association (APMA). *The Australian Pharmaceutical Industry Code of Conduct.* Sydney: APMA, c. 2001.

Australian and New Zealand Council for the Care of Animals in Research and Teaching. Promoting awareness of the three Rs. *ANZCCART News* 1998; 11(1): 1–5.

Bigby M, Gadenne A-S. Understanding and evaluating clinical trials. *Journal of the American Academy of Dermatology* 1996; 34(4): 555–90.

Bochner F, Burgess NG, Martin ED. Approaches to rationing drugs in hospitals: an Australian perspective. *Pharmacoeconomics* 1996; 10(5): 467–74.

Bowman WC, Harvey AL. *The discovery of drugs. Proc. Royal College of Physicians of Edinburgh* 1995; 25(1): 5–24.

British Medical Association and the Royal Pharmaceutical Society of Great Britain. *British National Formulary 41.* London: BMJ Books, 2001.

British Pharmacopoeia Commission. *British Pharmacopoeia 2005.* Vol. 1. London: The Stationery Office, 2005.

Cartwright FF, Biddiss MD. *Disease and History. Man-Made Problems of the Present and Future.* London: Hart-Davis, 1972 [ch. 9].

Collins DJ, Lapsley HM. *The Social Costs of Drug Abuse in Australia in 1988 and 1992.* National Drug Strategy Monograph no 30. Canberra: AGPS, 1996.

CSIRO. *Beyond Science: Managing Projects for Success.* Melbourne: CSIRO, 1998.

Davies CA. Keeping advertisers honest–an overview of the regulation of the advertising of medicines and medical devices in Australia. *Australian Prescriber* 2004; 27(5): 124–7.

Dhanesuan N, Sharp JA, Blick T, Price JT, Thompson EW. Doxycycline-inducible expression of SPARC/Osteonectin/BM40 in MDA-MB-231 human breast cancer cells results in growth inhibition. *Breast Cancer Research and Treatment* 2002; 75(1): 73–85.

Drews J. Drug discovery: a historical perspective. *Science* 2000; 287(17 March): 1960–4.

Dwyer P, Newgreen DB. Regulation of drugs. In Linden-Laufer S (ed.). Ch. 20: Health and guardianship. In: *The Laws of Australia.* Sydney: Law Book Company, 1998.

Ekins S, Waller CL, Swaan PW. Progress in predicting human ADME parameters in silico. *Journal of Pharmacological and Toxicological Methods* 2000; 44(1): 251–72.

Fastier FN. *Drugs and the Law in New Zealand.* Dunedin: Amidine Publications, 1998.

Galbally R. *Review of Drugs, Poisons & Controlled Substances Legislation: Options Paper and Final Report.* Woden, ACT: Therapeutic Goods Administration, 2000 and 2001.

Gazarian M. Why are children still therapeutic orphans? *Australian Prescriber* 2003; 26(6): 122–3.

Goldsworthy PD, McFarlane AC. Howard Florey, Alexander Fleming and the fairy tale of penicillin. *Medical Journal of Australia* 2002; 176: 176–8.

Handen JS (ed). *Industrialization of Drug Discovery: From Target Selection Through Lead Optimization.* Boca Raton: Taylor & Francis, 2005.

Harman RJ. *Development and Control of Medicines and Medical Devices.* London: Pharmaceutical Press, 2004.

Harrison R (ed.). *Biomedical, Biotechnology and Pharmaceutical Innovation: Australia's Opportunities.* Sydney: CL Creations & Health Media, 2000.

Irvine R, McPhee J, Kerridge IH. The challenge of cultural and ethical pluralism to medical practice. *Medical Journal of Australia* 2002; 176: 174–5.

Kerridge IH, Lowe M, McPhee J. *Ethics and Law for the Health Professions.* Sydney: Federation Press, 2005.

Komesaroff PA. Ethical perspectives on the communication of risk. *Australian Prescriber* 2003; 26(2): 44–5.

Komesaroff PA, Cohen A. The growth of ethics in medicine over the past 50 years. *Medical Journal of Australia* 2001; 174: 41–44.

Komesaroff PA, Kerridge IH. Ethical issues concerning the relationships between medical practitioners and the pharmaceutical industry. *Medical Journal of Australia* 2002; 176: 118–21.

Le Fanu J. *The Rise and Fall of Modern Medicine.* London: Little Brown, 1999 [ch. 3].

Lexchin J. Click, click: the internet and prescription drugs. *Australian Prescriber* 2000; 23(4): 73–4.

Lopert R, Henry D. The Pharmaceutical Benefits Scheme: economic evaluation works . . . but is not a panacea. *Australian Prescriber* 2002; 25(6): 126–7.

Mackay K. Showing the blue card: reporting adverse reactions. *Australian Prescriber* 2005; 28(6): 140–2.

McEwen J. What does TGA approval of medicines mean? *Australian Prescriber* 2004; 27(6): 156–8.

McNeill PM, Dowton SB. Declarations made by graduating medical students in Australia and New Zealand. *Medical Journal of Australia* 2002; 176: 123–5.

McPhee J. Perceptions of risk–a legal perspective. *Australian Prescriber* 2002; 25(5): 114–5.

Manderson D. *From Mr Sin to Mr Big, A History of Australian Drug Laws.* Oxford: Oxford University Press, 1993.

Meunier JC. Utilizing functional genomics to identify new pain treatments: the example of nociceptin. *American Journal of Pharmacogenomics* 2003; 3(2): 117–30.

Moran M. Why are global drug prices so high . . . and other questions. *Australian Prescriber* 2003; 26(2): 26–7.

Moulds RFW. Drugs and poisons scheduling. *Australian Prescriber* 1997; 20(1): 12–13.

National Drugs and Poisons Schedule Committee. *Standard for the Uniform Scheduling of Drugs and Poisons no. 16.* Woden ACT: National Drugs and Poisons Schedule Committee, 2001.

National Health and Medical Research Council. *NHMRC Statement on Human Experimentation and Supplementary Notes 1992.* Canberra: NHMRC, 1992.

Petrie A, Sabin C. *Medical Statistics at a Glance* 2nd edn. Malden, MA: Blackwell, 2005.

Pharmaceutical Society of Australia. *Australian Pharmaceutical Formulary and Handbook.* 20th edn. Curtin ACT: Pharmaceutical Society of Australia, 2006.

Roughead EE. The Australian Pharmaceutical Manufacturers Association Code of Conduct: guiding the promotion of prescription medicines. *Australian Prescriber* 1999; 22(4): 78–80.

Steinbock B, Arras JD, London AJ. *Ethical Issues in Modern Medicine* 6th edn. Boston: McGraw-Hill, 2003.

Therapeutic Goods Administration, Dept of Health and Ageing. *Drugs Designated as Orphan Drugs.* Woden ACT: Australian Government, 2006.

Trent RJ. *Molecular Medicine: An Introductory Text.* Amsterdam: Elsevier Academic Press 2005.

United Nations. *United Nations Convention Against Illicit Traffic in Narcotic Drugs and Psychotropic Substances.* Vienna: 20 December 1988 [1993] ATS 4.

United Nations. *United Nations Single Convention on Narcotic Drugs.* New York: 30 March 1961 [1967] ATS 31.

United States Pharmacopeial Convention. *USP DI: Drug Information for the Health Care Professional.* 18th edn. Rockville: United States Pharmacopeial Convention, 1998.

Vane JR. Inhibition of prostaglandin synthesis as a mechanism of action for aspirin-like drugs. *Nature New Biology* 1971; 231: 232–9.

Vitry A. Is Australia free from direct-to-consumer advertising? *Australian Prescriber* 2004; 27(1): 4–6.

Walter G, Konthur Z, Lehrach H. High-throughput screening of surface displayed gene products. *Combinatorial Chemistry & High Throughput Screening* 2001; 4(2): 193–205.

Zhang L, Demain AL (eds). *Natural Products: Drug Discovery and Therapeutic Medicine.* Totowa, NJ: Humana Press, 2005.

ON-LINE RESOURCES

Adverse Drug Reactions Advisory Committee (ADRAC). *Australian Adverse Drug Reactions Bulletin.* Canberra: Therapeutic Goods Administration [published 4 times per year]: www.tga.gov.au/adr/aadrb/htm

Australian and New Zealand Council for the Care of Animals in Research and Teaching (ANZCCART): www.adelaide.edu.au/ANZCCART/

Medicines regulation and the TGA (Sept. 2004): www.tga.gov.au/docs/html/medregs.htm

New Zealand Drug Regulatory Information: www.medsafe.govt.nz/reg.htm

Standard for the Uniform Scheduling of Drugs and Poisons (SUSDP): www.tga.health.gov.au/ndpsc/susdp.htm

Therapeutic Goods Administration. Access to unapproved therapeutic goods: clinical trials in Australia. Canberra: TGA, 2001: www.tga.gov.au/docs/html/clintrials.htm

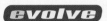 More weblinks at http://evolve.elsevier.com/AU/Bryant/pharmacology/

CHAPTER 5

Molecular Aspects of Drug Action and Pharmacodynamics

CHAPTER FOCUS

Drugs have been one of the mainstays of therapeutics for centuries. Belief in their 'magical' powers has now been supplanted by scientific understanding of the basis of drug action. This knowledge has enabled health-care professionals to use drugs more effectively and safely and to develop new drugs that produce more selective effects with diminished adverse effects. An understanding of the molecular targets for drug action and of the relation between the concentration of a drug and the pharmacological response it produces underpins many aspects of the use of drugs.

OBJECTIVES

- To describe the molecular targets at which drugs bind.
- To discuss the concept of drug selectivity.
- To discuss the molecular mechanisms by which drugs produce a functional response.
- To explain why some receptors lose responsiveness to drugs over time.
- To define the term pharmacodynamics.
- To explain the difference between a drug that acts as a receptor agonist and a drug that acts as a receptor antagonist.
- To define the terms drug potency and maximal drug efficacy.

KEY TERMS

agonist
antagonist
desensitisation
downregulation
drug potency
G-protein-coupled receptors
maximal drug efficacy
molecular target
pharmacodynamics
receptor
selectivity
specificity
tachyphylaxis
upregulation

KEY ABBREVIATIONS

GPCRs G-protein-coupled receptors
cAMP cyclic adenosine monophosphate

FOR centuries the curative and palliative power of medicinal products was embedded in the belief that their actions were brought about by 'magic'. Thanks to the work of Paul Ehrlich (1845–1915) and others, the myths of magical forces were dispelled and foundations were laid for the concept that the action of a drug involves a chemical interaction between the drug and a biological target.

Drugs do not confer any new functions on a tissue or organ in the body; they modify existing physiological, biochemical or biophysical functions. Their effects can be recognised by alterations to known functions or processes. For example, when an antihypertensive drug is prescribed for a person with hypertension, the health-care professional can monitor the effectiveness of the drug by repeated measurements of the person's blood pressure. Drugs can act by combining with a small molecule (e.g. antacids neutralise gastric acid), producing an alteration of cell membrane activity (e.g. local anaesthetics) or combining with receptors (e.g. atropine reduces the rate of salivation by interacting with receptors on salivary glands). With the exception of drugs that act on DNA, all drugs act by binding to a protein, the **molecular target** or site of action.

MOLECULAR TARGETS FOR DRUG ACTION

An ideal drug would interact with only one molecular target, at one site, and have only one effect. Such a drug would be described as having complete **specificity**; unfortunately, no drugs can lay claim to that title. Most drugs show **selectivity**: that is, they show a preference for a molecular target. For example, isoprenaline interacts with β_1 receptors in the heart, causing tachycardia, and β_2 receptors in the lungs, causing bronchodilation. In contrast, salbutamol is a selective β_2 bronchodilator, and greater site (in this case tissue) selectivity is achieved when the drug is inhaled. At higher doses, salbutamol causes muscle tremor by interacting with β_2 receptors in skeletal muscle—selectivity for β_2 receptors is retained but tissue selectivity is lost.

Selectivity of a drug depends on its chemical structure, molecular size and electrical charge. Changes in any of these parameters can dramatically increase or decrease the binding of a drug to its molecular target, altering its therapeutic efficacy or toxicity.

To understand how drugs act we need to understand the sites at which they bind, the molecular mechanisms by which an extracellular signal alters an intracellular pathway and causes a functional change in a cell, and why under some circumstances the response to drugs decreases with time.

Not all drugs act in exactly the same manner, but, in general, drugs act on four main types of proteins. These are called regulatory proteins because they mediate the actions of hormones, neurotransmitters and autocoids. The four types of regulatory proteins are:

- carriers
- enzymes
- ion channels
- receptors.

Carriers

Ions and small molecules that lack sufficient lipid solubility to enable them to diffuse across biological membranes must be transported. Examples of carriers include those that transport glucose, move sodium and calcium ions out of cells and transport sodium/potassium/chloride in the loop of Henle of the kidney nephron. Other important carriers include those that are involved in the uptake of chemicals acting at nerve terminals, such as noradrenaline, 5-hydroxytryptamine (5-HT, serotonin) and glutamate. These specific carriers are often targets for drugs. The tricyclic antidepressants and cocaine are examples of drugs that inhibit carrier-mediated uptake of noradrenaline, an important transmitter in the sympathetic nervous system (see Chapter 12).

Enzymes

Enzymes are indispensable biological catalysts that control all the biochemical reactions of the cell. A drug can inhibit the action of a specific enzyme and so alter a physiological response; for example, neostigmine combines with the enzyme acetylcholinesterase to prevent the breakdown of acetylcholine at the neuromuscular junction. This drug is used to manage the muscle weakness caused by myasthenia gravis.

Drugs that interact with enzymes are thought to do so by virtue of their structural resemblance to an enzyme's substrate molecule (the substance acted on by an enzyme). A drug may resemble an enzyme's substrate so closely that the enzyme combines with the drug instead of the substrate. Drugs resembling enzyme substrates are often termed 'antimetabolites' and can either block normal enzymatic action or result in the production of other substances with different biochemical properties. An example of an antimetabolite is the anticancer drug methotrexate.

Several commonly used drugs that target enzymes are listed in Table 5-1 along with the numbers of the chapters in which the individual drugs are discussed.

Ion channels

Cell membranes are complex lipoprotein structures that regulate the flow of ions and metabolites in a highly selective manner through ion channels, thereby maintaining an electrochemical gradient between the interior and exterior of the cell. A variety of drugs target ion channels. These

TABLE 5-1 Common enzyme-targeting drugs

ENZYME	DRUG	CHAPTER
Acetylcholinesterase	Neostigmine	13
Angiotensin-converting enzyme	Captopril	25
Cyclo-oxygenase	Ibuprofen	55
Dihydrofolate reductase	Trimethoprim	51
3-Hydroxy-3-methylglutaryl coenzyme A reductase	Simvastatin	26
Thymidine kinase	Aciclovir	52
Topoisomerase II	Ciprofloxacin	51
Xanthine oxidase	Allopurinol	55

**CLINICAL INTEREST BOX 5-1
DRUGS AND THE THEORY OF RECEPTORS**

John N Langley (1852–1926) first came up with the idea that drugs act on receptors when he was studying the effects of atropine and pilocarpine on saliva flow in cats. The term 'receptor' or 'receptive substance' is generally attributed to the Nobel laureate Paul Ehrlich. When studying more than 900 compounds in search of a drug to treat syphilis, he observed that many of the compounds produced antimicrobial effects with a high degree of selectivity. These observations led in 1913 to his proposal that the interaction of a drug with its receptor is akin to that of a lock and key, and that only certain drugs would fit into the receptor and activate it.

Knowledge of cell receptors is now a mainstay of pharmacology research and drug development as numerous drugs are targeted to act on specific receptors.

---

include the diuretic amiloride (see Chapter 28), which blocks entry of sodium into renal tubular cells, and the very large group of calcium channel-blocking drugs, such as verapamil, nifedipine and diltiazem (see Chapter 25).

Receptors

Receptors form a large group of proteins that are targets for drugs. However, the term 'receptor' is widely and loosely used. Some authors when referring to receptors mean any molecular drug target, for example a peptide, a membrane component, an enzyme, or even a cell or organ. Throughout this text the term 'receptor' refers specifically to "cellular macromolecules that are concerned directly and specifically in chemical signalling between and within cells. Combination of a hormone, neurotransmitter, drug or intracellular messenger with its receptor(s) initiates a change in cell function" (International Union of Pharmacology 1998).

Structural specificity is an essential postulate of the receptor theory of drug action. In essence, a certain portion of the drug molecule selectively combines or interacts with the receptor to produce a pharmacological effect. The relationship of a drug to its receptor has often been likened to that of the fit of a key in a lock. The drug represents the key that fits into the lock, or receptor. Thus a complementary spatial relationship exists between a certain portion of the drug molecule and the receptor site.

Families of receptors

There are four major families of receptors. Type 1: Ligand-gated ion channels; these include the nicotinic acetylcholine receptor (Chapter 13) and the type A gamma-aminobutyric acid (GABA$_A$) receptor (Chapter 14). Type 2: G-protein-coupled receptors (GPCRs); discussed in the following section. Type 3: Kinase-linked receptors; these transmembrane receptors are similar in structure to the GPCRs but have different transduction mechanisms. Receptors of this type include insulin receptors and the various types of receptors acted on by growth hormones and cytokines. Type 4: Nuclear receptors; these receptors regulate gene transcription. Although called 'nuclear' they are often located in the cytosol and require binding of various other molecules prior to translocation to the nucleus where they interact with specific response elements located on genes, e.g. steroid hormone receptors (Chapter 40). Types 1–3 are found bound in the cell membrane while Type 4, the nuclear receptors that affect gene transcription (e.g. the oestrogen receptor), are located in the cytosol. Specific examples of the membrane-bound receptors include the nicotinic acetylcholine receptor, which is discussed in detail in Chapter 13 and is the site of action of neuromuscular blocking drugs, and the large family of guanine nucleotide protein-coupled receptors. These receptors, more commonly referred to as **G-protein-coupled receptors** (GPCRs), include the receptors that are perhaps more familiar to healthcare professionals as muscarinic acetylcholine receptors, the receptors for adrenaline and noradrenaline (adrenoceptors), dopamine receptors, opiate receptors and many more. As GPCRs are important sites exploited in pharmacotherapy, a brief summary of how they influence cell functioning follows.

G-protein-coupled receptors and second messengers

Once a drug binds to a receptor, many different types of response can be elicited. This depends on the mechanism of coupling of the receptor to the intracellular system

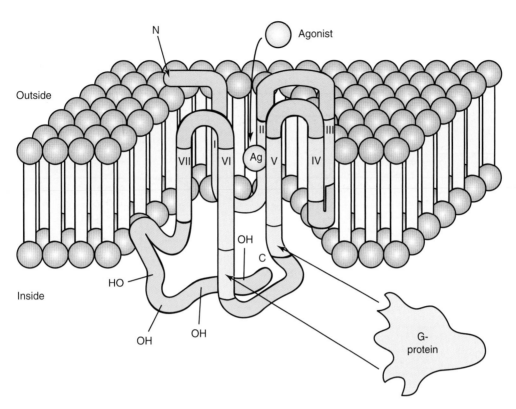

FIGURE 5-1 Membrane localisation of a typical G-protein-coupled receptor. The receptor's amino (N) terminal is above the plane of the membrane and is extracellular; the carboxyl (C) terminal is located inside the membrane and is intracellular. The terminals are connected by a polypeptide chain that traverses the membrane seven times. The segments located within the membrane are designated by roman numerals (I–VII). The agonist (Ag) approaches the receptor from the extracellular fluid and binds to a site surrounded by the transmembrane regions of the receptor protein. G-proteins (G) interact with cytoplasmic regions of the receptor, especially with portions of the third cytoplasmic loop between transmembrane regions V and VI. *Source*: Katzung, *Basic and Clinical Pharmacology*, 2004. Reproduced with permission of The McGraw-Hill Companies.

that produces the functional response. GPCRs consist of an extracellular (amino) terminal that projects above the membrane, a polypeptide chain shaped like a serpent that traverses the membrane seven times (designated I–VII) and an intracellular (carboxyl) terminal (Figure 5-1). Interaction with the receptor occurs when a chemical approaches the receptor from the extracellular fluid and binds to a site within the membrane-spanning regions. This leads to an interaction between the associated G-protein and the cytoplasmic portion of the third membrane-spanning loop. There are many different types of G-proteins and, through a series of reactions, the activated G-protein changes the activity of a second messenger specific to the type of G-protein (Figure 5-2).

Second messengers

For a cell to respond to an external stimulus (e.g. binding of a drug or hormone to a receptor), the signal has to be communicated from the exterior of the cell to the respective response elements within the cell. This mechanism of communication often involves a second messenger system.

cAMP

One of the most studied second messengers is cyclic adenosine monophosphate (cAMP), which mediates effects such as the breakdown of fat, conservation of water by the kidney and the rate and force of contraction of the heart. Cyclic AMP exerts most of its effects through a series of protein kinases that ultimately involve phosphate and ATP (Figure 5-2). The breakdown of cAMP by the enzyme phosphodiesterase terminates its action. Inhibition of phosphodiesterase is the mechanism by which caffeine and theophylline exert their effects. The cAMP second messenger system is linked to the action of β-adrenoceptors and many other receptors.

PHOSPHOINOSITIDES AND CALCIUM

Another well-studied second messenger system involves hydrolysis of a minor component of cell membranes, splitting it into two second messengers, diacylglycerol and inositol triphosphate (Figure 5-2). The diacylglycerol is confined to the cell membrane where it activates protein kinase C, which causes changes in the activity of other enzymes that ultimately produce the functional response (e.g. increased glandular secretions). The inositol triphosphate diffuses through the

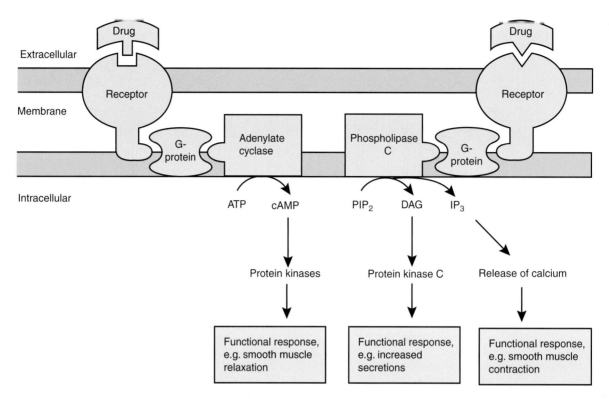

FIGURE 5-2 Schematic representation of activation of G-protein-coupled receptors by drugs. The second messenger systems involved include (1) cAMP, which activates various protein kinases linked to cellular functions (e.g. smooth muscle relaxation), and (2) activation of phospholipase C, which cleaves phosphatidylinositol-4, 5-bisphosphate (PIP$_2$) to form diacylglycerol (DAG), which activates protein kinase C, and inositol triphosphate (IP$_3$), which releases intracellular calcium. ATP = adenosine triphosphate.

cytoplasm and causes the release of calcium from storage sites. The increased intracellular calcium then regulates the activity of other enzymes, producing a response such as increased contractility. These particular second messengers are important for producing the effects mediated by α-adrenoceptors and muscarinic receptors.

Receptor desensitisation and turnover

Receptor populations are not static and receptors may undergo several changes, including loss of responsiveness or a decrease or increase in the number of receptors. The term used clinically to describe loss of responsiveness after repeated exposure to a drug that stimulates the receptor is **tachyphylaxis**. It is rapid in onset and the individual's initial response to the drug cannot be reproduced, even with larger doses of the drug. Transdermal nitroglycerin used in the treatment of angina is an example of a drug that requires an intermittent dosing schedule (12 hours on, 12 hours off) to limit the problem of tachyphylaxis.

The term **desensitisation** refers more specifically to a decrease in the response of the receptor–second messenger system and is a common feature of many receptors. The

mechanisms underlying receptor desensitisation are complex and include (1) an uncoupling of the receptor from its second messenger system, (2) altered binding of the drug to the receptor, and (3) a decrease in receptor numbers.

The total number of receptors in the cell membrane at any one time can change. A decrease in receptor number is called **downregulation** and can contribute to desensitisation and loss of response. An increase in receptor number is referred to as **upregulation** and can cause receptor supersensitivity. For example, upregulation of receptors often occurs after chronic use of drugs that block receptors; when the drug is abruptly removed the person may experience increased responsiveness to stimuli (e.g. rebound hypertension).

Because the binding of a drug to a receptor produces a functional response, it is appropriate at this stage to consider the relationship between the concentration of the drug and the response.

PHARMACODYNAMICS

Pharmacodynamics is the study of the interaction between a drug and its molecular target and of the pharmacological response: *what the drug does to the body*.

Drugs that bind to a receptor are termed agonists or antagonists. An **agonist** binds to (occupies) and activates the receptor and produces the same response as the endogenous ligand. Some drugs are considered partial agonists as they produce less than the maximal effect even when all receptors are occupied. An **antagonist** binds to the receptor and blocks access of the endogenous ligand, thus diminishing the normal response. Drugs may act as competitive (reversible) or irreversible antagonists. (Drugs that are antagonists are commonly called 'blockers'.)

Drugs that are receptor agonists

When a drug is administered, the response usually increases in proportion to the dose until the receptors are saturated. Increasing the dose further at this stage does not produce any further increase in response. When plotted on an arithmetic scale, the relation between the concentration of the drug and the response elicited is hyperbolic (Figure 5-3). This relationship is described by the equation

$$E = \frac{E_{max} \times C}{C + EC_{50}}$$

E = the effect observed at a drug concentration of C
E_{max} = the maximal response that the drug can produce
EC_{50} = concentration at which the drug produces 50% of its maximal response.

How does knowledge of the concentration–response relationship for a drug serve a useful purpose?

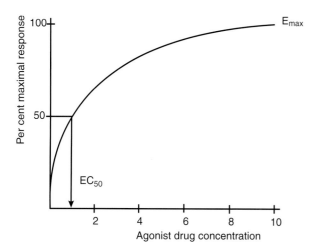

FIGURE 5-3 A drug concentration–response curve plotted on an arithmetic scale. The EC_{50} is the drug concentration at which 50% of the maximal response is observed. E_{max} is the maximal response when all the receptors are occupied.

Drug potency

Drugs are often referred to as 'potent' or 'very potent', but what does this mean and how is it calculated? If we use the relationship described previously, then the EC_{50} reflects the affinity or attraction between the drug and the receptor, and is a measure of **drug potency**. Plotting the concentration–response data for several drugs using a semi-logarithmic scale allows us to easily determine the relative potencies of the drugs (Figure 5-4). The sigmoid shape of the curves on a logarithmic plot includes a linear portion that occurs between 20% and 80% of the maximal response. This section "most often applies to drugs at therapeutic concentrations and increasing drug concentration above 80% maximal response achieves very little in terms of extra therapeutic effects, but increases the risk of adverse effects" (Birkett 2002).

Maximal drug efficacy

Another term that is also commonly used to describe drugs is their **maximal efficacy** (often simply called efficacy). Again, the concentration–response curves allow us to determine the maximal efficacy of a drug, i.e. the maximum response a drug can produce (E_{max}).

Several drugs may have the same potency (EC_{50}) but differ in their efficacy (Figure 5-5). Conversely, as shown in Figure 5-4, drugs may differ in their potency but have the same maximal efficacy. This is important clinically because the effectiveness of a drug depends on its maximal efficacy and not on its potency. To illustrate this point, let us assume that the three drugs in Figure 5-5 are used as bronchodilators in the treatment of asthma. The question could be asked: Does it matter which drug is used if they are equipotent as bronchodilators? Knowing the concentration–response curves for the various drugs would provide the answer. Drugs A and B would provide a greater clinical response (bronchodilation) than drug C as they have greater efficacy.

Drugs that are receptor antagonists

We also need to consider drugs that act as receptor antagonists. Drugs of this type bind to the receptor without eliciting a response (they have no efficacy) and prevent the binding of the endogenous agonist. An example of a receptor antagonist is propranolol, a β-adrenoceptor antagonist (commonly called a β-blocker) that blocks the action of circulating adrenaline and slows the heart rate. Antagonists can be divided into two types: those that compete with the endogenous agonist, and those that bind to the receptor in an irreversible manner.

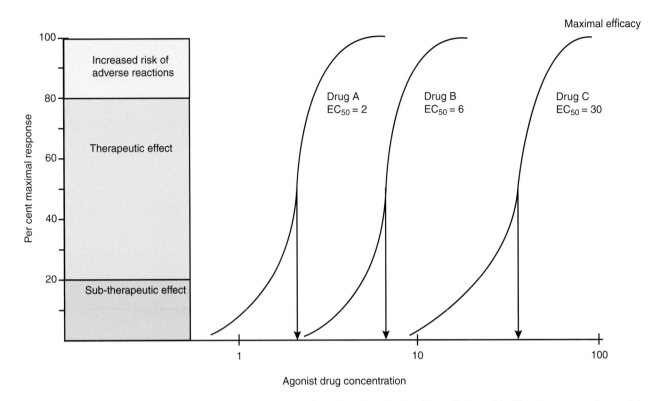

FIGURE 5-4 Theoretical concentration–response curves on a logarithmic scale for drugs A, B and C. The drugs are all agonists acting on the same receptor and eliciting the same response. Drug A ($EC_{50} = 2$) is three times more potent than drug B ($EC_{50} = 6$), which is five times more potent than drug C ($EC_{50} = 30$). Drugs A, B and C all differ in their potency but have the same maximal efficacy.

Competitive (reversible) antagonists

Competitive antagonists interfere with the binding of the endogenous agonist: that is, they 'compete'. Their action can be overcome by increasing the concentration of the agonist. In essence, the agonist displaces the antagonist but the maximal response produced by the agonist does not change. On a concentration–response curve of an agonist in the presence of a competitive antagonist, the curve is shifted to the right. This indicates that a much higher concentration of agonist is needed to produce 50% of the maximal response (Figure 5-6). For example, higher concentrations of adrenaline are needed to overcome the competitive blockade of β-adrenoceptors by propranolol.

Competitive (irreversible) antagonists

Irreversible antagonists have limited therapeutic usefulness, as they make the target receptor permanently unavailable for binding of the endogenous agonist. Used experimentally to

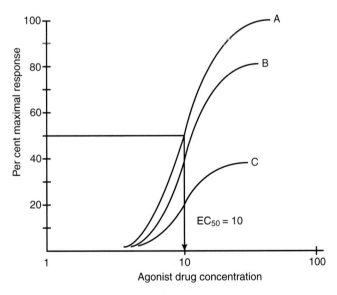

FIGURE 5-5 Concentration–response curves for three drugs A, B and C, all with the same potency ($EC_{50} = 10$) but different maximal efficacies. In this example, drugs B and C are classed as partial agonists as they produce less than the maximal effect achieved with the full agonist drug A.

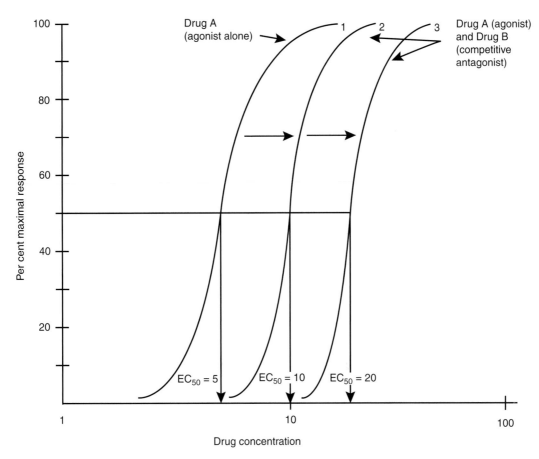

FIGURE 5-6 Competitive antagonism of the response produced by drug A (curve 1) by increasing concentrations (curves 2 and 3) of the competitive antagonist drug B. Note the shift of the concentration–response curve to the right without a change in the maximal efficacy of drug A.

investigate receptor function, their action is usually prolonged and is not terminated until the receptors 'die' and are replaced by new receptors. Examples of chemicals in this class include some inhibitors of acetylcholinesterase and chemicals such as nerve gases (see Chapter 13).

The magnitude of a pharmacological effect depends on the concentration of a drug at its molecular target or site of action. Factors that influence this include the absorption, distribution, metabolism and excretion of the drug. These aspects are discussed in detail in Chapter 6.

Non-competitive antagonists

Non-competitive antagonists block the response to an agonist at some point within the cascade of intracellular events. Examples of drugs in this category include the calcium channel blockers, which bind to the calcium channel and prevent the influx of calcium through the open channel. When another drug (agonist) binds to the calcium channel, the loss of calcium influx caused by the calcium channel blocker prevents smooth muscle contraction, which normally results from the binding of the agonist.

KEY POINTS

- Drugs do not confer any new functions on a tissue or organ in the body; they modify existing physiological, biochemical or biophysical functions.
- With the exception of many cancer chemotherapeutic drugs that act on DNA, all drugs act by binding to proteins, which are the molecular targets or sites of action.
- An ideal drug would interact with only one molecular target, at one site, and have only one effect, i.e. it would be specific. Most drugs show selectivity, i.e. they show a preference for a molecular target.
- Selectivity of a drug for any molecular target depends on its chemical structure, molecular size and electrical charge.

- There are four main types of regulatory proteins that drugs act on: carriers, enzymes, ion channels and receptors.
- A large group of proteins that are targets for drugs are receptors, which are cellular macromolecules directly concerned with chemical signalling to initiate a change in cell function.
- Many receptors are coupled through G-proteins linked to second messengers that produce the functional response to agonist binding.
- Receptors can lose responsiveness (tachyphylaxis), become desensitised, or be downregulated or upregulated.
- Pharmacodynamics is the study of the interaction between a drug and its molecular target and the pharmacological response: what the drug does to the body.
- An agonist binds to (occupies) and activates a receptor producing the same response as the endogenous ligand. Some drugs are partial agonists as they produce less than the maximal effect even when all receptors are occupied.
- An antagonist binds to a receptor and blocks access of the endogenous ligand, thus diminishing the normal response. Drugs may act as competitive (reversible) or irreversible antagonists. (Drugs that are antagonists are commonly called 'blockers'.)
- When a drug is administered, the response usually increases in proportion to the dose until the receptors are saturated. Increasing the dose further does not produce any further increase in response.
- The concentration at which a drug produces 50% of its maximal response is called the EC_{50}.
- The EC_{50} reflects the affinity or attraction between the drug and the receptor, and is a measure of drug potency.
- The maximal efficacy of a drug is the maximum response a drug can produce.
- The clinical effectiveness of a drug depends on its maximal efficacy and not on its potency.
- Competitive antagonists interfere with the binding of the endogenous agonist, i.e. they 'compete', and their action can be overcome by increasing the concentration of the agonist.
- Competitive irreversible antagonists have limited therapeutic usefulness as they bind irreversibly to the receptor, making it permanently unavailable for binding of the agonist. Their action is usually prolonged and is not terminated until the receptors are replaced by new receptors.

REVIEW EXERCISES

1. What are the four main types of regulatory proteins that drugs act on?
2. Why are some drugs receptor agonists while others are receptor antagonists?
3. Of what value clinically is knowledge of a drug's concentration–response relationship?

REFERENCES AND FURTHER READING

Birkett DJ. Pharmacodynamics—the concentration–effect relationship. In: Birkett DJ. *Pharmacokinetics Made Easy*. Sydney: McGraw-Hill, 2002 [ch. 11].

Brody TM. Concentration–response relationships. In: Brody TM, Larner J, Minneman KP (eds). *Human Pharmacology, Molecular to Clinical*. 3rd edn. St Louis: Mosby, 1998 [ch. 3].

Brody TM, Garrison JC. Sites of action: receptors. In: Brody TM, Larner J, Minneman KP (eds). *Human Pharmacology, Molecular to Clinical*. 3rd edn. St Louis: Mosby, 1998 [ch. 2].

International Union of Pharmacology. *The IUPHAR Compendium of Receptor Characterization and Classification*. Foxton, UK: The International Union of Pharmacology, IUPHAR Media Ltd, Burlington Press, 1998.

Katzung BG (ed.). *Basic and Clinical Pharmacology*. 9th edn. New York: The McGraw-Hill Companies, Inc, 2004 [ch. 2].

Rang HP, Dale MM, Ritter JM, Moore PK. How drugs act: general principles. In Rang HP, Dale MM, Ritter JM, Moore PK. *Pharmacology*. 5th edn. Edinburgh: Churchill Livingstone, 2003 [ch. 1].

Rang HP, Dale MM, Ritter JM, Moore PK. How drugs act: molecular aspects. In Rang HP, Dale MM, Ritter JM, Moore PK. *Pharmacology*. 5th edn. Edinburgh: Churchill Livingstone, 2003 [ch. 2].

evolve More weblinks at http://evolve.elsevier.com/AU/Bryant/pharmacology/

CHAPTER 6

Drug Absorption, Distribution, Metabolism and Excretion

CHAPTER FOCUS

To meet the knowledge challenge created by the numerous drugs already marketed combined with the many new drugs released annually, health-care professionals must develop an understanding of the fundamental principles of drug absorption, distribution, metabolism and excretion. From these processes stems the theoretical framework that provides the basis for the design of drug dosage regimens.

OBJECTIVES

- To discuss the influence of the pharmaceutical and pharmacokinetic phases on the concentration of drug that reaches its molecular target.

- To cite the main variables that affect drug absorption.

- To explain the concept of oral bioavailability of a drug.

- To discuss the contribution of pharmacogenetics and enzyme induction and inhibition to interindividual variability in drug metabolism.

- To explain the processes involved in renal excretion of drugs.

KEY TERMS

absorption
active transport
bioavailability
bioequivalence
conjugation
diffusion
dissolution
distribution
elimination
excretion
first-pass effect
functionalisation
ionised
loading dose
metabolism
pharmacogenetics
pharmacokinetics
un-ionised
volume of distribution

KEY ABBREVIATION

CYP   cytochrome P450

FOR a drug to produce an effect, it must reach its molecular target (see Chapter 5). This leads us to the fundamental principles of drug absorption, distribution, metabolism and excretion. With the exception of some drugs that are used solely for a local effect (e.g. ointments used for skin rashes), most drugs are administered outside the vascular system (extravascularly). Before they can be distributed to their site of action, drugs must be absorbed from the point of application into the systemic circulation. The concentration of drug that finally reaches its molecular target is influenced by various processes that may be divided broadly into three phases: pharmaceutical, pharmacokinetic and pharmacodynamic (discussed in Chapter 5). The sequential order of these phases is depicted in Figure 6-1.

PHARMACEUTICAL PHASE

Pharmaceutics is the study of the ways in which various drug formulations influence the pharmacokinetics and pharmacodynamics of a drug. An oral drug may be in a solid form (tablet, capsule or powder) or in liquid form (solution or suspension).

Disintegration of solid dosage forms must occur before **dissolution**, a process by which a drug goes into solution and becomes available for absorption. The drug dosage form is important because the more rapid the rate of dissolution, the more rapidly the drug is presented to the membrane for absorption. Oral drugs in liquid form are more rapidly available for gastrointestinal absorption than those in solid form (Figure 6-2 and Box 6-1).

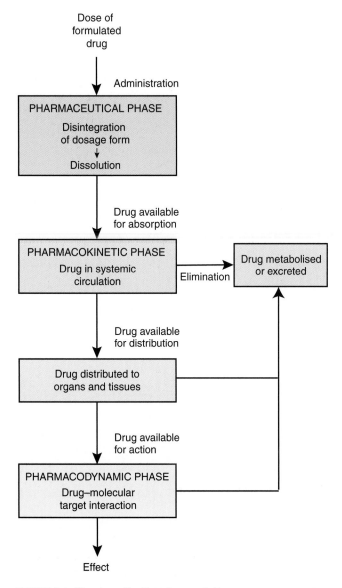

FIGURE 6-1 Phases affecting drug activity.

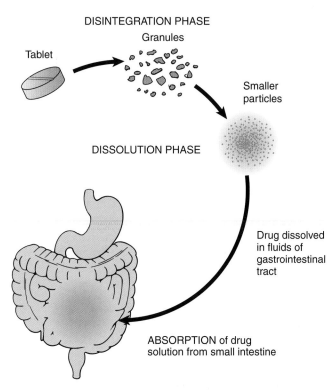

FIGURE 6-2 The pharmaceutical phase.

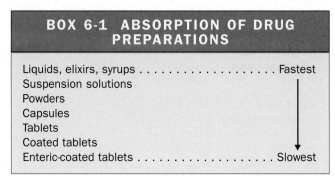

BOX 6-1   ABSORPTION OF DRUG PREPARATIONS

Liquids, elixirs, syrups . . . . Fastest
Suspension solutions
Powders
Capsules
Tablets
Coated tablets
Enteric-coated tablets . . . . Slowest

PHARMACOKINETIC PHASE

The concentration that a drug attains at its site of action is influenced by the rate and extent to which a drug is:
• absorbed into body fluids
• distributed to the sites of action
• metabolised into inactive or active metabolites
• excreted from the body by various routes (Figure 6-3).

The study of the kinetics of a drug during the processes of absorption, distribution, metabolism and excretion, or simply 'what the body does to the drug', is collectively described by the term **pharmacokinetics**. As there are many definitions that are relevant to the field of pharmacokinetics, these are compiled in Box 6-2.

Drug absorption

Absorption is defined as the process by which unchanged drug proceeds from the site of administration into the blood. It is an important factor for all routes of administration with the exception of the intravenous route, where the drug is administered directly into the systematic circulation and does not require absorption from the site of administration.

Absorption across biological membranes

For absorption to occur, it is necessary for a drug to cross a membrane and enter the blood vessels on the other side. The membrane typically consists of a lipid bilayer that contains protein molecules irregularly dispersed throughout it. These protein molecules themselves may act as carriers, enzymes, receptors or antigenic sites. Lipid(fat)-soluble drugs can easily pass through the lipid membrane, while ionised or water-soluble drugs have difficulty crossing cell membranes. The membrane, which contains aqueous channels (pores), permits the passage of small water-soluble substances such as urea, alcohol, electrolytes, and water itself.

When free to move to their sites of action, drug molecules are transported from one body compartment to another by way of the plasma; however, free movement can be somewhat limited because membranes enclose also these various sites. Whether the barrier to drug transport consists of a single layer of cells, such as the intestinal epithelium of the villi, or several layers of cells, such as skin, in order for a drug to gain access to the interior of a cell or a body compartment it has to penetrate cell membranes. All the physiological processes mediating absorption, distribution, metabolism and excretion are predicated on three drug transport systems: membrane openings or pores, passive transport, and active or carrier transport.

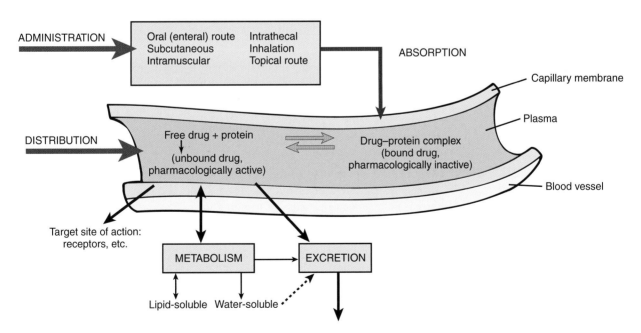

FIGURE 6-3 Schema of the pharmacokinetic phases, showing absorption, distribution, metabolism and excretion of drugs. Note that within any body compartment drug molecules are either free or in the bound state; however, only free (unbound) drug reaches the site of action, is metabolised and excreted. Within the systemic circulation the drug–protein complex represents bound drug and because the molecule is large it moves within the vascular system but is retained within the blood vessel until it dissociates into free drug, which then crosses biological membranes.

BOX 6-2 KEY PHARMACOKINETIC DEFINITIONS

- **Absorption**—the process by which unchanged drug proceeds from the site of administration into the blood
- **Bioavailability**—the proportion of the administered dose that reaches the systemic circulation as intact drug
- **Bioequivalence**—where two formulations of the same drug attain similar concentrations in blood and tissues at similar times, with no clinically important differences between their therapeutic or adverse effects
- **Distribution**—the process of reversible transfer of a drug between one location and another (one of which is usually blood) in the body
- **Elimination**—the irreversible loss of drug from the body by the processes of metabolism and excretion
- **Excretion**—the loss of chemically unchanged drug or metabolites from the body, e.g. in urine, bile, expired air or faeces
- **Metabolism**—the process of chemical modification of a drug
- **Volume of distribution**—the volume in which the amount of drug in the body would need to be uniformly distributed to produce the observed (measured) concentration in blood

---

MEMBRANE OPENINGS OR PORES

These openings or pores are very small, so only a few of the smallest drugs (<100 daltons) can be transported by this method.

PASSIVE TRANSPORT—DIFFUSION

Most drugs cross membranes by a process of **diffusion**, which is the transfer of drug from a region of higher concentration to a region of lower concentration until equilibrium is established at the membrane. No energy is required for this process, which is a passive process.

CARRIER-MEDIATED TRANSPORT

Carrier-mediated transport is necessary for the transport of amino acids, glucose, some vitamins, neurotransmitters, metal ions and some drugs. Moderate-sized ions and water-soluble drugs are transported by carriers that form complexes with the drug molecules on the membrane surface to carry them through the membrane and then dissociate from them. In the case of **active transport** this requires an energy source: active transport involves the movement of drug molecules against the concentration gradient (from areas of low concentration to areas of high concentration) or, in the case of ions, against the electrochemical potential gradient, as with the sodium–potassium pump.

Carrier-mediated transport of drugs is important in the kidney, the gastrointestinal tract, biliary tree and the blood–brain barrier. Often referred to as 'drug transporters', these proteins can function as either uptake transporters or efflux transporters. The most studied of the efflux transporters is P-glycoprotein (P-gp; also called MDR1, 'multi-drug resistance'), which was first discovered in tumour cells and is associated with the multi-drug resistance phenomenon observed clinically in patients treated with cancer chemotherapeutic drugs for long periods of time. This drug resistance results from overexpression of P-gp, which leads to an increased efflux of the cytotoxic drug from the cancer cell, thus lowering the intracellular concentration of such drugs as paclitaxel, vincristine and doxorubicin (Chapter 49). In addition to cytotoxic drugs, P-gp transports digoxin. P-gp is found in the adrenals, brain, intestine, kidney, liver, placenta and testes.

The major family of uptake transporters are the organic anion transporting polypeptides (OATP). The first human OATP (OATP1A2) was isolated from liver but it is also found in brain, lung, kidney and testes. OATP1A2 transports a diverse range of compounds including bile acids, thyroid hormones, steroid sulfates, the antihistamine fexofenadine and opioid peptides. OATP1A2 may be important for regulating permeability of the blood–brain barrier to solutes. In the liver OATP1B1 appears to play a major role in the hepatic uptake of bile acids, sulfate and glucuronide conjugates and of drugs such as methotrexate and the lipid-lowering drug pravastatin.

As knowledge of drug transporters continues to grow it is becoming increasingly apparent that drug transporters are subject to induction and inhibition by coadministered drugs (see the Drug interactions section in Chapter 9).

Variables that affect drug absorption

The rate and extent to which a drug is absorbed are influenced by the following variables.

Nature of the absorbing surface (cell membrane) that the drug must traverse. The drug molecule may pass through a single layer of cells (e.g. intestinal epithelium), in which case transport is faster than if it traverses several layers of cells (e.g. skin). The size of the surface area of the absorbing site is also an important determinant of drug absorption. Generally, the more extensive the absorbing surface, the greater the drug absorption and the more rapid its effects. Anaesthetics are absorbed immediately from the pulmonary epithelium because of the vast surface area of the lung. Absorption from the small intestine, which also offers a massive absorbing area, is more rapid than from an equivalent smaller absorbing surface, such as the stomach.

Blood flow. The circulation to the site of administration is a significant factor in the absorption of drugs. A rich blood supply (e.g. the sublingual route) enhances absorption, whereas a poor vascular site (e.g. the subcutaneous route) delays it. An individual in shock, for example, may not respond to intramuscularly administered drugs because of poor peripheral circulation. Drugs injected intravenously, on the other hand, are placed directly into the circulatory system and are available immediately. Food increases splanchnic blood flow and enhances absorption of orally administered drugs. Conversely, in hypovolaemic states absorption of drugs may be slowed due to decreased splanchnic blood flow.

Solubility of the drug. To be absorbed, a drug must be in solution; the more soluble the drug, the more rapidly it will be presented for absorption. Because cell membranes contain a fatty-acid layer, lipid solubility is a valuable attribute of drugs absorbed from certain areas, e.g. the gastrointestinal tract and the placenta. Chemicals and minerals that form insoluble precipitates in the gastrointestinal tract, such as barium salts, or drugs that are not soluble in water or lipids are not absorbed (e.g. the bile acid-binding resin cholestyramine).

Ionisation. In general, drugs exist as weak acids or weak bases and in body fluids they are either ionised or un-ionised. The **ionised** (charged polar) form is usually water-soluble (lipid-insoluble) and does not diffuse readily through the cell membranes of the body. By contrast, the **un-ionised** (non-polar) form is more lipid-soluble (less water-soluble) and is more apt to cross the cell membranes. The extent of ionisation is determined by the pH of the environment. Remember that reference to a 'weak' or 'strong' acid refers to the tendency of the acid to dissociate (break up) into hydrogen ions (H^+) and anions. This dissociation is often referred to as the pK_a, which describes the strength of weak acids. In general, acids with lower pK_a values (e.g. acetic acid, pK_a 4.75) are stronger acids that those with higher pK_a values (e.g. carbonic acid, pK_a 6.1). In simple terms the pK_a is the pH at which half the chemical (this can be a drug or an endogenous chemical such as an electrolyte) is in its ionised form. (The pH scale measures the concentration of hydrogen ions, and the higher the hydrogen ion concentration the lower the pH.) An acidic drug (e.g. aspirin, pK_a 2.98) is relatively un-ionised in an acid environment such as the stomach but a basic drug tends to ionise in the same acid environment. In contrast, absorption of a basic drug is enhanced in a more basic site such as the small intestine, while the acidic drug tends to be more ionised (Figure 6-4). Despite the varying states of ionisation, little drug absorption occurs in the stomach and most occurs in the small intestine.

Formulation. Drug formulation can be manipulated by pharmaceutical processing to achieve desirable absorption characteristics. An active drug can be combined with a resin or other substance from which it is slowly released, or prepared in a vehicle that offers relative resistance to the acidic environment of the stomach (e.g. enteric coating). Enteric coatings on drugs are used:

- to prevent decomposition of chemically sensitive drugs by gastric secretions (e.g. penicillin G and erythromycin are unstable in an acid pH), thus ensuring bioavailability

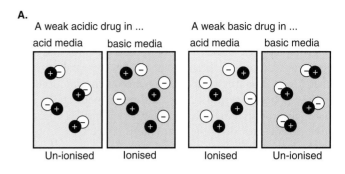

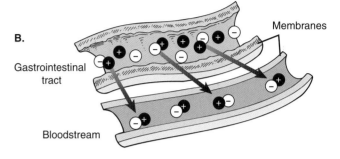

FIGURE 6-4 Effect of pH on drug ionisation and transport. **A.** Effects of pH on the ionisation state of a drug that is either a weak acid or a weak base. **B.** Effects of pH on the transport of drug molecules through membranes. Only un-ionised lipid-soluble drugs cross biological membranes.

- to prevent dilution of the drug before it reaches the intestine
- to prevent nausea and vomiting induced by the drug's effect in the stomach
- to provide delayed release of the drug.

Routes of drug administration

The route of drug administration can affect both the rate at which onset of action occurs and the magnitude of the therapeutic response that results. Drugs are given for either local or systemic effects. The local effect of a drug usually occurs at the immediate site of application, in which case absorption is a disadvantage. When a drug is given for a systemic effect, absorption is an essential first step before the drug appears in the circulation and is distributed to a location distant from the site of administration.

A drug may enter the circulation either by being injected there directly (intravenously) or by absorption from other extravascular sites. The routes of drug administration (see Figure 6-3) fall into the following major categories:

- oral (also called enteral)
- parenteral—subcutaneous, intramuscular, intravenous, intrathecal or epidermal
- inhalation
- topical.

Oral route

Oral, or enteral, ingestion is the most commonly used method of giving drugs. It is also the safest, most convenient and most economical route of administration. However, the frequent changes in the gastrointestinal environment produced by food, emotion, physical activity and other medications may make absorption unreliable and slow. Drugs may be absorbed from several sites along the gastrointestinal tract.

ABSORPTION FROM THE ORAL CAVITY

Although the oral cavity possesses a thin lining, a rich blood supply and a slightly acidic pH, little absorption occurs in the mouth. Despite its small surface area, the oral mucosa is capable of absorbing certain drugs as long as they dissolve rapidly in the salivary secretions (i.e. drugs given by the sublingual and buccal routes). In sublingual administration the drug is placed under the tongue to permit tablet dissolution in salivary secretions. Glyceryl trinitrate, used for treating angina, is administered in this manner and the recipient is advised to refrain as long as possible from swallowing saliva containing the tablet form of the drug. Because glyceryl trinitrate is un-ionised, with high lipid solubility, the drug readily diffuses through the lipid mucosal membranes. Drugs absorbed sublingually enter the systemic circulation directly without entering the portal system, thus bypassing the liver and escaping first-pass metabolism (see later). Accordingly, absorption is rapid and the effects of the drug may become apparent within 2 minutes. In buccal administration the drug (tablet) is placed between the teeth and the mucous membrane of the cheek. Some hormones and enzyme preparations are administered by this route and are rapidly absorbed.

ABSORPTION FROM THE STOMACH

Although the stomach has a rich blood supply and a relatively large surface area it is not an important site of drug absorption. The length of time a substance remains in the stomach is a significant variable in determining the extent of gastrointestinal absorption. Generally, lowering the gastric emptying rate decreases the rate of drug absorption. This is why many drugs are administered on an empty stomach, with sufficient water to ensure dissolution and rapid passage into the small intestine. (Drugs that cause gastric irritation are usually given with food.) After solid-dose drug administration the recipient should be encouraged to sit upright for at least 30 minutes to shorten gastric emptying time (the time required for the drug to reach the small intestine) and also to reduce the potential for tablets or capsules to lodge in the oesophageal area. Prolongation of emptying time increases the risk of destruction of acid-labile drugs (e.g. erythromycin base).

ABSORPTION FROM THE SMALL INTESTINE

The small intestine is highly vascularised and, with its many villi, which have more permeable membranes, it presents a significantly larger absorption area than the stomach. It is the major site for absorption of orally administered drugs that pass from the stomach into this region and are absorbed primarily in the upper part of the small intestine. The intestinal fluid is alkaline (pH 7–8), which strongly influences the rate of absorption of the un-ionised basic drugs. Increased intestinal motility caused, for example, by diarrhoea or cathartics may decrease exposure to the intestinal membrane and thereby diminish absorption, leading to therapeutic failure from low systemic drug concentration. Prolonged exposure, on the other hand, allows more time for absorption, and hence the possibility of increased plasma concentration and adverse drug reactions.

ABSORPTION FROM THE RECTUM

The surface area of the rectum is not very large, but drug absorption does occur because of extensive vascularity. Rectal suppositories are used for both local and systemic effects. Disadvantages to rectal drug administration include erratic absorption because of rectal contents, local drug irritation with some medications, and uncertainty of drug retention.

Parenteral route

The parenteral route refers to the administration of drugs by injection. Intravenous administration is the most rapid route of drug administration, with high concentrations being achieved quickly in the systemic circulation. Absorption from subcutaneous or intramuscular injection sites is faster than via the oral route but is less reliable, as local blood flow and diffusion through the tissue influences the pattern of absorption.

SUBCUTANEOUS (SC)

A subcutaneous injection of a drug is given beneath the skin into the connective tissue or fat immediately underlying the dermis. This site can be used only for drugs that are not irritating to the tissue; otherwise severe pain, necrosis, and sloughing of tissue may occur. The rate of absorption is slow and can provide a sustained effect.

INTRAMUSCULAR (IM)

Intramuscular administration refers to the injection of a drug into muscle. Absorption occurs more rapidly than with subcutaneous injection because of greater tissue blood flow.

INTRAVENOUS (IV)

The intravenous route produces an immediate pharmacological response because the desired amount of drug is injected directly into the bloodstream, thereby circumventing the absorption process. Intravenous drugs should generally be administered slowly to prevent adverse effects.

INTRATHECAL

Intrathecal drug administration means that the drug is injected directly into the spinal subarachnoid space, bypassing the blood–brain barrier. Many compounds cannot enter the cerebrospinal fluid or are absorbed in this region only very slowly. When rapid central nervous system (CNS) effects of drugs are desired, as with spinal anaesthesia or in treatment of acute infection of the CNS, this route may be used.

EPIDURAL

Epidural drug administration refers to the injection of a drug within the spinal canal on or outside the dura mater that surrounds the spinal column. This is sometimes called extradural or peridural. For other parenteral routes, see Box 6-3.

Inhalation

To ensure that normal gas exchange of oxygen and carbon dioxide is not interrupted in the lungs, drugs must be in the form of gases or fine mists (aerosols) when they are administered by inhalation. The lungs provide a large surface area for absorption and the rich capillary network adjacent to the alveolar membrane tends to promote ready entry of medications into the bloodstream. Drugs such as bronchodilators and antibiotics are administered by various inhalation devices (nebulisers, puffers) that propel the agents into the alveolar sacs, producing primarily local effects but at times— due to absorption—unwanted systemic effects.

Topical route

Absorption of drugs applied topically to the skin and mucous membranes of various structures in the body is generally rapid, for example cutaneous application, nasal sprays, eye-drops and inhalation (e.g. volatile anaesthetics, inhaled steroids).

SKIN

Drugs applied to the skin are used to produce either a local or a systemic effect through the use of ointments or transdermal patches. Only lipid-soluble compounds are absorbed through the skin, which acts as a lipid barrier. To prevent adverse effects from undesired systemic absorption of toxic chemicals, only an intact skin surface should be used. Massaging the skin enhances absorption of the drug because capillaries become dilated and local blood flow is increased as a result of the warmth created by the friction of rubbing.

BOX 6-3 OTHER PARENTERAL ROUTES

Drugs may be injected into other cavities of the body:
- intra-articular—drug delivery into the synovial cavity of a joint to relieve joint pain and reduce inflammation
- intraosseous—delivery into the bone marrow
- intraperitoneal—administration into the peritoneal cavity
- intrapleural—administration to the pleura

Transdermal administration is usually done with a patch that may contain a 1-, 3- or 7-day supply of medication, depending on the drug product. Examples of drugs that are applied transdermally are oestrogen and glyceryl trinitrate.

EYES

Ophthalmic administration of drugs produces a local effect on the conjunctiva or anterior chamber. Eyeball movements promote the distribution of drug over the surface of the eye.

EARS

Otic administration of drops into the auditory canal may be chosen to treat local infection or inflammatory conditions or to help remove wax in the external ear.

NOSE

Nasal drops or sprays containing medications may be applied or sprayed directly onto the nasal mucosa.

Drug bioavailability

After a drug crosses the membranes of the gastrointestinal tract, it is transported in the blood in capillaries of the gut wall, finally ending up in the portal vein. The portal vein then carries the blood containing the drug to the liver. The liver is the main site of drug metabolism (discussed in a later section) and, depending on whether the drug is metabolised or not, a variable amount of drug is extracted by the liver. The amount of drug reaching the systemic circulation then depends on:
- the amount absorbed from the gastrointestinal tract. This is designated as f_g and equals the fraction of the dose absorbed. When $f_g = 1$ the drug is completely absorbed; when $f_g = 0$ the drug is not absorbed
- the amount escaping extraction (first-pass metabolism) by the liver. This is designated f_H and equals the difference between the amount of drug entering the liver and the amount of drug exiting the liver.

Together these terms provide an indication of the **bioavailability** of a drug, which is defined as the proportion of the administered dose that reaches the systemic circulation intact. It is usually expressed as a percentage. The symbol for bioavailability is **F**. The fraction of drug not extracted by the liver is defined as 1− (hepatic extraction ratio) or 1−E_H (Figure 6-5):

$$\text{Bioavailability } F = f_g \times f_H$$

Drug bioequivalence

The term **bioequivalence** is used clinically when referring to two formulations of the same drug. This is an important concept because, once the patent expires on a drug, other pharmaceutical companies can produce a generic equivalent of the original patented drug with a new proprietary (trade)

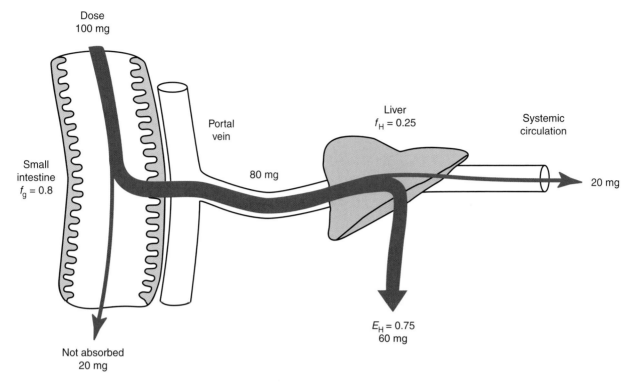

FIGURE 6-5 Factors affecting bioavailability. In this example, 80 mg of the original 100 mg dose is absorbed intact into the portal circulation (fraction absorbed is 0.8). The hepatic extraction ratio is 0.75, i.e. 60 mg is extracted in the first pass through the liver and 20 mg escapes extraction and is available for distribution via the systemic circulation. The bioavailability is $F = f_g \times f_H$, which is $0.8 \times 0.25 = 0.2$ (20%). (*Source*: Birkett 2002, reproduced with permission.)

<table>
<tr><td colspan="2">

**CLINICAL INTEREST BOX 6-1
NAMED BRAND AND A GENERIC
EQUIVALENT**

Diazepam (Valium) was developed under patent by the pharmaceutical company Roche. Patents are usually held for 17–20 years and if the drug is highly profitable a company may try to extend the patent period. During the patent period owned by Roche no other pharmaceutical company could produce or sell diazepam.

By the mid-1960s the annual sale of diazepam exceeded US$250 millions and by the mid-1970s around 60 million prescriptions were dispensed each year. The Roche patent expired in 1980 and by 1984 three other pharmaceutical companies had begun marketing generic diazepam under different trade names. Sales of generic diazepam now exceed the sales of Valium.

</td></tr>
</table>

name (see Clinical Interest Box 6.1). The bioavailablity of the new generic product is tested against the original market leader formulation (brand) to determine its relative bioavailability. Drugs are considered to be bioequivalent if they attain similar concentrations in blood and tissues at similar times and if there are no clinically important differences between their therapeutic or adverse effects (Birkett 2002).

TABLE 6-1 Drug distribution to body compartments

BODY COMPARTMENT	EXAMPLE OF DRUG DISTRIBUTED
Total body water (0.6 L/kg)	Small water-soluble molecules (e.g. ethanol)
Extracellular water (0.2 L/kg)	Larger (generally charged) water-soluble molecules (e.g. gentamicin)
Blood (0.08 L/kg); plasma (0.04 L/kg)	Highly protein-bound and large molecules (e.g. warfarin, heparin)
Bone (0.07 L/kg)	Ions (e.g. fluoride and calcium)
Fat (0.2–0.35 L/kg)	Highly lipid-soluble molecules (e.g. chloroquine)

*After Holford NHG. Pharmacokinetics and pharmacodynamics: Rational dosing and the time course of drug action. In: Katzung BG (ed.). *Basic and Clinical Pharmacology*. 9th edn. New York: Lange Medical Books, 2004 [ch. 3]. Reproduced with permission of the McGraw-Hill companies.

Drug distribution

After a drug reaches the systemic circulation it can be distributed to various sites within the body (Table 6-1). **Distribution** is defined as the process of reversible transfer of a drug between one location and another (one of which is usually blood) in the body (see Figure 6-3). Most of the drug is first distributed to organs that have good blood supply (e.g. heart, liver and kidneys) and initially the local concentration in these organs may be high. Drugs are also distributed more slowly to organs with poor blood supply, which include skeletal muscles and fat.

The rate at which a drug enters the different compartments of the body depends on the permeability of capillaries for the drug's molecules, and perfusion. As already discussed, lipid-soluble drugs can readily cross capillary membranes to enter most tissues and fluid compartments, whereas lipid-insoluble drugs require more time to arrive at their point of action. Cardiovascular function also affects the rate and extent of distribution of a drug, specifically, cardiac output (the amount of blood pumped by the heart each minute) and regional blood flow (the amount of blood supplied to a specific organ or tissue).

Plasma protein binding

On entry into the circulatory system, a proportion of free drug molecules bind to proteins to form drug–protein complexes. Acidic drugs bind mainly to albumin, while basic drugs bind to α_1-acid glycoprotein contained in the blood. The extent of binding depends on the affinity or attraction of the drug for the protein. Some drugs are highly bound, e.g. warfarin is 99.9% bound to albumin while less than 15% of paracetamol is bound to albumin. Protein binding decreases the concentration of free drug in the circulation and limits its distribution, as the drug–protein molecule is too large to diffuse out through the membrane of the blood vessel (see Figure 6-3). Protein binding is a reversible and dynamic process, with bound and unbound drug in equilibrium:

Free drug + protein ⇌ drug–protein complex

As free drug is removed from the circulation (e.g. by distribution, metabolism, excretion), the drug–protein complex dissociates so that more free drug is released to replace what is lost. This is very important, as it is only the free or unbound drug that exerts a pharmacological effect.

EXTENT OF DRUG BINDING

The extent of plasma protein binding is commonly expressed as a percentage, which represents the proportion of total drug bound. Among the highly protein-bound drugs is propranolol, which is about 93% protein-bound. Accordingly, a ratio exists between free and bound drug. In the case of propranolol this means that in a given period of time, 93% is bound to plasma proteins and only 7% of free drug is available for distribution and to exert a pharmacological effect and to be metabolised and excreted. Generally, acidic drugs (e.g. warfarin) are bound to albumin while basic drugs (e.g. quinine) bind to α_1-acid glycoprotein. Examples of highly protein-bound drugs include NSAIDS >99%, alfentanil 92%, amiodarone 99.9% and candesartan 99.8%. Drugs with low protein binding include cephalexin 14%, clonidine 20%, codeine 7% and fluconazole 11%.

COMPETITION FOR PLASMA PROTEIN BINDING SITES

Because albumin and other plasma proteins provide a number of binding sites, two drugs can compete with one another for the same site and displace each other. Although this does occur it is now generally accepted that competition between drugs for plasma protein binding rarely leads to an increased drug effect.

HYPOALBUMINAEMIA

Hypoalbuminaemia, or low levels of albumin in the blood, may be caused by hepatic damage such as cirrhosis or by failure of the liver to synthesise enough plasma proteins. The decrease in albumin concentration results in an increase in the amount of free drug available for distribution to tissue sites. When an individual is given the usual dosage of a drug in the presence of decreased plasma protein binding, more of the free form of drug is available to exert a pharmacological effect. This may also result in toxicity, and the drug dosage should be reduced.

Tissue binding
BODY FAT

Lipid-soluble drugs have a high affinity for adipose tissue, which is where these drugs are stored. Moreover, the relatively low blood flow in fat tissue makes it a stable reservoir for a limited number of drugs and also for some environmental chemicals (e.g. DDT). For example the lipid-soluble barbiturate anaesthetic thiopentone is initially rapidly distributed to brain, producing anaesthesia, but then redistributes to and accumulates in fatty tissue at levels 6–12 times those in the plasma. Continued administration of thiopentone causes a progressively longer period of anaesthesia as the drug accumulates in the body. This is one of the reasons why thiopentone is used for the induction of anaesthesia and not for surgical anaesthesia.

BONE

Some drugs have an unusual affinity for bone; for example, the antibiotic tetracycline accumulates in bone after being absorbed onto the bone-crystal surface. This site serves as a storage site for tetracycline, which later can interfere with bone growth when it accumulates in skeletal tissues of the fetus (by crossing the placenta from the mother) or young children. Distribution of tetracycline to the teeth in a young child results in discoloration. Brownish pigmentation of permanent teeth may also result if this drug is given during the prenatal period or early childhood.

Barriers to drug distribution

Specialised structures can serve as barriers to the passage of drugs at certain sites in the body, such as the blood–brain barrier and the placental barrier.

BLOOD–BRAIN BARRIER

The blood–brain barrier allows distribution of only lipid-soluble drugs (e.g. general anaesthetics and barbiturates) into the brain and cerebrospinal fluid. The barrier is made up of a layer of endothelial cells covered by a fatty sheath of glial cells joined by continuous tight intercellular junctions; normally drugs that are strongly ionised and poorly soluble in fat cannot enter the brain. In some circumstances, such as meningitis, the blood–brain barrier can become 'leaky', and this allows access of drugs that would not normally be able to penetrate the brain. The use of penicillin systemically to treat bacterial meningitis is an example of taking advantage of the inflammatory disruption of the blood–brain barrier.

PLACENTAL BARRIER

The membrane layers that separate the blood vessels of the mother and the fetus constitute the placental barrier. In addition, tissue enzymes in the placenta can metabolise some agents (e.g. catecholamines) by inactivating them as they travel from the maternal circulation to the embryo. Despite the thickness of the structure, it does not afford complete protection to the fetus. Unlike the blood–brain barrier, the non-selective passage of drugs across the placenta to the fetus is a well-established fact. Although lipid-soluble substances preferentially diffuse across the placenta, the barrier is also permeable to a great number of water-soluble drugs. Consequently, many drugs intended to produce a therapeutic response in the mother may also cross the placental barrier and exert harmful effects on the developing embryo (see Chapter 8). Among the drugs easily transported across the placenta are steroids, narcotics, anaesthetics, and some antibiotics.

Volume of distribution of a drug

Common reference is often made to the **volume of distribution** of a drug. It is defined as the volume in which the amount of drug in the body would need to be uniformly distributed to produce the observed concentration in the blood.

The volume of distribution of a drug (V) is calculated by dividing the total amount of drug in the body by the blood or plasma concentration of the drug.

$$V = \frac{\text{total amount of drug in body } (A)}{\text{drug concentration } (C)}$$

This is an abstract term and it is not a real volume. For example, if a drug is tightly bound to plasma proteins most, of it will remain within the circulatory system and it will have a volume of distribution similar to that of the blood volume. If, however, it is distributed out of the circulatory system and binds to tissue proteins, less remains in the blood and the drug will appear to be distributed in a larger volume. This is illustrated in Figure 6-6 using a bucket filled to its maximum capacity of 5 L, which is its actual volume.

If the volume of distribution is an 'imaginary volume', of what use is it clinically? First, it provides an indication of

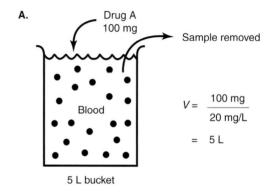

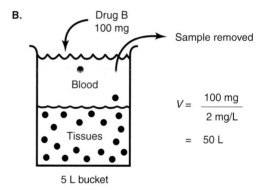

FIGURE 6-6 In this example the volume of the full bucket is 5 L and the amount of drug placed in each bucket is 100 mg. After the drug has distributed a 'blood' sample is removed from each bucket and the concentration of the drug measured. **A.** Bucket A is filled with 'blood' to represent the circulatory system. Drug A binds tightly to plasma proteins and remains within the circulation. The concentration of drug measured in the 'blood' sample is 20 mg/L and the calculated volume of distribution of Drug A is 5 L, the same as the volume of the bucket. **B.** Bucket B is filled with a mixture of 'blood' and 'tissues' to represent the intravascular and extravascular compartments. Drug B moves from the 'blood' and distributed to the 'tissues' where it binds strongly to tissue proteins. The concentration of drug measured in the 'blood' sample is 2 mg/L and the calculated volume of distribution of Drug B is 50 L, 10 times greater than the volume of the bucket!

accumulation of drugs in extravascular (tissue) compartments (e.g. fat, muscle). Second, it is a major determinant of the half-life of a drug (see later section). Third, on occasion it is necessary to achieve a high plasma concentration quickly to produce the desired therapeutic response. To do this a **loading dose** is administered to 'fill up' the volume of distribution. The size of the loading dose is calculated by knowing the volume of distribution of the drug:

Loading dose = volume of distribution
        × desired plasma concentration

Using Drug B from Figure 6-6 as an example, if the volume of distribution is 50 L and the desired plasma concentration is 2 mg/L, then the loading dose is 50 L × 2 mg/L = 100 mg. Some examples of volumes of distribution are: warfarin 8 L, frusemide 12 L, theophylline 35 L, digoxin 420 L, cyclosporin 1596 L and fluoxetine 2450 L. The larger the volume, the more widespread (tissue-bound) the drug is within the body. The volume of distribution changes with age, body composition and disease states, and differs between males and females. For example in infants <1 year of age V is approximately 75%–80% of body weight; in adult males it is approximately 60% of body weight and in adult females 55% of body weight.

Drug metabolism

Drug **metabolism**, or biotransformation, is the process of chemical modification of a drug and is almost invariably carried out by enzymes. Most drugs (around 70%) undergo metabolism to some extent, and in some but not all cases the products of metabolism have less biological activity than the parent drug. An exception to this is the use of prodrugs, which are inactive until converted to the active drug in the liver. Examples of prodrugs are the antihypertensive drug losartan and the anti-inflammatory drug sulindac. In general, metabolism results in the formation of a more water-soluble compound or metabolite, which can then be excreted. Metabolism thus clears the parent compound and promotes urinary excretion. The liver is the primary site of drug metabolism but with certain drugs, other tissues (e.g. kidneys, lungs and intestinal mucosa) may also be involved in this process to a limited extent.

Classification of drug metabolism reactions

The vast majority of drugs are metabolised in the liver by **functionalisation** and/or **conjugation** reactions. In many texts these are referred to as phase I and phase II reactions, respectively. A drug may initially be metabolised via a functionalisation reaction and then undergo further metabolism via conjugation. These reactions are not necessarily sequential and can occur simultaneously. Some drugs may simply be metabolised by either one of these individual processes.

FUNCTIONALISATION (PHASE I) REACTIONS
These reactions involve the introduction of a polar functional group into the molecule and include oxidation, hydrolysis, or reduction (Table 6-2). These chemical reactions produce more water-soluble metabolites. In some cases the metabolites are more pharmacologically active than the parent compound and, uncommonly, may be more toxic (e.g. acrolein, the toxic metabolite of cyclophosphamide, and N-acetyl-p-benzoquinone imine, the toxic metabolite of paracetamol). The major family of enzymes associated with these reactions is the cytochrome P450 (CYP) family.

CONJUGATION (PHASE II) REACTIONS
These involve the union of a suitable functional group present in the drug molecule with the polar group of an endogenous substance in the body (e.g. glucuronic acid, sulfate, acetyl-coenzyme A or glutathione). The conjugated molecule becomes more polar or more water-soluble, enhancing urinary excretion. The relationship between drug metabolism and renal excretion is illustrated in Figure 6-7. Conjugation reactions are catalysed by a variety of different transferase enzymes, including the uridine diphosphate (UDP)-glucuronosyltransferases, sulfotransferases, N-acetyltransferases and glutathione transferases (Table 6-3).

TABLE 6-2 Functionalisation (phase I) reactions		
ENZYME	**CHEMICAL REACTION**	**DRUG SUBSTRATE → DRUG METABOLITE**
CYP	Oxidation	Phenytoin → hydroxphenylhydantoin S-warfarin → 7-hydroxywarfarin Propranolol → 4-hydroxypropranolol
Esterases	Hydrolysis	Aspirin → salicylic acid Clofibrate → clofibric acid Succinylcholine → succinic acid
CYP	Reduction	Halothane → chlorotrifluoroethane

TABLE 6-3 Conjugation (phase II) reactions

ENZYME	ENDOGENOUS COFACTOR	REACTION	DRUG SUBSTRATE → DRUG METABOLITE
UDP-glucuronosyltransferases	UDP glucuronic acid	Glucuronidation	Morphine → morphine–3-glucuronide Naloxone → naloxone–3-glucuronide Codeine → codeine-6-glucuronide
Sulfotransferases	Sulfate	Sulfation	Salbutamol → salbutamol sulfate Paracetamol → paracetamol sulfate
N-acetyltransferases	Acetyl-CoA	Acetylation	Isoniazid → acetylisoniazid Clonazepam → 7-acetamidoclonazepam
Glutathione transferases	Glutathione	Glutathione conjugation	Paracetamol → paracetamol–glutathione conjugate

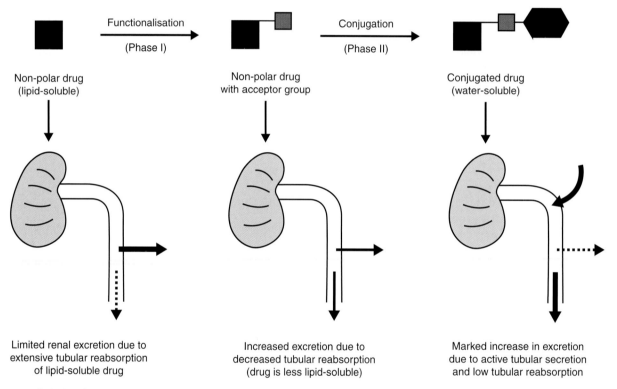

FIGURE 6-7 Relation between drug metabolism and renal excretion. Metabolism via functionalisation and conjugation reactions results in decreasing lipid solubility, increasing water solubility and progressive enhancement of urinary excretion. *Source*: Birkett 1979, reproduced with permission.

Drug-metabolising enzymes
CYTOCHROME P450

The enzymes of greatest importance in functionalisation reactions are the large cytochrome P450 family of enzymes, abbreviated CYP. CYPs are found in the smooth endoplasmic reticulum of cells and are particularly abundant in liver cells (hepatocytes). These key enzymes are involved not only in drug metabolism but also in the metabolism of environmental pollutants, dietary chemicals and in the synthesis and metabolism of steroids, hormones and fatty acids. There are more than 50 human cytochrome P450 isoforms (forms of the same protein); of these, 18 isoforms are able to metabolise drugs and foreign chemicals. These are divided into gene families and those most involved in drug metabolism in humans are in families 1, 2 and 3. Individual isoforms are given a number and a letter to denote their divergent evolution. The human isoforms of greatest importance to drug metabolism are CYP1A2, CYP2A6, CYP2C8, 2C9 and 2C19, CYP2D6, CYP2E1 and CYP3A4. Table 6-4 lists some common therapeutic drugs and the CYP that metabolises them.

TABLE 6-4 Common drugs metabolised by cytochrome P450 isoforms

CYTOCHROME P450 ISOFORM	DRUGS METABOLISED
CYP1A2	Caffeine, clozapine, tacrine, ropivacaine
CYP2A6	Nicotine
CYP2C8	Paclitaxel, chloroquine, rosiglitazone
CYP2C9	Tolbutamide, phenytoin, ibuprofen, diclofenac, S-warfarin, celecoxib
CYP2C19	Omeprazole, sertraline, proguanil, diazepam
CYP2D6	Amitriptyline, fluoxetine, haloperidol, codeine, metoprolol, perhexiline, nortriptyline
CYP2E1	Alcohol, enflurane, halothane
CYP3A4	Simvastatin, felodipine, tacrolimus, saquinavir, carbamazepine, cyclosporin, erythromycin, calcium channel blockers

TRANSFERASE ENZYMES

Like cytochrome P450, the transferase enzymes exist as families of isoforms that differ in terms of the drugs they metabolise. There are at least 12 UDP-glucuronosyltransferases that metabolise drugs, six isoforms of sulfotransferases and two isoforms of N-acetyltransferases (NATs), of which only one (NAT2) seems to be important in drug metabolism.

Interindividual variability in drug metabolism

Large differences can occur between individuals in the rates of metabolism of many drugs. Metabolism therefore becomes very important in determining the therapeutic and toxic responses to many drugs. This variability can be due to a range of factors, including:

- genetics
- environmental factors, e.g. coadministered drugs, diet etc
- age (discussed in Chapter 8)
- disease states
- hormonal changes.

GENETIC FACTORS (PHARMACOGENETICS)

The effect of genetics on drug action and elimination is referred to as '**pharmacogenetics**'. Genetic factors cause the greatest variability in enzyme activity, and this is particularly true when a single enzyme is responsible for the metabolism of a drug. If metabolism of a drug is under the control of one gene, a mutation in the gene may give rise to a genetic

CLINICAL INTEREST BOX 6-2 POLYMORPHISM IN NEW ZEALAND MAORI

In New Zealand Maori subjects phenotyped for polymorphisms of debrisoquine (CYP2D6) and proguanil (CYP2C19) metabolism, 5% were identified as poor metabolisers of debrisoquine and 7% as poor metabolisers of proguanil. The data for debrisoquine were similar to those reported for Caucasian populations (5%–10%) but the percentage of poor metabolisers was higher than that found in Asian populations (0.7%–2%). For proguanil, the incidence of the poor metaboliser phenotype in Maori was higher than that for Caucasian populations but lower than the usual ranges (15%–35%) reported in Asian populations. The authors concluded that the risk of adverse drug reactions in Maori with respect to CYP2D6 and CYP2C19 would be similar to that established for Caucasian populations (Wanwimolruk et al 1995).

Similar studies were performed in South Pacific Polynesians residing in the South Island of New Zealand. The incidence of poor metaboliser phenotypes for debrisoquine and proguanil in the South Pacific Polynesians was similar to those reported in Asian populations (Wanwimolruk et al 1998).

CLINICAL INTEREST BOX 6-3 GRAPEFRUIT JUICE–DRUG INTERACTIONS

Food–drug interactions are potentially an everyday occurrence. Many scientific findings have been serendipitous and perhaps none more so than an unexpected observation during a clinical study that the grapefruit juice that was used to mask the taste of ethanol led to an increase in the oral bioavailability of the drug being studied. Subsequent research indicated that the effect was due to the inhibition of CYP3A4 activity in the intestine, which resulted in a reduction of presystemic metabolism and subsequent increased bioavailability. This interaction is most clinically relevant with certain calcium channel blockers, saquinavir, cyclosporin, midazolam, triazolam and verapamil, and may be important with cisapride.

Although the active components in grapefruit juice responsible for the inhibition of enzyme activity have not yet been fully identified, the effect is observed with a single glass of juice and can persist for 24 hours: "Since grocers do not take a drug history, physicians, pharmacists and other health professionals should educate patients about consumption of grapefruit juice with medications" (Bailey, Arnold & Spence 1998).

polymorphism (the occurrence of two or more distinct types in a population), which is recognised in a population as individuals often described as 'poor metabolisers' and 'extensive (i.e. normal) metabolisers'. Studies conducted more than 30 years ago demonstrated that identical twins resembled each other in terms of how they metabolised a drug, whereas fraternal twins (developed from separate eggs) showed variations similar to the general population. This was consistent with fraternal twins having different patterns of inheritance.

The incidence of genetic polymorphisms varies; pseudocholinesterase deficiency, which affects the metabolism of the muscle relaxant suxamethonium, has a frequency of 1 in 2500 and is considered uncommon. In contrast, a deficiency in CYP2D6, which metabolises many clinically used drugs, has a frequency of 7%–10% in Caucasians and ~1% in Asian populations. The CYP2D6 polymorphism is of considerable clinical significance because CYP2D6 metabolises many clinically used drugs that have narrow therapeutic indices. Examples include:

- antianginals—perhexiline
- antiarrhythmics—flecainide, propafenone
- antidepressants—clomipramine, doxepin, fluoxetine, desipramine, nortriptyline, paroxetine, venlafaxine
- antipsychotics—haloperidol, perphenazine, risperidone, thioridazine
- opioids—codeine, dextromethorphan, oxycodone.

Of greater incidence is a deficiency in *N*-acetyltransferase, which occurs in around 50% of Caucasians. This is important in relation to the metabolism of isoniazid, used in the treatment of tuberculosis. Polymorphism in the *N*-acetyltransferase system divides the population into 'rapid acetylators' and 'slow acetylators'. The rapid acetylators metabolise a greater proportion of a drug dose and thus do not achieve a therapeutic plasma concentration, whereas the slow acetylators may appear more sensitive to the drug and experience serious adverse effects.

ENVIRONMENTAL FACTORS

The basis for many drug–drug interactions during metabolism is related to the induction or inhibition of enzyme activity.

INDUCTION. The extent of induction depends on the number of isoforms or enzyme systems that have their activity changed. Cigarette smoke increases the activity of CYP1A2 and thus increases the metabolism of caffeine, theophylline and imipramine. Other examples of the clinical consequences of enzyme induction include the need for higher doses of antiepileptic drugs in people treated with combinations of antiepileptic drugs, as many of these drugs are enzyme inducers, and the risk of contraceptive failure in women receiving phenobarbitone or rifampicin, because of the increased metabolism of oral contraceptive steroids.

INHIBITION. This most commonly occurs because of competition, i.e. two different drugs compete for metabolism by the same isoform or enzyme system. This invariably results in a decrease in metabolism of one of the drugs. The clinical consequences of inhibition of drug metabolism include a decreased rate of elimination from the body, resulting in an increased plasma concentration and risk of toxicity. Examples include inhibition of metabolism of the anticoagulant warfarin by cimetidine, resulting in haemorrhage, and death from inhibition of metabolism of the cancer chemotherapy agent azathioprine by the xanthine oxidase inhibitor allopurinol.

DISEASE STATES

In people with cardiac failure, liver perfusion and oxygenation may be decreased and this can reduce the activity of drug-metabolising enzymes. In liver disease the effects are harder to predict, as they depend on the disease type and severity, all of which can influence drug metabolism. In general, in severe cirrhosis and viral hepatitis the clearance of drugs metabolised by the cytochrome P450 system is decreased.

HORMONAL FACTORS

Although gender-related differences have been observed for drug-metabolising enzymes in other species, differences in humans appear to be minor and clinically insignificant. However, hormonal factors during pregnancy can have an important effect on drug metabolism, particularly during the third trimester. Induced activity of many CYP isoforms and of UDP-glucuronosyltransferase occurs, particularly during the third trimester. For example, it is well established that doses of the anticonvulsant drugs carbamazepine (metabolised by CYP3A4) and phenytoin (metabolised by CYP2C9) must be increased during the course of pregnancy to maintain plasma concentrations in the therapeutic range. Following birth, doses decline to pre-pregnancy requirements. CYP2D6 activity is also induced during pregnancy. In contrast, there is evidence suggesting that the metabolism of caffeine (a CYP1A2 substrate) declines during pregnancy. Thus, although induction occurs most commonly, effects of pregnancy on drug metabolism are not always predictable.

Hepatic first-pass effect

As discussed previously, orally administered drugs that are absorbed travel first through the portal system and the liver before entering the systemic circulation. Depending on whether the drug is metabolised or not, a variable amount of drug can be extracted by the liver before the drug ever reaches the systemic circulation (Figure 6-5). Consequently, often only a small fraction of the dose is available for distribution and to produce a pharmacological effect. For such medications the oral drug dose is calculated to compensate for this **first-pass effect**. For example, morphine has a significant hepatic first-pass effect—30 mg oral morphine is equivalent to 10 mg morphine administered IM/IV/SC (*Australian Medicines Handbook* 2006). The hepatic first-pass effect described here helps to explain why the intravenous doses of some drugs are so much smaller than the oral doses.

Excretion of drugs and drug metabolites

A drug continues to exert a pharmacological effect (in some cases a toxicological effect) in the body until it is eliminated. In pharmacokinetic terms, **elimination** is defined as the irreversible loss of drug from the body (at the site of measurement) by the processes of metabolism and excretion (Rowland & Tozer 1989). For example, after administration, a drug may be metabolised by the liver but its metabolites may remain in the body. However, the parent drug is considered to have been eliminated from the body. The terms 'elimination' and 'excretion' are often used interchangeably but **excretion** applies solely to the loss of (chemically) unchanged drug or metabolites from the body in urine, bile, expired air or faeces. The term 'unchanged' in this context may appear confusing but it refers to the immediate chemical species that is being excreted, which can be either a parent molecule or a metabolite. In this regard, the liver, being the major site of drug metabolism, is the main organ of elimination, while the kidneys are the main organs of excretion.

ROUTES OF EXCRETION

KIDNEYS. Some drugs are excreted unchanged in the urine, while other drugs are so extensively metabolised that only a small fraction of the parent drug is excreted unchanged. The process of excretion is accomplished primarily through glomerular filtration, active tubular secretion and passive reabsorption (Figure 6-8). For example, free unbound drugs and water-soluble metabolites are filtered by the glomeruli (the glomerular filtration rate is around 120 mL/min), whereas protein-bound substances do not pass through this structure. Most of the 120 mL water from the plasma filtered at the glomerulus is reabsorbed during its passage through the renal tubule and only about 1–2 mL finally appears as urine. As the water is reabsorbed, a concentration gradient is established between the drug in the tubular fluid and the unbound drug in the blood, i.e. the drug in the urine is concentrated relative to that in the blood. If the drug is lipid-soluble enough to pass through the membranes it will be reabsorbed from the tubular fluid back into the systemic circulation. If urine flow rate is high there is less of a concentration gradient and less drug is reabsorbed. Conversely, if the urine is more concentrated due to a low urine flow rate there is more of a concentration gradient and more drug is reabsorbed. The water-soluble compounds, on the other hand, are not reabsorbed and are excreted in the urine (Figure 6-7).

Urinary pH varies between 4.6 and 8.2 and affects the amount of drug reabsorbed in the renal tubule by changing the degree of ionisation. Weak acids are excreted more readily in alkaline urine and more slowly in acidic urine; the reverse is true for weak bases. By altering the pH of urine, excretion of certain drugs can be increased, preventing prolonged action of a toxic compound, or decreased, prolonging the effect of a drug. In the case of drug overdoses involving weak organic acids such as aspirin or phenobarbitone, alkalinisation of the urine can result in increased urinary drug excretion. Urine may be alkalinised by administering sodium bicarbonate. By contrast, high doses of vitamin C or ammonium chloride acidify the urine and promote the excretion of basic drugs such as quinidine and amphetamines.

The proximal tubule is the main site of active secretion, and both acidic and basic drugs are secreted into the lumen via their specific 'acid' and 'base' pumps. Examples of drugs secreted via the acid pump include penicillin and probenecid; those secreted via the base pump include ranitidine and procainamide. Another technique to reduce the rate of excretion of a drug is to competitively inhibit tubular secretion; for example, probenecid may be used to block tubular secretion and hence the renal excretion of penicillin. This prolongs the effect of the antibiotic by maintaining a higher therapeutic plasma concentration.

Another factor that affects renal excretion of drugs and drug metabolites is renal function, which is poorly developed in neonates and tends to decrease in the elderly. Also, when a person has chronic renal failure, excretion of drugs is almost non-existent and, in people with cardiac failure, reduced blood flow to the kidneys may decrease renal excretion of unchanged drugs and drug metabolites.

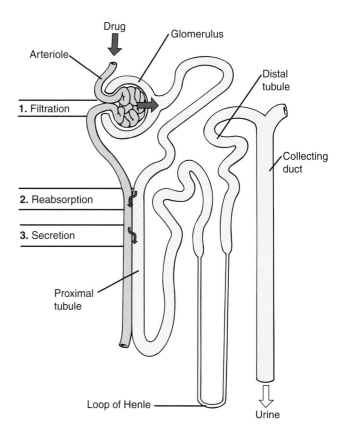

FIGURE 6-8 The drug excretion process, illustrating: 1. glomerular filtration; 2. tubular reabsorption; and 3. active secretion.

BILIARY EXCRETION. After metabolism by the liver, drug metabolites may be transported into the bile, passed into the duodenum and excreted in faeces. Often, drug metabolites such as glucuronides are hydrolysed after the bile mixes with the intestinal fluid and the free drug is then reabsorbed and returned to the liver. This process is called enterohepatic cycling and for some drugs this 'cycling' produces a supply of recirculating drug that contributes to the overall pool of drug in the body. Examples of drugs that undergo significant enterohepatic cyling are morphine and ethinyloestradiol.

EXPIRED AIR. Gases and volatile liquids (general anaesthetics) are administered and excreted via the lungs, generally in intact form. On inspiration, these agents enter the bloodstream and after crossing the alveolar membrane are distributed by the general circulation. The rate of loss depends on the rate of respiration; therefore, exercise or deep breathing, which causes a rise in cardiac output and a subsequent increase in pulmonary blood flow, promotes excretion. By contrast, decreased cardiac output, such as that occurring in shock, decreases pulmonary drug excretion. Other volatile substances, such as ethyl alcohol and paraldehyde, are highly soluble in blood and are excreted in limited amounts by the lungs. These compounds can be detected easily because the individual exhales the gases into the atmosphere.

SWEAT AND SALIVA. Drug excretion through sweat and saliva is relatively unimportant because this process depends on diffusion of lipid-soluble drugs through the epithelial cells of the glands, which is slow relative to other forms of excretion and represents only a minor proportion of total excretion. The excretion of drugs and metabolites in sweat may be responsible for adverse effects such as dermatitis and several other skin reactions.

BREAST MILK. Many drugs or their metabolites cross the epithelium of the mammary glands and are excreted in breast milk. The risk to the infant of exposure to these drugs during breastfeeding depends on the maternal plasma drug concentration and the amount of milk ingested by the infant. Breast milk is acidic (pH 6.5), therefore basic compounds with low plasma protein binding and high lipid solubility such as narcotics (e.g. morphine and codeine) achieve high concentrations in this fluid. A major concern arises over the transfer of such drugs from mothers to their breastfed babies, which can result in adverse effects such as sedation and failure to thrive (Ilett et al 1997).

KEY POINTS

- The concentration of drug that finally reaches its molecular target is influenced by various processes, which may be divided broadly into pharmaceutical, pharmacokinetic and pharmacodynamic phases.
- The concentration that a drug attains at its site of action is influenced by the rate and extent to which the drug is absorbed into body fluids, distributed to the sites of action, metabolised into active or inactive metabolites and excreted from the body by various routes.
- The study of the kinetics of a drug during the processes of absorption, distribution, metabolism and excretion, or simply 'what the body does to the drug', is collectively described by the term 'pharmacokinetics'.
- Absorption is defined as the process by which unchanged drug proceeds from the site of administration into the blood. It is an important factor for all routes of administration with the exception of intravenous administration.
- Variables that affect drug absorption include the nature of the absorbing membrane, blood flow, solubility of the drug, degree of ionisation and formulation characteristics.
- Routes of drug administration include oral, parenteral, inhalation and topical.
- Bioavailability of a drug is defined as the proportion of the administered dose that reaches the systemic circulation intact.
- Distribution is defined as the process of reversible transfer of a drug between one location and another (one of which is usually blood) in the body.
- On entry into the circulatory system, free drug molecules bind to proteins to form drug–protein complexes. Protein binding decreases the free drug concentration and limits tissue distribution. As free drug is removed from the circulation, the protein–drug complex dissociates so that more free drug is released.
- Only free or unbound drug exerts a pharmacological effect.
- The volume of distribution of a drug is defined as the volume in which the amount of drug in the body would need to be uniformly distributed in order to produce the observed concentration in blood.
- Drug metabolism, or biotransformation, is the process of chemical modification of a drug and is almost invariably carried out by enzymes.
- The vast majority of drugs are metabolised in the liver by functionalisation and/or conjugation reactions. The major drug-metabolising enzymes are the cytochrome P450 and UDP-glucuronosyltransferase families.

- Large differences may occur between individuals in the rate of metabolism of drugs. This variability may be due to genetic, environmental, age or disease-related factors.
- The major organs for the excretion of unchanged drugs and drug metabolites are the kidneys.
- The process of renal excretion is accomplished primarily through glomerular filtration, active tubular secretion, and passive reabsorption.
- The application of the kinetics principles associated with the processes of absorption, distribution, metabolism and excretion form the basis for the design of drug dosage regimens.

REVIEW EXERCISES

1. Discuss four variables that affect drug absorption.
2. Of what value is knowledge of the volume of distribution of a drug?
3. Select two examples involving hepatic drug metabolism and explain the importance of each of them in clinical practice.
4. What is meant by the term first-pass metabolism and how does it influence bioavailability?
5. Why are there large interindividual variations in drug metabolism?
6. Explain how urinary pH influences passive reabsorption of drugs.

REFERENCES AND FURTHER READING

Australian Medicines Handbook 2006. Adelaide: AMH, 2006.
Bailey DG, Arnold MO, Spence JD. Grapefruit juice–drug interactions. *British Journal of Clinical Pharmacology* 1998; 46: 101–10.
Birkett DJ. Bioavailability and first-pass clearance. In: Birkett DJ. *Pharmacokinetics Made Easy.* Sydney: McGraw-Hill 2002 [ch. 5].
Birkett DJ, Grygiel JJ, Meffin PJ, Wing LMH. Fundamentals of Clinical Pharmacology; 4. Drug biotransformation. *Current Therapeutics* 1979; 6: 129–38.
Birkett DJ. Volume of distribution. In: Birkett DJ. *Pharmacokinetics Made Easy.* Sydney: McGraw-Hill, 2002 [ch. 2].
Holford NHG. Pharmacokinetics and pharmacodynamics: rational dosing and the time course of drug action. In: Katzung BG (ed.). *Basic and Clinical Pharmacology.* 9th edn. The McGraw-Hill Companies, 2004 [ch. 3].
Ilett KF, Kristensen JH, Wojnar-Horton RE, Begg EJ. Drug distribution in human milk. *Australian Prescriber* 1997; 20: 35–40.
Kim RB. Transporters and drug discovery: why, when and how. *Molecular Pharmaceutics* 2006; 3(1):26–32.
Levy RH, Thummel KE, Trager WF et al (eds). *Metabolic Drug Interactions.* Philadelphia: Lippincott Williams & Wilkins, 2000.
Rang HP, Dale MM, Ritter JM, Moore PK. Absorption and distribution of drugs. In: Rang HP, Dale MM, Ritter JM, Moore PK. *Pharmacology.* 5th edn. Edinburgh: Churchill Livingstone, 2003 [ch. 7].
Rowland M, Tozer TN. *Clinical Pharmacokinetics: Concepts and Applications.* 2nd edn. Philadelphia: Lea & Febiger, 1989.
Wanwimolruk S, Pratt EL, Denton JR et al. Evidence for the polymorphic oxidation of debrisoquine and proguanil in a New Zealand Maori population. *Pharmacogenetics* 1995; 5: 193–8.
Wanwimolruk S, Bhawan S, Coville PF et al. Genetic polymorphism of debrisoquine (CYP2D6) and proguanil (CYP2C19) in South Pacific Polynesian populations. *European Journal of Clinical Pharmacology* 1998; 54: 431–5.

evolve   More weblinks at http://evolve.elsevier.com/AU/Bryant/pharmacology/

CHAPTER 7

Pharmacokinetics and Dosing Regimens

CHAPTER FOCUS

The choice of a drug for an individual patient is influenced by many factors, and using the correct dose is essential both for achieving the desired pharmacological effect and for limiting adverse effects. An understanding of pharmacokinetic principles allows selection of the right dose and prediction of the effects of disease states, drug interactions and environmental factors on dosing regimens. The importance of the key pharmacokinetic concepts of clearance, volume of distribution and half-life are illustrated in this chapter by the use of examples relevant to the clinical situation.

OBJECTIVES

- To describe the plasma drug concentration–time profiles following intravenous and oral drug administration.

- To discuss the key pharmacokinetic concepts of clearance, volume of distribution and half-life.

- To explain the importance of each of these individual pharmacokinetic parameters.

- To explain the relationship between half-life and the steady-state plasma drug concentration.

KEY TERMS

area under the plasma concentration versus time curve
clearance
half-life
loading dose
steady state
therapeutic range
volume of distribution

KEY ABBREVIATIONS

AUC   area under the plasma concentration versus time curve

CL   systemic clearance

C_{ss} steady-state plasma drug concentration

F   bioavailability

MDR   maintenance dose rate

$t_{1/2}$ half-life

V   volume of distribution

RATIONAL use of drugs is based on the assumption that a particular concentration of a drug will have the desired therapeutic effect and that adverse effects will be negligible. For many drugs there is a sufficient relationship between plasma drug concentration and clinical response for dosing regimens to be designed to maintain the concentration within a **therapeutic range**. Although therapeutic ranges are derived from data on populations of individuals, not everyone responds in the same way. Some individuals might not experience a therapeutic effect when the plasma drug concentration is at the top of the range, and others might experience toxicity when the plasma drug concentration is within the therapeutic range. The therapeutic range is generally considered to reflect the range of drug concentrations having a high probability of producing the desired therapeutic effect and a low probability of producing adverse effects. It should be possible to individualise the dosing regimen of any drug to achieve the desired plasma concentration for any individual by considering their characteristics (e.g. age, health status, liver and kidney function) and the pharmacokinetics of the drug. Unfortunately, the theory does not always work in practice.

After administration, each drug will have its own pharmacokinetic profile that is influenced by factors such as the route of administration, changes in the disease state of the individual, the person's genetic make-up and environmental factors. Despite these potential confounding factors, in general the aim is to achieve a constant (**steady-state**) plasma drug concentration that maintains the desired pharmacological response. This can be achieved through continuous administration (e.g. IV infusion) or through multiple dosing via other routes, most commonly the oral route. The size of the dose and the dosing frequency constitute a dosing regimen. As can be appreciated from Chapter 6, pharmacokinetics plays a major role not only in

establishing the initial dosing regimen but also in adjusting the regimen to deal with a lack of response or to reduce symptoms of toxicity.

PLASMA CONCENTRATION–TIME PROFILE OF A DRUG

Measuring the plasma concentration–time profile of a drug graphically demonstrates the relationship between the plasma drug concentration and therapeutic response or toxicity over time. For example, the theoretical drug in Figure 7-1 has been administered as a single oral dose. It has an onset of action of approximately 2 hours, a peak plasma concentration at 5 hours, and a 6-hour duration of action (the length of time the plasma drug concentration remains within the therapeutic range). In this case the processes of absorption, distribution and elimination (i.e. metabolism and excretion) influence the plasma concentration–time profile of the drug.

Administration of a drug by the IV route as a single bolus dose followed by an infusion, as a single bolus dose alone or as an infusion alone all give different plasma concentration–time profiles that are influenced by distribution and elimination but not absorption (Figure 7-2).

How does this knowledge help the establishment of appropriate dosing regimens? Buried within these plasma drug concentration–time profiles are the key pharmacokinetic parameters of clearance, volume of distribution and half-life. The clearance of a drug and its volume of distribution are determined by the characteristics of the patient and the drug, whereas half-life is a composite parameter that is related directly to the volume of distribution and inversely to

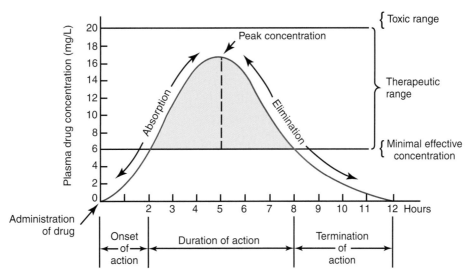

FIGURE 7-1 Plasma concentration–time profile for a theoretical drug administered as a single oral dose.

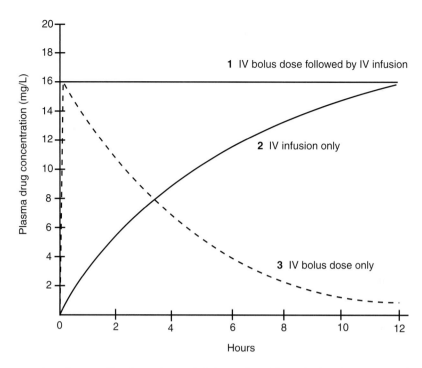

FIGURE 7-2 Plasma concentration–time profiles for a drug administered as (1) a single IV bolus dose followed by an IV infusion, (2) an IV infusion only, and (3) a single IV bolus dose.

clearance. Each of these parameters will be discussed in the context of their clinical relevance. Key pharmacokinetic definitions used throughout this chapter are listed in Box 7-1.

Area under the plasma concentration versus time curve (AUC)

The **area under the plasma concentration versus time curve** is exactly what the description implies. It can be used to calculate both the clearance of a drug after IV administration and the bioavailability of a drug. The latter is calculated by comparing the respective AUC values after IV and oral administration of the same dose of the same drug.

The AUC is defined as the 'total area under the curve that describes the concentration of the drug in the systemic circulation as a function of time (from zero until infinity)'. The value of AUC is determined by dividing the area under the curve into equal-sized strips, then estimating the area of each strip as that of a trapezium, then adding up all the results. This is commonly called 'the trapezoidal rule' and is illustrated in Figure 7.3. Generally, the larger the AUC, the smaller the clearance, because of the relationship

$$CL = \frac{dose}{AUC}$$

The AUC may also be used to determine the bioavailability of a drug (Chapter 6). Usually a group of subjects will be given the

same IV and oral dose of the same drug on separate occasions. After each drug dose, blood samples are collected for many hours (e.g. 24 hours). The plasma concentration versus time curve is plotted for each dose and the AUC calculated for each curve. Fortunately most pharmacokinetic programs calculate the AUC automatically, and manual calculation by the trapezoidal rule is not necessary! As the bioavailability of an IV dose is 100% by definition, if the AUC of the oral dose is half of the AUC of the IV dose, then the bioavailability of the oral formulation is 50%.

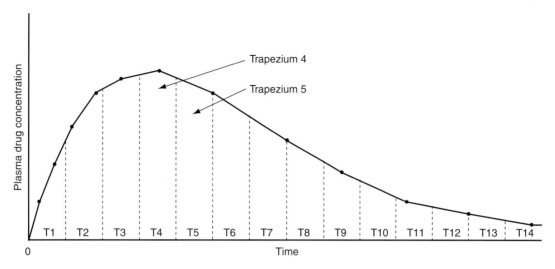

FIGURE 7-3 Plasma drug concentration versus time curve after an oral dose of a drug. The AUC is determined by calculating the area of each trapezium and summing the values. AUC = Area T1 + Area T2 + Area T3 + Area T4 . . . + Area T*n*

CLEARANCE

Clearance (CL) describes the ability of an individual organ or the body to eliminate a drug. If referring to the whole body, clearance reflects the sum of all the clearance processes relevant to the particular drug (Figure 7-4). For example:

$$CL_{Total\ body} = CL_{Hepatic} + CL_{Renal} + CL_{Other}$$

For a particular drug and a specific individual, providing they remain physiologically stable, clearance is constant. Thus the rate at which a drug is eliminated from the body varies directly with the plasma drug concentration (C).

$$Elimination\ rate\ (mg/h) = CL\ (L/h) \times C\ (mg/L)$$

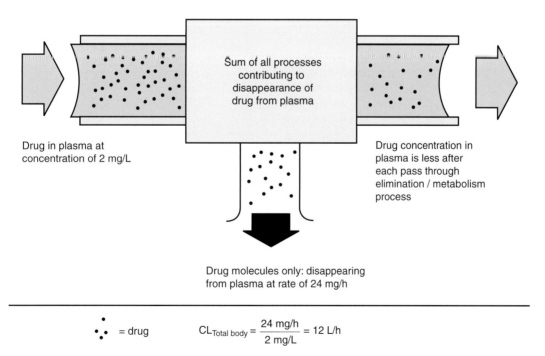

FIGURE 7-4 Concept of total body clearance of a drug from plasma. Only some drug molecules disappear from plasma on each pass of blood through kidneys, liver or other sites contributing to drug disappearance (elimination). In this example, it requires 12 L plasma to account for the amount of drug disappearance each hour (24 mg/h) at the concentration of 2 mg/L. Total body clearance is thus 12 L/h. *Source*: Brody et al 1998. Reproduced with permission.

Hepatic clearance

If a drug is described as having a hepatic clearance of 30 L/h, what does this mean if hepatic blood flow is 90 L/h? It does not mean that the liver irreversibly removes (clears) drug from only 30 L of blood and not from the other 60 L of blood that passes through it. What it does mean is that one-third (30/90) of the drug molecules entering the liver in blood are cleared by the liver in one pass. Clearance of drug occurs as a result of metabolism and in this case the capacity of the drug-metabolising enzymes is such that only one-third of the drug is removed from the blood. If the drug were not metabolised at all then hepatic clearance would be zero; conversely, if all the drug were metabolised then clearance would equal hepatic blood flow, 90 L/h.

Some drugs are classified in relation to liver blood flow as having low or high hepatic clearance. Low hepatic clearance is normally regarded as <12 L/h and high clearance as >60 L/h. Examples of drugs in these categories are shown in Table 7-1. Low hepatic clearance does not mean that the drug is then cleared by the kidneys; it indicates that the capacity of the hepatic enzymes involved in the metabolism of the drug is low. Hepatic clearance generally accounts for the clearance of lipid-soluble drugs.

Renal clearance

The kidneys are the major organs for the clearance of polar water-soluble drugs. Renal drug clearance is the net effect of glomerular filtration, secretion and passive reabsorption. Examples of drugs principally cleared by the kidneys include the penicillin and cephalosporin antibiotics. For most drugs, changes in renal function do not necessitate an adjustment in drug dosage. Only when renal function is reduced to less than half and the drug is more than 50% cleared by the kidneys is dosage adjustment necessary. Digoxin and gentamicin are examples of drugs cleared by the kidneys and for which the dosing regimen needs to be changed in individuals with renal impairment.

TABLE 7-1 Examples of drugs with low and high hepatic clearances

LOW HEPATIC CLEARANCE	HIGH HEPATIC CLEARANCE
Carbamazepine	Lignocaine
Diazepam	Morphine
Theophylline	Pethidine
Valproic acid	Propranolol

The importance of clearance

Continued drug administration eventually leads to a situation in which the rate of drug administration equals the rate of elimination, i.e. rate in equals rate out and the plasma drug concentration remains constant. This is called **steady state**. At steady state:

$$\text{Elimination rate} = \text{maintenance dose rate}$$

Clearance determines the maintenance dose rate (MDR) required to achieve the target plasma concentration at steady state (C_{ss}).

$$\text{Maintenance dose rate (MDR)} = \text{Clearance (CL)} \times \text{target steady-state plasma drug concentration } (C_{ss})$$

$$\text{MDR (mg/h)} = \text{CL (L/h)} \times C_{ss} \text{ (mg/L)}$$

A sample calculation for a theoretical drug is shown in Box 7-2.

BOX 7-2 MAINTENANCE DOSE CALCULATION

Let us consider a drug for which the target plasma concentration at steady state is 12.5 mg/L. As the individual to be given the drug has an acute condition, it is decided to administer the drug initially as an IV infusion. The clearance of the drug is 8 L/h. With IV administration, the bioavailability is 1 (100%).

$$\begin{aligned} \text{MDR} &= \text{CL} \times C_{ss} \\ &= 8 \text{ L/h} \times 12.5 \text{ mg/L} \\ &= 100 \text{ mg/h} \end{aligned}$$

Thus the infusion rate should be 100 mg/h.

As the person's condition improves, it is decided to switch to an oral dosing regimen, but it is essential to maintain the plasma drug concentration. The oral formulation has a bioavailability (F) of 0.8 (80%) and the recommended dosing interval is 8-hourly. Thus the oral maintenance dose can be calculated.

$$\begin{aligned} \text{Maintenance dose} &= \frac{\text{MDR} \times \text{dosing interval}}{\text{F}} \\ &= \frac{100 \text{ mg/h} \times 8 \text{ h}}{0.8} \\ &= 1000 \text{ mg} \end{aligned}$$

A formulation close to the ideal dose would then be prescribed. In this case the drug is available as a 500 mg capsule, so two capsules would be administered 8 hourly. If the drug were to be given 12-hourly, the dose would be 1500 mg (3 capsules).

VOLUME OF DISTRIBUTION

The **volume of distribution** is the volume in which the amount of drug in the body would need to be uniformly distributed to produce the observed concentration in blood (see Chapter 6) and is important for determining the **loading dose**. In the example described in Box 7-2, the medical condition was acute and a loading dose was administered to produce a rapid pharmacological effect. Figure 7-2 shows that if an infusion alone were used it would take around 8 hours to achieve the desired plasma drug concentration (curve 2). In contrast, an IV bolus dose would raise the plasma drug concentration to the desired level almost immediately (Figure 7-2, curve 3).

The loading dose is the initial amount of drug required to fill the volume of distribution. It is calculated from the relationship between the volume of distribution and the target plasma concentration. Using the example in Box 7-2, the volume of distribution of the drug was known to be 40 L and the target plasma drug concentration was 12.5 mg/L.

Loading dose = volume of distribution × target
plasma concentration
= 40 L × 12.5 mg/L
= 500 mg

Thus the loading dose would be 500 mg. As rapid intravenous administration is often undesirable because high plasma concentrations can occur before the distribution phase, loading doses may be given over a period of minutes or even hours.

HALF-LIFE

Use of the term **half-life** ($t_{1/2}$) when referring to drugs is very common. The elimination half-life is defined as the time taken

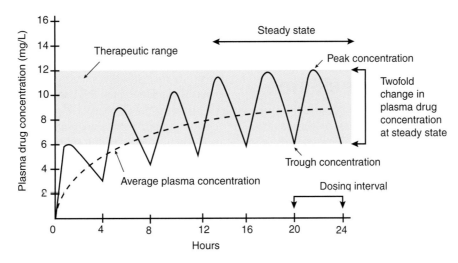

FIGURE 7-5 In this example, the drug has a half-life of 4 hours and is administered orally every 4 hours. After one half-life the average plasma concentration is 50% of the eventual steady-state concentration, which is reached after 3–5 half-lives. Once steady state is reached, the plasma drug concentration will fluctuate twofold between doses if dosing continues on the half-life.

CLINICAL INTEREST BOX 7-1   THE DILEMMA OF THE MISSED DOSE

Often the question is raised 'What do I do if I forget to take my medication?'. Inevitably, on one or more occasions, an individual will miss a dose of their drug. The simple issue of what to do if this occurs is rarely explained to patients, and an unintentionally missed dose is construed too readily as non-compliance. For some drugs (e.g. a lipid-lowering drug), a missed dose is of little consequence, but for others a missed dose can result in a decrease in the therapeutic plasma concentration and subsequent clinical manifestations (e.g. epilepsy). Pregnancy as a result of missing a dose of the oral contraceptive pill is well recognised.

Knowledge of the drug's half-life is useful for making a recommendation if a dose is missed. In general when the clinical effect of a drug is related to its half-life, a single missed dose for a drug with a long half-life is less of a problem than for a drug with a short half-life, for which the therapeutic effect will be lost rapidly. For some drugs (e.g. the oral contraceptive pill), specific recommendations exist for when a single dose is missed. A double dose should usually not be taken to make up for the dose missed because with many drugs (e.g. warfarin) this can cause adverse effects. The normal dosing regimen should be resumed and the next prescribed dose taken at the normal time (Gilbert et al 2002).

for the blood or plasma drug concentration to fall by one-half (50%). The pharmacokinetic parameters that determine half-life are clearance and volume of distribution:

$$t_{1/2} = \frac{0.693 \times V}{CL}$$

The half-life is the major determinant of:
- the duration of action of a drug after a single dose: if a drug is administered as a single dose, the longer the half-life of the drug the longer the plasma drug concentration will remain within the therapeutic range
- the time taken to reach steady state with chronic dosing: in general it takes 3–5 half-lives to reach the desired steady-state plasma drug concentration (Figure 7-5)
- the dosing frequency required to avoid massive fluctuations in plasma drug concentration during the dosing interval: once steady state has been reached, the half-life and the dosing interval determine the extent to which the plasma drug concentration fluctuates. If a drug is given orally every half-life, then the concentration will fall by one-half between doses and the plasma drug concentration will remain within the therapeutic range between doses (Figure 7-5).

Factors influencing half-life

The two factors that influence half-life are volume of distribution and clearance. Changes in either of these pharmacokinetic parameters will alter the half-life of a drug. It can be seen from Figure 7-6 that if two drugs have the same clearance but different volumes of distribution, then the half-life is shorter for the drug with the smaller volume of distribution. Similarly, if the two drugs have the same volume of distribution but different clearances, then the half-life is shorter for the drug with the higher clearance. This simple relationship explains why the half-life of a drug can change in individuals with heart failure because of decreased volume of distribution and decreased liver blood flow, and in persons with liver or kidney disease because of changes in clearance. Changes in half-life may necessitate changes in the dosing regimen.

Great importance is often placed on the half-life of a drug, but in fact it is a very poor indicator of the efficiency of drug elimination and hence the plasma drug concentration at steady state. For example, the half-life might be unaltered if both the volume of distribution of a drug and its clearance changed in the same direction. Under these circumstances, toxicity could occur if the usual maintenance dose rate were maintained (Box 7-3).

SATURABLE METABOLISM

The last situation to consider is saturable metabolism, which is particularly relevant to some hepatic drug-metabolising enzymes. Anyone who has consumed alcohol to excess will have experienced the consequences of saturable hepatic metabolism. How often the comment is made that 'It was the last drink that made me drunk' and how true that is! Saturable metabolism is the situation in which the enzyme metabolising the particular drug reaches its maximum capacity and the rate of metabolism cannot increase further as the dose increases. At that stage, metabolism is said to be saturated and a small change in dose can cause a large increase in the plasma drug concentration. This is illustrated in Figure 7-7. The drugs that

---

BOX 7-3   THE DANGER OF RELYING ON HALF-LIFE

This example illustrates how the half-life ($t_{1/2}$) of a commonly prescribed drug called *Pill* can remain the same while the plasma drug concentration increases to toxic levels. The pharmacokinetic data (which are theoretical) for *Pill* have been obtained from standard drug information sources.

Pill Volume of distribution = 50 L
Clearance = 8 L/h
Maintenance dose rate = 25 mg/h (200 mg 8-hourly)
Therapeutic plasma concentration range = 2.5–5 mg/L

Healthy person with stable physiology

$$t_{1/2} = \frac{0.693 \times 50 \text{ L}}{8 \text{ L/h}}$$

$t_{1/2}$ = 4.3 h
Steady-state plasma drug concentration =

$$\frac{25 \text{ mg/h}}{8 \text{ L/h}}$$

$$= 3.1 \text{ mg/L}$$

This concentration is in the middle of the therapeutic range.

Unhealthy person with unstable physiology
In this person the volume of distribution and clearance for *Pill* have decreased.

Volume of distribution = 20 L
Clearance = 3.2 L/h

$$t_{1/2} = \frac{0.693 \times 20 \text{ L}}{3.2 \text{ L/h}}$$

$t_{1/2}$ = 4.3 h (half-life is the same as for the healthy person)

If the maintenance dose rate is kept at 25 mg/h
Steady-state plasma drug concentration =

$$\frac{25 \text{ mg/h}}{3.2 \text{ L/h}}$$

$$= 7.8 \text{ mg/L}$$

This concentration is much higher than the upper limit of the therapeutic range (5 mg/L) and severe adverse reactions are highly likely.

In this example, relying on the half-life is of no value. Clearly the dosing regimen should be changed.

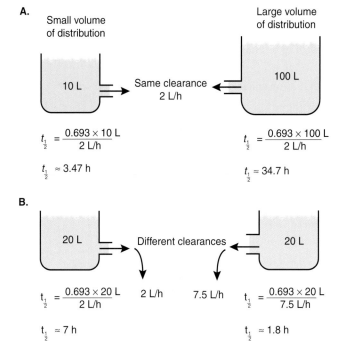

$$t_{\frac{1}{2}} = \frac{0.693 \times 10\ \text{L}}{2\ \text{L/h}}$$

$$t_{\frac{1}{2}} \approx 3.47\ \text{h}$$

$$t_{\frac{1}{2}} = \frac{0.693 \times 100\ \text{L}}{2\ \text{L/h}}$$

$$t_{\frac{1}{2}} \approx 34.7\ \text{h}$$

$$t_{\frac{1}{2}} = \frac{0.693 \times 20\ \text{L}}{2\ \text{L/h}}$$

$$t_{\frac{1}{2}} \approx 7\ \text{h}$$

$$t_{\frac{1}{2}} = \frac{0.693 \times 20\ \text{L}}{7.5\ \text{L/h}}$$

$$t_{\frac{1}{2}} \approx 1.8\ \text{h}$$

FIGURE 7-6 Effects of volume of distribution and clearance on half-life. In **A.** the drugs have the same clearance but differing volumes of distribution, and half-life differs about 10-fold. In **B.** the drugs have the same volume of distribution but clearances differ about fourfold. In both examples the half-life alters in relation to the change in volume of distribution or the change in clearance.

exhibit saturable metabolism include phenytoin, salicylic acid and, of course, ethanol.

It is important to have an understanding of basic pharmacokinetic principles, as they inform the clinical use of drugs and should allow for the rational design of dosing regimens.

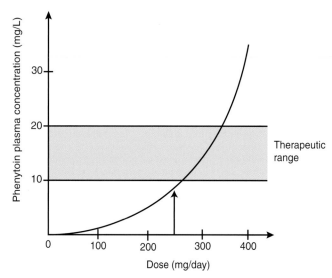

FIGURE 7-7 Illustration of the saturable metabolism of the antiepileptic drug phenytoin. Note that a small increment in dose above 250 mg/day results in a disproportionately large increase in phenytoin plasma concentration.

KEY POINTS

- Rational use of drugs is based on the assumption that a particular concentration of a drug will have the desired therapeutic effect and that adverse effects will be negligible.
- For many drugs there is a sufficient relationship between plasma drug concentration and clinical response that dosing regimens are designed to maintain the concentration within a therapeutic range.
- The therapeutic range is generally considered to reflect the range of drug concentrations having a high probability of producing the desired therapeutic effect and a low probability of producing adverse effects.
- Pharmacokinetics plays a major role not only in establishing the initial dosing regimen but also in adjusting the regimen to deal with a lack of response or to reduce symptoms of toxicity.
- The key pharmacokinetic parameters are clearance, volume of distribution and half-life.
- Clearance determines the maintenance dose rate required to achieve the target plasma concentration at steady state.
- The loading dose is the initial amount of drug required to fill the volume of distribution.
- Half-life is the major determinant of the duration of action of a drug after a single dose, the time taken to reach steady state with chronic dosing, and the dosing frequency required to avoid massive fluctuations in plasma drug concentration during the dosing interval.
- The factors influencing half-life include volume of distribution and clearance.
- Saturable metabolism refers to the situation in which the enzyme metabolising the particular drug reaches its maximum capacity. The rate of metabolism cannot increase further with increasing dose.

REVIEW EXERCISES

1. What are the key pharmacokinetic parameters that aid in the design of a rational dosing regimen?

2. What is meant by the terms low and high hepatic clearance?

3. How is a maintenance dose rate calculated for a drug administered intravenously and for one administered orally?

4. What is the importance of half-life and what does it fail to indicate?

REFERENCES AND FURTHER READING

Birkett DJ. *Pharmacokinetics Made Easy*. Sydney: McGraw-Hill, 2002.

Brody TM, Larner J, Minneman KP. *Human Pharmacology: Molecular to Clinical*. 3rd edn. St Louis: Mosby, 1998.

Gilbert A, Roughead L, Sansom L. I've missed a dose; what should I do? *Australian Prescriber* 2002; 25: 16–18.

Holford NHG. Pharmacokinetics and pharmacodynamics: rational dosing and the time course of drug action. In: Katzung BG (ed.). *Basic and Clinical Pharmacology*. 9th edn. New York: The McGraw-Hill Companies, 2004 [ch. 3].

Rang HP, Dale MM, Ritter JM, Moore PK. Drug elimination and pharmacokinetics. In: Rang HP, Dale MM, Ritter JM, Moore PK. *Pharmacology*. 5th edn. Edinburgh: Churchill Livingstone, 2003 [ch. 8].

Rowland M, Tozer TN. *Clinical Pharmacokinetics Concepts and Applications*. 2nd edn. Philadelphia: Lea & Febiger, 1989.

Somogyi A. Clinical pharmacokinetics and dosing schedules. In: Brody TM, Larner J, Minneman KP (eds). *Human Pharmacology: Molecular to Clinical*. 3rd edn. St Louis: Mosby, 1998.

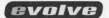 More weblinks at http://evolve.elsevier.com/AU/Bryant/pharmacology/

CHAPTER 8

Individual and Lifespan Aspects of Drug Therapy

CHAPTER FOCUS

The administration of drugs to pregnant women, children and the elderly varies because of numerous factors specific to each of these groups. Such variations may be individual and are altered by both physiological and pathophysiological factors present at different ages. Drug therapy in pregnant women may increase the risk of fetal abnormalities; in children, miscalculated doses of common drugs may cause adverse reactions; and in the elderly, polypharmacy may contribute to drug toxicity. Optimising drug therapy across the lifespan of an individual is a challenging process and requires a thorough understanding by health-care professionals of the effects of ageing on pharmacodynamic and pharmacokinetic processes.

OBJECTIVES

- To describe the physiological changes that occur during pregnancy and their effects on drug pharmacokinetics (i.e. absorption, distribution, metabolism and excretion).

- To discuss the important variables that should be considered if administering drugs to pregnant women.

- To discuss the Australian Drug Evaluation Committee (ADEC) pregnancy categories and their relationship to the safety of drugs in pregnancy.

- To discuss the transfer of drugs across the placenta and the handling of drugs by the fetus.

- To review the issues relating to drug use while breastfeeding.

- To discuss the factors that influence drug use and misuse in the elderly.

- To review the physiological changes of ageing that may affect drug pharmacokinetics and pharmacodynamics, and list an example for each effect.

KEY TERMS

ADEC pregnancy categories
carcinogen
fetal alcohol syndrome
mutagen
phocomelia
polypharmacy
teratogen

KEY ABBREVIATIONS

ADEC Australian Drug Evaluation Committee
BSA   body surface area
FAS   fetal alcohol syndrome

DRUG therapy in the pregnant woman, infant, child and the elderly patient may differ from that in the rest of the adult population; for example, drugs taken by the pregnant woman may reach the fetus via the maternal circulation and cause birth defects. Drugs consumed by a breastfeeding woman may be excreted in milk; if the drug levels are high enough this can cause adverse effects in the breastfed infant. Children and the elderly are often more sensitive to medications; in infants, this is because they have an immature organ system, whereas in the elderly, organ function may be compromised or impaired. Management of drug therapy throughout the lifespan of an individual must vary in line with the changes that occur to normal homeostatic systems through ageing.

DRUG USE DURING PREGNANCY

During pregnancy, any chemical or drug substance consumed and absorbed may reach the fetus by way of the maternal circulation or be transferred to the neonate via breast milk. Drug use during pregnancy should be avoided or limited to only those women who absolutely require treatment and where the benefit to the mother is considered greater than the risk to the fetus. All women should be counselled to avoid exposure to all unnecessary drugs (including complementary medicines) and chemicals throughout their pregnancies. With the recent trends towards higher birth rates in the older age groups of 35–39 and 40–44 years, it is likely that many more women will already be on medications for existing chronic medical conditions when they become pregnant. This will increase the risk of exposure of the fetus to maternal drugs. Similarly, many women may require drug therapy as a result of the pregnancy, e.g. to treat nausea and vomiting.

If it is necessary to administer drug therapy, the most important variables to be considered include:
• fetal gestational age at the time of exposure
• duration of therapy planned
• any other drugs administered concurrently
• the drug dose, dosing intervals and duration of treatment.
These should be adjusted carefully to avoid harmful effects.

A major problem with drug use is that the effects on the embryo may occur before a woman is aware she is pregnant. Women of childbearing age who are not using contraceptives and who are sexually active should be prescribed drugs carefully and should be instructed to use over-the-counter medications cautiously if they are contemplating pregnancy. Education and prevention are considered the best therapy.

Drug pregnancy categories
Even though many drugs cross the placenta, the potential for inducing adverse fetal effects depends on the drug type,
drug concentration and fetal age. Drugs taken during the first trimester may cause congenital malformations; those taken during the second and third trimesters may result in perturbation of functional and growth development, while those administered close to labour may affect the birth process and the neonate.

The Australian Drug Evaluation Committee (**ADEC**) has established seven **pregnancy categories** (A, B1, B2, B3, C, D and X) to indicate the level of risk to the fetus of drugs used at the recommended therapeutic doses (Table 8-1). Although this schedule is useful clinically, a range of drugs in use today have not been rated and many of the studies have been performed only in animals. In this scheme, which is used throughout Australasia, category A drugs are considered the least problematic, while drugs in category X are considered the most dangerous and should not be used in pregnancy or when contemplating pregnancy.

Any contemplation of the use of drug therapy in a pregnant woman should include consideration of the risk–benefit ratio. This ratio is evaluated based on the mother's condition and the potential beneficial effect of the drug(s) on the mother and the risk to the developing fetus. It is important to appreciate that no drug can really be labelled as totally safe. Typically, information on drugs not included in the ADEC categories provides non-specific warnings such as 'safe use in pregnancy has not been established', or 'it is not known whether . . . can cause fetal harm when administered to a pregnant woman or can affect reproduction capacity'. Statements of this type led Koren et al to conclude that "these typical disclaimers, although understandable from the medicolegal standpoint, put large numbers of women and their physicians in difficult situations" (Koren et al 1998).

Many historical examples highlight the problems of drug use in pregnancy and the issues faced by pregnant women and health-care providers. The use of the oestrogen diethylstilboestrol (DES) during pregnancy initially did not cause any problems; however, during the 1970s, it was linked to an increased risk of vaginal and cervical cancer in female offspring, and to genital abnormalities in both male and female offspring. It has been postulated that DES taken by the mother during the first trimester of pregnancy accumulated in the fetus, which was unable to metabolise it, resulting in problems later in life. The incidence was low (0.01%–0.1%) (Food and Drug Administration 1985) but the origin of the problem—a drug taken during developmental stages in pregnancy that has the potential to cause problems in offspring in later life—is still a concern.

The first trimester is when the developing embryo is most vulnerable to the teratogenic effects of various drugs and chemicals. Health-care professionals should keep in mind that drugs in this context include prescription and over-the-counter drugs, complementary medicines, alcohol, drugs of abuse, and any other chemical substance that the mother is exposed to during this time.

CATEGORY	DEFINITION
TABLE 8-1 ADEC drugs-in-pregnancy risk categories	
A	Drugs which have been taken by a large number of pregnant women and women of childbearing age, without any proven increase in the frequency of malformations or other direct or indirect harmful effects on the fetus having been observed
B1	Drugs which have been taken by only a limited number of pregnant women and women of childbearing age without an increase in the frequency of malformation or other direct or indirect harmful effects on the human fetus having been observed. Studies in animals have not shown evidence of an increased occurrence of fetal damage
B2	Drugs which have been taken by only a limited number of pregnant women and women of childbearing age without an increase in the frequency of malformations or other direct or indirect harmful effects on the human fetus having been observed. Studies in animals are inadequate or may be lacking, but available data show no evidence of an increased occurrence of fetal damage
B3	Drugs which have been taken by only a limited number of pregnant women and women of childbearing age without an increase in the frequency of malformations or other direct or indirect harmful effects on the human fetus having been observed. Studies in animals have shown evidence of an increased occurrence of fetal damage, the significance of which is considered uncertain in humans
C	Drugs which, owing to their pharmacological effects, have caused, or may be suspected of causing, harmful effects on the human fetus of neonate without causing malformations. These effects may be reversible. Accompanying texts should be consulted for further details
D	Drugs which have caused, are suspected to have caused, or may be expected to cause, an increased incidence of human fetal malformations or irreversible damage. These drugs may also have adverse pharmacological effects. Accompanying texts should be consulted for further details
X	Drugs which have such a high risk of causing permanent damage to the fetus that they should not be used in pregnancy or when there is a possibility of pregnancy

Note: For drugs in the B1, B2 and B3 categories, human data are lacking or inadequate and subcategorisation is therefore based on available animal data. **The allocation of a B category does NOT imply greater safety than the C category**. Drugs in Category D (e.g. anticonvulsants) are not absolutely contraindicted in pregnancy; moreover, in some cases the D category has been assigned on the basis of 'suspicion'.

Due to legal considerations in this country, sponsor companies have, in some cases, applied a more restrictive category than can be justified on the basis of the available data.

In some cases there may be discrepancies between the published Product Information and the information in this booklet due to the process of ongoing document revision.

These categories are subject to ongoing revision and amendment. Readers are asked to consult: www.tga.gov.au/docs/html/medpreg.htm

Reproduced from Australian Drug Evaluation Committee. *Prescribing Medicines in Pregnancy*. 4th edn. Canberra: Government Publishing Service, 1999. Copyright Commonwealth of Australia, reproduced by permission.

Embryo development

Drugs can exert a beneficial therapeutic effect in the fetus, cause predictable adverse effects in the fetus or act as **teratogens**, **mutagens** or **carcinogens** (see Box 8-1). Each embryo undergoes precisely programmed steps from cell proliferation to differentiation to organogenesis. The critical periods for drug effects on the fetus are the first 2 weeks of rapid cell proliferation, when exposure to drugs can be lethal to the embryo, and weeks 3–12 of pregnancy, the period of organogenesis (Figure 8-1). This is when the extremities (arms, fingers, legs and toes), central nervous system (CNS), muscles and organs are developing most rapidly (Ward & Mirkin 1998).

Thalidomide is a well-known example of a drug with teratogenic effects during organogenesis. It was used widely,

BOX 8-1 DEFINITIONS

- Teratogen: a substance that causes transient or permanent physical or functional disorders in the fetus without causing toxicity in the mother
- Mutagen: a physical or chemical agent that causes genetic material (DNA) to undergo a detectable and heritable structural change. All mutagens are teratogens but not all teratogens are mutagens (Ward & Mirkin 1998).
- Carcinogen: any agent that by either direct or indirect actions causes a normal cell to become a neoplastic cell

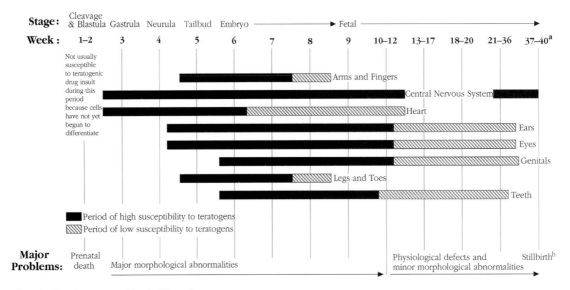

aAverage time from fertilisation to parturition is 39 weeks.
bDrugs administered during this period may cause neonatal depression at birth (or other effects directly related to the pharmacological effect of the administered drug).

FIGURE 8-1 Variation in tetratogenic susceptibility of organ systems during stages of human intrauterine development. Reprinted, by permission, from *Problems in Pediatric Drug Therapy*. 4th edn. p. 92. © 2002 by the American Pharmaceutical Association.

mostly in Europe, as a sedative–hypnotic drug from the 1950s to the early 1960s. Children whose mothers received this drug during pregnancy displayed abnormal limb development (**phocomelia**), a rare birth defect characterised by the absence or malformation of arms or legs. When administered after the 10th–12th week of pregnancy, physiological or behavioural alterations and growth delays were more likely. Thalidomide is currently available in Australia for use in certain malignancies. The history of this product is well recognised and every precaution is instituted if it is prescribed currently for a woman of childbearing age.

The abuse of cocaine during pregnancy has resulted in spontaneous abortions, fetal hypoxia, premature delivery and congenital abnormalities (skull defects, cardiac abnormality), and cerebral infarction or stroke. At birth, the newborn may exhibit symptoms of cocaine drug withdrawal (irritability, increased respiratory and heart rates, diarrhoea, irregular sleeping patterns, and poor appetite). It has been reported that long-term behavioural patterns of infants born to cocaine-abusing women may also occur, such as poor attention spans and a decrease in organisational skills (Hall et al 1990).

Drug transfer to the fetus
MATERNAL PHARMACOKINETICS
Many physiological changes that occur during pregnancy affect the pharmacokinetics of drugs. Although pregnancy does not directly affect drug absorption from the gastro-intestinal tract, it does delay gastric emptying and decreases motility, which can increase or decrease drug absorption;

for example, drugs that require an acidic environment for absorption may have a delayed absorption pattern because of the typical decrease in production of hydrochloric acid in the stomach during pregnancy.

Drug absorption from other sites may be increased; for example, an increase in pulmonary drug absorption and an increase in cutaneous or topical drug absorption may be seen secondary to a greater minute ventilation pattern and a larger surface area and blood flow during pregnancy (Ward & Mirkin 1998).

Changes in the woman's body mass and fluid distribution may also change the volume of distribution of a drug. During pregnancy, there is an increase in maternal plasma volume (30%–50%) and a 25% increase in body fat. The latter may affect the distribution of drugs that are deposited in fatty tissues and can result in a fall in their plasma concentrations. Maternal renal blood flow and glomerular filtration rate also increase during the first 8 months of pregnancy, while hepatic drug-metabolising enzyme activity can either increase or decrease during pregnancy.

The effects of these changes on drug therapies are difficult to predict, as the alterations can vary enormously between individual pregnant women. Although induction or inhibition of drug metabolism has been reported this really depends on the specific cytochrome P450 enzymes involved. For example, in pregnant women metabolism of caffeine is decreased but the metabolism of the anticonvulsant phenytoin is increased, often necessitating an increase in dosage during pregnancy. The changes in renal function, which in general cause increased elimination rates for drugs excreted by the kidneys,

---

CLINICAL INTEREST BOX 8-1
FETAL ALCOHOL SYNDROME

Alcohol consumption during pregnancy can cause tragic effects on the fetus. As many people do not consider alcohol a drug, its danger during pregnancy may be overlooked. Alcohol easily crosses the placenta to enter the fetal bloodstream, which can result in *fetal alcohol syndrome* (FAS), a series of congenital abnormalities.

The symptoms of FAS include small head (microcephaly), low birth weight, mental and growth retardation, impaired coordination, irritability in infancy, hyperactivity in childhood, cardiac murmurs, cleft lip or palate, hernias and many other neurological and structural abnormalities (see picture).

As even limited amounts of alcohol during pregnancy may have tragic effects on a developing fetus, the only safe approach is total abstinence.

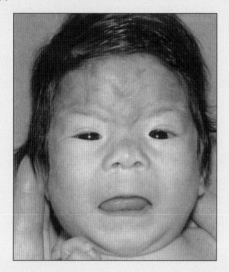

Source: Streissguth et al 1991.

---

also lead to the need for an increase in dose (Theis & Koren 1997). If drugs are absolutely necessary during pregnancy, they should be carefully selected and titrated to the desired clinical response.

FETAL PHARMACOKINETICS

Although the placenta functions to protect the fetus, many drugs ingested during pregnancy cross it. The fetus is then at risk of the pharmacological and teratogenic effects of the drug. The transfer of a drug across the placenta depends on the physicochemical properties of the drug, protein binding and lipid solubility. Transfer of drugs primarily involves simple diffusion, although other transport processes may also be involved to a much lesser degree. In pregnancy, low-molecular-weight drugs (250–500) freely cross the placenta, while drugs of molecular weight over 1000 (e.g. heparin) cross very poorly. In late gestation, the enhanced uteroplacental blood flow and the thinner membranes that separate maternal blood flow and placental capillaries result in an increased placental transfer of un-ionised, lipophilic (lipid-soluble) non-protein-bound drugs. Disease states such as pregnancy-induced hypertension or diabetes mellitus can also affect drug transfer.

Most drugs cross the placenta by simple diffusion; therefore fetal plasma drug concentrations may equal maternal concentrations. Certain drugs are contraindicated during pregnancy or are used only when the risk–benefit situation has been carefully reviewed and discussed with the woman. Examples of drugs considered to be teratogenic in humans, along with the critical time periods and potential defects, are given in Table 8-2.

Drug metabolism in the fetus

Drug effects in the fetus can be more significant and prolonged than in the mother because the fetus in general has immature liver drug-metabolising enzymes and thus metabolises drugs differently from adults. The expression of these enzymes varies depending on the developmental stage: activity can be detected at 5–8 weeks, and by 12–14 weeks the fetus has about 30% of the capacity of adults, while full maturation of drug-metabolising capacity is not evident until 1 year after birth (Gow et al 2001). The limited ability of the fetus to metabolise drugs may in some circumstances be detrimental. Increased exposure of the fetus to a drug or its metabolites can occur if the metabolite produced by the fetus is toxic and binds to fetal proteins, or if metabolism by the fetal liver results in the formation of a water-soluble metabolite that does not readily cross the placenta. Under these circumstances, drugs and drug metabolites accumulate in amniotic fluid, resulting in increased fetal exposure.

Enhanced exposure to drugs can also occur because the fetus has a slower overall rate of drug excretion, as the only connection to the environment is via the placenta. Drugs that are 'excreted' by the fetal kidneys may pass into the amniotic fluid and be reabsorbed by the fetus, thus increasing its exposure. Not every drug causes detrimental effects on the fetus but unfortunately some do. At this stage, our knowledge of the role of fetal drug-metabolising enzymes and a possible link with teratogenesis is incomplete.

Several chronic medical disorders in the mother often need to be treated during pregnancy. Diabetes, hypertension, epilepsy and asthma, for example, require close monitoring and careful selection of therapies to minimise or reduce fetal abnormalities and disease complications.

The use of alcohol and drugs of abuse should be avoided by pregnant women, as they can be extremely harmful to the fetus and newborn. Drugs given before delivery, such as barbiturates, or opioid analgesics, may result in withdrawal symptoms in the neonate. These symptoms include hyperactivity, increased irritability, persistent crying, convulsions, and sudden death. Table 8-3 lists drugs that are associated with neonatal withdrawal symptoms.

TABLE 8-2 Drugs and teratogenic effects in humans

DRUGS	CRITICAL TIME PERIOD	POTENTIAL DEFFECT
Alcohol (chronic use)	<12 weeks >24 weeks	Heart defects, CNS abnormalities Delay in development, low birth weight
Androgens	>10 weeks	External female genitalia masculinisation
Angiotensin-converting enzyme (ACE) inhibitors and angiotensin II receptor antagonists	1st–3rd trimester	Renal dysgenesis, defects in skull ossification, prolonged renal failure and hypotension in neonates
Carbamazepine	<30 days after conception	Neural tube defects
Cocaine	2nd–3rd trimester 3rd trimester	Abruptio placentae Premature labour and delivery, intracranial bleeding
Cyclophosphamide	1st trimester	CNS malformations, secondary cancer
Isotretinoin	>15 days after conception	Hydrocephalus, CNS abnormalities, fetal death
Lithium	<2 months	Ebstein's anomaly and other heart defects
Methotrexate	6–9 weeks after conception	Skull ossification defect, limb and craniofacial defects
Phenytoin	1st trimester	Craniofacial defects, underdevelopment of phalanges or nails, impaired neurological development
Tetracycline	>20 weeks	Stained teeth, bone growth defect
Valproic acid	<1 month after conception 1st trimester	Neural tube defects Craniofacial defects
Vitamin A (high doses and parenteral)	1st trimester	Fetal abnormalities including urinary tract malformations, growth retardation
Warfarin	1st–3rd trimester	CNS and skeletal defects, low birth weight (<10th percentile), hearing loss

Modified from: Jennings 1996; Jacqz-Aigrain & Koren 2005.

DRUG USE DURING LACTATION

Data on infant drug absorption, distribution, metabolism and excretion are scant and conflicting. Almost all forms of drugs in maternal circulation can be readily transferred to the colostrum and breast milk. Because drugs or their metabolites are handled by different pathways in the infant and the fetus, the impact of maternal medications on the infant is probably less, as the drug is diluted in the maternal circulation and the amount of milk swallowed is often small. However, immaturity of the neonate's hepatic and renal systems may limit the infant's capacity for further metabolism and excretion.

In general, the proven benefits of continuing breastfeeding must be weighed on an individual basis against the risks of exposure of the infant to maternal medications. Although the mammary glands are a relatively insignificant route for maternal drug excretion and the drug level in breast milk is usually less than the actual maternal dose, the infant's actual dose depends largely on the volume of milk consumed. Thus a single measurement of a drug in human milk will not accurately reflect the total dose the infant receives.

The drug concentration in the maternal circulation depends on the relationship of several factors: dosing and route of administration, the drug's distribution, its protein binding, and maternal metabolism and excretion. The mammary alveolar epithelium consists of a lipid barrier with water-filled pores; thus it is more permeable to drugs during the colostrum stage of milk production (first week of life). Drug factors that enhance drug excretion into milk are higher degree of ionisation, low molecular weight, greater fat solubility, and higher concentration. Transfer of a drug or its metabolites into milk occurs by both passive diffusion and carrier-mediated transport.

It is believed that absorptive processes in the infant's gastrointestinal tract and drug distribution are similar to those in the adult and that lipid-soluble drugs are well absorbed.

TABLE 8-3 Drugs associated with neonatal withdrawal symptoms

	SYMPTOMS	
DRUG	**General**	**Central nervous system**
Alcohol	Irritability, poor sleep pattern, diaphoresis	Crying, hyperactivity, increased sensitivity to sound, hypertonicity, tremor, seizures
Cocaine	Tremulousness, poor sleep pattern	Hypotonia, hyperreflexia
Antihistamines		
Diphenhydramine	Tremulousness	
Barbiturates		
Phenobarbitone	Irritability, poor sleep pattern, diaphoresis, skin abrasions	Excessive crying, hyperreflexia, increased sensitivity to sound, hypertonicity, tremor, seizures
Benzodiazepines		
Diazepam	Hypothermia	Hyperactivity, hypotonia, hypertonia, apnoea/tremor, hyperreflexia
Opiates		
Codeine	Irritability, wakefulness, yawning, tearing, fever	Coarse tremors, seizures, twitching
Heroin	Diaphoresis	Hyperactivity (high-pitched cry), hypertonicity
Pethidine	Skin excoriations, voracious sucking	
Methadone	Poor sleep pattern	Hyperreflexia, increased sensitivity to sound, photophobia, apnoeic spells
Morphine	Hypothermia	
Dextropropoxyphene	Irritability, fever	Hyperactivity, tremor, high-pitched cry

Modified from: Levy & Spino 1993.

The infant's age (and therefore the amount of drug-containing milk consumed) and the relative immaturity of the infant's important organs bear greatly on the outcome. The following factors are also relevant:

- if the drug is fat-soluble, it may be more highly concentrated in breast milk at the end of feeding and at midday
- because the infant's total plasma protein concentration is lower compared with the adult's, more free drug may be available to the circulation
- metabolic reactions in the infant's liver are slower than in the older child's and consequently drug metabolism may likewise be delayed
- drug excretion is delayed in the neonate because it is largely via the kidneys, where immature glomerular filtration and tubular functioning persist for months.

The extreme variability among drug effects and the infant's capacity to handle exposure to a drug often makes it difficult to decide whether the mother should take a drug and whether or not she should breastfeed.

If human milk contains small fixed amounts of substances absorbed by the mother, it is usually recommended that breastfeeding be temporarily interrupted (usually for 24–72 hours) and the breasts pumped to remove drug-containing milk. Less often, it is advisable to stop breastfeeding altogether. Taking medications after a feed may also lead to reduced traces of drug in breast milk before the next feed and hence to reduced effects on the infant. If diagnostic radioisotope testing is to be done, breastfeeding is interrupted until all the radioactive substance is absent from milk samples. Breastfeeding is also contraindicated:

- when the drug is so toxic that minute amounts may profoundly affect the infant
- when the drug has high allergenic potential
- when the mother's renal function deteriorates (which augments drug excretion into breast milk)
- when serious pathological conditions require prolonged administration of high doses of drugs (e.g. cancer chemotherapy).

BOX 8-2 EXAMPLES OF DRUGS THAT SHOULD BE AVOIDED DURING BREASTFEEDING

Amiodarone	Combined oral contraceptives	Ergotamine	Nicotine (smoking)
Aspirin (high-dose)	Cyclophosphamide	Gold salts	Phenindione
Atenolol	Cyclosporin	Heroin	Sotalol
Bromocriptine	Diazepam	Lithium	Tetracyclines
Caffeine	Doxorubicin	Marijuana	Theophylline
Cocaine	Ephedrine hydrochloride	Methotrexate	*Source*: Ito 2000; Rubin 1998.

Also, it is recommended that certain drugs be avoided while breastfeeding because they may either cause adverse effects in the infant or suppress lactation (Box 8-2).

DRUG METABOLISM IN CHILDREN

Neonates

Administering drugs to children requires special knowledge and approaches. Newborns require special consideration because they lack many of the protective mechanisms of older children and adults. Their skin is thin and permeable, their stomachs lack acid and their lungs lack much of the mucous barrier. Neonates regulate body temperature poorly and become dehydrated easily. After the transition from in utero to life, neonates are solely dependent on their own enzyme processes to metabolise drugs and chemicals. Their livers and kidneys are immature and cannot manage foreign substances as well those of older children and adults; for example, phenobarbitone plasma half-life is 70–500 hours in neonates (younger than 7 days), 20–70 hours in infants (younger than 1 month), 20–80 hours in children 1–15 years of age, and 60–180 hours in young adults (Walson 1997). Specific pharmacokinetic factors affecting medication use in neonates are reviewed in Table 8-4.

Infant–child

When the infant is 1 year old, most pharmacokinetic patterns (other than hepatic) are similar to those in an adult. Liver drug-metabolising enzyme activities are increased, so children metabolise drugs at a faster rate than adults, as illustrated with the example of phenobarbitone. This alteration is primarily due to the infant's liver being larger in proportion to body weight compared with an adult's (Walson 1997). The child reaches adult parameters at puberty, so drugs primarily eliminated by hepatic metabolism may require dosage or frequency adjustments because of a shorter plasma half-life. Such variations must be individually determined and carefully monitored.

Renal excretion is decreased in neonates and reaches adult parameters for glomerular filtration rate between 3 and 6 months, while tubular function does not mature until the infant is around 12 months old. For drugs excreted primarily by the kidneys, the plasma half-life will be prolonged during the first week of life (the lower the renal drug clearance, the longer the drug half-life in the body). Elimination rate increases rapidly over the next few weeks. Later in childhood, renal function may exceed adult parameters, and if ignored, may result in drug underdosing (Walson 1997).

Many drugs that are safe and effective for adults may not have been tested for use with children, nor have doses been established because of the complex medicolegal issues involved in experimentation on children. Often a standard paediatric medication dosage is non-existent and doses are usually calculated according to the weight or body surface area of the child. Calculation formulae based on the child's weight and age related to the adult, and on adult dose, are inaccurate and should not be used. Children are not small adults and their pharmacodynamic and pharmacokinetic differences will definitely affect the amount of drug needed to produce a therapeutic effect. An infant's body composition is about 75% water (adults have 50%–60%) and an infant has less fat content than the adult, therefore, water-soluble drugs are generally administered in larger doses to infants and children in proportion to body weight than to adults. A good example of this is the water-soluble drug gentamicin, an intravenous antibiotic. Recommended dosages (IM/IV) from the *Australian Medicines Handbook 2006* are:

• children 1 month–10 years: 7.5 mg/kg once daily
• children over 10 years: 6 mg/kg once daily
• adults: 4–7 mg/kg once daily.

Although pharmaceutical companies are increasing their marketing of paediatric drug products, many medications are

**CLINICAL INTEREST BOX 8-2
DRUG USE IN PREGNANCY AND
BREASTFEEDING**

In 1998 the National Drug Strategy Household Survey of Australians aged 14 years and over was conducted. At the time of the 1998 survey, 75% of women who were pregnant or breastfeeding reported consuming alcohol, 24% tobacco, 18% marijuana, 21% any illicit drug and 8% any illicit drug other than marijuana (Higgins et al 2000).

TABLE 8-4 Factors influencing drug dosing in neonates

PHYSIOLOGICAL PROCESS	CHANGES IN NEONATES	TYPE OF DRUGS AFFECTED
Absorption		
Gastric pH	Increased to 6–8 for first 24 hours; then usually a 10–15-day achlorhydria	Acid-labile drugs such as oral penicillin are better absorbed. Oral forms of phenobarbitone or phenytoin have reduced bioavailability
Gastric emptying time	Prolonged, usually 6–8 hours	Oral absorption of penicillin increase; that of phenytoin and phenobarbitone decrease
Distribution		
Total body water (TBW) content Adipose (fat) content	75–79% 5–12%	Average adults have about 60% TBW and 25%–45% fat. There are vast differences in drug distribution across the age span. Water-soluble drugs have a larger volume of distribution in newborns; fat-soluble drugs have considerably less. Drug dosage adjustments are largely based on this factor
Protein binding	Decreased	Highly protein-bound drugs require dose adjustment to avoid toxicity
Metabolism		
Liver metabolism	Decreased drug-metabolising enzyme activity	Potent or potentially toxic drugs requiring liver metabolism are slowly metabolised; lower doses are necessary for such drugs (especially chloramphenicol and theophylline, among others)
Excretion		
Glomerular filtration Tubular secretion	Decreased Decreased	Drugs excreted by filtration or secretion will accumulate in the neonate; dose adjustments are necessary (especially for aminoglycosides and digoxin)

still available only in the standard adult dosages; therefore, health-care professionals must be able to calculate and formulate such products to the correct paediatric dosage. If the calculated dose in mg/kg exceeds the usual adult dose, the recommended adult dose should be used instead (AMH 2006).

Body surface area as a basis for drug dosage

It was suggested years ago that drug dosages be calculated on size or the proportion of body surface area (BSA) to weight. Although BSA has been proposed to be a more accurate indicator of drug clearance and thus dosage, large inter-individual variations and difficulty in calculations challenge this premise. For some drugs, body weight is sufficient, whereas for others, BSA may be more accurate. Nomograms for the estimation of BSA from weight and height are available (Figure 8-2) and can also be found in common drug guides such as the *MIMS Annual*. When specific dosage information

is not available, specialist information should be sought from the drug information services in major hospitals.

Although rules have been devised for converting adult dosage schedules to those for infants and children, it must be emphasised that no rules or charts are adequate to guarantee safety of dosage at any age, particularly in the neonate. No method takes into account all variables, particularly individual tolerance differences. The calculated dose is a guide for initiating therapy but the severity of the primary disorder, the presence of coexisting conditions, clinical response and therapeutic drug monitoring all contribute to ascertaining the optimal dose.

Topical medication use in children

Children have a large skin surface area in proportion to total body weight. Their skin, especially that of neonates, is particularly thin and permeable and has limited protective oil. Although adults absorb more medication through intact skin than was previously believed, children are even more at risk

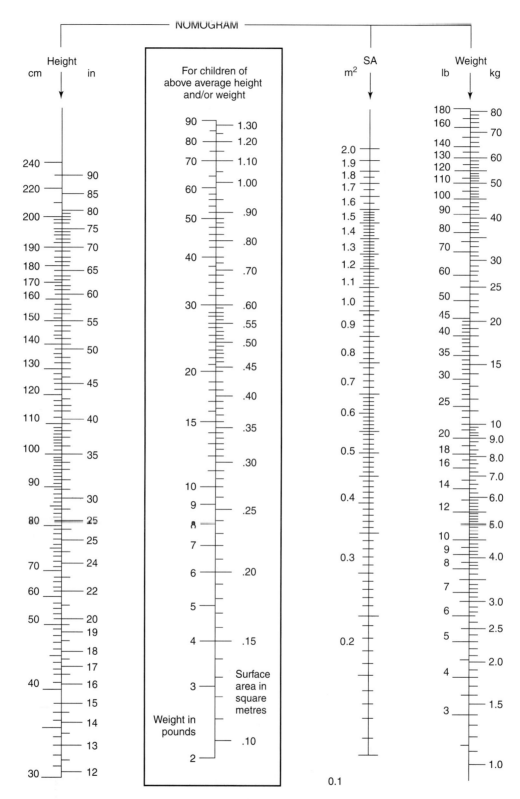

FIGURE 8-2 Nomogram for calculating drug doses in children. Body surface area is indicated where a straight line that connects height (on the left) and weight (on the right) intersects the SA column or, if the patient is above average size, from weight alone (enclosed area). *Source*: Barone 1996.

than adults from systemic absorption of topical medications. The discoveries that hexachlorophene could cause encephalopathy in newborns and that topically applied boric acid can cause systemic poisoning testify to the hazard of applying drugs to children's skin, especially in prolonged contact or over broken skin areas.

A dearth of pharmacokinetic and pharmacodynamic information on drug use in children remains a problem for health-care professionals. There are numerous reasons why pharmaceutical companies and medical researchers are unwilling to study the effects of drugs in children but "many paediatricians argue that it is unethical not to undertake drug trials in children. It is not acceptable that children require medicines which have not been properly tested" (Stephenson 2001).

DRUG USE IN THE ELDERLY

Australians and New Zealanders can, on average, expect to live long (75–80 years) and relatively healthy lives. Life-expectancy has in general increased in all developed countries (75 years) but it is not uniform across all population groups (64 years in less developed countries). The elderly represent a significant proportion of the population, and in general they:

- consume a high proportion of all prescribed drugs and over-the-counter medications
- take three times more drugs than younger persons
- frequently take multiple medications
- are admitted to hospitals with adverse drug reactions more frequently than younger adults (see Chapter 9).

Because the elderly are the most rapidly increasing segment of the population, an understanding of age-related alterations in pharmacokinetics and pharmacodynamics is necessary. Furthermore, the higher incidence of chronic diseases in the elderly often results in an increase in the number of prescriptions, over-the-counter medications and home remedies prescribed or self-selected. The age of specialisation has in some ways added to this problem because multiple physicians may prescribe a variety of medications, often without rationalising the number of drugs the patient is currently taking. This practice is often referred to as **polypharmacy**, the indiscriminate use of numerous medications concurrently.

Polypharmacy can be a dangerous practice that may increase the risk of drug interactions and adverse reactions and the need for, or prolongation of, hospitalisation. To minimise the risks associated with use of multiple medications and adverse drug reactions in this population, an understanding of the ageing process and the associated changes in pharmacokinetics and pharmacodynamics is essential.

Physiological changes of ageing

Ageing persons undergo a variety of physiological changes that may increase their sensitivity to drugs and drug-induced adverse reactions (Figure 8-3). The loss in body weight (decreased volume of drug distribution) in many elderly patients may require initiation of therapy at a lower adult dose or re-evaluation of dosages of medications already in use. The criterion for dosage should be shifted from age to weight. Some older patients weigh no more than the average large child and some weigh a lot less, yet they are often prescribed the larger adult doses.

Pharmacokinetics are altered in the ageing patient (Box 8-3) because of reduced gastric acid and slowed gastric motility, resulting in unpredictable rates of dissolution and absorption of drugs. Changes in absorption may occur when acid production decreases, altering the absorption of weakly acidic drugs such as barbiturates; however, few studies of drug absorption have shown clinically significant changes occurring with advanced age.

Changes in body composition, such as increased proportion of body fat and decreased total body water, plasma volume and extracellular fluid, have been noted in the elderly. The increased proportion of body fat increases the body's ability to store fat-soluble compounds such as phenothiazines and barbiturates and thus increases the accumulation of those drugs. The reduced lean body mass affects drug distribution by decreasing the volume in which the drug circulates, thereby causing higher peak levels. The risk of toxicity with hydrophilic or water-soluble drugs increases as total body water decreases. Digoxin, theophylline and the aminoglycosides are examples of hydrophilic drugs that may accumulate and cause an adverse reaction or toxicity.

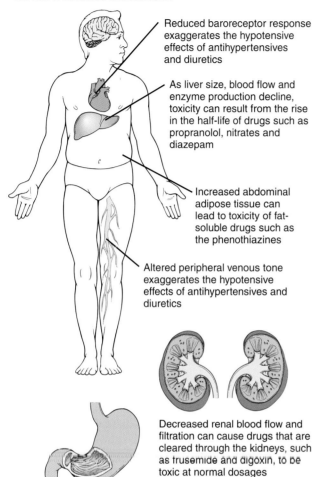

The blood–brain barrier is more easily penetrated by fat-soluble drugs such as the β-blockers, raising the risk of dizziness and confusion

Reduced baroreceptor response exaggerates the hypotensive effects of antihypertensives and diuretics

As liver size, blood flow and enzyme production decline, toxicity can result from the rise in the half-life of drugs such as propranolol, nitrates and diazepam

Increased abdominal adipose tissue can lead to toxicity of fat-soluble drugs such as the phenothiazines

Altered peripheral venous tone exaggerates the hypotensive effects of antihypertensives and diuretics

Decreased renal blood flow and filtration can cause drugs that are cleared through the kidneys, such as frusemide and digoxin, to be toxic at normal dosages

Slower gastric emptying time plus an increase in the pH of gastric juices increases the risk of stomach irritation with such drugs as aspirin

FIGURE 8-3 How pharmacokinetics change with age. *Source*: Goodman & Gorlin 1977, courtesy Dr Charles Linder, Medical College of Georgia.

Decreased plasma albumin for highly protein-bound drugs may lead to increased amounts of free drug in the circulation. Warfarin, phenytoin and diazepam are a few examples of highly protein-bound drugs.

Liver drug metabolism is also affected by ageing. Drugs that undergo functionalisation (Phase I) reactions (reduction, oxidation, hydroxylation or demethylation) may have a decreased metabolism, while conjugative metabolism (glucuronidation, acetylation, sulfonation etc) is not affected by ageing. Some drugs that may have decreased hepatic metabolism in the elderly are the nitrates, barbiturates, propranolol and lignocaine (Jinks & Fuerst 1995). Disorders common

to the ageing person, such as congestive heart failure, may impair liver function and decrease the metabolism of drugs, increasing the risk of drug accumulation and toxicity.

Renal function may be impaired because of loss of nephrons, decreased blood flow and decreased glomerular filtration rate. A reduction in renal function is also secondary to heart failure. Decreased renal clearance may cause increased plasma drug concentrations and longer half-lives of drugs and active metabolites that the kidney usually excretes. Drugs that are highly dependent on the kidneys for excretion include the aminoglycosides, ciprofloxin, digoxin, lithium and numerous other drugs.

Alterations in pharmacokinetics

It has been estimated that 70%–80% of all adverse drug reactions in the elderly are dose-related. The physiological changes previously discussed may result in decreases in drug metabolism, distribution in the body and renal excretion; therefore higher blood and tissue levels of potent medications may result in an increased incidence of adverse drug reactions. The half-life of diazepam increases from 20 hours in a 20-year-old to 90 hours in individuals in their 80s because of the increase in volume of distribution of the drug in the body of the elderly person. For drugs primarily excreted by the kidneys, reduced or impaired renal function may result in drug accumulation and perhaps toxicity—up to two-thirds of the elderly have some degree of "age-related renal insufficiency" (McCue et al 1992). When appropriate, determining creatinine clearance and therapeutic drug monitoring will help optimise dosing in the elderly with compromised renal function.

BOX 8-3 POTENTIAL ALTERED PHARMACOKINETICS IN THE ELDERLY

ABSORPTION
- Increase in gastric pH
- Altered gastric emptying and intestinal blood flow
- Decrease in first-pass metabolism in the liver

DISTRIBUTION
- Altered body composition (decrease in lean body mass, increase in adipose [fat] stores)
- Decrease in total body water
- Decrease in plasma albumin
- Decrease in blood flow and cardiac output

METABOLISM
- Decrease in oxidative metabolism (cytochrome P450 system)
- Decrease in hepatic blood flow

EXCRETION
- Decrease in glomerular filtration rate; most persons lose 10% of renal function per decade after age 50

Modified from: Trends & Analysis 1995.

TABLE 8-5 Commonly prescribed medications in the elderly

DRUGS	ADVERSE REACTIONS
Aminoglycoside antibiotics (gentamicin etc)	Ototoxicity (hearing impairment or loss), renal impairment or failure
Analgesics, opioids	Confusion, constipation, urinary retention (morphine and others), nausea, vomiting, respiratory depression
Anticholinergics, antispasmodics, especially antihistamines, antiparkinsonian drugs, atropine etc	Blurred vision, dry mouth, constipation, confusion, urinary retention, nausea, delirium
Anticoagulants (heparin, warfarin)	Bleeding episodes, haemorrhage, increase in drug-interaction potential
Antihypertensive medications	Sedation, orthostatic hypotension, sexual dysfunction, CNS alterations, nausea
Aspirin, aspirin-containing products	Tinnitus, gastric distress, ulcers, gastrointestinal bleeding
Digoxin, especially at higher dosages	Nausea, vomiting, cardiac arrhythmias, visual disorders, mental status changes, hallucinations
Diuretics (thiazides, frusemide etc)	Electrolyte disorders, rash, fatigue, leg cramps, dehydration
Hypnotics/sedatives (diazepam etc)	Confusion, daytime sedation, gait disturbances, lethargy, increased forgetfulness, depression, delirium
H_2-receptor antagonists (ranitidine etc)	Confusion, depression, mental status alterations
Non-steroidal anti-inflammatory drugs (NSAIDs)	Gastric distress, gastrointestinal bleeding, ulceration
Psychotropics (neuroleptic agents)	Sedation, confusion, hypotension, drug-induced parkinsonian effects, tardive dyskinesia
Tricyclic antidepressants (amitriptyline, doxepin and others)	Confusion, cardiac arrhythmias, seizures, agitation, anticholinergic effects, tachycardia etc

Alterations in pharmacodynamics

Changes in target-organ or receptor sensitivity in the elderly may result in a greater or lesser than normal drug effect. The reason for this alteration is unknown but it may be due to a decrease in the number of receptors at the site or an altered receptor response to the medication. The elderly often exhibit a decreased response to β-agonists and antagonists, but they have a greater response (CNS depression) with diazepam. It has also been reported that the muscarinic receptor density in the cortex tends to decrease with ageing, so the elderly are often very sensitive to anticholinergic medications. Often noted adverse effects of anticholinergic drugs include confusion, dry mouth, blurred vision, constipation and urinary retention (Lucas et al 1995). See Chapter 11 for additional information on anticholinergic drugs.

There is also believed to be a loss in responsiveness or an age-related decline in dopamine receptors in the elderly. The number of receptors may vary or the alteration may be in different areas of the CNS, which may result in altered drug responses or an increased risk of drug-induced Parkinson's disease (Lucas et al 1995).

In summary, the elderly are perceived to have a greater sensitivity to drugs, especially to CNS-acting medications. If monitoring and dosage adjustments are not instituted, the elderly may encounter more adverse reactions than younger persons.

Medication use in the elderly

Potent medications available to treat the elderly often have a narrow index between effectiveness and toxicity. Effective use of medicines in the elderly is problematic with numerous reports of adverse drug reactions resulting in hospitalisations, less than optimum treatment when guidelines are available and discrepancies with drugs prescribed occurring after discharge from hospital. Box 8-4 lists drugs that should be avoided in the elderly. This list was derived from a previously published list (Beers et al 1991) and is limited to drugs that should be avoided entirely in the geriatric patient. Long-acting benzodiazepines, for example, have been associated with daytime sedation and an increased risk of falls, while the antidepressant amitriptyline has been reported to have a higher incidence of anticholinergic adverse effects and orthostatic hypotension than other drugs of that category. The prescribing of such medications in the aged person increases the risk of adverse drug reactions, and perhaps injury.

Table 8-5 lists medications commonly prescribed for the elderly, with the most common adverse reactions reported. "Although all systems are altered by the ageing process, the central nervous system and the cardiovascular system appear to be the most affected", according to Lucas et al (1995). To reduce the potential for adverse reactions, it has been recommended that CNS-acting medications be reduced to around 50% of the usual adult recommended dose (Lucas et al 1995). Titration of the dose slowly to achieve a therapeutic effect reduces the potential for drug-induced adverse reactions.

Overprescribing and inappropriate prescribing in the elderly are common problems often exacerbated by unrecognised changes in pharmacokinetics and pharmacodynamics occurring as a consequence of the ageing process. Practical points in prescribing medications for the elderly (adapted from Pillans & Roberts 2001) include:
- non-pharmacological approaches
- frequent medication review
- avoiding polypharmacy, and use of the simplest drug regimen

---

BOX 8-4   DRUGS THAT SHOULD BE AVOIDED IN THE ELDERLY

Category	Drug Examples
Analgesics	Dextropropoxyphene
Antidepressant	Amitriptyline
Antihypertensives	Propranolol, methyldopa
Hypnotic/sedative	Diazepam
Muscle relaxants	Orphenadrine
Non-steroidal anti-inflammatory drugs (NSAIDs)	Indomethacin

- discontinuing drugs when the need no longer exists
- considering any new symptoms as possible adverse drug reactions
- careful choice of drug from within a drug class to reduce risk of adverse reactions
- use of the lowest dose to achieve the desired effect
- providing simple written and verbal instructions to aid compliance.

Optimising drug therapy across a person's lifespan is a challenging process and requires a through understanding by health-care professionals of the effects of ageing on pharmacodynamic and pharmacokinetic processes.

KEY POINTS

- This chapter reviews the effects of drug therapy on the fetus, neonate, infant, child, and elderly.
- Drug use during pregnancy should be avoided or limited to only those women who absolutely require treatment and when the benefit to the mother is considered greater than the risk to the fetus.
- Although many drugs cross the placenta, the potential for inducing adverse fetal effects depends on the drug type, drug concentration and fetal age.
- The Australian Drug Evaluation Committee (ADEC) has established seven pregnancy categories (A, B1, B2, B3, C, D and X) to indicate the level of risk to the fetus of drugs used at the recommended therapeutic doses.
- Drugs can exert a beneficial therapeutic effect in the fetus or cause predictable adverse effects in the fetus or act as a teratogen, mutagen or carcinogen.
- The transfer of drugs across the placenta depends on the physicochemical properties of the drug, protein binding and lipid solubility.
- Drug effects in the fetus can be more significant and prolonged than in the mother because the fetus in general has immature liver drug-metabolising enzymes and thus handles drugs differently to adults.
- Drug factors that enhance drug excretion into breast milk are high degree of ionisation, low molecular weight, fat solubility, and concentration.
- The disposition of drugs in children differs from that in adults because of factors such as growth, maturation of drug-metabolising enzymes, plasma and tissue binding, and physiological maturation of organ systems.
- Ageing produces changes in pharmacokinetics and pharmacodynamics, and the elderly are at an increased risk of adverse drug reactions.
- Practical points for decreasing inappropriate drug use in the elderly include frequent medication review, simplified drug regimens, use of low doses and the provision of simple written and verbal instructions.

REVIEW EXERCISES

1. Discuss the factors that must be considered when evaluating the risk–benefit ratio of prescribing a drug for a pregnant woman.
2. Discuss the physiological changes during pregnancy that affect drug transfer to the fetus.
3. Explain why the body surface area nomogram may be used for calculating drug dosages in children.
4. As a health-care professional working with a geriatric population, name three or more interventions that could be used to prevent complications and improve drug therapy in this population.

REFERENCES AND FURTHER READING

Australian Drug Evaluation Committee. *Prescribing Medicines in Pregnancy*. 4th edn. Canberra: Government Publishing Service, 1999.

Australian Medicines Handbook 2006. Adelaide: AMH, 2006.

Barone MA. *The Harriet Lane Handbook*. 14th edn. St Louis: Mosby, 1996.

Beers MH, Ouslander JG, Rollingher I et al. Explicit criteria for determining inappropriate medication use in nursing home residents. *Archives of Internal Medicine* 1991; 151: 1825–32.

Chambers HF. Antimicrobial agents. Ch 47 in: Hardman JG, Limbird LE, Gilman AG (eds). *Goodman & Gilman's The Pharmacological Basis of Therapeutics*. 10th edn. New York: McGraw-Hill, 2001.

Food and Drug Administration. Recommendations of DES Task Force. *FDA Drug Bulletin 1985*; 15: 40–2.

Gow PJ, Ghabrial H, Smallwood RA et al. Neonatal hepatic drug elimination. *Pharmacology and Toxicology* 2001; 88: 3–15.

Hall WC, Talbert RL, Ereshefsky L. Cocaine abuse and its treatment. *Pharmacotherapy* 1990; 10: 47–65.

Higgins K, Cooper-Stanbury M, Williams P. *Statistics on Drug Use in Australia 1998*. Australian Institute of Health and Welfare cat. no. PHE 16. Canberra: AIHW (Drug Statistics Series), 2000.

Ito S. Drug therapy for breast-feeding women. *New England Journal of Medicine* 2000; 343: 118–26.

Jacqz-Aigrain E, Koren G. Effects of drugs on the fetus. *Seminars in Fetal & Neonatal Medicine* 2005; 10: 139–47.

Jennings JC. Guide to medication use in pregnant and breastfeeding women. *Pharmacy Practice News* 1996; 23: 10.

Jinks MJ, Fuerst RH. Geriatric drug use and rehabilitation. In: Young LY, Koda-Kimble MA (eds). *Applied Therapeutics: The Clinical Use of Drugs*. 6th edn. Vancouver: Applied Therapeutics, 1995.

Kapusnik-Uner JE, Sande MA, Chamber HF. Antimicrobial agents. In: Hardman JG, Limbird LE, Molinoff PB et al (eds). *Goodman & Gilman's The Pharmacological Basis of Therapeutics*. 9th edn. New York: McGraw-Hill, 1996.

Koren G, Pastuszak A, Ito S. Drugs in pregnancy. *New England Journal of Medicine* 1998; 338: 1128–37.

Levy M, Spino M. Neonatal withdrawal syndrome: associated drugs and pharmacologic management. *Pharmacotherapy* 1993; 13: 202–11.

Loose-Mitchell DS, Stancel GM. Estrogens and progestins. Ch. 58 in: Hardman JG, Limbird LE, Gilman AG (eds). *Goodman & Gilman's The Pharmacological Basis of Therapeutics*. 10th edn. New York: McGraw-Hill, 2001.

Lucas DS, Noyes MA, Stratton MA. Principles of geriatric pharmacotherapy. *Clinical Consult* 1995; 14: 1–8.

McCue JD, Tessier FG, Gaziano P. *Geriatric Drug Handbook for Long-Term Care*. Baltimore: Lippincott, Williams & Wilkins, 1992.

Pagliaro LA, Pagliaro AM (eds). *Problems in Pediatric Drug Therapy*. 4th edn. Washington: American Pharmaceutical Association, 2002.

Pillans PI, Roberts MS. How to optimise use of medications in the elderly. *Medicine Today* 2001; 2: 60–4.

Rubin P. Drug treatment during pregnancy. *British Medical Journal* 1998; 317: 1503–6.

Stephenson T. Medicines for children—the last century and the next. *Archives of Disease in Childhood* 2001; 85: 177–9.

Streissguth AP, Aase JM, Clarren SK, et al. Fetal alcohol syndrome in adolescents and adults. *Journal of the American Medical Association* 1991; 265: 1961–7.

Theis JGW, Koren G. Maternal and fetal clinical pharmacology. Ch. 2 in: Speight TM, Holford NHG (eds). *Avery's Drug Treatment*. 4th edn. Auckland: Adis International, 1997.

Trends & Analysis. Long-term care of elderly patients: chronic disease comorbidity and other considerations. *The Consultant Pharmacist* 1995; 10: 583.

Walson PD. Paediatric clinical pharmacology and therapeutics. Ch. 3 in: Speight TM, Holford NHG (eds). *Avery's Drug Treatment*. 4th edn. Auckland: Adis International, 1997.

Ward RM, Mirkin BL. Perinatal/neonatal pharmacology. Ch. 65 in: Brody TM, Larner J, Minneman KP (eds). *Human Pharmacology: Molecular-to-Clinical*. 3rd edn. St Louis: Mosby, 1998.

Willcox SM, Himmelstein DU, Woolhandler S. Inappropriate drug prescribing for the community-dwelling elderly. *Journal of the American Medical Association* 1994; 272: 292–6.

evolve   More weblinks at http://evolve.elsevier.com/AU/Bryant/pharmacology/

CHAPTER 9

Adverse Drug Reactions and Drug interactions

CHAPTER FOCUS

The use of medications to alleviate ailments and to combat diseases has been common for centuries. Along with the development of therapeutic remedies came knowledge of the poisonous qualities of the ingredients. In modern times this evolved into the concept of adverse drug reactions and knowledge that in some instances these are dose-related (type A adverse drug reactions) but under other circumstances are unpredictable (type B adverse drug reactions). With the increasing use of multiple drug therapies, drug interactions are now a cause for concern because a drug interaction may result in loss of efficacy (decreased effect) or the development of toxicity (enhanced effect). Many studies have confirmed that adverse drug reactions and drug interactions are major clinical problems, accounting for a significant number of hospital admissions, extended hospital stays and substantial costs to the health-care system. It is important that health-care professionals be aware of the adverse reaction and drug interaction profiles of drugs and be ever vigilant for the occurrence of adverse outcomes.

OBJECTIVES

- To discuss the current classification of adverse drug reactions and the subdivisions within the main categories.

- To illustrate, using examples of drugs, the different types of adverse drug reactions.

- To discuss the various risk factors for developing an adverse drug reaction.

- To discuss the four types of immunological responses to drugs or their metabolites.

- To discuss the clinical implications of drug interactions.

- To outline strategies for limiting adverse drug reactions and drug interactions.

KEY TERMS

adverse effect
adverse drug reaction
adverse drug event
drug interactions
type A adverse drug reaction
type B adverse drug reaction
type C adverse drug reaction
type D adverse drug reaction

KEY ABBREVIATIONS

ADR   adverse drug reaction
ADE   adverse drug event

HERBS and medicinal products have been used for treating ailments and diseases for centuries. Ebers Papyrus (1550 BC) lists more than 700 remedies and describes in detail the procedures for preparing and administering them. Some of the individuals treated would certainly have suffered an adverse reaction, especially with the use of lizard's blood, domestic animal excreta, tortoise bile, cat uterus, and perhaps with the more reasonable ingredients of castor oil, squill and opium.

The relationship between a remedy and a poison was entrenched in the early teachings of the Chinese and Mayans. People learnt to avoid medicinal substances that were poisonous. The ancient Greeks later described the concept of a medicine and a poison in scientific terms, and in 1758 William Withering described both the therapeutic benefits and the adverse effects of digitalis. Throughout the centuries, the use of medicinal products has gone hand in hand with reports of adverse reactions.

DEFINITIONS

An **adverse drug reaction (ADR)** has been defined as "any response to a drug which is noxious, unintended, and which occurs at doses normally (and appropriately) used in man for the prophylaxis, diagnosis, or therapy of disease" (World Health Organization 1984). This definition has been in use for the last 22 years and at various times has been modified slightly, because some have considered that the word 'noxious' is perhaps not correct in the context of the definition. An alternative definition has been proposed: "an appreciably harmful or unpleasant reaction, resulting from an intervention related to the use of a medicinal product, which predicts hazard from future administration and warrants prevention or specific treatment, or alteration of the dosage regimen, or withdrawal of the product" (Edwards & Aronson 2000). Clinical responses to an ADR include modifying the dose, discontinuing the drug, hospitalising the patient or providing supportive measures. This definition does not encompass the situations of drug overdose, drug withdrawal, drug abuse or error in administration. The latter is included within the definition of an adverse drug event.

An **adverse drug event (ADE)** is defined as an "injury resulting from medical intervention related to a drug" (Bates et al 1995): simply stated, an adverse event occurs while a person is taking a drug, but it is not necessarily 'due to the drug'. Examples of ADEs include under- or overmedication resulting from misuse or malfunction of infusion pumps or devices; aspiration pneumonia resulting from drug overdose; and errors in ordering, dispensing or administration. These incidents are usually investigated and may be attributed to simple mistakes such as picking up the wrong syringe, giving treatment to the wrong body site or giving the wrong treatment. Under WHO guidelines, these types of incidents are not classed as ADRs.

The term 'side-effect' is often used by health-care professionals and often appears in drug advertisements and consumer information. In general the reference is to a type A ADR, but the term is often interpreted by individuals to mean that the adverse reaction is insignificant (non-deleterious) or medically trivial and in general acceptable. These inferences are often wrong, and in an ideal world this term is best avoided! The term **'adverse effect'** is preferable, and generally relates to an unwanted effect that occurs via a different mechanism to the pharmacological effect and may or may not be dose-related. As an example, anaphylaxis with penicillin is both an adverse effect and an adverse drug reaction. The difference is that an adverse effect is "seen from the point of view of the drug, whereas an adverse reaction is seen from the point of view of the patient" (Edwards & Aronson 2000). Throughout the literature, however, despite a difference in their definitions, in the disciplines of pharmacology, pharmacy and clinical toxicology the terms adverse effect and adverse drug reaction are used interchangeably.

HISTORY OF ADVERSE DRUG REACTIONS

Public concern about ADRs arose in the late 19th century because of the number of sudden deaths associated with the use of chloroform. This led to the development of investigative committees such as the Food and Drug Administration (FDA) in the USA, which establishes the safety of new drugs before marketing. Despite regulatory frameworks, there have been many notable incidences of ADRs that have resulted in withdrawal of the offending drug (Table 9-1). Public interest in the safety of drugs has increased as a result of better communication between patients and health-care professionals.

INCIDENCE OF ADVERSE DRUG REACTIONS

During 2002/03 there were 174.4 million government-subsidised prescriptions and approximately 42 million non-subsidised prescriptions dispensed in Australia (Australian Institute of Health and Welfare 2004). The 1995 National Health Survey on medication use showed that as the proportion of people using medications grew with age, so did total medications. Most people under 44 years used only one type of medication, but this increased to three or more medications in people older than 85 (Australian Bureau of Statistics 2000). Taking multiple types of drugs contributes to the incidence

TABLE 9-1 Notable incidences of adverse drug reactions necessitating withdrawal of the drug

YEAR	DRUG	USE	ADVERSE DRUG REACTION
1922	Salvarsan	Treatment of syphilis	Liver damage
1937	Sulfanilamide	Elixir	Liver damage
1961	Thalidomide	Sedative	Congenital malformations
1982	Benoxaprofen	NSAID	Liver/kidney damage
1983	Zomepirac	NSAID	Anaphylaxis
1992	Temafloxacin	Antibiotic	Blood dyscrasias
1997	Dexfenfluramine	Anorectic	Pulmonary hypertension and cardiac valve disorders
1998	Terfenadine	Antihistamine	Ventricular arrhythmia
2000	Troglitazone	Hypoglycaemic	Liver damage
2004	Rofecoxib	COX-2 selective NSAID	Cardiovascular events

of ADRs. In addition to prescribed medications and those bought over the counter, Australians have embraced the use of complementary and alternative medicines. The trend has been the strongest with women, and includes the use of herbal medicines, aromatherapy oils and ginseng. In 2000 it was estimated that in Australia the average expenditure per person per year on alternative medicines was $315, or $1.67 billion for the whole of Australia (AIHW 2004).

ADRs occur in people of all ages and are twice as common in women. They are a major cause of morbidity and mortality, especially in the elderly. A survey conducted in a major New South Wales teaching hospital found that 30% of elderly patients were taking 6–10 types of medications and 13% took more than 10 types each day (Nair 1999). A review of Australian studies published over the period 1988–1996 found that 2.4%–3.6% of all hospital admissions were reported to be drug-related, and 6%–7% of emergency admissions, 12% of all admissions to medical wards and 15%–22% of all emergency admissions among the elderly were drug-related. Between 32% and 69% of drug-related admissions were reported as definitely or possibly preventable (Roughead et al 1998). The drugs most commonly implicated were antihypertensives, anticoagulants, cardiovascular drugs, cytotoxics and non-steroidal anti-inflammatory drugs (NSAIDs). Cytotoxic and anticoagulant agents were also the drugs most often involved in serious ADRs in general practice settings in France (Lacoste-Roussillon et al 2001).

Little attention has been paid to the incidence of ADRs in neonates, infants, children and adolescents. Before release of a new drug, few if any studies are undertaken in children because of questions of ethics, responsibility, cost and regulations. This often leads prescribers to estimate dosage and hence increases the risk of ADRs. A recent analysis of prospective paediatric studies from the UK, USA and Spain

reported that the incidence of ADRs in hospitalised children was 9.53%. The overall rate of hospital admissions due to ADRs was 2.09%, of which 39.3% involved life-threatening reactions. In the outpatient setting the overall incidence of ADRs in children was 1.46% (Impicciatore et al 2001). These data clearly show ADRs as a significant health issue in children.

CLASSIFICATION OF ADVERSE DRUG REACTIONS

The current classification system is not ideal, and not every ADR may fit perfectly into one of the categories. It is generally accepted that there are two main categories of ADR, type A (augmented) and type B (bizarre), and two subordinate categories, type C (continuous) and type D (delayed). Type D ADRs have been further subdivided into two classes: time-related reactions and withdrawal effects (type E). Unexpected failure of therapy has now been proposed as a sixth category (type F).

Type A (augmented) ADRs are characterised by:
- predictability from the known pharmacology of the drug (often an exaggeration of effect)
- relationship to dose
- common occurrence (about 80% of ADRs)
- usually mild
- high morbidity and low mortality
- reproducibility in animals.

Factors predisposing to type A reactions include the dose, pharmaceutical variation in drug formulation, pharmacokinetic variation (e.g. renal failure), pharmacodynamic variation (e.g. altered fluid and electrolyte balance) and drug–drug interactions (e.g. inhibition of metabolism of one drug by another concomitantly administered drug). Examples include:

- sedation with the use of antihistamines
- bleeding with anticoagulants
- hypoglycaemia from the use of insulin
- hypokalaemia with the use of diuretics.

Type B (bizarre) ADRs are characterised by:
- unpredictability
- no relationship to dose
- uncommon occurrence (about 20% of ADRs)
- increased severity
- high morbidity and high mortality
- lack of reproducibility in animals.

These reactions are less common but often cause death. Factors contributing to type B reactions include pharmaceutical variation, receptor abnormalities, unmasking of a biological deficiency (e.g. glucose-6-phosphate dehydrogenase deficiency), abnormalities in drug metabolism (e.g. slow acetylators of the antituberculosis drug isoniazid), drug allergy (see next section) and drug–drug interactions (e.g. rare incidence of hepatitis) (Pirmohamed et al 1998). Examples include interstitial nephritis with the use of NSAIDs and eosinophilia with the use of anticonvulsants such as carbamazepine and phenytoin.

Type C (continuous) ADRs are characterised by occurrence as a consequence of long-term use. Examples of reactions in this category include:
- adaptive changes (e.g. development of drug tolerance and physical dependence)
- appearance of tardive dyskinesia in persons treated long-term with neuroleptic drugs for schizophrenia
- rebound phenomena (e.g. rebound tachycardia after the abrupt discontinuation of β-blockers and acute adrenal insufficiency after abrupt withdrawal of corticosteroids).

Type D (delayed) ADRs are characterised by the appearance of delayed effects. These may be acceptable if the benefit of drug therapy outweighs the risk, as in the case of irreversible infertility in young persons receiving cytotoxic drugs for malignancies. In general, however, they are considered unacceptable. Examples include carcinogenesis (e.g. the association of lymphoma with immunosuppressive drugs) and teratogenesis.

Type E ADRs are fortunately uncommon and are related to withdrawal of a drug. They include opiate withdrawal syndrome and myocardial ischaemia after abrupt cessation of β-blockers.

Type F ADRs, classed as unexpected failure of therapy, are increasingly common and are often caused by a drug interaction, e.g. inadequate dose of the oral contraceptive when a drug that induces the metabolism of oestrogen is administered concomitantly.

Drug allergy

A drug allergy, or hypersensitivity, is a type B ADR. Drug allergies are characterised by:

- occurrence in a small number of individuals
- the requirement for previous exposure to either the same or a chemically related drug
- the rapid development of an allergic reaction after re-exposure
- the production of clinical manifestations of an allergic reaction (deShazo & Kemp 1997).

The diagnosis of a drug allergy is often difficult to establish because there are no reliable laboratory tests that can identify the relevant drug, and in some cases the symptoms can imitate infectious disease symptoms. The situation may be easier if the drug administered is notorious for producing an allergic reaction (e.g. penicillin), but it is difficult if the drug used is seldom reported to produce an allergic reaction. Some drugs can produce a pseudoallergic reaction, i.e. one resembling an allergic reaction but for which there is no immunological basis. An example of a pseudoallergic reaction is the release of histamine by opioids.

Allergic reactions to drugs generally follow the Type I–IV classification (see Chapter 54). Table 9-2 lists the types of reactions, the main clinical manifestation and examples of drugs commonly implicated.

RISK FACTORS FOR DEVELOPING AN ADVERSE DRUG REACTION

Risk factors for ADRs are specific to both the person and the drug.

Factors relating to the person include:
- age: the elderly and neonates have a higher incidence
- gender: women appear to be more susceptible
- concurrent disease: an association between viral infections, drug use and skin reactions has been described
- genetic factors: deficiency of an enzyme involved in the metabolism of a drug may increase the risk of an ADR
- history of prior drug reaction: some individuals appear to be more susceptible to allergic drug reactions, including people with a history of atopic disease (e.g. asthma, hay fever, eczema).

Factors specific to the drug include:
- chemical characteristics: large molecules such as heparin can themselves be immunogenic, and smaller drug molecules or their metabolites can combine with body proteins to form antigens that elicit an allergic response

TABLE 9-2 Allergic drug reactions

TYPE/REACTION	CLINICAL MANIFESTATIONS	EXAMPLES OF DRUGS
I Immediate hypersensitivity	Urticaria, anaphylaxis, angio-oedema, bronchospasm	Penicillins, streptomycin, local anaesthestics, neuromuscular blocking drugs, radiological contrast media
II Antibody-dependent cytotoxic	Cytopenia, vasculitis, haemolytic anaemia	Quinine, quinidine, rifampicin, metronidazole
III Complex-mediated	Serum sickness, vasculitis, interstitial nephritis	Anticonvulsants, antibiotics, hydralazine, diuretics
IV Cell-mediated or delayed hypersensitivity	Contact sensitivity	Local anaesthetic creams, antihistamine creams

- route of drug administration: topical and oral routes generally involve a lower incidence of drug allergy; topical application tends to cause a delayed hypersensitivity reaction
- dose: many ADRs are dose-related
- duration and frequency: prolonged and frequent therapy can increase the likelihood of an ADR.

The role of genetics in predisposing individuals to ADRs has been known since the late 1950s through the discovery of enzyme deficiencies such as pseudocholinesterase and the link to succinylcholine apnoea. With increased understanding of the human genome, we are moving slowly towards an era of pharmacogenetics and the prescribing of medications tailored to individual genotypes. However, genotyping would remove only one of the factors contributing to the risk of ADRs, leaving age, a history of atopy, polypharmacy and inappropriate prescribing to deal with.

DRUG–DRUG INTERACTIONS

A drug–drug interaction (commonly shortened to '**drug interaction**') occurs when the intensity of a drug's pharmacological effect is altered by another drug: that is, the effect(s) of a drug are increased or decreased by the concurrent or previous administration of another. Drug interactions are a concern because they may result in loss of efficacy (diminished effect) or the development of toxicity (enhanced effect). Moreover, drug interactions often are unanticipated or go unrecognised.

Frequency of drug interactions

The exact frequency of drug interactions is unknown, although anecdotal evidence suggests that they are relatively common

and result in a significant number of hospital admissions. The possibility of a drug interaction exists whenever two or more medications are prescribed to an individual, and the likelihood of an interaction will grow as the number of medications used increases. Individuals at greatest risk of a drug interaction are:

- the severely ill, who typically receive multiple drugs
- individuals receiving chronic therapy, often comprising a cocktail of drugs (e.g. in the treatment of either HIV infection or cancer)
- the elderly, who tend to have multiple pathologies and often receive multiple drugs concurrently.

Drug interactions are of greatest concern with drugs that have a narrow therapeutic index. Even a small change in the concentration of the drug available at the target site (e.g. receptor, enzyme) can lead to a major alteration in response. For example:

- enhanced anticoagulation (bleeding) with warfarin resulting from concomitant use of the antiarrhythmic drug amiodarone, which inhibits the metabolism of warfarin
- bradycardia with digoxin resulting from concomitant administration of the antiarrhythmic drug quinidine, which decreases renal or biliary excretion of digoxin.

Interactions involving drugs with a wide therapeutic index (e.g. penicillin antibiotics, β-adrenoceptor antagonists) cause fewer problems. Knowledge of the mechanisms of drug interactions is essential to enable health professionals to prevent interactions occurring (wherever possible) and to systematically analyse potentially new drug interactions. Indeed, analysis of known and potential interactions is critical in the planning of a therapeutic regimen.

Although drug interactions may have deleterious effects, they may also be used to advantage. For example, antimicrobial drugs with different mechanisms of action are commonly used in combination for increased effectiveness in treating bacterial infections. Similarly, combinations of drugs are commonly used in cancer chemotherapy and in the treatment of tuberculosis.

Classification of drug interactions

Drug interactions are broadly classified, according to their pharmacological mechanism, into either pharmacodynamic or pharmacokinetic interactions.

Pharmacodynamic drug interactions

Pharmacodynamic drug interactions may be 'direct' or 'indirect'. *Direct* pharmacodynamic interactions involve effects at a common target, additively (and possibly potentiation) or antagonism due to actions at different sites in an organ. An example of antagonism at a common receptor site is the concurrent use of a β_2-adrenoceptor agonist (used in the treatment of asthma; e.g. salbutamol) and a non-selective β-adrenoceptor antagonist (used in the treatment of hypertension; e.g. propranolol). Both these drugs have opposing effects at the same receptor (i.e. the β_2-adrenoceptor). Unintentional interactions of this type should not occur because they are so obvious!

Examples of direct pharmacodynamic interactions involving drugs with different mechanisms of action include the following:
- Monoamine oxidase (MAO) inhibitors, which are used in the treatment of depression and which increase the amount of noradrenaline stored in nerve terminals, interact dangerously (to cause marked hypertension) with 'sympathomimetic' drugs such as ephedrine that cause the release of stored noradrenaline. The tyramine present in foods such as cheese, yeast extracts and Chianti-type wines produces a similar response in patients treated with MAO inhibitors.
- Warfarin causes anticoagulation by inhibition of the vitamin K-mediated synthesis of clotting factors. The risk of bleeding is increased by coadministration of aspirin, which decreases platelet aggregation by inhibiting the biosynthesis of thromboxane A_2.
- Combinations of CNS depressants enhance drowsiness, even when they act at different sites within the CNS, e.g. combinations of alcohol (ethanol), 'sedating' histamine-1-receptor antagonists (antihistamines), benzodiazepine hypnosedatives/anxiolytics, tricyclic antidepressants, and antipsychotic drugs.

An *indirect* pharmacodynamic interaction occurs when the pharmacological effects of one drug alter the response to another drug, even though the two effects are not themselves directly related. Common examples include the following:
- Certain diuretics (e.g. frusemide or hydrochlorothiazide) lower the blood potassium concentration. This will enhance the toxic effects of the cardiac glycoside digoxin, which is used in the treatment of atrial fibrillation and cardiac failure, and of type III antiarrhythmic drugs (e.g. amiodarone) that prolong the cardiac action potential.
- Apart from reducing renal blood flow, non-steroidal anti-inflammatory drugs promote the retention of salt and water by reducing prostaglandin-mediated effects on the action of antidiuretic hormone and the reabsorption of chloride ions. This, in turn, may reduce the effectiveness of antihypertensive drugs.

Pharmacokinetic drug interactions

The plasma concentration of a drug may be altered by interactions occurring during absorption, distribution, metabolism and excretion:
- **Absorption.** Absorption interactions involve a change in either the rate or the extent of absorption. Drugs that change the rate of gastric emptying (i.e. the time it takes for the contents of the stomach to empty into the small bowel) will alter the rate of absorption of coadministered drugs. Muscarinic receptor antagonists (e.g. hyoscine) delay gastric emptying and gastrointestinal motility. This combination of effects delays drug absorption from the gastrointestinal tract. Many drugs, including tricyclic antidepressants and histamine-1-receptor antagonists that possess antimuscarinic properties (sometimes referred to as 'anticholinergic adverse effects') delay the absorption of coadministered drugs. Gastric emptying rate is slowed by opioid drugs, including morphine and pethidine, and hence the time to peak plasma concentration is generally increased for a drug coadministered with an opioid. Coadministered drugs may also decrease the extent of drug absorption. Whereas changes in the rate of absorption generally affect only the time for onset of action, changes in extent of absorption can alter response. For example, cholestyramine is a bile acid-binding resin used in the treatment of hypercholesterolaemia. Unfortunately, cholestyramine also binds other drugs, reducing the amount of drug that is absorbed. As cholestyramine reduces the absorption of corticosteroids, digoxin, thyroxine and warfarin (and probably other drugs), these drugs should be administered either several hours before or after the cholestyramine dose.
- **Distribution.** As many drugs circulate in the blood bound (at least in part) to the proteins albumin and α_1-acid glycoprotein, they may compete for the same binding sites. Displacement from plasma protein of one drug by another is common, and this leads to an increase in the unbound, pharmacologically active, concentration of the drug in the blood. Although it is still widely believed that the increase in unbound concentration arising from 'displacement interactions' may precipitate drug toxicity, this is rarely the case. Following a drug displacement interaction, the concentration of unbound drug in blood does indeed increase. However, the unbound drug is available for distribution into tissues, leading to an increase in the volume of distribution, and for clearance

by glomerular filtration and/or metabolism. There is, however, a decrease in total drug concentration (i.e. bound plus unbound drug) because of the higher clearance.

- **Metabolism.** As discussed in Chapter 6, administration of some drugs can lead to decreased (inhibited) or increased (induced) activity of drug-metabolising enzymes such as cytochrome P450 (CYP). Many important drug interactions arise from altered metabolism, and the clinical importance of the interaction will depend on the change in clearance and the therapeutic index of the altered drug. A 10% change in clearance is unlikely to be important, but a 30% change in the clearance of a narrow-therapeutic-index drug like warfarin can have serious implications. Importantly, just as there is considerable interindividual variability in the clearance of metabolised drugs, there is significant variability in the magnitude of the change in clearance associated with any metabolic drug interaction.

  Induction results in increased enzyme activity and drug metabolism, hence the steady-state blood concentration will decrease with the possibility of therapeutic failure. Drugs known to cause induction are generally non-selective in their effects on CYP isoforms. Examples include:
  - the antituberculosis drug rifampicin, which appears to induce all CYP- and UDP-glucuronosyltransferase (UGT) isoforms, therefore potentially decreasing the blood concentration of all coadministered drugs that are metabolised by these enzymes
  - the anticonvulsant drugs phenobarbitone, phenytoin and carbamazepine, which induce CYP2C9 and CYP3A4, and possibly other isoforms of CYP and UGT. Epileptic patients receiving these drugs are prone to drug interactions and their consequences (e.g. unwanted pregnancy due to enhanced metabolism of oral contraceptive steroids)
  - chronic consumption of ethanol (alcohol), which induces CYP2E1, although there are relatively few clinically used drugs that are metabolised by this isoform.

  Inhibitory drug interactions are relatively common, and inhibition of metabolism increases steady-state blood concentration and the likelihood of drug toxicity. Some drugs, notably cimetidine, inhibit the activity of most CYP isoforms (although UGT is unaffected). Conversely, probenecid inhibits most UGT isoforms (without affecting CYP). Most inhibitory interactions are relatively selective for one or a limited number of isoforms, as they most commonly arise from competition for metabolism at the enzyme active site. It is generally not correct to refer to a drug as 'an inhibitor of drug metabolism'. Rather, a drug will normally selectively inhibit the metabolism of other drugs for a limited number of isoforms, and this specificity of interactions is used to predict and

interpret metabolic drug interactions. Some selective inhibitors of CYP isoforms are shown in Table 9-3. As an example, fluoxetine causes interactions with many drugs metabolised by CYP2D6 (e.g. other antidepressants, perhexiline), which generally requires a reduction of the dose. The clearances of drugs metabolised by CYP3A4 are similarly decreased by the commonly used antibiotic erythromycin, again generally requiring a dose reduction.

Metabolic drug interactions also occur with other drug-metabolising enzymes. Probenecid is a 'universal' inhibitor of drug glucuronidation, and there is evidence to suggest that rifampicin, phenobarbitone, phenytoin and carbamazepine may induce numerous UGT isoforms. For example, fluconazole appears to inhibit only UGT2B7 (which metabolises morphine and zidovudine). In the case of morphine, a rise in the plasma concentration may result in respiratory depression.

A potentially fatal interaction occurs when azathioprine and allopurinol are coadministered. Allopurinol is an inhibitor of the enzyme xanthine oxidase, and is used in the treatment of gout and gouty arthritis. Azathioprine (used mainly in the treatment of cancer) is converted to an active metabolite, 6-mercaptopurine, which is subsequently cleared by xanthine oxidase. Coadministration of azathioprine and allopurinol leads to accumulation of 6-mercaptopurine, resulting in potentially life-threatening bone marrow suppression.

- **Excretion.** Interactions may occur between drugs that are excreted by active transport systems in the kidney. The mechanism of such interactions is simply 'competition' for the same transporter. For example, the renal clearance of methotrexate is impaired by coadministration of probenecid or salicylates (and possibly other NSAIDs).

TABLE 9-3 Drug inhibitors of cytochrome P450 isoforms

CYP ISOFORM	INHIBITORS
CYP1A2	Fluvoxamine, propranolol
CYP2C8	Gemfibrozil, trimethoprim
CYP2C9	Amiodarone, fluconazole, gemfibrozil, sulfonamide antibiotics
CYP2C19	Fluvoxamine, moclobemide
CYP2D6	Fluoxetine, paroxetine, perphenazine, quinidine, quinine, thioridazine
CYP3A4	Clarithromycin, diltiazem, erythromycin, indinavir, itraconazole, ketoconazole, nelfinavir, ritonavir, roxithromycin, verapamil

Metabolic drug interactions involving nutrients and herbal medicines

Although there is wide appreciation of drug interactions, interactions between nutrients and/or food components and herbal remedies are often not considered and, in fact, may be discounted. Chemicals present in food may alter the activity of drug-metabolising enzymes. Notable in this regard are chemicals present in grapefruit (but not orange) juice that inhibit the activity of CYP3A4 present in the gastrointestinal tract. (CYP3A4 is localised in both liver and small bowel.) The enzyme present in the small bowel appears to contribute significantly to the first-pass metabolism of numerous CYP3A4 substrates. Thus, the bioavailability of a number of drugs, such as cyclosporin, felodipine, midazolam, triazolam and verapamil, increases significantly when they are taken with grapefruit juice, which enhances the potential for toxicity.

Currently there is intense interest in the effects of herbal medicines on drug metabolism and the consequences of herb–drug interactions. Herbal medicines are used widely, given the perception that 'natural' products are a safe and effective alternative to pharmaceuticals. As plant products, herbal medicines typically contain hundreds of different chemicals, it is not surprising that some of these will alter the activity of drug-metabolising enzymes. In the USA the seven top-selling herbal medicines in descending order are *Ginkgo biloba*, St John's wort, ginseng, kava, saw palmetto, garlic and echinacea (Bressler 2005).

Important in terms of drug interaction is St John's wort, which is taken to treat the symptoms of depression. St John's wort contains chemicals called hyperforins, which mimic the effects of rifampicin as an inducer of CYP isoforms. Thus the clearances of amitriptyline, carbamazepine, cyclosporin, HIV protease inhibitors, warfarin and several other drugs have been shown to be increased in subjects taking St John's wort, with risk of therapeutic failure. Furthermore, unwanted pregnancy has been reported as a problem in women who use oral contraceptive steroids and St John's wort. There is evidence to suggest that other herbal products may interact (pharmacodynamically or pharmacokinetically) with 'pharmaceutical' drugs, and studies are investigating the mechanisms involved and quantifying the magnitudes of any interactions.

Interactions between herbal medicines and conventional drugs are no longer just a theoretical possibility, and it is likely that their incidence is more common than anticipated initially. It is essential that a patient's exposure to herbal medicines be determined when assessing the potential for drug interactions (refer to Appendix 3).

STRATEGIES FOR LIMITING ADVERSE DRUG REACTIONS AND DRUG INTERACTIONS

Hospital admissions for ADRs are a significant and expensive health problem worldwide. The evidence from numerous studies indicates that ADRs may be impossible to avoid completely, but given the high predictability of many ADRs, there is significant room for improvement in reducing the incidence of ADRs. Strategies for limiting ADRs include:

- careful history-taking, including drug allergies, types of allergies, and use of prescribed, over-the-counter and alternative medications
- considering non-drug treatment
- correct and appropriate dosing using the lowest effective dose
- frequent review of therapeutic goals and drug regimens
- being familiar with potential ADRs of a drug to avoid misinterpretation of an ADR as a symptom of a new medical condition
- avoiding polypharmacy and keeping the drug regimen simple

**CLINICAL INTEREST BOX 9-1
CENTRE FOR ADVERSE REACTIONS MONITORING (CARM)**

Pharmaco-vigilance activities in New Zealand include the reporting of adverse drug reactions. Based in Dunedin, the Centre for Adverse Reactions Monitoring (CARM) collects and evaluates adverse reaction reports from health professionals. These are reported for medicines, herbal products and dietary supplements, and are held in a database of over 50,000 reports. Individual patients who suffer from life threatening adverse reactions have CARM warnings or danger alerts recorded against their National Health Index (NHI) numbers; the information is accessible through hospital systems and contributes to the safe use of medicines.

Anonymised data from various pharmaco-vigilance sources in New Zealand are fed into the database of the World Health Organisation's International Drug Monitoring Programme based in Uppsala, Sweden. CARM also provides feedback to the Medicines Adverse Reactions Committee which in turn makes recommendations to Medsafe, the regulatory medicines authority in New Zealand.
Adapted from: http://carm.otago.ac.nz/CARM.asp, accessed 17 January 2006.

- careful communication with the patient and/or carer to inform them of the risks and benefits of the proposed treatment and the need for adherence to the recommended dosing schedule.

There is an overwhelming amount of information published on drug interactions, and sources such as the *Australian Medicines Handbook* and the website of Professor D Flockhart, School of Medicine, Indiana University (http://medicine. iupui.edu/flockhart), are excellent. Continued education of health professionals is essential, as new drugs enter the marketplace on an annual basis. Specific strategies for limiting drug interactions (in addition to those listed above) include:

- avoiding the combination entirely
- spacing the dosing time to avoid the interaction
- close laboratory or clinical monitoring for early evidence of the interaction
- improving patient education on drug interactions.

KEY POINTS

- An adverse drug reaction is defined as any response to a drug that is noxious and unintended, and that occurs at doses normally (and appropriately) used for the prophylaxis, diagnosis or therapy of disease.
- Public interest in the safety of drugs has increased as a result of better communication between patients and health-care professionals.
- Taking multiple drugs contributes to the incidence of ADRs.
- Adverse drug reactions occur in people of all ages and are twice as common in women. They are a major cause of morbidity and mortality, especially in the elderly.
- There are two main categories of adverse drug reactions, type A (predictable) and type B (unpredictable), and two subordinate categories, type C (a consequence of long-term use) and type D (delayed reactions).
- The type B adverse drug reactions include immunological reactions such as drug allergy and hypersensitivity.
- The diagnosis of a drug allergy can often be difficult to establish because there are no reliable laboratory tests that can identify the relevant drug, and the symptoms can sometimes imitate infectious disease symptoms (e.g. fever).
- Risk factors for developing an ADR include age, gender, presence of concurrent disease, genetics, a history of prior drug reaction, the drug dose, and the duration and frequency of drug use.
- Drug interactions are broadly classified according to their pharmacological mechanisms: that is, pharmacodynamic or pharmacokinetic.
- Pharmacodynamic drug interactions may be 'direct' or 'indirect'.
- Direct pharmacodynamic interactions involve effects at a common target, or additively (and possibly potentiation) or antagonism due to actions at different sites in an organ.
- A pharmacodynamic interaction occurs when the pharmacological effects of one drug alter the response to another drug, even though the two types of effects are not themselves directly related.
- A pharmacokinetic drug interaction can alter the concentration of drug in the systemic circulation through interactions occurring at any stage: that is, during absorption, distribution, metabolism or excretion.
- Strategies for reducing the incidence of ADRs and drug interactions include careful history-taking, considering non-drug treatment, correct and appropriate dosing, frequent review of therapeutic goals and drug regimens, avoiding polypharmacy, and careful communication with the patient or carer.

REVIEW EXERCISES

1. What is the definition of an adverse drug reaction?
2. Discuss the four categories of adverse drug reactions and provide examples of drugs implicated.
3. Discuss the mechanistic bases of the four types of drug allergies.
4. Discuss the clinical implications of an inhibitory drug interaction involving a drug with a narrow therapeutic index.

REFERENCES AND FURTHER READING

Australian Bureau of Statistics. *Year Book Australia 2000*. No. 82, Canberra: ABS, 2000.

Australian Institute of Health and Welfare. *Australia's Health 2004*. Canberra: AIHW, 2004.

Bates DW, Cullen DJ, Laird N, Petersen LA, Small SD et al. Incidence of adverse drug events and potential adverse drug events: implications for prevention. *Journal of the American Medical Association* 1995; 274: 29–34.

Bressler R. Herb–drug interactions: interactions between kava and prescription medications. *Geriatrics* 2005; 60: 24–5.

deShazo RD, Kemp SF. Allergic reactions to drugs and biologic agents. *Journal of the American Medical Association* 1997; 278: 1895–906.

Edwards IR, Aronson JK. Adverse drug reactions: definitions, diagnosis, and management. *Lancet* 2000; 356: 1255–9.

Grahame-Smith DG, Aronson JK. Adverse reactions to drugs. In: Grahame-Smith DG, Aronson JK (eds). *Oxford Textbook of Clinical Pharmacology and Drug Therapy*. 2nd edn. Oxford: Oxford University Press, 1992 [ch. 9].

Hansten PD. Drug interaction management. *Pharmacy World Science* 2003; 25: 94–7.

Impicciatore P, Choonara I, Clarkson A, Provasi D, Pandolfini C, Bonati M. Incidence of adverse drug reactions in paediatric in/out-patients: a systematic review and meta-analysis of prospective studies. *British Journal of Clinical Pharmacology* 2001; 52: 77–83.

Lacoste-Roussillon C, Pouyanne P, Haramburu F, Miremont G, Begaud B. Incidence of serious adverse drug reactions in general practice: a prospective study. *Clinical Pharmacology and Therapeutics* 2001; 69: 458–62.

Nair B. Older people and medications: what is the right prescription? [editorial]. *Australian Prescriber* 1999; 22: 130–1.

Pirmohamed M, Breckenridge AM, Kitteringham NR, Park BK. Adverse drug reactions. *British Medical Journal* 1998; 316: 1295–8.

Roughead EE, Gilbert AL, Primrose JG, Sansom LN. Drug-related hospital admissions: a review of Australian studies published 1988–1996. *Medical Journal of Australia* 1998, 168(8): 405–8.

World Health Organization. Collaborating Centers for International Drug Monitoring. Geneva: WHO, 1984 (WHO publication DEM/NC/84:153 (E)).

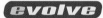 More weblinks at http://evolve.elsevier.com/AU/Bryant/pharmacology/

CHAPTER 10

Overview of the Autonomic Nervous System

CHAPTER FOCUS

The peripheral nervous system is subdivided functionally and anatomically into two divisions: the autonomic nervous system and the somatic nervous system (Chapter 13). The autonomic nervous system, which comprises the parasympathetic, sympathetic and enteric nervous systems, is responsible for regulation of the internal viscera such as the heart, blood vessels, digestive organs, kidneys and reproductive organs. An understanding of the peripheral nervous system and in particular the autonomic nervous system is central to understanding the actions of many major drug groups that either mimic or block the actions of autonomic neurotransmitter chemicals.

OBJECTIVES

- To describe the major physiological and anatomical differences between the parasympathetic and sympathetic divisions of the autonomic nervous system.

- To describe the sequence of events that culminates in the generation of a nerve action potential.

- To explain the process of neurochemical transmission.

- To identify the different types of receptors in the autonomic nervous system and their respective neurotransmitters.

- To describe the synthesis, function and inactivation of the primary neurotransmitters acetylcholine and noradrenaline.

KEY TERMS

acetylcholine
acetylcholinesterase
action potential
adrenaline
adrenergic neuron
alpha (α)-adrenoceptors
autonomic ganglion
autonomic nervous system
autonomic (visceral) reflexes
beta (β)-adrenoceptors
catecholamine
dopamine
cholinergic neuron
enteric nervous system
exocytosis
homeostasis
muscarinic receptor
neurochemical transmission
neuroeffector junction
neuron
neurotransmitter
nicotinic receptor
noradrenaline
parasympathetic nervous system
sympathetic nervous system
synapse

KEY ABBREVIATIONS

A	adrenaline
ACh	acetylcholine
AChE	acetylcholinesterase
ANS	autonomic nervous system
CNS	central nervous system
COMT	catechol-O-methyltransferase
DA	dopamine
DOPA	dihydroxyphenylalanine
M	muscarinic
MAO	monoamine oxidase
N	nicotinic
NA	noradrenaline
PNMT	phenylethanolamine-N-methyltransferase
PNS	peripheral nervous system

THE two principal divisions of the nervous system are the central nervous system (CNS) and the peripheral nervous system (PNS). The CNS consists of the brain and the spinal cord, which together integrate and correlate the vast array of incoming sensory information and generate the appropriate response signals for propagation to the periphery. The CNS is connected to the peripheral parts of the body by the PNS, which consists of the cranial nerves and the spinal nerves and their branches. The PNS is divided further on a functional and anatomical basis into two subdivisions: the autonomic and the somatic nervous systems. The afferent (incoming) fibres of both systems carry sensory information to the CNS, which is integrated at various levels within the brain. The information that flows out from the CNS is conducted along efferent (outgoing motor) neurons of either the autonomic efferent system or the somatic efferent system. These systems innervate various organs and tissues (commonly called effectors) that produce a physiological response when stimulated by the appropriate nerves (Figure 10-1). Innervation of skeletal muscle is principally coordinated by the somatic nervous system, discussed in Chapter 13.

The **autonomic nervous system** (**ANS**) primarily maintains the internal environment of the body at an optimal level (**homeostasis**) and cannot function independently of the CNS. The activities regulated by the ANS are not under direct conscious control and include the contraction and relaxation of smooth muscle, regulation of heartbeat, and glandular secretions (Figure 10-2). All of these processes interact in many vital physiological tasks. Digesting a meal and maintaining blood pressure are examples of processes internally regulated by the ANS. The simplest means by which these types of activities are adjusted are **autonomic (visceral) reflexes**.

The first component of the reflex arc is the receptor, which detects changes such as a rise or fall in temperature or in pressure in blood vessels, or distension in the viscera. These changes are responsible for producing a stimulus in the receptor. Information from the sensitised receptor is then transmitted via a sensory (afferent) neuron to the CNS, the site of integration. The preganglionic, autonomic efferent (motor) neuron then conveys nerve impulses from the CNS to ganglia and onwards to the effector, which produces the appropriate alteration of activity of muscles and glands.

The information carried to the CNS (sensory input) and instructions sent from the CNS (motor output) constitute a feedback control mechanism. Information fed back to the CNS from a receptor is modulated so that nerve impulses may vary in frequency and pattern according to the degree of activity required of the effector. The control of visceral function is involuntary, so the feedback mechanism must include all the components of a control system essential to performing the reflex act, the sole purpose of which is to prevent extreme changes in function that may create a disturbance in the internal environment.

Several centres in the CNS integrate all ANS activities. There is evidence that the hypothalamus, in particular, performs such integrating activities. It contains centres that regulate body temperature, water balance, carbohydrate and fat metabolism, and also integrates information concerned with emotional behaviour, the waking state and sleep. The medulla oblongata integrates the control of blood pressure, respiration and cardiac function; a series of 'vital centres', including the vasomotor centre, respiratory centre and cardiac centre, respectively, coordinate these activities. The midbrain, limbic system, cerebellum and cerebral cortex are all involved in the control of physiological functions regulated by the ANS. An understanding of autonomic reflexes is integral to appreciating the actions of autonomic drugs, especially those that evoke significant compensatory 'reflex' responses.

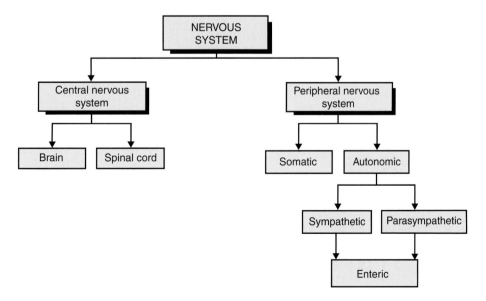

FIGURE 10-1 Divisions of the nervous system.

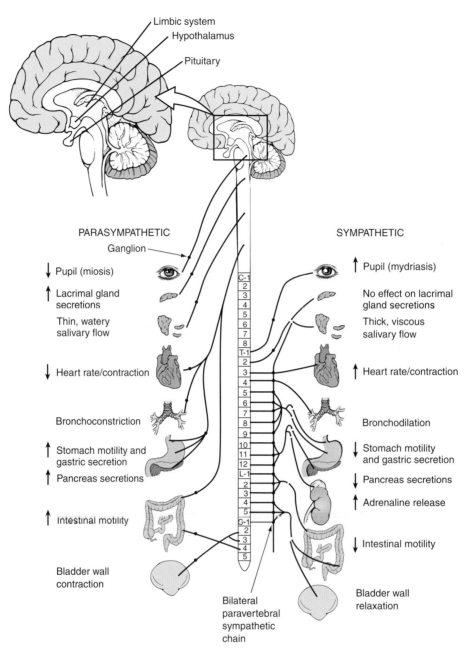

FIGURE 10-2 A schematic diagram of the autonomic nervous system.

DIFFERENCES BETWEEN THE PARASYMPATHETIC AND SYMPATHETIC NERVOUS SYSTEMS

The ANS is organised into three subdivisions (Figure 10-1):
- the **parasympathetic nervous system**
- the **sympathetic nervous system**
- the **enteric nervous system**.

Most organs receive dual innervation from the parasympathetic and sympathetic systems. In many instances the systems produce opposite effects but they may also produce the same effect, e.g. in salivary glands stimulation from both systems produces secretion. The noticeable exceptions are the lacrimal (tear) glands of the eye, and bronchial smooth muscle, which receive only parasympathetic fibres, and, in contrast, the arrector pili muscles attached to hair follicles in the skin, adipocytes (fat cells), kidneys and blood vessels, which are innervated solely by sympathetic fibres. The opposing actions of the two systems balance one another; for example, a rise in parasympathetic activity is accompanied by a fall in sympathetic input (Table 10-1).

Physiological differences

The parasympathetic system functions mainly to conserve energy and restore body resources. This includes reducing heart rate, increasing gastrointestinal activity and secretion of digestive enzymes associated with increased digestion and absorption. In contrast, the sympathetic system dominates the body during emergency and stress situations and is often called the 'fight-or-flight' system. The sympathetic response to physical or emotional stress involves expenditure of energy and includes an increase in the blood sugar concentration, heart activity and blood pressure (Table 10-1). The concept of these two extreme situations (rest and flight) in humans is outdated, as in everyday life the ANS functions continually and the balance of sympathetic and parasympathetic control depends on the needs of a particular organ at any given time.

Unlike the parasympathetic and sympathetic systems, the enteric nervous system consists of a collection of neural plexuses (networks) in the walls of the gastrointestinal tract that can function independently of the CNS. Incoming nerves from the parasympathetic and sympathetic systems serve primarily to modulate the intrinsic activity of the enteric neural network, which controls motility, secretion and the microcirculation of the gastrointestinal tract.

Anatomical differences

The parasympathetic and sympathetic efferent pathways consist of two **neurons** (nerve cells) and an **autonomic ganglion**, which is a collection of neuronal cell bodies. The first neuron is known as the preganglionic neuron and extends from the cell body in the CNS to the autonomic ganglion. The second neuron is called the postganglionic neuron and extends from the autonomic ganglion to the effector organ, gland or cell. The parasympathetic preganglionic fibres emerge with the cranial nerves (III, VII, IX and X) and at the sacral spinal levels from about S2 through S4 (Figure 10-2). The 10th cranial nerve (X), or vagus nerve, has extensive branches that supply fibres to the heart, lungs and almost all the abdominal organs. The parasympathetic ganglia are located close to the effectors that produce the physiological response, and consequently the preganglionic axon tends to be long (Figure 10-2).

The sympathetic system is also called the thoracolumbar system because its preganglionic fibres originate in the spinal cord from thoracic segment T1 to the lumbar segment at L2 level (Figure 10-2). The sympathetic ganglia lie on either side of the vertebral column in two chains, called the paravertebral sympathetic chains; hence the sympathetic preganglionic neurons tend to be short (Figure 10-2). The only exception

to the two-neuron arrangement is the adrenal medulla, which is supplied directly by a preganglionic neuron. The major characteristics that differentiate the parasympathetic and sympathetic nervous systems are summarised in Table 10-2.

ACTION POTENTIAL GENERATION AND NEUROCHEMICAL TRANSMISSION
Neurons

Communication throughout the nervous system occurs through a highly integrated network of neurons and neuroglia (support cells). Neurons are the cells that transmit electrical impulses (also called action potentials), and they have three basic parts (Figure 10-3):

- **the cell body**, which contains a nucleus (genetic information), cytoplasm and other common organelles such as mitochondria and lysosomes, and Nissl bodies, which are clumps of rough endoplasmic reticulum. The synthesis of new proteins for the various components of the cell body, and for growth and repair of neurons, is carried out in the Nissl bodies. Most neuron cell bodies are located within the brain and spinal cord, where they are protected by the bones of the cranium and vertebral column, respectively

- **dendrites**, which are short, highly branched processes extending out from the cell body, giving it a tree-shaped appearance. The branching network of dendrites increases the surface area available to receive incoming electrical signals from other neurons. When the signal is received via the dendrites it is directed inwards towards the cell body

- **the axon**, which arises from a cone-shaped region of the cell body, called the axon hillock. Each neuron has only one axon, which narrows from the axon hillock to form a narrow, cylinder-shaped projection that is the same size for its whole length. Very long axons are called nerve fibres* and can be up to a metre or more in length, for example the motor neuron extending from the spine to the foot. Axons are the conducting network that generate nerve impulses and transmit them away from the cell body to other neurons, muscle fibres, secretory glands and organs. At the end of the axon, extensive branching into axon terminals occurs, the distal ends of which resemble a bulb or button. Within these nerve terminals

---

*Not to be confused with a 'nerve' proper, which is a group of many nerve fibres bundled together and which connects the CNS to other parts of the body.

TABLE 10-1 Responses to autonomic nerve impulses

EFFECTOR ORGANS	PARASYMPATHETIC		SYMPATHETIC	
	Response	Receptor	Response	Receptor
Heart				
Sinoatrial node	$\downarrow$ Heart rate	M_2	$\uparrow$ Heart rate	β_1, β_2
Atrioventricular node	$\downarrow$ Conduction velocity	M_2	$\uparrow$ Automaticity $\uparrow$ Conduction velocity	β_1, β_2
Atria	$\downarrow$ Force	M_2	$\uparrow$ Force $\uparrow$ Conduction velocity	β_1, β_2
Ventricles	No effect	—	$\uparrow$ Force of contraction $\uparrow$ Conduction velocity $\uparrow$ Automaticity	β_1
Arterioles (smooth muscle)				
Coronary	Dilation	—	Constriction and dilation	$\alpha_1, \alpha_2, \beta_2$
Skin and mucosa	Dilation	—	Constriction	α_1, α_2
Skeletal muscle	No innervation	—	Constriction and dilation	α_1, β_2
Cerebral	Dilation	—	Slight constriction	α_1
Mesenteric	No innervation	—	Constriction and dilation	α_1, β_2
Renal	No innervation	—	Constriction and dilation	$\alpha_1, \alpha_2, \beta_1, \beta_2$
Veins (systemic)	No innervation	—	Constriction and dilation	$\alpha_1, \alpha_2, \beta_2$
Lung				
Bronchial muscle	Bronchoconstriction	M_3	Bronchodilation (no sympathetic innervation)	β_2 (dilated by circulating adrenaline)
Bronchial glands	Secretion	M_3	No effect	—
Gastrointestinal tract				
Motility	$\uparrow$ Motility	M_3	$\downarrow$ Motility	$\alpha_1, \alpha_2, \beta_2$
Sphincters	Relaxation	M_3	Contraction	α_2, β_2
Exocrine glands	$\uparrow$ Secretion Gastric acid secretion	M_3 M_1	No effect	
Salivary glands	Copious watery secretion		Thick, viscous secretion	α_1, β
Gallbladder and ducts	Contraction		Relaxation	β_2
Kidney (renin secretion)	No effect	—	Decrease and increase	α_1, β_1
Urinary bladder				
Detrusor muscle	Contraction	M_3	Relaxation	β_2
Sphincter	Relaxation	M_3	Contraction	α_1
Eye				
Radial muscle, iris	No effect	—	Contraction (mydriasis)	α_1
Sphincter muscle, iris	Contraction (miosis)	M_3		
Ciliary muscle	Contracted for near vision	M_3	Relaxed for vision (slight)	β_2
Liver	Glycogen synthesis		Glycogenolysis, gluconeogenesis	α_1, β_2

(Continued)

TABLE 10-1 Responses to autonomic nerve impulses—cont'd

| EFFECTOR ORGANS | PARASYMPATHETIC | | SYMPATHETIC | |
	Response	Receptor	Response	Receptor
Skin				
Sweat glands	No effect	—	↑ Sweating	α_1, mainly cholinergic
Arrector pili muscle	No innervation	—	Piloerection (gooseflesh)	α_1
Lacrimal glands	↑ Secretion	M_3	No innervation	—
Nasopharyngeal glands	↑ Secretion	M_3	No innervation	—
Male sex organs	Erection	M_3	Ejaculation	α_1

α = alpha receptor, β = beta receptor, M = muscarinic receptor.

are the vesicles containing the **neurotransmitter**, which, when released, influences the activity of other neurons or effectors. Within the ANS, the axons of preganglionic neurons terminate in autonomic ganglia, which also contain the cell body of the postganglionic neuron.

Myelination

Most axons are covered with a whitish lipid–protein coating called the myelin sheath. The myelin sheath is formed by Schwann cells that wrap themselves around the axon, forming as many as 100 concentric circles (Figure 10-4). Myelin protects the neuron, insulates it from other neurons and aids the speed of conduction of electrical impulses. Gaps (nodes of Ranvier) occur at regular intervals in the myelin sheath and speed conduction, as the electrical impulse is forced to jump from one node to the next. Unmyelinated fibres also exist but impulses tend to be conducted very slowly (around 1 m/s or less). In the ANS, the preganglionic neuron is myelinated while the postganglionic neuron is unmyelinated.

Generation of nerve impulses

Neurons communicate with each other via generation of an electrical signal or **action potential**. Although the human body is electrically neutral, having the same number of positive and negative charges, the inside (cytoplasmic side) of the membrane of a resting neuron is negatively charged with respect to the outside. This potential or voltage difference is called the resting membrane potential and is in the order of –40 to –90 mV, typically –70 mV. Neurons exhibiting a membrane potential are referred to as polarised. The principal ions involved in generating the membrane potential are potassium and sodium. Movement of sodium into the neuron and the movement of potassium out of the neuron occur principally via voltage-gated sodium and potassium channels.

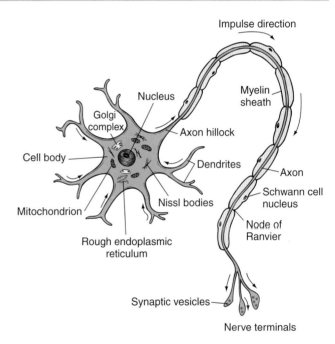

FIGURE 10-3 Structural components of a neuron.

Under normal (resting) conditions, a slow inward leakage of sodium ions occurs. These are pumped out of the neuron by a sodium–potassium pump that expels three sodium ions for each two potassium ions imported. This pump maintains the resting membrane potential at around –70 mV (Figure 10-5).

An action potential (Figure 10-6) occurs when:
- a stimulus causes the voltage-gated sodium channels to start to open
- sodium ions start to move inwards, making the interior less negative
- the membrane reaches a threshold voltage of about –55 mV
- sodium channels then rapidly open and sodium rushes

TABLE 10-2 Differentiating characteristics between the parasympathetic and sympathetic nervous systems

CHARACTERISTIC	PARASYMPATHETIC NERVOUS SYSTEM	SYMPATHETIC NERVOUS SYSTEM
Origin	Craniosacral	Thoracolumbar
Innervation	Cardiac muscle, smooth muscle, glands, viscera	Cardiac muscle, smooth muscle, glands, viscera
Autonomic ganglia	Near or within the wall of the effector	Near the CNS
Length of fibres	Preganglionic (long) Postganglionic (short)	Preganglionic (short) Postganglionic (long)
Ratio of preganglionic to postganglionic fibres	Branching is minimal (1:4), very discrete, fine responses	High degree of nerve branching (1:11, 1:17)
Response	Discrete	Diffuse
Chemical transmitter at autonomic ganglia	Acetylcholine	Acetylcholine
Chemical transmitter at postganglionic nerve endings	Acetylcholine	Noradrenaline (most cases); adrenaline and noradrenaline (adrenal medulla); acetylcholine for sweat glands

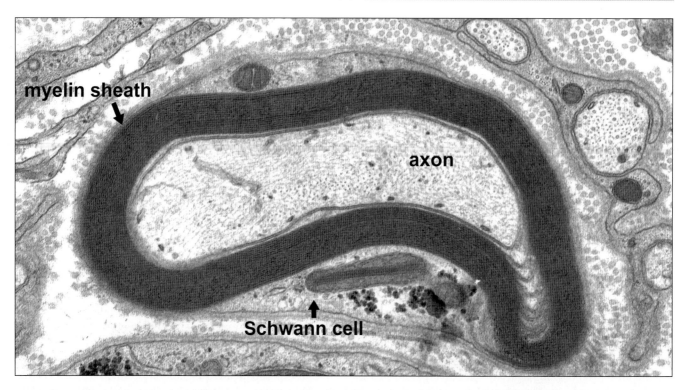

FIGURE 10-4 Electron micrograph of a peripheral myelinated nerve (human skin). Transverse section. The myelin sheath (which is formed by the Schwann cells) completely encircles the axon. Magnification X 38 000. Reproduced with permission of John W Stirling, Electron Microscope Unit, South Path, Flinders Medical Centre, Adelaide, Australia.

inwards, causing depolarisation (the membrane potential moves from −55 mV to 0 mV to +30 mV)
• sodium channels start to close and inflow of sodium ions slows

• voltage-gated potassium channels open and outflow of potassium accelerates (the membrane potential moves from +30 mV to 0 mV to −70 mV), causing the membrane to repolarise.

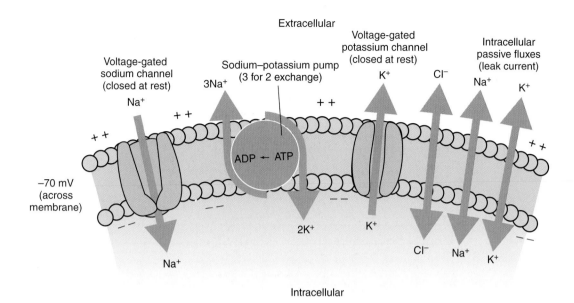

FIGURE 10-5 Primary determinants of the resting membrane potential. At rest the small build-up of positive ions along the outside of the membrane and negative ions along the inside of the membrane gives rise to the resting membrane potential of about −70 mV.

After an action potential is initiated it self-propagates along the full length of the axon in one direction only, away from the cell body towards the nerve terminals. Nerve fibres conduct electrical impulses only along the axon but communication throughout the neuronal network relies completely on the conversion of these impulses into chemical signals at synapses or effector junctions.

Neurochemical transmission

The passage of a nerve impulse from one neuron to another neuron (e.g. at autonomic ganglia) or from a neuron to an effector via a chemical signal is called **neurochemical transmission**. When the action potential reaches the presynaptic nerve terminal, the electrical signal is converted to a chemical signal by release of a **neurotransmitter**, which acts as a chemical messenger enabling nerve cells to communicate signals to the structures they innervate. The site at which communication between neurons occurs is called a **synapse**. Communication between a neuron and an effector occurs at a **neuroeffector junction**. In the parasympathetic and sympathetic nervous systems, synapses occur at ganglia, which are the sites of synapses between the preganglionic and postganglionic neurons and between the postganglionic neuron and the effector tissue or organ. The presence of a specific chemical at these synapses determines the type of information a neuron can receive and the range of responses it can yield in return. Receptors on the postsynaptic membrane bind the transmitter, which initiates a postsynaptic response that can be either excitatory or inhibitory. There are many specific neurotransmitters and these will be discussed in the context of the relevant pharmacology in the appropriate chapters.

TRANSMITTERS IN THE PERIPHERAL NERVOUS SYSTEM

For correct transmission across synapses to occur the neurotransmitter must be synthesised, stored and released, activate receptors and finally be inactivated. Many autonomic drugs affect one of these individual events, so it is essential to understand the basic mechanisms involved in neurotransmission.

There are multiple neurotransmitters in the ANS but the two about which most is known are **acetylcholine** (ACh) and **noradrenaline** (NA). Nerves that release ACh are called **cholinergic neurons** and are involved in cholinergic transmission. ACh is the neurotransmitter released from:
- preganglionic neurons in both the parasympathetic and sympathetic systems
- postganglionic parasympathetic nerve fibres
- sympathetic postganglionic neurons that innervate sweat glands.

Nerves that contain NA or **adrenaline** (from the adrenal medulla) are known as **adrenergic neurons** and are associated with adrenergic transmission. NA acts as the neurotransmitter between sympathetic postganglionic nerves and the organs they innervate (Figure 10-7).

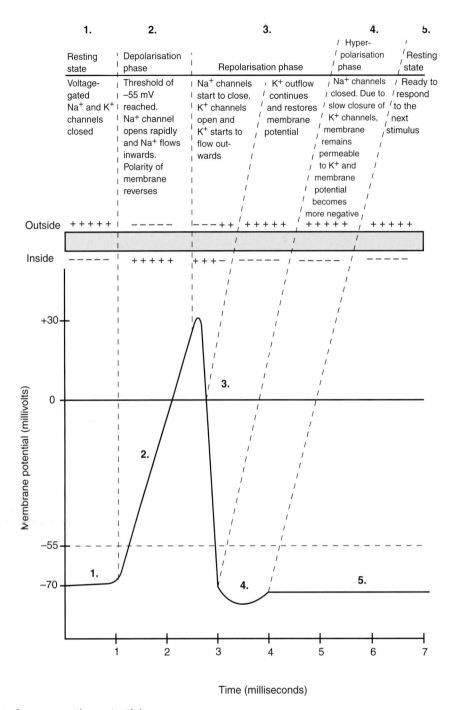

FIGURE 10-6 Phases of a nerve action potential.

Acetylcholine and cholinergic transmission
Synthesis and storage

ACh is synthesised in the cytoplasm of the nerve terminal from free choline and acetyl coenzyme A (acetyl-CoA) via the action of the enzyme choline acetyltransferase. Once synthesised, the ACh is packaged into synaptic vesicles or granules, which are located in the nerve terminal (Figure 10-8).

Release and action

The arrival of an action potential at the nerve ending facilitates the entry of calcium, which induces the synaptic vesicles containing ACh to attach to specific docking sites on the synaptic membrane and release the neurotransmitter molecules (via a process called **exocytosis**) into the synaptic cleft. The whole process of vesicle docking, cycling and exocytosis is under the control of various trafficking proteins. Once free, ACh diffuses across the synaptic cleft and attaches

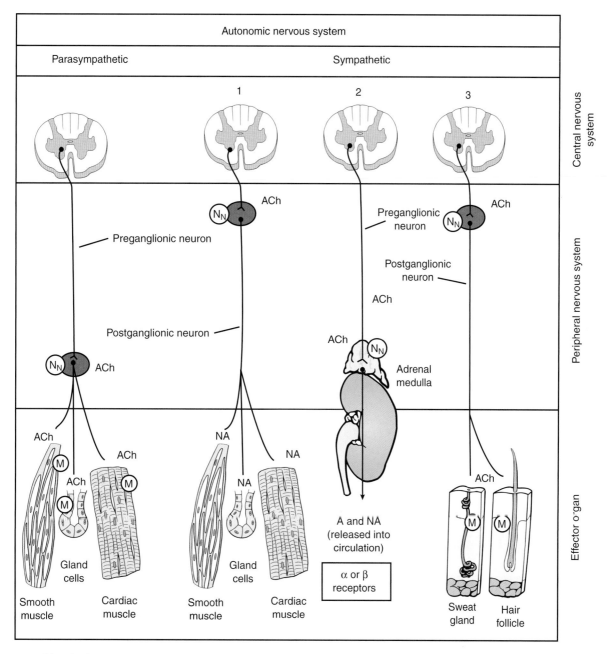

FIGURE 10-7 Chemical neurotransmitters and receptor sites in the autonomic nervous system. A = adrenaline; ACh = acetylcholine; NA = noradrenaline; N_N = neuronal nicotinic receptor; M = muscarinic receptor.

to specialised postsynaptic receptors on the membrane of the next neuron or effector. The binding of ACh to the receptor increases the permeability of the postsynaptic membrane to sodium and potassium ions, causing a depolarising action that results in excitation or inhibition of neural, muscular or glandular activity (Figure 10-8).

Acetylcholine receptors

Sir Henry Dale, investigating the pharmacological properties of ACh in 1914, distinguished two actions that were reproduced by the alkaloids muscarine and nicotine. As the effects of muscarine mimicked the parasympathetic nervous system, he termed the receptors 'muscarinic', while those in autonomic ganglia and at the skeletal neuromuscular junction were termed 'nicotinic' (N). In the periphery, **muscarinic (M) receptors** are located in smooth muscle, cardiac muscle and glands, while in the CNS, M receptors are involved in motor control, memory, and cardiovascular and temperature regulation.

Five distinct subtypes of M receptors have been identified, of which three are relevant pharmacologically. These subtypes

CLINICAL INTEREST BOX 10-1 MULTIPLE SCLEROSIS

Multiple sclerosis (MS) is a chronic inflammatory disorder of the CNS and is characterised by loss of axons and patchy loss of myelin sheaths. Current evidence indicates that the tissue damage results from an abnormal antibody-mediated immune response to antigens located on the surface of the myelin sheath. The cause of this is unknown but it is thought to involve a complex interplay between genetic and environmental factors (Wingerchuck et al 2001).

In most people (about 80%), the course of the disease is characterised initially by relapses and periods of symptomatic remission. The symptoms include trunk and limb paraesthesias (numbness, 'pins and needles'), muscle weakness, clumsiness, balance and coordination difficulties, extreme fatigue, sensitivity to heat, and bladder and bowel disturbances. Progression of the disease may occur during the periods of symptomatic remission and about 15% of affected individuals experience progressive neurological dysfunction.

Multiple sclerosis was first described in Australia by Dr James Jamieson in 1886 and affects mainly adults aged 20–50 years. In 1996 the estimated prevalence of MS in Australia was 39 per 100,000, with female representation twice that of males (Australian Institute of Health and Welfare 2000). Interestingly, increasing distance from the equator increases prevalence, and in Tasmania the prevalence of MS is around seven times higher than in Queensland (McLeod et al 1994). Pharmacological management is aimed at the prevention and treatment of exacerbations, and includes the use of corticosteroids, immunosuppressive agents, interferons and glatiramer (a synthetic analogue of 'myelin basic protein'). Symptomatic management often involves the use of antispasticity drugs, anticonvulsants, tricyclic antidepressants and anticholinergic drugs (van Oosten et al 1998).

are classified broadly as the neural type (M_1), the cardiac and presynaptic type (M_2) (discussed in Chapter 11) and the glandular or smooth muscle type (M_3) (Table 10-1). Nicotinic receptors are classed as either neuronal (N_N) or muscle (N_M) type. The neuronal **nicotinic receptors** (N_N) are in the ganglia of both the parasympathetic and sympathetic systems and the adrenal medulla.

Inactivation

To ensure that the action of released ACh is brief (1–2 ms), after acetylcholine has exerted its effect on the postsynaptic receptors the excess amount is inactivated rapidly by the

CLINICAL INTEREST BOX 10-2 NEUROTRANSMITTERS

To date, over 50 different chemicals have been identified as neurotransmitters or as putative neurotransmitters. These include acetylcholine, adrenaline, noradrenaline, dopamine, 5-hydroxytryptamine (5-HT, also commonly called serotonin), histamine, γ-aminobutyric acid, glycine, aspartate, glutamate, nitric oxide and numerous peptides such as substance P and the endorphins and enkephalins. Some neurons synthesise and release only one type of neurotransmitter but equally many synthesise and release multiple transmitters. The pathology of many diseases has been linked to neurotransmitter–receptor dysfunction, including Parkinson's disease, myasthenia gravis, Alzheimer's disease, depression and schizophrenia. An estimated 36,000 Australians are afflicted with Parkinson's disease (Australian Institute of Health and Welfare 2000).

enzyme **acetylcholinesterase** (AChE). This enzyme, which is bound to the basement membrane of the nerve terminal, is a target for drugs, insecticides and nerve gases. As a result of the action of AChE, ACh is metabolised to choline and acetate, which have no transmitter action and are recycled for synthesis of ACh (Figure 10-8).

Noradrenaline and adrenergic transmission

The term **catecholamine** refers to a group of chemically related compounds containing a catechol nucleus and an amine group in the side chain: **noradrenaline** (NA), **adrenaline** (A) and **dopamine** (DA). Although a precursor for the synthesis of NA and A, DA has a principal role as a neurotransmitter in the brain and is important in diseases such as Parkinson's and schizophrenia (see Chapters 19 and 21).

Synthesis and storage

The catecholamines produced by the sympathetic nervous system and the adrenal medulla include NA and A. The complex pathway for synthesis of these catecholamines is mediated by different enzymes located in the postganglionic nerve terminals and in the chromaffin cells of the adrenal medulla. Chromaffin cells are specialised cells in the adrenal medulla that secrete both NA and A. An abnormal secretion of catecholamines occurs in phaeochromocytoma, a rare chromaffin cell tumour.

The formation of NA begins with tyrosine, which is an amino acid derived from proteins in the diet. Tyrosine is taken up by adrenergic neurons and converted into dihydroxyphenylalanine (DOPA), which in turn is decarboxylated to

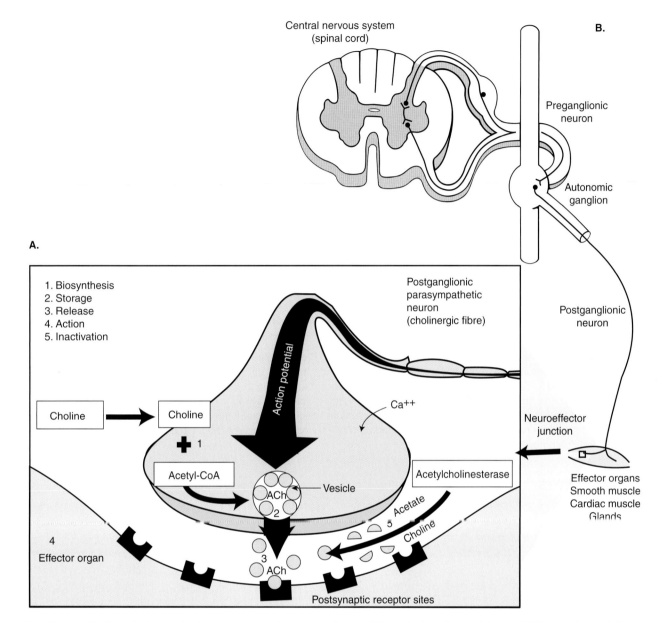

FIGURE 10-8 A. Cholinergic transmission at a neuroeffector junction. **1.** Biosynthesis of acetylcholine (ACh): choline is taken up by the axon terminal and ACh is synthesised from choline and acetyl-CoA. **2.** Storage: after synthesis, ACh is stored in the vesicle until the arrival of a nerve impulse. **3.** Release: an action potential arriving at the nerve terminal causes the vesicle to attach itself to the membrane and release ACh, which then diffuses across the synaptic cleft and combines with the receptors on the effector cell. **4.** Action: the interaction of ACh with the receptors results in a response. **5.** Inactivation of ACh: at the synaptic cleft, ACh is hydrolysed by the enzyme acetylcholinesterase. **B.** Schematic representation of the relation between a neuron in the CNS, a preganglionic neuron and an effector organ innervated by a postganglionic parasympathetic neuron.

DA. DA is then taken up into the storage vesicles, or granules, where it is transformed into the neurotransmitter NA by the enzyme DA β-hydroxylase (Figure 10-9).

In the adrenal medulla, the enzyme phenylethanolamine N-methyltransferase (PNMT) converts NA to A. On stimulation, both A and NA are released from the adrenal medulla and carried by the systemic circulation to all parts of the body.

Release and action

In a manner similar to that of cholinergic transmission, the arrival of an action potential at the nerve terminal of the postganglionic neuron causes an influx of calcium ions, fusion of vesicles with the cell membrane, and release of stored NA into the junctional cleft. NA then diffuses across the cleft to the receptor sites on the postjunctional membrane of neuro-effector cells (smooth muscle, cardiac muscle or glands) (Figure 10-9).

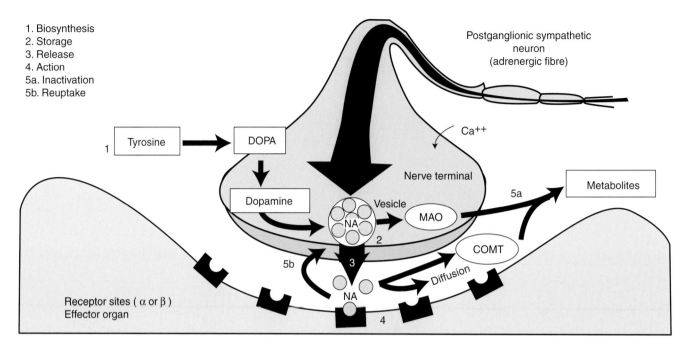

FIGURE 10-9 Adrenergic transmission at a neuroeffector junction. **1.** Biosynthesis and storage of noradrenaline (NA): tyrosine is taken up by adrenergic neurons and metabolised to dopamine, which is taken up by the storage vesicles. Inside the vesicles dopamine is converted to noradrenaline. **2.** Release: an action potential arriving at the nerve terminal causes the vesicle to attach itself to the membrane and release NA, which then diffuses across the synaptic cleft and combines with the receptors on the effector cell. **3.** Action: the interaction of NA with the receptors results in a response. **4.** The action of NA is terminated by reuptake of NA into the nerve terminal, enzymatic degradation by monoamine oxidase (MAO) and catechol-*O*-methyltransferase (COMT) and by diffusion away from the receptors.

Adrenoceptors

The adrenoceptors that are stimulated by the endogenous catecholamines NA and A consist of two subtypes: **alpha (α)** and **beta (β)**. α-Adrenoceptors are then further divided into α_1 and α_2 subtypes, and β-adrenoceptors into the three subtypes β_1, β_2 and β_3.

The α-adrenoceptors are differentiated primarily by neuronal location: α_1 receptors are located on the postsynaptic membrane, while α_2 receptors are located on presynaptic nerve terminals. These inhibitory α_2 autoreceptors are pharmacologically distinct from the postsynaptic α_1 receptors and control the amount of NA released through a negative feedback mechanism. α_2 Receptors are also found on liver cells, platelets and blood vessel smooth muscle cells. By contrast, β receptors show wide tissue distribution: β_1 receptors are located primarily in the heart, β_2 receptors are found on smooth muscle of the bronchioles, arterioles and various other visceral organs in the body, while β_3 receptors are localised to adipose tissue (Table 10-1).

Inactivation

The uptake and degradation of catecholamines differs substantially from that of ACh. Once NA has activated the adrenoceptor, its action must be rapidly terminated to prevent prolongation of its effects, which could lead to a loss of regulatory control of visceral function. The inactivation of NA occurs by reuptake of the NA into nerve terminals, enzymatic degradation and diffusion.

Catecholamines are metabolised by two enzymes, monoamine oxidase (MAO) and catechol-*O*-methyltransferase (COMT). (Two types of MAO have been identified, MAO-A and MAO-B, and these are discussed in Chapter 19.) Free NA within the cytoplasm of the nerve terminal is metabolised by MAO, which is bound to the surface membrane of intraneuronal mitochondria. COMT, which is located in both neuronal and non-neuronal tissues, metabolises both NA and the metabolites produced by the action of MAO.

The reuptake of NA plays a more significant role than enzymatic transformation in catecholamine inactivation. The reuptake processes, called uptake 1 (neuronal) and uptake 2 (extraneuronal), function collectively to accumulate catecholamines against a concentration gradient. NA is removed from the junctional sites by these active transport processes and is returned to the sympathetic nerve terminal and storage vesicles. In this way, an adequate supply of NA is provided by reuptake as well as by synthesis. Finally, a small portion of NA released at the synaptic cleft diffuses away, enters the systemic circulation and is metabolised elsewhere in the body (Figure 10-9).

The ANS plays a pathophysiological role in diseases of the cardiovascular, respiratory and gastrointestinal systems, and the use of drugs to modulate autonomic function is widespread. The following chapters discuss the way in which drugs affect the cholinergic and adrenergic divisions of the ANS.

KEY POINTS

- The principal divisions of the nervous system are the central nervous system (CNS) and the peripheral nervous system (PNS).
- The PNS has two subdivisions: the autonomic nervous system (ANS) and the somatic nervous system (SNS).
- The ANS regulates the function of smooth muscle, cardiac muscle and glandular secretions, which are not under direct conscious control.
- The ANS is organised in three subdivisions: the parasympathetic, sympathetic and enteric nervous systems.
- The parasympathetic system functions to conserve energy, while activity of the sympathetic system increases in stress situations.
- Autonomic reflexes play a key role in maintaining homeostasis.
- The enteric nervous system receives parasympathetic and sympathetic inputs but can function independently of the CNS to modulate motor and secretory functions of the gastrointestinal tract.
- Parasympathetic and sympathetic efferent (motor) pathways consist of preganglionic neurons that extend from cell bodies in the CNS to the autonomic ganglia, and postganglionic neurons that extend from the ganglia to various effector organs.
- Communication throughout the nervous system occurs through a highly integrated network of neurons.
- A neuron is composed of a cell body, dendrites and axon. Neurons communicate with each other or with effectors via generation of an electrical signal or action potential.
- Information transferral (signal transmission) at synapses is facilitated by neurotransmitters.
- Neurotransmitters are stored in presynaptic vesicles, released by exocytosis and have their actions terminated by metabolism, reuptake into nerve terminals and diffusion.
- The principal neurotransmitters in the ANS are acetylcholine (ACh) and noradrenaline (NA).
- ACh is the transmitter between pre- and postganglionic neurons in both the parasympathetic and sympathetic systems, and between postganglionic parasympathetic nerves and effector organs.
- NA acts as the neurotransmitter between sympathetic postganglionic nerves and effector organs.
- Acetylcholine receptors are classed as either nicotinic (N_N, N_M) or muscarinic (M_1, M_2, M_3).
- The subtypes of adrenoceptors are alpha (α_1, α_2) and beta (β_1, β_2, β_3).

REVIEW EXERCISES

1. Describe the physiological and anatomical differences between the parasympathetic and sympathetic nervous systems.
2. Describe the components of an autonomic reflex arc.
3. Describe the basic process of neurochemical transmission.
4. Give examples of the opposing actions of the parasympathetic and sympathetic systems.
5. Name the principal neurotransmitters in the ANS and list their respective receptor subtypes.

REFERENCES AND FURTHER READING

Australian Institute of Health and Welfare. *The Seventh Biennial Health Report of the Australian Institute of Health and Welfare.* Canberra: AIHW, 2000.

Byrne JH. Neuromuscular and synaptic transmission. Ch. 6 in: Johnson LR (ed.). *Essential Medical Physiology.* 2nd edn. Philadelphia: Lippincott-Raven, 1997.

Goyal RK, Hirano I. Mechanisms of disease: the enteric nervous system. *New England Journal of Medicine* 1996; 334(17): 1106–15.

Hoffman BB, Lefkowitz RJ, Taylor P. Neurotransmission: the autonomic and somatic motor nervous systems. Ch. 6 in: Hardman JG, Limbird LE (eds). *Goodman & Gilman's The Pharmacological Basis of Therapeutics.* 9th edn. New York: McGraw-Hill, 1996.

Marieb E. Fundamentals of the nervous system and nervous tissue. Ch. 11 in: Marieb E (ed.). *Human Anatomy and Physiology*. 4th edn. Menlo Park, CA: Benjamin Cummings Publishing, 1998.

McLeod JG, Hammond SR, Hallpike JF. Epidemiology of multiple sclerosis in Australia. *Medical Journal of Australia* 1994; 160: 117–22.

Rang HP, Dale MM, Ritter JM, Moore PK. *Pharmacology*. 5th edn. Edinburgh: Churchill Livingstone, 2003 [chs 9–12].

Tortora GJ, Grabowski SR. *Principles of Anatomy and Physiology*. 9th edn. New York: Harper Collins, 2000 [ch. 17].

Van Oosten BW, Truyen L, Barkhof F, Polman CH. Choosing drug therapy for multiple sclerosis. *Drugs* 1998; 56(4): 555–69.

Weisbrodt NW. Autonomic nervous system. Ch 9 in: Johnson LR (ed.). *Essential Medical Physiology*. 2nd edn. Philadelphia: Lippincott-Raven, 1997.

Wingerchuck DM, Lucchinetti CF, Noseworthy JH. Multiple sclerosis: current pathophysiological concepts. *Laboratory Investigation* 2001; 81(3): 263–81.

ON-LINE RESOURCES

Australian Institute of Health and Welfare: www.aihw.gov.au
Multiple Sclerosis Australia: www.msaustralia.org.au
The World of Multiple Sclerosis: www.ifmss.org.uk

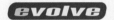 More weblinks at http://evolve.elsevier.com/AU/Bryant/pharmacology/

CHAPTER 11

Drugs Affecting Cholinergic Transmission

CHAPTER FOCUS

The parasympathetic component of the autonomic nervous system uses principally acetylcholine as the neurotransmitter. The action of acetylcholine on muscarinic receptors leads to responses primarily in the gastrointestinal and respiratory tracts, bladder, heart, eye and glands. This chapter reviews clinically relevant drugs that mimic, intensify or block the action of acetylcholine on muscarinic receptors in the parasympathetic system.

OBJECTIVES

- To discuss the muscarinic actions of acetylcholine.

- To explain the differences between the tertiary amine and quaternary ammonium muscarinic antagonist drugs.

- To describe the major adverse reactions of muscarinic agonist and antagonist drugs.

- To discuss the limitations of drugs affecting cholinergic transmission.

KEY DRUGS

atropine
bethanechol
hyoscine

KEY TERMS

choline esters
cholinomimetic alkaloids
ganglion-blocking drugs
muscarinic receptor agonists
muscarinic receptor antagonists
parasympatholytics
parasympathomimetics

AUTONOMIC drugs can mimic, enhance or block the effects of the parasympathetic and sympathetic divisions (see Chapter 12) of the autonomic nervous system. Following is a brief summary of the clinically relevant drugs.

Muscarinic receptor agonists, also referred to as parasympathomimetic drugs (e.g. bethanechol), mimic the action of acetylcholine on the parasympathetic nervous system. Muscarinic receptor antagonists, also referred to as parasympatholytic, or anticholinergic, drugs (e.g. atropine), block the action of acetylcholine and hence the effect of parasympathetic nervous system stimulation. Adrenoceptor agonists, also referred to as sympathomimetic drugs (e.g. isoprenaline), mimic the action of adrenaline and noradrenaline on the sympathetic nervous system. Adrenoceptor antagonists, also referred to as sympatholytic drugs (e.g. propranolol, a β-blocker), block the action of the sympathetic nervous system.

DRUGS ACTING AT MUSCARINIC RECEPTORS

As discussed in Chapter 10, acetylcholine plays an important role in the transmission of nerve impulses in the parasympathetic division of the autonomic nervous system.

Acetylcholine has two major actions on the nervous system:
- stimulant effects on the ganglia, adrenal medulla and skeletal muscle
- stimulant effects at postganglionic nerve endings in cardiac muscle, smooth muscle and glands.

The first action resembles the effects of nicotine, such as tachycardia, elevated blood pressure and peripheral vasoconstriction, and is referred to as the nicotinic effect of acetylcholine. The second action of acetylcholine at the postganglionic nerve endings is like that of muscarine (an alkaloid obtained from the toadstool *Amanita muscaria*) and is referred to as the muscarinic effect of acetylcholine. See Figure 10-7 to review nicotinic and muscarinic sites.

Although acetylcholine is important physiologically, it has no therapeutic value because its actions are very brief, due to rapid hydrolysis by acetylcholinesterase, and no selective purpose can be achieved through its use because it has many sites of action (Table 11-1). This lack of selectivity, which is due to the widespread distribution of muscarinic receptors, is common to many of the drugs discussed in this chapter.

Muscarinic receptor agonists

Muscarinic receptor agonists mimic the action produced by stimulation of the parasympathetic nervous system and are often referred to as **parasympathomimetics**. These drugs are divided into two groups: **choline esters**, which are chemically similar to the neurotransmitter acetylcholine and include bethanechol, carbachol and methacholine, and **cholinomimetic alkaloids** and synthetic analogues, which include muscarine, pilocarpine and oxotremorine. Only three of these drugs are used clinically: bethanechol is used systemically for urinary and gastrointestinal symptoms (see Drug Monograph 11-1), and carbachol and pilocarpine are used for the treatment of glaucoma (see Chapter 35).

Bethanechol and carbachol are quaternary amines, so they are poorly absorbed orally. Their actions are similar to, although longer-acting than, those of the physiological mediator acetylcholine, and their effect is blocked by atropine. The adverse effects of these drugs, which include bradycardia, hypotension, sweating, salivation, vomiting, diarrhoea and intestinal cramps, are a consequence of parasympathetic stimulation (Table 11-1).

Muscarinic receptor antagonists

Muscarinic receptor antagonists are often referred to as **parasympatholytic**, antimuscarinic or anticholinergic drugs because they competitively block the action of acetylcholine at muscarinic receptors. When the neuron is stimulated, the acetylcholine liberated from the terminal cannot bind to the receptor site and fails to produce a cholinergic effect. (See Figure 10-7 for muscarinic receptor sites.) These drugs

TABLE 11-1 Acetylcholine: muscarinic actions

SITE	MUSCARINIC ACTION*
Cardiovascular	
Blood vessel	Dilation
Heart rate	Slowed
Blood pressure	Decreased
Gastrointestinal	
Tone	Increased
Motility	Increased
Sphincters	Relaxed
Glandular secretions	Increased salivary, lacrimal, intestinal and sweat secretion
Eye	Pupil constriction and decreased accommodation

*Usual sites for therapeutic effects.

DRUG MONOGRAPH 11-1 BETHANECHOL

Bethanechol acts on muscarinic receptors on the detrusor muscle of the urinary bladder and smooth muscle of the gastrointestinal tract. In the bladder, the resulting contraction of the smooth muscle is sufficiently strong to initiate micturition and empty the bladder. In the gastrointestinal tract, the drug stimulates gastric motility, increases gastric tone and often restores impaired peristaltic activity of the oesophagus, stomach and intestine. It also promotes defecation. Unlike acetylcholine, bethanechol is not degraded by acetylcholinesterase and its effects therefore are more prolonged than those of acetylcholine. Therapeutic doses in normal human subjects have little effect on heart rate, blood pressure or the peripheral circulation.

INDICATIONS More effective drugs have generally replaced bethanechol, but it is available for treating postoperative and postpartum non-obstructive urinary retention and for neurogenic atony of the urinary bladder associated with retention.

PHARMACOKINETICS Despite being poorly absorbed from the gastrointestinal tract, bethanechol chloride is effective orally. It does not penetrate the blood–brain barrier in therapeutic doses but its distribution to other tissues has not been documented. Onset of action is within 30–90 minutes of oral administration, peak effect occurs within 90 minutes and duration of action is up to 6 hours, depending on the dose administered. When the drug is administered subcutaneously, the onset of action is within 5–15 minutes, peak effect occurs within 15–30 minutes and the duration of action is about 2 hours. Routes of metabolism and excretion are unknown.

DRUG INTERACTIONS The following effects can occur when bethanechol is given with the drugs listed below:

Other muscarinic agonists or anticholinesterase medications	Enhanced cholinergic effects and perhaps toxicity. Monitor closely for adverse effects or if possible avoid this combination of medications
Ganglion-blocking agents	Can result in severe abdominal distress followed by a precipitous fall in blood pressure. Avoid or a potentially serious drug interaction could occur
Procainamide or quinidine	Can antagonise the effects of bethanechol

ADVERSE REACTIONS Adverse reactions are presented in Table 11-2.

WARNINGS AND CONTRAINDICATIONS Use is contraindicated in people with known bethanechol hypersensitivity, Parkinson's disease, asthma, epilepsy, vagotonia, hypotension, severe bradycardia, coronary artery disease, gastrointestinal (GI) obstruction, hyperthyroidism and peptic ulcer. No data are available regarding excretion in breast milk or safety during pregnancy, so avoid use.

DOSAGE AND ADMINISTRATION The oral dosage for adults (preferably given when the stomach is empty) is 10–30 mg orally or sublingually, 3–4 times daily.

CLINICAL INTEREST BOX 11-1 TREATMENT OF ALZHEIMER'S DISEASE

In Australia, dementia is a leading cause of disease burden. Current projections show an increase in the number of Australians affected by dementia, including Alzheimer's disease, from ~161,300 in 2002 to ~242,700 in 2020 (AIHW 2004). The effect of Alzheimer's disease on the individual and carers is considerable. Significant effort is being undertaken to improve drug treatment. The decline in cognitive function in Alzheimer's disease is causally related to deficits in neurotransmitter function, particularly cholinergic neurons. Several clinical trials are in progress using selective muscarinic receptor (M_1) agonists, as it has been speculated that these drugs might ameliorate the progressive deterioration of cognitive ability. Muscarinic M_1 agonists with desirable penetration of the blood–brain barrier that are in advanced clinical trials for the treatment of Alzheimer's disease include cevimeline, milameline, talsaclidine, sabcomeline and xanomeline (Eglen et al 1999).

are categorised either as tertiary amines, which are lipid-soluble, absorbed from the gastrointestinal (GI) tract and the conjunctiva, and penetrate the blood–brain barrier; or as quaternary ammonium compounds, which exhibit poor lipid solubility, poor penetration of the blood–brain barrier and poor absorption from the GI tract and conjunctiva.

The best-known muscarinic antagonists are atropine and hyoscine. *Atropa belladonna* (deadly nightshade) contains mainly atropine whereas *Hyoscyamus niger* (henbane) and *Datura stramonium* (jimsonweed) contain hyoscine. Atropine (see Drug Monograph 11-2) is the prototype muscarinic antagonist and its use for more than half a century is

DRUG MONOGRAPH 11-2 ATROPINE

Atropine has very little effect on the actions of acetylcholine at nicotinic receptor sites but can produce a wide range of pharmacological effects because of the widespread distribution of parasympathetic cholinergic nerves in the body. The main effects are summarised below.

EYES The pupil is dilated (mydriasis) and relaxation of the ciliary muscle causes failure of accommodation (cycloplegia). Pupil dilation may reduce outflow of aqueous humour, causing a rise in intraocular pressure, a hazardous situation for people with narrow-angle glaucoma. These effects in the eye are brought about by both local and systemic administration of atropine, although the usual single therapeutic dose of atropine given orally or parentally has little effect on the eye. After the pupil is dilated photophobia occurs, and when the drug has reached its full effect the usual reflexes to light and accommodation disappear.

SKIN AND MUCOUS MEMBRANES Low doses of atropine inhibit secretion in lacrimal, bronchial, salivary and sweat glands. This produces the characteristic drying of the mucous membranes of the mouth, nose, pharynx and bronchi, and causes the skin to become hot and dry.

RESPIRATORY SYSTEM Atropine relaxes the smooth muscle of the bronchial tract but is less effective than adrenaline as a bronchodilator and is rarely used for asthma.

CARDIOVASCULAR SYSTEM When very low doses of atropine are administered, the heart rate is temporarily slowed because of a central action that augments vagal activity (paradoxical bradycardia). Larger doses block the effect of vagal stimulation on the sinoatrial node and atrioventricular junction, causing an increased heart rate. In therapeutic doses, atropine has little or no effect on blood pressure because most vascular beds lack significant cholinergic innervation.

GASTROINTESTINAL TRACT The effect of atropine on the secretions of the pancreas and intestinal glands is not therapeutically significant but atropine (in larger doses) incompletely inhibits GI motility.

URINARY TRACT Atropine slightly relaxes smooth muscle of the urinary tract, and therapeutic doses decrease the tone of the fundus of the urinary bladder. It also causes constriction of the internal sphincter, which can produce urinary retention, particularly in the elderly.

CENTRAL NERVOUS SYSTEM Atropine has prominent effects on the CNS and in large doses causes excitement and maniacal behaviour. These behavioural effects suggest the existence of important cholinergic pathways and receptors within the CNS.

Small or moderate doses of atropine have little or no cerebral effect. Large or toxic doses cause restlessness, wakefulness and talkativeness, which can develop into delirium and finally stupor and coma. A rise in temperature is sometimes seen, especially in infants and young children, probably as a result of suppression of sweating. Atropine has been used to treat the extrapyramidal effects (tremor, involuntary movements and rigidity) of Parkinson's disease by reducing cholinergic transmission.

PHARMACOKINETICS Atropine is readily absorbed after oral and parenteral administration; it is also absorbed from mucous membranes. After intramuscular administration, peak plasma concentration is reached within 30 minutes. The duration of action is 4–6 hours but ocular effects can last longer. About 50% of the drug is bound to plasma proteins but it readily crosses the placental barrier and the blood–brain barrier. Atropine is metabolised primarily in the liver but about 30%–50% is excreted unchanged in the urine.

DRUG INTERACTIONS AND ADVERSE REACTIONS
The antimuscarinic effect of drugs such as tricyclic antidepressants, some antihistamines (e.g. promethazine) and the phenothiazines (e.g. chlorpromazine) may be additive with atropine. The reduction in gastric motility caused by atropine can also impair the absorption of other drugs. For adverse reactions see Table 11-2.

WARNINGS AND CONTRAINDICATIONS Avoid use in people with atropine hypersensitivity or known hypersensitivity to other muscarinic antagonists. Atropine is contraindicated in myasthenia gravis, severe cardiac disease, GI obstructive disease, narrow-angle glaucoma, acute haemorrhage, prostatic hypertrophy, urinary retention, pyloric obstruction, ulcerative colitis, toxaemia of pregnancy and febrile conditions, and in debilitated patients with intestinal atony or paralytic ileus. Caution should be exercised in any situation where there is a higher likelihood of adverse effects, e.g. Down syndrome, the elderly, people with autonomic neuropathy and hepatic and renal disease.

DOSAGE AND ADMINISTRATION Atropine is used in a variety of circumstances including before surgery, to treat anticholinesterase poisoning, to treat bradycardia during resuscitation and for asystole. For atropine sulfate injection in general, the paediatric dose is 0.01 mg/kg IM, IV or SC not exceeding 0.4 mg, every 4–6 hours if necessary, and the adult parenteral dose is 0.4–0.6 mg IM, IV or SC to a total of 2 mg. As a premedication to prevent excessive salivation and respiratory tract secretions in adults during anaesthesia, 0.4–0.6 mg may be given IM or SC about 1 hour before anaesthesia or IV immediately before induction.

TABLE 11-2 Drugs affecting the parasympathetic nervous system: adverse reactions

DRUG	ADVERSE REACTIONS
Muscarinic agonist	
Bethanechol	Abdominal pains or upset, increased salivation and sweating, nausea or vomiting, flushed skin, blurred or disturbed vision, unsteadiness, headache and diarrhoea
Muscarinic antagonists	
Atropine and hyoscine	Inhibition of sweating, constipation, dry mouth, throat and skin, blurred vision, urinary retention, headache, photophobia, drowsiness, weakness, nausea or vomiting, urticaria, dermatitis and eye pain from raised intraocular pressure. In addition, euphoria, amnesia and insomnia are reported more often with hyoscine
Glycopyrrolate (synthetic antispasmodic)	Abdominal distension, headache, dizziness, constipation, nausea, vomiting, sedation, dry mouth, nose, throat and skin, blurred or disturbed vision, dysuria, weakness, hypotension and decreased sexual ability
Ganglion-blocking drug	
Trimetaphan	Adverse effects are dose-related: anorexia, nausea, vomiting, constipation, dilated pupils, dry mouth, impotence, pruritus, hives, hypotension, tachycardia, angina and urinary retention

testimony to its therapeutic effectiveness. With the exception of some degree of selectivity for the heart and GI tract, all the muscarinic antagonists produce peripheral effects similar to those observed with atropine. The M_1 selective antagonist pirenzipine (not available in Australia and New Zealand) inhibits gastric acid secretion but has little effect elsewhere in the body.

Hyoscine hydrobromide

Similar to atropine, hyoscine is a muscarinic receptor antagonist. Hyoscine's peripheral effects are similar to those of atropine but, due to greater permeation of the blood–brain barrier, it has marked effects on the central nervous system (CNS). At therapeutic doses, it depresses the CNS and causes drowsiness, euphoria, memory loss, relaxation, sleep and relief of fear. It does not increase blood pressure or respiration.

Because of its depressant action on vestibular function, it is used for motion sickness, to prevent nausea and vomiting, and as an adjunct medication with general anaesthesia to reduce respiratory tract secretions. Hyoscine's pharmacokinetics are similar to those of atropine. For adverse reactions see Table 11-2.

For travel sickness the adult oral dose is 0.3–0.6 mg 30 minutes before travel and repeated 3–4 hours later if required, to a maximum dosage of 1.2 mg/day. The dosage for children varies: age 2–7 years, a maximum of 0.15–0.3 mg/daily; and over 7 years of age, a maximum of 0.6 mg/daily. The elderly are more sensitive to this drug at the usual adult dosage; sensitivity can manifest as confusion, blurred vision and ataxia.

Synthetic and semisynthetic substitutes for atropine

The usefulness of atropine is limited by the fact that it is a complex drug and because it produces effects in a range of organs or tissues simultaneously, owing to the widespread distribution of muscarinic receptors. When it is administered for its antispasmodic effects, it also produces prolonged effects in the eye, causing dilated pupils and blurred vision. It also causes dry mouth and possibly tachycardia. Atropine does have some desirable effects, and a large number of drugs have been synthesised in an effort to take advantage of the antispasmodic effect of atropine without its other effects.

Many products are marketed as antispasmodic and anticholinergic agents but their formulations are either modifications of a belladonna alkaloid or include one or more of the natural alkaloids as their active ingredients. The pharmacological properties are therefore similar to previously reviewed substances (see Table 11-3). One of the more commonly used systemic agents is glycopyrrolate.

GLYCOPYRROLATE

This is a synthetic muscarinic receptor antagonist with effects similar to those of atropine. Unlike atropine, it is unable to easily cross lipid membranes (such as the blood–brain barrier) and hence has minimal CNS effects. It is also less likely to produce pupillary or ocular effects. Glycopyrrolate is indicated as an antimuscarinic drug to reduce salivary, tracheobronchial and pharyngeal secretions preoperatively, to prevent bradycardia induced during anaesthesia, and to prevent or reduce the peripheral effects of acetylcholinesterase inhibitors (neostigmine or pyridostigmine).

TABLE 11-3 Muscarinic antagonists: clinical use and route of administration

DRUG	CLINICAL USE	ROUTE OF ADMINISTRATION
Atropine	Mydriatic, cycloplegic, antisecretory	IV, IM, SC, topical (eye-drops)
Benztropine	Parkinson's disease	Oral, IV, IM
Benzhexol	Parkinson's disease	Oral
Biperiden	Parkinson's disease	Oral
Cyclopentolate	Mydriatic, cycloplegic	Topical (eye-drops)
Glycopyrrolate	Antisecretory	IM, IV
Homatropine	Mydriatic, cycloplegic	Topical (eye-drops)
Hyoscine butylbromide	Antispasmodic	Oral, IM, IV
Ipratropium bromide	Bronchodilator	Inhalational
Mebeverine*	Antispasmodic	Oral
Orphenadrine	Parkinson's disease	Oral
Oxybutynin**	Antispasmodic (urge incontinence)	Oral
Propantheline bromide	Antispasmodic (urge incontinence)	Oral
Tolterodine	Antispasmodic (urge incontinence)	Oral
Tropicamide	Mydriatic, cycloplegic	Topical (eye-drops)

* Has multiple mechanisms of action and is not solely a muscarinic antagonist.
** Has calcium channel-blocking activity at high doses.

Following an IV dose, the onset of action occurs within about 1 minute, and following an IM dose, about 15–30 minutes. Vagal blocking action lasts 2–3 hours and the antisialagogue effect (inhibition of the flow of saliva) can last up to 7 hours. Glycopyrrolate is predominantly excreted by the kidneys unchanged.

To reduce excessive salivation and respiratory tract secretions in adults during anaesthesia, the dose is 0.2–0.4 mg IV or IM, or 0.004–0.005 mg/kg of body weight to a maximum of 0.4 mg given 30–60 minutes before anaesthesia. For children aged 1 month to 12 years, 0.004–0.008 mg/kg of body weight to a maximum of 0.2 mg IV or IM, is given 30–60 minutes before anaesthesia.

GANGLION-BLOCKING DRUGS

The major neurotransmitter at all autonomic ganglia is acetylcholine. **Ganglion-blocking drugs** block the action of acetylcholine at autonomic ganglia by competing with acetylcholine at the synapse. This results in reduced impulse transmission from preganglionic to postganglionic neurons in both the sympathetic and parasympathetic systems. Because of the profound physiological effects (hypotension, loss of cardiovascular reflexes) elicited by ganglion-blocking drugs, they are now clinically obsolete.

PREGNANCY SAFETY

ADEC Category	Drug
A	Atropine
B1	Benzhexol, oxybutynin
B2	Bethanechol, benztropine, biperiden, hyoscine, hyoscine hydrobromide, glycopyrrolate, orphenadrine, propantheline
B3	Tolterodine

DRUGS AT A GLANCE 11: Drugs affecting cholinergic transmission

Therapeutic group	Pharmacological group	Key examples	Key pages
Parasympathomimetics	Muscarinic receptor agonists	bethanechol	179
		carbachol	178
		pilocarpine	178
Parasympatholytics (anticholinergic drugs)	Muscarinic receptor antagonists	atropine	180
		hyoscine	181
		glycopyrrolate	181
		tolterodine	182

KEY POINTS

- The cholinergic receptor sites that are stimulated by acetylcholine are either nicotinic or muscarinic.
- Nicotinic receptors appear in the ganglia of the parasympathetic and sympathetic systems, adrenal medulla and skeletal muscle (somatic motor system), whereas muscarinic receptors are located at postganglionic sites in smooth muscle, cardiac muscle and glands.
- Muscarinic agonists are also referred to as parasympathomimetic drugs (e.g. bethanechol) and they mimic the action of acetylcholine on the parasympathetic nervous system.
- Muscarinic antagonists are also referred to as parasympatholytic or anticholinergic drugs (e.g. atropine) and they block the action of acetylcholine and hence the effect of parasympathetic nervous system stimulation.
- Muscarinic agonists such as bethanechol are used systemically for non-obstructive urinary retention and for atony of the urinary bladder associated with retention. Carbachol and pilocarpine are used for the treatment of glaucoma.
- Adverse reactions to bethanechol include abdominal pains or upset, increased salivation and sweating, nausea or vomiting, flushed skin, blurred or disturbed vision, unsteadiness, headache and diarrhoea.
- Muscarinic antagonists such as atropine and synthetic substitutes are used clinically as antispasmodics, mydriatics and cycloplegics. They are also used as preanaesthetic drugs to decrease respiratory secretions.
- Ganglion-blocking drugs are indicated for the management of severe and malignant hypertension. With the exception of trimetaphan, they are now clinically obsolete.

REVIEW EXERCISES

1. Bethanechol is contraindicated for use in people with asthma, severe bradycardia, gastrointestinal obstruction and peptic ulcer. Discuss why this drug has these contraindications by reviewing the response elicited by acetylcholine at muscarinic receptors on the heart, lungs, intestines and parietal cells.
2. Discuss the effects of atropine in the body, particularly on smooth muscle, cardiac muscle, exocrine glands and the eye.
3. Give four indications for atropine.

REFERENCES AND FURTHER READING

Australian Institute of Health and Welfare. *Australia's Health 2004*. Canberra: AIHW, 2004.
Australian Medicines Handbook 2006. Adelaide: Australian Medicines Handbook, 2006.
Brown JH, Taylor P. Muscarinic receptor agonists and antagonists. In: Hardman JG, Limbird LE, Gilman AG (eds). *Goodman & Gilman's The Pharmacological Basis of Therapeutics*. 10th edn. New York: McGraw-Hill, 2001 [ch. 7].
Dollery C (ed.). *Therapeutic Drugs*. Vol. 1. London: Churchill Livingstone, 1991.
Eglen RM, Choppin A, Dillon MP, Hegde S. Muscarinic receptor ligands and their therapeutic potential. *Current Opinion in Chemical Biology* 1999; 3: 426–32.
Eglen RM, Watson N. Selective muscarinic receptor agonists and antagonists. *Pharmacology and Toxicology* 1996; 78: 59–68.

Rang HP, Dale MM, Ritter JM, Moore PK. *Pharmacology*. 5th edn. Edinburgh: Churchill Livingstone, 2003 [ch. 10].
United States Pharmacopeial Convention. *USP DI: Drug Information for the Health Care Professional*. 18th edn. Rockville: US Pharmacopeial Convention, 1998.

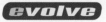 More weblinks at http://evolve.elsevier.com/AU/Bryant/pharmacology/

CHAPTER 12

Drugs Affecting Noradrenergic Transmission

CHAPTER FOCUS

The sympathetic (adrenergic) nervous system is the second major subdivision of the autonomic nervous system. This system acts in concert with the parasympathetic nervous system to regulate the heart, secretory glands, and vascular and non-vascular smooth muscle. Drugs that stimulate or block α- and β-adrenoceptors are very common in clinical practice today. Understanding the physiological responses mediated by adrenergic receptors aids in rationalising the pharmacological and adverse effects of drugs affecting noradrenergic transmission.

OBJECTIVES

- To explain the major effects mediated by stimulation of α_1-, α_2-, β_1- and β_2-adrenergic receptors.

- To list the three main classes of adrenergic drugs.

- To discuss adrenaline's mechanism of action, indications, significant drug interactions and adverse reactions.

- To describe the effects of the three naturally occurring catecholamines on the cardiovascular, respiratory and gastrointestinal systems.

- To explain the basis of the antihypertensive, antianginal and antiarrhythmic effect of β-adrenoceptor antagonists.

KEY DRUGS

adrenaline
dobutamine
dopamine
ephedrine
noradrenaline
prazosin

KEY TERMS

α-adrenoceptor agonist
α-adrenoceptor antagonist
β-adrenoceptor agonist
β-adrenoceptor antagonist
catecholamines
chronotropic effect
dromotropic effect
inotropic effect
intrinsic sympathomimetic activity
sympathomimetic drugs

ADRENERGIC DRUGS

DRUGS affecting noradrenergic transmission include:

- direct-acting sympathomimetic drugs (adrenoceptor agonists) that mimic the effects of either noradrenaline released from sympathetic nerve terminals, or adrenaline released from the adrenal medulla on α- and β-adrenoceptors
- indirect-acting sympathomimetics that either facilitate the release of noradrenaline from, or block the uptake of noradrenaline into, nerve terminals
- adrenoceptor antagonists (blockers), also referred to as sympatholytic drugs, which block the action of the sympathetic nervous system.

Direct-acting sympathomimetics

These **sympathomimetic drugs** (also called **adrenoceptor agonists**) are designed to directly stimulate α- and β-adrenoceptors, mimicking the effects of sympathetic stimulation, such as increasing cardiac output, vasoconstriction of arterioles and veins, regulation of body temperature, bronchial dilation, and a variety of other effects. (For additional information on the effects of the sympathetic nervous system, see Chapter 10.) The prototype drugs of this class are the **catecholamines** and many modifications have been made to the basic structure to obtain drugs with greater selectivity for α- and β-adrenoceptor subtypes. Examples of synthetic catecholamines are isoprenaline and **dobutamine**.

Catecholamines

There are three naturally occurring catecholamines in the body: **dopamine, noradrenaline** and **adrenaline**. Dopamine is the precursor for the synthesis of noradrenaline and adrenaline and has a major role as a neurotransmitter in certain areas of the central nervous system. (For information on CNS transmission, see Chapter 14.) Noradrenaline is released from sympathetic nerve terminals, while adrenaline is a circulating catecholamine released from the adrenal medulla.

There is evidence that the α receptors exist in two primary locations, pre- and postsynaptic. The α_2 receptors are found on presynaptic nerve terminals, postsynaptically on vascular and smooth muscle cells, and on sites remote from the nerve terminals, such as platelets and leucocytes. The presynaptic α_2 receptor controls the amount of noradrenaline released per nerve impulse, which is regulated by a feedback mechanism. When the concentration of noradrenaline in the synaptic cleft reaches a high level, it stimulates the α_2 receptors, which prevent the further release of noradrenaline (Figure 12-1). This feedback prevents excessive and prolonged stimulation of postsynaptic α_1-adrenoceptors on effector organs such as the

eye, arterioles, veins, males sex organs and bladder neck (Box 12-1). The α_1-adrenoceptors are generally located close to the nerve terminal so that the action of released noradrenaline is almost immediate.

Beta-adrenoceptors are subdivided into three types:

- **β_1 receptors**, which are primarily located on the heart
- **β_2 receptors**, which mediate the actions of catecholamines on smooth muscle, especially bronchioles, arterial smooth muscle and skeletal muscle
- **β_3 receptors**, which are located on adipose tissue and mediate lipolysis.

Noradrenaline acts principally on α-, β_1- and β_3-adrenoceptors, with negligible activity at β_2 receptors. In contrast, adrenaline acts on all α and β receptor subtypes, with significantly greater effects on α receptors at higher doses. Isoprenaline, a synthetic catecholamine, acts only on β receptors.

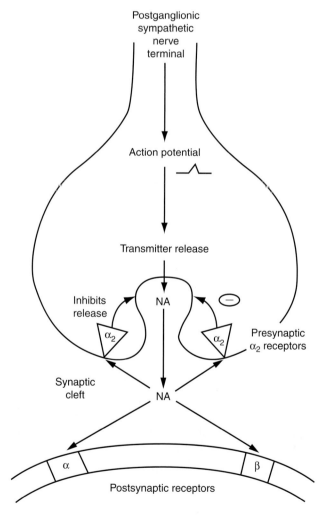

FIGURE 12-1 Control of noradrenaline release by presynaptic α_2 receptors.

The most important responses mediated by α-receptor stimulation in humans include:

- vasoconstriction of arterioles in the skin and splanchnic area, resulting in a rise in blood pressure
- pupil dilation
- relaxation of the gut.

β-adrenergic stimulation includes:

- increase in heart rate and contractility
- vasodilation of arterioles supplying skeletal muscles
- bronchial relaxation
- uterine relaxation.

The effects of both α- and β-receptor stimulation often result in a summation of action when they are interrelated. Most arteries and veins contain both α and β receptors, and a change in blood pressure will depend on the degree of vasoconstriction in the skin and splanchnic area, and the extent of vasodilation in skeletal muscle blood vessels, along with changes in heart rate (Table 12-1).

Specific drugs that stimulate or block α and β receptors are available and many of these drugs are discussed in specific chapters in the context of the relevant pharmacology. The extent of sympathetic innervation or the presence of adrenoceptors on various organs will determine the magnitude of response to an individual adrenergic drug. With the exception of central α_2 receptors, which are discussed in Chapter 25, these agents all act at peripheral autonomic sites.

ADRENALINE

Adrenaline stimulates α and β receptors, although its primary action is on the β receptors of the heart, smooth muscle of the bronchi, and the blood vessels. At low doses adrenaline has predominantly β-receptor actions, but with increasing doses an increase in α-receptor activity is observed.

CARDIAC EFFECTS. Adrenaline produces a significant increase in myocardial contraction (positive **inotropic effect**) as a result of increased influx of calcium into cardiac fibres. The strong myocardial contractions result in more complete emptying of the ventricles and an increase in cardiac work, oxygen consumption and cardiac output. It has been shown experimentally and clinically that 0.5 mg adrenaline given IV and circulated by cardiac compression or massage may stimulate spontaneous and vigorous cardiac contractions. Even if the heart is in ventricular fibrillation, adrenaline increases fibrillation vigour and frequently promotes successful electric defibrillation. In these situations the drug may be injected repeatedly; however, adrenaline cannot be used repeatedly to improve the function of a failing heart (congestive heart failure) because it increases oxygen consumption by cardiac muscle. The production of strong contractions provides the rationale for the use of adrenaline in cardiac arrest.

A significant increase in cardiac rate (positive **chronotropic effect**) occurs as a result of the increased rate of membrane depolarisation in the pacemaker cells in the sinus node during diastole. Action potential threshold is reached sooner, pacemaker cells fire more often and heart rate increases. Adrenaline may also produce spontaneous firing of Purkinje fibres, which may cause them to exhibit pacemaker activity. This effect can cause ventricular extrasystoles and increase the susceptibility of ventricular muscle to

---

BOX 12-1 OVERVIEW OF ADRENERGIC RECEPTOR STIMULATION

RECEPTOR	EFFECT	LOCATION
α_1	Vasoconstriction of peripheral blood vessels Dilation (contraction) of pupil Increased contractility of heart (inotropic effect)	
α_2	Inhibition of transmitter release Aggregation of platelets Contraction of smooth muscle	
β_1	Increased heart rate (chronotropic effect) Increased contractility of heart (inotropic effect)	
β_2	Relaxation of uterus Glycogenolysis Dilation of bronchial smooth muscle	

TABLE 12-1 Adrenergic receptor type and responses

EFFECTOR ORGANS	ADRENERGIC RECEPTOR TYPE	RESPONSE
Heart		
Cardiac muscle (atria, ventricles)	β_1, β_2	Increased force of contraction (inotropic action)
Sinoatrial node	β_1, β_2	Increased heart rate (chronotropic action)
Atrioventricular node	β_1, β_2	Increased automaticity and conduction velocity
Blood vessels		
Arterioles		
Coronary	α_1, α_2, β_2	Constriction, dilation*
Cerebral	α_1	Constriction (slight)
Pulmonary	α_1, β_2	Constriction, dilation*
Mesenteric visceral	α_1, β_2	Constriction,* dilation
Renal	α_1, α_2, β_1, β_2, dopaminergic	Constriction,* dilation
Skin, mucosa	α_1, α_2	Constriction
Skeletal muscle	α_1, β_2	Constriction, dilation
Veins	α_1, α_2, β_2	Constriction, dilation
Lung		
Bronchial smooth muscle	β_2	Bronchodilation
Gastrointestinal tract		
Smooth muscle (motility, tone)	α_1, α_2, β_2	Decreased
Sphincter	α_1, β_2	Contraction
Gallbladder and ducts	β_2	Relaxation
Liver	β_2	Glycogenolysis
Spleen capsule	α_1, β_2	Contraction,* relaxation
Pancreas: insulin secretion	α_2	Decreased
Adipose tissue	β_3	Lipolysis
Urinary bladder		
Detrusor muscle	β_2	Relaxation
Sphincter	α_1	Contraction
Kidney		
Ureter	α_1	Contraction
Secretion (renin)	α_1; β_1	Decreased; Increased
Uterus		
Pregnant	α_1	Contraction
Non-pregnant	β_2	Relaxation
Male sex organs	α_1	Ejaculation
Skin		
Pilomotor muscles	α_1	Contraction
Sweat glands	α_1, cholinergic	Increased secretion
Eye		
Radial muscle, iris (pupil size)	α_1	Contraction: pupil dilation (mydriasis)
Ciliary muscle	β_2	Relaxation for far vision

*Predominant response.

fibrillation. An improvement in atrioventricular conduction (positive **dromotropic effect**) may also occur in conduction abnormalities.

VASCULAR EFFECTS. Vascular effects of adrenaline depend on the dose and the vascular bed affected. Low doses of adrenaline decrease total peripheral vascular resistance and lower blood pressure. In large doses adrenaline activates α receptors in the greater peripheral vascular system, which increases resistance and raises blood pressure. The dominant net response is often vasodilation; for example, during situations of high sympathetic demand, the release of adrenaline from the adrenal medulla constricts blood vessels in the skin and splanchnic areas but dilates those of skeletal muscles, thus shunting blood to the areas needed for fight-or-flight type responses.

Renal artery constriction and resistance occurs with adrenaline, and renal blood flow may be substantially reduced. Direct action on β_1 receptors on juxtaglomerular cells increases the secretion of renin.

CENTRAL NERVOUS SYSTEM EFFECTS. Adrenaline in therapeutic doses is not a CNS stimulant. Signs of restlessness, tremors and anxiety may be secondary to the effects of adrenaline on skeletal muscle, the cardiovascular system and changes in metabolism. Beneficial cerebral effects from adrenaline in persons with hypotension are thought to be the result of increased systemic pressure with a resultant improvement in cerebral blood flow.

SMOOTH MUSCLE EFFECTS. Generally, adrenaline relaxes smooth muscle of the gastrointestinal tract. The stomach is relaxed and the amplitude and tone of intestinal peristalsis are reduced. In theory, this may retard gastrointestinal emptying and propulsion of food; however, this effect is rare in humans with therapeutic doses of catecholamines.

In the urinary bladder, adrenaline causes trigone and sphincter constriction via α-receptor stimulation and detrusor relaxation (β-agonist activity), which may cause a delay in the desire to void and hence urine retention.

Adrenaline inhibits uterine contraction during the last months of pregnancy, and the β_2 agonists such as salbutamol are used to prevent premature labour.

RESPIRATORY EFFECTS. Adrenaline is a powerful bronchodilator and relieves respiratory distress due to allergens such as bee venom. In asthma it is likely that beneficial effects also occur through the effect of adrenaline on mast cells and on bronchial mucosa (see Chapter 31).

METABOLIC EFFECTS. Adrenaline inhibits insulin secretion and decreases the uptake of glucose by peripheral tissues, thus raising blood glucose levels. It stimulates lipolysis in adipose tissue which results in an increase in free fatty acids in blood; thus in response to high sympathetic drive there is an abundant supply of fuel and energy. Adrenaline also has a calorigenic effect, primarily as a result of increased metabolism, which increases oxygen consumption (Figure 12-2).

INDICATIONS. Adrenaline is used:
• for the emergency treatment of acute anaphylactic shock and severe acute reactions to drugs, animal serums, insect stings and other allergens, to relieve bronchospasm, urticaria, angio-oedema, and swelling of the mucosa.

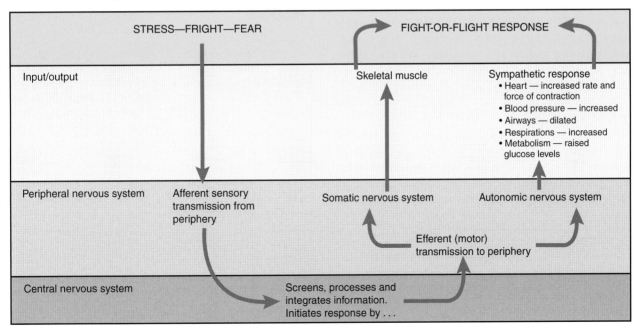

FIGURE 12-2 Nervous system response to high sympathetic drive.

Pulmonary congestion is also alleviated by constriction of mucosal blood vessels

- as an adjunct to local anaesthetics. Concurrent administration of adrenaline with local anaesthetics reduces circulation to the site, which results in a slowing of vascular absorption. This promotes the local effect of the anaesthetic and prolongs its duration of action
- as a haemostatic agent to control superficial bleeding from arterioles and capillaries in the skin, mucous membranes or other tissues
- in ocular surgery to control bleeding, induce mydriasis and conjunctival decongestion and to lower intraocular pressure
- to provide inotropic support in acute exacerbations of chronic heart failure and in situations of acute heart failure and septic shock
- to treat cardiac arrest.

Adrenaline should not be given orally because it is rapidly metabolised in the mucosa of the gastrointestinal tract and liver by catechol-*O*-methyltransferase (COMT) and monoamine oxidase (MAO). It is well absorbed after IM or SC injection.

Adrenaline has a rapid onset of action—3–5 minutes after inhalation or between 6 and 15 minutes after SC injection. The duration of action is 1–3 hours by inhalation and 1–4 hours after IM or SC injection. In severe anaphylaxis, asthma or cardiac arrest, doses may need to be repeated every 5–20 minutes, depending on the dosage used and the person's response. Adrenaline comes in two strengths: 1:1000, which is 1 mg adrenaline in 1 mL; and 1:10,000 which is 1 mg in 10 mL. When giving adrenaline intravenously the more dilute formulation (1:10,000) is used.

See the table Drug Interactions 12-1 for adrenaline. Adverse reactions include increased nervousness, restlessness, insomnia, tachycardia, tremors, sweating, hypertension, nausea, vomiting, pallor and weakness. With inhalation devices, adverse reactions include bronchial irritation and coughing (with high doses), dry mouth and throat, headaches and flushing of face and skin. High doses may cause ventricular arrhythmias.

Adrenaline is used with caution in persons with diabetes mellitus, closed-angle glaucoma, hypertension, ischaemic heart disease, hyperthyroidism and Parkinson's disease. When used in end-artery areas, such as fingers, toes or penis, the reduced blood supply to the area may result in ischaemia and gangrene. Avoid use in persons with known hypersensitivity to adrenaline (or sympathomimetics), organic brain damage, coronary insufficiency or shock.

NORADRENALINE (ACID TARTRATE)

Noradrenaline has a high affinity for α receptors and, because the blood vessels of the skin and mucous membrane contain α receptors, noradrenaline produces vasoconstriction in these tissues. The blood vessels (both arteriolar and venous beds)

DRUG INTERACTIONS 12–1 Adrenaline	
Drug	**Possible effect and management**
Halogenated anaesthetics such as halothane, enflurane, isoflurane etc	May sensitise the heart, increasing risk of severe arrhythmias. Monitor closely, as a reduction in dose of adrenaline (sympathomimetics) is usually necessary
Non-selective β-adrenoceptor antagonists (β-blockers)	With β-receptor blockade, α-receptor-mediated vasoconstriction predominates, resulting in hypertension, severe bradycardia and possibly heart block. Avoid combination or monitor very closely
α-adrenoceptor antagonists (α-blockers)	With α-receptor blockade, β-receptor-mediated effects predominate, producing hypotension
Digitalis glycosides	Digitalis sensitises the myocardium to the effects of adrenaline; the additive effect of the adrenaline increases the risk of arrhythmias. Avoid or a serious drug interaction may occur
Oxytocics	Concurrent use may produce severe hypertension
Tricyclic antidepressants, MAO inhibitor antidepressants, cocaine	Potentiate the effect of adrenaline. Concurrent use may result in arrhythmias, tachycardia and hypertension or hyperpyrexia. Avoid or a serious drug interaction may occur

in the visceral organs, including the kidneys, also contain predominantly α receptors. Consequently, noradrenaline causes vasoconstriction and a reduced blood flow through the kidneys and other visceral organs. Although noradrenaline activates β_1 receptors on the heart, changes in diastolic and systolic pressure, peripheral vascular resistance coupled with compensatory vagal reflexes results in no change in heart rate and cardiac output. Stimulation of α and β_1 receptors with noradrenaline is dose-related. At low doses (<0.002 mg/min), β_1 receptors are stimulated; at doses higher than 0.004

mg/min stimulation of α receptors increases total peripheral resistance. Titration of the dose in steps of 0.002–0.004 mg/min is based on haemodynamic response.

The main therapeutic effect of noradrenaline results from peripheral arteriolar vasoconstriction in all vascular beds. Both systolic and diastolic pressures are elevated, causing a rise in mean arterial pressure. Of importance during shock is constriction of the venous capacitance vessels, which reduces splanchnic and renal blood flow. This is brought about by severe restriction of tissue perfusion in these regions. In persistent hypotension after blood volume deficit has been corrected, noradrenaline helps to raise the blood pressure to an optimal level and establishes a more adequate circulation. Noradrenaline is selectively used for restoring blood pressure in acute hypotensive states such as sympathectomy, myocardial infarction, phaeochromocytomectomy, and blood transfusion reaction. It is also used as adjunct therapy in cardiac arrest.

Noradrenaline is administered only by intravenous infusion because oral noradrenaline is destroyed in the gastrointestinal tract and subcutaneous noradrenaline is poorly absorbed owing to local vasoconstriction at the site of injection. Onset of action is rapid by intravenous infusion and distribution is mainly to heart, spleen and glandular tissues. The half-life is short and ranges from about 30 seconds to 3 minutes. The drug is extensively metabolised in the liver and other tissues but the most significant clearance occurs by uptake into sympathetic nerves and other extraneuronal tissues. Most of the dose is excreted in urine as metabolites.

Noradrenaline's drug interactions are similar to those of adrenaline and include interactions with halogenated inhalational anaesthetics, β-adrenergic blocking agents, digitalis glycosides, tricyclic antidepressants, MAO inhibitors, cocaine and oxytocics. Adverse reactions include anxiety, dizziness, pallor, tremor, insomnia, headache, palpitations and, infrequently, hypertension and bradycardia.

Use noradrenaline with caution in patients with atherosclerosis, mesenteric and peripheral vascular thrombosis or other occlusive vascular diseases, metabolic acidosis, hypoxia or hyperthyroidism. Avoid use in persons with hypertension, hypersensitivity to sodium metabisulfite (the preservative in the solution, Box 12-2), hypovolaemia, myocardial infarction and ventricular arrhythmias. Noradrenaline solution should be protected from light and should not be used if brown coloration is present.

ISOPRENALINE (HYDROCHLORIDE)

Isoprenaline, a synthetic catecholamine, is a non-selective β-**adrenoceptor agonist**—it stimulates β1 and β2 receptors. The β1-receptor activity produces an increase in the force of myocardial contraction and heart rate. The β2-receptor response of the smooth muscle of the bronchi, skeletal muscle, gastrointestinal tract, and blood vessels of the splanchnic bed is relaxation. This drug also stimulates insulin secretion through β-receptor activation of pancreatic islet cells, and causes the release of free fatty acids from adipocytes.

Haemodynamically, the β_1 activity of the heart increases cardiac output and venous return to the heart. However, peripheral vascular resistance is reduced and in normal individuals this may cause a significant drop in blood pressure with excessive dosage. Isoprenaline is used as a cardiac stimulant in Stokes–Adams syndrome and serious episodes of heart block. It may also be used as adjunctive therapy in treatment of hypovolaemic states, septic shock, congestive heart failure and cardiogenic shock.

Oral absorption of isoprenaline is erratic and this route is no longer recommended. Following IV administration, the plasma level of isoprenaline declines in a biphasic manner. The first phase corresponds to rapid uptake in smooth muscle and cardiac tissue (around 5 minutes), while the second phase, which reflects widespread metabolism, lasts for more than 2.5 hours. Isoprenaline is metabolised by COMT in the gastrointestinal tract, liver and lungs and is excreted in the urine, predominantly as unchanged drug (60%).

Drug interactions with isoprenaline include β-blockers, which antagonise the therapeutic effect of isoprenaline (may precipitate asthma), and entacapone, which inhibits metabolism of isoprenaline and hence dose reduction of isoprenaline is necessary. Also avoid concurrent administration of isoprenaline with other sympathomimetic amines, as additive effects may occur and cardiotoxicity may result.

The range of adverse reactions for isoprenaline is similar to that for adrenaline. Use isoprenaline with caution in the elderly and in persons with diabetes mellitus, hyperthyroidism and ischaemic heart disease. Isoprenaline is contraindicated in the presence of tachycardia, ventricular arrhythmias and myocardial infarction, and in persons with known hypersensitivity to isoprenaline.

BOX 12-2 SULFITE SENSITIVITY

Sulfite is contained in the commercially available formulations of:
- adrenaline
- dobutamine
- dopamine
- metaraminol
- noradrenaline.

These drugs should not be administered to individuals with a known sensitivity to sulfite agents (sulfur dioxide, potassium or sodium bisulfite, potassium or sodium metabisulfite, sodium sulfite).

Symptoms of sulfite sensitivity include:
- skin: clamminess, flushing, pruritus, urticaria, cyanosis
- respiratory: bronchospasm, shortness of breath, wheezing, laryngeal oedema, respiratory arrest
- cardiovascular: hypotension, syncope
- CNS: severe dizziness, loss of consciousness
- other: anaphylaxis, death.

Drugs used for shock

During circulatory shock, the autonomic nervous system plays an essential compensatory role in an attempt to restore normal circulation; therefore many sympathomimetic drugs are used to manage this condition. Although there are other agents, the five drugs that are widely used for circulatory shock are adrenaline, noradrenaline, dopamine (which all produce vasoconstriction to varying degrees), dobutamine and isoprenaline. The use of isoprenaline in shock is limited by β_2-mediated vasodilation that may worsen the hypotension (Table 12-2).

DOPAMINE

Dopamine is a catecholamine that occurs as the immediate precursor of noradrenaline (see Figure 10-9). It acts both directly on various receptors and indirectly by releasing noradrenaline. Dopamine stimulates dopaminergic receptors, β_1 receptors and, in high doses, α_1 and α_2 receptors. Its actions are dose-dependent and very complex.

Unlike noradrenaline, in low doses (0.5–2 mcg/kg/min), dopamine acts mainly on dopaminergic (D_1) receptors to cause vasodilation of the renal and mesenteric arteries. Renal vasodilation increases renal blood flow, usually with greater urine and sodium excretion.

In low to moderate doses (usually 2–10 mcg/kg/min), dopamine acts directly on the β_1 receptors on the myocardium and indirectly by releasing noradrenaline from myocardial storage sites. These actions increase myocardial contractility and stroke volume, thereby increasing cardiac output. Systolic blood pressure and pulse pressure may rise, with either no effect or a slight elevation in diastolic blood pressure. Nevertheless, total peripheral resistance is usually unchanged. Coronary blood flow and myocardial oxygen consumption increase, while heart rate increases only slightly at low doses.

With higher doses of dopamine (10 mcg/kg/min or more), α receptors are stimulated, increasing peripheral resistance.

As a consequence, higher doses may reduce urinary output, eliminating the benefit of D_1-mediated renal vasodilation.

Unlike noradrenaline, dopamine aids perfusion of vital splanchnic organ systems. The combination of cardiac and vascular effects has led to dopamine's successful use in the treatment of circulatory shock and refractory heart failure. Dopamine is used to correct haemodynamic imbalances associated with shock syndrome caused by myocardial infarction, trauma, endotoxin septicaemia, open heart surgery, renal failure and chronic cardiac decompensation (as in congestive heart failure).

Dopamine is administered by IV infusion. The drug has a rapid onset of action (2–5 minutes) and a short duration of action (5–10 minutes). It is widely distributed throughout the body and is actively taken up into sympathetic nerves but does not cross the blood–brain barrier and therefore does not act on central dopaminergic receptors. Dopamine is rapidly metabolised to inactive metabolites by COMT and MAO in the liver, kidney and plasma, these metabolites are excreted in the urine.

Adverse reactions include headaches, nausea, vomiting, angina, respiratory difficulties, decreased blood pressure and, less frequently, hypertension, irregular or ectopic heart beats, tachycardia and palpitations. For drug interactions, warnings and contraindications, see discussion of adrenaline (above).

DOBUTAMINE

Dobutamine, a synthetic catecholamine used primarily in cardiogenic shock, acts directly on heart muscle to increase the force of myocardial contraction. This response is attributed to the direct stimulation of cardiac β_1 receptors. At the same time, dobutamine produces comparatively little increase in heart rate or peripheral vascular resistance. By enhancing stroke volume, this agent is an effective positive inotropic drug. Because of its minimal influence on heart rate and blood pressure (both major determinants of myocardial oxygen

TABLE 12-2 Comparative information on drugs used for shock

DRUG	RECEPTOR SITE EFFECTS*			ORGAN RESPONSE†		
	β_1	β_2	α_1	Kidneys	Cardiac	BP
Adrenaline (high dose)	+ +	0	+++	D	I	I/D
Dobutamine	+++	+	0/+	0	I	0/I
Dopamine (high dose)	+ +	0	+++	I		0/I
Isoprenaline	+++	+++	0	I/D	I	#
Noradrenaline	+	+	+++	D	0/D	I

*Receptor site effects: α_1 = vasoconstriction; β_1 = inotropic effect, blood vessel effects; β_2 = vasodilation.
†Organ response: kidneys = renal perfusion; cardiac = cardiac output; BP = blood pressure.
+ = minimal effect; ++ = moderate effect; +++ = greatest effect; 0 = no effect; I = increased; D = decreased; # = usual doses maintain or raise systolic pressure.

demand), it is valuable for use in individuals with low cardiac output. Dobutamine does not have any effect on dopamine receptors and does not cause vasodilation in the kidney.

Dobutamine is administered intravenously in the short-term management of patients requiring inotropic support, as in those with congestive heart failure, cardiogenic shock due to myocardial infarction, or after cardiac surgery. Its beneficial effects include a progressive increase in cardiac output and a decrease in pulmonary capillary wedge pressure, thereby improving ventricular contraction. The onset of action of dobutamine is within 1–2 minutes and it has a duration of action of about 10 minutes. Its plasma half-life is less than 3 minutes, as it is rapidly metabolised by liver COMT to form methyldobutamine, which is conjugated with glucuronic acid and excreted in the urine. The glucuronide metabolite has no significant cardiovascular activity.

Drug interactions are similar to those of adrenaline with regard to α- and β-blockers, general anaesthetics and oxytocin. Additive vasodilatory effects also occur with the coadministration of nitroprusside. In combination with milrinone there is an increased potential for tachycardia and arrhythmias. Adverse reactions include nausea, headache, respiratory distress, angina, palpitations, tachycardia, hypertension and, commonly, ventricular ectopic beats. Hence dobutamine is contraindicated in persons with atrial fibrillation, ventricular arrhythmias and phaeochromocytoma.

Indirect-acting sympathomimetics

Indirect acting sympathomimetics trigger the release of noradrenaline and adrenaline from their storage sites in the adrenal medulla and sympathetic neurons; these neurotransmitters then activate α and β receptors. Some of these drugs also stimulate the receptors directly but they are primarily considered to be indirect-acting drugs. Agents in this class include ephedrine (Drug Monograph 12-1), metaraminol, phenylephrine (Figure 12-3) and the amphetamines (Chapter 20).

Metaraminol

Metaraminol is a vasopressor agent with both direct (primarily) and indirect effects on the sympathetic system. It acts indirectly by causing the release of noradrenaline, and directly via an action on β and $α_1$ receptors, although it has predominantly more α activity. In general it is less potent than noradrenaline.

Metaraminol has a positive inotropic effect, constricts blood vessels, increases peripheral resistance, elevates both systolic and diastolic blood pressure and improves cardiac contractility. Adverse reactions are dose-related. Overdosage may cause severe hypertension, sinus arrhythmias, myocardial infarction and cardiac arrest.

Metaraminol is used for the treatment of acute hypotensive states occurring with spinal anaesthesia and as an adjunct in the treatment of hypotension due to haemorrhage, cardiogenic shock or septicaemia. This drug is infrequently used in anaesthesia and intensive care.

ADRENOCEPTOR ANTAGONISTS
α-adrenoceptor-antagonists

α-adrenergic antagonists compete with catecholamines at α-receptor sites and inhibit sympathetic stimulation. The main groups of drugs are:
- $α_1$-selective antagonists such as prazosin, tamsulosin and terazosin
- non-selective ($α_1$ and $α_2$) antagonists such as phenoxybenzamine, phentolamine and labetalol
- ergot alkaloids, which usually act as partial α-adrenergic antagonists. These have many actions but the α-blocking effect is not used therapeutically. Ergot alkaloids are used in the treatment of migraine, which is discussed in Chapter 21.

$α_1$-adrenoceptor antagonists

The principal uses of prazosin (Drug Monograph 12-2), terazosin and tamsulosin are for the treatment of hypertension and for symptomatic relief of urinary obstruction in benign prostatic hypertrophy. Selective blockade of postsynaptic α_1 receptors results in a decrease in peripheral vascular resistance because of inhibition of catecholamine-induced vasoconstriction. Only a minor increase in heart rate occurs because these drugs have negligible α_2-adrenoceptor activity.

As the smooth muscle in the neck of the urinary bladder has α receptors, blockade results in reduced resistance to urinary flow.

Non-selective (α_1 and α_2) antagonists

These agents include phenoxybenzamine, phentolamine and labetalol.

PHENOXYBENZAMINE (HYDROCHLORIDE)

Phenoxybenzamine is a long-acting, irreversible α_1- and α_2-adrenergic-blocking agent that abolishes or decreases the receptiveness of α receptors to adrenergic stimuli. At higher doses it also antagonises the action of acetylcholine, histamine and 5-hydroxytryptamine (5-HT, serotonin) because it covalently binds to the various receptors. This covalent interaction with α receptors results in a long duration of action and a progressive decrease in peripheral vascular resistance. A reflex increase in heart rate occurs that may be exacerbated by blockade of presynaptic α_2 receptors, which

results in release of noradrenaline, which in turn causes tachycardia. Phenoxybenzamine is used in the management of phaeochromocytoma and the preparation of patients with this condition for surgery.

Oral absorption of the drug is variable and the onset of action occurs in 1–2 hours. The clinical effect of the drug can persist for 3–4 days and this most probably relates to turnover time of the receptor. The half-life is in the order of 24 hours, with metabolism in the liver and excretion via urine and faeces.

Avoid concurrent use of phenoxybenzamine with other sympathomimetics, such as adrenaline, as unopposed stimulation of β_2 receptors will exacerbate the hypotension and reflex tachycardia. Adverse reactions include dizziness (postural hypotension), miosis, tachycardia, nasal congestion, confusion, dry mouth, headache and inhibition of ejaculation. Use with caution in persons with heart failure, coronary artery disease, respiratory infections or renal impairment. The drug is contraindicated when hypotension is undesirable, e.g. after cerebrovascular accident and myocardial infarction.

PHENTOLAMINE (MESYLATE)

Phentolamine competitively blocks α_2 (presynaptic) and α_1 (postsynaptic) receptors equally. The action occurs at both arterial and venous vessels. This direct relaxation of vascular smooth muscle lowers total peripheral resistance, inducing a marked reflex tachycardia. This drug is used to prevent or control hypertensive episodes in the individual with

---

DRUG MONOGRAPH 12-1 EPHEDRINE (SULFATE)

Ephedrine has both a direct and an indirect sympathomimetic action. It acts indirectly by stimulating the release of noradrenaline from presynaptic nerve terminals and also acts directly on both α and β receptors. Like adrenaline and noradrenaline, ephedrine has positive inotropic and chronotropic activities, but it is a less effective vasoconstrictor.

INDICATIONS Parenteral ephedrine has been used in hypotensive patients who do not respond to fluid replacement and as a vasopressor agent in hypotensive states secondary to spinal anaesthesia. Ephedrine has been used to produce bronchodilation in bronchial asthma and reversible bronchospasm, but generally more $\beta2$-selective drugs are used.

PHARMACOKINETICS Absorption of the drug is rapid after IM or SC administration. Onset of action occurs within 10–20 minutes of IM administration. The duration of the pressor effects and cardiac responses after parenteral administration of ephedrine is 1 hour and the half-life of the drug is 3–11 hours. Most of the drug (55%–75%) is excreted unchanged in urine with the remainder metabolised in the liver.

DRUG INTERACTIONS, WARNINGS AND CONTRA-INDICATIONS See discussion of adrenaline.

ADVERSE REACTIONS These include a range of cardiac effects (e.g. palpitations, angina, bradycardia, tachycardia, hypotension and hypertension, arrhythmias), gastrointestinal effects (e.g. nausea, vomiting) and CNS effects (e.g. nervousness, insomnia, fear, irritability, confusion, delirium and euphoria).

These are similar to those for adrenaline, although ephedrine is not available in aerosol form, so coughing and local irritation are not reported. In addition, ephedrine may cause mood changes and hallucinations.

DOSAGE AND ADMINISTRATION For vasopressor effects the adult ephedrine dose IM or SC is 25–50 mg, repeated if necessary. If an immediate effect is desired it may be administered IV at a dose of 10–25 mg, which may be repeated every 5–10 minutes if required. In children the dose recommended is 3 mg/kg/day via the IV or SC route, administered as 4–6 divided doses.

phaeochromocytoma, especially preoperatively and during surgery.

Phentolamine is administered IM and IV. Its half-life is around 19 minutes after IV administration but the haemodynamic response may persist for up to 12 hours. About 13% of the drug is excreted in urine unchanged. Drug interactions, adverse effects and warnings and contraindications are similar to those of phenoxybenzamine.

LABETALOL

Labetalol acts on both α_1 and β receptors and competitively antagonises the action of catecholamines. It is a complex drug that selectively blocks α_1, β_1 and β_2 receptors but also partially stimulates β_2 receptors and inhibits the neuronal uptake of noradrenaline (similar to the action of cocaine). Blockade of α_1 receptors leads to a fall in peripheral vascular resistance, while blockade of β_1 receptors prevents the reflex sympathetic stimulation of the heart. Labetalol is indicated for the treatment of hypertension.

Rapid absorption occurs after oral administration, and peak plasma concentration occurs within 20–90 minutes. Bioavailability is highly variable (11%–86%), due primarily to extensive presystemic metabolism. Labetalol is extensively metabolised to glucuronide conjugates that are excreted in urine (55%–60%) and faeces (12%–27%).

Drug interactions, adverse effects, warnings, contra-indications, dosage and administration are discussed in the following section in the context of the predominant β-blocking activity of labetalol.

β-adrenoceptor-antagonists

β-adrenoceptor antagonists, commonly referred to as β-blockers, competitively block the actions of catecholamines (Figure 12-3). The main group is the β_1-selective blockers that are frequently referred to as cardioselective blockers because these agents block β_1 receptors on the heart. At high doses, however, β_1 selectivity diminishes and the adverse effects of β_2 blockade then need to be considered. Drugs that block both types of receptors, β_1 and β_2, are referred to as non-selective β-adrenoceptor antagonists. The use of all of these drugs is contraindicated in people with asthma because of inhibition of bronchodilation mediated by β_2 receptors.

A further differentiation of β-blockers relates to a property called **intrinsic sympathomimetic activity** (ISA). The ISA property was initially believed to be advantageous when compared with agents that possessed only β-blocking effects. It was suggested that fewer serious adverse effects would occur with such agents but, clinically, the significance of this property has not been proved. Intrinsic sympathomimetic activity causes partial stimulation of the β receptor, although this effect is less than that of a pure agonist. For example, if a person has a slow heart rate at rest, the partial agonists may help to increase the heart rate, but if the person has a rapid heart rate or tachycardia from exercise, these agents may help to slow the heart rate, primarily due to the predominant β-blocking effect. It is believed that the only role for the ISA property might be in treating patients who experience severe bradycardia from non-ISA medications (Carter et al 1995).

DRUG MONOGRAPH 12-2   PRAZOSIN

Prazosin was the first of the α_1-selective antagonists developed in the 1970s. In 2005 around 475,000 pre-scriptions for prazosin were written in Australia. Blockade of α_1 receptors in arterioles and veins leads to a decrease in peripheral vascular resistance, reducing venous return to the heart. Unlike other vasodilator drugs, prazosin does not produce a reflex tachycardia.

PHARMACOKINETICS Prazosin is well absorbed after oral administration, with bioavailability in the order of 50%–70%. Peak concentration occurs about 1–3 hours after an oral dose and, as the drug is highly bound to plasma proteins, less than 5% is free in the circulation. The plasma half-life ranges from 2.5 to 3.5 hours and more than 90% of the drug is metabolised in the liver. Both the metabolites and unchanged drug (about 10%) are excreted in urine.

An increase in plasma half-life (about 7 hours) and bioavailability (2–3-fold) occurs in persons with congestive cardiac failure. Some of the metabolites of prazosin also have antihypertensive activity, which may contribute to the effect of the drug.

DRUG INTERACTIONS The first dose of prazosin may

cause hypotension. The risk of this first-dose phenomenon may be increased by β-blockers, diuretics and calcium channel blockers.

ADVERSE REACTIONS Common adverse reactions include postural hypotension, dizziness, headaches, drowsi-ness, fatigue, nasal congestion and urinary urgency.

WARNINGS AND CONTRAINDICATIONS Care should be exercised in persons with pre-existing renal disease (which may exacerbate the first-dose effect), liver disease (which may necessitate a dosage reduction) and the elderly (who are often more likely to suffer orthostatic hypotension). Prazosin is contraindicated in heart failure associated with mechanical obstruction such as aortic stenosis and in persons with known sensitivity to prazosin.

DOSAGE AND ADMINISTRATION For the treatment of hypertension, the dosage initially is 0.5 mg twice daily for 3–7 days, increasing to 1 mg 2–3 times daily. The maintenance dose range is 3–20 mg daily in 2–3 divided doses and the optimal response may take up to 6 weeks to occur.

Table 12-3 classifies adrenergic blocking drugs by receptor activity. The prototype of the β-adrenoceptor antagonists is propranolol and it is the drug against which all others are compared.

Mechanism of action

β-adrenoceptor antagonists competitively block β-receptor sites located on the heart, smooth muscle of the bronchi and blood vessels, kidney, pancreas, uterus, brain and liver. Cardiac muscle contains principally β_1 receptors, while smooth muscle sites contain primarily β_2 receptors.

Cardiovascular effects

Pharmacologically, blockade of β_1 receptors on the heart decreases rate, conduction velocity, myocardial contractility and cardiac output. The antianginal effects produced by β-blockers are primarily a result of the reduction in myocardial oxygen requirements because of the diminished heart rate and myocardial contractility. Their antihypertensive actions result from decreased cardiac output, without a reflex increase in peripheral vascular resistance, diminished sympathetic outflow from the vasomotor centre in the brain to the peripheral blood vessels, and reduced renin release by the kidney. Antiarrhythmic activity is associated with

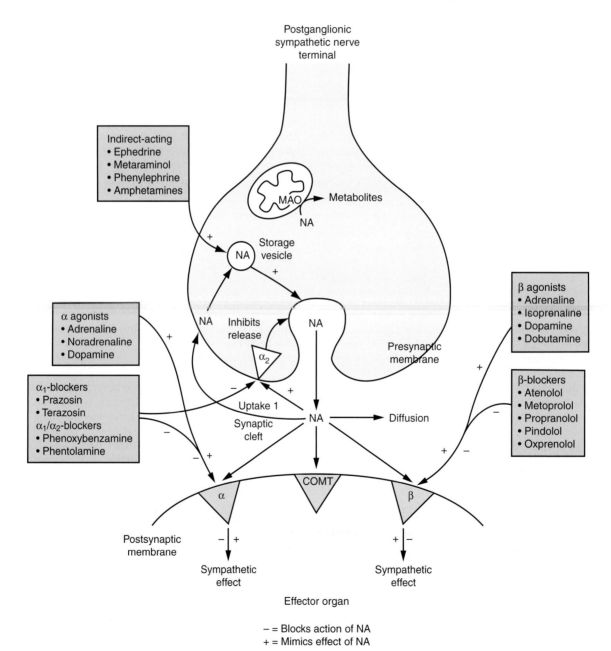

FIGURE 12-3 Site of action of drugs affecting noradrenergic transmission.

TABLE 12-3 Classification of β-blockers

Selective β₁-adrenoceptor antagonists

Atenolol, betaxolol, bisoprolol, esmolol, metoprolol

Non-selective β₁- and β₂-adrenoceptor antagonists

Carvedilol,* labetalol,* levobunolol, propranolol, sotalol, timolol

Non-selective β₁- and β₂-adrenoceptor antagonists with ISA activity

Pindolol, oxprenolol

*Also α₁ antagonists.

Source: Carter et al 1995; Olin 1998.

CLINICAL INTEREST BOX 12-2 WITHDRAWAL OF A β-BLOCKING AGENT

Abrupt cessation of β-blockers can cause a rebound phenomenon that exacerbates hypertension, angina or ventricular arrhythmias and may precipitate a myocardial infarction. It is recommended that the dose of a β-blocking agent be reduced gradually (Therapeutic Guidelines Cardiovascular Writing Group 2003). The person should be advised to avoid vigorous physical exercise or activity during this time to decrease the risk of a myocardial infarction or cardiac dysrhythmia. If withdrawal signs occur (angina or chest pain, sweating, rebound hypertension, dysrhythmias, tremors, tachycardia or respiratory distress), these may be controlled by temporary reinstitution of the drug.

---

depression of sinus node function, slowing of conduction in the atria and the atrioventricular (AV) node and an increased refractory period of the AV node. Sotalol also prolongs the action potential duration and is used specifically as an antiarrhythmic drug.

Various mechanisms may be involved in the prevention of vascular headaches, such as prevention of arterial vasodilation, inhibition of platelet aggregation and increased oxygen release to tissues.

Metabolic effects

Catecholamines are involved in the regulation of lipid and carbohydrate metabolism and, in response to hypoglycaemia, promote glycogen breakdown and mobilisation of glucose. Blockade of β receptors prevents an adequate response to hypoglycaemia in people with insulin-dependent diabetes and may also mask the symptoms. Non-selective β-blockers raise plasma triglyceride levels and lower high-density lipoprotein levels, raising concern that this may be undesirable in people with hypertension.

Indications

β-blocking drugs are used to treat angina pectoris, hypertension, Fallot's tetralogy, tremors and tachycardia associated with anxiety and hyperthyroidism; to prevent or treat cardiac arrhythmias, myocardial infarction (acute and in the long term), vascular headaches, phaeochromocytoma and glaucoma (topical eye-drops); and as an adjunct to conventional therapy for heart failure (the only approved drugs in this setting are carvedilol, bisoprolol and metoprolol).

Pharmacokinetics

For the pharmacokinetics and usual adult dose range of β-blockers, see Table 12-4. These drugs are either metabolised in the liver or excreted as unchanged drug by the kidneys. This allows the use of different agents in pre-existing conditions of hepatic or renal impairment; for example, a drug such as metoprolol is metabolised by the liver, which is more suitable for use in persons with renal impairment, whereas atenolol is more suitable in a person with hepatic disease because it is predominantly cleared by the kidneys. When these agents are discontinued they should be withdrawn slowly to avoid inducing a potentially serious withdrawal syndrome. (See Clinical Interest Box 12-2 for information on withdrawal of a β-blocking agent.)

Drug interactions

See table Drug Interactions 12-2 for the drug interactions of β-blockers.

Common adverse effects of β-blockers include insomnia, nightmares, depression, nausea, diarrhoea, dizziness, fatigue, hypotension, heart failure, heart block, bradycardia, cold hands and feet, bronchospasm and shortness of breath. Use β-blockers with caution in persons with liver or renal function impairment, heart failure, diabetes, hyperlipidaemia, peripheral vascular disease, hyperthyroidism, myasthenia gravis or phaeochromocytoma. β-blockers are contraindicated in persons with drug hypersensitivity, cardiogenic shock, heart block, bradycardia, severe hypotension, and asthma and chronic obstructive airways disease. For pregnancy safety, see the Pregnancy Safety box at the end of this chapter.

DRUG INTERACTIONS 12–2 Beta-blockers

Drug	Possible effect and management
Adrenaline	Severe hypertension and bradycardia may occur. Use with extreme caution and monitor closely
Antidiabetic agents, oral hypoglycaemic agents, insulin	May mask symptoms of and prolong hypoglycaemia. Symptoms of hypoglycaemia such as increased heart rate and lowered blood pressure may be blocked, making monitoring difficult. Monitoring of blood glucose levels and dosage adjustments of the hypoglycaemic agent may be necessary
Digoxin	May have an additive effect, increasing atrioventricular conduction time. Monitor heart rate and use with caution
Calcium channel blockers (diltiazem and verapamil)	Enhanced cardiac-depressant effects, further decreasing rate, contractility and conduction
Clonidine	Combination may produce severe adverse reactions. Each drug is associated with withdrawal symptoms such as rebound hypertension. Avoid combination
MAO inhibitors	Combination may result in hypotension and bradycardia. Use with caution and monitor closely
NSAIDs	Antihypertensive effect of β-blockers may be reduced. Monitor blood pressure and avoid concurrent use

TABLE 12-4 Pharmacokinetics and adult dose range of β-adrenoceptor antagonists*

DRUG	ORAL BIOAVAILABILITY (%)	HALF-LIFE (h)	ELIMINATION	ADULT DOSE RANGE
Atenolol	About 50	6–7	Renal (85%–100%)	25–100 mg/day
Betaxolol	Ophthalmic preparation	14–22	Liver/renal (>80%)	Eye-drops
Bisoprolol	About 80	9–12	Hepatic (50%)/renal (50%)	1.25–10 mg/day
Carvedilol	25	6–10	Hepatic (>75%)	6.25–50 mg/day
Esmolol	Parenteral	0.15	Red cell cytosolic esterases	Varies
Labetalol	About 20	6–8	Hepatic (95%)	200–800 mg/day
Levobunolol	Ophthalmic preparation	6–7	Hepatic (50%)	Eye-drops
Metoprolol	About 40	3–5	Hepatic (90%)	50–300 mg/day
Oxprenolol	24–60	1–3	Hepatic (95%)	80–320 mg/day
Pindolol	About 75	3–4	Hepatic (50%)/renal (50%)	10–30 mg/day
Propranolol	About 25	3–6	Hepatic (>99%)	40–320 mg/day
Sotalol	About 100	7–18	Renal (90%)	80–320 mg/day
Timolol	Ophthalmic preparation	5–6	Hepatic (85%)	Eye-drops

*Consult approved product information for individual drugs and specific indications.

PREGNANCY SAFETY

ADEC Category	Drug
A	Adrenaline, ephedrine, isoprenaline
B1	Phentolamine
B2	Dobutamine, phenoxybenzamine
B3	Dopamine
C	Atenolol, betaxolol, bisoprolol, carvedilol, esmolol, labetalol, levobunolol, oxprenolol, metaraminol, metoprolol, pindolol, propranolol, sotalol, timolol
Unclassified	Noradrenaline

DRUGS AT A GLANCE 12: Drugs affecting noradrenergic transmission

Therapeutic group	Pharmacological group	Key examples	Key pages
Sympathomimetics	Adrenoceptor agonists	adrenaline	187
		dobutamine	192
		dopamine	192
		ephedrine	194
		isoprenaline	191
		noradrenaline	190
Sympatholytics	α-adrenoceptor antagonists	phenoxybenzamine	194
		phentolamine	194
		prazosin	195
	β-adrenoceptor antagonists	atenolol	195–198
		carvedilol	195–198
		esmolol	195–198
		labetalol	195–198
		metoprolol	195–198
		propranolol	195–198
		sotalol	195–198

KEY POINTS

- A comprehensive understanding of the autonomic nervous systems is necessary to understand the principal functions of each system, the primary receptor effects and the pharmacological agents that enhance, mimic or block activity.
- The sympathetic nervous system is responsible for major physiological changes in the body in response to high demand or stressful situations.
- Drugs that affect this system are either adrenergic (sympathomimetic) drugs (i.e. they mimic the effects of sympathetic nerve stimulation) or adrenergic-blocking (sympatholytic) drugs (i.e. drugs that compete at receptor sites to inhibit

adrenergic sympathetic stimulation). These agents may be direct-acting or indirect-acting drugs and affect α- and/or β-adrenoceptors.

- Adrenaline is an important drug (a direct-acting catecholamine) that stimulates α, β_1 and β_2 receptors. It is commonly used in the treatment of asthma, emergency treatment of anaphylactic shock and cardiac arrest, treatment of local haemostasis, and in management of simple open-angle glaucoma.
- Noradrenaline has a high affinity for α receptors and is thus a potent peripheral arteriolar vasoconstrictor. It raises both systolic and diastolic pressure.
- Dobutamine is used for patients with low cardiac output because it directly stimulates the β_1-adrenergic receptors of the heart. Dopamine's effects are dose-related and in the lower dose range this agent causes vasodilation of the renal and mesenteric arteries. Both these agents have been used for the treatment of circulatory shock.
- The indirect-acting sympathomimetics include ephedrine and metaraminol.
- The adrenergic-blocking agents (sympatholytic) are classified by their receptor activity, i.e. α- and/or β- receptor competitive blocking effects. The main groups of α antagonists are the α_1-selective antagonists such as prazosin and terazosin, the non-selective α_1 and α_2 antagonists such as phenoxybenzamine, phentolamine and labetalol, and the ergot alkaloids (which have a blocking effect not used clinically).
- The classification of β-blocking drugs includes the selective β_1 (cardioselective) agents such as atenolol and metoprolol, the non-selective β-blocking agents such as propranolol, and the non-selective β-blocking agents with ISA activity, such as pindolol and oxprenolol.

REVIEW EXERCISES

1. Compare and contrast the pharmacological effects of adrenaline, dopamine, dobutamine and noradrenaline on the cardiovascular system.
2. Describe the pharmacological effects of noradrenaline in the treatment of acute hypotensive episodes. What receptors are affected?
3. Discuss the pharmacological effects of β-adrenergic-blocking agents when used to treat angina pectoris and hypertension.

REFERENCES AND FURTHER READING

Australian Medicines Handbook 2006. Adelaide: AMH, 2006.
Benowitz NL, Pentel P, Leatherman J. Drug use in the critically ill. Ch. 13 in: Speight TM, Holford NHG (eds). Avery's Drug Treatment. 4th edn. Auckland: Adis International, 1997.
Cardiovascular Expert Group. Therapeutic Guidelines: Cardiovascular 2003. Melborne: Therapeutic Guidelines Limited, 2003.
Carter BL, Furmaga EM, Murphy CH. Essential hypertension. In: Young LY, Koda-Kimble MA (eds). Applied Therapeutics: The Clinical Use of Drugs. 6th edn. Vancouver: Applied Therapeutics, 1995.
Dollery C (ed.). Therapeutic Drugs. Vols 1 and 2. London: Churchill Livingstone, 1991.
Gonzalez JP, Clissold SP. Ocular levobunolol: a review of its pharmacodynamic and pharmacokinetic properties and therapeutic efficacy. Drugs 1987; 34: 648–61.
Hoffman BB. Catecholamines, sympathomimetic drugs, and adrenergic receptor antagonists. Ch. 10 in: Hardman JG, Limbird LE, Gilman AG (eds). Goodman & Gilman's The Pharmacological Basis of Therapeutics. 10th edn. New York: McGraw Hill, 2001.
Moore KE. Drugs affecting the sympathetic nervous system. Ch. 10 in: Brody TM, Larner J, Minneman KP (eds). Human Pharmacology, Molecular to Clinical. 3rd edn. St Louis: Mosby, 1998.
Olin BR. Facts and Comparisons. Philadelphia: JB Lippincott, 1998.
Rang HP, Dale MM, Ritter JM, Moore PK. Pharmacology. 5th edn. Edinburgh: Churchill Livingstone, 2003 [ch. 11].
Ravel R. Adrenal function tests. Ch. 30 in: Ravel R. Clinical Laboratory Medicine. 6th edn. St Louis, Mosby, 1995.
United States Pharmacopoeial Convention. USPDI: Drug Information for the Health Care Professional. 18th edn. Rockville: USPDI, 1998.

evolve More weblinks at http://evolve.elsevier.com/AU/Bryant/pharmacology/

CHAPTER 13

Overview of the Somatic Nervous System and Drugs Affecting Neuromuscular Transmission

CHAPTER FOCUS

The somatic nervous system is the division of the peripheral nervous system that coordinates consciously controlled functions such as movement, posture and respiration. In this system a single motor neuron connects the central nervous system to the skeletal muscles, which are the effector organs. Blockade of neuromuscular transmission by drugs is used as an adjunct to anaesthesia for producing muscle relaxation. In clinical practice, anticholinesterase agents are used for reversing neuromuscular blockade. Poisoning from organophosphate anticholinesterase agents can also occur as a result of their use as pesticides and chemical warfare agents.

OBJECTIVES

- To discuss the nicotinic actions of acetylcholine.
- To explain the process of neuromuscular transmission.
- To explain the differences between non-depolarising and depolarising neuromuscular blocking drugs in terms of their pharmacological effects and adverse reactions.
- To discuss the major signs and symptoms of an overdose of an anticholinesterase agent.

KEY DRUGS

neostigmine
pancuronium
suxamethonium

KEY TERMS

acetylcholinesterase
anticholinesterase agents
depolarising drugs
neuromuscular blocking drugs
neuromuscular junction
non-depolarising drugs
somatic nervous system

KEY ABBREVIATIONS

NMJ neuromuscular junction
ACh acetylcholine
AChE acetylcholinesterase

THE second major division of the peripheral nervous system is the **somatic nervous system** (Figure 10-1), which coordinates consciously controlled functions, including movement, posture and respiration. In this system, a single motor neuron connects the central nervous system (CNS) to the skeletal muscles, which are the effector organs of the somatic nervous system. Often called the voluntary nervous system, this system allows us to consciously control our skeletal muscles and hence movement. Initiating and controlling both gross movements (such as jumping or walking) and precise movements (such as those done with our hands) involves the motor cortex, which initiate and control movement, the basal ganglia, which integrate and establish our muscle tone, and the cerebellum, which ensures our movements are smooth and coordinated. Integration of these systems aids in the maintenance of normal posture and balance.

Once the primary motor area of the cerebral cortex initiates a voluntary movement, nerve impulses propagate from the motor cortex through upper motor neurons that cross over in the medulla oblongata to the other side; thus, muscles on the right side of the body are controlled by the left motor cortex, and the right side of the brain controls the muscles on the left side of the body. The upper motor neurons terminate in the anterior grey horn of the spinal cord at each spinal segment. In many instances, the upper motor neurons synapse first with interneurons, which act as the connection with the lower motor neurons; they in turn innervate skeletal muscles of the trunk and limbs (Figure 13-1). The lower motor neurons are the final common pathway that connects the CNS to the skeletal muscles.

THE NEUROMUSCULAR JUNCTION

The synapse between the lower motor (somatic) neuron and the skeletal muscle is called the **neuromuscular junction**

(NMJ). At the NMJ, the motor neuron divides, forming a cluster of synaptic end bulbs that contain vesicles carrying the neurotransmitter acetylcholine (ACh). Following arrival of a nerve action potential, ACh is released from the vesicles and diffuses across the synaptic cleft to act on postsynaptic nicotinic receptors on the motor end-plate of the muscle fibre. As muscle fibres tend to be long, the NMJ is usually near the centre of the fibre. This allows the impulse to spread evenly towards the ends of the muscle fibres and ensures that contraction occurs simultaneously throughout the length of the muscle. As each nerve impulse produces only one muscle contraction, the action of ACh is rapidly terminated (within 1 ms) by acetylcholinesterase, which is attached to the collagen fibres. The release and metabolism of acetylcholine occur by the same mechanisms as those described for the parasympathetic nervous system (Chapter 10). The difference is that in the somatic nervous system acetylcholine acts on postsynaptic nicotinic receptors on the motor end-plate, whereas the postsynaptic receptors in the parasympathetic system are muscarinic receptors.

Motor end-plate nicotinic receptors

Nicotinic receptors mediate the effect of ACh on skeletal muscles, and they are the main biological targets of the tobacco alkaloid nicotine. The receptor is classed as an ion channel and is composed of five subunits arranged in a circular manner with the ion channel in the centre. The human adult skeletal muscle receptor subunits are designated using a Greek letter: there are two alpha (α) subunits and one beta (β), one delta (δ) and one epsilon (ϵ) subunit. The bulk of the receptor faces the extracellular surface. The density of the receptors is very high on the motor end-plate. When two molecules of ACh bind (one molecule to each of the α subunits), the channel opens immediately and sodium ions flow through, causing depolarisation of the motor end-plate. This triggers the muscle action potential,

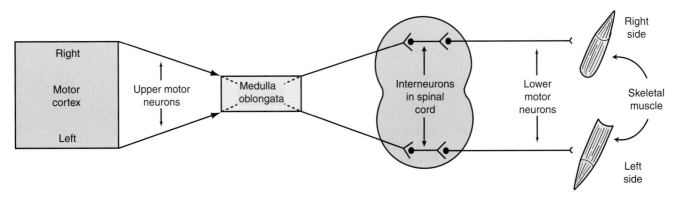

FIGURE 13-1 Diagrammatic representation of motor pathways from the right and left sides of the motor cortex innervating skeletal muscles on the opposite sides of the body.

causing muscle contraction (Figure 13-2). Contraction occurs because of a sliding filament mechanism involving actin and myosin (see Chapter 23).

There are many sites at which drugs and toxins can interrupt neuromuscular transmission. These include blockade of action potential generation in the motor neuron, inhibition of release of ACh (Clinical Interest Box 13-1), and blockade of postsynaptic receptors. The pharmacological agents of clinical relevance are those used principally as adjuncts to anaesthesia, and include drugs acting at postsynaptic receptors,

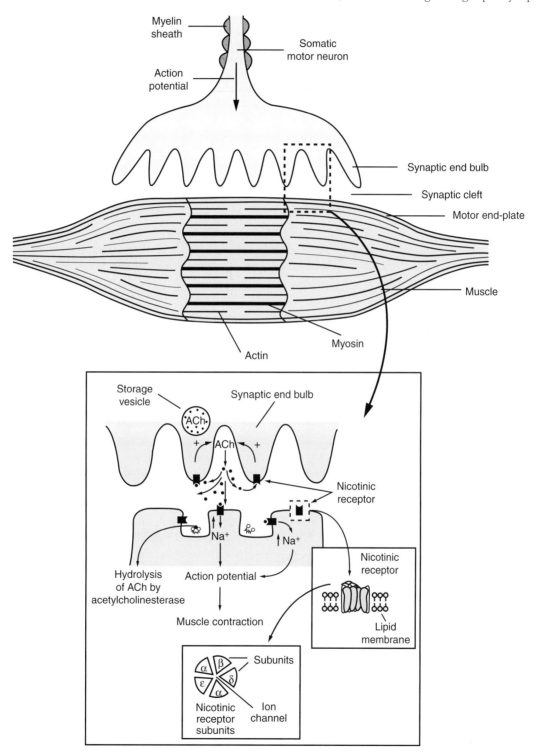

FIGURE 13-2 The neuromuscular junction, showing release of acetylcholine, which acts on both presynaptic and postsynaptic nicotinic receptors. The insets show enlargements of the relevant structures.

CLINICAL INTEREST BOX 13-1 COSMETIC USE OF BOTULINUM TOXIN, AN INHIBITOR OF ACETYLCHOLINE RELEASE

Although botulinum toxin is commonly associated with outbreaks of lethal food poisoning, it has been used since the 1970s for the treatment of facial dystonias (see Chapter 21 and Drug Monograph 35-3). Botulinum acts presynaptically, blocking the release of ACh and causing generalised muscle weakness. The muscle weakness produced slowly recovers over several months with the growth of new nerve terminals.

Different types of botulinum toxin exist and highly localised injections of small quantities of botulinum toxin type A (Botox) are widely used for cosmetic correction. The cosmetic use of botulinum toxin followed the observation by Jean Carruthers in 1987 that Botox reduced frown lines. Its use has now extended from frown lines to crow's feet, horizontal forehead creases, eyebrow shaping and chin dimpling (Klein & Glogau 2000). The drug was approved in

Australia in 1994 for the treatment of blepharospasm but it is also used widely in private cosmetic clinics for wrinkle treatment. The popularity of Botox continues to grow with an ever-increasing number of 'stars' having Botox injections prior to high-profile public appearances. Botox is often termed a 'cosmeceutical' and the aim is to use a sufficient dose at the right anatomical facial site to accomplish muscle weakening without muscle paralysis. Using the incorrect dose or imprecision in the injection site may result in a mask-like or frozen face or ptosis (eyelid drooping). Such is the social acceptability of Botox that it is now being used for vertical lip lines, flaring nostrils and to soften nasolabial folds. Unwanted paralysis is the biggest drawback and may not always be predictable. Drug interactions can also occur and the action of Botox is prolonged by concomitant use of aminoglycoside or spectinomycin antibiotics.

---

commonly referred to as neuromuscular blocking drugs, and anticholinesterase agents, which are also used for a variety of other therapeutic purposes. In addition, anticholinesterase agents are used as insecticides and chemical warfare agents, which can lead to situations of acute human exposure.

NEUROMUSCULAR BLOCKING DRUGS

The **neuromuscular blocking drugs** are principally of two types. The competitive drugs, or **non-depolarising drugs**, competitively block the action of ACh at postsynaptic and presynaptic nicotinic receptors, blocking the normal feedback loop that increases ACh release under conditions of enhanced stimulation. In contrast the **depolarising drugs**, which are nicotinic receptor agonists, maintain the depolarised state

---

CLINICAL INTEREST BOX 13-2 SITES OF ACTION OF TOXINS ON SOMATIC MOTOR NEURONS AND THE MOTOR END-PLATE

Many toxins impede skeletal muscle contraction, by mechanisms that include blocking conduction of motor neuron action potentials, disrupting neurotransmitter storage vesicles, depleting the nerve ending of ACh, preventing release of ACh, and blocking motor end-plate nicotinic receptors (Figure 13-3). Many of these toxins are found in food (e.g. botulinum), in spider venom (e.g. Australian redback and funnel-web spiders) and in the venom of the blue-ringed octopus (see Chapter 59).

---

of the motor end-plate, thus preventing transmission of another action potential. The agents that most typify the NMJ drugs are tubocurarine for the non-depolarising drugs, and suxamethonium for the depolarising drugs.

Non-depolarising blocking drugs

Curare is synonymous with the South American arrow-tip poisons that were used by indigenous people along the Amazon and Orinoco Rivers for killing animals. The pharmacologist Claude Bernard investigated the muscle paralysing effect of curare in 1856. He showed that the drug prevents response of skeletal muscle to nerve stimulation but does not inhibit contraction from a direct stimulus, nor does it block nerve conduction. These elegant experiments established the concept of nerve–muscle conduction, and in 1942 curare was introduced for promoting muscle relaxation during general anaesthesia. This heralded the search for other curare-like drugs. Although tubocurarine (the active constituent of curare) is no longer in clinical use, various synthetic drugs have been produced. These include atracurium, cisatracurium, mivacurium, pancuronium, rocuronium and vecuronium. As these drugs are quaternary ammonium compounds, they are poorly absorbed and do not readily cross the blood–brain barrier or placenta; the latter is an advantage when operating on pregnant women.

Effects on skeletal muscle

In general, the non-depolarising drugs produce rapid blockade characterised by motor weakness that progresses to total flaccid paralysis. Small muscles (e.g. those of the eyelid) are affected first, proceeding through to the limbs, neck, trunk and finally the diaphragm and intercostal muscles. With paralysis of the respiratory muscles, respiration ceases and mechanical ventilatory support is required. Return to normal muscle function varies markedly between individuals and between individual muscle groups. Normally function returns first to the respiratory system, the diaphragm and intercostal muscles; pharyngeal and facial muscles recover more slowly.

Effects on mast cells

Typically the non-depolarising neuromuscular blocking agents cause histamine release from mast cells. This often manifests as harmless cutaneous reactions (flushing and rash) but more severe symptoms can occur, including hypotension and bronchospasm. The effect is not related to an action at nicotinic receptors but is more likely due to the highly basic nature of these drugs. The tendency to cause histamine release varies among these drugs, with tubocurarine eliciting the greatest release and pancuronium, vecuronium and rocuronium showing lesser tendencies. The most frequently implicated drug is suxamethonium, and severe anaphylactoid reactions are more frequent in women.

Drug Monograph 13-1 describes pancuronium, and the main characteristics of the other non-depolarising NMJ blockers are summarised in Table 13-1.

Depolarising blocking drugs

Currently the only depolarising neuromuscular blocking drug in clinical use is **suxamethonium**. In contrast to tubocurarine, which blocks nicotinic receptors and produces flaccid muscle paralysis, suxamethonium acts as an agonist at the nicotinic receptors on the motor end-plate. Binding to the receptor results in persistent stimulation and maintains the depolarised state of the motor end-plate. Loss of electrical excitability ensues because the sodium channels remain open and the motor end-plate can no longer respond to an electrical stimulus (Figure 13-4). With suxamethonium, initial muscle fasciculations (twitching) occur because as each end-plate is depolarised it produces a localised action potential in the muscle fibre. As each fibre has only one motor end-plate when depolarised individually it is not sufficient to produce complete muscle contraction. These fasciculations subside quickly and neuromuscular blockade follows.

ANTICHOLINESTERASE AGENTS

Acetylcholinesterase (AChE) hydrolyses the neurotransmitter acetylcholine, forming choline and acetate (Figure 10-8). The enzyme is bound to the postsynaptic membrane and the active site, which resembles a deep gorge, contains

---

DRUG MONOGRAPH 13-1 PANCURONIUM

Pancuronium is a potent competitive antagonist of acetylcholine at nicotinic receptors on the skeletal muscle motor end-plate (Figure 13-4). Interruption of neuromuscular transmission requires occupancy of >70% of the nicotinic receptors while blockade requires >95% occupancy.

INDICATIONS As an adjunct to general anaesthesia to provide muscle relaxation during surgery.

PHARMACOKINETICS Pancuronium is widely distributed following IV administration and within 5 minutes high concentrations can be found in the kidney, liver and spleen. As the drug is highly water-soluble, urinary excretion begins almost immediately and up to 25% is excreted as unchanged drug. The remainder of the drug is cleared via hepatic metabolism and biliary excretion, both of which can be depressed in persons with liver disease. The half-life is >30 minutes. In the presence of pre-existing renal disease clearance can be reduced and the half-life prolonged.

DRUG INTERACTIONS Potentiation of effect can occur with inhalation anaesthetics, suxamethonium, antibiotics such as the aminoglycosides (which themselves cause blockade), diazepam, calcium channel blockers, lithium, propranolol and magnesium salts. A decrease in effect can occur with adrenaline, anticholinesterase agents such as neostigmine, high-dose corticosteroids, and the chloride salts of calcium, sodium and potassium.

ADVERSE REACTIONS These are uncommon but a slight increase in heart rate, cardiac output and blood pressure can occur. A life-threatening anaphylactoid reaction can occur but the incidence is less than 1 in 10,000 anaesthetics.

WARNINGS AND CONTRAINDICATIONS Care should be exercised with the use of pancuronium in people with hypertension or impaired hepatic or renal function. The drug is contraindicated in people with known hypersensitivity to pancuronium or the bromide ion (pancuronium is administered as a bromide salt).

DOSAGE AND ADMINISTRATION Pancuronium is administered IV and the usual dose range is 0.05–0.1 mg/kg in adults and in children >1 month of age. The incremental dose range is 0.01–0.02 mg/kg.

TABLE 13-1 Comparative information on non-depolarising neuromuscular blocking drugs

DRUG	ONSET OF BLOCKADE (MINUTES)	DURATION OF BLOCKADE (MINUTES)	ADEC PREGNANCY CATEGORY	COMMENTS
Atracurium	2–6	<30	C	Transient hypotension. Histamine release at higher clinical doses
Cisatracurium	2–7	10–35	C	Low incidence of flushing, hypotension and bronchospasm
Mivacurium	1–4	~15	B2	Reports of skin rash, transient bronchospasm, hypotension and tachycardia
Pancuronium	4–6	120–180	B2	See Drug Monograph 13-1
Rocuronium	1–3	30–40	B2	Limited adverse effects. No significant tachycardia or hypotension
Vecuronium	2–4	30–40	C	Limited adverse effects. Allergic cross-sensitivity with pancuronium

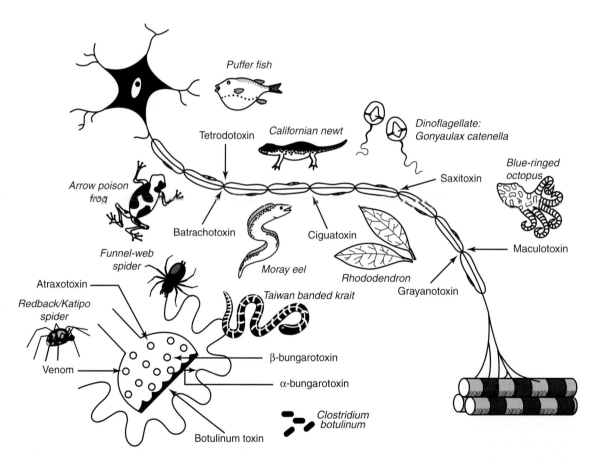

FIGURE 13-3 Summary diagram illustrating the sites of action of various toxins on somatic motor neurons and the motor end-plate. Tetrodotoxin, saxitoxin and maculotoxin prevent conduction in the axon by blocking the sodium channels; batrachotoxin, ciguatoxin and grayanotoxin block conduction by opening the sodium channels and thereby depolarising the axon membrane. *Latrodectus* spider spp (redback [AUST]/katipo [NZ]) venom, atraxotoxin and β-bungarotoxin disrupt the vesicles and deplete the nerve ending of acetylcholine. Botulinum toxin prevents the release of acetylcholine by acting on the axon terminal membrane. α-bungarotoxin combines specifically with the acetylcholine receptors on the muscle side of the junction. *Source*: Bowman 1973; published with permission from the *Pharmaceutical Journal*.

DRUG MONOGRAPH 13-2 SUXAMETHONIUM

INDICATIONS Suxamethonium is an analogue of acetylcholine and is the only truly short-acting muscle relaxant. It is used when brief muscle relaxation is required (e.g. electroconvulsive therapy, tracheal intubation, short surgical procedures and orthopaedic manipulations). In addition to its muscle relaxant properties suxamethonium affects the cardiovascular system, causing bradycardia.

PHARMACOKINETICS The onset of action of suxamethonium is rapid and the estimated half-life is on the order of 2–4 minutes. Blockade persists for about 10 minutes and the drug is rapidly hydrolysed by butyrylcholinesterase (also known as pseudocholinesterase or plasma cholinesterase). In some individuals with atypical butyrylcholinesterase, blockade can persist for an extended period. Hydrolysis results in formation of the metabolite succinylmonocholine, which is excreted in the urine.

DRUG INTERACTIONS Many drugs enhance the neuromuscular blocking activity of suxamethonium (e.g. lignocaine, non-penicillin antibiotics, β-blockers, quinidine, lithium carbonate, high-dose corticosteroids and some cancer chemotherapy drugs). Current sources should be consulted for a more extensive list.

ADVERSE REACTIONS Suxamethonium can cause profound and complex effects on the cardiovascular system, including bradycardia, tachycardia, arrhythmias, hypertension and cardiac arrest. Because of loss of

potassium from the motor end-plate, an increase in plasma potassium concentration can occur and this is important in situations of extensive burns and massive trauma and in people with muscular disorders. In rare situations suxamethonium can precipitate malignant hyperthermia, an often fatal condition characterised by intense muscle spasm and a rapid rise in body temperature. Although the action of suxamethonium is short, in some individuals prolonged apnoea occurs as a result of a butyrylcholinesterase deficiency, the use of anticholinesterase drugs that inhibit the action of butyrylcholinesterase or the presence of liver disease, which can cause a low butyrylcholinesterase concentration.

WARNINGS AND CONTRAINDICATIONS Care should be taken with the use of suxamethonium in people with electrolyte disturbances, low butyrylcholinesterase concentration, renal disease and concomitant digitalis therapy. The drug is contraindicated in people with a known or suspected familial history of malignant hyperthermia and in cases of extensive burns or multiple traumas.

DOSAGE AND ADMINISTRATION Dosage is individualised depending on the circumstances of use and the degree of relaxation required. The drug is usually administered IV but the IM route may be used when a suitable vein is not accessible. Under no circumstances should suxamethonium be administered to a conscious person.

within its structure three crucial amino acids: a serine and a histidine, which form the esteratic site, and a glutamate, termed the anionic site. Together, these three amino acids are crucial for hydrolysis of acetylcholine and are the targets for the reversible and irreversible acetylcholinesterase inhibitors (Figure 13-4). **Anticholinesterase agents** are used for conditions such as glaucoma, Alzheimer's disease and myasthenia gravis, and to reverse neuromuscular blockade after anaesthesia. In addition, acetylcholinesterase is the biological target of pesticides and chemical warfare agents.

Three broad categories of anticholinesterase agents exist:
- short-acting drugs, e.g. edrophonium (not used clinically)
- medium-acting drugs, e.g. **neostigmine** (used for myasthenia gravis and reversal of NMJ blockade; see Drug Monograph 13-3), pyridostigmine (for myasthenia gravis) and physostigmine (for the reversal of the CNS effects of anticholinesterase agents)
- irreversible drugs, e.g. pesticides and chemical warfare agents.

The main pharmacological and toxicological effects of these agents are explained by enhanced levels of acetylcholine (Table 13-2). See also Clinical Interest Box 13-3.

TABLE 13-2 Therapeutic and toxicological effects of anticholinesterase agents

SITE	EFFECT
NMJ	Inhibition of AChE leads to an increased number of ACh molecules, which antagonise the action of the competitive non-depolarising NMJ blockers. This results in reversal of blockade
Postganglionic, parasympathetic synapses	Increased ACh leads to increased salivation, tears, gastrointestinal tract and bronchial secretions, augmentation of motor activity of bowel, bronchoconstriction, bradycardia, hypotension and constricted pupils
CNS	Stimulation and depression (larger doses)

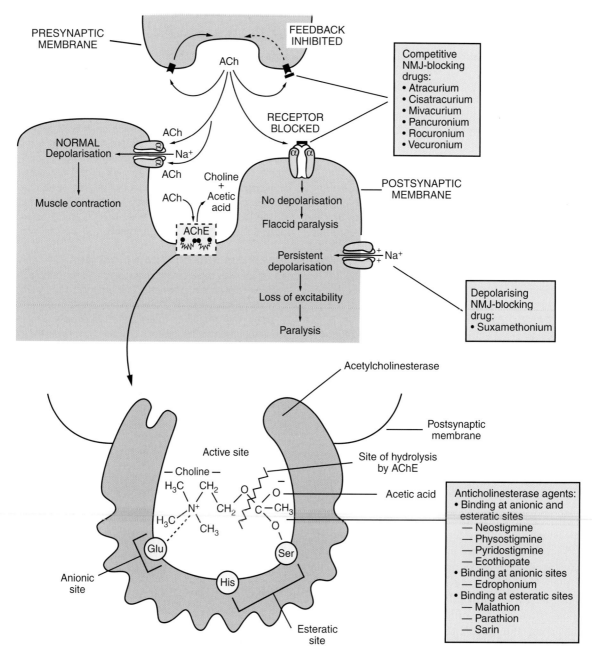

FIGURE 13-4 Sites of action of neuromuscular blocking drugs and anticholinesterase agents. Schematic representation of postsynaptic membrane of motor end-plate showing nicotinic receptors and acetylcholinesterase. The enlargement shows acetylcholine within the active site of acetylcholinesterase. The critical amino acids forming the catalytic site are indicated: Glu = glutamate, His = histidine, Ser = serine. The zigzag line indicates the site of hydrolysis of acetylcholine, yielding choline and acetic acid.

Irreversible anticholinesterase agents

With the exception of ecothiopate, which was formerly used in the treatment of glaucoma, most irreversible inhibitors of acetylcholinesterase (AChE) are pesticides of the organophosphate class or chemical warfare agents such as the nerve gases sarin, tabun and soman. The organophosphate pesticides

(e.g. parathion and malathion) are widely used in agriculture, horticulture and urban gardening and are a common cause of poisoning in humans. The organophosphate pesticides inhibit acetylcholinesterase by forming a very stable complex principally with the esteratic site. This phosphorylated form of the enzyme is not degraded and return of AChE activity is dependent on synthesis of new enzyme.

Nerve gases are also organophosphate anticholinesterase

DRUG MONOGRAPH 13-3 NEOSTIGMINE

Neostigmine is a reversible inhibitor of acetylcholinesterase, forming a carbamylated enzyme complex at the active site. This complex is hydrolysed slowly by AChE over the following 3–4 hours.

INDICATIONS Neostigmine is most commonly used for the reversal of neuromuscular blockade induced by non-depolarising NMJ blockers such as pancuronium. In addition to its use as an adjunct to anaesthesia, it is used for the treatment of myasthenia gravis.

PHARMACOKINETICS Neostigmine is a quaternary ammonium compound. It is poorly absorbed from the gastrointestinal tract and does not cross the blood–brain barrier. The plasma half-life is on the order of 0.5–1.5 hours and the drug is predominantly excreted in the faeces (>50%) and urine (about 30%). It is metabolised principally by plasma cholinesterases and kinetics of the drug are unlikely to be affected by liver disease.

DRUG INTERACTIONS The anticholinesterase effect of neostigmine is diminished by corticosteroids. Many of the drug interactions are more relevant to the situation where the drug is used to treat myasthenia gravis, rather than to its predominant use in reversing neuromuscular blockade.

ADVERSE REACTIONS These often relate to the overdose situation and resemble a cholinergic crisis, with many of the symptoms as listed in Table 13-2.

WARNINGS AND CONTRAINDICATIONS The drug should be used with care in people with a history of asthma, cardiac disease, hypotension or peptic ulceration. Safety of neostigmine in pregnancy has not been established (ADEC Category B2).

DOSAGE AND ADMINISTRATION For reversal of neuromuscular blockade in adults, 50–70 mcg/kg to a maximum of 5 mg is administered IV over 1 minute after or with atropine (0.6–1.2 mg).

CLINICAL INTEREST BOX 13-3 CHEMICAL WARFARE AGENTS

Chemicals (chlorine and phosgene) hazardous to humans were first used as 'weapons of mass destruction' during World War I. Since that time refinement of chemical processes has resulted in the continued production of chemical weapons. Organophosphorus nerve agents such as tabun, sarin, cyclosarin and soman were manufactured during WW II and sarin and soman have been stockpiled in a number of countries including the USA. Another class of nerve gases is the V class, which are organophosphate esters of various 2-aminoethanethiols of which VX is the most lethal. It is estimated that the lethal dose in humans is 0.3 mg/person via the inhalational route and 5 mg/person via dermal absorption (Szinicz 2005). These agents are inhibitors of acetylcholinesterase and the antidote carried by military personnel is atropine, which antagonises the persistent stimulation of muscarinic receptors and pralidoxime, an acetylcholinesterase-reactivating drug.

Sulfur mustard, which is classed as a vesicant, was explicitly developed as a chemical warfare agent and was first used in battle in 1917. The most recent use of sulfur mustard was in the Iran–Iraq War in the 1980s, where it is estimated that over 100,000 Iranians were injured by the chemical and approximately one-third are still suffering from late effects (Kehe & Szinicz 2005). Sulfur mustard has a different mechanism of action from the nerve gases and it is generally accepted that following exposure the sulfur mustard is metabolised to reactive intermediates, which then alkylate DNA, RNA and proteins, resulting in subsequent failure of cellular functions. Clinical manifestations include respiratory tract damage, chronic obstructive lung disease, eye lesions, bone marrow depression and cancer. Currently there is no antidote to sulfur mustard.

agents. A great deal of interest has been rekindled since the terrorist attack in Japan and use of nerve gases during the Gulf War. These agents are highly volatile and their vapours pose a significant health problem. Toxicity occurs as a result of irreversible inactivation of AChE leading to an accumulation of acetylcholine. Persistent stimulation by ACh at presynaptic and postsynaptic receptors occurs initially, followed finally by paralysis of cholinergic neurotransmission. This ultimately affects the somatic, autonomic and central nervous systems.

The signs and symptoms of poisoning from pesticides and nerve gases can be categorised according to whether excessive stimulation occurs at muscarinic or nicotinic receptors. For example, muscarinic effects include bronchoconstriction, nausea, vomiting, abdominal pains, incontinence and bradycardia. Nicotinic effects would occur more from stimulation of the somatic nervous system (e.g. skeletal muscle twitching, weakness and flaccid paralysis), and from the release of catecholamines from the adrenal medulla (Sidell & Borak 1992).

DRUGS AT A GLANCE 13: Drugs affecting neuromuscular transmission

Therapeutic group	Pharmacological group	Key examples	Key pages
Neuromuscular blocking drugs	Non-depolarising blocking drugs	atracurium	206
		pancuronium	205
		vecuronium	206
	Depolarising blocking drugs	suxamethonium	207
Drugs that inhibit cholinesterase	Anticholinesterases	neostigmine	209
		physostigmine	207
		pyridostigmine	207

KEY POINTS

- The somatic nervous system coordinates consciously controlled functions such as posture, movement and respiration.
- The synapse between the lower motor (somatic) neuron and the skeletal muscle is called the neuromuscular junction.
- The transmitter at the neuromuscular junction is acetylcholine, which acts on both presynaptic and postsynaptic nicotinic receptors.
- Released acetylcholine is hydrolysed rapidly by acetylcholinesterase.
- The neuromuscular blocking drugs are principally of two types: competitive non-depolarising drugs and depolarising nicotinic receptor agonists.
- Non-depolarising drugs such as pancuronium competitively block the action of ACh. They produce rapid blockade at the motor end-plate, which is characterised by initial motor weakness that progresses to flaccid paralysis.
- Non-depolarising blockers characteristically cause a release of histamine that may manifest as a rash or in more severe cases, as hypotension and bronchoconstriction.
- The only depolarising nicotinic receptor agonist in clinical use is suxamethonium.
- Acetylcholinesterase is the biological target for anticholinesterase drugs, pesticides and chemical warfare agents such as nerve gases.
- The anticholinesterase drug neostigmine is commonly used to reverse neuromuscular blockade produced by non-depolarising blockers; it is also used as an adjunct to anaesthesia.
- Irreversible anticholinesterase agents are, in general, organophosphates. They are used as pesticides (e.g. parathion and malathion) and chemical warfare agents (e.g. tabun, sarin, soman).
- Toxicity occurs as a result of accumulation of ACh and excessive stimulation of the somatic, autonomic and central nervous systems.

REVIEW EXERCISES

1. Discuss briefly the role of the somatic nervous system.
2. Why is pancuronium referred to as a non-depolarising neuromuscular junction blocker? How does it work?
3. Explain why neostigmine effectively reverses blockade of a non-depolarising blocker but worsens the neuromuscular blockade produced by suxamethonium.
4. List the major symptoms of organophosphate poisoning.

REFERENCES AND FURTHER READING

Atchinson WD. Neuromuscular blocking agents. In: Brody TM, Larner J, Minneman KP (eds). *Human Pharmacology: Molecular to Clinical.* 3rd edn. St Louis: Mosby, 1998 [ch. 10].

Bowman WC. Therapeutically useless drugs from unusual sources. *Pharmaceutical Journal* 1973; 211: 219–23.

Dollery C (ed.). *Therapeutic Drugs.* London: Churchill Livingstone, 1991 [vols 1, 2].

Feldman S, Karalliedde L. Drug interactions with neuromuscular blockers. *Drug Safety* 1996; 15: 261–73.

Kehe K, Szinicz L. Medical aspects of sulphur mustard poisoning. *Toxicology* 2005; 214: 198–209.

Klein A, Glogau RG. Botulinum toxin: beyond cosmesis. *Archives of Dermatology* 2000; 136: 539–41.

Lukas RJ, Changeux JP, Le Novere N et al. International Union of Pharmacology: current status of the nomenclature for nicotinic acetylcholine receptors and their subunits. *Pharmacological Reviews* 1999; 51: 397–401.

Naguid M, Magboul MA. Adverse effects of neuromuscular blockers and their antagonists. *Drug Safety* 1998; 18: 99–116.

Rang HP, Dale MM, Ritter JM, Moore PK. *Pharmacology.* 5th edn. Edinburgh: Churchill Livingstone, 2003 [ch. 10].

Sidell FR, Borak JB. Chemical warfare agents: II. Nerve gases. *Annals of Emergency Medicine* 1992; 21: 865–71.

Szinicz L. History of chemical and biological warfare agents. *Toxicology* 2005; 214: 167–81.

Taylor P. Anticholinesterase agents. In: Hardman JG, Limbird LE, Goodman AG (eds). *Goodman & Gilman's The Pharmacological Basis of Therapeutics.* 10th edn. New York: McGraw Hill, 2001 [ch. 8].

Taylor P. Agents acting at the neuromuscular junction and autonomic ganglia. In: Hardman JG, Limbird LE, Goodman AG (eds). *Goodman & Gilman's The Pharmacological Basis of Therapeutics.* 10th edn. New York: McGraw Hill, 2001 [ch. 9].

Tortora GJ, Grabowski SR. *Principles of Anatomy and Physiology.* 9th edn. New York: John Wiley & Sons, 2000 [ch. 15].

evolve More weblinks at http://evolve.elsevier.com/AU/Bryant/pharmacology/

UNIT IV
Drugs Affecting the Central Nervous System

CHAPTER 14

Overview of the Central Nervous System

CHAPTER FOCUS

The central nervous system (CNS), comprising the brain and spinal cord, regulates all body functions; therefore its activities allow the person to adapt, both consciously and subconsciously, to the internal and external environment. A broad knowledge of the anatomy and physiology of the CNS is necessary for the understanding of the various pharmacological agents used to treat diseases and illnesses that affect this system.

OBJECTIVES

- To present an overview of the physiology and anatomy of the CNS, identifying the locations and functions of the major components of the brain.

- To describe the blood–brain barrier and its physiological effects and clinical implications.

- To name and describe major functional systems of the CNS.

- To describe the generation and propagation of action potentials and the steps involved in synaptic transmission.

- To list the major groups of chemicals identified as CNS neurotransmitters, and their general functions.

- To describe how imbalances in levels of neurotransmitters may occur in various CNS disorders, and how drugs may modify neurotransmission.

KEY TERMS

acetylcholine
action potential
afferent pathway
amino acids
basal ganglia
blood–brain barrier
brainstem
catecholamines
central nervous system
cerebellum
cerebrum
cranial nerves
depolarisation
efferent pathway

extrapyramidal system
glial cell
grey matter
hypothalamus
ion channel
limbic system
membrane potential
monoamines
neurotransmitter
peripheral nervous system
reticular activating system
spinal cord
synapse
white matter

KEY ABBREVIATIONS

ACh	acetylcholine
ANS	autonomic nervous system
CNS	central nervous system
CSF	cerebrospinal fluid
DA	dopamine
EAA	excitatory amino acid
5-HT	5-hydroxytryptamine (serotonin)
ICP	intracranial pressure
NA	noradrenaline
NMDA	N-methyl-D-aspartate
PNS	peripheral nervous system
RAS	reticular activating system

THE nervous system consists of the **central nervous system** (CNS) and the **peripheral nervous system** (PNS; see Figure 14-1). When a drug is described as having a central action, this means that it has an action on the brain or the **spinal cord** (see Clinical Interest Box 14-1). The specific response caused by a drug depends on many factors, including specific attributes of the drug, the personality and emotional and physiological state of the individual, any concurrent disease or drug therapy, and even the environment in which the drug is administered.

Drugs affecting the CNS are of particular importance in pharmacology. Not only are they often prescribed for treatment of common clinical conditions (pain, headache, anxiety, epilepsy, sleeplessness, depression, psychoses) but they are also the commonest self-administered drugs—as analgesics, tobacco, alcohol and caffeine. Unfortunately, it is not easy to study CNS-active drugs in the laboratory and extend the results to human medicine. This is partly because animals may respond very differently from humans (and cannot tell us how they are feeling or thinking). Also, actions at the cellular level may bear little obvious relationship to

effects on the whole person in terms of complex functions such as emotions, memory, thought processes, personality and behaviour. Consequently some of the most commonly used CNS-active drugs, such as general anaesthetics and drugs affecting mood and behaviour, are those about which we understand the least in terms of their mechanisms of action.

Composed of the brain and spinal cord, the CNS essentially controls all functions in the body. The PNS consists of all nervous tissue outside the brain and spinal cord—cranial and spinal nerves; somatic, sensory, autonomic and enteric neurons; and ganglia and receptors. (The PNS is discussed in greater detail in Unit III.) The PNS is the network that transmits information to and from the CNS. Sensory information is transmitted via **afferent pathways**,* alerting the CNS to internal and external changes, such as muscle tension, blood vessel alterations, pain, fever, sound, smell,

---

*A little Latin (or Italian) knowledge is helpful here: afferent comes from the Latin *ad ferens*, carrying towards, and efferent from *ex ferens*, carrying away from.

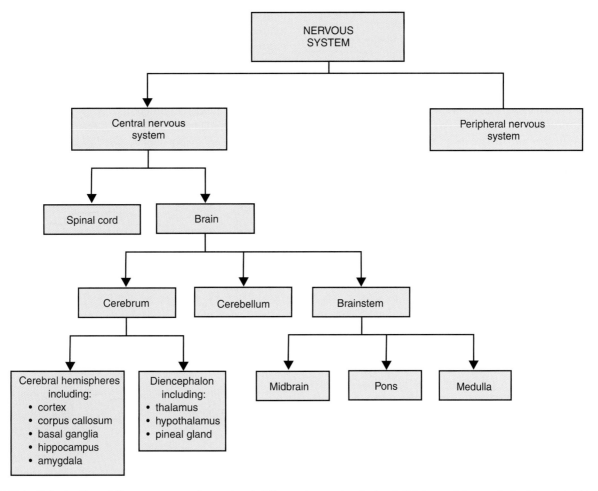

FIGURE 14-1 Organisation of the nervous system, showing the major anatomical subdivisions of the central nervous system. (Details of the peripheral nervous system subdivisions are shown in Figure 10-1.)

taste, touch and sight. This information is integrated in the CNS and messages are then relayed via peripheral **efferent pathways** to appropriate cells or tissues to produce the necessary actions and adjustments. Information concerning these actions and adjustments is again fed back into the CNS, permitting continuous adjustments to be made in various tissues to ensure effective control of body functions (i.e. homeostasis).

BRAIN

The human brain weighs about 1400 g and is estimated to contain around 100 billion neurons, each of which connects with around 10,000 others (on average) in branching networks (see Figure 10-3). The brain is suspended in cerebrospinal fluid (CSF), and surrounded and protected by membranes called the meninges. CSF helps keep the brain in a very stable environment, acts as a fluid shock-absorber, and circulates compounds such as neurotransmitters and other mediators. The brain can be divided and discussed in various ways; a simplified approach is to consider the major component areas (see Figure 14-2):
- the **brainstem** (continuous above the spinal cord), consisting of medulla oblongata, pons and midbrain, and including the reticular formation
- the **cerebellum**

- the diencephalon (comprising the thalamus, hypothalamus and pineal gland)
- the two cerebral hemispheres, each subdivided by fissures into parietal lobe, frontal lobe, occipital lobe and temporal lobe.

In the following sections, the major areas of the brain are described briefly, especially those areas affected by drug therapies. The 'special senses' and drugs affecting the eye or the ear are discussed in Chapters 35 and 36.

Brainstem

The **brainstem** is composed of the midbrain, pons and medulla oblongata, and is the source of cranial nerves III–XII (see Table 14-1); the exceptions are the olfactory and optic nerves, which have origins in the nasal mucosa and retina respectively. It is the most primitive part of the brain, and is essential for life. It has enormous strategic importance, with major long-fibre tracts running through it, conveying sensory fibres from the peripheral nervous system, and motor fibres from the cerebral cortex; fibres from the cerebellum are also channelled through the brainstem. The medulla, pons, and midbrain contain many important correlation centres (**grey matter**), as well as ascending and descending pathways (**white matter**). Tests for brain death, e.g. after severe CNS trauma or anoxia, all involve testing of brainstem functions, such as gag and cough reflexes, ocular and vestibular reflexes and spontaneous breathing. Brain death is defined as irreversible cessation of brainstem functions.

The midbrain contains nerve tracts to and from the cerebrum. It is the source of the third (oculomotor) and fourth (trochlear) **cranial nerves**; centres for visual and auditory

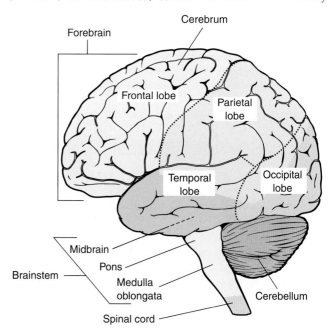

FIGURE 14-2 The human brain, left lateral view.

TABLE 14-1 The cranial nerves*

CRANIAL NERVE	TYPE OF NERVE	FUNCTION
I Olfactory	Sensory	Sense of smell
II Optic	Sensory	Vision; afferent limb of pupillary light reflex
III Oculomotor	Motor (mainly), parasympathetic	Movement of eye and eyelid muscles, accommodation, pupillary constriction and efferent limb of pupillary light reflex; proprioception of muscle position
IV Trochlear	Motor	Eye muscle for downward and inward motion of eye
V Trigeminal	Motor, automatic	Chewing, lateral jaw movement; lacrimation
	Sensory	Sensations of the face, scalp, oral cavity, teeth and tongue; taste
VI Abducent	Motor	Eye movements
VII Facial	Motor and parasympathetic	Facial expressions; secretion of saliva and tears, vasodilator
	Sensory	Taste and proprioception
VIII Acoustic (or vestibulo-cochlear)	Sensory	Hearing, balance
IX Glossopharyngeal	Motor and parasympathetic	Swallowing; salivation, vasodilation
	Sensory	Taste, throat and tongue sensations; chemoreceptors and pressure receptors
X Vagus	Motor and parasympathetic	Voice production, swallowing; increased peristalsis and GIT secretions; slowing heart, constriction of airways
	Sensory	Gag reflex; sensations of throat, larynx, thoracic and abdominal viscera; chemoreceptors
XI Spinal accessory	Motor (mainly)	Head and shoulder movements; swallowing
XII Hypoglossal	Motor (mainly)	Tongue movements, neck muscles

* Note that the **cranial nerves** are anatomically part of the PNS, not the CNS; they are included in this chapter for convenience.
There are many mnemonics to help students remember the order and names of the cranial nerves, some more memorable (and funnier) than others. A 'clean' and relatively memorable version is: 'On Old Olympus' Towering Top, A Finn and German Viewed a Hop'.
The problem then becomes one of associating the right anatomical name (e.g. olfactory, optic or oculomotor) with the right word (On, Old or Olympus).
Drug effects or toxicity have been reported to affect various cranial nerve functions. For example, ototoxicity, or eighth cranial nerve damage, has been reported with aminoglycoside antibiotics. Vincristine, an antineoplastic agent, may produce ptosis (by damage to cranial nerve III), trigeminal neuralgia (cranial nerve VII), facial palsy (cranial nerve V) and jaw pain. GIT = gastrointestinal tract.

reflexes are also located here. The midbrain serves as a relay station between higher areas of the brain and the spinal cord.

The pons helps bridge the left and right sides of the cerebellum, which hangs off the pons by thick tracts of fibres called the cerebellar peduncles. All information to and from the cerebellum passes through the pons, which also contains ascending sensory and descending motor tracts, as well as nuclei associated with the fifth, sixth, seventh and eighth cranial nerves. The lower pons and medulla contain centres that control involuntary respiratory regulation; the upper pons and medulla contain the **reticular activating system**.

The medulla oblongata contains several vital centres: the respiratory, vasomotor, cardiac and vomiting centres. (Such centres are referred to as vital because they are necessary for survival—see Clinical Interest Box 14-2). Other essential functions also originate here, such as sneezing, coughing and swallowing reflexes. Within the pyramids of the medulla, the large motor tracts from the motor areas of the cerebral cortex to the spinal cord cross over. This is known as the decussation of the pyramids and explains why damage at a high level to motor areas (e.g. a stroke) causes motor impairment or paralysis on the contralateral side.

CLINICAL INTEREST BOX 14-2 RAISED INTRACRANIAL PRESSURE (ICP)

- The brain is enclosed within a rigid sphere of skull bones, with only slight room for expansion; thus any increase in the volume of the components inside the skull (brain tissue, interstitial fluid, blood within vessels, or CSF within the ventricles) will raise the pressure inside the skull and put pressure on the other components.
- Common causes of raised ICP are generalised oedema or a space-occupying lesion, which could be a tumour, infection, haemorrhage, haematoma, hydrocephalus or abscess.
- Clinical manifestations include headache (which worsens with coughing or leaning forward), drowsiness, vomiting, confusion and papilloedema. Raised ICP can lead to blindness (from compression of optic nerves) or death (from compression of vital centres in the brainstem).
- Localised expansion of the brain may cause the brainstem to herniate through a foramen (hole) in the skull; compress nerves; compress blood vessels, causing ischaemia; or damage blood vessels, leading to rupture and bleeding, hence further raising ICP. This is a life-threatening condition and urgent treatment is required.
- Treatment may be surgical, to reduce pressure, or pharmacological, with corticosteroids to relieve inflammation, osmotic dehydrating agents to reduce oedema, or diuretics to reduce fluid load.

If the respiratory centre is depressed by drugs it will discharge fewer impulses down nerve pathways to the muscles of respiration, and respiration will be depressed. Other centres in the medulla that respond to certain drugs are the cough and vomiting centres.

Cerebellum

Located in the posterior cranial fossa behind the brainstem, the **cerebellum** contains more neurons than all the rest of the brain, with centres for muscle coordination, maintenance of posture, and muscle tone. It receives afferent impulses from the vestibular nuclei, as well as the cerebrum, and plays an important role in the maintenance of posture and skilled muscular activity. The cerebellum is an error-detector for all movements, and a lesion or damage to it leads to ataxia (postural instability). Drugs that disturb the cerebellum or vestibular branch of the eighth cranial nerve cause dizziness and loss of equilibrium.

Thalamus

The thalamus is composed of sensory nuclei and serves as the major relay centre for impulses to and from the cerebral cortex. With only a few important exceptions (including olfaction, the sense of smell), all information from the periphery is transmitted via the thalamus before being consciously perceived or processed; thus sensations such as pain, temperature, touch and other sensory impulses are relayed via the thalamus to the cerebral cortex.

The thalamus enables the individual to have impressions of pleasantness or unpleasantness, plays a role in acquisition of knowledge, and also appears to play a part (with the reticular activating system [see later in this chapter]) in arousal or alerting signals. Drugs that depress cells in the various portions of the thalamus may interrupt the free flow of impulses to the cerebral cortex; this is one way in which pain may be relieved.

Hypothalamus

The **hypothalamus** lies below the thalamus and is a major controller of homeostatic mechanisms; it is vital for maintaining many body functions. It is a major link between the mind and the body, and between higher centres in the brain and the autonomic nervous system (ANS) and the endocrine system. Functions of the hypothalamus can be summarised as:

- control of the ANS, including regulation of smooth muscle tone, body temperature, cardiovascular and gut functions
- control of the pituitary gland and regulation of release of anterior pituitary gland hormones—thereby controlling most endocrine functions, including growth, reproduction and sexual functions—and thyroid and adrenal cortex hormones
- regulation of emotional and behavioural patterns, partly through the appetite centre and pleasure or reward centres
- regulation of hunger and thirst, carbohydrate and fat metabolism and water balance
- regulation of circadian rhythms and sleep.*

Drugs may affect these functions of the hypothalamus. An example is the use of antidepressants to treat the symptoms of depression: tricyclic antidepressants often also reverse the symptoms, of weight loss, anorexia, decreased libido and insomnia, associated with depression. Some of the

---

*Circadian rhythms and sleep patterns are determined by complex interactions among the hypothalamus, pineal gland (which secretes melatonin) and tracts (linked to the retina) that sense light. This system becomes confused by long-distance air travel, Arctic/Antarctic extremes of day/night cycles, and by total blindness.

sleep-producing drugs are thought to depress hypothalamic centres. Other psychotherapeutic agents may cause a range of hypothalamic side-effects, including breast engorgement, lactation, amenorrhoea, appetite stimulation and alterations in temperature regulation.

Cerebrum

The **cerebrum**, the largest and uppermost section of the brain, is the highest functional area, where memory storage and sensory, integrative, emotional, language and motor functions are controlled. The cerebrum consists mainly of two hemispheres (right and left) connected by thick fibrous tracts. Each hemisphere is involved in functions and sensations of the opposite side of the body, i.e. contralateral control. The superficial, massively folded layer of the cerebrum is called the cerebral cortex (Latin: bark, rind), or grey matter of the brain, and covers the four lobes into which each hemisphere is divided. (These lobes are named for the bones of the skull under which they lie: frontal, parietal, occipital and temporal.) The white matter is so-called as it is largely made up of myelinated axons, whereas the grey matter comprises dendrites, cell bodies and supportive tissues.

The cortex can be broadly classified into motor areas and sensory areas. The frontal lobe contains the motor and speech areas, and areas for intellectual functions, affective behaviour (mood) and abstract thinking. The sensory areas are located in the parietal lobe, the visual cortex in the occipital lobe, and the auditory cortex and memory areas in the temporal lobe. Association areas, which deal with complex integrative functions, lie near these lobes and act in conjunction with them. In addition, large parts of the cortex are concerned with higher mental activity—reasoning, creative thought, judgement and memory.* The limbic lobe is the most primitive component of the cerebral cortex (see Limbic system, below) and is responsible for emotions, activities and drives required for the survival of the species.

Important areas in the cerebrum include the **basal ganglia**, which coordinate gross automatic muscle movements and regulate muscle tone, and the **limbic system**, which is involved in emotional aspects of behaviour related to survival. Even simple tasks require simultaneous interactions among many parts of the brain, plus general functions of consciousness, attention and decision making. In right-handed people (about 90% of the population), the left hemisphere is dominant, and controls speech and language, ability with sequential mathematical problems, and aggressive or cheerful

moods, while the right hemisphere is more concerned with emotional inflections of speech, consciousness, appreciation of music, three-dimensional relationships and introspective depressed moods.

Drugs that depress cortical activity (CNS depressants such as alcohol) may decrease acuity of sensation and perception, inhibit motor activity, decrease alertness and concentration, depress higher mental functions such as cognition and memory, and even promote drowsiness and sleep. Drugs that stimulate the cortical areas (CNS stimulants such as caffeine or amphetamines) may cause more vivid impulses to be received and greater awareness of the surrounding environment. Increased muscle activity and restlessness may also occur.

CNS functional systems

Specific types of signals are processed in particular brain regions, described not so much by anatomical boundaries as by overall functional aspects. Generally, sensory areas receive and interpret information from sensory receptors such as those for touch, temperature, pain and proprioception; motor areas integrate all voluntary movements, including speech; and association areas have complex integrative functions in memory, emotions, willpower, intelligence and personality. Four major CNS functional systems affected by CNS-active drugs include the reticular activating system, the limbic system, the extrapyramidal system and the basal ganglia.

Reticular activating system

The **reticular activating system** (RAS) is a diffuse system of nuclei in the reticular formation of the brainstem (see Figure 17-3) that permits a two-way communication among the spinal cord, thalamus and cerebral cortex. The primary functions of the RAS are:

- consciousness and arousal effect, requiring an external signal such as a pain stimulus, an alarm clock or bright light†
- an alerting mechanism, important in self-preservation, e.g. waking up at night because of feeling cold or hearing a loud noise
- a filter process that allows for concentration on a specific stimulus at a given time
- involvement in regulation of muscle tone and spinal reflexes
- an important centre for pain perception
- important centres for cardiovascular regulation via descending sympathetic pathways.

*Some of the greatest mysteries of medicine relate to the higher workings of the cerebrum, e.g. how memory works and how personality is formed and controlled. There is a widely held view that our brains are not sufficiently powerful for us ever to understand how they function.

†The alerting reaction is not, however, stimulated by smell; hence the need for electronic smoke alarms in buildings to detect smoke and change the chemical stimulus to one to which the RAS responds, e.g. sound or light.

Inactivation of the RAS results in sleep, and injury or disease to the RAS may produce a lack of consciousness or a comatose state; in deep coma, even reflexes are lost.

Many drugs act on the RAS. Anaesthetics dampen its activity and induce sleep, whereas amphetamines stimulate or activate the system. Lysergic acid diethylamide (LSD) and other hallucinogenic agents may act on the RAS by interfering with its ability to filter out stimuli; therefore the person taking this substance is bombarded by stimuli. In contrast, it is proposed that chlorpromazine enhances the filtering activity of the RAS, making it useful in reducing hallucinations in the psychotic patient or people taking LSD.

Limbic system

The **limbic system** is a border of subcortical structures that surround the corpus callosum around the top of the brainstem (Figure 14-3). Among the components of the limbic system are the olfactory bulbs, hippocampus, cingulate gyrus, hypothalamic nuclei and the amygdala.

The limbic system is extremely complex in its functioning, interacting with other parts of the brain to influence or normalise expressions of emotions, such as anger, fear, anxiety, pleasure and sorrow, or to affect the biological rhythms, sexual behaviour and motivation of a person. In addition, learning and memory have been associated with the hippocampus.

Drugs affecting the limbic system include the benzodiazepines and morphine. The benzodiazepines are believed to suppress the limbic system, preventing it from activating the reticular formation and thus causing drowsiness and sleep, especially in patients with anxiety. Morphine is thought to alter subjective reactions to pain as well as abolishing pain stimuli received by special areas within the limbic system.

Extrapyramidal system

The **extrapyramidal system** is a series of indirect motor pathways located in the CNS that are outside the main motor pathways that traverse the pyramids in the thalamus (hence the term extrapyramidal). The term embraces many pathways or tracts (with complicated names such as the lateral reticulospinal tract and the rubrospinal tract) that innervate mainly muscles in the limbs, head and eyes. This system is associated with coordination of muscle group movements and posture. Antipsychotic agents that block dopamine receptors may produce adverse effects related to this system; these are referred to as extrapyramidal effects and may mimic the signs of parkinsonism (see Chapters 19 and 21, and Clinical Interest Box 19-2).

Basal ganglia

The **basal ganglia** are a series of paired nuclei in each cerebral hemisphere; the main components are the corpus striatum

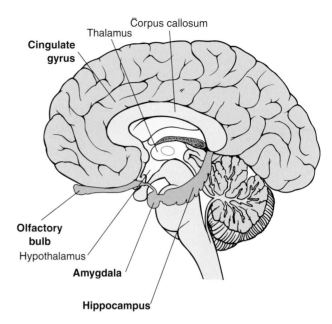

FIGURE 14-3 Components of the limbic system (in bold).

(made up of the caudate nucleus and putamen) and the globus pallidus. The substantia nigra and the red nuclei of the midbrain are sometimes included as components of the basal ganglia. They are connected with the cerebral cortex, thalamus and hypothalamus, and regulate the tone and characteristics of all voluntary movements; thus damage to the basal ganglia, such as occurs commonly in Parkinson's disease, can lead to increased muscle tone, rigidity and tremors.

Spinal cord

The **spinal cord** is a thick band of nerve fibres surrounded by the three meningeal membranes that surround the entire CNS, and lies within the spinal canal formed by the protective vertebrae. It functions in the transmission of impulses to and from all parts of the brain and is also a centre for reflex activity. Ascending tracts of afferent nerves conduct impulses up from peripheral receptors and nerves to the brain, and descending tracts conduct efferent impulses down from the brain to **synapse** with peripheral motor and autonomic nerves.

A cross-section of the spinal cord (Figure 14-4) reveals an internal mass of grey matter (cell bodies, dendrites, axon terminals, unmyelinated axons and neuroglia) enclosed by white matter (tracts or columns of myelinated nerve fibres). The butterfly-shaped grey matter is divided into horns; the afferent (sensory) nerve fibres are located in the dorsal, or posterior, section, while the efferent (motor and autonomic) nerve fibres exit from the ventral, or anterior, horns. When a pain impulse reaches the dorsal horn, for example, the impulse will be transmitted towards the brain along specialised tracts (lateral spinothalamic tracts) to the thalamus, which then

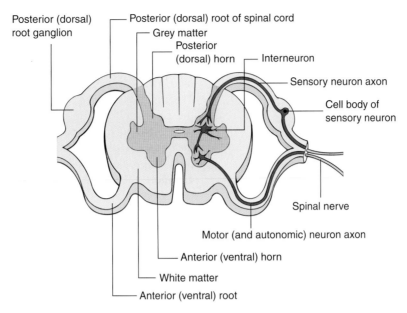

FIGURE 14-4 Transverse section of the spinal cord; neural components of a spinal reflex are shown in darker blue on the right-hand side.

distributes the message to other areas of the brain. The brain responds by means of the descending efferent fibre pathways to inhibit or modify other incoming pain stimuli (see the discussion of the gate theory of pain in Chapter 16). Through this pathway, the perception of pain can be blunted by stress, stoic determination or the 'heat of battle'. Small doses of spinal stimulants may increase reflex excitability; larger doses may cause convulsions.

Some sensory afferent neurons synapse with motor efferents in the grey matter of the spinal column, forming reflex arcs. An example is the flexor (withdrawal) reflex, which is important in preventing injury. If the hand touches a hot object, for example, then before the ascending impulse reaches the brain and allows conscious thought about dangers, synapses between sensory neurons onto ipsilateral motor efferents within the spinal dorsal horn (via interneurons) relay signals back to the appropriate muscle groups, initiating movement to pull the hand away.

The blood–brain barrier

The **blood–brain barrier** is a selectively permeable filter between the blood circulation and the cells of the brain and spinal cord, which tends to exclude from the CNS large water-soluble molecules, microorganisms and other toxins. The existence of a barrier between the blood and the brain, preventing easy passage of molecules from the systemic circulation into the CNS, was first postulated to account for the fact that acidic dyes (after being injected IV into animals to stain tissues for histological studies) did not stain the brain cells. Other clinical evidence was that many antimicrobial

drugs useful in peripheral infections were ineffective in treating infections of the CNS.

The blood–brain barrier is now attributed to tight junctions between endothelial cells in the cerebral capillaries, a covering formed from the foot-like processes of the **glial cells** (astrocytes) that encircle the brain's capillary walls, and the almost complete absence of pinocytotic vesicles in the capillary endothelial cells.

The barrier presumably evolved for protective functions, as it prevents passage of many potentially toxic large molecules into the CNS and keeps the brain and spinal cord in a remarkably stable internal environment. This barrier function is not absolute but is selectively permeable, as it will allow small molecules (such as water, alcohol, oxygen and carbon dioxide), lipid-soluble substances and gases to penetrate but excludes water-soluble and large molecules. There is also active transport and secretion of compounds between the brain and blood: nutrients such as D-glucose and precursors to neurotransmitter substances (such as choline and the amino acids phenylalanine, tyrosine and L-dopa) pass across or are actively transported. Such selective processing allows the brain a degree of security against the toxic effects of some ingested poisons or drugs on the CNS, while substances essential to energy supply or metabolic pathways are permitted. The barrier also effectively prevents active compounds such as neurotransmitters released in one site in the CNS or in the periphery from being taken up into the bloodstream, transported to other CNS sites and acting inappropriately. Some of the important clinical implications of the existence of the blood–brain barrier are summarised in Clinical Interest Box 14-3.

CLINICAL INTEREST BOX 14-3
CLINICAL ASPECTS OF THE
BLOOD–BRAIN BARRIER

- The barrier is broken down in most focal injury to the brain, e.g. in inflammation, convulsions, trauma, tumours or infection; this has the useful effect that drugs that might not otherwise pass across into the brain, such as many antibiotics, are more likely to penetrate infected or inflamed tissue.
- The barrier is underdeveloped at birth; hence infants are at risk of CNS side-effects from any drugs administered, or indeed from drugs taken by the mother during pregnancy or while breastfeeding.
- A consequence of the previous point is that infants are at risk of accumulating in the brain bilirubin, a breakdown product of cell metabolism; the neonate's liver is too immature to deal with large amounts of bilirubin, which can pass across into the brain and cause permanent brain damage. (Such infants are often placed under a UV lamp, as the energy from the UV source helps break down bilirubin and prevent its accumulation.)
- As a general summary rule, drugs that do pass the blood–brain barrier are uncharged compounds (not ionised), have high lipid solubility and are not highly protein-bound.
- A focus of current research is on methods to increase the permeability of the blood–brain barrier to specific therapeutic agents, such as antibiotics or the antineoplastic agents needed to treat localised brain infections or brain tumours.

Nerve cells and action potentials

The two major cell types in the CNS are **glial cells** (neuroglia) and neurons, or nerve cells. The functions of the glial cells are not fully understood although this type of network might serve to support and assist neurons in the transfer and integration of information in the CNS, and in maintaining nutrients, forming myelin, protecting against disease and helping form the blood–brain barrier. Recent studies indicate that glial cells play a role in neural plasticity (protection from or recovery after injury) and may also be crucial to memory formation. Neurons in the CNS have the same basic structure as those in the PNS: dendrites, cell body, axon and nerve terminals (see Figure 10-3).

Neurotransmission

The process of conveying messages from one neuron to another (or, in the PNS, to an effector cell such as a muscle or gland cell) involves chemical transport of the message across the synapse (gap) between them. Most information transmitted in the CNS is due to alterations in electrical currents. The electrical properties of nerve cells are generated by various ions, pumps and channels located in the cell membrane (see Chapter 10 and Figure 10-5 for more detail). The pumps maintain an electrical difference or potential across the cell membrane by maintaining imbalances in the ionic concentrations of sodium, potassium and chloride across the membrane. They are capable of actively moving charged ions from one side of the membrane to the other side through **ion channels** (membrane pores) that allow the passage of specific ions. Channels are described as voltage-gated if they open in response to changes in **membrane potential** (voltage), e.g. during the generation and conductance of action potentials. By comparison, a ligand-gated channel opens and closes in response to a specific chemical stimulus (a ligand is something that binds, e.g. a neurotransmitter, hormone or drug that binds to a specific receptor or channel).

The movement and concentration of ions in and around the cell are the primary determinants affecting the membrane potential of the nerve cells. In the resting state, sodium and chloride are found in large amounts outside the cell, while potassium is in high concentration within the cell. The concentration gradients are stabilised by the sodium–potassium adenosine triphosphatase (ATPase) pump, which trades three sodium ions from the intracellular fluid for two potassium ions from the extracellular fluid. Overall, there is a small build-up of negative ions (phosphate and proteins) in the cytosol inside the cell membrane, and an equal build-up of positive ions (mainly sodium) just outside the membrane. This helps to maintain the resting membrane potential, i.e. the voltage difference across the membrane, normally at about −70 mV, as the inside of the cell is negative compared with the extracellular fluid.

An important property of a nerve cell therefore is that it is polarised (electrically charged) in the resting state. However, a depolarising potential or other stimulus may reduce the membrane potential, i.e. depolarise the cell, to a critical level. This **depolarisation** will result in the rapid opening of voltage-gated sodium channels, allowing sodium to flow into the cell, which causes further depolarisation of the nerve cell along its length; this reduction in membrane potential generates an **action potential** (see Figure 10-6). Voltage-gated potassium channels open slightly later, allowing potassium ions to rush out of the cell, producing repolarisation. As the action potential moves very rapidly along the membrane of an axon, the nerve impulse is propagated along the nerve towards the terminals.

Many drugs act either directly on the ion channels or via receptors that affect ion channels; for example, local anaesthetics enter nerve cells and physically block sodium channels, which effectively reduces sodium influx, preventing generation of the action potentials and conduction of nerve impulses, especially in neurons that carry messages from pain receptors.

Cardiac glycoside drugs stimulate the heart via actions on the sodium–potassium pump on cardiac muscle cells.

Synaptic transmission in the CNS

The CNS can be envisioned as an incredibly complex series of wired connections among neurons, with an estimated 100 billion neurons in a human brain. The connections, however, are incomplete—between each nerve terminal and the next cell is a gap, or synapse, and electrical impulses cannot jump directly across. Instead, chemical messengers cross the gap from the terminal end of the first neuron (the presynaptic side) to receptors in the membrane of the cell on the post-synaptic side, which may be a neuron or (in the PNS) another cell that carries out some function stimulated by the nerve (an effector cell). This process is known as **neurochemical transmission** and the chemical messenger is termed a **neuro-transmitter**. Neurotransmission is described in more detail in Chapter 10 and Figures 10-7 to 10-9 in the context of transmission in the PNS. Neurotransmission in the CNS is a similar process but there are many more connections: each CNS neuron may synapse directly or indirectly with around 10,000 others.

Criteria for neurotransmitter status

The criteria for a chemical to be classed as a central neuro-transmitter are:

- the chemical precursor(s) to the transmitter molecule must be present in the neuron or capable of being transported across the blood–brain barrier and neuronal membrane into the neuron
- the transmitter must be synthesised (if not already present) in the presynaptic (first) neuron; this process requires that the precursor chemicals and enzymes for synthesising the transmitter also be present
- the transmitter is taken up into and stored in packages (vesicles) in an inactive form in the nerve terminal
- electrical stimulation of the neuron releases quanta (bursts) of active transmitter into the synapse in a calcium-dependent manner
- there are appropriate receptors on the postsynaptic (second) neuron, specific for the transmitter
- interaction of the substance with its receptor induces changes in the electrical membrane potential of the postsynaptic neurons, and thereby a physiological response (e.g. propagation of an action potential)
- there is a system for removal of transmitter from the synapse (e.g. a reuptake process, an enzyme to degrade the transmitter, or rapid diffusion away from the receptors)
- experimental application of the substance at the synapse produces an identical response to that of stimulating the neuron.

CNS neurotransmitters

There are about 40 different types of CNS neurons (classified by **neurotransmitter**) that use chemical transmitters for rapid communication across synapses. Some of the chemicals that have been identified as acting as CNS neurotransmitters are:

- amino acids—excitatory: glutamate, aspartate; inhibitory: glycine, γ-aminobutyric acid (GABA); also possibly alanine, taurine, serine
- **monoamines**—noradrenaline (NA), adrenaline, dopamine* (DA), serotonin (5-HT [5-hydroxytryptamine]), and possibly histamine
- **acetylcholine** (ACh)
- neuroactive peptides—gastrointestinal peptides such as substance P and cholecystokinin (CCK); hypothalamic releasing factors, including somatostatin; opioids such as enkephalins and endorphins; and other hormones and peptides including oxytocin,* calcitonin, bradykinin and neuropeptide Y.

Pathways (tracts) of neurons containing a particular trans-mitter have been identified and tracked through brain areas —see Figure 14-5. For example, there are dopaminergic pathways (neurons that use dopamine as a transmitter) from the substantia nigra to the striatum, involved in motor control; from the ventral tegmental area to the limbic system and the frontal cortex, involved in cognition and emotion; and from the hypothalamus to the pituitary, controlling release of pituitary hormones. Drugs that affect dopamine transmission will therefore have major actions and/or side-effects on motor control, thought processes and emotions, and endocrine functions. Dopamine receptors have been classified into several subtypes (D_{1-5}); availability of specific agonists or antagonists for the different receptor types will be beneficial clinically and assist research into dopaminergic mechanisms.

ACETYLCHOLINE

Acetylcholine (ACh) is the best known chemical transmitter of nerve impulses; however, not all parts of the CNS contain ACh. (In the PNS, ACh is the neurotransmitter at all autonomic ganglia, at parasympathetic [and sympathetic cholinergic] neuroeffector junctions, and at the neuromuscular junction.) CNS areas with high concentrations of cholinergic neurons are the reticular formation, the basal forebrain, basal ganglia and anterior spinal roots. In the CNS, ACh may be involved in cognition, memory, consciousness and motor control. Levels appear to be low in Huntington's disease and in dementias such as Alzheimer's disease.

---

*Researchers at Cornell University in New York have identified three brain neurotransmitters involved in human love: dopamine, phenylethylamine and oxytocin. These transmitters are apparently released in the early stages of courtship, and for about 18 months—long enough for a couple to meet, fall in love, mate and produce a child.

MONOAMINES

The **monoamine** transmitters are NA,[†] DA, adrenaline,[†] 5-HT and (probably) histamine. DA is particularly involved in motor control, behaviour, reward systems and endocrine control and is present in high concentrations in the ventral tegmental area, the substantia nigra and the caudate nucleus (see Figure 14-5). Cell bodies for noradrenergic neurons are found in the pons and medulla. NA is present in central autonomic pathways, particularly in the hypothalamus and medullary centres, and is involved in central autonomic control, arousal, mood and reward systems. Important 5-HT pathways run between the midbrain and cortex, with extensive innervation of virtually all parts of the CNS. Cell bodies are especially prevalent in the raphe nuclei of the brainstem. 5-HT is involved in cognition, behaviour, sleep–wake cycles, mood, vomiting and pain (especially in the aetiology of migraine).

Although the effects of **catecholamines** (NA, DA and adrenaline) injected into the CNS are slight in comparison with their effects in the autonomic nervous system, rises in levels of catecholamines and 5-HT do cause cerebral stimulation. Drugs, such as reserpine, that release catecholamines and reduce amine concentration in the brain have a depressing or sedative action. Methyldopa lowers the 5-HT and noradrenaline levels and this, too, has a cerebral depressing effect. Centrally acting α_2-adrenoceptor stimulants such as clonidine paradoxically reduce blood pressure, by inhibiting peripheral sympathetic stimulation. The roles of monoamine transmitters in psychiatric disorders (schizophrenia and depression) and the effects of psychotropic drugs on aminergic transmission are discussed in greater detail in Chapter 19.

AMINO ACID TRANSMITTERS

Amino acids are probably the most ancient (from an evolutionary viewpoint) type of neurotransmitter, being particularly prevalent in the spinal cord. For example, GABA is an important inhibitory transmitter in many interneurons in the spinal cord, and in the cerebellum and hippocampus. GABA is involved particularly in motor control, in spasticity and in sleep/wakefulness. Inhibitory control is necessary to avoid such excessive excitation as occurs during seizures and epilepsy.

The excitatory amino acids (EAA)—glutamate, aspartate, cysteic acid and homocysteic acid—are present in virtually all regions, and are thought to be implicated in the neuronal injury involved in many neurological disorders. Monosodium glutamate (MSG), a flavour enhancer present in many Asian foods and meals, causes in susceptible people the 'Chinese restaurant syndrome', with CNS stimulation, flushing and nausea. Other excitotoxins may be involved in chronic degenerative diseases such as Huntington's chorea, in dysfunction

---

[†]Note that in the American literature, noradrenaline and adrenaline are known as norepinephrine and epinephrine, respectively.

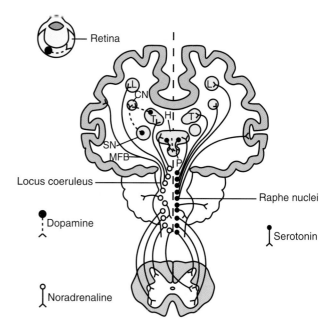

FIGURE 14-5 Major pathways of monoamine-containing fibres. Both sides of the brain and spinal cord are the same but, for simplicity, dopamine- and noradrenaline-containing neurons are shown on the left, and 5-hydroxytryptamine-containing neurons on the right. CN = caudate nucleus; H = hypothalamus; L = limbic system; MFB = medial forebrain bundle; P = pituitary; SN = substantia nigra; T = thalamus. *Source*: Bowman & Rand 1980; used with permission.

after CNS viral infections and in neurological syndromes linked to plant neurotoxins.

NEUROPEPTIDES

Neuroactive peptides are derived from secretory proteins formed in the cell body; they may be considered as neuromodulators, neurohormones or neurotransmitters. Peptides may cause excitation or inhibition of target neurons. The parenteral or intracerebral injection of these chemicals causes potent behavioural effects. Some of these peptides also exist in tissues other than the CNS, primarily in the gastrointestinal tract cells, or in the hypothalamus or pituitary gland.

There are several families of neuropeptides. Peptides in the same family contain long stretches of identical amino acid chains. Examples are vasopressin and oxytocin, the secretins, the tachykinins, the somatostatins and the opioid peptides. (The opioids, including enkephalins and endorphins, are considered in greater detail in Chapter 16, in the context of pain and analgesic drugs.) Many of the neuropeptides that have been demonstrated to be present in the brain have at present no specific pharmacological antagonists, so it is difficult to identify their functions. In the process of co-transmission, neuroactive peptides and classic neurotransmitters may be released simultaneously from the same neuron, e.g. ACh and vasoactive intestinal peptide (VIP), noradrenaline and neuropeptide Y, or dopamine and cholecystokinin.

OTHER CNS NEUROTRANSMITTERS

Other chemicals that may act as neurotransmitters or neuromodulators include prostaglandins and purine nucleotides such as adenosine and ATP. There may indeed be many other chemicals with neurotransmitter functions in the CNS but these are as yet unidentified.

RECEPTORS FOR NEUROTRANSMITTERS

The effect of a transmitter at any synapse is determined by the nature of the receptor to which it binds; thus ACh may have fast excitatory effects at nicotinic receptors, and slower effects via G-proteins and second messengers at muscarinic receptors. There are at least three types of glutamate receptor and seven main types of 5-HT receptors, with a bewildering number of subtypes. Some transmitters may have inhibitory effects, e.g. by hyperpolarising postsynaptic membranes or by inhibiting further release of transmitter from the presynaptic terminal by actions on autoreceptors (see below). The $GABA_A$ receptor has sites for binding GABA and also sites that bind benzodiazepines, barbiturates, neurosteroids and picrotoxin, a GABA antagonist. Several types of receptors for EAA have been identified, including receptors for NMDA (N-methyl-D-aspartate) and kainate (a constituent of seaweed); these may be involved in the aetiology of epilepsy (see Chapter 14).

Release of some transmitters can be modulated by the transmitter acting back on autoreceptors located on the presynaptic side of the nerve ending and on the dendrites and axons (analogous to α_2-adrenoreceptors in the sympathetic nervous system; see Figure 12-1). The mechanisms by which a transmitter inhibits its own release have not been fully elucidated and may be different from postsynaptic transduction mechanisms. Presynaptic receptors may also be involved in modulating the release of other transmitters; for example, noradrenaline release can be inhibited by agonists acting on muscarinic, opioid and dopamine receptors and can be facilitated by agonists on β_2-adrenergic, ACh-nicotinic and angiotensin II receptors. There are also presynaptic dopamine autoreceptors that inhibit dopamine synthesis and release and slow the firing of dopaminergic neurons; these may be involved in the on–off effects in levodopa therapy for Parkinson's disease. The presynaptic inhibitory and facilitatory receptors on the same nerve terminals are thought to allow for fine-tuning of transmitter release in various physiological (and pharmacological) situations.

Neurotransmitter imbalances in disease states

In many disorders of the CNS, it appears there are imbalances between levels of different neurotransmitters in particular parts of the brain. In some conditions, chemical analysis of areas of the brains of patients who have died from a disease has shown that tracts or neurons had degenerated in particular areas. In a (simplistic) attempt to describe an overview of these

conditions, the following scheme can be proposed (see Figure 14-6). The effects of monoamines (NA, DA, adrenaline, 5-HT) are envisaged to balance (as on a see-saw) the effects of ACh, particularly on motor control, mood and thought processes. Thus in depression there is a relative deficiency of NA and 5-HT in areas of the brain related to mood (affect). The depressed mood can be improved by antidepressant drugs

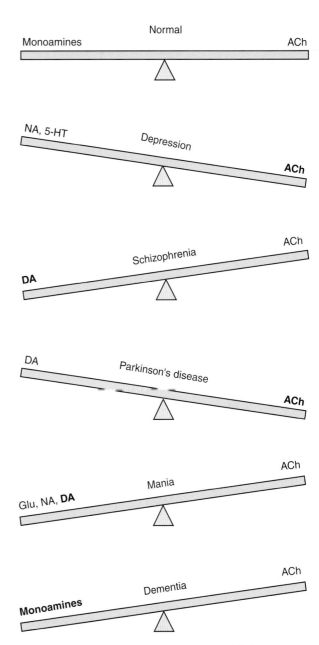

FIGURE 14-6 Neurotransmitter balances in CNS disorders. In the normal state, effects of monoamine transmitters are balanced by those of acetylcholine. In various CNS disorders, imbalances occur and pharmacological management attempts to bring the levels back into balance. 5-HT = 5-hydroxytryptamine (serotonin); ACh = acetylcholine; DA = dopamine; Glu = glutamate; NA = noradrenaline.

such as the selective serotonin reuptake inhibitors (SSRIs), tricyclic antidepressants (TCAs) and monoamine oxidase inhibitors (MAOIs), all of which, by differing mechanisms, increase the levels of monoamines at synapses in the CNS. By contrast, in Parkinson's disease there appears to be damage to dopamine-containing neurons and a relative deficiency of DA or excess of ACh. The main drugs used in treatment of Parkinson's disease either raise the levels of DA or block the actions of ACh (atropinic drugs). This concept (and Figure 14-6) will be referred to again in later chapters on clinical use of drugs in neurological and psychiatric disorders.

How drugs modify neurotransmission

The stages of neurochemical transmission, including the synthesis, storage, release and inactivation of transmitters, have been described in some detail, as have also the processes of generation and propagation of action potentials. In between are the complicated mechanisms whereby a transmitter activates a specific receptor and initiates a chain of events in the postsynaptic cell. These may include second messenger systems, G-proteins, ion channels, intracellular enzymes, transport systems (carriers and pumps), transcription factors that activate genes, the genes that code for synthesis of all the proteins involved, the enzymes involved in the biosynthetic pathways, and the receptors themselves.

Virtually every step in these processes and every enzyme or receptor involved can potentially malfunction or be affected by other chemicals, i.e. by drug actions. It is therefore not surprising that there are many pathological conditions in which impaired neurotransmission may be implicated, many drugs that have actions (therapeutic and/or adverse effects) on the CNS, and even more situations in which we do not as yet know how the physiological, pathological or pharmacological effects occur. However, wherever possible in the following chapters, the clinical use of drugs will be related back to the level of the synapse and to the drugs' effects on neurochemical transmission.

KEY POINTS

- The CNS is a complex system that monitors and regulates all body functions, allowing adaptation to changes in both the internal and external environments.
- Essentially, the CNS integrates information it receives from the PNS and then transmits messages via the PNS to organs and tissues in the body to maintain homeostasis.
- The CNS is composed of the brain (cerebrum, cerebellum and brainstem) and the spinal cord. Component anatomical areas and functional systems have specific and interrelated neurophysiological effects.
- Four of the major CNS functional systems are the reticular formation, limbic system, extrapyramidal system and basal ganglia. These are responsible for many functions: consciousness and attention; personality, emotions and behaviour; learning, memory and decision making; sensory perception; and motor control, muscle tone and coordination. All of these systems may be affected by drugs.
- The blood–brain barrier maintains the CNS in a highly stable chemical environment, allowing passage of required nutrients, transmitters and lipid-soluble substances while excluding large water-soluble and potentially toxic compounds. The barrier is less efficient in young infants and in conditions of focal damage to CNS tissue.
- Neurons have important characteristics in terms of the resting electrical potential maintained across neuronal membranes. Ionic pumps and ion channels maintain the polarised state of the nerve cell.
- Action potentials generated in nerve cells are propagated along axons to nerve terminals, where a synapse intervenes between adjacent neurons.
- Messages are transmitted across synapses by neurotransmitters, chemicals that are synthesised, stored, then released at nerve terminals to cross the synapse and initiate an action at receptors in the postsynaptic neurons to increase or decrease their activity.
- Of the many chemicals proposed as neurotransmitters in the CNS, the most important are acetylcholine, the catecholamines (dopamine, noradrenaline and adrenaline), 5-HT, some amino acids, and neuroactive peptides.
- In many clinically important neurological and psychiatric disorders, imbalances in levels of neurotransmitters have been proposed as aetiological or pathological factors.
- Most drugs used for their actions in the CNS have effects via modification of neurotransmission.

REVIEW EXERCISES

1. List the major component areas of the brain, and their main functions.
2. Name the areas of the brain that perform the following functions:
   - registers pain sensations, temperature, touch and other sensory impulses and relays this information on to the cerebrum
   - maintains many of the body functions and controls the autonomic and endocrine systems
   - is the source of most of the cranial nerves, with the exception of the olfactory and optic nerves.
3. Describe the anatomical basis and function of the blood–brain barrier and its clinical implications for drug therapy.
4. Describe the reticular activating system and give two examples of how it works to protect the individual.
5. Describe the location and functions of the limbic system and the basal ganglia. Name and describe the actions of drugs that affect each of these systems.
6. Describe (with diagrams) the process of neurotransmission in the CNS and explain how drugs may modify the process.
7. List the major groups of CNS neurotransmitters, giving examples for each group and describing important pathways in which the transmitter is involved.

REFERENCES AND FURTHER READING

Bowman WC, Rand MJ. *Textbook of Pharmacology*. 2nd edn. Oxford: Blackwell, 1980 [ch. 6].
Cooper JR, Bloom FE, Roth RH. *The Biochemical Basis of Neuropharmacology*. 8th edn. New York: Oxford University Press, 2002.
Ge S, Song L, Pachter JS. Where is the blood–brain barrier—really? *Journal of Neuroscience Research* 2005; 79(4): 421–7.
Kandel ER, Schwartz JH, Jessell TM. *Essentials of Neural Science and Behavior*. New Jersey: Prentice Hall, 1995 [ch. 16].
Nolte J. *The Human Brain: An Introduction to its Functional Anatomy*. 4th edn. St Louis: Mosby, 1999.
Pardridge WM. The blood–brain barrier: bottleneck in brain drug development. *NeurRx* 2005; 2(1): 3–14.
Stahl SM. *Essential Psychopharmacology: Neuroscientific Basis and Practical Applications*. 2nd edn. Cambridge: Cambridge University Press, 2000 [chs 1–4].
Tortora GJ, Grabowski SR. *Principles of Anatomy and Physiology*. 9th edn. New York: HarperCollins, 2000 [chs 12–15].
Youngson RM. *Collins Dictionary: Medicine*. 2nd edn. Glasgow: HarperCollins, 1998.

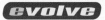 More weblinks at http://evolve.elsevier.com/AU/Bryant/pharmacology/

CHAPTER 15

Anaesthetics

CHAPTER FOCUS

The discovery of anaesthesia and the development of new anaesthetic drugs have proven invaluable in limiting pain and suffering during surgical procedures, and have resulted in many advances in modern surgical techniques. The two major categories of anaesthetic agents are the general anaesthetics, which depress consciousness and cause generalised loss of sensation, and the local anaesthetics, which interfere with the conduction of sensory nerve impulses to the central nervous system. Many other drugs are also used during surgery, to maintain the patient in a stable physiological state and relieve or prevent pain, anxiety and post-operative nausea.

OBJECTIVES

- To describe the effects and mechanisms of action of general anaesthetics and the stages of anaesthesia for surgery.

- To outline the clinical use of general anaesthetics and the adjunct drugs and special considerations important in particular patient groups.

- To describe the main inhalation anaesthetics (gas and volatile liquids) and intravenous anaesthetics.

- To describe the chemistry, effects, mechanisms of action and pharmacokinetics of typical local anaesthetic drugs.

- To discuss the indications and contraindications for the use of local anaesthetics, and the techniques by which they are administered.

- To describe the actions of local anaesthetics in the body and their adverse and toxic effects.

- To list the most significant drug interactions with anaesthetic agents and suggest management of adverse effects and interactions.

KEY DRUGS

atracurium
bupivacaine
cocaine
halothane
lignocaine
midazolam
nitrous oxide
propofol
remifentanil
sevoflurane
suxamethonium

KEY TERMS

anaesthesia
balanced anaesthesia
epidural anaesthesia
general anaesthesia/anaesthetic
infiltration anaesthesia
inhalation anaesthetic
intravenous general anaesthesia
intravenous regional anaesthesia (Bier's block)
local anaesthesia/anaesthetic
malignant hyperthermia
maximum safe dose
nerve block
neuroleptanalgesia
neuromuscular blocking agent
premedication
regional anaesthesia
spinal (subarachnoid) anaesthesia
stages of anaesthesia
topical local anaesthesia
volatile liquid anaesthetic

KEY ABBREVIATIONS

CNS	central nervous system
EMLA	eutectic mixture for local anaesthesia
GA	general anaesthesia/anaesthetic
IV	intravenous
IVRA	intravenous regional anaesthesia
LA	local anaesthesia/anaesthetic
MAC	minimum alveolar concentration (for anaesthesia)
N_2O	nitrous oxide
PABA	p-aminobenzoic acid
SC	subcutaneous
TIVA	total intravenous anaesthesia
w/v	weight in volume

ANAESTHESIA is the loss of the sensations of pain, pressure, temperature or touch, in a part or the whole of the body. Anaesthetic drugs cause unconsciousness or insensitivity to pain, by a reversible action, i.e. cells return to normal when the drug is eliminated from the cells. The two major classifications for these agents are **general anaesthetics** and **local anaesthetics**. **General anaesthetics** induce a state of unconsciousness and general loss of sensation, with varying amounts of analgesia, muscle relaxation, amnesia and loss of reflexes. **Local anaesthetics** block nerve conduction in a body region or localised area when applied locally or to nerve pathways. Drugs used specifically to suppress the pain sensation are known as analgesics; they are dealt with in Chapter 16, as is the physiology of pain. (It is important to differentiate between analgesia and anaesthesia, as a drug may be a good analgesic but a poor anaesthetic, and vice versa.)

Before the era of modern medicine, successful surgery was virtually impossible, owing to the devastating effects of pain, blood loss and infection. Until the development of effective analgesics and anaesthetics (see Clinical Interest Box 15-1), surgery was a painful, exceedingly rapid procedure, during which the patient was usually tied or held down, or rendered unconscious by hypoxia or concussion. Nowadays, anaesthetists are said to be the medical profession's best clinical pharmacologists, as they administer a wide range of specific drugs in highly technical surroundings and often emergency or intensive care situations, continually monitoring the patient for pharmacological effects, adverse reactions and drug interactions.

GENERAL ANAESTHESIA

The requirements that anaesthesia for surgery be of rapid onset, extendable for the duration of the surgical procedure, then rapidly reversible, mean that only central nervous system (CNS) depressants that have short half-lives and can be continually administered are useful as general anaesthetics. (Hence depressants such as alcohol, long-acting barbiturates and most benzodiazepines are not useful.) General anaesthesia is usually induced by intravenous injection of a solution of anaesthetic agent, and then maintained by inhalation of a gas or gas/volatile liquid mixture.

Depressant effects of general anaesthetics

General anaesthetics depress all excitable tissues of the body at concentrations that produce anaesthesia. The pattern of depression is similar for all general anaesthetics: irregular and descending, with higher cortical functions (conscious thought, memory, motor control, perception of sensations) depressed first and the medullary centres depressed last.

Unconsciousness is usually produced. The medulla is spared temporarily, which is fortunate as it contains the vital centres concerned with maintenance of cardiovascular and respiratory control.

Stages of general anaesthesia

The four stages of CNS depression during general anaesthesia were first described in detail by American anaesthetist Dr Arthur Guedel,* who observed the effects on the eyes of slowly advancing unconsciousness induced with early anaesthetics such as ether and chloroform. However, the **stages of anaesthesia** vary with the choice of anaesthetic, speed of induction and skill of the anaesthetist. It is now recognised that stage 2 (excitation) can be dangerous, so the current practice is to induce general anaesthesia rapidly with an intravenously administered anaesthetic, then maintain the stage of surgical anaesthesia (stage 3) by inhalation of an anaesthetic gas.

Stage 1: Analgesia

* Begins with the onset of anaesthetic administration and lasts until loss of consciousness.
* Senses of smell and pain are abolished first; vivid dreams and auditory or visual hallucinations may be experienced; speech becomes difficult and indistinct; numbness spreads gradually, hearing is the last sense lost (hence a quiet environment should be maintained).
* There is adequate analgesia for venepuncture, minor dental or obstetric procedures.

Stage 2: Excitement

Since the advent of balanced anaesthesia, the signs and duration of this stage have been reduced. Stages 1 and 2 constitute the stage of induction.

* Stage 2 varies greatly with individuals and depends on the amount and type of premedication, the anaesthetic agent used and the degree of external sensory stimuli.
* Most reflexes are still present and may be exaggerated, particularly with sensory stimulation such as noise;

---

*Dr Guedel (1883–1956) became known as 'the motorcycle anaesthetist of World War I' as he roared through the mud of the battle fields in France doing the rounds of the six field hospitals for which he was responsible. His painstaking observations of changes in pupil dilation and eyeball oscillation in response to general anaesthetics, in the days before electronic monitoring equipment, allowed surgeons to operate safely while the patient was anaesthetised with open-drop ether, administered by nurses and orderlies trained by Guedel (after Calmes 2002).

CLINICAL INTEREST BOX 15-1   HISTORY OF ANAESTHESIOLOGY

Early techniques for pain relief included:
- cold, ice packs; nerve or carotid artery compression; knocking the patient out
- appeal to higher authorities: conjurers, priestesses, the church, kings, witches
- pharmacological means: opium poppy, mandragora, hemp and 'soporific sponge'.

In the 15th and 16th centuries:
- 'sweet vitriol' (later named 'aether') was described by Cordus and Paracelsus
- sleeping draughts (opium) and hypnotism were used to relieve pain.

In the 18th century:
- gases were prepared and studied: CO_2, O_2, N_2O
- Humphrey Davy, a famous English chemist, reported effects of nitrous oxide (N_2O)
- ether inhalation was recommended to relieve pain.

In the 19th century:
- morphine had been purified in 1806 and was used for analgesia, both orally and by (primitive) hypodermic syringe
- Claude Bernard, the French physiologist, experimented with curare, chloroform, alcohol and ether, described the stages of CNS depression, developed a theory of the mechanism of anaesthesia and suggested premedication with morphine to reduce the dose of anaesthetic required
- in the 1840s ether 'frolics' were held to test its effects, and ether was used in dentistry, surgery and obstetrics
- the psychedelic effects of N_2O were demonstrated in itinerant medical shows and the gas was used as a dental anaesthetic (especially in the USA)
- chloroform was studied (especially in Britain) and various halogenated hydrocarbons synthesised and tested; James Simpson, an Edinburgh obstetrician, encouraged use of chloroform
- in 1853 Queen Victoria used chloroform during childbirth (of her 7th child), thus giving it the royal seal of approval
- because of the flammability of ether and the toxicity of chloroform, administration devices were developed, including inhalers, cylinders for compressed gases and valves

- hepatotoxicity and a spate of deaths under chloroform anaesthesia led to a royal commission into its use and the recommendation that premedication with atropine could prevent the cardiovascular depression induced by vagal stimulation
- in the 1850s, cocaine was brought to Europe from Central America, where it had been used for thousands of years, and was studied (by Sigmund Freud, among others); it was noted to 'numb the tongue'; the active ingredient isolated in 1860 was proposed as a local anaesthetic
- in the 1880s and 1890s, cocaine was used for corneal anaesthesia, in dentistry and general surgery, and for spinal and epidural anaesthesia, but because of its toxicity safer chemical analogues were developed, including benzocaine
- Meyer and Overton developed theories on the mechanism of action of anaesthetics, based on the lipid solubility of series of hydrocarbon compounds.

In the 20th century:
- in 1905 procaine (Novocaine) was developed and found to be non-addictive
- in the 1910s, Guedel described the stages of eye responses to general anaesthetics
- in the 1940s and 1950s amide derivatives such as lignocaine, prilocaine and bupivacaine were synthesised and shown to be less allergenic
- ether was supplanted by halothane (1957) and later by isoflurane and sevoflurane
- the muscle relaxants suxamethonium (1952) and pancuronium (1967) were introduced, as well as the IV induction agent propofol (1986)
- screening for and management of malignant hyperthermia markedly reduced mortality from this condition
- improved monitoring of patients and of adverse effects increased the safety of anaesthesia
- simultaneously, studies were being carried out on new analgesics and local anaesthetics (LAs)
- in 1984 EMLA cream was formulated, a potent lignocaine/prilocaine mixture, effective topically.

---

swallowing reflex is abolished and there is risk of aspiration.
- The patient may struggle, shout, laugh, swear or sing; autonomic activity, muscle tone, eye movement, dilation of pupils and rapid and irregular breathing increase (irregular respiration may cause uneven inhalation of anaesthetic); vomiting and incontinence sometimes occur.

Stage 3: Surgical anaesthesia

The third stage is divided into four planes of increasing depth of anaesthesia. The anaesthetist continually monitors

the patient's respirations, eye movements, pupil size and the degree to which reflexes (such as responses to painful stimuli) are present, to determine which plane a patient is in, before giving approval to begin the procedure. Most operations are done with the patient in plane two or in the upper part of plane three.
- Respiration is initially full and regular; as anaesthesia deepens, respiration becomes more shallow and more rapid, then paralysis of the intercostal muscles occurs, followed by increased abdominal breathing, hence respiration needs to be assisted.
- A loss of reflexes occurs in a cephalocaudal direction

(from the head downwards): the conjunctival reflex is lost; the pupils constrict to about their size in natural sleep, then the reaction to light is lost and the pupils dilate as plane four is approached; the gag and laryngeal reflexes are lost.
- The muscle tone decreases as reflexes are progressively abolished (most abdominal surgery cannot be performed until the abdominal reflexes are absent and the abdominal wall relaxed); body temperature drops and skin becomes cold, wet and pale.
- The pulse is initially full and strong, but by plane four the blood pressure drops and the pulse weakens.

Stage 4: Medullary paralysis (toxic stage)

This is the stage of impending overdose and medullary paralysis, characterised by respiratory arrest and vasomotor collapse.
- Respiration ceases before the heart action, so artificial respiration and/or reduction of the gaseous agent are required in the reversal of this stage.

These stages may appear complicated, so the scheme has been simplified to the following three levels: anaesthesia is inadequate, surgical or deep, or more simply still, 'the patient is awake, asleep, or nearly dead'.

Mechanism of action of general anaesthetics

General anaesthetics (GAs) vary widely in their chemical structures and in the concentration necessary for each to produce a given state of anaesthesia. Although GAs have been studied and used for more than 150 years and many theories of anaesthesia have been proposed, no theory satisfactorily explains the basic mechanisms of action. As there appears to be no simple chemical structure–activity relationship among different GAs, it is assumed that there is no 'GA receptor'. Any theory of GA action must take into account the clearest fact emerging from mechanism studies: the potency of anaesthetic effect is strongly correlated with the lipid solubility of the compound, with very lipid-soluble compounds being very potent. Indeed, the inverse correlation between lipid solubility and dose (expressed as minimal alveolar concentration to achieve anaesthesia) has been said to be one of the most powerful correlations in biology, extending over a 100,000-fold dose range, across species ranging from goldfish to humans.

Three main theories of **general anaesthesia** have been proposed:
- the lipid theory: this proposes that GAs dissolve in the membranes of central neurons, causing altered function,

possibly via volume expansion or increased fluidity of the membrane
- the protein theory: this proposes that GAs interact with hydrophobic parts of modulatory proteins, including receptors and ion channels, leading to a change in ion conductance (this is an extension to the theory originally proposed in the 19th century by Claude Bernard)
- the 'crystal hydrate' theory: popular in the 1960s, this proposes that GAs somehow cause water molecules in the neuronal membrane to form cage-like structures, thus increasing stability of the membranes and decreasing ion movements.

There is still much ongoing research into the mechanisms of action of GAs. At the cellular and receptor level, GAs have been shown to:
- decrease the functions of excitatory neurotransmitters, including ACh (nicotinic), 5-hydroxytryptamine (5-HT, serotonin), glutamate and N-methyl-D-aspartate (NMDA)
- increase the functions of inhibitory transmitters, including GABA (A receptors) and glycine
- affect sodium and potassium channels and interact with peptidergic transmission, opioid receptors, the nitric oxide–cyclic GMP transduction pathway and reactive oxygen species.

Overall, GAs affect a wide range of processes in CNS neurons, the most sensitive areas being sensory pathways from the thalamus to the cortex, and the hippocampus (hence the amnesia caused by GAs). Immobility is mediated primarily via multiple molecular targets in the spinal cord. The current best theory of GA actions is that they modulate the activity of transmitter-gated ion channels.

Pharmacokinetic aspects

For anaesthesia to be rapidly controllable, it is important that the concentration of anaesthetic in blood (and hence CNS tissues) should equilibrate rapidly with the concentration in the lungs. This increases the speeds of both induction and recovery of anaesthesia. The depth of anaesthesia depends on the partial pressure of the anaesthetic gas in the brain. Study of the ideal pharmacokinetics of anaesthetic gases is complicated, involving consideration of the solubility of the agent both in blood and tissues (the blood–gas partition coefficient) and in lipids (the oil–gas partition coefficient), as well as physiological factors that determine the efficiency of respiration and circulation. In summary, it can be concluded that:
- high lipid solubility enhances anaesthetic potency
- high lipid solubility delays recovery, as the agent forms a depot in fat tissues in the body (following a two-compartment pharmacokinetic model) and may take hours to be cleared from the body, leading to a 'hangover' effect

- high blood–gas partition coefficient (solubility of agent in blood) implies a longer time for equilibration of gas to tissues, as higher levels have to be reached
- low blood and tissue solubility speeds equilibration of the agent from the lungs to the blood and tissues and hence shortens onset time and recovery time
- alveolar ventilation is important in equilibration of the agent into the blood, especially for agents having high blood solubility
- overall, the optimal anaesthetic agent has low blood and tissue solubility, with high potency; sevoflurane and desflurane are good examples (Figure 15-1), whereas nitrous oxide is weak but rapid and ether is potent but slow.

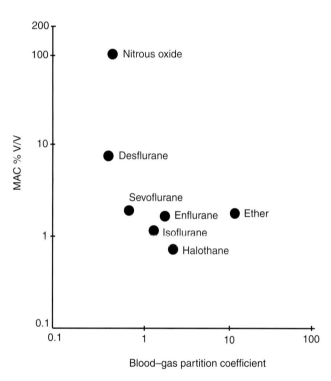

FIGURE 15-1 Potency and solubility of inhaled general anaesthetics. The minimal alveolar concentration [% v/v] required to produce anaesthesia in 50% of patients [MAC] is plotted against the solubility of the anaesthetic drug in blood (expressed as blood–gas partition coefficient). Drugs with a high blood solubility (such as ether) are relatively slow in onset of and recovery from anaesthesia, whereas drugs that have lower blood solubility (desflurane, nitrous oxide) are rapid in onset and recovery. The most potent anaesthetics (halothane, isoflurane) are those with low MAC values, whereas nitrous oxide requires >100% concentration for anaesthesia and is usually used at 50% concentration as an analgesic and carrier gas. Note: Data are plotted with logarithmic scale on each axis. Data from: Speight & Holford 1997; Oberoi & Phillips 2000.

Clinical aspects

Thanks to recent advances in drugs, monitoring devices and delivery systems, general anaesthesia is now very well tolerated in virtually all patients, allowing new surgical techniques to be made available to all ages of patients. However, most drugs used are both potent and potentially toxic, so patients must be monitored and managed well before, during and after the operation, and drugs and techniques must be chosen carefully.

Endotracheal intubation

Because most patients will be administered an anaesthetic by inhalation, the first rule of anaesthesiology is keep a clear airway. Airway obstruction will lead to anoxia and impaired gas intake, and hence to decreased absorption of anaesthetic drug and the risk of the patient regaining consciousness too early. Obstruction can be caused by the tongue falling back, laryngeal spasm, airways disease or mechanical faults. For these reasons, most patients will be intubated, i.e. have an endotracheal tube passed via the larynx into the upper part of the trachea (see Figure 32-6), to maintain a reliable airway. The tube is usually cuffed to help prevent inhalation of secretions or vomit. A dose of a skeletal muscle relaxant (see below, Adjuncts to anaesthesia) is normally administered to facilitate intubation. A typical set-up of equipment for administration of gas and volatile liquid anaesthetics via the mouth and larynx is shown diagrammatically in Figure 15-2.

Balanced anaesthesia

Maintaining the patient insensible to pain, while supporting life functions and balancing mechanisms for fluid, electrolyte and metabolic homeostasis, requires the administration of many drugs concurrently by non-oral routes. Analgesia, relief of anxiety, muscle relaxation, amnesic effects, suppression of reflexes, physiological stability and rapid, maintained, reversible anaesthesia are not produced safely by a single anaesthetic drug. The induction of anaesthesia by using a combination of drugs, each for its specific effect, rather than by using a single drug with multiple effects, is termed **balanced anaesthesia** (see Clinical Interest Box 15-2).

A typical drug regimen to cover a surgical procedure might be:
- for premedication: midazolam/atropine/morphine (see later section)
- for induction: IV thiopentone or propofol
- for maintenance: inhaled N_2O/sevoflurane
- for analgesia: morphine, fentanyl or remifentanil (see Clinical Interest Box 15-3)
- for neuromuscular blockade: suxamethonium or vecuronium
- to reduce postoperative vomiting: metoclopramide or ondansetron.

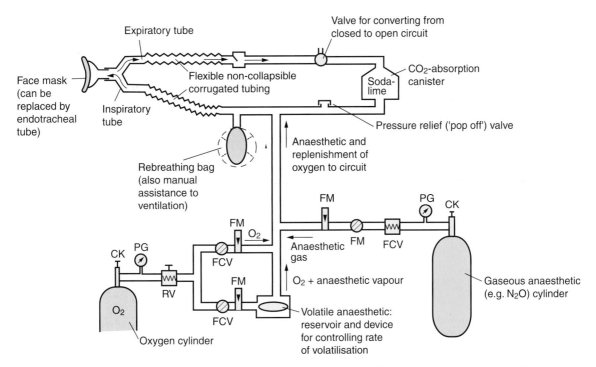

FIGURE 15-2 A diagrammatic representation of the arrangement and workings of a typical general anaesthetic machine. Gases from the cylinders are admitted by opening the cylinder keys (CK), and the pressures are measured with gauges (PG). The pressures are lowered by reduction valves (RV) and the flows of gases are controlled by flow control valves (FCV) and monitored by flowmeters (FM). Gases other than those shown may be available (e.g. 5% CO_2 in O_2) and there may be additional volatilisers for generating anaesthetic vapour in the replenishment line or in the circuit. *Source*: Bowman & Rand 1980; used with permission.

CLINICAL INTEREST BOX 15-2   DRUGS IN THE ANAESTHETIC DRUG TROLLEY

A typical anaesthetic drug trolley may contain supplies of the following drugs, for use by the anaesthetist (only two or three examples of each type are given here):
- induction agents (thiopentone, propofol)
- local anaesthetics (lignocaine, bupivacaine)
- muscle relaxants (suxamethonium, vecuronium)
- sedatives (midazolam)
- reversal drugs (neostigmine, flumazenil, naloxone)
- resuscitation agents (adrenaline, atropine)
- cardiovascular drugs (antihypertensives, antiarrhythmics, sympathomimetics, inotropic agents, antianginal drugs)
- renal drugs (vasodilators, diuretics)
- electrolyte replacements (calcium, potassium, bicarbonate)
- antiasthma drugs (salbutamol, hydrocortisone)
- antiemetics (ondansetron, prochlorperazine)
- analgesics (morphine, parecoxib, tramadol, fentanyl)
- blood substitutes (dextrans, platelets)
- anticoagulants (heparin, warfarin)
- vasoconstrictors (vasopressin, sympathomimetics)
- stabilising agents (clonidine, dexmedetomidine)
- saline solutions (normal saline, dextrose saline)
- miscellaneous (eye-drops, nasal drops, non-opioid analgesics).

The anaesthetist must be continually monitoring the operation, the patient's progress and the drugs' effects while adjusting doses, watching for adverse drug reactions and interactions and considering the implications of any concurrent diseases and drug regimens.

It would be a useful pre-examination exercise for the student to play anaesthetist and consider the actions, indications for use and adverse effects of all the above drugs and attempt to predict any potentially major drug interactions and problems in elderly or renal-impaired patients.

The specific drugs and dosages used depend on the procedure to be carried out, the physical condition of the patient and the patient's responses to the medications. The advantages of balanced anaesthesia include a safer induction, quicker recovery and lower reported incidence of postoperative nausea, vomiting and pain.

Neuroleptanalgesia and day surgery procedures

An anaesthetic technique formerly frequently used, but now dropping out of favour, is **neuroleptanalgesia**, or neuroleptanaesthesia. This is a state of deep sedation, analgesia and

---

**CLINICAL INTEREST BOX 15-3
REMIFENTANIL: A RAPID-ACTING
OPIOID FOR USE DURING GENERAL
ANAESTHESIA**

Remifentanil (Ultiva) is a potent short-acting analgesic used as an adjunct during induction and maintenance of general anaesthesia and for pain in the immediate post-operative period. This drug is administered by IV infusion or bolus and allows a marked reduction in dose of the main anaesthetic agent.

A selective mu (μ) opioid receptor agonist, remifentanil has a rapid onset of action and is metabolised and inactivated by non-specific esterases in blood and tissues, with an elimination half-life of 10–20 minutes. Its effects last for between 5 and 10 minutes after the drug is discontinued, so rapid titration of analgesic effects is possible. To control postoperative pain, adequate alternative analgesia should be instituted before discontinuation of remifentanil. Adverse effects include cardiovascular depression and muscle rigidity. (See a current reference text or package insert for additional information.)
Source: AMH 2005; Padley 2004.

---

amnesia produced by a combination of a neuroleptic agent (i.e. an antipsychotic, see Chapter 19), such as droperidol, and a narcotic analgesic, most commonly fentanyl. Neuro-leptanalgesia was used for minor surgical procedures requiring the patient's cooperation, such as endoscopies. However, there was a high incidence of postoperative sedation and restlessness, and newer anaesthetic, anxiolytic and analgesic agents are considered to provide better pain relief and recovery. A typical current IV sedative/analgesic regimen for minor day procedures such as colonoscopy is propofol and midazolam (for induction/sedation) and fentanyl (for analgesia). Patients must be warned not to drive or operate machinery for at least 24 hours.

Adverse effects and toxicity of general anaesthetics

Although each individual drug has its particular adverse effects, there are adverse effects that are common to all GAs because they are all general CNS depressants and depress the cardiovascular and respiratory systems and reflexes. GAs may also cause postoperative convulsions, headache, nausea and vomiting, kidney or liver toxicity (hepatotoxicity especially with chloroform and halothane) and hypersensitivity reactions. They are relatively contraindicated during pregnancy (see Pregnancy Safety box); however, maintenance of the mother's health is important to the wellbeing of the fetus.

Studies on chemical series of halogenated hydrocarbon compounds have shown that, overall, fluorinated compounds are more potent and less toxic than others, and that volatile anaesthetics with low solubility in blood, which are not subject to metabolism, have faster onset and shorter recovery times. Two recently introduced drugs, sevoflurane and desflurane, appear to have optimal properties as anaesthetics, compared with earlier agents such as ether, chloroform and halothane (Figure 15-1).

Malignant hyperthermia

Malignant hyperthermia, or hyperpyrexia, is a rare but potentially fatal condition occurring in susceptible patients with an inherited abnormality in muscle membranes. It appears to be precipitated by the combination of a depolarising neuromuscular blocking agent (suxamethonium) with a halogenated GA agent. Trigger drugs include all volatile GAs, xanthines (including caffeine), phenothiazines and possibly sympathomimetics; safe drugs include the benzodiazepines and barbiturates. It is a syndrome of acute accelerated metabolism in skeletal muscle, with rapid fever, acidosis, hyperkalaemia, muscle rigidity and dysfunction of many organ systems.

The predisposition to the condition is diagnosed by muscle biopsy and in-vitro testing with caffeine and halothane. While it occurs in only 1 in 6000 to 200,000 persons due to mutations in the ryanodine receptor gene, mortality is 70% if specific treatment is not given. Emergency treatment consists of substituting the volatile GA agent with propofol infusion, actively cooling the patient and administering dantrolene (a direct inhibitor of muscle contractions), bicarbonate, an antiarrhythmic agent and appropriate electrolyte and fluid replacements. The patient needs to be cared for in an intensive care unit for at least 24 hours.

Other surgery-related problems

Many other problems unrelated to the anaesthetics used can occur during surgical procedures, such as:
- oxygen toxicity, if the oxygen concentration is too high (see Chapter 32)
- hypovolaemia and haemoconcentration, due to lack of fluid intake and blood loss, exacerbated by use of vasoconstrictors and non-steroidal anti-inflammatory drugs; decreased renal blood flow can lead to acute tubular necrosis
- acidosis, due to build-up of acid metabolic products during long procedures
- hypovolaemic shock, due to blood loss and decreased tissue perfusion, with low blood pressure, increased heart rate, pallor and sweating; irreversible damage to vital organs can be pre-empted with an early IV line for administration of adequate fluids, and treatment of acidosis, hypotension and oliguria
- awareness can occur during apparently adequate anaesthesia, leading to enduring memories of the events during the procedures, with potential adverse psychological sequelae

- occupational hazards: the patient may suffer injury or burns from equipment-related problems, and fire is a potential problem because of the use of electrocautery in the presence of flammable gases and volatile liquids.

In addition, the staff in the operating theatre are subject to potentially harmful levels of waste gases, even though exhaust gases are extracted from anaesthetic circuits (see Clinical Interest Box 15-4).

Significant drug interactions

Among the dangers facing a surgical patient is an unexpected drug interaction occurring in preparation for or during anaesthesia. Interactions can occur not only among the many drugs likely to be used during surgery, but also with any drugs the patient has been taking for concurrent illness, whether prescribed, over-the-counter, complementary therapies, or for social rather than medical purposes. Anaesthetists must always be familiar with the significant interactions between anaesthetics and the maintenance drug therapies used in a wide range of illnesses and must monitor the surgical patient closely.

As a general guideline, if a drug is needed for treatment preoperatively, it should be continued through surgery. Unnecessary drugs are discontinued for a period at least five times the half-life of the drug before surgery. Drugs having significant interactions with anaesthetic agents are replaced, where possible, with an alternative medication before surgery. An overview of potentially significant drug interactions during anaesthesia follows; reference texts should be consulted for likely effects of specific combinations.

Anticoagulants such as heparin and warfarin are usually discontinued 6 and 48 hours (respectively) before surgery to reduce the risk of haemorrhage.

CLINICAL INTEREST BOX 15-4
WASTE ANAESTHETIC GASES AS AN OCCUPATIONAL HEALTH HAZARD

Chronic exposure of staff in the operating room to waste anaesthetic gases can present a significant occupational health hazard. Studies have demonstrated an increased incidence of spontaneous abortions among women exposed to nitrous oxide, as well as among wives of men who are exposed. In addition, impaired mental performance and neurological, hepatic and renal disorders have been seen in chronically exposed people.

Operating theatre staff should protect themselves by avoiding the area within about 20 cm of the patient's mouth and nose when the breath contains exhaled anaesthetic agents. Health-care institutions need to be active in ensuring that all exhaust gases are scavenged and vented to the outside air and in establishing exposure monitoring programs to detect unsafe levels caused by faulty equipment or unsafe practices.

CNS depressants such as alcohol, antihistamines, antianxiety agents, opioids and hypnotics intensify the CNS-depressant effects.

Antiarrhythmics may reduce cardiac conduction and heart rate, increase peripheral vasodilation and potentiate the effects of neuromuscular blocking agents such as pancuronium.

Some antihypertensive agents such as calcium channel blockers and β-blockers can have synergistic effects with GAs, causing enhanced cardiovascular suppression and arrhythmias.

Corticosteroids taken chronically produce adrenal gland suppression, which may result in hypotension during surgery and lack of ability to respond to stress; corticosteroid dosages are usually increased in the perioperative period.

Cholinesterase inhibitors and exposure to organophosphate insecticides may prolong suxamethonium neuromuscular blockade.

Many antibiotics, particularly aminoglycosides, tetracyclines and polymyxins, can potentiate neuromuscular blockade, necessitating reduction in the dose of the neuromuscular blocking agent and careful monitoring of patients with neuromuscular disorders.

Not all drug interactions are adverse: the additive CNS-depressant effects of opioid analgesics and GAs can be useful in allowing lower doses of the GA, provided the interaction is anticipated and monitored.

Special anaesthesia considerations

Many disease states and risk factors can alter an individual's response to anaesthesia. The preoperative assessment of the patient's health status by the health-care professional should consider acute and chronic medical conditions.

YOUNG AGE

The physical characteristics of a neonate predispose the infant to upper airway obstruction or laryngospasm during anaesthesia or resuscitation. A large body water compartment, immature liver and kidneys, a rapid metabolic rate and undeveloped blood–brain barrier all contribute to the susceptibility to adverse reactions to CNS-active drugs and the need for careful monitoring of the infant or paediatric patient. Drug dosages and administered fluids must be carefully calculated, using recommended paediatric dose regimens. Halothane and nitrous oxide are commonly used in paediatrics because the incidence of hepatitis in children is considered low. Neonates are usually more sensitive to the non-depolarising muscle-relaxing agents (see Chapter 8).

ADVANCED AGE

Ageing results in a generalised decline in organ function, decreased organ reserve capacities, and often the existence of chronic disease processes and polypharmacy with drugs taken to treat concurrent diseases, the latter results in greater potential for drug interactions and adverse effects. Generally, an increased and prolonged drug effect is seen in the elderly and drug-induced confusion is more likely (especially after midazolam). Mortality rates for elderly patients undergoing major surgery may be four to eight times higher than those for younger people.

PREGNANCY AND CHILDBIRTH

Because CNS-active drugs are lipid-soluble, they are likely to cross the placenta and reach significant levels in the fetal bloodstream. Hence inhaled and IV GAs, LAs, analgesics and sedatives must be dosed and monitored carefully if used during pregnancy. For analgesia during childbirth, nitrous oxide ('gas') is commonly self-administered by the mother. Opioid analgesics used during childbirth can lead to respiratory depression in the neonate, so doses are kept to a minimum and effects may need to be reversed by administration of naloxone to the infant. Caesarean section may require general anaesthesia, but can often be carried out under epidural anaesthesia with lignocaine and fentanyl, which allows the mother to remain conscious throughout the birth.

Before any drug is used, the expected drug benefits should be considered against the possible risk to the fetus (see the Pregnancy Safety box).

OBESITY

Overweight and obese patients may have cardiac insufficiency, respiratory problems, atherosclerosis, hypertension, or an increased incidence of diabetes, liver disease or thrombophlebitis. In such patients, obtaining the desired depth of anaesthesia and muscle relaxation may be a problem. Generally, highly fat-soluble anaesthetics, especially those with toxic metabolites such as methoxyflurane, should be avoided.

SMOKING

Individuals who smoke have increased risks of coronary heart disease, peripheral vascular disease and compromised lung function (e.g. bronchitis, emphysema or carcinoma). Postoperative complications are six times more common in smokers than in non-smokers. Smoking also increases a patient's sensitivity to muscle relaxants.

ALCOHOL INTAKE

People who are heavy or regular drinkers of alcohol may have a variety of associated disease states, including liver dysfunction, pancreatitis, gastritis and oesophageal varices. Anaesthetic requirements may be increased because of the increase in liver drug-metabolising enzymes and the development of cross-tolerance. Alcoholic patients need to be monitored closely during the postanaesthetic period for alcohol withdrawal syndrome, as its onset may be delayed by the administration of analgesics. Diazepam or other sedatives may be required to prevent withdrawal symptoms.

CONCURRENT DISEASE CONDITIONS

Whenever possible, concurrent diseases should be treated and pathologies corrected before operation. Implications of common diseases for drug use in anaesthesia are summarised below.

CARDIOVASCULAR DISEASES. Heart failure, recent heart attack, major vascular surgery, arrhythmias, valve disease and hypertension predispose patients to stress-induced tachycardia, hypoxia and ischaemia, myocardial infarction and stroke, and cardiac complications post-surgery; epidural analgesia is protective in the postoperative period.

RESPIRATORY DISEASES. Asthma and chronic obstructive airways diseases impair inhalation of anaesthetics and exacerbate hypoxia and respiratory depression from CNS depressants and opioids; pre- and postoperative physiotherapy, bronchodilators and epidural analgesia assist postoperative care and coughing.

ENDOCRINE DISEASES. Diabetic patients require careful blood glucose control and those on oral hypoglycaemic agents are switched to insulin before the operation; patients on corticosteroids or with thyroid disease are monitored carefully for responses to stress.

RENAL DISEASE. Patients may have problems with anaemia, blood pressure control, fluid and electrolyte balance and impaired drug clearance; severe kidney dysfunction leads to marked increases in drug half-lives—active opioid metabolites are retained, and non-narcotic analgesics (NSAIDs) can further damage kidneys.

LIVER DISEASE. In mild cirrhosis, there is CNS tolerance to depressant drugs, but in severe alcoholic cirrhosis, hepatic metabolic pathways may be impaired, the blood–brain barrier may be more permeable and encephalopathy may be present, so CNS depressants should be avoided; blood clotting and drug protein binding may also be impaired.

Preoperative management and premedication

The preoperative visit to the patient by the anaesthetist and care of the patient by other health-care professionals should include the taking of a thorough medical history and attempts to ascertain any relevant information such as drug allergies and concurrent disease. Questions (in words the patient can understand) are asked about:

- respiratory and circulatory systems, kidney and liver functions
- diabetes, fits and faints, bleeding problems
- previous drug reactions and drug use (including alcohol and tobacco)
- fasting period (solids and fluids)
- current conditions and medications
- possibility of pregnancy and/or infectious disease.

Preoperative management also includes general aspects such as correct identification of the patient and obtaining written consent; providing information on the proposed procedures, risks and equipment; allaying of anxieties; and teaching of exercises for breathing, coughing and movement postoperatively.

Premedication (i.e. preoperative medication) was introduced in the early days of anaesthetic practice to prevent or treat some of the problems associated with the early inhaled GAs such as ether and chloroform. It is no longer considered essential and is often omitted or prescribed only when specifically indicated. Rationales for 'premed' include: to allay anxiety (allows lower doses of anaesthetics); to decrease secretions (salivary, gastric and bronchial); to reduce postoperative vomiting; to overcome CNS depression; and to provide prophylactic analgesia and sedation. Table 15-1 gives an overview of the common agents; Clinical Interest Box 15-3 discusses remifentanil, a rapid-acting opioid used during general anaesthesia.

Adjuncts to anaesthesia: muscle relaxants

Many surgical procedures, especially those on the abdomen, require inhibition of voluntary muscle tone and reflexes to stop muscles contracting when stimulated, to provide surgeons with easier access or to aid intubation. This can be achieved with deep general anaesthesia or with nerve block regional anaesthesia, but both these techniques carry risks. More simply, selective skeletal muscle relaxants can be administered once the patient is lightly anaesthetised and adequate analgesia provided. Artificial mechanical ventilation must be administered as the respiratory muscles are paralysed by **neuromuscular blocking agents**. The two main groups of drugs used are summarised below.

Non-depolarising neuromuscular blockers:
- are competitive antagonists of acetylcholine (ACh) nicotinic receptors at the neuromuscular junction (NMJ)
- do not directly depolarise the end-plate

- cause a flaccid paralysis, lasting 20–30 minutes
- are reversible with anticholinesterase drugs such as neostigmine
- are based on the natural arrow-poison curare
- examples: **pancuronium** (see Drug Monograph 13-1), **atracurium**.

Depolarising neuromuscular blockers:
- activate the nicotinic ACh receptor at the NMJ, depolarising the end-plate
- cause initial muscle twitching, then paralysis, lasting 3–5 minutes
- are useful for short procedures (e.g. intubation and electroconvulsive therapy)
- are enhanced rather than reversed by anticholinesterase drugs
- example: **suxamethonium** (= succinylcholine) (suxamethonium is a powerful trigger of malignant hyperpyrexia; see Drug Monograph 13-2).

The pharmacology of these drugs is considered in detail in Chapter 13.

Postoperative aspects

There are many potential complications following surgical operations. Nausea and vomiting can be induced by pain, drugs (especially opioids), suggestion, irritation, ketosis or dehydration. Refraining from food is sometimes helpful; if nausea and vomiting are severe, antiemetics (metoclopramide, ondansetron) can be given. Postoperative pain is common particularly after procedures involving the thorax or abdomen, episiotomy and haemorrhoidectomy. Adequate pain relief must be maintained to facilitate recovery and ease of coughing and defecation; remifentanil and non-steroidal anti-inflammatory agents (such as parecoxib) are useful.

Respiratory depression often follows the use of narcotic analgesics (opioids); treatment may be with the opioid antagonist naloxone. Chest complications are exacerbated in

TABLE 15-1 Premedication agents and adjuncts to anaesthetics

DRUG CLASSIFICATION	AGENTS FREQUENTLY USED	DESIRED EFFECT
Opioid analgesics	Morphine, fentanyl	Sedation to decrease anxiety; provide analgesia and decrease amount of anaesthetic used
Benzodiazepines	Midazolam, flunitrazepam	Antianxiety, sedative, rapid induction, amnesia
Phenothiazines	Prochlorperazine, promethazine	Sedative, antihistaminic, antiemetic, decreased motor activity
Anticholinergics	Atropine, glycopyrrolate	Inhibition of secretions; reduced vomiting and laryngospasms
Skeletal muscle relaxants	Suxamethonium (depolarising); atracurium (non-depolarising)	Muscular relaxation; aid intubation

smokers and patients with chronic airways diseases and by sputum retention, dehydration, ongoing use of opioids and pain that inhibits coughing. Physiotherapy and rehydration are helpful. The inactivity caused by long surgical procedures and prolonged bed-rest predisposes to thrombosis; early ambulation and antithrombotic drugs (aspirin) help prevent thrombosis and embolism.

More general aspects of postoperative care include monitoring of cardiovascular and respiratory functions and fluid balance, supportive nursing, and provision of adequate information. Doses of concurrent drugs may need to be lower than usual in the postoperative period, until the patient's functioning returns to normal.

Types of general anaesthetics

General anaesthetics are usually divided into two groups: (1) the **inhalation anaesthetics**, which include gases and volatile liquids; and (2) **intravenous general anaesthetics**, such as thiopentone and propofol.

Inhalation anaesthetics

Inhalation, or volatile, **anaesthetics** are gases or liquids that can be administered by inhalation when mixed with oxygen. These rapidly reach a concentration in the blood and brain sufficient to depress the CNS and cause anaesthesia. This is expressed as the minimum alveolar concentration (MAC) for anaesthesia and is inversely related to potency as an anaesthetic (Figure 15-1). Inhalation anaesthetics have the following characteristics:

- they are complete anaesthetics and thus can abolish superficial and deep reflexes
- they provide controllable anaesthesia, as depth of anaesthesia is readily varied by changing the inhaled concentration
- as the route of administration (and most excretion) is via the airways, lung function is critical to effective use of inhaled agents
- the agents are all good anaesthetics, but may not have useful analgesic actions, so they are used in combination with an adjunct analgesic such as fentanyl
- rapid recovery can occur as soon as administration ceases, as the anaesthetic is excreted in expired air
- allergic reactions to these agents are uncommon.

Early inhaled anaesthetics included ether and chloroform as volatile liquids, and cyclopropane and nitrous oxide as gases; of these only **nitrous oxide** is still in clinical use today (in developed countries with advanced facilities) (see Drug Monograph 15-1).

DRUG MONOGRAPH 15-1
NITROUS OXIDE

Nitrous oxide, commonly referred to simply as 'gas', has the chemical formula N_2O. (It should not be confused with nitric oxide [NO], now recognised as a gas generated in many body cells and involved in vasodilation and immune responses and as a chemical mediator in the CNS in neurotransmission and neurodegeneration.)

INDICATIONS Nitrous oxide is the most commonly used agent for dental surgery, minor surgery and obstetric analgesia. It is a powerful analgesic but a weak anaesthetic, so is often combined with other (volatile) anaesthetics to enhance its effects, when it is also used extensively in major surgery. It is presented as a compressed gas in a 50:50 mixture with oxygen (Entonox), in blue cylinders (see Clinical Interest Box 32-1 and Figure 32-1).

PHARMACOKINETICS Nitrous oxide is inhaled and absorbed via the lungs; it has low solubility in blood and tissues, so has a rapid onset of action and recovery time. It is excreted 100% unchanged through the lungs.

ADVERSE EFFECTS AND DRUG INTERACTIONS It is non-irritant and virtually without odour. Its few adverse effects consist primarily of mild cardiac depression and postoperative nausea, vomiting or delirium; it has no known significant drug interactions. There is abuse potential, and escaped gas contributes to the greenhouse effect. It is considered safe in pregnancy and in fact is very widely used as an inhaled analgesic in childbirth, as it can be inhaled during painful contractions then released, and does not accumulate or cause respiratory depression in the neonate.

WARNINGS AND CONTRAINDICATIONS There is a risk of hypoxia if inadequate oxygen is provided. At the termination of nitrous oxide anaesthesia, the rapid movement of large amounts of nitrous oxide from the circulation into the lungs may dilute the oxygen in the lungs (diffusion hypoxia). To prevent this, the anaesthetist usually administers 100% oxygen to clear the nitrous oxide from the lungs.

DOSAGE AND ADMINISTRATION For general anaesthesia, the recommended dosage is 70% nitrous oxide with 30% oxygen for induction and 30%–70% nitrous oxide with oxygen for maintenance. In obstetrics, women self-administer a mixture of N_2O/O_2 : 50/50, and in dental procedures a 25% concentration may be used.

Volatile liquid anaesthetics

When **volatile liquid anaesthetics** such as ether or chloroform were first used, they were administered by placing a pad soaked in the liquid over the patient's mouth and nose, so that the fumes of the liquid were inhaled. This unpleasant procedure caused struggling, skin reactions, uncertain levels of dosage and absorption and a slow progression through the stages of anaesthesia. The more civilised technique used now involves controlled vaporisation of the volatile liquid into a flow of gas (oxygen with or without nitrous oxide), so that a known concentration of volatile agent in oxygen is administered via a mask or endotracheal tube.

Chloroform is hepatotoxic and ether and cyclopropane are highly flammable; these agents have now been replaced by safer anaesthetics. In 1956 **halothane**, a non-flammable agent, largely replaced the older volatile liquids. However, halothane has been associated with hepatic dysfunction and failure, so safer analogues of the halogenated hydrocarbon series have been developed: methoxyflurane, desflurane, enflurane, isoflurane and sevoflurane (see Table 15-2). **Sevoflurane** has become the drug of choice for most procedures owing to its fast action and low toxicity (see Drug Monograph 15-2).

Intravenous anaesthetics

Intravenous anaesthetic agents are used for induction or maintenance of general anaesthesia, to induce amnesia and as adjuncts to inhalation-type anaesthetics. The major groups include ultrashort-acting barbiturates (thiopentone) and non-barbiturates (propofol and ketamine). The benzodiazepine **midazolam** is mainly a sedative-antianxiety agent, but is considered here as it is frequently used as an adjunct to IV anaesthesia. Intravenous anaesthetics are valuable in allaying emotional distress because many patients fear having a tight mask placed over the face while they are fully conscious. These anaesthetics reduce the amount of inhalation anaesthetic required. Clinical Interest Box 15-5 lists the advantages and disadvantages of intravenous anaesthetics.

The intravenous anaesthetics are rapidly taken up by brain tissue because of their high lipid solubility. For example, equilibrium between brain and blood levels occurs within one arm–brain circulation time (patients are usually asked to count backwards from 10 as the agent is injected; they rarely reach 4 or 3). Shortness of action results from the drug being quickly redistributed into the fat depots of the body. The amount of body fat affects drug action: the greater the amount of body fat, the briefer the effect of a single IV dose. With prolonged administration or large doses, however, prolonged drug action results in delayed recovery. This is caused by saturation of fat depots and the slow rate of drug release back into the circulation to be eliminated (10%–15% per hour).

TABLE 15-2 Volatile liquid anaesthetic agents

AGENT	MAC (%)	INDUCTION/RECOVERY	METABOLISM	EXCRETION	ADVERSE REACTIONS AND NOTES
Halothane	0.8	Medium	Up to 20% by liver	60%–80% unchanged via lungs; remainder via kidneys	Halothane hepatitis, liver damage, respiratory depression, arrhythmias, hangover effect; used less now
Desflurane	6.7	Fast	Minimal	Primarily via lungs	Airway irritation; low boiling point, requires vaporiser
Enflurane	1.4	Medium	About 2.5% by liver	80% unchanged via lungs; remainder via kidneys	Respiratory depression, convulsions, raises intracranial pressure; potential fluoride toxicity
Isoflurane	1.2	Medium	Less than 1% by liver	Via lungs	Marked respiratory depression; pungent odour
Sevoflurane	2.1	Fast	5%	Primarily via lungs	Well tolerated, drug of choice; possible risk of fluoride toxicity

*MAC = minimum alveolar concentration (percent in oxygen) for anaesthesia; inversely proportional to potency. May need higher concentrations in some patients: generally highest in very young children, lowest with increasing age, pregnancy, hypotension or concurrent use of CNS depressants. Note that all the volatile agents are non-flammable liquids, are absorbed through the lungs, may cause some cardiovascular depression and are potential triggers for malignant hyperthermia (especially halothane and enflurane).

DRUG MONOGRAPH 15-2
SEVOFLURANE

Sevoflurane is non-irritant and has a pleasant smell and a rapid onset of action and recovery, so it is suitable for inhalation anaesthesia, particularly in children and in day surgery.

INDICATIONS Sevoflurane is indicated for induction and maintenance of general anaesthesia during surgery.

PHARMACOKINETICS Sevoflurane has a faster uptake, distribution and rate of elimination than isoflurane and halothane (but slightly slower than desflurane). About 5% is metabolised in the liver to an inactive derivative that is rapidly eliminated. Inorganic fluoride, released during metabolism of sevoflurane, has an elimination half-life in the range 15–23 hours.

ADVERSE EFFECTS Cardiac and respiratory depression and shivering and salivation can occur, as well as postoperative nausea and vomiting.

DRUG INTERACTIONS Few significant interactions have been reported. Concurrent administration of other CNS depressants (opioid analgesics, benzodiazepines, inhaled anaesthetics) allows reduction in sevoflurane dosage.

WARNINGS AND CONTRAINDICATIONS Sevoflurane is contraindicated in patients with susceptibility to malignant hyperthermia and used with caution in those with renal failure. A fluoro-ether derivative of sevoflurane (known as compound A), formed after passage of the exhaust gas over lime absorbers for carbon dioxide, is potentially toxic. Levels can be minimised by using high gas-flow rates.

DOSAGE AND ADMINISTRATION Sevoflurane is administered from a vaporiser in a stream of oxygen, with or without nitrous oxide. While the induction dose is individualised, the usual inhalation dose for maintenance is up to 5% in adults and 7% in children; surgical anaesthesia is achieved in less than 2 minutes.

CLINICAL INTEREST BOX 15-5
ADVANTAGES AND DISADVANTAGES OF INTRAVENOUS ANAESTHETICS

Advantages: They
- rapidly induce unconsciousness
- are readily controllable
- have amnesic effects
- reduce the amount of inhalational agent required
- allow prompt recovery with minimal doses
- are simple to administer and provide pleasant induction (most patients prefer an IV line to a mask)
- do not pose hazard of fire or explosion.

Disadvantages: They
- cause tissue irritation (swelling, pain, ulceration, tissue sloughing and necrosis) if drug or vehicle infiltrates tissue
- cause thrombosis and gangrene if arterial injection occurs
- cause hypotension, laryngospasm and respiratory failure with overdosage or prolonged administration
- have minimal muscle relaxation and analgesic effects
- are subject to elimination by hepatic metabolism and renal excretion
- commonly cause hypersensitivity reactions (to drug or vehicle)

Intravenous anaesthetic agents present an interesting pharmaceutical problem: an IV anaesthetic agent must be highly lipid-soluble (to cross the blood–brain barrier and act) yet sufficiently water-soluble to be formulated as an injectable solution. This problem has been solved for some drugs with very low water solubilities by formulating them as oil-in-water emulsions (similar to milk), e.g. diazepam or **propofol** in a soya oil/egg lecithin/glycerol emulsion.

TOTAL INTRAVENOUS ANAESTHESIA (TIVA)

It is possible to carry out surgical procedures under total intravenous anaesthesia (i.e. using the IV agent throughout the operation with no inhaled agents). Both thiopentone and **propofol** are used this way. A constant plasma drug level is achieved with a bolus initial dose, then an infusion that can be altered depending on the patient's responses. There are automated, computer-controlled infusion pumps that can be programmed to take into account the mathematically modelled pharmacokinetic parameters of the drug, patient parameters such as weight, age, liver and renal functions, the desired blood concentrations of drug, adjunct analgesics and type of surgical operation.

ULTRASHORT-ACTING BARBITURATES

Ultrashort-acting barbiturate-type agents include thiopentone, which is a CNS depressant that produces hypnosis and anaesthesia without analgesia, and hence is often combined with a muscle relaxant and analgesic in balanced anaesthesia. Thiopentone also has anticonvulsant effects and reduces intracranial pressure; it is particularly useful in emergency anaesthesia. General anaesthesia with ultrashort-acting barbiturates is believed to result from suppression of the reticular activating system.

The most common adverse effects during the recovery period are shivering and trembling and additive effects with other CNS depressants. Less frequently reported are nausea, vomiting, prolonged somnolence and headache. Serious adverse reactions include emergence delirium (increased excitability, confusion, hallucinations), cardiac arrhythmias or depression, allergic responses and respiratory depression.

NON-BARBITURATES

Non-barbiturate intravenous anaesthetic agents include the short-acting hypnotics propofol and ketamine, and the benzodiazepines **midazolam**, diazepam and lorazepam. **Propofol** will be considered as the prototype drug of this group (see Drug Monograph 15-3). Ketamine is an effective analgesic as well as anaesthetic and is useful for brief procedures such as changing burns dressings; it can be administered IV, IM or orally. It has been called a dissociative anaesthetic as it causes analgesia and amnesia without loss of respiratory function or reflexes; it produces a cataleptic state in which the patient appears to be awake but is detached from the environment and unresponsive to pain. Because dreams and hallucinations can occur, it is sometimes subject to abuse, so it has recently been moved to SUSDP Schedule 8.

The opioids fentanyl, sufentanil and alfentanil are sometimes included in this classification as they can be used in high doses to induce anaesthesia. However, they are probably best considered as opioid analgesics (see Chapter 16).

BENZODIAZEPINES (MIDAZOLAM, DIAZEPAM, LORAZEPAM)

Benzodiazepines are given intravenously as premedication (antianxiety and sedative effects), for induction of anaesthesia, for their amnesic actions and for seizure control. (This group of drugs is considered in detail in Chapter 17.) Diazepam and lorazepam are not water-soluble, so their non-aqueous solutions (emulsions) can cause local irritation; they have very long elimination half-lives and are long-acting, with prolonged recovery times.

Midazolam is water-soluble and thus is less irritating locally. Intravenously midazolam has a rapid onset of action (2–4 minutes) and a short elimination half-life of about 1–2 hours. It is metabolised in the liver and excreted by the kidneys. It is commonly used in conjunction with propofol and fentanyl in day-surgery procedures.

Concurrent use of benzodiazepines with alcohol or CNS-depressant drugs may result in hypotension and respiratory depression; a reduction in drug dosage and close monitoring are indicated.

LOCAL ANAESTHESIA

Local anaesthesia refers to the direct administration of an agent to tissues to induce the absence of pain sensation in a part of the body. Unlike general anaesthesia, local anaesthesia does not depress consciousness. As most sensations, including consciousness, are not lost, the term 'anaesthesia' (total lack of sensation) is strictly speaking inappropriate, and some pharmacologists prefer the term 'local analgesia'. However, 150 years of usage sanction the terms 'local anaesthesia' and 'local anaesthetic'. **Local anaesthetic** (LA) drugs reversibly prevent both the generation and conduction of impulses in excitable membranes, particularly in sensory nerves, and hence decrease the sensitivity to pain. They are used in many surgical procedures and for pain relief.

An ideal LA would produce nerve blockade only in sensory nerves when administered topically or parenterally (by injection) and would be rapidly reversible, non-toxic to both local tissue and major organs, with rapid, painless onset of action for a reasonable operating time. While no LA is perfect, the two most commonly used are **lignocaine** (also known as lidocaine or Xylocaine) and the longer-acting **bupivacaine**.

DRUG MONOGRAPH 15-3 PROPOFOL

Propofol is a rapidly acting, non-barbiturate hypnotic, formulated in an emulsion for IV injection or infusion. It has no analgesic effects. Propofol can be used for total intravenous anaesthesia. Its mechanism of action is not known for certain; the CNS depression is probably mediated through GABA receptors.

INDICATIONS It is used for the induction and maintenance of general anaesthesia and for conscious sedation.

PHARMACOKINETICS It has a rapid onset of action within 40 seconds and the duration of effect is only 3–5 minutes, owing to redistribution from the brain to other body tissues. It has a more rapid redistribution time than thiopentone, hence a shorter recovery period and fewer hangover effects. The elimination half-life is 3–8 hours.

ADVERSE EFFECTS This agent is a respiratory and cardiac depressant and can produce apnoea, bradycardia and hypotension, depending on dose, rate of administration and drugs concurrently administered. Nausea, vomiting and involuntary muscle movement are commonly reported.

DRUG INTERACTIONS Sedative effects of other CNS depressants are increased; there are no other clinically significant interactions with drugs likely to be used in anaesthesia.

WARNINGS AND CONTRAINDICATIONS Pain on injection can occur; there is potential for abuse.

DOSAGE AND ADMINISTRATION IV dose for adults and children over 3 years is 2–2.5 mg/kg. Dosage regimens for total intravenous anaesthesia are calculated and controlled by the infusion system.

Local anaesthetic drugs were developed following the introduction of the natural compound cocaine into medicine and ophthalmic surgery in the 1870s and 1880s (as described in Clinical Interest Boxes 15-1 and 15-6). The main problems with cocaine were its acute toxicity and dependence properties, so other benzoic acid esters were studied for LA activity. Benzocaine (active only topically), procaine and amethocaine were all found to be clinically useful. The amide compound, lignocaine, was developed in 1943. It rapidly became widely used and is still considered the prototype LA (see Drug Monograph 15-4). A new series of longer-acting agents (the bupivacaine family) is used when longer duration of activity is required, and more recently a combination of lignocaine and prilocaine (EMLA: eutectic mixture for local anaesthesia) has been formulated as a cream and a patch for topical application (see under Formulations of LAs).

Topical local anaesthesia may also be achieved by freezing, as low temperatures in living tissues produce diminished sensation (hence the use of ice-packs to relieve pain, as in the first-aid acronym RICE: Rest, Ice, Compression, Elevation). This form of anaesthesia is sometimes used for minor operative procedures. However, tissues that are frozen too intensely for too long can be destroyed. Ethyl chloride is a volatile liquid formerly used to produce this effect by evaporative cooling.

Local anaesthetic drugs
Chemistry and dissociation of LA drugs

Chemically, LA drugs are closely related compounds: they generally have at one end an aromatic (phenyl) group, joined through an intermediate chain of carbons to an amine (nitrogen-containing) group. The aromatic group helps make that end of the molecule lipid-soluble (lipophilic) and the amine group makes the other end water-soluble (hydrophilic). This property appears to be essential, as it allows the LA molecules to align themselves and act within nerve cell membranes (which can be considered as protein–lipid–protein bilayers).

The intermediate carbon chains contain either an ester link (CO–O) or an amide link (CO–N), which has some important clinical implications. The ester-type local anaesthetics (cocaine, procaine, amethocaine and benzocaine) are metabolised rapidly by plasma esterase enzymes to p-aminobenzoic acid (PABA) metabolites, which are mainly responsible for allergic reactions in some patients; ester LAs are not often used now. The amide anaesthetics (such as lignocaine, prilocaine, bupivacaine and ropivacaine) are not metabolised to PABA derivatives, and allergic reactions induced by these anaesthetics are rare.

As the LAs are all amines (except benzocaine), they can exist in solution as the uncharged amine form (analogous to ammonia, NH_3) or as the charged quaternary amine form (like the ammonium ion, NH_4^+). The forms are in equilibrium, as shown in the dissociation reaction below:

$$H^+ + NR_3 \rightleftharpoons N^+R_3H$$

The proportion of each form depends on the chemistry of the individual LA molecule and the pH of the solution or tissue it is in. Clinically this is important for the following reasons:

- the basic form (NR_3, where R stands for any radical) is non-ionised, non-polar and lipid-soluble; it is the form that can diffuse across membranes and enter cells
- the cation form (N^+R_3H) is ionised, polar and water-soluble; it is the active form of the LA that blocks sodium ion channels
- at physiological pH (around 7.4) sufficient basic form is present for it to enter cells, where it can pick up a hydrogen ion (H^+) to become charged and able to act

---

CLINICAL INTEREST BOX 15-6
COCAINE—THE ORIGINAL LOCAL ANAESTHETIC

- Cocaine comes from the leaves of the plant *Erythroxylon coca*; it has been used for about 2000 years in Central America, where the leaves are chewed or sucked to relieve pain, cause central stimulation and facilitate heavy work at high altitudes.
- The dried leaves of *Erythroxylon coca* contain about 1% pure cocaine alkaloid, extractable as flaky crystals, hence the street name 'snow'.
- The famous Austrian physician and psychotherapist Sigmund Freud described how 50–100 mg cocaine injected SC decreased fatigue, sleep and appetite, increased power and caused euphoria; Freud's friend Koller introduced cocaine as a local anaesthetic (in the eye); however, it led to corneal damage, as protective reflexes were suppressed.
- The peripheral actions of cocaine are as a local anaesthetic; it also inhibits reuptake of noradrenaline into nerve terminals, hence has indirect sympathomimetic effects, including vasoconstriction.
- Unlike all other LAs, cocaine has marked central actions: initially it acts as a stimulant, causing excitement, talkativeness, tremors and vomiting, and increases respiration; it induces powerful psychological dependence, with 'reward' feelings and exhilaration.
- The toxic effects are psychosis, hallucinations and paranoia, then CNS depression, with cardiotoxicity and respiratory depression.
- Cocaine is still occasionally used medically in Australia in nasal and ophthalmic surgery and for intubation.
- Cocaine was present in the (secret) formula of Coca Cola until 1908 when the US government insisted that it be excluded; however, the company won the right to keep the name (which implies the presence of cocaine).

- at very acid pH (in inflamed tissue), the equilibrium shifts to the right and virtually all LA molecules exist in the charged (cation) form, and hence cannot enter cells to act; this explains why LAs are less effective in inflamed tissues.

**DRUG MONOGRAPH 15-4
LIGNOCAINE**

Lignocaine (also known as lidocaine or Xylocaine) is an amide-type local anaesthetic and has antiarrhythmic properties because it stabilises all potentially excitable membranes and prevents the initiation and propagation of nerve impulses.

INDICATIONS Lignocaine is used commonly for production of local anaesthesia by topical, infiltration, nerve block, epidural or spinal routes. It is also used to treat or prevent ventricular arrhythmias.

PHARMACOKINETICS Onset of action is rapid and duration of nerve blockade is 1–1.5 hours. After absorption into the general circulation or after IV injection, the drug is redistributed rapidly to tissues, especially the heart. Metabolism occurs in the liver and excretion via the kidneys; less than 10% is excreted unchanged. The elimination half-life is 90–120 minutes.

ADVERSE EFFECTS Excessive dosage, rapid absorption or delayed elimination can lead to toxic depressant effects in the central, autonomic and peripheral nervous systems, and cardiovascular and respiratory systems. Allergic reactions are rare.

DRUG INTERACTIONS Other antiarrhythmics and alcohol may potentiate the effects of lignocaine. The clearance of lignocaine may be reduced by β-blockers and cimetidine and enhanced by enzyme inducers.

WARNINGS AND CONTRAINDICATIONS Reduced doses should be given to children, elderly patients and those with cardiac, neurological, liver or kidney disease; cardiovascular function should be monitored during IV administration. Lignocaine is contraindicated in patients with hypersensitivity to amide LAs, inflammation or sepsis at the site of injection, severe shock or hypotension, diseases of the CNS or supraventricular arrhythmias.

DOSAGE AND ADMINISTRATION For local anaesthesia, the lowest effective dosage should be used, depending on the area to be anaesthetised, technique to be used, vascularity of the tissues and patient factors. The typical maximum safe dose is quoted as 3 mg/kg (solution without adrenaline). When used as an anti-arrhythmic, plasma levels should be monitored, with not more than 300 mg infused during 1 hour.

Mechanism of action

Local anaesthetics reversibly prevent the generation and conduction of impulses in excitable membranes and thus decrease sensitivity to pain. The basic mechanism of action of these drugs has been studied in detail: they enter the cell, bind to a modulatory site in the voltage-dependent sodium channel (see Figure 10-5), block the sodium channel and interfere with the transient opening of these channels, thus preventing the transient inrush of sodium. Hence threshold potential is not reached, the cell membrane is not depolarised, the development of the action potential and its propagation are prevented, and the nerve is blocked.

It is important to remember that all potentially excitable membranes are affected, so LAs have actions not only on sensory nerve cells but also on autonomic and motor nerves, muscle cells (cardiac, smooth, skeletal), secretory cells and neurons in the CNS.

The susceptibility of a nerve to LA action depends on the fibre diameter, myelination, tissue pH and length of nerve fibre exposed to LA solution. Local anaesthetics are capable of abolishing all sensation, but pain fibres are affected preferentially because they are thinner, unmyelinated and more easily penetrated by these drugs. Sympathetic fibres are blocked first, then loss of pain is followed in sequence by loss of response to temperature, proprioception (position of body parts), touch and pressure. Most motor fibres can also be anaesthetised when an adequate concentration of the drug is present over sufficient time. This sequence can be remembered by recalling the experience of having an injection (i.e. of LA) at the dentist's surgery. Loss of pain occurs very rapidly, allowing the dental procedures within about 5 minutes. Some time later there may still be lingering loss of sensations of pressure, heat and pain, so it can be dangerous to attempt to drink a hot drink or chew food. Loss of sense of proprioception accounts for the phenomenon of feeling as if the face is grossly swollen when in fact it looks normal.

The LA drugs are said to be ion channel modulators or membrane stabilisers. Other drug groups with similar actions are the antiarrhythmic agents and anticonvulsants (lignocaine is in fact used for these effects). Natural toxins, such as those of the puffer fish (tetrodotoxin), blue-ringed octopus (maculotoxin) and marine organisms (saxitoxin), also block nerve transmission, particularly in skeletal muscle, often causing fatal paralysis (see Figure 13-3).

Pharmacokinetics

The purpose of giving a local anaesthetic is to localise its action in the tissue or nerve pathway into which it is injected. It is only later that the drug is absorbed from the tissues into the bloodstream and distributed around the body, where it may have effects in other systems and be metabolised and excreted (see Figure 15-3). This is in contrast to the more usual situation of an orally administered drug, which is

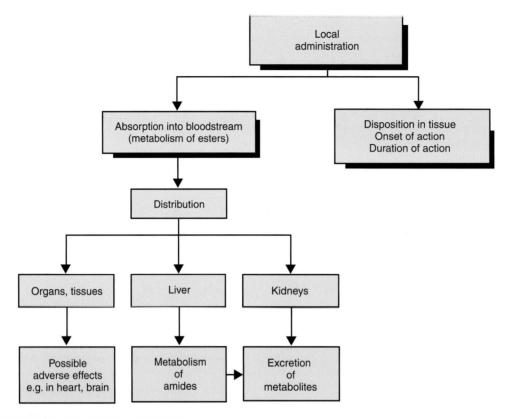

FIGURE 15-3 Pharmacokinetics of local anaesthetics.

absorbed from the gastrointestinal tract and passes through the liver before being distributed via the bloodstream to the tissues where it acts.

An injected LA will first undergo local disposition (i.e. move around) in the tissue. The onset of action is determined by the speed with which it diffuses into nerve cells, which depends largely on its lipid solubility, which depends in turn on the pH of the tissue and the degree of ionisation of the LA molecules (a function of the pK_a [negative logarithm of ionisation constant] of the drug). Binding of the LA to tissue proteins and the presence of a vasoconstrictor in the solution help retain the drug in the tissues for longer action. Other potential factors include the volume and concentration of solution injected, speed of injection and local blood flow.

Action is terminated by diffusion away, dilution and uptake into the vasculature, i.e. systemic absorption from the tissue. Lipid solubility is again the major determining factor and a vasoconstrictor, by decreasing blood flow in the area, will decrease the rate of absorption into the general circulation. Studies have shown that the peak plasma concentration of lignocaine (plain, i.e. without adrenaline) is reached about 20 minutes after injection; this is when systemic adverse effects are most likely to occur. During distribution around the body, effects may occur in other tissues, the drug may bind in tissues and it may be transferred across the blood–brain barrier or the placenta. Ester LAs (procaine and benzocaine) are rapidly

metabolised by esterase enzymes in the plasma, red cells and liver and have few systemic adverse effects. Rapid metabolism of amide LAs occurs en route through the liver; this first-pass effect explains why LAs are inactive if taken orally. Inactive metabolites are excreted via the kidneys.

Overall, the onset and duration of action of an injected LA depends on all the above factors and on the patient's cardiovascular and liver functions. The half-lives of LAs are generally short (1–2 hours); **bupivacaine** has a high lipid solubility and is highly protein-bound so it has a longer duration of action. The choice of a local anaesthetic for a particular procedure depends largely on the duration of drug action desired. Table 15-3 summarises the properties of several commonly used short-, intermediate- and long-acting local anaesthetic drugs.

Clinical aspects
Indications and contraindications for use of local anaesthetics

Local anaesthetics are indicated for surgical procedures when the patient's cooperation and consciousness are required or desired, for minor superficial and body surface procedures when general anaesthesia would be hazardous, and for sympathetic blockade or postoperative analgesia.

TABLE 15-3 Properties of commonly used local anaesthetics

NAME	TYPE/METABOLISM	USES	TOXICITY/NOTES
Short-acting (30–60 min)			
Procaine	Ester/plasma	Infiltration, nerve block, spinal	Least toxic LA; low lipid solubility; slow onset; potency 0.5 × lignocaine
Benzocaine	Ester/plasma	Topical: drops, gel, lozenges, paint, suppositories	Relatively non-toxic; very low potency; only active topically
Intermediate duration (1–3 h)			
Lignocaine	Amide/liver	Infiltration, nerve block, spinal epidural, IV, topical	Prototype LA, potency = 1; more cardiotoxic than prilocaine; rapid onset
Prilocaine	Amide/liver	Infiltration, nerve blocks, caudal, epidural, IV	Lower systemic toxicity than lignocaine; equipotent with lignocaine; products of liver metabolism may cause methaemoglobinaemia
Lignocaine/ prilocaine cream (EMLA)	Amides/liver	Topical (venepuncture, cannulation, minor skin surgery)	Local irritation; risk in infants <6 months (methaemoglobinaemia); toxic if swallowed by small children
Mepivacaine	Amide/liver	Infiltration, nerve blocks, caudal, epidural	Less toxic than lignocaine; equipotent with lignocaine; avoid use in pregnancy
Articaine	Amide/liver	Dental	Combined with adrenaline 1:100,000 provides 1–3 hour regional anaesthesia; no significant advantages over lignocaine
Long duration (3–10 h)			
Bupivacaine, levobupivacaine, ropivacaine	Amides/liver	Infiltration, caudal, epidural, nerve blocks	More cardiotoxic than lignocaine; potency 4 × lignocaine; slow onset; adrenaline not needed; less motor blockade
Amethocaine (tetracaine)	Ester/plasma	Topical anaesthesia	Potency 5 × lignocaine; slow onset; high systemic toxicity; useful for analgesia for venous cannulation

Contraindications to the use of local anaesthesia include extensive surgery that would require potentially toxic doses, known allergy or hypersensitivity to the LA agent, lack of cooperation from the patient, and local inflammation, infection or ischaemia at the injection site. As usual, precautions may be required in paediatric, elderly or pregnant patients and in patients with liver disease.

Dosage

The lowest effective dose should be used, noting that **maximum safe doses** are only guides (see Clinical Interest Box 15-7). Because a dose that is safe when injected SC may be toxic if injected IV, the dose should be injected slowly, with frequent aspirations (applying suction to syringe) to avoid intravascular injection.

Use of a vasoconstrictor

Most local anaesthetics produce vasodilation by direct action on blood vessels and by anaesthetising sympathetic vasoconstrictor fibres. This can cause rapid absorption of the drug; when the rate of absorption exceeds the rate of elimination, toxic effects can occur. Hence vasoconstrictors, such as adrenaline or felypressin, are sometimes formulated in with the LA solution to prolong the contact of the drug with local tissue, prolong the anaesthetic's duration of action and decrease systemic absorption and risk of systemic toxicity. Another example is the combination of phenylephrine, an α-adrenoceptor agonist, with lignocaine in a nasal spray for use in nasal/pharyngeal anaesthesia.

Vasoconstrictors are not used for nerve blocks in areas where there are end arteries (fingers, toes, ears, nose or penis) because ischaemia may develop, resulting in gangrene.

CLINICAL INTEREST BOX 15-7 CALCULATING THE SAFE DOSE OF A LOCAL ANAESTHETIC

The strength of a solution of a local anaesthetic formulated for injection is usually expressed in % terms, e.g. lignocaine 2% w/v. This means that there are 2 g solid drug dissolved in 100 mL solution. It follows that each 1 mL contains 20 mg lignocaine. Adrenaline concentration is usually expressed differently, e.g. as 1 in 200,000. This means that 1 g is present in 200,000 mL solution, or 1 mg in 200 mL.

Doses of LAs depend on many factors, including the drug, type of regional anaesthesia intended, weight and state of the patient, and whether a vasoconstrictor is present.

The minimum dose that results in effective anaesthesia should be used. The average dose of a local anaesthetic is usually quoted in mL solution, rather than mg/kg body weight; thus for a brachial plexus block in an average 70 kg adult, 20–40 mL of a 1% lignocaine solution is the maximum recommended.

The maximum safe dose of lignocaine plain (i.e. without adrenaline) is about 3 mg/kg. Thus for an average 70 kg adult, 210 mg will be the maximum dose, which is contained in 21 mL of 1% solution, supplied in 5 mL ampoules, so no more than 4.2 5 mL ampoules should be needed. (If calculations show that 42 or 420 ampoules are required, warning bells should ring and the calculations should be checked.)

As a vasoconstrictor localises the LA in tissues and prevents a rapid bolus of drug being absorbed into the bloodstream, larger doses can be used than are safe in the absence of the vasoconstrictor. Thus the maximum dose of lignocaine in the presence of adrenaline is 7–8 mg/kg.

Dosages quoted from: Padley 2004; AMH 2005.

The dose of vasoconstrictor must be carefully determined to prevent ischaemic necrosis at the injection site. Other potential risks include cardiovascular stimulation (from stimulation of cardiac β_1-adrenoceptors by adrenaline), so caution is required in patients with cardiovascular or thyroid disease or those taking antidepressants.

Some LAs do not require the use of a vasoconstrictor: cocaine has vasoconstrictor actions (due to its sympathomimetic effects) and bupivacaine and related drugs have long contact times in tissues, allowing tissue binding and prolonging their actions.

Formulations of local anaesthetics

For infiltration and nerve block techniques, the LA must be formulated in an injectable form, i.e. as a parenteral solution. Such solutions must be sterile, particle-free, stable, and preferably isotonic and buffered to the pH of body solutions. Particular cases are those of LA solutions with added vasoconstrictor (e.g. adrenaline, usually added in the strength 1 in 80,000 or 1 in 200,000: see Clinical Interest Box 15-7) and heavy solutions (for spinal anaesthesia) such as Marcain Spinal 0.5% Heavy Injection, a hyperbaric bupivacaine solution containing glucose at 80 mg/mL. Parenteral solutions may also be formulated with an opioid analgesic, such as fentanyl or pethidine.

For topical administration, almost every dose form known to pharmaceutical science has been used, including creams, jellies, paints, lotions, ointments, adhesive ointments, sprays, dressings, lozenges, eye/ear-drops, viscous solutions, emulsions and suppositories. Some interesting topical combination formulations are lignocaine with chlorhexidine in a gel, for use as a lubricant in urological procedures, and lignocaine with benzalkonium chloride in a skin spray, for sunburn relief.

Interestingly, there are no formulations for oral administration and systemic absorption (although there are topical formulations for mouth and gastric ulcers). This is because LAs are rapidly metabolised in the first-pass effect, and because it would be impossible to localise their effects once absorbed into the systemic circulation.

Adverse drug reactions and drug interactions

Because local anaesthetics are potentially toxic drugs, a patient's age, weight, physical condition and liver function must be taken into account in determining drug dosage. Adverse reactions can occur very quickly, so patients must never be left alone. Most reactions to local anaesthetics result from overdosage, inadvertent IV administration, rapid absorption into systemic circulation, or individual hypersensitivity or allergic response. The lowest effective dose should be used and IV injections must be avoided by aspirating gently and injecting slowly.

Procaine is considered the least toxic LA and cocaine the most toxic. In order of increasing toxicity, the common LAs are procaine, prilocaine, mepivacaine, lignocaine, etidocaine, bupivacaine, tetracaine, cinchocaine, cocaine.

Adverse reactions can be classified as:
- local complications at site of injection, e.g. inflammation, haematoma, nerve injury, abscess formation, necrosis
- psychogenic reactions: hyperventilation or vasovagal syncope (fainting) secondary to the injection stress (these may occur before injection)
- adverse drug reactions specific to the individual LA, e.g. prilocaine causing methaemoglobinaemia and cyanosis
- systemic effects of the vasoconstrictor, e.g. sympathetic or central stimulation
- local effects of the vasoconstrictor, such as ischaemia, necrosis, gangrene

- reactions specific to epidural and spinal LAs: headache, hypotension, infections, neuropathies, paraesthesias and autonomic dysfunction
- allergies and hypersensitivity reactions, such as rash, bronchospasm, anaphylaxis (more common with esters than amides; can also occur in response to preservatives in the solution)
- systemic effects of the LA after absorption: numbness of tongue, CNS stimulation (visual disturbances, irritability, convulsions, due to blockade of inhibitory pathways) then depression, relaxation of smooth and skeletal muscle, cardiovascular depression, respiratory depression.

Adverse reactions may require treatment. For minor reactions, conservative resuscitation and first-aid efforts are effective. For major reactions, oxygen, assisted ventilation and IV infusion of fluids and drugs to counteract convulsions, cardiovascular and respiratory depression may be necessary.

Significant drug interactions

Significant drug interactions are limited but this does not preclude a variety of unexpected responses, so close observation is needed. Prior or concurrent administration of CNS-depressant drugs such as antiarrhythmic agents may result in additive CNS depression effects. Adjust dosages and monitor closely. Anticholinesterase drugs may inhibit the metabolism of ester-type LAs (procaine).

Anaesthetics containing a vasoconstrictor are used with caution in patients receiving drugs that alter blood pressure, such as antihypertensives, monoamine oxidase inhibitors and tricyclic antidepressants. The combination may produce hypertension. Cardiac arrhythmias may occur when catecholamine vasoconstrictors (e.g. adrenaline) are used in patients receiving general anaesthesia with cyclopropane or halothane.

Techniques for local anaesthesia

There are several techniques by which LAs are administered (see Figure 15-4 and Table 15-4). They can be applied to an area or injected into tissues where they produce their effect in the immediate area only, hence the term 'local anaesthesia'. They can also be injected around a nerve or nerve trunk (e.g. nerve block, spinal or epidural techniques) to produce anaesthesia in a large region of the body (**regional anaesthesia**).

Topical or surface anaesthesia

The use of surface, or topical, anaesthesia is restricted to mucous membranes, damaged skin surfaces, wounds and burns. **Topical local anaesthesia** is used to relieve pain and itching and to anaesthetise mucous membranes of the eye,

nose, throat or urethra for minor surgical procedures, to facilitate instrumentation, and before venepuncture or split skin grafting. Many dose forms are available, including eye- and ear-drops, solutions, ointments, gels, creams, sprays or powders.

Topical anaesthetics do not effectively penetrate unbroken skin, except for the combination cream EMLA (eutectic mixture for local anaesthesia), which contains 25 mg/g each of lignocaine and prilocaine. Cocaine in a 4%–10% solution is still used topically for nasal anaesthesia.

A number of local anaesthetic agents cannot be injected, because they are too insoluble (benzocaine) or too toxic (cocaine, tetracaine). However, because they are only slowly absorbed, they can usually be used safely on open wounds, ulcers and mucous membranes. They occasionally cause dermatitis and allergic sensitisation, which necessitate their discontinuance. Absorption is increased from mucous membranes and broken skin (e.g. abrasions, trauma and ulcers), leading to the possibility of systemic effects; deaths have occurred from absorption via the urethra. When they are used in the oral cavity (mouth and pharynx), interference with swallowing may occur and aspiration is a risk. The patient is assessed for a returning gag reflex by gentle touching of the back of the pharynx with a tongue blade. All food and fluids are withheld until the reflex returns.

Infiltration anaesthesia

Infiltration anaesthesia is the use of local anaesthetics in an area that circles the operative field; it is produced by injecting dilute solutions (0.1%) of the agent into the skin and then subcutaneously into the region to be anaesthetised. Adrenaline is often added to the solution as a vasoconstrictor to intensify the anaesthesia in a limited region and to prevent excessive bleeding and systemic effects. Repeated injection extends the anaesthesia as long as needed. The sensory nerve endings are anaesthetised, but not motor nerves. This method of administration is used for minor surgery such as for skin lesions, skin incision and drainage or excision of a cyst, and sometimes for more major procedures including dental extractions.

Intravenous regional anaesthesia (Bier's block)

Intravenous regional anaesthesia (IVRA) is a specialised technique for anaesthesia of the upper limb; the technique is as follows (see Figure 15-5):
- a tourniquet is placed on the upper part of the arm to be anaesthetised
- a vein distal to the tourniquet is cannulated, e.g. a vein in the dorsum of the hand
- the field of operation is exsanguinated by wrapping an Esmarch bandage up the arm or by elevation for 4–5 minutes

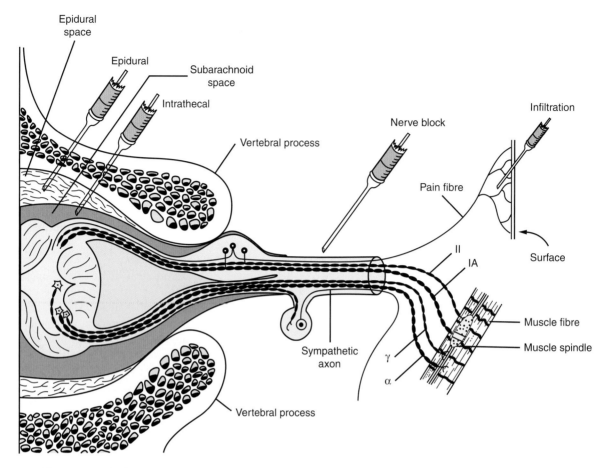

FIGURE 15-4 The routes of administration of local anaesthetic drugs. Half of a cross-section of the spinal column is shown with a spinal nerve composed of examples of the main types of efferent and afferent fibres. II = group II afferent axon from flower spray ending of muscle spindle; IA = group IA afferent axon from annulospiral ending of muscle spindle; γ = γ-efferent axon to intrafusal fibres of muscle spindle; α = α axon (lower motoneuron) to extrafusal muscle fibres. Note that intrathecal injection into the subarachnoid space (spinal anaesthesia) is usually made in the lumbar region below the termination of the spinal cord. *Source*: Bowman & Rand 1980; used with permission.

- the tourniquet is inflated to a pressure greater than the patient's pulse pressure to occlude arterial flow (e.g. to 150 mmHg above systolic pressure) and kept inflated; the Esmarch bandage is then removed
- the LA solution (prilocaine or lignocaine, without adrenaline or preservative) is injected slowly IV distal to the cuff
- the procedure is then carried out
- after the procedure the tourniquet must be released only gradually to avoid a large bolus of LA entering the systemic circulation; during this time the patient's pulse, blood pressure and ECG are monitored.

The tourniquet is kept tight during the operation (and for a minimum of 20 minutes) to reduce blood flow to and from the area, which localises the LA and facilitates tissue binding. It is proposed that the injected LA diffuses from the vein into adjacent arteries and thence into the tissues, causing rapid analgesia and muscle relaxation within 10–15 minutes; the whole limb distal to the cuff is anaesthetised, allowing major surgery. This technique is considered safer than a major nerve block of the upper limb. It is not used in children, who do not tolerate well the discomfort of the tourniquet, but is very useful in emergency situations, e.g. treatment of Colles' fracture, and in Third World countries.

In theory, Bier's block can also be used for the lower limb but the large muscle masses in the leg make the method unsatisfactory in practice.

Nerve (conduction) block anaesthesia

For a **nerve block**, the local anaesthetic is injected into the vicinity of a nerve trunk and inhibits the conduction of impulses to and from the area supplied by that nerve, the region of the operative site. The injection can be made at some distance from the surgical site. A single nerve may be blocked,

TABLE 15-4 Local anaesthetic techniques

METHOD	TISSUE AFFECTED	DOSE FORM USED	EXAMPLES OF DRUGS USED	THERAPEUTIC INDICATIONS
Topical	Sensory nerve endings in mucous membranes and dermis	Solution, ointment, cream, powder, eye-drops, spray etc	Cocaine, benzocaine, lignocaine, amethocaine, prilocaine	Relief of pain or itching; examination of conjunctiva; minor surgery; instrumentation
Infiltration	Sensory nerve endings in subcutaneous tissues or dermis	Injection	Procaine, prilocaine, lignocaine, mepivacaine	Minor surgery; skin lesions
Nerve block	Nerve trunk	Injection	Articaine, procaine, prilocaine, lignocaine, bupivacaine, mepivacaine	Dental, eye and limb surgery; sympathetic block; obstetrics; postoperative pain relief
Epidural block	Spinal roots	Injection	Lignocaine, bupivacaine, levobupivacaine, ropivacaine	Thoracic and abdominal surgery; labour pain; caesarean section; postoperative pain relief
Spinal (subarachnoid) block	Spinal roots	Injection	Bupivacaine, levobupivacaine, lignocaine	Abdominal surgery; surgery of the lower extremities; muscle relaxation
Intravenous regional anaesthesia	Upper limb	Injection	Prilocaine	Surgery on upper limb

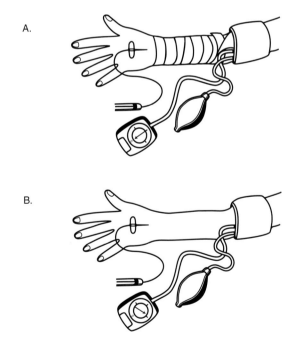

FIGURE 15-5 Technique for Bier's block: IV regional anaesthesia of the upper limb. **A.** Cuff has been positioned, IV cannula inserted and limb exsanguinated by winding an Esmarch bandage proximally up the arm. **B.** Cuff has been inflated and the bandage removed, allowing injection of local anaesthetic.

or the anaesthetic may be injected where several nerve trunks emerge from the spinal cord (paravertebral block). During peripheral nerve block, motor nerves are usually blocked as well as sensory pathways. A concentrated solution is required because of the thickness of nerve trunk fibres. This method of anaesthesia is often used for foot and hand surgery, eye surgery, for pudendal block for obstetric procedures, and for postoperative pain relief.

EPIDURAL AND SPINAL ANAESTHESIA

Two specialised types of central nerve blocks are the epidural and spinal blocks, in which spinal roots are blocked where they emerge from the spinal canal. These techniques are used for abdominal, pelvic and lower limb surgery. Autonomic nerves can also be blocked, so there is a risk of autonomic adverse effects. To increase analgesia, an opioid such as morphine, pethidine or fentanyl is often also administered by these techniques. Central nerve block is contraindicated if there is systemic anticoagulation or coagulation abnormality or if there is raised intracranial pressure.

EPIDURAL (EXTRADURAL) ANAESTHESIA. An epidural is an injection of LA into the space between the dura mater and the ligamentum flavum, at spinal cord levels C7–T10 (see Figure 15-4). The 'space' is actually filled with loose adipose tissue, lymphatics and blood vessels; the solution tends to remain localised at the level at which it is injected. It is commonly used for obstetrics, urology, and thoracic, abdominal and perineal surgery. The solution does not contact the spinal cord or CSF, so there is less risk of CNS infection than with spinal injection. Postoperative urinary retention is common, as parasympathetic nerves are blocked.

Caudal anaesthesia is an epidural procedure in which the anaesthetic solution is injected into the caudal canal, the sacral part of the vertebral canal containing the cauda equina or the bundle of spinal nerves that innervate the pelvic viscera. It is used in obstetrics and for pelvic or genital surgery.

SPINAL (SUBARACHNOID) ANAESTHESIA. In **spinal anaesthesia** (also called **subarachnoid**, intradural or intrathecal block), the LA is injected into the CSF in the subarachnoid space, below the level of termination of the spinal cord, i.e. at L3–4 or L4–5, and affects the lower part of the spinal cord and nerve roots. As the needle and solution come into contact with the CSF, sterility and aseptic procedures are required to prevent infections such as meningitis.

The LA can spread through the spinal canal, so the specific gravity of the LA solution and the patient's position determine the level of anaesthesia. For example, for low spinal anaesthesia, the patient is placed in a flat or Fowler's position and a solution with a specific gravity greater than that of cerebrospinal fluid is used, as it tends to diffuse downward.

The onset of anaesthesia usually occurs within 1–2 minutes of injection. The duration is 1–3 hours, depending on the anaesthetic used. Spinal anaesthesia is used for surgical procedures on the lower abdomen, inguinal area or lower extremities, and is often the method of choice for elderly patients or those with severe respiratory problems or liver, kidney or metabolic disease.

Marked hypotension, decreased cardiac output and respiratory depression tend to occur because of depression of medullary centres and sympathetic pathways; they are considered disadvantages of this method. Postoperatively, headache is the most common complaint and may be accompanied by difficulty in hearing or seeing. Headache may be postural and occur only in the head-up or sitting or standing position. This symptom is thought to be the result of the opening in the dura made by the large spinal needle. The opening may persist for days or weeks, permitting loss of cerebrospinal fluid and risk of infection (meningitis). Paraesthesias such as numbness and tingling may occur after spinal anaesthesia; they are usually limited to the lumbar or sacral areas and disappear within a relatively short time. The success and safety of spinal anaesthesia depend primarily on the anaesthetist's skill and knowledge.

Saddle block is a type of subarachnoid block sometimes used in obstetrics and for surgery involving the perineum, rectum, genitalia and upper parts of the thighs. The patient sits upright while the heavy anaesthetic solution is injected after a lumbar puncture. The person remains upright for a short time, until the anaesthetic has taken effect and anaesthetised the sacral nerves. (The body parts that contact a saddle when horse-riding become anaesthetised, hence the name.)

PREGNANCY SAFETY

ADEC Category	Drug (common formulation)
A	Bupivacaine, EMLA, enflurane, halothane, lignocaine, mepivacaine, nitrous oxide, prilocaine, suxamethonium, thiopentone
B1	Ropivacaine
B2	Methohexitone, mivacurium, pancuronium, procaine, rocuronium, sevoflurane
B3	Articaine, desflurane, isoflurane, ketamine, levobupivacaine
C	Atracurium, cisatracurium, methoxyflurane, propofol, vecuronium

DRUGS AT A GLANCE 15: Anaesthetics

Therapeutic group	Pharmacological group	Key examples	Key pages
General anaesthetics			pp. 227–9
Induction agents (IV)	Barbiturates	thiopentone	p. 238
	Non-barbiturates	propofol	pp. 238, 9
Maintenance agents (inhaled)	Inhaled general anaesthetics		
	· Gases	nitrous oxide	p. 236
	· Volatile liquid anaesthetics	sevoflurane	pp. 237, 8
		halothane	p. 237
Premedication			pp. 234, 5
Sedative–antianxiety agents	Benzodiazepines	midazolam	pp. 235, 7, 9
Antisecretory agents	Antimuscarinics	atropine	p. 235
Adjuncts			pp. 231, 5
Analgesics	Opioids	morphine	p. 235
Skeletal muscle relaxants	Competitive, non-depolarising relaxants	pancuronium	p. 235
	Depolarising relaxants	suxamethonium	p. 235
Antiemetics	Dopamine antagonists	metoclopramide	p. 235
	5-HT antagonists	ondansetron	p. 235
Local anaesthetics	Esters	procaine, amethocaine	p. 243
	Amides	lignocaine	pp. 241, 3
		prilocaine	p. 243
	Long-acting	bupivacaine	p. 243
		ropivacaine	p. 243

COX = cyclo-oxygenase; 5-HT = 5-hydroxytryptamine.

KEY POINTS

- General anaesthesia is the loss of all sensations and consciousness; it can be achieved by inhalation or injection of rapidly acting, reversible CNS depressants, which are lipid-soluble agents that act by modulation of transmitter-gated ion channels.

- Inhalation agents include the gas nitrous oxide and volatile agents such as sevoflurane; IV anaesthetics include propofol and thiopentone.

- Balanced anaesthesia is the use of a combination of agents to achieve unconsciousness, analgesia, muscle relaxation and amnesia. Premedication may include an antianxiety agent (midazolam) and atropine to suppress secretions. Antiemetics and opioids are used for postoperative nausea and pain.

- Common adverse effects and interactions are the potentiation of CNS depression and the risk of malignant hyperthermia from suxamethonium plus a general anaesthetic.

- Local anaesthesia is used to render a specific part or region of the body insensitive to pain. Local anaesthetics such as lignocaine block action potential transmission in all excitable tissues, especially in sensory nerves.

- The local anaesthetic drug acts locally in the tissue to which it is administered before being absorbed into the general circulation.

- A vasoconstrictor agent may be added to the solution to localise and prolong the action of the drug and minimise systemic adverse effects.

- Local anaesthesia is achieved by topical application or by subcutaneous infiltration of the selected operative area.

Regional anaesthesia is the injecting of a local anaesthetic drug near a peripheral nerve trunk (nerve block) or around the spinal column to anaesthetise spinal nerve roots (epidural or subarachnoid techniques).

● Adverse drug reactions include allergies (especially to the ester-type drug procaine) and systemic effects on the heart, CNS and respiratory system if large amounts of the drug are absorbed.

● An awareness of drug actions, adverse effects, toxicity, potential drug interactions and the particular precautions required for young, old, pregnant and ill patients is necessary for the safe and effective use of the various anaesthetic agents.

REVIEW EXERCISES

1. Discuss the actions, mechanism of action and clinical uses of:
   * inhalation general anaesthetics
   * intravenous general anaesthetics
   * premedication agents
   * neuromuscular blocking agents
   * local anaesthetics (esters and amides).

2. Discuss the use and advantages of intravenous anaesthetics in general anaesthesia. What are some of the disadvantages with using intravenous anaesthetics?

3. Describe the different techniques for administering local anaesthetics, the situations in which they are used and the appropriate drugs and formulations.

4. Discuss the differences between ester- and amide-type local anaesthetics, giving examples.

REFERENCES AND FURTHER READING

Ali SZ, Taguchi A, Rosenberg H. Malignant hyperthermia. Best practice and research *Clinical Anaesthesiology* 2003; 17(4): 519–33.
Analgesic Expert Group. *Therapeutic Guidelines: Analgesic, version 4*. Melbourne: Therapeutic Guidelines Limited, 2002.
Australian Medicines Handbook 2005. Adelaide: AMH, 2005.
Bailey AR, Jones JG. Patients' memories of events during general anaesthesia. *Anaesthesia* 1997; 52: 460–76.
Belelli I, Pistis I, Peters JA, Lambert JJ. General anaesthetic action at transmitter-gated inhibitory amino acid receptors. *Trends in Pharmacological Sciences* 1999; 20: 496–502.
Bissonnette B, Swan H, Ravussin P, Un V. Neuroleptanesthesia: current status. *Canadian Journal of Anaesthesia* 1999; 46: 154–68.
Bowman WC, Rand MJ. *Textbook of Pharmacology*. 2nd edn. Oxford: Blackwell, 1980 [chs 7, 16].
Calmes SH. Arthur Guedel, MD, and the eye signs of anesthesia. *American Society of Anesthesiologists Newsletter* 2002; 66(9): 17–9.
Caswell A. (ed.). *MIMS Annual June 2005*. Sydney: CMPMedica Australia, 2005.
Cousins MJ, Bridenbaugh PO. *Neural Blockade in Clinical Anaesthesia and Management of Pain*. 3rd edn. Philadelphia: Lippincroft-Raven, 1998.
de Jong RH. *Local Anaesthetics*. St Louis: Mosby, 1994.
Dodds C. General anaesthesia: practical recommendations and recent advances. *Drugs* 1999; 58: 453–67.
Fischer HBJ, Pinnock CA. *Fundamentals of Regional Anaesthesia*. Cambridge: Cambridge University Press, 2004.
Krasowski MD, Harrison NL. General anaesthetic actions on ligand-gated ion channels. *Cellular and Molecular Life Sciences* 1999; 55: 1278–303.
Muravchick S. The aging process: anaesthetic implications. *Acta Anaesthesiologica Belgica* 1998; 49: 85–90.
Oberoi G, Phillips G. *Anaesthesia and Emergency Situations: A Management Guide*. Sydney: McGraw-Hill, 2000.
Padley AP. *Westmead Pocket Anaesthetic Manual*. 2nd edn. Sydney: McGraw-Hill; 2004.
Phillips GD. Defining moments in medicine: anaesthesia. *Medical Journal of Australia* 2001; 174: 17–18.
Richards CD. What the actions of anaesthetics on fast synaptic transmission reveal about the molecular mechanism of anaesthesia. *Toxicology Letters* 1998; 100–101: 41–50.
Rudolph U, Antkowiak B. Molecular and neuronal substrates for general anaesthetics. *Nature Reviews Neuroscience* 2004; 5: 709–20.
Schug S, Dodd P. Perioperative analgesia. *Australian Prescriber* 2004; 27(6): 152–4.
Speight TM, Holford NHG (eds). *Avery's Drug Treatment*. 4th edn. Auckland: Adis, 1997.
Suruda A. Health effects of anaesthetic gases. *Occupational Medicine* 1997; 12: 627–34.

ON-LINE RESOURCES

New Zealand medicines and medical devices safety authority: www.medsafe.govt.nz

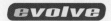 More weblinks at http://evolve.elsevier.com/AU/Bryant/pharmacology/

CHAPTER 16

Analgesics

CHAPTER FOCUS

Pain is a universal symptom experienced by nearly everyone at some point in life; yet each person's experience is individual and subjective. Pain is more distressing and disabling than almost any other patient symptom. Fortunately, the distressing and incapacitating nature of pain is mostly unnecessary because the potent analgesics currently available are safe and effective when properly selected and administered, based on individual patient needs and responses and on individual drug pharmacokinetics. As pain is the symptom patients most commonly fear, the health-care professional needs to be knowledgeable about types of pain and interventions that are useful in controlling or preventing pain.

OBJECTIVES

- To describe components of pain and how they contribute to overall suffering.

- To discuss physiological theories of pain and the transmitters and chemical mediators involved.

- To define acute and chronic pain, giving examples of each.

- To describe pain of nociceptive, neurogenic and psychogenic origins, giving examples.

- To discuss the clinical management of pain, with guidelines for assessment and choice of appropriate analgesic drugs and adjunct techniques.

- To discuss the special issues related to the use of analgesics in children and the elderly.

- To describe the actions of opioid agonist analgesics, antagonists, and agonist–antagonist agents, and their clinical use.

- To discuss the relationship between prostaglandin effects in tissues and the use of non-steroidal anti-inflammatory drugs in inflammation and pain relief.

KEY DRUGS

aspirin
codeine
fentanyl
morphine
naloxone
paracetamol

KEY TERMS

acute pain
adjuvant analgesic
analgesic
chronic pain
cyclo-oxygenase
endorphin
enkephalin
equianalgesic dose
gate control theory
neurogenic pain
neuropathic pain
nociceptive pain
non-steroidal anti-
  inflammatory drug

opioid
opium
pain
prostaglandins
psychogenic pain
receptors (opioid)
salicylate
stepwise management
  of pain
substance P
tolerance

KEY ABBBREVIATIONS

COX	cyclo-oxygenase
glu	glutamate
5-HT	5-hydroxytryptamine (serotonin)
LT	leukotriene
M6G	morphine-6-glucuronide
NMDA	N-methyl-D-aspartate
NSAID	non-steroidal anti-inflammatory drug
PCA	patient-controlled analgesia
PG	prostaglandin
TENS	transcutaneous electrical nerve stimulation

PAIN is defined by the International Association for the Study of Pain as 'an unpleasant sensory and emotional experience associated with actual or potential tissue damage, or described in terms of such damage'. This complicated definition emphasises both the dual aspects of pain (sensory and emotional) and that there may not be actual tissue damage, only potential damage. More simply, pain is what the experiencing person says it is; in other words, only the person suffering the pain can tell how much pain is being experienced. Understanding pain and the actions of analgesics (pain-relieving drugs) in treating it requires first an understanding of how it is generated.

PHYSIOLOGY OF PAIN
Pain and suffering

Because of its highly subjective nature, **pain** is difficult to study objectively. It can be viewed as having two components: the physical component, or the sensation of pain (nociception), which involves peripheral and central nerve pathways; and the psychological component, or the emotional response to pain, which involves factors such as a person's anxiety level, previous pain experiences, age, sex and culture.

People have a relatively constant pain threshold under normal circumstances; for example, heat applied to the skin at an intensity of 45°–48°C will initiate the sensation of pain in almost all people. By contrast, pain tolerance—the point beyond which pain becomes unbearable—varies widely among individuals and in a single person under different circumstances. Figure 16-1 shows factors affecting pain perception and tolerance.

A scheme illustrating pain and suffering and the various issues that influence suffering in a terminally ill patient is shown in Figure 16-2. As this model shows, physical pain is only part of the overall suffering and is not interchangeable with suffering. A person may suffer without physical pain or may have physical pain without suffering. Suffering may be defined as multiple issues that must be endured and which prevent a person from living without fear or pain. Suffering may include physical pain, emotional fears (fear of the unknown, fear of dying, fear of dying alone, lack of social supports, loss of independence or integrity), social conflicts (unresolved conflicts with family and friends) and spiritual despair. Such problems are often tackled by interdisciplinary teams in hospices and pain management programs.

Theories of pain

Noxious stimuli in the periphery are detected by nociceptors (pain receptors) and the signals transmitted to the spinal cord via A-delta (δ) fibres (mediating sharp, transient fast pain), or C-fibres (mediating burning, aching, slow, visceral pain) (see Figure 16-3A). These primary afferent fibres synapse in the dorsal horn of the spinal cord. The second-order neurons cross over and continue upwards in the anterolateral spinothalamic tracts (Figure 16-3B) to the thalamus and the cerebral cortex, where the messages are perceived as pain. Efferent pathways from the cortex descend via the periaqueductal grey matter to the dorsal horn areas in the cord, and may modify afferent impulses.

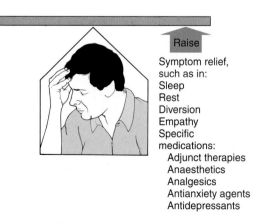

FIGURE 16-1 Factors affecting pain tolerance; those on the left tend to lower the tolerance, making pain worse or more likely to occur.

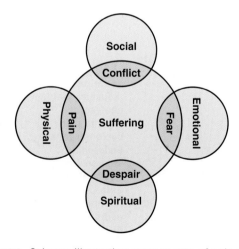

FIGURE 16-2 Scheme illustrating components of pain and suffering.

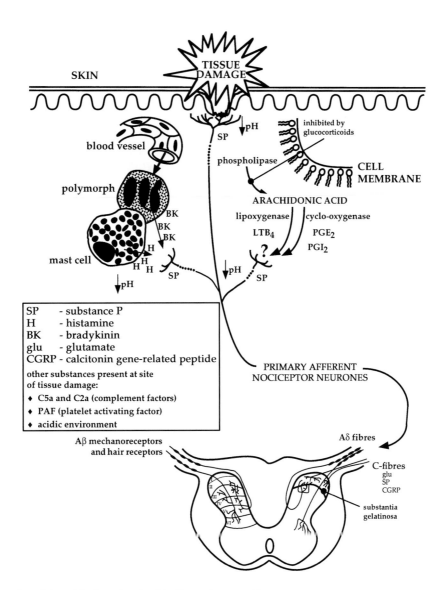

FIGURE 16-3A Diagram of peripheral factors involved in the pain sensation.

The gate control theory

Several theories of pain transmission and pain relief have been proposed. The **gate control theory**, proposed by Melzack and Wall in 1965, proposes that a mechanism in the dorsal horn of the spinal cord (the spinal 'gate') can modify the transmission of painful sensations from the peripheral nerve fibres to the thalamus and cortex of the brain. The gate is influenced by descending inhibition from the brain, involving control systems with noradrenaline, 5-HT, substance P and enkephalins in particular as neurotransmitters.

Facilitation in the dorsal horn area results in greatly increased sensitivity (hyperalgesia, or 'opened gate'), which spreads beyond the injured area. Substance P, glutamate and nitric oxide are thought to be involved as transmitters.

Conversely, techniques of afferent stimulation to relieve pain, such as transcutaneous electrical nerve stimulation (TENS), acupuncture, and rubbing or 'itching' the skin, are thought to act through inhibitory circuits within the dorsal horn to diminish nociceptive transmission through the C-fibres, thus decreasing pain ('closing the gate'). (Descending pathways that may also 'gate' impulse transmission in the dorsal horn area are shown on the left-hand side of Figure 16-3B.)

Endogenous opioids

There are high concentrations of receptors for the body's natural opioids, the **endorphins** and **enkephalins**, in many areas of the CNS, particularly in the periaqueductal grey matter of the midbrain, in the limbic system and at interneurons

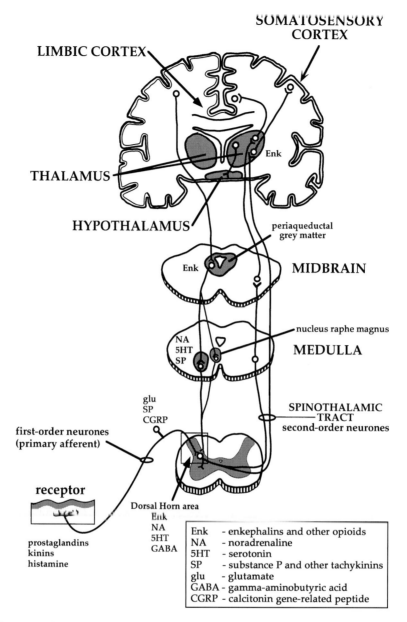

FIGURE 16-3B Diagram of nerve pathways and some neurotransmitters involved in pain sensation. Ascending afferent pathways are shown on the right-hand side and descending efferent pathways on the left. Diagrams by Victor Iwanov, University of Melbourne; reproduced from *Therapeutic Guidelines: Analgesic.* 4th edn; with permission.

in the dorsal horn areas. These areas are known to be involved in pain transmission or perception. The enkephalins (pentapeptides), endorphins (larger polypeptides: the name implies 'endogenous morphines') and dynorphin are thought to be the body's natural pain-relieving chemicals and to act by enhancing inhibitory effects at opioid receptors (see later discussion). One main group of analgesic drugs, the opioids, such as morphine and codeine, cause their effects by mimicking the actions of endorphins and enkephalins on opioid receptors. Endorphin release in the body is higher

after acupuncture and TENS, and both effects may be reversed by the use of naloxone, an opioid antagonist. It has been proposed that the analgesic response associated with the use of a placebo may result from an increased release of endorphins in the body.

Prostaglandins

Damage to tissue may directly activate sensory nerves and also sets in train the process of inflammation (see Figure

16-3A), in which a large number of inflammatory mediators are released (so many in fact that this has been referred to as the 'inflammatory soup'). Of particular importance in the context of pain mechanisms is arachidonic acid, a compound produced from damaged cell membranes that is metabolised by the cyclo-oxygenase enzyme system to tissue hormones called **prostaglandins** (PGs), which lower the threshold of nociceptors to other mediators. (These mechanisms are discussed in greater detail in Chapters 54 and 55.) The second main group of analgesic agents, the non-steroidal anti-inflammatory drugs (NSAIDs), owe their analgesic effects to inhibition of the production of PGs.

Tachykinins

Another group of modulators in the nociceptive pathway are the tachykinins (fast-acting polypeptides), including substance P and neurokinins A and B. Tachykinins are involved in inflammatory and neurogenic pain (see below). Competitive antagonists at neurokinin receptors are being developed and studied as potential new analgesic agents.

These theories of pain are the basis for many pharmacological and non-drug regimens of pain relief, including opioids, NSAIDs, local anaesthetics, γ-aminobutyric acid (GABA) agonists, N-methyl-D-aspartate (NMDA) antagonists, tachykinin antagonists, TENS, acupuncture, and the Lamaze (psychoprophylaxis) technique for pain relief.

Pain classification

Pain can be classified in various ways, e.g. on the basis of its time course as acute or chronic (see Table 16-1). Pain may also be classified on the basis of its origin, i.e. as nociceptive, neurogenic or psychogenic.

Acute and chronic pain

Acute pain, a state in which an individual experiences the sensation of severe discomfort, has a sudden onset, often with a protective function and an obvious cause, and usually subsides with treatment. Examples of acute pain include the pain of myocardial infarction, burn, appendicitis and kidney stones.

Chronic pain, such as that accompanying cancer or rheumatoid arthritis, is a persistent or recurring pain that continues for more than 3 months, or after completion of healing, and may be difficult to treat effectively. A person with chronic severe pain experiences an adaptation process (see Table 16-1); patients are likely to become trapped within a chronic pain cycle in which ineffective treatments increase anxiety and contribute to the pain persisting. The primary goal of treatment thus becomes not total relief from pain, but minimisation of pain-related disabilities and avoidance of unnecessary investigations and ineffective therapies. Regular medication with NSAID analgesics and addition of an antidepressant are advised. Opioids must be used with caution in the management of chronic non-malignant pain, due to the possible adverse drug reactions.

TABLE 16–1 Comparisons between acute and chronic pain		
	ACUTE PAIN	**CHRONIC PAIN**
Onset	Usually sudden	Longer duration
Characteristics	Generally sharp, localised, may radiate	Dull, aching, persistent, diffuse
Signs and symptoms		
Physiological response	Raised blood pressure, respiratory and heart rates; sweating, pallor, dilated pupils; increased muscle tension	Often absent: normal blood pressure, respiratory and heart rates, and pupil size; dry skin
Emotional/behavioural responses	Increased anxiety and restlessness; focus on pain, rubs affected part; cries, grimaces, moans	Person may be depressed, withdrawn, expressionless and exhausted; physical inactivity or sleep; no report of pain unless questioned
Therapeutic goals	Relief of pain; prevent transition to chronic pain; sedation often desirable	Prevention of pain; improve quality of life; sedation not usually wanted
Drug administration	Usually opioids	Paracetamol, NSAIDs, opioids and/or adjuvants
Timing	Start as soon as possible; assess regularly; patient-controlled analgesia is useful	Regular preventive schedule
Dose	Standard dosages are often adequate	Individualise according to patient response
Route	Parenteral (IV or SC)	Oral

Nociceptive pain

Nociceptive pain arises from stimulation of superficial or deep nociceptors by noxious stimuli such as tissue injury or inflammation. Somatic nociceptive pain originates especially in the skin, mucosal surfaces, bones and joints, pleura and peritoneum. It is described as being throbbing, burning, stinging, or a dull ache. Examples are the pain from a skin ulcer, arthritis, bony metastases of cancer, or minor surgery. Somatic pain responds best to treatment with NSAIDs.

Visceral nociceptive pain originates in organs such as the liver and pancreas, and large muscle masses. It is described as being deep, diffuse and nagging, and may be associated with nausea and vomiting, or sweating. The pain may be referred to another area of the body (which has sensory nerves running to the same segment of the spinal cord), such as the pain of a myocardial infarction that may be felt initially in the arm or shoulder. Examples include pain from bowel obstruction, abdominal tumours, ischaemic muscle or major surgery. Visceral pain usually responds well to opioid analgesics.

Muscle spasm nociceptive pain originates in skeletal or smooth muscle, is mediated by PGs and is worse on movement or when smooth muscle is stretched (colic). Biliary colic, bowel obstruction, spinal cord damage and some types of acute low-back pain exemplify muscle spasm pain. Muscle relaxants and NSAIDs are usually the analgesics of choice.

Neurogenic pain

Neurogenic pain arises from a primary lesion, alteration or dysfunction in the peripheral or central nervous system (PNS, CNS). It may be due to nerve compression, for example by a prolapsed intervertebral disc. Neuropathic neurogenic pain is caused by peripheral nerve injury rather than stimulation. This pain has been described as burning, shooting and/or tingling and is often associated with paraesthesia and allodynia (pain due to a stimulus that does not usually cause pain, e.g. pressure from clothing). This type of pain, caused for example by post-herpetic neuralgia, limb amputation, trigeminal neuralgia, diabetic neuropathy or cancer tumour invasion, may be accompanied by sympathetic nervous system dysfunction. **Neuropathic pain** responds less well to opioid analgesics and often requires the addition of adjunct medication to the patient's drug regimen (e.g. an anticonvulsant, such as gabapentin, local anaesthetic or tricyclic antidepressant).

Psychogenic pain

Psychogenic pain has psychological, psychiatric or psychosocial causes as its primary aetiology. Anxiety, depression and fear of dying have been known to cause severe pain. It is a CNS syndrome and may have no obvious somatic source but is very real and distressing to the sufferer and may lead to anger and depression. In such patients, drug therapy alone does not usually bring relief; a multimodal approach with psychotherapy is indicated.

Specific pain syndromes

Other more specific types of pain are treated whenever possible with specific therapies known as directed analgesia. Tension headaches, for example, usually respond to over-the-counter analgesics such as aspirin and paracetamol, sinus headaches to NSAIDs plus a decongestant, trigeminal neuralgia to carbamazepine, pain from osteoporotic fractures may be helped by the osteoblastic actions of calcitonin, while migraine headaches may require more potent drugs such as sumatriptan or ergotamine (see Chapter 21). Cancer pain relief requires a multimodal approach of palliative care (see Chapter 49), possibly involving analgesics and anaesthetics, other cancer therapies (radiotherapy, hormones, surgery, chemotherapy), neurosurgical techniques, physical therapies (splints, electrotherapy, occupational therapy), complementary and alternative medicine methods, and psychological support and therapy for patients and their carers.

Breakthrough pain

When pain occurs between doses of regular analgesics in patients with severe chronic pain, this is referred to as 'breakthrough pain'. It is usually managed with extra doses of short-acting oral or transdermal opioids (see section on breakthrough pain in Chapter 49).

PAIN MANAGEMENT

Assessing pain

As 'pain is what the patient says hurts', it is important to assess from the patient's experience the time course, type, site and extent of pain and its associations and effects. The Pain Assessment Chart shown in Figure 16-4, or the 'PQRST' approach (Analgesic Expert Group 2002), helps the patient describe the pain:

- P: palliative or provocative factors—what makes the pain better or worse?
- Q: quality—what is the pain like: burning, nagging, shooting?
- R: radiation—where does it hurt? Does the pain go anywhere else?
- S: severity—how severe is it? How much does it hurt?
- T: timing—does the pain come and go? What brings it on? How long has it hurt?

With respect to locating the pain, a body chart such as that shown in Figure 16-4 (1: Location) can be helpful. For an estimate of the severity of the pain, scales such as those in Figure 16-5 help patients indicate the intensity and distress levels of the pain. For children, a pictorial scale can be used, with faces to 'show how much it hurts' (Figure 16-6).

Regular reassessment of pain is essential, to monitor both the disease process and analgesic therapy and to assess whether other analgesic or adjuvant therapy is required.

Undertreatment of pain

Even though effective pain management techniques are available, the wide application of such approaches has been slow and many patients still suffer pain. Some of the reasons for undertreatment of pain are summarised in Clinical Interest Box 16-1.

The undertreatment of patients in pain is well documented in the literature and has resulted in litigation. Despite health-care providers being legally as well as morally responsible for pain relief, undertreatment and improper use of analgesics continue to be major problems in both acute and chronic pain settings.

Tolerance to analgesics

Drug **tolerance** is defined as the gradual decrease in the effectiveness of a drug given repeatedly over a period of time; if tolerance develops, higher doses are required to achieve the same effect. Morphine and the opioids provide

Date ______

Client's Name ______ Age ______ Room ______

Diagnosis ______ Physician ______

Nurse ______

I. Location: Client or nurse mark drawing

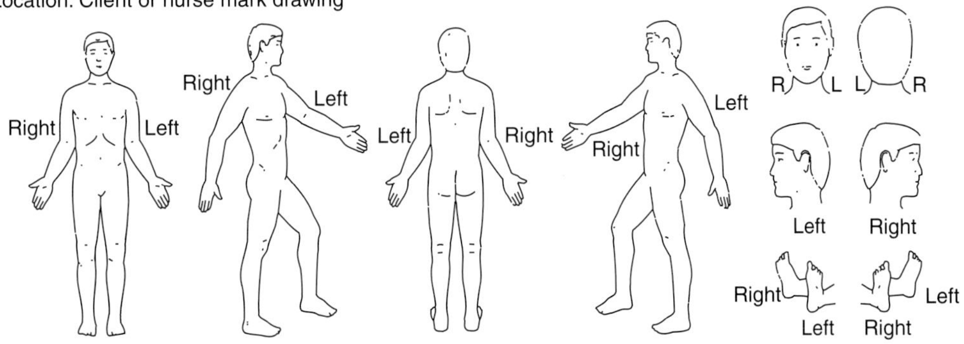

II. Intensity: Client rates the pain. Scale used ______
- Present: ______
- Worst pain gets: ______
- Best pain gets: ______
- Acceptable level of pain: ______

III. Quality: (Use client's own words, e.g., prick, ache, burn, throb, pull, sharp) ______

IV. Onset, duration variations, rhythms: ______

V. Manner of expressing pain: ______

VI. What relieves the pain? ______

VII. What causes or increases the pain? ______

VIII. Effects of pain: (note decreased function, decreased quality of life)
- Accompanying symptoms (e.g., nausea) ______
- Sleep ______
- Appetite ______
- Physical activity ______
- Relationship with others (e.g., irritability) ______
- Emotions (e.g. anger, suicidal, crying) ______
- Concentration ______
- Other ______

IX. Other comments: ______

X. Plan: ______

FIGURE 16-4 Pain assessment chart. Developed by McCaffery & Pasero 1999; from Salerno 1999.

I. Pain Intensity Scale

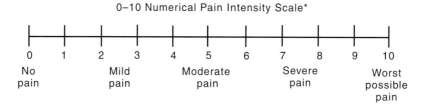

II. Pain Distress Scale

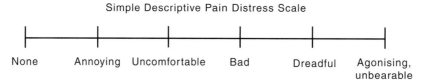

FIGURE 16-5 Scales for rating the intensity and distress of pain. *Adapted from*: Salerno 1999; Carr et al 1992.

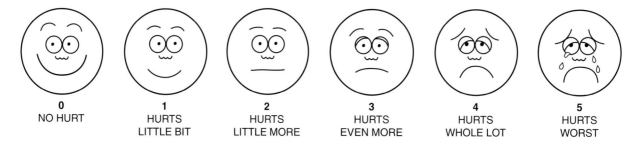

FIGURE 16-6 Faces Pain Scale. The gradation in 'hurt' or 'pain' is explained to the child, with increasing pain from left to right. The child is asked to point to the face that shows how much she/he hurts now. *Source*: Wong et al 2001; reproduced with permission.

the classic example of this. If this is not recognised and higher doses are not given, patients may be undertreated with opioid analgesics. The dose of an opioid may therefore be gradually increased to large amounts (doses potentially fatal in 'opioid-naïve' individuals) to control pain in persons with cancer, without producing the adverse effects of respiratory depression or excessive sedation. Tolerance develops to the analgesic effects and to the sedation, nausea and vomiting that opioids cause. Unfortunately, tolerance does not develop to the accompanying constipation, confusion, nightmares and hallucinations, so these adverse reactions may become more of a problem as doses are increased. A change to another opioid (fentanyl) sometimes helps with the adverse CNS effects.

Principles of pain management

Some important principles in pain management are summarised below.

- Treat the cause of pain where possible: as usual, the primary cause of a condition should be treated if possible, not just the symptom.
- Make accurate diagnosis and assessment of pain extent and type, to ensure appropriate analgesic prescription. Traditional analgesics (NSAIDs and opioids) are used for nociceptive pain; anticonvulsants and antidepressants with opioids for neuropathic pain; and a 'whole patient', multimodal approach for psychogenic or cancer pain.
- Keep the patient pain-free: it is now recognised that patients recover faster if pain is relieved, and they should not have to suffer pain before being allowed the next dose of analgesic—pain should be anticipated and prevented rather than reacted to. Analgesic effect should be optimised, starting with a low dose and titrating the dose upwards depending on patient's response and adverse effects. In prescription notation, the dose should be 'qs' (sufficient quantity) to prevent pain, not 'prn' (only when necessary).
- Dose at regular specified intervals: particularly for chronic pain, analgesics should be given on a regular fixed-time

basis to avoid pain, to optimise blood levels and analgesia, and to reduce the conditioning reaction in which periods of pain lead to drug-seeking behaviours (i.e. dose qid or qqh, not prn) (see Clinical Interest Box 16-2).

- Avoid the chronic pain stress cycle and 'sick role': minimise pain-related disability, with review of all related factors, and reassurance and explanations. An antidepressant may help stabilise sleep patterns and enhance analgesia, whereas sedatives and tranquillisers may impair participation in pain management programs.
- Prevent adverse effects of opioids: adverse effects should be prevented rather than allowed to occur and then

CLINICAL INTEREST BOX 16-1
FEARS OR MYTHS ABOUT PAIN AND PAIN MANAGEMENT

Many mistaken ideas contribute to the mismanagement of pain:

- *fear of inducing addiction*. This leads to patients being inadequately treated for pain and thus developing a pattern of drug-seeking behaviours ('pseudoaddiction') to achieve adequate pain control. The risk of addiction in hospitalised persons receiving opioids at regular intervals is minimal.
- *fear of tolerance* (the need to increase the dose of an analgesic to maintain the desired effect). Tolerance is not usually seen in 'opioid-naïve' patients with severe acute or chronic pain for which there is a physical cause such as trauma, tumour growth or surgery. Usually, an increase in pain in such people is due to disease progression or complications.
- *fear of inducing respiratory depression*. With careful assessment, prescribing and monitoring, the potential for this adverse effect is low. In patients with advanced cancer or terminally ill patients, very large amounts of opioids are often necessary to control pain but tolerance develops to the respiratory depression effects.
- *underassessment of pain*, and personal biases on the administration of pain medications. There may be a vast discrepancy between the physician's and the patient's estimate of pain severity. Women, especially those under 50, people over 70 of both sexes, and minority groups are often undertreated for pain.
- *fear of legal regulation of opioids*. Opioids have the potential for abuse and illegal diversion; therefore laws strictly monitor and regulate their availability, prescription and use. Regulations restricting prescribing have resulted in undertreatment of pain, even in patients with severe pain from cancer.
- *the wish to reserve stronger analgesics for later use*, in case pain becomes more severe. In practice, it is important for patients to be reassured that it will be possible to treat more severe pain with higher doses and/or combinations of analgesic methods.

treated. Constipation is a common problem and requires a bowel management program with attention to high-fibre diet, high fluid intake and laxatives. Postoperative orders for an antiemetic and analgesic may prevent the patient from vomiting and opening up a wound. Respiratory depression may be problematic in patients with asthma or chronic obstructive airways disease. Tolerance and dependence can occur even after 1 week on continuous opioid therapy, and higher doses may be needed. Addiction is not usually a problem with medical use of opioids and is not an issue in terminal care of cancer patients.

- **Stepwise management**: doses should be stepped up the 'analgesic ladder' (Figure 16-7) as required for increasing pain or development of tolerance:
  — Step 1: for mild pain, start with non-opioids (soluble aspirin, paracetamol) with or without adjuvant drugs (antidepressants, anticonvulsants, antipsychotics, antispasmodics)
  — Step 2: for mild to moderate pain, substitute or add a low-dose opioid (morphine as slow-release tablets or capsules, fentanyl patches or tramadol capsules, injection or sustained-release tablets)
  — Step 3: for moderate to severe pain, increase the dose of opioid, with adjuvant drugs.
- Develop a patient management plan: integrate analgesia into a comprehensive patient management plan, with a multidisciplinary approach, combination therapy, and involvement of a pain-control team if appropriate.

ANALGESIC DRUGS AND METHODS
Routes of administration

If it is possible to deliver an **analgesic** drug directly to the site of pain or to the sensory nerve pathway, this will localise the effects, minimise the dose required and reduce the time to onset of action. Examples are the epidural administration of local anaesthetics and opioids, intra-articular administration of corticosteroids, and topical administration of local anaesthetics and NSAIDs. Generally, however, analgesics must be administered systemically to circulate to the required site of action, whether in the painful tissues or in the CNS.

Oral route

The oral route is preferred as being the simplest and most acceptable and has the advantage of minimising the risk of IV drug-related problems. Opioid drugs may undergo significant hepatic metabolism after oral administration (first-pass effect), so higher doses are required than for

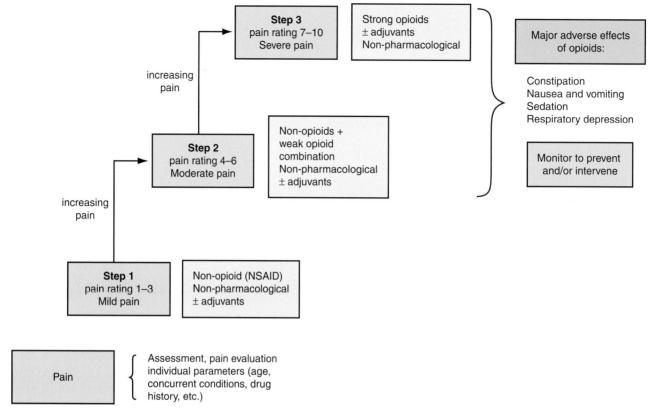

FIGURE 16-7 Flowchart for the 'stepwise' pharmacological management of pain. *Adapted from*: Salerno & Willens 1996. Adjuvants may include antidepressants, anti-inflammatories, antianxiety agents and local anaesthetics; non-pharmacological techniques include physiotherapy, acupuncture, counterirritants, psychotherapeutic methods, and complementary and alternative therapies. NSAID: non-steroidal anti-inflammatory drugs

parenteral administration; however, as the metabolites may be pharmacologically active, they contribute to the analgesic effects. Sustained-release preparations help prolong the half-life of morphine from 3–4 hours to 12–24 hours, and are useful for stable, chronic pain.

Continuous infusion of opioids

Continuous opioid infusions by SC or IV routes may be used when there is intractable vomiting, severe pain that is not relieved by oral, rectal or intermittent parenteral opioid dosing, or for pain management in the postoperative period.

Opioids may be infused by a microdrip infusion set and pump or by a patient-controlled analgesia (PCA) infusion pump unit. PCA is commonly ordered in a hospital setting, usually after surgery or for chronic cancer pain. It is a microprocessor-controlled injector programmed to deliver a predetermined IV opioid dose when the patient triggers the pump mechanism. This dose is based on the prescriber's order of a specific analgesic dose and a lock-out interval (5–20 minutes), which protects the patient from overdosing. Figure 16-8A illustrates a portable wrist model of a PCA unit,

and Figure 16-8B shows a pump that can be programmed for continuous drug administration, patient-activated drug release or clinician-activated drug release. The unit may record all patient dosing attempts so that the prescriber can evaluate the individual's need for the analgesic.

Other routes for systemic absorption

The rectal route (e.g. paracetamol suppositories) is useful in patients who cannot swallow or who are vomiting, and for slower absorption. Transdermal administration is effective for chronic administration of lipid-soluble drugs: fentanyl patches are available for patients who cannot tolerate oral morphine (see Clinical Interest Box 16-6). Additional analgesics may be prescribed to cover rising levels of pain ('breakthrough' pain).

Nitrous oxide and other gaseous and volatile general anaesthetics are administered by inhalation. IM and SC injection routes are common for opioid analgesics, the latter having a slower onset of action because the tissues are less vascular.

Intravenous injection is obviously the fastest route for rapid pain control, as it avoids the absorption phase. Relatively poor lipid solubility delays the onset of analgesia when morphine is administered by epidural or intrathecal injection. The risk of inducing respiratory depression is greater by the intrathecal route than by epidural administration, so patients must be monitored for at least 24 hours after administration by the intrathecal route.

Endpoints of treatment

Pain assessment charts and scales (Figures 16-4 to 16-6) are useful for monitoring pain intensity during treatment and to assess need for ongoing analgesia. Doses are titrated depending on clinical responses and adverse effects; depth of respiratory depression is correlated with depth of sedation. The aim is to maintain comfort for the patient, avoiding peaks and troughs of pain relief and relapses.

Analgesic use in special groups
Pregnancy, labour and delivery

During pregnancy, the analgesic of choice for mild to moderate pain is paracetamol or codeine. In late pregnancy, NSAIDs should be avoided because of increased risk of bleeding (especially after aspirin), adverse effects on the fetal respiratory system, and prolongation of gestation and labour. A concern with the use of opioids during pregnancy (particularly in an addicted woman) is that these agents may lead to physical drug dependence in the fetus, causing severe withdrawal reactions in the neonate after birth. Pregnant women dependent on an opioid and/or enrolled in methadone maintenance programs may present with fetal

distress syndrome in utero and often deliver an underweight baby at birth. Such infants are usually lethargic, with difficulty breathing, high-pitched cry, and poor feeding and sleeping patterns; the infant will require small doeses of morphine postnatally to prevent potentially fatal opiate withdrawal effects and may require special-care nursing for weeks while being weaned off the opioids.

During labour, most women experience pain. Ideally, the analgesic used will provide pain relief without any interference with labour and without increasing the risk or danger to the mother or fetus. While there is no ideal analgesic available for use during childbirth, inhaled nitrous oxide is commonly used. For more severe pain, epidural administration of combined local anaesthetic and opioid is effective and allows the mother to remain conscious even through caesarean section.

Opioid drugs may lengthen or shorten the time of labour but the primary concern with their use is neonatal respiratory

---

CLINICAL INTEREST BOX 16-2
WORLD HEALTH ORGANIZATION
GUIDELINES ON ANALGESIC USE

The World Health Organization guidelines on clinical use of analgesics are that analgesics should be prescribed:
- by the ladder (non-opioid, + adjuvant, + low-dose opioid, then higher-dose opioid)
- by the clock (regularly, to keep patient pain-free)
- by the mouth (oral rather than parenteral)
- for the individual (depending on response, type and extent of pain, other medical conditions)
- with attention to detail (dosage adjustments, assessment, monitoring, adverse effects.

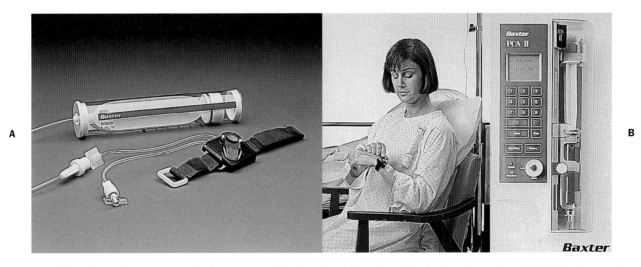

FIGURE 16-8 Examples of continuous infusion pumps. **A.** Portable wrist model. **B.** Patient-controlled analgesia (PCA): pump is designed for patient- or clinician-activated medication delivery. Courtesy of Baxter Healthcare Corporation, Deerfield, IL.

depression. Morphine is a potent analgesic but has been associated with greater neonatal respiratory depression than pethidine and has a slower onset of action. Both drugs cross the placenta to enter fetal circulation. Naloxone, an opioid antagonist, should always be available to treat the mother or neonate if excessive CNS or respiratory depression occurs.

If an opioid analgesic or methadone is administered to a woman who is breastfeeding, the next scheduled feeding should be 4–6 hours after the drug, to minimise the quantity of drug passed on to the infant.

Analgesic use in children

Children are often untreated or inadequately treated for pain, due to an incorrect belief that children do not 'feel pain' in the same way that adults do, which results in needless suffering. Assessing pain in young children is more difficult than in an older child or adult. At a minimum, it should be based on knowledge of the procedure or event that caused the pain, as well as the child's non-verbal behaviour. Even when children can verbalise their feelings they may be somewhat reluctant to report pain, often fearing that the results (diagnostic test, examination or injection) will be more painful than the pain they are experiencing.

Medicating a child under 2 years who cannot verbally report pain is justified if the child displays increased irritability, restlessness, crying, anorexia and decreased activity. The approach to a child should be individualised, based on the child's age and stage of development and the various assessment tools available, such as figure drawings to identify the area that hurts, and scales that rate pain intensity (Figure 16-6). Some general rules for analgesic use in children follow.

- As with adults, it is best to medicate a child early for pain rather than waiting until the pain is severe.
- Young infants are especially sensitive to CNS adverse effects, including respiratory depression.
- In some situations the pain of a local anaesthetic injection may be more severe than that of a quick procedure (such as venepuncture or bladder aspiration); local anaesthetic cream (EMLA, see Chapter 15) is useful in such cases.
- Children may deny pain to avoid receiving an injection; therefore the health-care professional should be aware of alternative analgesic dose forms, such as suppositories and liquid preparations.
- Aspirin should not be used in children because of its association with Reye's syndrome.
- Paracetamol is the analgesic of choice, but children are often underdosed.
- Preterm neonates are often given parenteral opiate analgesia to minimise fluctuations in heart rate and blood pressure after frequent invasive procedures such as heel-pricks for blood sampling.
- Non-organic (psychogenic?) pain in children usually resolves spontaneously but may mask more serious problems such as child abuse or depression.
- Non-pharmacological means of analgesia and reassurance are important.

Analgesic use in the elderly

Analgesic use in the elderly usually requires careful adjustments in dosage and dosing interval according to the person's liver and kidney function, therapeutic response, and development of undesirable adverse effects (increased pain, confusion, excessive untoward CNS effects or respiratory depression). The elderly often have enhanced drug responses and may not tolerate adverse effects as well as younger patients. Elderly persons may have multiple medical problems and several medications prescribed for them (polypharmacy).

The elderly often report pain differently from younger persons, because of the belief that pain is a part of old age, because they do not want to be a bother to their carer, or because they deny their discomfort as a cultural and ethnic issue. In such instances, non-verbal communication and behaviours should be carefully assessed, such as increased irritability, loss of appetite, decrease in activity, crying easily or tightly gripping an object. Cognitive impairment, dementia and confusion may make pain assessment in these people difficult; methods are available for assessing pain in patients with dementia.

The elderly may have impaired circulatory function, which results in slower absorption of drugs administered by the IM and SC routes. Administering additional doses in such a situation may result in unpredictable or increased drug absorption, which increases the potential for adverse reactions.

Specific analgesics that may be inappropriate for use in the elderly because of high risk of toxicity include dextropropoxyphene and pethidine; safer analgesics are available. All NSAIDs are relatively dangerous in the elderly because of gastrointestinal, renal and cardiovascular adverse effects; those with long half-lives, such as naproxen, piroxicam and tenoxicam, must be avoided.

Opioid analgesics

The prototype **opioid** analgesic, still most commonly used clinically, is morphine, so most discussion here will be based on the actions and clinical uses of morphine. Other opioids will be mentioned briefly, highlighting the main aspects in which they differ from morphine.

Mechanism of action of opioids

The mechanism of the analgesic action of opioids is still not totally clear despite decades of intensive study. At the spinal level, morphine stimulates opioid receptors and thus inhibits release of substance P from dorsal horn neurons.

(Substance P is a neurokinin present especially in nociceptive primary afferent neurons—see Figures 16-3A and B—and is involved in mediating pain, inflammation, smooth muscle contraction, a slow excitatory response, and stimulation of many exocrine glands.)

At supraspinal levels, opioids act to close the gate in the dorsal horn, thus inhibiting afferent transmission (see Figure 16-3B). Opioids are also capable of altering perception and emotional responses to pain because opioid receptors are widely distributed in the CNS, especially in the limbic system, thalamus, hypothalamus and midbrain. Pain perception is inhibited, which enhances the analgesic effect of morphine. Patients have reported they could still feel the pain, but it no longer worried them.

Opioid receptors

The endogenous opioid peptides involved in nociception and sensory pathways have been described (above). High-affinity binding sites for the enkephalins and endorphins are located in the membranes of central neurons (also in peripheral tissue, especially in the gut), and are responsive to various opioids. On the basis of their actions at these **opioid receptors**, drugs may be classed as opioid agonists (natural or synthetic agents that have a full morphine-like effect), antagonists, or partial agonists (e.g. buprenorphine, having a less than maximal effect at mu (μ) receptors.

Opioid receptors are G-protein-coupled receptors, activation of which inhibits adenylate cyclase and reduces cyclic adenosine monophosphate (cAMP) levels. Hyperpolarisation of presynaptic neurons leads to reduced neuronal excitability and inhibition of release of excitatory (pain) transmitters, leading to inhibitory effects at the cellular level. Effects that appear to be excitatory are probably actually due to suppression of firing of inhibitory neurons. Tolerance to opioid effects is thought to be due to both a gradual loss of inhibitory functions and an increase in excitatory signalling. Withdrawal effects may be due to a rebound increase in cAMP formation which has been activated by chronic administration of opioid via delta opioid receptors.

Subtypes of opioid receptors have been classified according to their responses to the actions of different agonists and antagonists (just as there are several subtypes of noradrenaline receptors). The primary opioid receptors concentrated in the CNS are named by the Greek letters μ (m; mu), κ (k; kappa) and δ (d; delta). (A new member, the 'opioid receptor-like 1 receptor', discovered in the Human Genome Project, is being studied as a potential target for new agents involved in analgesia, anxiety and drug addiction.) Analgesia has been associated with all three receptors, with less known about the δ receptor. What were formerly thought to be specific sigma (σ) opioid receptors are now considered general 'psychotomimetic receptors', primarily associated with unwanted effects such as dysphoria, hallucinations and confusion.

The agonist analgesics (e.g. morphine or hydromorphone) activate both the μ and κ receptors, while the partial agonist agents such as buprenorphine activate κ receptors (agonist effect) and have minimal effects on the μ receptors (antagonist effect). The partial agonist drugs may induce the undesirable effects associated with σ-receptor activity. A summary of opioid receptor responses is shown in Table 16-2.

Pharmacological effects of opioids

Considering the widespread distribution of opioid receptors in both peripheral and central tissues, it is not surprising that opioids have a broad spectrum of actions. (Aspects of opioid actions relevant to drug dependence and social pharmacology are discussed in Chapter 22.)

CENTRAL EFFECTS
Effects of opioids in the CNS include:
- analgesia—the main clinical use
- suppression of the cough reflex—another useful effect, e.g. codeine or pholcodine cough linctuses
- suppression of the respiratory centre—a major adverse effect leading to toxicity; the commonest cause of death from overdose
- sedation and sleep, hence the term narcotic analgesics; a useful clinical effect if pain is keeping the patient awake, but not helpful with daytime activities
- euphoria, the feeling of contentedness and wellbeing, which contributes to the analgesic actions
- dysphoria (unpleasant feelings, hallucinations, nightmares)
- miosis (pupillary constriction); 'pinpoint pupils' are a diagnostic sign of an addict
- nausea and vomiting—mediated through the chemoreceptor trigger zone; tolerance develops to these effects
- prolongation of labour—not usually a problem clinically
- hypotension and bradycardia, which occur after large doses, mediated by the medulla
- tolerance and dependence or addiction, mediated by μ receptors; tolerance develops after a few doses of morphine; physical dependence is shown by a marked withdrawal syndrome after an addicted person misses doses for 1–2 days.

PERIPHERAL EFFECTS
Effects of opioids in the PNS include:
- effects on opioid receptors in the gut, leading to decreased motility and increased tone in smooth muscle; severe constipation is a common adverse effect; these effects may be useful in treating diarrhoea
- spasms of sphincter muscles, which can lead to delayed gastric emptying, biliary colic or urinary retention
- suppression of some spinal reflexes

• release of histamine, causing bronchoconstriction and itching* (this effect of morphine is not mediated by opioid receptors).

Pharmacokinetic aspects of opioids

Opioids generally are not well absorbed after oral administration and have a low and variable bioavailability due to extensive first-pass metabolism in the liver.† Even after parenteral administration there is variability in plasma concentrations and rates of elimination, so doses need to be individualised.

People with liver damage may accumulate active drug and are very sensitive to the depressant effects of opioids. The toxic pethidine metabolite norpethidine may cause convulsions. Because methadone is not metabolised to glucuronides, it may be a safer alternative in liver disease. Codeine (the 3-methyl ether of morphine) is actually a prodrug, being rapidly metabolised in most people to morphine. In the 6%–10% of the (Caucasian) population who lack the enzyme to metabolise codeine, it has no analgesic effect. Renal disease can extend the half-lives of opioids that are excreted in an active form, and lead to respiratory depression, especially from methadone, morphine-6-glucuronide (M6G) and norpethidine.

---

*The severe itching can cause the symptom of formication (a word that must be read and spelt carefully!)—the sensation of having ants crawling over the body.

†Hence opium was traditionally smoked, while on the street scene morphine and heroin are usually injected ('shot up'), so that addicts get 'more bang for their bucks'—an interesting example of pharmacokinetic principles being put into common practice.

TABLE 16-2 Selected opioid receptor responses

RECEPTOR	DRUG EXAMPLES	RESPONSE
mu (μ)	Strong agonist: morphine, fentanyl, methadone, hydromorphone, β-endorphin	Supraspinal analgesia, euphoria, respiratory depression, sedation, constipation, miosis, drug dependence
	Partial agonist: buprenorphine	
	Weak agonist: pethidine	
	Antagonist: naloxone, nalorphine	Reverses opioid effects, induces acute withdrawal in opioid dependency
kappa (κ)	Agonist: morphine, β-endorphin, dynorphin	Spinal and peripheral analgesia, sedation, miosis, dysphoria, respiratory depression
	Little or no activity: methadone, pethidine	
	Antagonist: naloxone	Reverses opioid effects, induces acute withdrawal in opioid dependency
delta (δ)	Agonist: enkephalins, β-endorphin	Spinal analgesia, respiratory depression, constipation

CLINICAL INTEREST BOX 16-4
OPIUM, OPIATES, OPIOIDS AND NARCOTICS

A note on terminology: **opium** is the dried extract of the seed capsules of the opium poppy, *Papaver somniferum* (meaning 'the poppy bringing sleep'). Opium contains many pharmacologically active alkaloids (nitrogenous compounds), including morphine, codeine and papaverine. The term 'opiate' strictly refers only to opium derivatives, whereas 'opioid' means any opium-like compound and includes endogenous pain-relieving transmitters and synthetic drugs that mimic the actions of the opiates.

The medicinal effects of opium (in particular the sedative, analgesic and antidiarrhoeal actions) have been known in many cultures for over 6000 years. Pharmacologists too have known (and experimented with) morphine and similar drugs for many decades, naming and classifying the morphine receptors, probably without stopping to wonder why evolution had endowed the human CNS with receptors for a poppy extract. It was not until 1975, when Hughes and Kosterlitz in Aberdeen succeeded in isolating from mammalian brain two pentapeptides that competed with and mimicked the actions of morphine, that the body's natural analgesic compounds, the enkephalins, were discovered. Since then, the receptors mediating pain relief have been referred to as opioid receptors rather than morphine receptors.

The term 'narcotic' has also suffered misuse and confusion: literally, it means a compound causing numbness or stupor; hence, 'narcotic analgesics' was the group name for the morphine-like drugs, which cause sedation and pain relief. (Morphine was named after Morpheus, the Greek god of sleep and dreams.) The term 'narcotic' was extended to refer to all drugs causing addiction and likely to be abused, and thence to all illicit drugs. It is probably best avoided in the medical context.

Morphine is not highly protein-bound (35%) and is relatively hydrophilic, so it crosses only slowly into the CNS. (By comparison, fentanyl and its analogues are highly lipophilic and so have rapid onset and short duration of action and can be administered transdermally.)

In the elderly and in infants under 1 year, doses need to be reduced because of increased CNS sensitivity and decreased clearance. In patients with hypovolaemia (e.g. from burns or trauma), IM medications are poorly absorbed.

Morphine remains the standard opioid, although in certain circumstances another drug may be chosen because of particular pharmacokinetic parameters or clinical requirements (see Table 16-3).

Opioid receptor agonists
OPIUM PREPARATIONS

Opium, the dried exudate from the opium poppy's seed capsules, contains about 25% by weight alkaloids, including morphine and small amounts of codeine and papaverine. The effects of opium result from the presence of morphine in the preparations, so the mechanism of action and pharmacokinetics are the same as or similar to those of morphine. Opium preparations are now mainly of historical interest (see Clinical Interest Box 16-5). Because of their addictive potential, opium and opioids are tightly controlled worldwide. Most opioids (except low-dose codeine, pholcodine, dextropropoxyphene and tramadol preparations) are 'Controlled Drugs' (Schedule 8) in Australia and New Zealand, requiring strict controls on storage and supply.

MORPHINE

Morphine is the prototype opioid analgesic and is still obtained from the opium poppy because of the difficulties encountered in synthesising it in the laboratory. Many analgesics are now available but none has been proven to be overall clinically superior to morphine. In fact, all new analgesics are compared with morphine, which remains the gold standard for potency and for therapeutic effects or adverse reactions.

Morphine is available in many dosage forms, including oral mixture, injection, tablets and controlled-release capsules, granules and tablets. Because the controlled-release preparations are very commonly used clinically (and interesting pharmacokinetically) they will be considered in detail here, in Drug Monograph 16-1; note that controlled-release preparations are not suitable for treatment of acute pain.

CLINICAL INTEREST BOX 16-5
IN PRAISE OF OPIUM

In the past, opium was almost literally 'the panacea for all ills', as it is effective in treating pain, diarrhoea, cough and sleeplessness. One of the synonyms for opium preparations was 'laudanum', meaning praiseworthy. A doctor's bag could have contained many opium preparations, such as Raw Opium, Tincture of Opium, Aromatic Chalk with Opium Mixture, Compound Aspirin and Opium Tablets, Gall and Opium Ointment, Ipecacuanha and Opium Powder (Dover's Powder), Opiate Squill Linctus, Opium Liniment, Opium and Atropine Suppositories, and Sedative Opium Solution.

Opium preparations were standardised in terms of their morphine content. It is now considered preferable to administer pure forms of single drugs (e.g. morphine) rather than crude extracts (e.g. opium) containing not only varying amounts of several active ingredients but also unknown amounts of contaminants.

TABLE 16-3 Overview of selected opioid dosage forms

DRUG/DOSE FORM	USUAL DOSE	DURATION OF ACTION (h)	NOTES
Morphine			For severe pain, acute and chronic pain; active metabolite
Oral			
Solution, tablets	5–30 mg	2–4	
Sustained-released preparations	10–200 mg	12–24	
IM/SC/IV	10 mg	4–6	The 'gold standard' analgesic
Epidural	0.2–5 mg	up to 24	
Buprenorphine			Chronic pain; partial agonist, low dependence liability
IM	0.4 mg	6–8	
Sublingual	0.2–8 mg	6–8	
Transdermal patch	5, 10 or 20 mcg/h	7 days	
Codeine			Weak opioid, mild to moderate pain, cough suppression
Oral	30–200 mg	4	
IM	15–60 mg	4	
Dextropropoxyphene			Weak opioid, avoid in long term, toxic active metabolite
Oral	30–100 mg	4–6	
Fentanyl			Highly potent; moderate to severe pain, anaesthesia
SC/IV	50–100 mcg	0.5–2	
Patch	2.5–10 mg	3 days	Patches release 25–100 mcg/h
Lozenge ('lollipop')	200–800 mcg	6-8	Absorbed via buccal mucosa
Hydromorphone			Less sedative
Oral	2–8 mg	4	
IM/IV	1–2 mg	4–5	
Methadone			Postoperative or chronic pain, maintenance of addiction; risk of accumulation
Oral	5–20 mg	4–24	
IM/IV	5–15 mg	4–24	
Oxycodone			Oral bioavailability 50%
Oral	5–30 mg	3–4	Controlled-release formulations have longer duration of action
IM	10 mg	4–6	
Rectal	30 mg	6–8	
Pethidine			Risk of excitement, not recommended, poor oral efficacy; useful in labour, renal and biliary colic pain; interactions with monoamine oxidase inhibitors
IV/IM/SC	25–100 mg	3–5	
Tramadol			Weak opioid; moderate to severe pain; amine uptake inhibitor
Oral	50–200 mg	3–6	
IM	50–100 mg	5–6	

NB: Doses for high-potency opioids buprenorphine and fentanyl are in mcg or fractions of a mg.
Adapted from: Information in *MIMS December 2005–January 2006.*

OTHER OPIOIDS

Doses of other opioids are compared to those of morphine and quoted in terms of **equianalgesic dose** to standard 10 mg morphine IM/SC or 30 mg orally.

CODEINE. Codeine (see Drug Monograph 32-7) is absorbed well after either oral or parenteral administration and is metabolised in the liver (in most people) to morphine. Oral administration is used for analgesic, antitussive and antidiarrhoeal effects. Codeine may also be injected SC or IM for treatment of mild to moderate pain. Constipation is a frequent adverse effect and may require treatment or may limit the clinical usefulness of this drug.

Codeine is often combined with a non-opioid analgesic such as aspirin or paracetamol in compound analgesic tablets to provide stronger relief than the NSAID alone can achieve. In Australia, tablets containing ≤ 10 mg codeine are available over the counter (Schedule 2 or 3 [Pharmacy Medicines, Pharmacist Only Medicines, respectively]), but at higher doses (30 mg) must be prescribed (S4 or S8 [Prescription Only Medicines, Controlled Drugs, respectively]).

DEXTROPROPOXYPHENE. Dextropropoxyphene is a synthetic analgesic structurally related to methadone, indicated for the treatment of mild to moderate pain. It has significant dysphoric effects, accumulation and cardiotoxicity can occur, and it has no marked advantages over safer analgesics such as codeine, aspirin or paracetamol, so its use is not recommended.

FENTANYL. Fentanyl is a very potent opioid with a short duration of action and a good adverse effect profile, so it has become popular for use as a component of anaesthesia in day-surgery procedures (see Chapter 15) and in breakthrough pain in cancer therapy. Fentanyl is formulated for IM or slow IV injection, as a lozenge ('lollipop') for absorption via the oral mucosa, and in combination with bupivacaine or ropivacaine for epidural administration for postoperative or obstetric analgesia.

Fentanyl is also available in a patch dosage form, with doses of 2.5–10 mg, indicated for severe pain associated with malignant neoplasia in patients experiencing problems with other opioids. (See Clinical Interest Box 16-6 for additional tips for transdermal administration of fentanyl.)

Related drugs are sufentanil, alfentanil and remifentanil. These are used as adjunct opioid analgesics in general anaesthesia, postoperatively and in intensive care situations (see Clinical Interest Box 15-3).

HEROIN. The case is often put for the legalisation of heroin for treatment of intractable pain because of its analgesic and euphoric effects. Some advocates believe it is more potent, faster-acting and produces a more prolonged analgesic and euphoric effect than other analgesics. Pharmacologically,

however, heroin is a prodrug: when it is administered, it is converted in the liver to morphine and morphine metabolites, and its analgesic effects are due to the morphine produced. Due to its greater lipid solubility, heroin crosses the blood–brain barrier faster than does morphine, inducing a greater 'rush'; hence it is preferred by opioid-dependent persons, however, it has a shorter duration of action.

Heroin is a popular illegal drug of abuse (Schedule 9), so an additional fear associated with legalising it is that there may be an increased risk for drug diversion, pharmacy burglaries and crime. As heroin offers few (if any) advantages over the already marketed opioids, it is Australian policy that legalisation and clinical use of heroin are not essential to optimal treatment of pain.

HYDROMORPHONE. Hydromorphone is a semisynthetic opioid with a faster onset but a shorter duration of action than morphine. It is prescribed for its analgesic and antitussive effects and is administered as tablets, oral liquid or injection.

METHADONE. Methadone (see Drug Monograph 22-2) is an effective analgesic with properties similar to those of morphine, with the exception of its extended half-life. The duration of action for methadone is usually listed at 4–6 hours, but with repeated oral dosing it may extend to 72 hours (perhaps even

---

CLINICAL INTEREST BOX 16-6
TIPS FOR TRANSDERMAL ADMINISTRATION OF FENTANYL

- Fentanyl patches are used to provide continuous opioid administration through the skin.
- Water should be used to clean the skin area before application. The patch should be applied intact.
- Avoid exposing the patch site to direct heat sources because increased fentanyl release, absorption and toxicity may result. Fentanyl serum levels may rise by one-third in a patient with a fever.
- The transdermal patch has a slow onset of action; therefore other shorter-acting analgesics should be administered as required when therapy is initiated.
- Dosage is based on the previous 24-hour requirement for SC fentanyl (or equianalgesic opioid dosage).
- Fentanyl has a long duration of action (up to 72 hours), so adverse effects are not easily reversed.
- Common adverse effects include rash and itching; constipation is less of a problem than after oral morphine or pethidine.
- Fentanyl patches should not be administered to children under 16 years, and should not be used in nursing mothers.
- Around 50% of the dose remains in the patch after 72 hours, so patches should be discarded with care.

DRUG MONOGRAPH 16-1
MORPHINE SULPHATE CONTROLLED-RELEASE TABLETS

As described earlier for opioids generally, morphine is a strong analgesic with central actions on pain perception, used in moderate to severe acute and chronic pain; it mimics the actions of enkephalins and endorphins at opioid receptors.

INDICATIONS Morphine is indicated for the treatment of opioid-responsive severe pain, such as after trauma or surgery or for cancer pain. It has additional pharmacological effects that are useful, e.g. it may be given to patients with lung cancer to treat pain aggravated by coughing and to suppress an unproductive nagging cough; the sedative and euphoriant actions are also useful. Morphine's gastrointestinal effects include increased tone and decreased peristalsis and glandular secretions, which usually result in the adverse effect of constipation; these actions are useful in treating diarrhoea.

PHARMACOKINETICS Morphine may be administered by many routes—PO, IM, IV, SC, epidural, intrathecal and rectal. It is rapidly absorbed and is subject to an extensive first-pass effect, leading to poor bioavailability (about 40% when taken orally), so the oral dose may need to be 2–6 times the parenteral dose (see Table 16-3). It is metabolised in the liver primarily to morphine-3-glucuronide (M3G) and morphine-6-glucuronide (M6G), an active metabolite.

Morphine is distributed widely in most body tissues but only a small fraction crosses the blood–brain barrier. Metabolites are excreted primarily via the kidneys, with 7%–10% undergoing enterohepatic circulation, which extends the half-life.

The mean elimination half-life is 2–3 hours but this is increased in slow-release preparations (tablets, capsules, granules, oral suspension), such that the peak morphine concentrations during chronic use occur 4–8 hours after dosing and therapeutic effects may extend for 16–24 hours.

DRUG INTERACTIONS The following effects may occur when morphine or opioids are given with the drugs listed below:

Drug	Possible effect and management
Alcohol or other CNS depressants (other opioids, anaesthetics, sedatives, psychotropics)	May result in enhanced CNS depression, respiratory depression and hypotension. Reduce dosage and monitor closely

Drug	Possible effect and management
Buprenorphine (partial agonist)	May result in additive effect of respiratory depression if given concurrently with low doses of μ- or κ-receptor agonists; avoid concurrent usage. Partial agonists given with an opioid agonist may reduce the analgesic effects of the full agonist or precipitate withdrawal symptoms
MAOIs: phenelzine, tranylcypromine; moclobemide and selegiline	MAOIs intensify the effects of opioids (especially pethidine and tramadol); caution should be taken and dosages of opioids reduced
Opioid antagonists (naltrexone, naloxone)	Will produce withdrawal symptoms in patients dependent on opioid medications. Avoid concurrent administration

ADVERSE REACTIONS The most serious adverse reactions reported are constipation, nausea and vomiting, itch, urinary retention, sedation and circulatory and respiratory depression. Addicts who overdose on opioids are likely to die from cessation of respiration (see Box 16-1).

Constipation requires treatment with a stool-softening or osmotic laxative. Many other effects also occur (see above). Tolerance occurs to analgesia as well as to depressant effects (but not to constipation), requiring higher dosages. Respiratory depression, dependence and withdrawal reaction are not usually problems when opioids are used clinically for relief of severe pain.

WARNINGS AND CONTRAINDICATIONS Avoid the use of opioids in patients with known opioid drug hypersensitivity, acute respiratory depression, acute alcoholism or head injury. Use opioids with caution in patients with acute asthma, chronic obstructive pulmonary disease (COPD) or any respiratory impairment, or a history of drug abuse, and in patients with elevated intracranial pressure (may rise), biliary colic or pancreatitis (may cause spasm of biliary tract muscle and sphincter), acute abdominal conditions or severe inflammatory bowel disease (risk of obscuring

DRUG MONOGRAPH 16-1
MORPHINE SULPHATE CONTROLLED-RELEASE TABLETS—CONT'D

the diagnosis, or risk of toxic megacolon). Doses need to be reduced in patients with endocrine abnormalities, renal or liver impairment, and in the elderly and children. Administration during pregnancy may result in dependence in the infant; use during labour may cause respiratory depression in the infant (treated with naloxone, see Pregnancy Safety box).

DOSAGE AND ADMINISTRATION See Table 16-3 for dosing information for opioid analgesics and for analgesic equivalent doses, useful for determining drug equivalencies when a prescriber changes a patient's drug or route of administration. Standard morphine doses are 10 mg IV/IM/SC or 30 mg orally. Initial doses for opioid-naive patients are much lower than doses required for patients in whom tolerance has developed.

longer in the elderly and in patients with renal dysfunction). To control pain, methadone is administered once or twice daily, based on the individual's response. Accumulation can occur and steady-state concentrations may not be reached for several days.

Because of its extended half-life, which reduces the need for frequent dosing, methadone is approved for use in opioid detoxification and maintenance treatment programs in individuals who are physiologically dependent on heroin, opium or other opioids. Oral administration in liquid form is preferred for detoxification and required for maintenance programs, as this removes the need for injections.

OXYCODONE. Oxycodone is a potent synthetic opioid about 10 times more potent than codeine. It is well absorbed through the rectal mucosa, making the suppository dosage form (30 mg) useful as a night-time analgesic and in patients unable to swallow. (*Note*: Suppositories should not be cut (divided up) to reduce the dosage, as the pieces may not contain an even distribution of the drug.)

PETHIDINE. Pethidine (known as meperidine in the USA) is an effective analgesic for short-term use but is unsuitable for oral administration because of low bioavailability. It is less apt than morphine to release histamine or to raise biliary tract pressure; it is thus often prescribed for patients with acute asthma, biliary colic or pancreatitis. A metabolite produced in the liver is neurotoxic and can accumulate, so pethidine is used only short-term, e.g. postoperatively, or in acute pain such as for obstetric analgesia. Concurrent use of MAO inhibitors may result in severe, unpredictable life-threatening reactions. Pethidine is often requested by illicit drug users (who may very effectively mimic the signs and symptoms of severe pain), and prescribers are warned of this danger.

PHOLCODINE. Pholcodine (see Drug Monograph 32-7), an opioid compound chemically similar to the opium derivative papaverine, is interesting in that it has virtually no analgesic effects but retains many morphine-like effects, including

suppressing cough and respiration and causing mild sedation, nausea and vomiting, dependence and constipation. It is used as a cough suppressant (see Chapter 32).

TRAMADOL. Tramadol is a relatively new centrally acting synthetic analgesic that is not chemically related to the opioids. It appears to bind to the μ opioid receptors and also inhibits the reuptake of noradrenaline and 5-HT; hence it is sometimes referred to as an opioid–SSRI (selective serotonin reuptake inhibitor) analgesic. It is indicated for the treatment of moderate to moderately severe pain and in neuropathic pain, but is less effective and more expensive than morphine; however, it may have a lesser potential for respiratory depression and drug dependency. Common adverse reactions include nausea, dizziness, hypertension and seizures; it's many drug interactions include serotonin syndrome.

Partial agonists

Partial agonists produce less than maximal effects at a receptor; for example, buprenorphine is a partial agonist at the μ receptors. Generally these drugs are less effective analgesics and have a lower dependency potential and less severe withdrawal symptoms than full opioid agonist medications; however, their clinical use is not recommended, as they may precipitate pain or withdrawal reactions in patients taking other opioids, and their actions may not be reversible with an antagonist (naloxone).

Opioid antagonists

The search for pure morphine antagonists produced naloxone and naltrexone, opioid antagonists that competitively displace opioid analgesics from their receptor sites, thus reversing their effects. Antagonism of endogenous opioids (enkephalins and endorphins) released during inflammatory reactions and acupuncture can lead to a state of hyperalgesia (exacerbated pain).

Antagonists block subjective and objective opioid effects and can precipitate withdrawal symptoms in people physically dependent on opioids. Naloxone and naltrexone are used to reverse the adverse or overdosage effects of opioid agonists (morphine, codeine, fentanyl, heroin, methadone etc). Respiratory difficulties in newborn babies, caused by opioids given to the mother for pain relief during childbirth, can also be treated. Respiratory depression induced by non-opioids (e.g. barbiturates), CNS depression or respiratory disease will usually not respond to opioid antagonist drug therapy.

In an opioid analgesic overdosage, the antagonist drugs will reverse the respiratory depression, sedation, pupillary miosis (constriction) and euphoric effects. The drugs are believed to work at all three receptor sites, but their greatest affinity is for μ receptors.

Naloxone, a short-acting antagonist administered parenterally, is used mainly for treatment of overdose or for reversal of opioid depressant effects (see Box 16-1); frequent doses may be necessary to prevent the person slipping back into the overdose state. The serum half-life of naloxone is approximately 0.5–1 hour, whereas that of morphine is 1.5–2 hours. Naltrexone, a long-acting antagonist given orally, is used mainly for treatment of alcohol or opioid dependence and for rapid opioid detoxification (see Chapter 22, and Drug Monograph 22-1). Adverse reactions include nausea, dizziness, nervousness, headache and fatigue.

Non-opioid analgesics—the NSAIDs

Pharmacological actions and clinical uses

The second main group of analgesic drugs is the non-opioid or non-narcotic analgesics, typified by aspirin (see Drug Monograph 16-2). As these drugs also have significant anti-inflammatory and antipyretic (antifever) actions but do not possess the steroidal chemical structure of endogenous and exogenous anti-inflammatory corticosteroids, they are also known as **non-steroidal anti-inflammatory drugs** (NSAIDs) or antipyretic analgesics.* The drugs also have antiplatelet actions, which inhibit platelet aggregation and thus decrease the risk of thrombosis. The main drugs in this classification include aspirin, paracetamol, ibuprofen, indomethacin,

---

*There is considerable confusion in terminology in this area, especially as to whether paracetamol (known as acetaminophen in North America) should be included among the NSAIDs. Admittedly, paracetamol has very little anti-inflammatory effect in many tissues, but aspirin, paracetamol and other NSAIDs all act by the same mechanism (inhibition of PG synthesis) and show varying levels of analgesic, anti-inflammatory, antipyretic and antiplatelet actions. Hence we are using the term NSAID in the broad sense and including aspirin (as the prototype NSAID) and paracetamol.

BOX 16-1 MANAGING OPIOID OVERDOSE

If an oral opioid overdose occurs, aspiration or gastric lavage is used to empty the stomach and activated charcoal is administered. If respiratory depression or any other life-threatening adverse effect is present, the treatment for these effects takes precedence.

For respiratory depression, establish a patent airway and controlled respiration, with oxygen. Administer naloxone to reverse the opioid-induced respiratory depression and sedation, by displacing the opioids at the receptor site. In opioid-dependent patients, naloxone can also induce acute drug withdrawal (agitation, tachycardia).

The IV route is the preferred method of administering naloxone; its effects are seen within 1 minute. Naloxone can also be given IM or SC; the onset of action is then seen within 2–5 minutes.

Naloxone is shorter-acting than most opioids; to prevent the recurrence of respiratory depression caused by long-acting opioids, it must therefore be administered by a continuous infusion or by repeated injections (IM or SC). (See Drug Monograph 22-1 for additional relevant information.)

---

diclofenac, and the newer specific cyclo-oxygenase-2 (COX-2) inhibitors such as celecoxib. Only aspirin and paracetamol will be considered in detail in this chapter; the NSAIDs are covered in Chapter 55 along with other drugs used for inflammatory conditions.

The non-opioid analgesics are effective for mild to moderate pain (Step 1 in the stepwise management of pain, Figure 16-7), and are often combined with opioid analgesics to enhance pain control in patients with moderate to severe pain (Step 2). These agents are some of the most commonly used of all drugs (see Clinical Interest Box 16-7): they are used for the treatment of mild to moderate pain, fever, and inflammation caused by rheumatoid arthritis, osteoarthritis, and various other acute and chronic musculoskeletal and soft tissue inflammations. The NSAIDs are also used to treat bone pain associated with metastatic cancer, usually in combination with an opioid analgesic. Aspirin is also used in very low doses to prevent thrombosis and reduce the risk of stroke or heart attacks. (Information on the over-the-counter dosage forms of these preparations is given in Chapter 3; on antithrombotic use in Chapter 30; and on anti-inflammatory actions in Chapters 54 and 55.)

Mechanism of action
INHIBITION OF PROSTAGLANDIN FORMATION

Despite salicylates having been used for thousands of years for the relief of pain, fever and inflammation, their mechanism of

The history of the development of analgesics is an interesting one in the realm of pharmacognosy (the study of properties of drugs obtained from plants and other natural sources). Extracts of bark from trees of the willow family (*Salicaceae*) were used medicinally in ancient times, but later fell into disuse. In the 18th century in England, cinchona bark, which was imported for use as an antimalarial, analgesic, antipyretic and anti-inflammatory agent, was very expensive, so local plants were tested as cheaper substitutes.

The Rev. Edward Stone, noting that many of his parishioners suffered from 'the ague' (fevers, shivering, rigor and rheumatism), trusted that the cure for their ills would be provided nearby. As willows flourish in damp areas, he tested extracts of willow bark, with great success. Salicin, the bitter glycoside of the *Salix* species, was extracted in 1827 and found to contain saligenin, an active ingredient from which salicylic acid was prepared. Sodium salicylate was first used in 1875, and acetylsalicylic acid was introduced into medicine in 1899 as aspirin. The trade name Aspro was popularised by the Nicholas drug company in Australia. Many derivatives of salicylic acid have been synthesised and trialled; some of those still in use are methyl salicylate (present in oil of wintergreen), salicylamide, choline salicylate. Aspirin remains the standard antipyretic analgesic worldwide.

In Australian indigenous bush medicine, several traditional remedies are available to relieve the symptoms of headaches. Often, inhalations of volatile oils obtained from the leaves of such plants as small leaf clematis (*Clematis microphylla*), stinkwood (*Ziera* spp.) or *Melaleuca* species are said to provide relief; their leaves may be crushed and the vapour inhaled, or leaves bound around the head to relieve pain.

spinal cord. The antipyretic action is due to inhibition of PG synthesis in the hypothalamus, the temperature-regulating centre of the body.

Common adverse drug reactions to NSAIDs include gastrointestinal tract disorders (dyspepsia, nausea and vomiting, diarrhoea/constipation and gastritis) due to suppression of mucoprotective PGs by systemically absorbed NSAIDs. Other common adverse effects include asthma attacks, skin reactions (rashes, urticaria), sodium retention and renal damage (due to inhibition of vasodilator PGs—particularly a problem in elderly patients on long-acting NSAIDs) and consequent heart failure and hypertension in predisposed individuals. Individual NSAIDs may cause specific adverse effects, e.g. salicylates generally can cause tinnitus, impaired haemostasis and acid–base imbalances, while large overdose of paracetamol can cause fatal acute liver damage if not promptly treated (see Box 16-2).

Aspirin and other salicylates

Aspirin is readily available, both over the counter and by prescription for some combination products. After absorption, administered salicylates are rapidly metabolised in the plasma to salicylic acid, which is the active form of salicylate drugs.*

Salicylates can also be absorbed after topical application to inflamed soft tissues (e.g. methyl salicylate [oil of wintergreen] is used in creams, ointments and liniments for relief of inflammatory pain such as from sporting injuries and arthritic conditions). Salicylic acid itself is too strong an irritant to be taken orally but is used topically in many dermatological preparations for its antimicrobial and keratolytic effects (see Chapter 56).

In addition to its analgesic, anti-inflammatory and antipyretic actions, aspirin decreases the risk of thrombosis in blood vessels by inhibiting the formation of thromboxanes, which mediate vasoconstriction and platelet aggregation. In low doses (75–150 mg/day, i.e. 1/4 to 1/2 tablet/day), aspirin decreases the risk of recurrence of stroke or myocardial infarction.[†] In this respect, the effect of aspirin is qualitatively different from that of the other NSAIDs, as it causes irreversible inhibition of platelet cyclo-oxygenase by acetylation of the

action was discovered only relatively recently (Vane 1971). Aspirin and the NSAIDs peripherally inhibit the synthesis and release of prostaglandins (PGs) by inhibiting the arachidonate **cyclo-oxygenase** (COX) enzymes (see Figure 55-1). As shown in Figure 16-3A, the products of arachidonic acid, such as PGs, play important roles in both pain and inflammation. This mechanism accounts for most of the therapeutic effects and also the adverse effects of the NSAIDs.

The analgesic effects of NSAIDs are particularly useful in relief of pain of inflammatory origin, as NSAIDs reduce the production at the site of injury of PGs that sensitise nociceptors to the algesic actions of bradykinin and other mediators of pain (see Figure 16-3). The analgesic action is thus said to be peripheral, and NSAIDs do not cause tolerance or dependence, or modify psychological reactions to pain. They may, however, also have a central analgesic action in the

*The term 'salicylates' refers to salts of salicylic acid. Just as sulfates (salts of sulfuric acid) will be ionised in biological fluids, so salicylic acid and its salts will be present as salicylate (negative ions) and hydrogen ions or other cations.

†This action and clinical use of aspirin have become so important (in view of the high incidence of heart attacks and strokes in our ageing population) that aspirin is now often considered as mainly a cardiovascular drug, and it has been recommended that all persons aged over 50 take half an aspirin tablet, i.e. about 150 mg aspirin, each day.

active site of the enzyme (Clinical Interest Box 30-2). Aspirin also appears to be effective prophylactically in decreasing the risk of bowel cancer. The benefits in reduced cardiovascular events must always be weighed against the risks of gastrointestinal or intracranial bleeding.

Paracetamol

Paracetamol (known as acetaminophen in the USA) is an effective antipyretic analgesic, producing these effects by inhibiting prostaglandin synthesis in the CNS. Although its anti-inflammatory effects are minimal, paracetamol does appear to inhibit COX in some tissues in some species, so its exact mechanisms of action are not clear. In normal doses, it is a safer OTC analgesic than aspirin (see Drug Monograph 3-1 and Clinical Interest Box 16-8), and is recommended particularly for treatment of mild pain and fevers in children. Paracetamol is an effective analgesic provided that adequate regular doses are maintained; typical adult dosage is two tablets to start, then one tablet (500 mg) every 3–6 hours.

Paracetamol is indicated for treatment of a wide range of conditions causing mild to moderate pain (especially of non-inflammatory origin), fever, migraine and tension headache, and some forms of arthritis (osteoarthritis). Aspirin or other NSAIDs are preferred in moderate to severe arthritis when there is a major inflammatory component, as in rheumatoid arthritis (see Chapter 55).

Pharmacokinetically, paracetamol taken orally is rapidly absorbed, reaching peak serum levels in 15–60 minutes; its elimination half-life is 1–3 hours. It is metabolised in the liver (see Figure 16-9), and glucuronide and sulfate metabolites are excreted by the kidneys. The usual maximum daily paracetamol dose for adults is 4 g/day (8 × 500 mg tablets); for children, the single dose is 15 mg/kg orally or rectally, with a maximum of 60–90 mg/kg/day. Paracetamol is available in infant, paediatric and adult strengths, as tablets, capsules, chewable tablets, elixirs and suppositories. Extended-release tablets are also now available, containing 655 mg paracetamol in a formulation that maintains therapeutically active levels of drug for up to 8 hours after oral administration. The dose is 2 tablets every 6–8 hours, with a maximum of 6 tablets in any 24 hours; as with most sustained-release preparations, the tablets must not be crushed.

Adverse effects are rare with paracetamol in normal therapeutic doses, although in some instances nausea and rash have occurred. Overdose can cause serious damage to the liver and kidneys, and hypoglycaemia. The hepatotoxic effects of very high levels of paracetamol are due to build-up of a toxic metabolite. This can occur after ingestion of 20 or more tablets (10 g), and an overdose is potentially fatal. Inadvertent overdose can also occur, for example by exceeding the recommended daily dose in attempts to manage incresing pain, or by additive effects of paracetamol present in more than one OTC preparation. (See Box 16-2 for management of paracetamol

BOX 16-2   MANAGING PARACETAMOL OVERDOSE

Patients are notoriously unreliable as to the amount taken and the time of ingestion, and may appear well for 1–2 days after a potentially fatal paracetamol overdose. As there is a specific antidote (acetylcysteine, which replaces depleted glutathione, see Figure 16-9), it is important that any patient with possible paracetamol overdose be tested for paracetamol plasma levels. Toxicity is probable if the patient has ingested more than 150 mg paracetamol per kg body weight (about 20 standard 500 mg paracetamol tablets for an average adult), or 10 g total paracetamol.

Symptoms
- Early symptoms are sweating, anorexia, nausea or vomiting, abdominal pain or cramping and/or diarrhoea, and usually occur 6–14 hours after ingestion and last for about 24 hours.
- Late symptoms are swelling, tenderness, or pain in the abdominal area 2–4 days after ingestion (indicates hepatic damage).
- Patients with previously impaired liver function (e.g. by alcohol abuse) are more susceptible to liver damage, and have a lowered threshhold for toxicity.

Treatment
- If less than 1 hour since overdose, gastric lavage is indicated or activated charcoal is administered.
- Obtain plasma for liver function tests and coagulation studies. Determine paracetamol serum levels at 4 hours or more after ingestion, then start acetylcysteine administration. Hepatotoxicity is likely if plasma paracetamol concentration is more than 200 mcg/mL at 4 hours, 150 mcg/mL at 6 hours, 100 mcg/mL at 8 hours, 50 mcg/mL at 12 hours, or 5 mcg/mL at 24 hours.
- Administer acetylcysteine IV in 5% glucose from 4 hours after overdose, with a loading dose, then maintenance dose continuing for 21 hours. (See *Australian Medicines Handbook 2005* or *MIMS Annual* for nomogram to determine likelihood of paracetamol toxicity from plasma levels, and dosage instructions.)
- Perform liver function tests and prothrombin time determinations to monitor hepatotoxicity. Institute supportive measures as indicated for bleeding disorders, renal failure, cardiac toxicity and hepatic encephalopathy.

overdose, and Drug Monograph 32-1 for use of acetylcysteine via a different formulation as a mucolytic agent in respiratory disorders.)

Compound analgesics

Simple analgesics (500 mg paracetamol, 300–500 mg aspirin) are sometimes formulated with other drugs (other NSAIDs, antihistamines, the mild opioid drug codeine, caffeine, or antacids) to combine the pharmacological actions of two or more drugs. Examples are Disprin Forte: 500 mg aspirin + 9.5 mg codeine, or Panadeine Forte: 500 mg paracetamol + 30 mg codeine. Codeine is also formulated with other NSAIDs such as ibuprofen.

Such combinations, however, suffer the disadvantages of all fixed-dose combinations: it is impossible to titrate the dose of either individual drug; the drug with the longer half-life may accumulate; and combinations are usually more expensive than taking the individual drugs at the appropriate intervals and dosages. Codeine and caffeine have been

thought to enhance the analgesic effects of aspirin; however, while codeine (60 mg) may have additive analgesic actions, caffeine provides no adjunctive analgesia.

There is little evidence that combinations (even buffered aspirin or aspirin–antacid preparations) offer any advantage over individual drugs. There are, however, at least three situations in which NSAID–other drug combinations are clinically useful:
• the administration of paracetamol with another NSAID; adequate analgesic doses of paracetamol may allow decreased dosing of the other (anti-inflammatory) NSAID, with a decrease in incidence of adverse effects

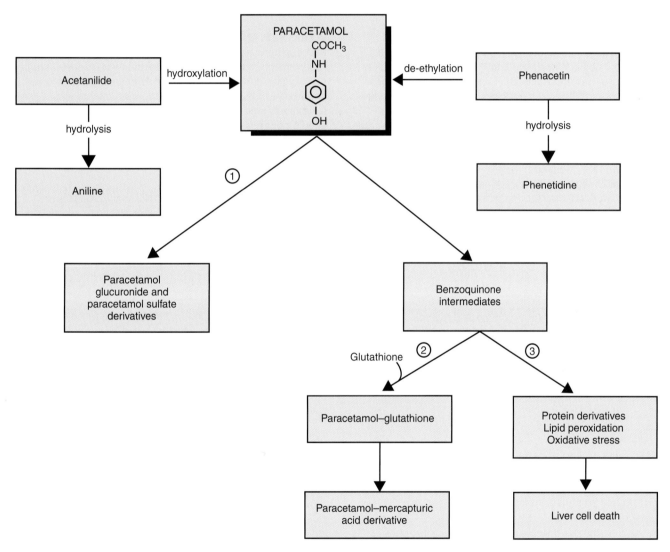

FIGURE 16-9 Metabolic pathways involving paracetamol. In normal doses, paracetamol is conjugated (pathway 1) to non-toxic glucuronide and sulfate derivatives. In higher doses, pathway 1 becomes saturated and a benzoquinone intermediate (BQI) is produced. Combination of the BQI with glutathione (GSH, a gamma-glutamyl-cysteinyl-glycine tripeptide involved in amino acid transport in cells) via pathway 2 produces mercapturic acid metabolites. In massive overdoses, GSH reserves are used up and BQIs are diverted via pathway 3, in which toxic derivatives cause potentially lethal reactions in liver cells. Paracetamol overdose is treated with acetylcysteine, a precursor of the natural compound GSH; this replenishes GSH supplies and avoids formation of toxic BQI metabolites.

DRUG MONOGRAPH 16-2 ASPIRIN

Aspirin has analgesic, antipyretic, anti-inflammatory and antiplatelet effects. Its commonest formulation is in tablets containing 300 mg aspirin.

INDICATIONS Aspirin is indicated for the treatment of pain and fever (in those over 18 years), headaches, rheumatic fever, rheumatoid arthritis and osteoarthritis, and in prevention of acute myocardial infarction (AMI) or reinfarction, and in prevention of stroke. The advantages of aspirin over paracetamol include its anti-inflammatory effects and its effectiveness in preventing AMI and thrombi.

PHARMACOKINETICS Aspirin taken orally is rapidly absorbed, partly from the stomach (as the drug is itself acidic), and also from the intestine. Peak serum levels of acetylsalicylic acid are reached within 20–40 minutes. Rapid metabolism by tissue and blood esterases occurs, hydrolysing aspirin to acetic acid and salicylate; the peak plasma salicylate level is reached in 2–4 hours. Salicylate is distributed throughout most body tissues and fluids, including synovial fluid and cerebrospinal fluid, and is 50%–90% bound to plasma proteins. Salicylate then undergoes hepatic metabolism to inactive metabolites. The plasma salicylate level required for analgesic and antipyretic effects is about 28 mg/L, whereas 100 mg/L is required for anti-inflammatory effects. Toxic effects (salicylism) are seen above about 200 mg/L.

COMMON ADVERSE EFFECTS Common adverse effects include gastrointestinal irritation or discomfort, and nausea or vomiting (see earlier section on adverse drug reactions). Taking aspirin with a full glass of water helps reduce these effects. Toxic reactions due to salicylate poisoning (salicylism) include tinnitus, vertigo and complicated effects on acid–base balance (both respiratory alkalosis and metabolic acidosis). See Box 16-3 for clinical management of aspirin overdose.

DRUG INTERACTIONS There are many potential drug interactions, in particular with other drugs affecting platelet function or the blood-clotting process; drugs eliminated mainly by renal excretion or drugs used to treat heart failure (as aspirin can impair renal function); antihypertensive agents (as aspirin can raise blood pressure); other NSAIDs (increased risk of gastric ulceration or bleeding); corticosteroids (may decrease salicylate concentration and clinical effect); probenecid (uricosuric effect may be reduced); valproate (concentration and effects of valproate may be enhanced, as may effects of aspirin on blood parameters). In most cases, low-dose aspirin (e.g. 100 mg daily) is safe with other drugs.

WARNINGS AND CONTRAINDICATIONS Precautions with aspirin use are required in heart failure and hypertension, renal impairment, severe liver disease, during surgery and in those predisposed to bleeding, peptic ulcer or asthma, or if previous serious adverse effects with salicylates have occurred, and during late pregnancy. It should not be used in children under 18 years, especially those with fever, because of the possibility of rare but potentially fatal Reye's syndrome (severe liver damage and encephalopathy).

DOSAGE AND ADMINISTRATION Aspirin products are available in tablet, effervescent tablet, capsule, enteric-coated, extended-release tablet and oral powder dosage forms. Aspirin should be taken after food, to minimise irritant effects in the gastrointestinal tract (this also has the effect of delaying absorption). The usual adult dose is 1–2 regular-strength tablets (300 mg) every 4–6 hours or as needed. Higher doses are required for anti-inflammatory effects. For prophylactic antiplatelet effects, much lower doses are sufficient, e.g. 75–150 mg/day (¼ to ½ standard tablet).

• combination of a simple analgesic (aspirin or paracetamol) with a mild opioid (codeine, at 8 or 30 mg), an intermediate step in the 'analgesic ladder'

• combination with misoprostol to minimise gastrointestinal adverse effects; misoprostol is a PG analogue and is thought to replace mucoprotective PGs in the gastrointestinal tract, reducing the risk of NSAID-induced ulcers. Misoprostol is available both by itself (200 mcg tablets) and formulated in combination with diclofenac sodium 50 mg for patients requiring an NSAID, in whom the risk of gastrointestinal complications is high.

NSAIDs and polypharmacy

Aspirin or paracetamol is often included in products that contain more than one ingredient, such as pain relievers, cough and cold remedies, sedatives, and medicines for allergy, menstrual or premenstrual problems. Taking more than one of these products at the same time, or with a prescribed NSAID, can lead to overdose and potential toxicity. In particular, elderly patients may be unaware that they are taking several NSAIDs concurrently,* for example for headache, fever,

---

*A tactful review of the family's drug cabinet, or questioning about all the medicines currently being taken, including those bought in pharmacies or supermarkets, often reveals a potentially toxic cocktail of many NSAID preparations.

BOX 16-3 MANAGING ASPIRIN OVERDOSE

The effects of severe overdose of aspirin can be dramatic and potentially fatal, especially in children. Treatment includes gastric lavage and forced alkaline diuresis, and close monitoring of vital functions is necessary. Fluid, electrolyte and acid–base imbalances must be corrected and hyperthermia, hyperglycaemia or hypoglycaemia treated.

Plasma salicylate concentration is monitored until it is lowered to a non-toxic level; for example, if large amounts of aspirin have been consumed and the salicylate concentration 2 hours after ingestion is 500 mg/L, this indicates a serious toxicity, whereas a plasma concentration of 800 mg/L is potentially fatal. If large amounts of delayed-release formulations have been taken, plasma salicylate concentration is not reliable for estimating degree of toxicity.

Exchange transfusion, haemodialysis or peritoneal dialysis may be necessary in cases of severe salicylate overdose. It is important to note that there is no specific antidote for aspirin poisoning, as there is for paracetamol (acetylcysteine).

CLINICAL INTEREST BOX 16-8 ADVANTAGES OF PARACETAMOL OVER ASPIRIN

Paracetamol offers several advantages over aspirin, including the following:
- Adverse effects and allergic reactions are rare with therapeutic doses.
- There is very low risk of gastric upset, peptic ulceration or bleeding, tinnitus or renal impairment, as reported more often with aspirin and other NSAIDs, hence it can be used when other NSAIDs are contraindicated.
- Plasma protein binding is negligible, hence there is no risk of displacement causing drug interactions.
- There are few serious adverse drug interactions; it may be used by patients taking anticoagulant medications.
- It may be used by children with mild fevers and colds and flu symptoms because it has not been associated with Reye's syndrome, as is the case with aspirin.
- It is safe to use during pregnancy and lactation.

CLINICAL INTEREST BOX 16-9 A CUP OF TEA, AN APC, AND ANALGESIC NEPHROPATHY

A 'classic' Australian compound analgesic formulation, APC powders or tablets, contained standard doses of aspirin, phenacetin and caffeine. Many people suffering repetitive strain injuries, headache or muscular or soft tissue pain followed the common advice 'Have a cup of tea, an APC, and a good lie-down', and took the compound analgesics regularly in high doses for relief of pain and inflammation (aspirin and phenacetin) and for mild CNS stimulation (caffeine).

Unfortunately, the caffeine withdrawal tended to cause a rebound headache and consequent dependence on the preparation; the aspirin and phenacetin components caused gastric upsets and pain; leading to more doses of APC being taken; and the chronic use of NSAID analgesics, especially phenacetin, caused chronic nephritis, renal tubular necrosis, and eventually chronic renal failure requiring regular dialysis or kidney transplantation. Compound analgesics have been blamed for the high incidence of analgesic nephropathy common in Australia for much of the 20th century. (Phenacetin has long been withdrawn from use.)

arthritis, cough and cold, and prophylaxis of AMI or stroke. The pharmacological and toxic effects are additive, and elderly patients with impaired renal function are particularly at risk of adverse drug reactions and interactions, especially from NSAIDs with long half-lives.

Other pharmacological analgesics
GABA ANALOGUES

New analgesics unrelated to opioids or NSAIDs are pregabalin and gabapentin. Pregabalin (an analogue of the neurotransmitter GABA, and related to the anticonvulsant drug gabapentin) reduces the release of various transmitters via interference with the calcium channels in nerve terminals. It is particularly useful in neuropathic pain such as occurs in diabetic neuropathy and post-herpetic neuralgia, but patient response is variable. Adverse reactions are mainly due to effects on CNS transmitters, and include dizziness, sedation and incoordination. It is also useful as adjunctive therapy in partial seizures. The related gabapentin, a new anticonvulsant drug (see Chapter 18), has also been shown to be effective in the relief of neuropathic pain.

CAPSAICIN

Capsaicin, an alkaloid found in chilli peppers, is formulated into topical creams that are indicated for the treatment of neuralgias, arthritic pain, and pain associated with cystitis and HIV infection. It is said to activate capsaicin receptors; on application it causes an initial release and then a depletion of substance P from nerve fibres, which results in a decrease in pain transmission.

Other drugs useful for their analgesic effects include:
- local anaesthetics, e.g. lignocaine, EMLA cream (see Chapter 15)

- general anaesthetics, e.g. halothane, nitrous oxide (see Chapter 15)
- ethanol or phenol injected near sensory nerve fibres, causing irreversible lesion of fibres and loss of pain transmission (rarely carried out now)
- cannabinoids, i.e. derivatives of the marijuana plant *Cannabis sativa*, main active ingredient Δ^9-tetrahydrocannabinol (THC; see Chapter 22); its psychopharmacological actions depend on the dose, route, setting and person, and include some analgesic effects mediated via δ and κ opioid receptors. THC enhances the analgesic potency of morphine, and this synergistic interaction is being exploited to develop analgesic regimens that allow lower doses of opioids to be used in pain syndromes resistant to opioids alone
- specific antimigraine drugs, including 5-hydroxy-tryptamine (5-HT, serotonin) agonists (sumatriptan) and antagonists (methysergide), and vasoconstrictors (ergot alkaloids).

New pharmacological approaches to pain management include research on drugs that enhance the inhibitory effects of adenosine on nociceptors, mimic the actions of analgesic neuropeptides (e.g. nociceptin/orphanin FQ, a novel peptide discovered in brain extracts as the natural ligand of the opioid receptor-like 1-receptor, identified during the elucidation of the human genome), or inhibit the enzymes that inactivate enkephalins or endorphins.

Adjuvant analgesics

Adjuvant (co-analgesic) medications are used in combination with opioid or NSAID analgesics to enhance pain relief or to treat symptoms that exacerbate pain. In some instances they are used alone to treat specifically identified pain. **Adjuvant analgesic** medications include a variety of drugs whose main clinical indications are in other conditions, such as anticonvulsants, antidepressants, antihistamines, corticosteroids, antiarrhythmics, psychostimulants, clonidine and capsaicin, as follows:

- Tricyclic antidepressants and membrane-stabilising agents, such as some anticonvulsants and antiarrhythmic agents, may be useful in neuropathic pain and are often used in combination with opioids for cancer-associated nerve pain; the mechanism is via blockade of sodium channels. The analgesic actions of nimodipine and gabapentin may be due to blockade of calcium channels.
- Corticosteroids are useful in relief of pain associated with inflammation, swelling and space-occupying lesions, e.g. for cancer pain that originates in a restricted area such as intracranially, alongside a nerve root, or in pelvic, neck or hepatic areas. Dexamethasone is prescribed to reduce intracranial pressure and for relief of pain caused by pressure on a nerve.
- Psychotropic drugs, including the phenothiazines and

benzodiazepines, may be useful for their sedating, antianxiety and muscle-relaxing properties.
- Bisphosphonates (which reduce bone turnover) are sometimes useful for metastatic or osteoporotic bone pain, and antispasmodics (which relax smooth muscle) for colic pain.
- Clonidine, a centrally acting α_2-adrenergic agonist and antihypertensive agent, has been tried for the treatment of pain associated with reflex sympathetic dystrophy, diabetic neuropathy, post-herpetic neuralgia, spinal cord injury, phantom pain, and pain in cancer patients who are opioid-tolerant. Clonidine is administered to enhance spinal anaesthesia via spinal injection, which minimises cardiovascular and other autonomic effects. It was formerly used as a preventive treatment in migraine, but clinical trials have failed to prove benefit. Clonidine is effective in treating opioid withdrawal reactions by reducing the symptoms due to autonomic hyperactivity.
- NMDA receptor channel modulators, such as dextromethorphan, phencyclidine and amantadine derivatives, are showing promise as analgesics in neuropathic pain by inhibiting NMDA receptors involved in pain transmission. Ketamine, a general anaesthetic (see Chapter 15), is an antagonist at NMDA receptors, and in subanaesthetic doses helps relieve chronic neuropathic pain; other NMDA receptor antagonists are being developed.

Non-pharmacological analgesic techniques

Non-pharmacological analgesic methods include:

- first aid techniques: RICE (**r**est, **i**ce, **c**ompression, **e**levation)
- physiotherapy: after the acute phase of traumatic injury, and in chronic conditions, exercise techniques that improve strength and flexibility, or muscle relaxation techniques and massage, can help prevent or relieve chronic pain
- counterirritants, e.g. scratching, liniments, rubefacients (substances that redden the skin by causing vasodilation)
- transcutaneous electrical nerve stimulation (TENS): a method of treating chronic pain by passing small electrical currents into the spinal cord or sensory nerves via electrodes applied to the skin; afferent stimulation of A-fibres is thought to reduce transmission from nociceptors through C-fibres
- acupuncture: a technique from traditional Chinese medicine in which needles are inserted into the skin at specific points to produce analgesia; acupuncture has been shown to release endorphins and may also act by blocking gates in the dorsal horn regions; there is further a major placebo effect

CLINICAL INTEREST BOX 16-10 HERBAL REMEDIES FOR PAIN

The most important herbal remedies for pain are, of course, morphine and codeine in opium extracts from the poppy *Papaver somniferum*, and salicin and salicylates from the bark of the willow tree *Salix alba* and from the herb meadowsweet (*Filipendula ulmaria*). Many other plants also produce herbal extracts that have analgesic properties, including the following, which have been clinically tested and proven:

- cloves, the dried flower buds of *Eugenia* species, containing the oil eugenol, which has analgesic, anti-inflammatory, antimicrobial and antiplatelet activities (among others); clove oil has long been used in dentistry to relieve dental pain and as an antiseptic; the mechanism of action is via depression of nociceptors and inhibition of prostaglandin synthesis
- feverfew, the leaves and flowering tops of the plant *Tanacetum parthenium*, containing many active ingredients including the terpene parthenolide; feverfew has been used for centuries in Europe to treat headaches, arthritis and fever, and has more recently been shown to be effective prophylactically against migraine headache; various mechanisms have been proposed and demonstrated

- kava kava, a beverage prepared by Pacific islands people from the root of *Piper methysticum*; the lipid-soluble lactones and flavonoids have mainly CNS effects (sedative and anxiolytic, via various transmitter receptors), as well as analgesic actions (via inhibition of COX enzymes) and local anaesthetic effects
- St John's wort, used since ancient times to rid the body of evil spirits, and treat neuralgia, neuroses and depression; the many pharmacologically active ingredients are now known to affect various CNS neurotransmitters, and the herb is mainly used for its antidepressant actions, which mimic those of the serotonin selective reuptake inhibitors such as fluoxetine; analgesic actions are due to modulation of both opioid receptors and COX enzyme expression
- other natural extracts and supplements with analgesic properties, such as devil's claw, ginger, ginseng, lemon balm, stinging nettle and shark cartilage.

Adapted from: Braun & Cohen (2007), which excellent resource contains details of herbal remedies' chemical components, pharmacological activities, clinical uses, adverse drug reactions and interactions, and practice points, and references to scientific studies on the plants' properties.

- psychotherapeutic methods for pain relief, including hypnosis, behaviour modification, biofeedback techniques, assertiveness training, art and music therapy, meditation, and the placebo effects induced by various other methods
- surgery; a variety of neurosurgical techniques used in treatment of chronic pain resistant to other management procedures; neurectomy (removal of part of a nerve), leucotomy (removal of part of the white matter of the CNS), sympathetic chain ablation and cortical ablation (removal of part of the cerebral cortex) have all been tried
- community support groups, education about the condition, family therapy and support, occupational therapy to assist with activities of daily living, and use of orthoses, all contributing to total patient care
- complementary and alternative medicine (CAM) in acute

pain. Methods shown to be effective in relieving pain and/or reducing required doses of analgesics include relaxation, music therapy, self-hypnosis, acupuncture, spinal manipulation, biofeedback and cognitive behaviour therapy (pyschotherapy in which learning and conditioning are employed to alter illogical beliefs through dialogue and self-evaluation of irrational thoughts)
- CAM in the treatment of chronic pain and cancer pain. The long-term effects of therapies have rarely been studied; methods showing some short-term pain relief include herbs and natural supplements (see Clinical Interest Box 16-10), relaxation therapy, aromatherapy, Chinese herbs, acupuncture, therapeutic touch, education, cognitive behaviour therapy and biofeedback; results with TENS are not conclusive. Such methods can help relieve symptoms (pain, anxiety and depression).

PREGNANCY SAFETY

Most analgesics are classified in Category C—opioids because they can cause respiratory depression in the newborn infant, and prolonged use during pregnancy can lead to withdrawal symptoms in the neonate; and NSAIDs because when given late in pregnancy, the inhibition of prostaglandin synthesis can cause premature closure of the fetal ductus arteriosus, fetal renal impairment, inhibition of platelet aggregation, and delayed labour and birth.

ADEC Category	Drug
A	Codeine, dextromethorphan, dihydrocodeine, paracetamol, pholcodine
B1	Naloxone
B3	Naltrexone
C	Alfentanil, aspirin, buprenorphine, dextropropoxyphene, fentanyl, hydromorphone, methadone, morphine, oxycodone, pentazocine, pethidine, tramadol

DRUGS AT A GLANCE 16: Analgesics

Therapeutic group	Pharmacological group	Key examples	Key pages
Opioid analgesics (narcotic analgesics)	Opioid receptor agonists	morphine fentanyl	pp. 263–6, 8 pp. 266, 7
	Opioid/SSRI	tramadol	pp. 266, 9
Opioid antagonists	Opioid receptor antagonists	naloxone naltrexone	pp. 269, 70
Non-opioid analgesics	Antipyretic analgesics (non-steroidal anti-inflammatory drugs, NSAIDs)	aspirin paracetamol	pp. 270, 1, 4 pp. 272, 3
	GABA analogues	gabapentin	p. 275
	Irritants	capsaicin	p. 275
	NMDA antagonists	ketamine	p. 276
Adjuvant drugs	Tricyclic antidepressants	nortriptyline	p. 276
	Membrane-stabilising agents, anticonvulsants	carbamazepine	p. 276
	Corticosteroids	dexamethasone	p. 276
	α_2-Adrenoceptor agonists	clonidine	p. 276

GABA = gamma-aminobutyric acid; NMDA = N-methyl-D-aspartate; SSRI = selective serotonin reuptake inhibitor.

KEY POINTS

- Pain is a major worldwide health problem, with sensory and emotional components contributing to suffering that disables and distresses people.
- Physiological theories of pain involve nociceptors, ascending afferent pathways of sensory nerves and spinothalamic tracts, and descending efferent pathways from the cortex, which modulate dorsal-horn 'gating' mechanisms.
- Many neurotransmitters and other chemical factors are involved in pain sensation; analgesic drugs in particular affect endorphins and prostaglandins as mediators.

- Pain may be classified by its time course and origin, and assessed by its severity.
- Pain is often inadequately or inappropriately treated because of attitudes, fears and biases of health-care professionals, patients and family.
- Clinical principles of pain management emphasise the importance of adequate regular doses of appropriate analgesics, stepping up the analgesic ladder as necessary, with adjunctive care.
- Many effective pharmacological and non-drug methods are available for the treatment and/or prevention of pain. Assessment tools, pain scales and clinical guidelines are the basis for an effective pain management program.
- The main group of strong analgesic drugs is the opioids, which act centrally on opioid receptors. Opioid antagonists are used to treat adverse effects, overdoses or dependence.
- The other main group is the non-narcotic analgesics, or non-steroidal anti-inflammatory drugs, such as aspirin and paracetamol. These act peripherally by inhibiting production of prostaglandins and may also have antipyretic and antiplatelet actions.
- The health-care professional needs to be informed on the pharmacodynamics and pharmacokinetics of these agents, and to be able to discuss choice of appropriate analgesic agents and to recognise adverse effects.
- An understanding of the effective control of pain in a wide variety of patient populations should be an ultimate goal of a health-care provider.

REVIEW EXERCISES

1. What are the primary myths or fears that interfere with health-care professionals providing adequate pain management?

2. Describe the aetiology and recommended drug therapy for nociceptive, neuropathic and breakthrough pain syndromes.

3. Mr Brown is a 59-year-old man with metastatic disease of unknown origin. He reports his pain as 9 on a scale of 1 (least pain) to 10 (most severe pain). His prescriber ordered Panadeine Forte (paracetamol 500 mg with codeine phosphate 30 mg) 1–2 tablets every 6 hours as required for pain. Two hours after receiving two tablets of this medication, Mr Brown is still in very severe pain. Was this order appropriate for the reported pain level? How might the prescription be improved? What adjuvant medications and non-pharmacological interventions would you suggest, and why?

4. Review at least four potential issues to be considered when selecting an analgesic for an elderly patient (among the areas to consider: the individual's current health problems, physiological changes in the body with age, pharmacokinetic parameters of various analgesics). Name three analgesics that should be avoided for use in the elderly patient, explaining the reasons.

5. Name the three primary opioid receptors in the CNS, and effects mediated through stimulation of these receptors.

6. Discuss factors associated with legislative approval of heroin for intractable pain.

7. Describe the transmitters and other chemical factors involved in the pain sensation and explain how the two main groups of analgesic drugs affect these mediators.

8. Describe the main pharmacological actions and common adverse effects of the opioids and of the non-narcotic analgesics.

9. Outline the stages in the stepwise management of pain.

10. Describe the main symptoms of overdose with the following drugs, and the management steps in treatment of overdose: aspirin; paracetamol; morphine or heroin.

REFERENCES AND FURTHER READING

Analgesic Expert Group. *Therapeutic Guidelines: Analgesic; version 4*. Melbourne: Therapeutic Guidelines, 2002.
Australian Medicines Handbook 2005. Adelaide: AMH, 2005.
Bashford GM. The use of anticonvulsants for neuropathic pain. *Australian Prescriber* 1999; 22 (6): 140–1.
Bowman WC, Rand MJ. *Textbook of Pharmacology*. 2nd edn. Oxford: Blackwell, 1980 [ch. 16].
Braun L, Cohen M. *Herbs and Natural Supplements: An Evidence-Based Guide*. 2nd edn. Sydney: Elsevier Mosby, 2007.
Buckle J. Use of aromatherapy as a complementary treatment of chronic pain. *Alternative Therapies in Health and Medicine* 1999; 5 (5): 42–51.
Carr DB, Goudas LC. Acute pain. *Lancet* 1999; 353 (9169): 2051–8.
Carr DB, Jacox AK, Chapman CR et al. *Acute Pain Management: Operative or Medical Procedures and Trauma. Clinical Practice Guideline.* AHCPR

Pub. no 92-0032. Rockville, MD: Agency for Health Care Policy and Research, Public Health Service, US Department of Health and Human Services, 1992.

Caswell A (ed.). *MIMS Annual 2005.* Sydney: CMPMedica Australia, 2005.

Chahl L. Opioids–mechanisms of action. *Australian Prescriber* 1996; 19 (3): 63–5.

Cichewicz DL. Synergistic interactions between cannabinoid and opioid analgesics. *Life Sciences* 2004; 74 (11): 1317–24.

Dickinson T, Lee K, Spanswick D, Munro FE. Leading the charge: pioneering treatments in the fight against neuropathic pain. *Trends in Pharmacological Sciences* 2003; 24 (11): 555–7.

Ducharme J. Acute pain and pain control: state of the art. *Annals of Emergency Medicine* 2000; 35 (6): 592–600.

Feekery C. Non-organic pain in childhood. *Australian Prescriber* 1999; 22 (5): 122–5.

Graziotti PJ, Goucke CR. The use of oral opioids in patients with chronic non-cancer pain: management strategies. *Medical Journal of Australia* 1997; 167 (1): 30–4.

Hassed C. Cancer and chronic pain. *Australian Family Physician* 1999; 28 (1): 17–21, 23–4.

Hewson P. Paracetamol: overused in childhood fever. *Australian Prescriber* 2000; 23 (3): 60–1.

Hicks CL, von Baeyer CL, Spafford P, van Korlaar I, Goodenough B. The Faces Pain Scale–revised: toward a common metric in pediatric pain measurement. *Pain* 2001; 93: 173–83.

Hunt SP, Koltzenberg M. *The Neurobiology of Pain.* Oxford: Oxford University Press, 2005.

Jeal W, Benfield P. Transdermal fentanyl: a review of its pharmacological properties and therapeutic efficacy in pain control. *Drugs* 1997; 53 (1): 109–38.

Kaye K. Trouble with tramadol. *Australian Prescriber* 2004; 27 (2): 26–7.

Lipman AG. The argument against therapeutic use of heroin in pain management. *American Journal of Hospital Pharmacy* 1993; 50 (5): 996–8.

McCaffery M, Pasero C. *Pain: Clinical Manual.* St Louis: Mosby, 1999.

McCarthy RL, Montagne M. The argument for therapeutic use of heroin in pain management. *American Journal of Hospital Pharmacy* 1993; 50 (5): 992–6.

McMahon SB (ed.). *Wall and Melzack's Textbook of Pain.* 5th edn. Philadelphia: Elsevier/Churchill Livingstone, 2005.

McQuay H. Opioids in pain management. *Lancet* 1999; 353 (9171): 2229–32.

Melzack R. The tragedy of needless pain. *Scientific American* 1990; 262 (2): 19–25.

Melzack R, Wall PD. Pain mechanisms: a new theory. *Science* 1965; 150: 971–9.

Meunier JC. Utilizing functional genomics to identify new pain treatments: the example of nociceptin. *American Journal of Pharmacogenomics* 2003; 3(2): 117–30.

Mitchell JA, Warner TD. Cyclo-oxygenase-2: pharmacology, physiology, biochemistry and relevance to NSAID therapy. *British Journal of Pharmacology* 1999; 128 (6): 1121–32.

Muth-Selbach US, Tegeder I, Brune K, Geisslinger G. Acetaminophen inhibits spinal prostaglandin E2 release after peripheral noxious stimulation. *Anesthesiology* 1999; 91 (1): 231–9.

Oberoi G, Phillips G. *Anaesthesia and Emergency Situations: A Management Guide.* Sydney: McGraw-Hill, 2000.

Padley A. *Westmead Pocket Anaesthetic Manual.* Sydney: McGraw-Hill, 2000.

Palliative Care Expert Group. *Therapeutic Guidelines: Palliative Care, version 2.* Melbourne: Therapeutic Guidelines, 2005.

Pasternak GW. Multiple opiate receptors: deja vu all over again. *Neuropharmacology* 2004; 47(Suppl1): 312–23.

Rang HP, Dale MM, Ritter JM, Moore PK. *Pharmacology,* 5th edn. Edinburgh: Churchill Livingstone, 2003 [chs 5, 50]

Ravenscroft PJ. Opioids: clinical applications in palliative care. *Australian Prescriber* 1996; 19 (3): 66–8.

Ripamonti C, Bruera E. Current status of patient-controlled analgesia in cancer patients. *Oncology (Huntington)* 1997; 11 (3): 373–80, 383–4.

Richards S. Which analgesia? Guidelines to pharmacological pain control. *Professional Nurse* 1997; 12 (9 Suppl.): 1–12.

Salerno E. *Pharmacology for Health Professionals.* St Louis: Mosby, 1999 [chs 3, 8].

Salerno E, Willens JS. *Pain Management Handbook.* St Louis: Mosby, 1996.

Speight TM, Holford NHG (eds). *Avery's Drug Treatment.* 4th edn. Auckland: Adis, 1997.

Spencer JW, Jacobs JJ. *Complementary and Alternative Medicine: An Evidence-Based Approach.* St Louis: Mosby, 1999.

Surratt CK, Adams WR. G protein-coupled receptor structural motifs: relevance to the opioid receptors. *Current Topics in Medicinal Chemistry* 2005; 5(3): 315–24.

Tuckwell K (ed.). *MIMS Disease Index.* 2nd edn. Sydney: MediMedia Australia, 1996.

Vane JR. Inhibition of prostaglandin synthesis as a mechanism of action for aspirin-like drugs. *Nature New Biology* 1971; 231: 232–9.

Vane JR. The fight against rheumatism: from willow-bark to COX-1 sparing drugs. *Journal of Physiology and Pharmacology* 2000; 51 (4 Part 1): 573–86.

Varga EV, Yamamura HI, Rubenzik MK, Stropova D, Navratilova E, Roeske WR. Molecular mechanisms of excitatory signaling upon chronic opioid agonist treatment. *Life Sciences* 2003; 74 (2–3): 299–311.

Virik K, Glare P. Pain management in palliative care: reviewing the issues. *Australian Family Physician* 2000; 29 (11): 1027–33.

Wade A (ed.). *Martindale: The Extra Pharmacopoeia.* 27th edn. London: Pharmaceutical Press, 1977.

Wong D, Hockenberry-Eaton M, Wilson D et al. *Wong's Essentials of Pediatric Nursing.* 6th edn. St Louis: Mosby, 2001.

Youngson RM. *Collins Dictionary: Medicine.* 2nd edn. Glasgow: HarperCollins, 1998.

Zhang WY, Po AL. Do codeine and caffeine enhance the analgesic effect of aspirin? A systematic overview. *Journal of Clinical and Pharmacological Therapeutics* 1997; 22 (2): 79–97.

evolve   More weblinks at http://evolve.elsevier.com/AU/Bryant/pharmacology/

CHAPTER 17

Antianxiety, Sedative and Hypnotic Drugs

CHAPTER FOCUS

Anxiety, worry and insomnia are health problems that occur commonly across the lifespan. When anxiety or fear is the result of a threat or danger, this is a normal physiological response to a threatening situation. However, excessive anxiety or panic that interferes with daily functioning and sleep is counterproductive and usually requires medical intervention and treatment. Insomnia is a common sleep disorder and is often a concern in the elderly. This chapter reviews the antianxiety, sedative and hypnotic drugs available to treat these disorders.

OBJECTIVES

● To describe the physiology of sleep across the lifespan, and how anxiety is related to sleep disorders.

● To explain the mechanisms of action, pharmacological effects and indications for the benzodiazepines.

● To discuss non-pharmacological approaches to sleep disturbances, and their importance in relation to hypnotic drug use in particular groups.

● To explain the mechanisms of action, indications, and significant adverse effects and drug interactions for older sedatives, including the barbiturates and chloral hydrate.

KEY DRUGS

barbiturates
benzodiazepines
chloral hydrate
diazepam
flumazenil

KEY TERMS

anterograde amnesic effect
antianxiety, or anxiolytic, agents
anxiety
γ-aminobutyric acid
hypnotics
insomnia
non-rapid eye movement (non-REM) sleep
rapid eye movement (REM) sleep
sedatives
sleep

KEY ABBREVIATIONS

CAM	complementary and alternative medicine
CNS	central nervous system
EEG	electroencephalograph
GABA	γ-aminobutyric acid
OTC	over-the-counter
REM	rapid eye movement

SLEEP is a recurrent, natural condition of inertia, reduced consciousness and reduced metabolism, during which an individual's overt and covert responses to stimuli are markedly reduced. During **sleep** a person is no longer in sensory contact with the immediate environment, and stimuli no longer attract attention or exert a controlling influence over voluntary and involuntary movements or functions. The purpose of sleep is unknown; however, prolonged sleep deprivation is harmful, causing depression, mental disturbances and hallucinations.

Drugs used to promote sleep include the **sedatives** and **hypnotics**; all are central nervous system (CNS) depressants. Sedatives reduce alertness, consciousness, nervousness or excitability by producing a calming or soothing effect. Hypnotics induce sleep. The major difference between a sedative and a hypnotic is the degree of CNS depression induced: the same drug might be used in small doses for a sedative effect and in larger doses for hypnotic effects. Barbiturates were previously used extensively as sedative–hypnotic agents, but because of their low selectivity and safety they have largely been replaced by the safer benzodiazepines, which have a specific anxiolytic (antianxiety) action.

PHYSIOLOGY OF SLEEP

Sleep is not just one level of unconsciousness. It consists of two basic stages that occur cyclically: **non-rapid eye movement (non-REM) sleep** and **rapid eye movement (REM) sleep**.

The stages of sleep are based on electrical activity that can be observed in the brain by means of an electroencephalograph (EEG). The EEG provides graphic illustrations of brain waves, which are an indication of the electrical activity occurring in the brain (see Figure 18-1).

During sleep, the individual moves first through the four stages of non-REM sleep (Figure 17-1). These are characterised on an electroencephalogram by alpha waves, which are slow and of low amplitude. The sleeper then passes into REM sleep, the fifth stage of sleep, characterised by rapid eye movements, dreaming and fast, low-amplitude waves on an EEG. Periods of REM and non-REM sleep alternate throughout the night. Infants spend a greater proportion of sleep time in REM sleep than do adults (Figure 17-2). REM sleep is not synonymous with light sleep. It takes a more powerful stimulus to arouse a person from REM sleep than from synchronous slow-wave sleep.

Sleep research indicates that there are psychological and physiological reasons for the body to maintain an equilibrium between the various stages of sleep. The physiological functions of the body tend to be depressed during non-dreaming and deep sleep; for example, all of the following are decreased or slowed: blood pressure (falls by 10–30 mmHg), pulse rate, metabolic rate, gastrointestinal tract activity, urine formation, oxygen consumption and carbon dioxide production, body temperature, respirations and body movement. In contrast, during REM dreaming sleep, body movements are more noticeable (moving of the arms and

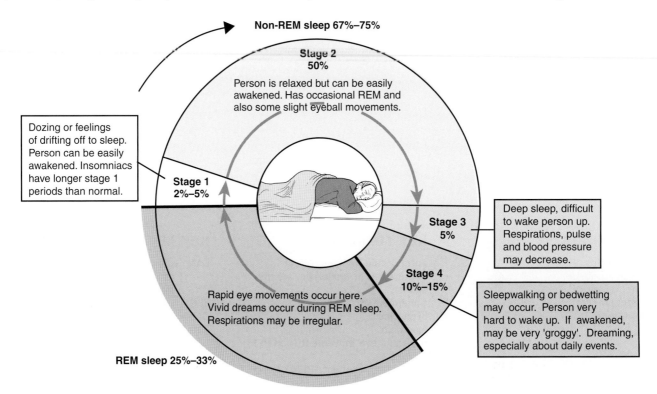

FIGURE 17-1 Stages of sleep.

legs, talking, crying or laughing) and eye movements show under the closed lids. When individuals are deprived of deep sleep, they become physically uncomfortable and depressive, tend to withdraw from their friends and society, and are less aggressive and outgoing.

Dreaming sleep is also important, as individuals deprived of dreaming sleep experience a range of undesirable effects: confusion, suspicion, withdrawal, anxiety, difficulty concentrating and increase in appetite with a definite weight gain. The longer dream deprivation continues, the greater the increase in REM sleep.

SLEEP DISORDERS

Each individual establishes his or her own normal sleep pattern. This can vary from night to night and is influenced by the individual's emotional and physical state. The sleep pattern is controlled from the ascending reticular activating system in the brain (see Figure 17-3, and section in Chapter 14 on CNS functional systems). **Insomnia** is the inability to obtain adequate sleep, whether from difficulty in falling asleep, frequent nocturnal waking or early awakening. Excessive intake of CNS stimulants such as caffeine-containing drinks can cause insomnia, as can anxiety disorders, depression, alcohol abuse, environmental factors (heat, cold, noise),

pain, cardiac or respiratory disorders, and jet-lag. Disorders of excessive daytime sleepiness may be due to inadequate sleep at night, excessive use of CNS depressants (including antidepressants, antihistamines and alcohol), narcolepsy (sudden sleep attacks) or sleep apnoea causing disturbed sleep at night. Box 17-1 lists some drugs that can cause insomnia or sedation.

Management of sleep disorders requires careful attention to specific sleep history and patterns, drug history including use of 'social' drugs such as caffeine and alcohol, and discussion of lifestyle and psychological factors that might impair good sleep cycles. Any physical or depressive disorders that might compromise sleep need treating. Non-pharmacological treatments include attention to sleep hygiene (see Clinical Interest Box 17-1) before hypnotic drugs are tried. Owing to the risk of dependence, hypnotic drugs should be used only for limited periods, preferably less than 2 weeks, such as to assist with impaired sleep cycles following jet-lag or shift-work changes, or as preoperative medication.

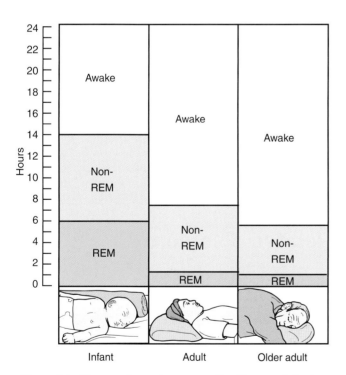

FIGURE 17-2 Sleep–wake cycles across the lifespan. Infants: approximately 40% of total sleep time is REM. Adults: 20% of total sleep time is REM. Older adults: total sleep time is slightly reduced; REM remains 20% of total. *Source*: Beare & Myers 1998.

CLINICAL INTEREST BOX 17-1
SLEEP HYGIENE

Sleep hygiene includes various non-pharmacological approaches to sleep promotion. Useful strategies include the following:

- Restrict use of caffeinated beverages within 8 hours of bedtime. Read labels, because many over-the-counter preparations contain caffeine (see Clinical Interest Box 22-11).
- Establish set times for retiring and getting up. Avoid daytime napping whenever possible. Try to make the bedroom quiet and dark; avoid clock-watching.
- Avoid smoking cigarettes within 8 hours of bedtime or during the night.
- Avoid heavy meals or alcohol just before bedtime.
- Exercising during the day helps sleep patterns, but avoid strenuous exercise or hard work before bedtime.
- Relax in the evening before retiring by reading, taking a warm bath, listening to relaxing music or using relaxation techniques.
- Try not to worry if unable to sleep, because anxiety will cause or add to insomnia. If you cannot sleep, get out of bed and go to another room until sleepy.
- Do not use the bedroom for wake-time activities such as eating or watching television.
- If recurrent and disturbing thoughts interfere with sleep, it might help to write them down and consider a plan of action to solve the problem.
- Home remedies that help induce sleep include drinking warm, non-caffeinated drinks, such as warm milk, or eating a snack high in carbohydrate and low in protein.

Adapted from: Salerno 1999; Psychotropic Expert Group *2003*.

BOX 17-1   DRUGS ASSOCIATED WITH INDUCING INSOMNIA OR SEDATION

Drugs liable to induce insomnia or sleep disturbances
ACE inhibitors (captopril etc)
Alcohol
β-adrenergic blocking agents (propranolol etc)
CNS stimulants (amphetamines, ephedrines)
Corticosteroids
Fluoroquinolones
Levodopa
Methyldopa
Metoclopramide
Monoamine oxidase inhibitors
Nicotine (cigarettes, gum, patches)
Phenytoin
Thyroid hormones
Xanthines (caffeine, theophylline)

Withdrawal from CNS depressants (induces insomnia)
Alcohol
Barbiturates
Benzodiazepines
Tricyclic antidepressants (amitriptyline, imipramine)
Hypnotic drugs
Opioids
Drugs liable to induce sedation or CNS depression
Alcohol
Antihistamines
Opioids
Antipsychotics (phenothiazines)
Tricyclic antidepressants (high doses)
Clonidine
Methyldopa
Cannabis
CNS depressants (benzodiazepines, antiepileptics, general anaesthetics, barbiturates)

ANXIETY

Anxiety is a state or feeling of apprehension, agitation, uncertainty and fear resulting from the experience or anticipation of some stress, threat or danger. It is usually a natural psychological and physiological response to a personally threatening situation, such as a threat to one's health, body, loved ones, job or lifestyle. Generally, this anxiety stimulates the person to take purposeful, constructive actions to counteract the threats and dangers of the anxiety-producing state. In its extreme form, anxiety can be characterised by autonomic nervous system responses including rapid heart rate, dry mouth, sweaty palms, insomnia, loss of appetite, muscle tremor, diarrhoea and dyspnoea. Anxiety is thought to be mediated in the limbic system of the cerebrum.

When a person is unable to cope with a persistently stressful situation because excessive anxiety interferes with daily functioning, help is necessary. Although many non-pharmacological treatments, such as counselling and behaviour modification therapies, are available, antianxiety agents are commonly prescribed for the treatment of anxiety. The **antianxiety**, or **anxiolytic**, **agents** reduce feelings of excessive anxiety, such as apprehension, fear and panic, and reduce the physiological responses. These drugs were previously called the minor tranquillisers to distinguish them from the antipsychotic drugs (major tranquillisers) used in treating schizophrenia. Because excessive anxiety frequently causes insomnia, effective treatment of anxiety usually improves sleep patterns. Thus anxiolytic drugs both directly and indirectly are also sedatives/hypnotics.

Related disorders

Generalised anxiety disorder is considered to exist when a patient has symptoms of excessive anxiety, worry, irritability, muscle tension and sleep disturbances about various events for a period of 6 months or longer. Other associated disorders include adjustment disorder with anxious mood, panic attacks, panic disorder, obsessive–compulsive disorder, phobic disorders and post-traumatic stress disorder. For most of these conditions drug therapy is not the preferred option. Recommended primary therapies include counselling, relaxation techniques, stress management and cognitive behaviour therapy. Short-term use of anxiolytic or antidepressant drugs is sometimes required.

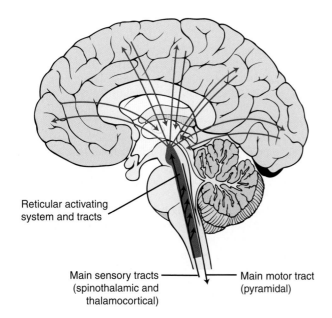

Reticular activating system and tracts

Main sensory tracts (spinothalamic and thalamocortical)

Main motor tract (pyramidal)

FIGURE 17-3 The reticular activating system.

DRUG USE IN SPECIFIC GROUPS

Paediatric drug use

Because young children are much more sensitive to the CNS-depressant effects of antianxiety, sedative or hypnotic drugs, use of these agents is not recommended and counselling and psychotherapy are usually tried first. Paradoxical reactions (reactions contrary to the expected reaction) have been reported with the use of antihistamine and barbiturate sedatives in children. These reactions include increased excitability, hostility, confusion, hallucinations and acute elevation of body temperature. However, sedation may be indicated for particular situations if the drug and dosage are carefully selected for the individual child. Antihistamines are generally safe for mild sedation. Indications for their use include treatment of convulsive disorders (see Chapter 18), as an adjunct pre-anaesthetic agent, or for sedation of a child in intensive care to minimise the risk of removal of catheters. Benzodiazepines should be avoided except for short-term use in specific conditions, such as night terrors or sleepwalking. Close monitoring and assessment by the health-care provider are required (see Paediatric Implications box).

Geriatric drug use

The elderly have more fragmented sleeping patterns than do younger adults. They tend to go to bed earlier, may have difficulty in falling asleep, wake up earlier, and may take multiple daytime naps. Primary sleep disorders, including sleep apnoea and restless legs syndrome, and other factors such as retirement, death of a close friend or spouse, social isolation and increased use of medications also contribute to disturbed sleep (see the Geriatric Implications box).

The elderly frequently use hypnotic drugs, about three times more pro rata than younger adults do. Drug interactions among multiple medications, altered pharmacokinetics (delayed elimination and hence increased accumulation) and increased sensitivity to CNS effects all compound to cause frequent problems (see Clinical Interest Box 17-2). Paradoxical reactions (i.e. increased excitability, rage, hostility, confusion and hallucinations) have been reported in patients with the barbiturates and, in rare instances, the benzodiazepines; these agents should be monitored.

Generalised anxiety is also an issue with elderly people and is often associated with depression. In this situation, antidepressant medication is more effective and safer than use of benzodiazepines, which carry an increased risk of over-sedation, confusion, falls, respiratory depression and short-term memory impairment.

Careful drug selection and dosage are necessary to avoid producing excessive CNS depression in the elderly. Because drug half-lives may be extended, agents with shorter half-lives and no active metabolites are safer for geriatric patients. The short-acting benzodiazepines are much safer than the barbiturates, which are less effective anxiolytic and hypnotic agents and commonly cause confusion and ataxia. Oxazepam, lorazepam, temazepam, alprazolam and triazolam have short to intermediate half-lives (see Table 17-1) and are usually recommended for elderly patients who require a benzodiazepine.

When possible, prescribers suggest that the elderly limit their intake of hypnotic drugs to three or four times a week, allowing patients to select the nights on which they need to take their medication. This schedule usually results in enhanced effectiveness, less daytime drowsiness or sedation, and a decreased potential for inducing tolerance to the medication. Regular and careful assessment, monitoring and re-evaluation of the need for hypnotics are recommended.

BENZODIAZEPINES

The benzodiazepines are among the most widely prescribed drugs in clinical medicine, primarily because of their advantages over the older hypnotic agents such as the barbiturates, chloral hydrate and alcohol. Their popularity results from their anxiolytic and hypnotic dose-related effects, which have the following advantages:
- lower fatality rates following acute toxicity and overdose
- lower potential for abuse
- more favourable adverse effect profiles
- fewer potentially serious drug interactions reported when administered with other medications.

Diazepam (well known as Valium, see Drug Monograph 17-1) is the prototype benzodiazepine. It was the most commonly prescribed benzodiazepine for many years, until newer and safer (shorter-acting) benzodiazepines were released, e.g. lorazepam and alprazolam. As the benzodiazepines have similar pharmacodynamic effects, they will be discussed as a group; pharmacokinetic differences are summarised in Table 17-1.

Pharmacological effects

Benzodiazepines do not exert a general CNS-depressant effect. Instead, selectivity is seen with the various members of this class. The general pharmacological effects of this class include antianxiety, muscle-relaxant, antiepileptic, hypnotic and memory-impairing actions.

TABLE 17-1 Pharmacokinetic overview: benzodiazepines

NAME	DURATION OF ACTION*	HALF-LIFE (h)	ACTIVE METABOLITES (HALF-LIFE [h])
Alprazolam	S	11–16	(10–15)
Bromazepam	M	12–24	(20)
Clobazam	L	18–48	(2–5 days)
Clonazepam	L	18–50	None
Diazepam	L	20–70	Desmethyldiazepam (30–100)
			Temazepam (9.5–12.4)
			Oxazepam (5–15)
Flunitrazepam	L	20–30	(10–16, 23–33)
Lorazepam	M	10–20	None
Midazolam	VS	1–3	(1–3)
Nitrazepam	L	25	None
Oxazepam	S	5–15	None
Temazepam	S	8–15	None
Triazolam	VS	1.5–5.5	None

*VS = very short-acting; S = short-acting; M = medium-acting; L = long-acting.

CLINICAL INTEREST BOX 17-2 FALLS AND FRACTURES IN THE ELDERLY

Studies in Sydney have shown that each year about 30% of people aged over 65 have a major fall, with the rate even higher in nursing homes. Many falls lead to fractures, particularly hip fractures with severe associated morbidity and mortality. Tracing links between medications and falls reveals:

- a twofold increased risk of falls and fractures in elderly persons taking psychotropic drugs
- a strong association with antidepressants
- benzodiazepine dosage appears to be related to risk of falls
- there is less evidence of association of falls with other drugs commonly taken by elderly persons, including cardiovascular drugs, non-steroidal anti-inflammatory drugs (NSAIDs) and diuretics
- antipsychotic drugs are more commonly prescribed in nursing homes than for elderly persons in other locations.

Given the high concentration of elderly patients with dementia in nursing homes and the lack of specific drugs effective in behavioural disturbance and dementias, it is not surprising that psychotropic agents are frequently prescribed. However, it is recommended that psychotropic drug use in the elderly be minimised, especially in nursing home residents.
Based on: Cumming 1998; Mant & Donnelly 1996.

Mechanism of action

Benzodiazepines act via effects on receptors for the inhibitory CNS neurotransmitter γ-aminobutyric acid (GABA). This is the main inhibitory transmitter in the brain, at about 30% of all CNS synapses, in many pathways and brain areas. The GABA$_A$ receptors are ligand-gated chloride channels in the membranes of postsynaptic cells and they mediate fast inhibition: when activated by GABA, there is an increase in chloride permeability and influx of chloride into the cell causing hyperpolarisation and decreased excitability of the neuron. There are several subtypes of GABA$_A$ receptors. In addition, GABA$_A$ receptors have several sites at which drugs can act. The natural endogenous ligand is (obviously) GABA but other endogenous ligands have been identified, including some neuropeptides and steroid metabolites. These could be considered the body's 'natural Valium', by analogy with endorphins being named as the body's endogenous morphine.

Benzodiazepines do not occupy the entire GABA$_A$ receptor, but act at a modulatory site (sometimes confusingly referred to as the benzodiazepine receptor) to facilitate GABA binding to the GABA$_A$ receptors and thus enhance chloride channel opening, leading to more neuronal inhibition. The limbic system, associated with the regulation of emotional behaviour, contains a highly dense area of benzodiazepine binding sites in the amygdala, suggesting that the antianxiety effects occur there. Patients with pathological anxiety

DRUG MONOGRAPH 17-1 DIAZEPAM

Diazepam (well known by the trade name Valium) is the prototype benzodiazepine and as such has anxiolytic, sedative–hypnotic, muscle relaxant and antiepileptic actions by facilitating GABA-mediated CNS inhibitory pathways. However, owing to its metabolism to active derivatives and hence very long duration of action, other benzodiazepines may be indicated when short-acting sedatives are required, or for the elderly.

INDICATIONS Diazepam is indicated for short-term (a few days) management of anxiety, acute withdrawal from alcohol, muscle spasm and spasticity, premedication and conscious sedation, and febrile seizures and epilepsy (as adjunctive treatment or for acute treatment of seizures).

PHARMACOKINETICS Diazepam is one of the longest-acting benzodiazepines as it is very lipid-soluble and is metabolised to active metabolites, some of which themselves are administered as benzodiazepines (see Table 17-1).

ADVERSE REACTIONS All benzodiazepines can cause excessive CNS depression, dependence and neurological dysfunction. Diazepam is likely to cause fatigue, drowsiness and muscle weakness. Less common adverse effects include disturbances of memory, GI tract function, genitourinary functions and vision, and skin reactions. Paradoxical CNS stimulation can occur. Tolerance develops readily.

DRUG INTERACTIONS Diazepam has additive CNS-depressant effects with all other CNS depressants including alcohol, other sedative–hypnotics, antihistamines, anaesthetics, antidepressants and antiepileptic agents. Anticholinergic effects of other drugs may be potentiated. Many drugs can inhibit the metabolism of diazepam and hence prolong its effects; examples are cimetidine and omeprazole.

WARNINGS AND CONTRAINDICATIONS Diazepam is contraindicated in people with chronic obstructive airways disease, severe respiratory or liver disease, sleep apnoea, myasthenia gravis, dependence on other substances or hypersensitivity to benzodiazepines. It should be prescribed only for short periods. Dependence develops readily and a long withdrawal period may be necessary to avoid withdrawal seizures. Diazepam should be used only with caution in people with glaucoma, impaired kidney or liver function, depression or other psychosis, elderly or very young persons, or during pregnancy or lactation.

DOSAGE AND ADMINISTRATION Dosage should be individualised depending on the person's liver and kidney functions, age and the indication for which the drug is prescribed. Diazepam is normally given orally, the dose being 1–10 mg up to 3 times daily. It can also be administered IV or IM or by suppository.

have reduced numbers of GABA–benzodiazepine receptor complexes.

Flumazenil (see later discussion) is an antagonist at the benzodiazepine binding site on the $GABA_A$ receptor. It decreases the binding of GABA so the chloride channels remain closed. Flumazenil is anxiogenic and is used to treat benzodiazepine overdoses. Barbiturates, another group of hypnotic/antiepileptic agents, act as channel modulators at a different site on the $GABA_A$ receptors, not at the benzodiazepine binding site.

Indications for use

The most common indications for benzodiazepines include anxiety disorders, preoperative medication, insomnia and sleep disturbances, seizure disorders, panic disorder (see Clinical Interest Box 17-3), alcohol withdrawal and muscle spasm. They are also used to induce amnesia during cardioversion and endoscopic procedures. The choice of benzodiazepine depends on pharmacokinetic characteristics (Table 17-1), with longer-acting (long half-life) agents such as diazepam preferred for treating anxiety and epilepsy, and short-acting agents such as temazepam and midazolam preferred for induction of

anaesthesia and sleep and treating insomnia. Medium-acting sedative drugs are useful for early-morning wakefulness.

Anxiety disorders

Alprazolam, bromazepam, diazepam, lorazepam and oxazepam are the benzodiazepines most commonly used as antianxiety agents. Alprazolam is also used as an adjunct medication to treat anxiety associated with depression.

Sleep disorders

Nitrazepam, flunitrazepam, clobazam, temazepam and triazolam are usually prescribed for sleep disorders such as insomnia. Generally, these drugs are indicated only for short-term treatment of insomnia (2–4 weeks), owing to the risk of dependence developing.

Seizure disorders

Clonazepam and clobazam are available orally as anticonvulsants (see Chapter 18). Parenteral diazepam is indicated for intractable, repetitive seizures, such as in status epilepticus.

CLINICAL INTEREST BOX 17-3
TREATMENT OF PANIC DISORDER

Panic is an acute condition characterised by intense fears, with palpitations, sweating, chest pain, sensations of choking or smothering and feelings of unreality or dizziness. It is often associated with agoraphobic fears about being in particular situations (alone, or in a crowd, on a bridge, in a vehicle).

Panic disorder involves recurrent and unexpected disabling panic attacks, with persistent concerns and behaviour changes.

Many patients respond to cognitive behavioural therapy and lifestyle changes, particularly control of caffeine and alcohol use.

Benzodiazepines are effective but the requirement for chronic administration and the likelihood of dependence and sedation limit their usefulness.

Antidepressants are effective but generally have significant unwanted adverse effects.

Oral diazepam may be used for short-term adjunctive therapy (1–2 weeks) with other antiepileptics for the treatment of convulsions.

Preoperative medication

Diazepam, lorazepam and parenteral midazolam are used preoperatively, particularly in day-surgery and endoscopic procedures, to reduce anxiety and help induce general anaesthesia and to reduce the dose of anaesthetic needed (see Chapter 15). They can also produce a useful **anterograde amnesic effect**, i.e. decrease the patient's memory of the procedure.

Muscular spasms

Benzodiazepines, especially diazepam, are useful as adjunct medications for treating skeletal muscle spasms caused by muscle or joint inflammation, or spasticity resulting from upper motor neuron dysfunction, such as cerebral palsy and paraplegia.

CNS depressant withdrawal

The benzodiazepines most often used for treatment of alcohol, barbiturate or benzodiazepine withdrawal syndromes are diazepam and oxazepam. These drugs are very useful for the acute agitation, tremors and other symptoms of acute withdrawal.

Pharmacokinetics

The pharmacokinetic properties of the benzodiazepines vary widely and determine the choice between the drugs in this group. For example, half-lives range from about 2 to 60 hours, and there are many metabolic interconversions to active metabolites with long half-lives (see Table 17-1).

The benzodiazepines, being lipid-soluble (lipophilic), are readily absorbed from the gastrointestinal (GI) tract; diazepam and flunitrazepam are the most rapidly absorbed drugs in this class and produce a prompt and intense onset of action. The benzodiazepines become widely distributed in the body and brain. After multiple doses, they accumulate in the body's fluids and tissues, which act as storage depots and account for the prolonged actions even after the drugs have been discontinued. These drugs are mostly highly protein-bound (>85%); protein binding is reduced in newborns, in alcoholic patients and in patients with cirrhosis or impaired liver function.

The GI tract and the liver are the sites of metabolism. Benzodiazepines are often hydroxylated or demethylated to active derivatives, including desmethyldiazepam, a long-acting metabolite (30–100 hours). The long-acting benzodiazepines with active metabolites are more apt to accumulate, especially in the elderly, resulting in higher risk of falls and hip fractures. Oxazepam and lorazepam are metabolised to inactive metabolites and are preferred agents in elderly patients and people with liver disease. Metabolites are generally excreted by the kidney.

The injectable benzodiazepines include diazepam and midazolam. The onset of sedative, anticonvulsant, antianxiety and muscle-relaxant effects of these agents after intravenous administration occurs at about 1–5 minutes.

Drug interactions

Significant drug interactions, such as enhanced CNS depressant effects, sedation and respiratory depression, can occur when benzodiazepines are used in combination with other CNS depressants, including alcohol, opioid analgesics, anaesthetics, antihistamines, psychotropic agents and antidepressants. Close monitoring is necessary because the dosage of one or both drugs may need adjustment.

Many drugs have the potential to inhibit the metabolism of benzodiazepines by the liver's cytochrome P450 enzymes, leading to enhanced CNS depression and respiratory depression. Such drugs include azole antifungals (ketoconazole and itraconazole), cimetidine, macrolide antibiotics (erythromycin) and some antivirals used against HIV infection. On the other hand, the antitubercular rifampicin and antidepressant St John's wort increase benzodiazepine metabolism, so higher dosage may be required.

Adverse reactions

As a group, the benzodiazepines commonly cause excess CNS depression: drowsiness, ataxia, diplopia, vertigo, lassitude, memory loss, slurred speech and loss of dexterity. Less frequently, headaches, decreased libido, anterograde amnesia, muscle weakness and hypotension can occur, as well as increased behavioural problems (anger and impaired ability to concentrate), seen mostly with children. Neurological reactions include paradoxical insomnia, increased excitability, hallucinations and apprehension. There is a greater risk of falls and motor vehicle accidents, particularly in the elderly. Rarely, the patient can experience blood disorders, impaired liver functions and allergic reactions. See Box 17-2 for the treatment of overdose.

Tolerance develops to the sedative effects, but less often to the anxiolytic effects. Dependence is common and leads to the overuse and abuse of these drugs (as 'mother's little helpers') when the causes of anxiety should really be addressed instead. Coping methods are better developed with behavioural therapies than with drugs. Dependence can develop after only a few days' use of benzodiazepines, and withdrawal from chronic use of the drugs can be difficult. Withdrawal is characterised by CNS stimulation: anxiety, sleep disorders, aching limbs, palpitations and nervousness; seizures can occur in people who previously were taking high doses.

Warnings and contraindications

Benzodiazepines are contraindicated in people with respiratory depression or sleep apnoea, severe hepatic impairment or myasthenia gravis. They should be used with caution in children and in the elderly, during pregnancy or lactation, in debilitated patients and in patients with hepatic and renal impairment. Triazolam, in particular, appears to be associated with amnesia, dependence, psychotic disturbances, impaired REM sleep, paradoxical rage, and excessive adverse effects in the elderly. It has been withdrawn in the United Kingdom and in Australia is recommended only for short-term treatment of insomnia.

Benzodiazepine antidote

Flumazenil, a specific benzodiazepine-receptor antagonist (see above, Mechanism of action), is indicated for the treatment of a benzodiazepine overdose or to reverse the sedative effects of benzodiazepines after surgical or diagnostic procedures. This drug will not reverse the effects of opioids or other non-benzodiazepine CNS-depressant drugs. Although it can reverse the sedative effects of benzodiazepines, reversal of the benzodiazepine-induced respiratory depression has not been demonstrated, so respiratory and cardiovascular support may be required.

It is administered intravenously, with antagonistic effects (reversal of sedation) occurring within 1–2 minutes and duration of action of about 1–3 hours. Because most benzodiazepines have a half-life longer than 1 hour, repeated injections of flumazenil are necessary. Flumazenil is metabolised in the liver and excreted by the kidneys.

Adverse reactions reported with this drug include headache, visual disturbance, increased anxiety, nausea and lightheadedness. Because it antagonises receptors at which the endogenous inhibitory neurotransmitter GABA acts, flumazenil can cause dangerous convulsions in patients taking benzodiazepines to control epilepsy, or in mixed overdoses with benzodiazepines and proconvulsant drugs such as antidepressants or CNS stimulants. Caution is advised when giving flumazenil to patients who are known to use benzodiazepines chronically, because moderate to severe withdrawal symptoms and seizures may be precipitated.

In practice, because benzodiazepines are considerably safer than earlier sedative–hypnotics, overdose is rarely a clinical emergency and flumazenil is indicated only to avoid intubation or intensive care admission.

OTHER ANTIANXIETY AND SEDATIVE/ HYPNOTIC AGENTS

Drugs related to benzodiazepines
Zopiclone

Zopiclone is a relatively new drug that is chemically unlike the benzodiazepines but has very similar pharmacological properties. It is a hypnotic indicated for short-term treatment of insomnia. It is rapidly absorbed, distributed and metabolised, with only one metabolite having weak CNS-depressant activity. The half-life is short (5–7 hours) but may be extended in the elderly and in people with impaired liver function.

The adverse reactions profile is similar to that of the benzodiazepines: CNS depression, possibility of dependence and withdrawal reactions. In addition, zopiclone can interfere with thyroid hormone balance. It alters taste sensation, causing bitter taste. Use during pregnancy or lactation and in children is not recommended.

Zolpidem

Zolpidem tartrate* is a non-benzodiazepine that is more selective in its binding to a subunit of the GABA$_A$ receptor than the benzodiazepines; thus it has pharmacological properties that are similar to those of benzodiazepines but lacks the anticonvulsant, muscle-relaxant and antianxiety properties associated with the benzodiazepines. It is approved for short-term treatment of insomnia. It has a rapid onset of action, short half-life and no active metabolites, so should be taken immediately before retiring. Adverse effects, drug interactions and precautions are similar to those of the benzodiazepines. In addition, zolpidem is likely to cause diarrhoea and myalgia and can cause hallucinations.

Buspirone

Buspirone is not closely related pharmacologically to the other drugs discussed in this chapter. It is an anxiolytic with less sedative effect than the benzodiazepines and little anticonvulsant or muscle-relaxant activity. The exact mechanism of action is unknown, but the drug has a high affinity for 5-hydroxytryptamine (5-HT, serotonin) receptors and a moderate affinity for brain dopamine D$_2$ receptors in the CNS. It does not affect GABA, nor does it have any significant affinity for the benzodiazepine receptors.

Buspirone is indicated for the treatment of anxiety disorders and is considered equivalent in efficacy to the benzodiazepines but usually with less sedation. It appears to have little risk of causing dependence and withdrawal reactions. Common adverse effects are CNS and GI tract disturbances. Due to its affinity for brain dopamine receptors, it can cause dopamine-mediated dysfunction, including parkinsonian symptoms and endocrine disturbances.

---

*Another example is zaleplon; these new hypnotics have been referred to as the 'z-drugs'.

Barbiturates

The **barbiturates** were once the most commonly prescribed class of medications for hypnotic and sedative effects. They are derivatives of barbituric acid, so named because it was discovered in 1863 on St Barbara's Day. The first active drug in this group, barbitone, was used medically in 1903 and thousands of 'me-too' barbiturates soon followed. With few exceptions, barbiturates have been replaced by the safer benzodiazepines and more specific antiepileptic agents. Phenobarbitone, the prototype drug for this classification, is now used mainly as an antiepileptic (see Chapter 18), and thiopentone to induce general anaesthesia (see Chapter 15).

The mechanism of action for barbiturates is non-selective depression of the CNS via enhancement of inhibitory systems that use GABA as a neurotransmitter. Barbiturates can also decrease excitatory neurotransmitter effects. Barbiturate depression of the ascending reticular formation decreases cortical stimuli, reducing the need for wakefulness and alertness. High doses of barbiturates can induce anaesthesia. Phenobarbitone exerts a selective action on the motor cortex even in small doses. This explains its use as an anticonvulsant.

Large doses, especially when administered intravenously, depress the respiratory and vasomotor centres. Elderly or debilitated patients are especially sensitive to the CNS-depressant effects and can exhibit confusion, disorientation and mental depression. Barbiturates have a much lower therapeutic index (safety margin) than do the benzodiazepines; they were the classic sleeping pills with which many people committed suicide or died after an inadvertent overdose. Drug interactions are frequent, especially with other CNS depressants including alcohol. The barbiturates are also the main group of drugs that induce hepatic drug-metabolising enzymes, thus enhancing the metabolism and inactivation of many other drugs, including anticoagulants, anticonvulsants, oral contraceptives and corticosteroids.

These agents have virtually dropped out of use as sedatives. They are occasionally provided for elderly patients who remain dependent on them following chronic use.

Miscellaneous sedatives and hypnotics
Older sedative–hypnotics
BROMIDES

Bromide salts such as potassium bromide were used in medicine as antiepileptic agents and as sedative–hypnotics from the mid-1850s (see Clinical Interest Box 17-4); a triple bromide mixture contained lithium, sodium and potassium bromides. The term bromide came to have a more general meaning: a conventional idea or trite remark—presumably by extension referring to an idea or remark so boring as to put someone to sleep. Bromide ion is absorbed in the body

CLINICAL INTEREST BOX 17-4 DEATH BY BROMIDE AND STRYCHNINE

Agatha Christie, the well-known English writer of detective fiction, was very knowledgeable about poisons, and worked in a Red Cross hospital dispensary during both World War I and World War II. The plot of her first detective novel, *The Mysterious Affair at Styles* (1920), depends on some interesting toxicological and pharmaceutical information. (People wishing to read the story without knowing the ending are advised to stop here.)

An elderly wealthy woman, suffering insomnia, was prescribed bromide powders to help her sleep.

She also took a daily dose of a tonic containing strychnine—low doses of strychnine used to be included in tonics partly because it is a CNS stimulant and because it tastes so bad that it should obviously do the patient some good.

The conspirators dropped a few bromide powders into the large, full bottle of tonic mixture. Because strychnine hydrochloride is incompatible with bromides, the strychnine precipitated as an insoluble bromide and settled to the bottom of the bottle.

The plotters then neglected to shake the bottle when they gave the old woman her dose of tonic, until the last dose contained all the strychnine from the bottle.

This last dose was poured into the woman's evening cup of coffee, which was sufficiently bitter to mask the taste of the strychnine, so she drank a lethal dose of strychnine (and probably of bromide too) and died from CNS stimulation, convulsions and paralysis of the respiratory muscles causing respiratory arrest.

Of course, to confuse the reader, there were several possible suspects, all of whom had enough medical/pharmaceutical knowledge to realise that 'addition of a bromide to a mixture containing strychnine would cause the precipitation of the latter', as pointed out by the detective Hercule Poirot in the denouement of the story.

The plot is certainly feasible from a pharmacological viewpoint: Strychnine Mixture (present in the British National Formulary as late as 1963) contained about 6.24 mg strychnine hydrochloride per 30 mL dose. A large bottle (say 500 mL) would contain more than 100 mg strychnine, a fatal dose.

CLINICAL INTEREST BOX 17-5 THE 'MICKEY FINN'

The combination of chloral or chloral hydrate with alcohol is very potent and potentially toxic. This mixture, used with criminal intent and known as a Mickey Finn, or knock-out drops, is particularly dangerous because not only are the CNS-depressant effects additive, but trichloroethanol also inhibits the metabolism of alcohol and prolongs its actions.

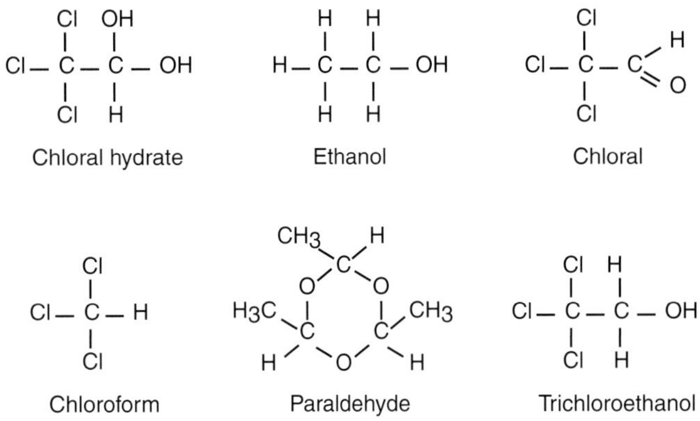

FIGURE 17-4 Chemical structures of some simple sedative drugs, showing close structural relationships between the sedative chloral hydrate, anaesthetic chloroform, depressant ethanol (alcohol), and sedative paraldehyde, which can be visualised as three molecules of ethanol joined in a cyclical ether formation. Most of these drugs are rarely used nowadays.

converted in the body to active trichloroethanol, which has a rapid, powerful hypnotic action. Its exact mechanism of action is unknown. It has a general CNS-depressant effect similar to that of alcohol.

Chloral hydrate was formerly frequently used as a sedative and hypnotic and as premedication, particularly in children and the elderly, as both oral and rectal forms are rapidly absorbed. It was considered relatively safe but can be toxic in overdose, especially in combination with alcohol (see Clinical Interest Box 17-5), causing cardiac and respiratory failure. Deaths have occurred with the use of this drug. It is still sometimes used as a mild hypnotic or preoperative sedative, particularly in children's hospitals to sedate children in intensive care units so that catheters are not pulled out; continuous monitoring is required. A mixture form is available, containing 1 g/10 mL sweetened with sucrose and saccharin.

and replaces chloride (biologically the more common halide ion) in extracellular fluids. Bromide acts in the CNS as a depressant and sedative, and in (not much) larger doses it depresses motor activity and reflexes. At toxic levels it causes ataxia, delirium, coma and death. It is particularly toxic as a cumulative poison so it has been replaced by safer drugs.

CHLORAL HYDRATE

Chloral hydrate is a simple chemical substance (trichloro-ethane-diol) related structurally to both chloroform and ethanol (see Figure 17-4). It is essentially a 'prodrug' that is

PARALDEHYDE

Paraldehyde is a polymer of acetaldehyde. It is a colourless liquid with a strong odour and taste. The CNS-depressant effects of paraldehyde are similar to those of alcohol,

CLINICAL INTEREST BOX 17-6 COMPLEMENTARY AND ALTERNATIVE SEDATIVES

For treating insomnia, the natural products valerian, kava kava, lavender, lemon balm, passionflower and L-tryptophan and low-energy electromagnetic fields applied to the oral mucosa have been shown to be clinically effective.

Melatonin, the natural hormone from the pineal gland, appears to reset the body's circadian rhythm clocks and is used by many people to help overcome jet-lag or adapt to altered shift-work hours. However, clinical evidence for effectiveness and mechanism is sparse. Other techniques that still require evidence of effectiveness include acupuncture and cranial electrostimulation.

CAM techniques used to alleviate stress include relaxation techniques (yoga, Qi Gong, exercise and meditation) and dance classes; evidence of clinical effectiveness is hard to validate because of the difficulties of conducting double-blind controlled studies.

In the treatment of anxiety, music therapy, massage, acupuncture and the Chinese herb suanzaorentang have been shown to be effective. Yoga, meditation, homeopathic remedies and 'electrosleep' have shown little efficacy.

barbiturates and chloral hydrate. It depresses various levels of the CNS, including the ascending reticular activating system. Paraldehyde is indicated for intramuscular administration as an anticonvulsant in status epilepticus and convulsive episodes arising from tetanus and from poisoning with convulsant drugs. Like alcohol, it is metabolised in the liver to acetaldehyde. Paraldehyde was used in the past as a sedative–hypnotic agent but has been superseded by safer and more effective drugs.

ANTIHISTAMINES

The antihistamines (histamine H_1-antagonists) have significant sedative effects as well as being useful in suppressing allergic reactions (see Chapter 55) and as antiemetics. Examples of antihistamines effective as sedatives are promethazine and diphenhydramine. They are readily available over the counter, and antihistamine mixtures are sometimes used as mild sedatives for children. When used as antiemetics to protect

children against travel sickness, their sedative effects can be useful (for parents).

DEXMEDETOMIDINE

Dexmedetomidine is a new sedative drug, related to the imidazole α_2-adrenoceptor agonists such as clonidine and with similar pharmacological properties. It is used specifically by IV infusion for post-surgical and intensive care sedation of intubated patients. It has cardiovascular and CNS adverse effects, but does not cause respiratory depression.

Complementary and alternative sedatives

Many natural products and techniques from the complementary and alternative medicine (CAM) paradigm have been used to attain sleep or relieve stress and anxiety (see Clinical Interest Box 17-6).

PAEDIATRIC IMPLICATIONS

Antianxiety agents and sedatives
- Young children are very susceptible to CNS-depressant effects of sedatives and hypnotics.
- To reduce or minimise potential adverse CNS-depressant effects, carefully follow the manufacturer's dosage instructions and whenever possible avoid concurrent administration of other CNS-depressant types of drugs, including those in over-the-counter medications.
- Monitor children for excessive sedation, lethargy and lack of coordination; if any of these effects are present, dosage adjustments may be necessary.
- In neonates, profound CNS depression can result because of the lower rate of drug metabolism by the immature liver.
- Paradoxical reactions (excitability, hallucinations) have been reported in children with the use of antihistamines and barbiturates.
- Although diazepam may be used in infants 6 months and over, this drug and other benzodiazepines should not be used to treat a hyperactive or psychotic child.
- Chronic use of clonazepam (an antiepileptic) can result in impaired physical, endocrine or mental functions in the developing child, which may not become apparent until years later.
- Buspirone and other new sedative drugs have not been studied in people under 18 years of age, so they are not recommended for use in this age group.

GERIATRIC IMPLICATIONS

Insomnia and hypnotic agents

* Sleep latency increases while REM and stage 4 sleep may be absent in the geriatric patient.
* Sleep disturbance is one of the most frequent concerns of the elderly.
* Individuals should be evaluated for pre-existing health conditions because various illnesses such as arthritic pain, hyperthyroidism, cardiac dysrhythmia, respiratory difficulties and paroxysmal nocturnal dyspnoea can alter sleep patterns.
* Hypnotics should be reserved to treat acute insomnia and, when prescribed, limited to short-term or intermittent use to avoid the development of tolerance and dependence.
* A hypnotic with a short duration of action is preferred because daytime sedation, ataxia, memory deficits and falls can result when longer-acting hypnotics are given.
* Encourage older patients to use non-pharmacological approaches to promote sleep.
* Be aware that the elderly, children and people with CNS dysfunction can experience a paradoxical reaction (CNS stimulation) to hypnotics and antihistamines. Common adverse effects with antihistamines (which may be prescribed but are also often in over-the-counter drugs) include dizziness, tinnitus, blurred or altered vision, gastrointestinal disturbance and dry mouth.

PREGNANCY SAFETY

ADEC Category	Drug
A	Chloral hydrate
B1	Buspirone, dexmedetomidine
B3	Flumazenil, zolpidem
C	All barbiturates; all benzodiazepines; zopiclone
D	Paraldehyde

DRUGS AT A GLANCE 17: Antianxiety, sedative and hypnotic drugs

Therapeutic group	Pharmacological group	Key examples	Key pages
Antianxiety sedative agents	Benzodiazepines • Long-acting • Short-acting	 diazepam alprazolam	 pp. 285–7, 89 pp. 286, 7
Other sedatives/hypnotics	Barbiturates	phenobarbitone	p. 290
	Others	zopiclone, buspirone	pp. 289, 90
		chloral hydrate	p. 291
		dexmedetomidine	p. 292

KEY POINTS

* Sleep disturbances and insomnia cause many physiological dysfunctions. They are common, particularly in the elderly.
* Anxiolytic, sedative and hypnotic medications can be used in the short term to treat insomnia.
* Benzodiazepines such as diazepam are the most common drugs used to treat anxiety and insomnia today; they act by facilitation of GABA-mediated CNS inhibitory pathways to cause sedation and muscle relaxation, and relieve anxiety and convulsions.

- Because of their safety and effectiveness and the variety of conditions in which benzodiazepines are effective, they have largely replaced the barbiturates, chloral hydrate and other earlier sedatives.
- Pharmacokinetic properties vary widely: half-lives range from 2 to 60 hours and many benzodiazepines are converted to pharmacologically active metabolites that prolong the sedative effects. Short-acting agents are used to induce anaesthesia or sleep and longer-acting agents to treat anxiety or epilepsy.
- Common adverse reactions include excessive CNS depression, tolerance and dependence. Drug interactions frequently occur with other CNS depressants and with drugs that affect the metabolism of benzodiazepines.
- Newer related agents are zolpidem and zopiclone; buspirone acts by different mechanisms and is less sedating.
- As geriatric patients are more sensitive to these agents than the younger adult and are at risk of accumulation of active drug and of falls, the use of non-pharmacological approaches to treat sleep disturbances and a limited use of short-acting benzodiazepines should be considered.
- Health-care professionals should be aware that both the paediatric and geriatric populations are at greater risk of paradoxical-type reactions (CNS stimulation rather than depression) from sedative drugs. It is recommended that prescriptions for these agents be limited, with close patient monitoring.
- Flumazenil, a specific benzodiazepine antagonist, is used in emergencies to treat overdose with benzodiazepines.
- Many other drugs can cause sedation and CNS depression, including anaesthetics, alcohol, antipsychotics and antidepressants, opioid analgesics and antihistamines. Insomnia can also be an adverse effect of drugs, especially CNS stimulants such as the amphetamines and caffeine-containing drinks.

REVIEW EXERCISES

1. Describe the physiology of sleep, and problems caused by insomnia or sleep deprivation.
2. Discuss guidelines for the use of hypnotics in the elderly and in long-term care facilities.
3. Review the mechanisms of action for the benzodiazepines and for flumazenil, and describe how flumazenil is used.
4. Describe common adverse effects of benzodiazepines, and explain how overdose is managed clinically.
5. Explain the major differences in action and effects between a benzodiazepine such as diazepam and buspirone.

REFERENCES AND FURTHER READING

Ancoli-Israel S. Insomnia in the elderly: a review for the primary care practitioner. *Sleep* 2000; 23 Suppl 1: S23–30.
Austin D, Blashki G, Barton D, Klein B. Managing panic disorder in general practice. *Australian Family Physician* 2005; 34(7): 563–71.
Australian Medicines Handbook 2005. Adelaide: AMH, 2005.
Beare PB, Myers JL. *Adult Health Nursing*. 3rd edn. St Louis: Mosby, 1998.
Bowman WC, Rand MJ. *Textbook of Pharmacology*. 2nd edn. Oxford: Blackwell, 1980 [ch. 8].
Braun L, Cohen M. *Herbs and Natural Supplements: An Evidence-Based Guide*. Sydney: Elsevier Mosby, 2005.
Buckley NA, Whyte IM, Dawson AH et al. Correlations between prescriptions and drugs taken in self-poisoning: implications for prescribers and drug regulation. *Medical Journal of Australia* 1995; 162: 194–7.
Carey DL, Day RO, Cairns DR et al. An attempt to influence hypnotic and sedative drug use. *Medical Journal of Australia* 1992; 156: 389–96.
Caswell A (ed.). *MIMS Annual June 2005*. Sydney: CMPMedica Australia, 2005.
Costa E. From GABA-A receptor diversity emerges a unified vision of GABAergic inhibition. *Annual Review of Pharmacology and Toxicology* 1998; 38: 321–50.
Cumming RG. Epidemiology of medication-related falls and fractures in the elderly. *Drugs and Aging* 1998; 12: 43–53.
Mant A, Donnelly NJ. Drug use in nursing homes: some new evidence. *Medical Journal of Australia* 1996; 65: 295–6.
Michael Kaplan E, DuPont RL. Benzodiazepines and anxiety disorders: a review for the practicing physician. *Current Medical Research and Opinion* 2005; 21(6): 941–50.
Norman TR, Ellen SR, Burrows GD. Benzodiazepines in anxiety disorders: managing therapeutics and dependence. *Medical Journal of Australia* 1997; 167: 490–5.
Psychotropic Expert Group. *Therapeutic Guidelines: Psychotropics, version 5*. Melbourne: Therapeutic Guidelines Limited, 2003.
Roy-Byrne PP. The GABA–benzodiazepine receptor complex: structure, function and role in anxiety. *Journal of Clinical Psychiatry* 2005; 66 Suppl 2: 14–20.
Salerno E. *Pharmacology for Health Professionals*. St Louis: Mosby, 1999 [ch. 10].
Spencer JW, Jacobs JJ. *Complementary/Alternative Medicine: An Evidence-Based Approach*. St Louis: Mosby, 1999.
Stahl SM. *Essential Psychopharmacology: Neuroscientific Basis and Practical Applications*. 2nd edn. Cambridge: Cambridge University Press, 2000 [ch. 8].
Teuber L, Watjens F, Jensen LH. Ligands for the benzodiazepine binding site—a survey. *Current Pharmaceutical Design* 1999; 5: 317–43.
Tiller JWG. The management of insomnia: an update. *Australian Prescriber* 2003; 26(4): 78–81.

Weinbroum AA, Flaishon R, Sorkine P et al. A risk–benefit assessment of flumazenil in the management of benzodiazepine overdose. *Drug Safety* 1997; 17: 181–96.
Whiting PJ. The GABA-A receptor gene family: new targets for therapeutic intervention. *Neurochemistry International* 1999; 34: 387–90.

ON-LINE RESOURCES

New Zealand medicines and medical devices safety authority: www.medsafe.govt.nz

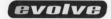   More weblinks at http://evolve.elsevier.com/AU/Bryant/pharmacology/

CHAPTER 18

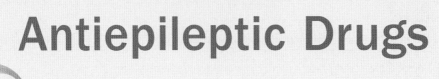

Antiepileptic Drugs

CHAPTER FOCUS

Epilepsy is a common neurological illness involving recurrent epileptic seizures that may affect parts or the whole of the cerebral hemispheres and cause muscle twitching and impaired consciousness. It affects one in every 200 adults in Western societies; mild seizures in children are much more common. This chapter discusses classifications of the types of epilepsy and the various antiepileptic drugs available to treat this disorder.

OBJECTIVES

- To outline the international classification of seizure disorders (epilepsies).

- To identify the major antiepileptic drug groups, including drug examples, mechanisms of action and primary indications.

- To discuss clinical aspects of therapy of epilepsies, including choice of drug, compliance, therapeutic monitoring and drug use in particular patient groups.

KEY DRUGS

carbamazepine
clonazepam
phenobarbitone
phenytoin
sodium valproate
topiramate

KEY TERMS

anticonvulsant
antiepileptic drug
epilepsy
focal seizure
generalised absence seizures
induction of metabolism
mixed seizures
non-linear pharmacokinetics
partial complex (psychomotor)
    seizures
primary, or idiopathic, epilepsy
secondary epilepsy
status epilepticus
tonic–clonic generalised (grand mal)
    epilepsy

KEY ABBREVIATIONS

AED   antiepileptic drug
CNS   central nervous system
EEG   electroencephalogram
GABA γ-aminobutyric acid
NMDA N-methyl-D-aspartate

EPILEPSY

EPILEPSY is a group of chronic neurological disorders characterised by sporadic, recurrent episodes of convulsive seizures resulting from occasional excessive disorderly discharges in neuronal pathways across the cerebral cortex. The seizures can lead to loss of consciousness, muscle jerking, sensory disturbances and abnormal behaviour. Although nearly 70% of seizures do not have an identifiable cause (**primary**, or **idiopathic**, **epilepsy**), around 30% have an underlying cause (**secondary epilepsy**) that is treatable, e.g. head injury, cerebrovascular infarct or haemorrhage, infection, brain tumour, drug toxicity or a metabolic imbalance. It is estimated that about 2% of a population will suffer seizures at some stage in their lives.

Classification of seizures

The choice of appropriate antiepileptic (anticonvulsant) drugs for treating individual patients depends on accurate diagnosis and classification of the seizure type. A full medical history, laboratory tests, a neurological examination and electroencephalogram (EEG) are necessary for classification. Computed tomography (CT) and magnetic resonance imaging (MRI) may also be used to detect anatomical defects or to locate small focal brain lesions. Identifying specific seizure types is critical to the development of a treatment plan. The aim of therapy is to avoid factors that tend to trigger attacks (see Clinical Interest Box 18-1) and to find the drug or drugs that will effectively control the seizures with a minimum of undesirable side-effects and restore physiological homeostasis.

The terminology currently used with epileptic seizures is shown in Clinical Interest Box 18-2, on the International Classification of Seizures. **Mixed seizures** are seen in some individuals who have more than one type of seizure disorder. In practice, many health-care providers still use the former common terms: grand mal, jacksonian, psychomotor and petit mal epilepsy; therefore we should be familiar with both seizure classifications.

Types of epilepsy

Partial simple motor (jacksonian) **epilepsy** is described as a type of **focal seizure**; it is associated with irritation of a specific part of the brain. A single body part such as a finger or an extremity may jerk, and such movements may end spontaneously or spread over the whole musculature. Consciousness may not be lost unless the seizure develops into a generalised convulsion.

Partial complex (psychomotor) seizures are characterised by brief alterations in consciousness, unusual stereotyped movements (such as chewing or swallowing movements) repeated over and over, changes in temperament, confusion, and feelings of unreality. These seizures may spread and evolve to generalised grand mal seizures, and are likely to be resistant to therapy with drugs.

Generalised absence* seizures, simple or complex (petit mal), are most often seen in childhood and consist of temporary lapses in consciousness that last a few seconds. Generally, children appear to stare into space or daydream, are inattentive and may exhibit a few rhythmic movements of the eyes (slight blinking), head or hands, but they do not convulse. They may have many attacks in a single day. The EEG records a 3/second spike-wave pattern (see Figure 18-1). Sometimes an attack of generalised absence seizures is followed by a generalised tonic–clonic seizure. When the child reaches adulthood, other types of seizures may occur.

Myoclonic seizures are characterised by bilaterally symmetrical muscle jerks, often with loss of consciousness.

Tonic–clonic generalised (grand mal) epilepsy is the type most commonly seen. Such attacks may be characterised by an aura and a sudden loss of consciousness and motor control. The aura is specific to the individual; it may consist of numbness, visual disturbance or a particular form of dizziness that warns the person of an approaching seizure. The person falls forcefully due to continuous tonic spasm (stiffening, increased muscle tone), which may be followed by a series of clonic (rapid, synchronous jerking) muscular contractions. The eyes roll upwards, the arms flex and the legs extend. The force of the muscular contractions causes air to be forced out of the lungs, which accounts for the cry that the person may make on falling. Respiration is suspended temporarily, the skin becomes sweaty and cyanotic, saliva flows, incontinence may occur, and the person may froth at the mouth and bite the tongue if it gets caught between the teeth. No pain is felt, as the person is deeply unconscious. When the seizure subsides, the individual regains partial consciousness, may complain of aching, and then tends to fall into a deep sleep.

Status epilepticus is a clinical emergency. It is the state of recurrent seizures for more than 30 minutes without an intervening period of consciousness. A 10%–20% mortality rate results from anoxia in this state. The major cause of status epilepticus is non-compliance with an antiepileptic drug regimen; other causes include cerebral infarction, central nervous system (CNS) tumour or infection, trauma, or low blood concentration of calcium or glucose.

---

*To be pronounced with a French accent! There are many French terms in neurology (such as grand mal, petit mal, migraine, Guillain–Barré syndrome, contre-coup, tic douloureux, Duchenne's muscular dystrophy, Gilles de la Tourette syndrome, and Charcot joint) due to the important early work in this area by French neuroscientists. Even nicotine is named after Jean Nicot, who popularised tobacco smoking in France in the 16th century as a treatment for headache.

CLINICAL INTEREST BOX 18-1
TRIGGERS OF EPILEPTIC SEIZURES

- Secondary, or organic, epilepsy frequently follows head injury or a focal lesion in the CNS, such as an infection or tumour, or birth damage or an endocrine disorder. These lesions may set off the high-frequency discharges in brain neuronal pathways that lead to the seizure.
- Idiopathic epilepsy has no known organic cause, but many factors are likely to act as triggers to an attack: hyperventilation, trauma, lack of sleep, poor nutrition, fever, stress, bright lights—especially flashing lights of a TV set or strobe lights such as in a disco—or changes in blood levels of hormones, fluids or electrolytes.
- A wide range of drugs has been implicated as potentially able to cause convulsions or lower the seizure threshold, including many common drugs (aspirin, antihistamines, antidepressants, antibiotics, local and general anaesthetics, vaccines, neuroleptic agents, oral contraceptives, narcotic analgesics, bronchodilators), social drugs (alcohol, caffeine, cocaine, cannabis) and even antiepileptic drugs themselves (clonazepam, sodium valproate).

Relation of age to seizures

A relation exists between age and onset of an epileptic seizure state. Most people with epilepsy have their initial seizure before the age of 20; however, seizures may have an onset at any age in life. Idiopathic (of no defined aetiology, or genetic in origin or cause) seizures are often diagnosed between the ages of 5 and 20. Onset before or after this age period is often from non-idiopathic (identifiable) causes and is termed 'symptomatic' (acquired, organic) epilepsy.

Neonates

Neonatal seizures occur in children younger than 1 month. Among the more common causes of neonatal seizures are congenital defects or malformation of the brain, infections (meningitis, encephalitis, abscess) within the CNS, hypoxia (in utero or during delivery), premature birth and defects in metabolism. These epileptic seizures are also referred to as organic or acquired.

Infants

In infants younger than 2 years, the seizure types most frequently diagnosed include generalised tonic–clonic seizures and partial seizures. The infantile spasm is not classified as a type of epileptic seizure itself. Among the more common causes of infant seizures are those reported above for neonatal seizures as well as infection, exposure to toxins (in utero,

caused by maternal exposure to or use, misuse or abuse of drugs), maternal exposure to X-rays, and postnatal trauma. Infantile spasms may lead to atonic epileptic seizures seen in later development (ages 2–5 years).

Children

In children 2–5 years of age the seizure types often diagnosed include generalised tonic–clonic seizures and atonic seizures. The causes are similar to those mentioned above for newborns

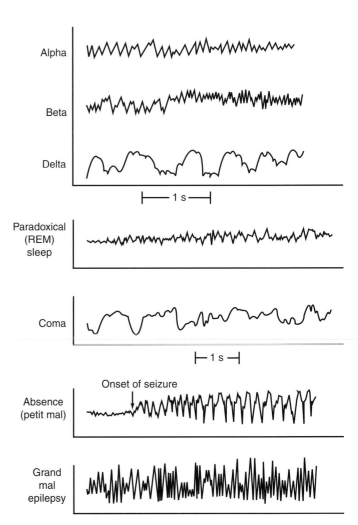

FIGURE 18-1 The electroencephalogram during sleep and in epilepsy.
Alpha waves: awake, eyes closed (8–13 cycles/second).
Beta waves: mental activity (14–30 cycles/second).
Delta waves: deep sleep (1–5 cycles/second).
REM sleep: EEG pattern similar to that for alpha waves when awake. **Coma:** similar to delta waves. **Epilepsy: generalised absence (petit mal) seizure:** EEG tracing shows spikes and waves (3 cycles/second). **Epilepsy: generalised tonic–clonic seizure (grand mal):** tracing shows spikes of clonic phase.
Adapted from: Tortora & Grabowski 2000; Vander et al 1998; Rang et al 2003.

CLINICAL INTEREST BOX 18-2 INTERNATIONAL CLASSIFICATION OF SEIZURES

PARTIAL SEIZURES

Simple (no impairment of consciousness)

- Motor symptoms (formerly called jacksonian)
- Sensory (hallucinations of sight, hearing or taste); somatosensory (tingling)
- Autonomic (autonomic nervous system responses)
- Psychic (personality changes)

Complex (impaired consciousness)

- Psychomotor symptoms (complex symptoms that may include an aura, automatism [e.g. chewing, swallowing movements], unreal feelings, bizarre behaviours, motor seizures)
- Cognitive symptoms (confusion); affective (bizarre behaviour); psychosensory (purposeless behaviours)
- Compound (tonic, clonic, or tonic–clonic seizures)

Partial seizures, secondarily generalised

- Unilateral or predominantly unilateral seizures (formerly called grand mal with aura)

GENERALISED SEIZURES (CONVULSIVE OR NON-CONVULSIVE; WIDESPREAD INVOLVEMENT OF BOTH CEREBRAL HEMISPHERES)

- Tonic–clonic seizures (formerly called grand mal)
- Tonic (sustained contractions of large muscle groups)
- Clonic (various dysrhythmic contractions in the body)
- Myoclonic (unaltered consciousness, isolated clonic contractions)
- Absence seizures (formerly called petit mal—brief loss of consciousness for a few seconds, no confusion, EEG demonstrates 3/second spike-wave patterns)
- Atonic (head-drop or falling-down symptoms)

INFANTILE SPASMS

and infants, with the addition of chronic diseases involving the CNS. The parents of the child may wrongly believe the child has a behavioural disorder rather than a treatable seizure disorder. Febrile convulsions are frequently associated with a fever from a source outside the CNS.

In children 6 years and over the seizure types that emerge most commonly on diagnosis are absence seizures and generalised tonic–clonic seizures, which may be idiopathic in origin. Sometimes the convulsive seizure is associated with a brain tumour, vascular disease, brain infection, head trauma (accident or sport), fever, growth of scar tissue, presence of a toxin or a poison, or drug withdrawal (See the Paediatric Implications box at the end of this chapter for more information.)

Young adults

Within the 16–25-year age group, generalised seizures may be idiopathic in origin. The partial seizure and less commonly seen generalised seizures may result from the use of alcohol, social or recreational drug use, drug abuse, misuse or withdrawal, or head injury.

Elderly

People over 60 are at greater risk of seizure episodes. In this population, osteoporosis and cerebrovascular disease are common and therefore seizures may lead to fractures, intracranial bleeding, neurological deficit, cognitive impairment and severe limitation in daily functioning. Common causes of seizures in the elderly include trauma, brain tumours, vascular disease, embolic stroke and Alzheimer's disease. (See the Geriatric Implications box at the end of this chapter for more information.)

ANTIEPILEPTIC THERAPY

Clinical aspects

Although secondary seizures usually respond to correction of the underlying condition and perhaps short-term use of antiepileptic agents, primary recurrent seizures require long-term antiepileptic drug therapy. The main goal of drug therapy is to control or prevent the recurrence of the seizure disorder while ensuring that unwanted effects of the treatment do not handicap the person more than further seizures would. Lifestyle aspects, including issues related to emergency management of seizures, employment, driving, sport, relationships and pregnancy, also need to be discussed with patients.

If possible, epilepsy is controlled with one antiepileptic drug (monotherapy) introduced slowly; if maximum tolerated doses of one drug are not effective, another drug is substituted. Only if seizure control cannot be achieved with any drug is a second drug added to the regimen. About 70% of patients can be well controlled with one drug; half of the remainder may require two to three drugs, and the rest may remain refractory to treatment or require surgery.

Choice of antiepileptic drug

As stated earlier, different types of seizure may respond to particular antiepileptic agents, hence the importance of accurate diagnosis of seizure type. The currently recommended drugs are listed in Table 18-1; other second-line agents may be tried if the first-line drugs are not successful in controlling seizures.

TABLE 18-1 Anticonvulsant agents for seizure disorders

First-line agents considered most effective with the least toxicity in treatment of seizure disorders in adults are as follows.*

GENERALISED TONIC–CLONIC (GRAND MAL)	ABSENCE SEIZURES (PETIT MAL)	SIMPLE OR COMPLEX PARTIAL	MYOCLONIC
Valproate	Ethosuximide	Carbamazepine	Valproate
Carbamazepine	Valproate	Phenytoin	Clonazepam
Lamotrigine	Clonazepam	Valproate	Phenobarbitone
Phenytoin	Lamotrigine	Lamotrigine	

Adapted from: AMH 2005; Neurology Expert Group 2002.
* For infantile spasms, tetracosactrin (ACTH) and prednisolone are the first-line drugs.

TABLE 18-2 Central nervous system effects of selected anticonvulsants

DRUG	BEHAVIOURAL ALTERATIONS	COGNITIVE EFFECTS
Barbiturates, especially phenobarbitone	May see a paradoxical effect, especially in children or the elderly (e.g. increased activity or excitement, irritability, altered sleep patterns, increased tiredness)	Impaired judgement, short-term memory impairment, decreased attention span
Carbamazepine	Increased irritability, insomnia, behavioural changes (especially in children), depression	Less than phenytoin, phenobarbitone or primidone
Clonazepam	Drowsiness, dizziness, ataxia, impaired speech and vision, hysteria; dependence and withdrawal symptoms after cessation; paradoxical reactions (excitement, insomnia, agitation)	Anterograde amnesia, memory impairment, confusion, impaired concentration
Phenytoin	Fatigue, increased clumsiness, confusion, mood alterations	Decreased attention span, decreased ability to solve problems, decreased learning
Sodium valproate	Sedation, ataxia, depression, increased appetite and weight; hyperactivity and aggression in children	Stupor (associated with excess dosage or polytherapy)

Adverse drug reactions and compliance

Adverse drug reactions are common with antiepileptic drugs; in particular, CNS depression is likely (see Table 18-2). While each drug has its own adverse-effect profile, common reactions include excessive sedation, ataxia and confusion; depression of the cardiovascular and respiratory centres; and adverse cognitive effects such as impaired memory and learning, which can impair progress of children in school. Paradoxical reactions (excitation rather than depression) sometimes occur with benzodiazepines and barbiturates, especially in children and the elderly. Effects on the gastrointestinal tract and haematological system, and hypersensitivity reactions including rashes, are also possible.

Good compliance with therapy is often difficult, as with many drug regimens for chronic conditions for which therapy may need to be lifelong. Lack of compliance can lead to drug withdrawal symptoms, including lack of seizure control and onset of convulsions. Therapeutic monitoring is usually carried out regularly (see below), partly to facilitate adjustment of doses and also to check compliance. Compliance is improved if the patient (and family and carers) understands the condition and the importance of regular therapy (see Clinical Interest Box 18-3).

Special situations
INFANCY

Febrile seizures in infancy occur commonly with mild infections and fevers. While distressing to parents, these do not indicate that the child will develop epilepsy. Paracetamol reduces fever symptoms in children but does not prevent febrile convulsions; in susceptible infants, phenobarbitone or sodium valproate prevents recurrences.

CLINICAL INTEREST BOX 18-3
EPILEPSY SUPPORT GROUPS

The National Epilepsy Association of Australia has affiliated groups with branches in major cities. The Epilepsy Foundation of Victoria, based in Camberwell, Melbourne, has as its mission the enhancement of the quality of life of people living with epilepsy.

The Foundation runs workshops, educational sessions, epilepsy awareness programs, clinics, parent support groups, family camps, forums and continuing education for health professionals.

Library facilities offer information on specific issues; loans of books, videos, periodicals, clippings collections and education kits; and publications including newsletters and brochures.

Publications are available on topics such as:
- epilepsy medications
- managing your epilepsy
- key points about epilepsy
- driving and epilepsy
- employing people with epilepsy
- sudden unexplained deaths in epilepsy.

EPILEPSY IN WOMEN

In some women, seizure frequency increases during menstruation. Antiepileptic drugs may reduce the effectiveness of the oral contraceptive pill, leading to breakthrough bleeding, pill failure and pregnancy.

Because many antiepileptic drugs are potentially teratogenic or can affect cognitive development (see Pregnancy Safety box at the end of this chapter), treatment of women of childbearing age must always include consideration of these risks if the woman becomes pregnant. Increasing the intake of folic acid (5 mg/day) before conception and for the first 3 months thereafter may decrease the risk of spina bifida in the fetus. Overall, seizure control is of the highest priority, as seizures during pregnancy pose a greater risk to mother and fetus than do antiepileptic drugs. (See Clinical Interest Box 18-4 for seizure prevention in eclampsia.)

Although breastfeeding is not usually contraindicated, CNS-depressant drugs may pass into breast milk, so the infant should be monitored for drowsiness or feeding difficulties.

TREATMENT OF CHILDREN OR ELDERLY PATIENTS

See the Paediatric and Geriatric Implications boxes at the end of this chapter.

Maintenance therapy

After a drug regimen is found that successfully controls seizures without significant adverse effects, it is continued until the patient has been seizure-free for 2–3 years. Plasma drug levels are occasionally monitored to check compliance (non-compliance being the commonest cause of failure of seizure control). Carers should watch for delayed adverse effects such as gum hypertrophy, poor school performance or liver failure.

Therapeutic monitoring

Plasma levels of antiepileptic drugs are monitored frequently. This is useful for establishing baseline data, predicting toxicity, detecting interactions that affect blood levels and checking compliance.

Published therapeutic plasma ranges of various anticonvulsant agents are used as a guide to therapy. This allows the prescriber to adjust dosages according to the individual's requirement, to reach the therapeutic range (see Figure 18-2) or to achieve seizure control without adverse effects. While the time needed to reach a steady-state drug level in plasma is usually five times the elimination half-life of the drug, dosage requirements of individual patients are unpredictable so therapeutic response is the best measure of success.

CLINICAL INTEREST BOX 18-4
ECLAMPSIA—TOXAEMIA OF PREGNANCY

Eclampsia is a serious complication of pregnancy in which dangerous seizures occur with a high maternal and fetal mortality.

It is always preceded by pre-eclampsia, a condition characterised by elevated blood pressure, oedema of the extremities (hands, feet and ankles) and proteinurea. This occurs in about 5% of all pregnancies; regular antenatal care with monitoring of maternal blood pressure and weight gain helps warn of impending pre-eclampsia.

Pregnancy-induced hypertension is associated with primigravidae (first-time mothers), diabetes, multiple pregnancy, and underlying renal or hypertensive disease.

The treatment plan for pre-eclampsia is to control the elevated blood pressure, prevent seizures, maintain renal function and generally provide optimal conditions for the fetus. This approach is primarily symptomatic because the only real cure for this syndrome is delivery of the baby.

The usual anticonvulsant drugs (diazepam, phenobarbitone or phenytoin) are administered parenterally to prevent convulsions and for sedation. Magnesium sulfate has useful CNS-depressant effects as well as reducing neuromuscular transmission and hence muscular contractions; however, decreased muscle tone and respiratory depression may be seen in the neonate.

The mother should be monitored for up to 2 days after delivery, as seizures may still occur in the immediate postpartum period.

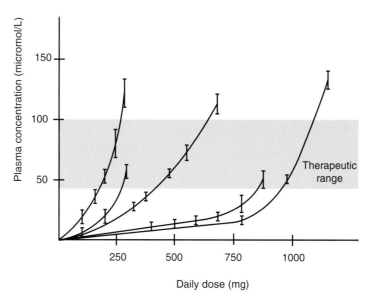

FIGURE 18-2 Non-linear relation between daily dose of phenytoin and steady-state plasma concentration in five individual human subjects. Although the therapeutic range is quite broad (40–100 micromol/L), the daily dose required varies greatly between individuals, and for any individual the dose has to be adjusted in small increments to keep within the acceptable plasma concentration range. Note: 1 mmol is equal to about 250 mg phenytoin.
Adapted from: Rang 2003 with permission; data redrawn from Richens & Dunlop 1975.

Adverse drug interactions

Drug interactions with antiepileptic drugs are common, variable and unpredictable; they need to be anticipated and monitored. Typically:

- barbiturates, clonazepam, ethosuximide, phenytoin and sodium valproate can cause raised plasma concentrations of other antiepileptic agents and of many other drugs, and increase toxicity; drug dosages may need to be lowered
- barbiturates, carbamazepine, phenytoin and sodium valproate can **induce drug-metabolising enzymes** and cause lowered plasma concentrations of other antiepileptic agents and even of themselves (and of other drugs, including hormones, cardiovascular drugs and antimicrobial agents) and reduce seizure control; drug dosages may need to be raised
- antidepressants, antipsychotics and antihistamines lower the convulsive threshold and alter anticonvulsant requirements.

Clearly, the possibilities for variable plasma drug concentrations and responses can make treatment confusing; a good general rule is 'see an antiepileptic, think drug interactions'. Clinical efficacy requires constant monitoring until the patient is stabilised on an effective drug regimen. (A reference text should be consulted for details of adverse effects or drug interactions of individual antiepileptic agents.)

Parenteral use of antiepileptics

Antiepileptic drugs (AED) are administered parenterally (usually IV or IM) in acute conditions involving seizures, such as eclampsia, status epilepticus, severe recurrent seizures, tetanus, seizure during neurosurgery and convulsant drug toxicity. Phenobarbitone, phenytoin and the benzodiazepines diazepam and lorazepam are given by injection. If it is impossible to administer the drugs by injection because of severe convulsions, the rectal route may be used.

Discontinuing anticonvulsant therapy

A diagnosis of epilepsy no longer implies a lifetime of drug therapy: studies have indicated that anticonvulsant drugs may be withdrawn from up to 70% of patients who are seizure-free for at least 2 years. In long-term studies, seizures recurred in 12%–36% of the patients who were monitored for more than 20 years after complete drug withdrawal. There are some risk factors that help in predicting which patients may have seizure recurrence after drug withdrawal. These include:

- an onset of seizures after 12 years of age
- a family history of seizure activity
- a 2–6-year period before seizure control
- a large total number of seizures
- requiring more than one AED
- an abnormal EEG even with therapy
- the presence of an organic neurological disorder or mental retardation.

Withdrawal from phenytoin or valproate is associated with a higher rate of recurrence than for other drugs.

Anticonvulsant medications should be tapered down slowly (in a non-emergency situation) to avoid the potential for inducing seizures and status epilepticus. If the patient is taking more than one anticonvulsant, each drug is withdrawn separately and slowly over several months.

Use of antiepileptics in neuropathic pain

Anticonvulsant agents are sometimes used in conditions other than epilepsy, notably in pain syndromes such as neuropathic pain (see Chapter 16) that do not respond to the usual analgesic drugs. In particular, carbamazepine is used in trigeminal neuralgia, sodium valproate in migraine headache, and some of the newer antiepileptics such as gabapentin in painful diabetic neuropathy and post-herpetic neuralgia.

Antiepileptic drugs
The ideal antiepileptic drug

Although there is no ideal **anticonvulsant** drug, the following characteristics would be highly desirable:
- highly effective but with a low incidence of toxicity
- effective against more than one type of seizure and for mixed seizures, in any environment
- long-acting and non-sedating, so that the patient is not inconvenienced by the need for multiple daily drug dosing or by excessive drowsiness
- not highly protein-bound and not involved in significant drug interactions
- well tolerated by patients and inexpensive, as patients may have to take it for years or for the rest of their lives
- not resulting in the development of tolerance to the therapeutic effects.

The major drugs used in the treatment of partial seizures and generalised tonic–clonic seizures are sodium valproate, phenytoin, carbamazepine, benzodiazepines (especially clonazepam) and the barbiturates (especially phenobarbitone). Newer miscellaneous anticonvulsants include gabapentin, lamotrigine, vigabatrin, tiagabine, topiramate and levetiracetam.

Mechanisms of action

While the aim of using a drug to prevent seizures is to decrease the likelihood of excessive neuronal transmission in CNS pathways, most CNS depressants are too sedating to be clinically useful in epilepsy. For those that are effective antiepileptic agents, the exact modes and sites of action are complex and incompletely understood. A common mechanism of action appears to relate to stabilisation of the nerve cell membrane by altering cation transport, especially that of sodium, potassium and calcium.

There are three main groups of **antiepileptic (anticonvulsant) drugs**:
- those that enhance gamma (γ)-aminobutyric acid (GABA)-mediated inhibition of neural activity, e.g. by facilitating GABA-mediated opening of chloride channels; by inhibiting GABA-transaminase, the enzyme that inactivates GABA; or by inhibiting the GABA reuptake processes. The benzodiazepines, barbiturates and some newer drugs (vigabatrin, tiagabine and topiramate) act by these mechanisms. Some GABA-ergic drugs are now being trialled in anxiety, affective disorders and pain conditions
- those that inhibit sodium channel function, thus blocking repetitive depolarisation of neurons. These drugs appear to block preferentially the excitation of cells that are firing repetitively; for example, phenytoin decreases abnormal seizure discharge by blocking sodium channels and perhaps calcium influx. Phenytoin thus suppresses seizures by stabilising cell membrane excitability and reducing the spread of seizure discharge. Carbamazepine also enhances inactivation of sodium channels, which alters neuronal excitability and decreases synaptic transmission. Other examples of drugs acting by this mechanism are sodium valproate and lamotrigine
- miscellaneous drugs with varying mechanisms, which are still being studied and assessed. This group includes ethosuximide, gabapentin and some drugs that are more commonly used in other clinical conditions but have useful membrane-stabilising actions (acetazolamide, sulthiame, adrenocorticotrophic hormone [ACTH]).

As no antiepileptic agent is ideal, there is considerable current research into new mechanisms of action of anticonvulsant drugs. As it is very expensive to carry out large-scale, high-powered clinical trials, particularly in a chronic condition like epilepsy in which the manifestations (seizures) occur occasionally and randomly, there is little level-one evidence on the efficacy and safety of the newer AEDs from randomised controlled clinical trials. As well as the mechanisms listed above, there is interest in compounds that may reduce CNS neuronal excitation by the excitatory amino acid transmitter glutamate.* Three types of glutamate receptors are of interest: NMDA (N-methyl-D-aspartate) receptors, kainate receptors, and AMPA (alpha-amino-3-hydroxy-5-methyl-4-isoxazole propionic acid) receptors. All are ionotropic receptors involving calcium channels. Antagonists of these receptors are being assessed for clinical efficacy in neurodegenerative conditions and in epilepsy, anxiety, hyperalgesia and psychosis.

---

*Glutamate is infamous for its involvement in the 'Chinese restaurant syndrome'. Many people are sensitive to the stimulant effects of monosodium glutamate (MSG), added to dishes of Asian food to enhance the flavours. Excessive amounts can cause flushing and nausea.

DRUG MONOGRAPH 18-1 TOPIRAMATE

Topiramate is a relatively new AED, which acts both by blocking sodium channels, thus reducing the frequency of action potentials, and by enhancing inhibitory neuronal activity at kainate-type GABA$_A$ receptors. It is considered safer than some of the older AEDs, however, the newer drugs are currently considerably more expensive. Its mechanism of action in migraine is unknown.

INDICATIONS Topiramate is indicated for monotherapy in newly diagnosed epilepsy, and in conversion to monotherapy, and as add-on therapy of partial onset seizures and primary generalised tonic–clonic seizures. It is also used for prophylaxis of migraine headaches in adults.

PHARMACOKINETICS Topiramate is administered orally, and is well and rapidly absorbed. It is distributed to the total body water, with low protein binding, reaching peak plasma concentration by 2–3 hours. It is not extensively metabolised, and metabolites are inactive. It is mainly cleared by the kidneys, with a long half-life of approximately 21 hours; steady-state is not reached for several days. Topiramate is not a potent inducer of drug-metabolising enzymes.

DRUG INTERACTIONS As with all AEDs, there are potential additive effects with other CNS depressants. The metabolism of topiramate may be increased by drugs that induce drug-metabolising enzymes, including other AEDs such as carbamazepine and phenytoin, necessitating dose increase. Topiramate may increase the concentration of phenytoin in plasma.

ADVERSE REACTIONS The most common adverse effects are due to CNS depression, and include ataxia and speech disorders; patients need to be warned against driving or operating machinery. Psychiatric disorders also occur, including anorexia, confusion, mood disturbances and depression, and amnesia. Other possible adverse effects include fatigue, diarrhoea, reduced sweating and hyperthermia, nephrolithiasis, myopia and secondary angle-closure glaucoma, and metabolic acidosis.

WARNINGS AND CONTRAINDICATIONS Precautions are required before prescribing to patients predisposed to the adverse effects, especially renal stone formation, psychiatric disturbances, metabolic acidosis or glaucoma. In patients with reduced renal function, topiramate's half-life may be even longer. The drug is classified B3 with respect to pregnancy safety, however, the risk to the baby of maternal seizures is much greater than the risk of malformations. Prophylactic dosing with folic acid 1 month before and 3 months after conception is advised.

DOSAGE AND ADMINISTRATION Topiramate is available as tablets and as 'sprinkle capsules', which may be opened and the contents sprinkled on soft food before swallowing without chewing. The usual starting dose in adults is 25 mg/day, taken at night, gradually increasing to 100 mg/day; dosage in children is 0.5–1 mg/kg/day, increasing to 3–6 mg/kg/day.

Drugs from the above groups will be discussed briefly, with more detailed drug monographs on topiramate and and phenytoin as important examples from groups 1 and 2 respectively.

Antiepileptics that enhance GABA inhibition

BENZODIAZEPINES

The benzodiazepines used as antiepileptic agents are those with long half-lives, such as clonazepam, diazepam, nitrazepam and clobazam. These drugs are discussed in detail in Chapter 17 as the standard sedative–hypnotic and antianxiety agents (see Drug Monograph 17-1). Their mechanism of action is to occupy specific benzodiazepine-binding sites in the GABA receptor and hence facilitate GABA-mediated inhibition of neural activity and suppress the propagation of seizure activity produced by foci in the cortex, thalamus and limbic areas. Dependence, tolerance and withdrawal reactions are common problems.

Clonazepam is a long-acting benzodiazepine used to treat absence seizures, myoclonic seizure disorders and status epilepticus. It has been used alone but more often it is prescribed as an adjunct to other anticonvulsants to establish seizure control. Diazepam can be given orally or IV, or rectally when IV injection is not possible, e.g. in prolonged convulsions in children. Clonazepam is given orally or by slow IV injection.

Drug interactions with other CNS depressants (including alcohol, which is contraindicated) are common. Severe withdrawal reactions and an increase in seizures may follow abrupt withdrawal of benzodiazepines. Dosage is usually individualised for each patient and increased as necessary. The elderly or debilitated persons and patients taking other CNS-depressant-type medications usually receive a smaller dose with a slower dosage increase.

VIGABATRIN

Vigabatrin also enhances GABA-mediated inhibition but by a very different mechanism: it is an irreversible inhibitor of

GABA transaminase, the enzyme that inactivates GABA, and thereby allows a build-up of the neurotransmitter in synapses. It is a relatively new drug, indicated for adjunctive (add-on) treatment, especially of complex partial seizures, focal epilepsy and infantile spasms. It has a specific adverse effect on vision: it can cause an irreversible visual field constriction in 20%–40% of patients taking the drug, so visual fields should be tested before starting therapy, then every 3–6 months. Vigabatrin may soon be withdrawn.

TIAGABINE AND TOPIRAMATE

Tiagabine is a GABA reuptake inhibitor and is indicated as adjunctive therapy in patients with partial seizures. Drug interactions may occur when tiagabine is given in combination with other anticonvulsants such as carbamazepine, phenytoin, primidone or phenobarbitone. It has been reported that tiagabine clearance is increased by nearly 60% when combined with these anticonvulsants; therefore tiagabine dosage increase may be necessary. Adverse reactions occur most commonly in the CNS and gastrointestinal tract.

Topiramate is another new antiepileptic (see Drug Monograph 18-1). Although the exact mechanism of action for topiramate is unknown, it has four useful properties:
- it appears to have a sodium channel-blocking action
- it potentiates the neurotransmitter inhibitory activity of GABA
- it antagonises kainate's ability to activate an excitatory glutamate receptor
- it is a weak carbonic anhydrase inhibitor (see under acetazolamide and sulthiame [below] for a description of the mechanism of action).

Topiramate is used as adjunctive therapy for partial and generalised seizures in adults. The main adverse reactions are CNS-depressant effects.

BARBITURATES

Barbiturates, especially phenobarbitone, have been used for many years for the treatment of generalised tonic–clonic and partial seizures, and for neonatal febrile convulsions and status epilepticus. This class is relatively inexpensive and efficacious but has a low therapeutic index (safety margin) because of its CNS-depressant side-effects. The mechanism of action of the barbiturates is discussed in Chapter 17. Barbiturates are now 'last resort' drugs in epilepsy.

PRIMIDONE. Primidone, while strictly speaking not a barbiturate, has two active metabolites, phenobarbitone and phenylethylmalonamide, which contribute to anticonvulsant activity. Primidone has been used for control of generalised tonic–clonic (grand mal) and complex seizures but is less well tolerated than phenobarbitone alone and so is dropping out of use.

CLINICAL INTEREST BOX 18-5 TITRATING PHENYTOIN DOSES

As explained in the caption to Figure 18-2, for each individual the dose of phenytoin may need to be adjusted (titrated) frequently and precisely to keep the plasma concentration within the therapeutic range. This is done through regular monitoring of drug level in samples of the patient's plasma and with the help of various formulations of phenytoin, which allow small changes in dose.

The average (adult) dose is about 300 mg/day, with a range of 200–500 mg/day; however, owing to the non-linear pharmacokinetics, a small increase in dose, say, from about 375 to 500 mg, may more than double the plasma concentration.

In Australia, phenytoin is available in several dose forms:
- ampoules for injection, 50 mg/mL, in 2 mL or 5 mL sizes
- capsules, 30 mg or 100 mg
- paediatric tablets (yellow chewable spearmint-flavoured triangles), 50 mg
- paediatric suspension, 30 mg/5 mL (liquid formulations allow easy adjustment of dose).

Antiepileptics that inhibit sodium channel functions

PHENYTOIN

The prototype hydantoin drug is phenytoin (diphenyl-hydantoin), which was developed from a search for an anticonvulsant that would cause less sedation than the barbiturates. Phenytoin is recommended for the treatment of all types of epilepsy except absence seizures. It blocks voltage-dependent sodium channels, decreasing the propagation of seizures. It is particularly interesting from the pharmacokinetic point of view, as it has **non-linear pharmacokinetic** parameters (see Figure 18-2 and Drug Monograph 18-2), which often make clinical use of phenytoin very difficult (see Clinical Interest Box 18-5).

Fosphenytoin is a phenytoin analogue, a prodrug that is rapidly converted to phenytoin in the body. It has been formulated to overcome the problems with parenteral pheny;toin (not very soluble and the injectable form is very alkaline and can cause venous irritation). Fosphenytoin is less alkaline and can be given IM for status epilepticus and to treat and prevent seizures associated with neurosurgery or head trauma.

CARBAMAZEPINE

Carbamazepine also blocks sodium channels, decreasing the propagation of seizures. The drug's effects are somewhat

DRUG MONOGRAPH 18-2   PHENYTOIN

INDICATIONS Phenytoin acts to reduce the maximal activity of brainstem centres responsible for the tonic phase of grand mal seizures. Phenytoin is more effective for grand mal and partial seizures than for petit mal seizures. It is also frequently prescribed in combination with phenobarbitone and may be prescribed for patients to prevent seizures after surgery on the brain, after head trauma and for status epilepticus.

PHARMACOKINETICS With most drugs, as the dose is increased the plasma drug concentration increases in a linear, arithmetic (direct) relationship; however, because of saturable metabolism, the **non-linear pharmacokinetics** of phenytoin means that with phenytoin the dose–plasma concentration relationship is not linear, and a small rise in dose may cause an unexpectedly large rise in plasma drug levels (see Figure 18-2). Oral absorption of phenytoin is slow and variable (poor in neonates); the time to peak serum level is 1.5–3 hours and half-life varies with dose and serum level, ranging from 7 to 42 hours, with an average of about 20 hours. It is inactivated in the liver and excreted in the bile and in urine.

DRUG INTERACTIONS There are many important drug interactions with phenytoin (see *Australian Medicines Handbook* Appendix A); examples are given below. In particular, many drugs may inhibit the metabolism of phenytoin and hence prolong the half-life, leading to neurotoxic effects.

Drug	Possible effect and management
Antacids, sucralfate and calcium	Concurrent use may decrease the absorption of phenytoin; administer 2–3 hours apart
Adrenocorticoids, oestrogens, oral contraceptives, anticoagulants (warfarin), loop diuretics, methadone, pethidine	An increase in metabolism of these drugs may result from phenytoin's **induction of microsomal enzymes**, which may decrease the therapeutic effects of these drugs; dosage adjustment may be necessary. Breakthrough bleeding and an increased risk of conception may occur with oestrogen-containing contraceptives

Drug	Possible effect and management
Carbamazepine	A decrease in therapeutic effect may occur with one or both drugs. Plasma drug levels should be closely monitored
Chloramphenicol, cimetidine, disulfiram, isoniazid, amiodarone, oral anticoagulants, allopurinol, omeprazole, imipramine, azole antifungals, sulfonamides	A decrease in phenytoin metabolism may cause an increased plasma drug concentration and toxicity of phenytoin. Dosage adjustment may be required
CNS depressants, alcohol	May result in enhanced CNS depression; monitor closely for respiratory depression and drowsiness

ADVERSE REACTIONS There are many dose-related neurotoxic effects (drowsiness, dizziness), also idiosyncratic reactions (hirsutism, gingival hyperplasia with bleeding, sensitive gum tissue, or overgrowth of gum tissue, acne and facial coarsening). Signs of overdose or toxicity include blurred or double vision, slurred speech, clumsiness, dizziness, confusion and hallucinations. In addition, signs of toxicity with intravenous phenytoin include cardiovascular collapse, CNS depression and hypotension. The rate of IV administration (25–50 mg/min) is critical, as severe cardiotoxic reactions and fatal outcomes have been reported with faster infusions.

WARNINGS AND CONTRAINDICATIONS Use with caution in pregnancy and in persons with drug allergies, diabetes mellitus, and liver or renal impairment. Women relying on oestrogen-containing contraceptives may require higher doses. Regular dental care is important to detect gum problems. Avoid use in persons with hydantoin hypersensitivity, and use caution with similar compounds such as phenobarbitone and carbamazepine.

DOSAGE AND ADMINISTRATION The usual adult dosage is 200–500 mg daily; however, careful monitoring and titration of dose is required.

similar to those of phenytoin. Carbamazepine is indicated in the treatment of generalised tonic–clonic seizures, partial complex seizures and psychomotor seizures, and for mixed seizure patterns. It is also indicated in the treatment of neuropathic pain, such as that associated with trigeminal neuralgia, and for bipolar disorder and mania.

PHARMACOKINETICS. Oral absorption is slow and onset of action may range from hours to days, depending on the individual. Due to autoinduction of metabolism (i.e. it induces higher levels of the enzymes that metabolise it), it may take a month to reach a stable therapeutic serum level. Carbamazepine is metabolised in the liver (it has one active metabolite) and excreted primarily by the kidneys.

DRUG INTERACTIONS. Again, there are many clinically significant drug interactions with carbamazepine. It boosts the metabolism and thus decreases the effectiveness of many drugs, including anticoagulants (warfarin), other anticonvulsants and carbamazepine itself, corticosteroids and oral contraceptives. Blood levels should be monitored whenever any of these medications is added or discontinued in persons receiving carbamazepine, as dosage adjustment may be necessary. Sodium valproate, however, may prolong the half-life of carbamazepine.

ADVERSE REACTIONS. These include CNS depression, possible severe allergic and skin reactions, depressed white cell counts and antidiuretic hormone-like effects.

OXCARBAZEPINE. Oxcarbazepine, an analogue of carbamazepine, has been developed to overcome some of the problems of the latter. Oxcarbazepine is less toxic and has fewer drug interactions; it is useful in adults and children with partial and generalised seizures uncontrolled by other drugs and has been used as both adjunctive and monotherapy. Hyponatraemia (low sodium concentrations) can develop, so it is recommended that plasma sodium concentration be monitored.

SODIUM VALPROATE

The mechanism by which **sodium valproate** exerts its anticonvulsant effects has not been fully established. It may enhance brain levels of GABA; it also may act by blocking sodium, potassium and/or calcium channels. By competitive inhibition it may prevent the reuptake of GABA by glial cells and axonal terminals.

INDICATIONS. As can be seen from Table 18-1, sodium valproate is one of the most generally useful anticonvulsants. It is indicated for use as sole or adjunctive therapy in the treatment of absence seizures, including petit mal seizures, and in patients with multiple seizure types, including partial (simple and complex), generalised, myoclonic or atonic seizures, and in bipolar disorder and migraine.

PHARMACOKINETICS. Sodium valproate is converted in the stomach to valproic acid, which is rapidly absorbed from the gastrointestinal tract. Valproate has variable onset time and half-life (6–16 hours), depending on the formulation administered.

ADVERSE EFFECTS AND DRUG INTERACTIONS. These include drowsiness, tremors, mild gastric distress, hair thinning, weight gain, irregular menstruation, and hepatotoxicity. Drug interactions occur, particularly with CNS depressants (alcohol, general anaesthetics, barbiturates), anticoagulants and aspirin (increased risk of bleeding), and with combinations of antiepileptic drugs because of drug metabolism interactions (levels should be monitored). Valproate causes an increased risk of congenital malformations, including spina bifida, and is in Pregnancy Safety Category D.

LAMOTRIGINE

Lamotrigine is believed to stabilise seizures by blocking sodium channels and thus inhibiting the release of excitatory neurotransmitters (glutamate and aspartate). It is indicated as adjunctive therapy for the treatment of partial seizures and generalised epilepsy. It has a long half-life (30 hours) that may be reduced by enzyme-inducing drugs and female sex hormones but increased by sodium valproate.

Early clinical experience with lamotrigine has shown that there is a high risk of severe potentially life-threatening skin reactions, including toxic epidermal necrolysis, in particular with high dosage or when drug interactions prolong the half-life. Any rashes or skin reactions should be carefully evaluated and recommended doses not exceeded.

Other antiepileptics
ETHOSUXIMIDE

This is the only surviving member of the succinimide group of antiepileptic agents. These agents produce a variety of effects; by decreasing calcium conductance in the motor cortex they increase the seizure threshold and reduce the EEG spike-and-wave pattern of absence seizures. Ethosuximide has a long half-life, allowing once-daily administration. Common and adverse reactions are disturbances in CNS and gastrointestinal functions. Other antiepileptic agents may increase the metabolism of ethosuximide, decreasing its effectiveness, or may change the pattern of seizures.

GABAPENTIN

Gabapentin is an antiepileptic that was designed as a GABA analogue but unexpectedly appears not to mimic the actions of GABA; the mechanism for its anticonvulsant action is not yet established; however, it raises brain GABA levels. It is indicated for the treatment of partial seizures with or without secondary generalisation; also for neuropathic pain, such as in diabetic neuropathy and post-herpetic neuralgia.

LEVETIRACETAM

Levetiracetam is a new antiepileptic introduced in Australia in 2001 and indicated as adjunctive therapy for patients whose partial onset seizures are not well controlled with other drugs. Its mechanism of action is as yet unknown. Common adverse effects include somnolence and headache, but long-term safety has not yet been established.

ACETAZOLAMIDE AND SULTHIAME

Acetazolamide is a carbonic anhydrase inhibitor usually prescribed for the treatment of open-angle glaucoma. Its membrane-stabilising activity may be due to inhibition of carbonic anhydrase in the CNS, resulting in an increase in carbon dioxide that retards neuronal activity. Systemic metabolic acidosis may also play a part in its action. It is occasionally used in combination with other anticonvulsant agents.

Sulthiame, another older antiepileptic drug, is also a carbonic anhydrase inhibitor.

MAGNESIUM SULFATE

Magnesium sulfate has a depressant effect on the CNS and reduces striated muscle contractions. It is used to treat toxaemia of pregnancy (see Clinical Interest Box 18-4).

ACTH AND PREDNISOLONE

The most effective treatment for infantile myoclonic spasms is corticotrophin (ACTH) IM or oral prednisolone. The mechanism of action is not understood but it is thought that the hormones may act as central neurotransmitters or neuromodulators. They improve the associated psychomotor retardation more effectively than do the usual antiepileptic agents.

PAEDIATRIC IMPLICATIONS

Anticonvulsants
- Be aware that neonates whose mothers received phenytoin during pregnancy may require vitamin K to treat hypoprothrombinaemia.
- Whenever possible, anticonvulsants other than phenytoin should be considered first: sodium valproate, lamotrigine, clonazepam and phenobarbitone are less likely to cause the adverse effects induced by the hydantoins.
- Young children receiving valproic acid, especially those up to 2 years of age or those receiving multiple anticonvulsant drugs, are at a greater risk of developing serious hepatotoxicity. This risk decreases with advancing age.

Problems related to phenytoin use in children
- Chewable phenytoin tablets are not indicated for once-daily administration.
- If skin rash develops with use of phenytoin, discontinue drug immediately and notify prescriber.
- Avoid intramuscular phenytoin injections.
- Young persons are more susceptible to gingival hyperplasia (gum overgrowth). Gingivitis or gum inflammation usually starts during the first 6 months of drug therapy, although severe hyperplasia is unlikely at dosages under 500 mg/day. A dental program of teeth cleaning and plaque control started within 7–10 days of initiating drug therapy helps to reduce the rate and severity of this condition.
- Coarse facial features and excessive body hair growth are more frequently reported as adverse drug reactions in young patients.
- Impaired school performance is reported with long-term high-dose phenytoin therapy (especially at high plasma concentrations).

GERIATRIC IMPLICATIONS

Anticonvulsants
- Seizures are very common in the elderly, often precipitated by stroke, systemic diseases or chronic neurological conditions. The prevalence of epilepsy is as high as 1% in the elderly; complex partial seizures are frequent.
- The prognosis for complete seizure control is good. Drug therapy should be initiated cautiously, with low doses.
- The elderly tend to metabolise and excrete anticonvulsants more slowly; thus drug accumulation and toxicity may occur. Monitor closely because dosage adjustments (lower doses) may be necessary.
- Serum albumin levels may be lower in geriatric patients, resulting in decreased protein binding of highly bound drugs, such as phenytoin and valproic acid. Monitor closely because lower drug doses may be necessary.
- Administer intravenous doses at a rate slower than the recommended rate for a younger adult.
- If skin rash develops with the use of phenytoin, discontinue drug immediately and notify the prescriber.
- Drug interactions are common because of the likelihood of multiple pathologies and polypharmacy.

PREGNANCY SAFETY

ADEC Category	Drug
B1	Gabapentin
B3	Acetazolamide, lamotrigine, levetiracetam, pregabalin, tiagabine, topiramate
C	Clonazepam, diazepam
D	Carbamazepine, ethosuximide, oxcarbazepine, phenobarbitone, phenytoin, primidone, sodium valproate, sulthiame, vigabatrin

Note that many of the commonly prescribed antiepileptics (carbamazepine, phenobarbitone, phenytoin, primidone, sodium valproate) are documented as causing higher incidence of birth defects if taken during pregnancy, particularly as combination therapy. Spina bifida, minor craniofacial defects, coagulation defects and developmental disabilities occur. Prophylactic administration of vitamin K and folic acid may reduce the risk of some effects.

DRUGS AT A GLANCE 18: Antiepileptic agents

Therapeutic group	Pharmacological group	Key examples	Key pages
Antiepileptic drugs (= anticonvulsants)	GABA inhibition enhancers • Benzodiazepines	clonazepam diazepam	pp. 300, 4 p. 304
	• Barbiturates • Others	phenobarbitone topiramate tiagabine	pp. 300, 5 pp. 304, 5 p. 305
	Sodium channel function inhibitors	phenytoin carbamazepine sodium valproate	pp. 300, 2, 5, 6 pp. 300, 305–7 pp. 300, 7
	Others	gabapentin levetiracetam	p. 307 p. 307

Note: See also Tables 18-1, 18-2.
GABA = gamma (γ)-aminobutyric acid.

KEY POINTS

- Epilepsy is characterised by sporadic recurrent episodes of convulsive seizures, and is classified by extent (generalised/partial) and signs exhibited (loss of consciousness; muscle tone and twitching).
- The seizures may be idiopathic, triggered by external events or internal changes, or secondary to head injury or focal brain damage.
- Different types of seizure are more likely at different life stages.
- Antiepileptic drug therapy to control seizures may be lifelong; choice of drug is determined by type of seizure, likely adverse drug reactions, other drugs that may interact, and individual aspects such as pregnancy and compliance.
- Therapeutic monitoring is regularly carried out by measuring drug concentration in plasma samples; this helps check whether levels are in the therapeutic range and monitors compliance.
- While all CNS-depressant drugs may reduce seizure incidence, most are too sedating to be useful. The major drugs used to treat seizures act by enhancing GABA-mediated inhibition of neural transmission, or inhibit neurotransmission by blocking sodium channel functions.
- Antiepileptic agents include barbiturates, benzodiazepines, phenytoin, carbamazepine, sodium valproate and miscellaneous drugs.

● The most common adverse effects are those of CNS depression. Drug interactions are common because of the effects of antiepileptic agents in increasing or decreasing the metabolism of other drugs. This information is crucial to the health-care professional providing care for epileptic patients.

REVIEW EXERCISES

1. Explain the differences between idiopathic and non-idiopathic seizures and their relation to epilepsy.
2. Explain the main mechanisms of action of antiepileptic drugs, giving examples.
3. List characteristics considered desirable in the ideal antiepileptic drug.
4. Discuss the mechanisms of action, indications, common adverse effects and major drug interactions for phenobarbitone, phenytoin and sodium valproate.
5. Explain the potential for antiepileptic agents to cause paradoxical reactions in children and the elderly.
6. Explain the clinical importance to the health-care professional of knowledge of a drug's adverse reactions, warnings and contraindications.
7. Explain the importance of the concepts of non-linear pharmacokinetics and induction of liver enzymes in the clinical use of antiepileptic drugs.

REFERENCES AND FURTHER READING

Ashton H, Young AH. GABA-ergic drugs: exit stage left, enter stage right. *Journal of Psychopharmacology* 2003: 17(2): 174–8.
Australian Drug Evaluation Committee. *Prescribing Medicines in Pregnancy: An Australian Categorisation of Risk of Drug Use in Pregnancy.* 4th edn. Canberra: Therapeutic Goods Administration, 1999.
Australian Medicines Handbook 2005. Adelaide: AMH, 2005.
Buchanan N. Medications which may lower seizure threshold. *Australian Prescriber* 2001; 24(1): 8–9.
Caswell A (ed.). *MIMS Annual June 2005.* Sydney: CMPMedica Australia, 2005.
Faught E. Epidemiology and drug treatment of epilepsy in elderly people. *Drugs & Aging* 1999; 15(4): 255–69.
Herkes GK. Epilepsy. *Medical Journal of Australia* 2001; 174: 534–9.
Kilpatrick CJ. Withdrawal of anti-epileptic drugs in seizure-free adults. *Australian Prescriber* 2004: 27(5): 114–17.
Lander C. Pregnancy and epilepsy: balancing the risks. *Medicine Today 2000;* July 2000: 20–4.
LaRoche SM, Helmers SL. The new anti-epileptic drugs: scientific review. *Journal of the American Medical Association* 2004; 291(5): 605–14.
Lees GJ. Pharmacology of AMPA/kainate receptor ligands and their therapeutic potential in neurological and psychiatric disorders. *Drugs* 2000; 59(1): 33–78.
Meldrum BS. Glutamate as a neurotransmitter in the brain: review of physiology and pathology. *Journal of Nutrition* 2000; 130 (4S Suppl.): 1007S–15S.
Morrell MJ, Flynn KL (eds). *Women with Epilepsy: A Handbook of Health and Treatment Issues.* Cambridge; Cambridge University Press, 2003.
Moshe SL. Mechanisms of action of anticonvulsant agents. *Neurology* 2000; 55 (5 Suppl. 1): S32–40, S54–58.
Neurology Expert Group. *Therapeutic Guidelines Neurology, version 2.* Melbourne: Therapeutic Guidelines Limited, 2002.
Rang HP, Dale MM, Ritter JM, Moore PK. *Pharmacology.* 5th edn. Edinburgh: Churchill Livingstone, 2003.
Richens A, Dunlop A. Serum-phenytoin levels in management of epilepsy. *Lancet* 1975: 2: 247–8.
Ross EL. The evolving role of antiepileptic drugs in treating neuropathic pain. *Neurology* 2000; 55 (5 Suppl. 1): S41–46, S54–58.
Smith RL. Withdrawing anti-epileptic drugs from seizure-free children. *Australian Prescriber* 2006; 29(1): 18–20.
Tortora GJ, Grabowski SR. *Principles of Anatomy and Physiology.* 9th edn. HarperCollins, New York, 2000 [ch. 14].
Vander A, Sherman J, Luciano D. *Human Physiology: The Mechanisms of Body Function.* 7th edn. McGraw-Hill, Boston; 1998 [ch. 13].

ON-LINE RESOURCES

Epilepsy Foundation of Victoria: www.epinet.org.au
New Zealand medicines and medical devices safety authority: www.medsafe.govt.nz

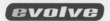 More weblinks at http://evolve.elsevier.com/AU/Bryant/pharmacology/

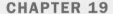

CHAPTER 19

Psychotropic Agents

CHAPTER FOCUS

To care properly for patients with schizophrenia, depression or mania, health-care professionals must be familiar with the functions of the central nervous system and its role in mood and emotions, the changes that occur in psychiatric disorders, and the mechanisms of action, main effects and adverse effects of psychotropic drugs. A thorough knowledge of the different drugs is required, as these are potent substances with the potential for inducing serious adverse reactions and drug interactions.

OBJECTIVES

● To discuss the relationships between neurotransmitter levels in the brain and mood, emotions and behaviour.

● To describe the epidemiology and pathogenesis of the major psychoses: schizophrenia and bipolar affective disorder.

● To discuss the pharmacological properties of the main groups of psychotropic drugs: antipsychotic agents used in schizophrenia, and antidepressants and lithium used in affective disorders.

● To understand the proposed mechanisms of action of psychotropic agents and their propensity for causing serious adverse effects and drug interactions.

KEY DRUGS

chlorpromazine
clozapine
fluoxetine
imipramine
lithium
moclobemide

KEY TERMS

affective disorders
anticholinergic effects
antidepressant
antipsychotic
atypical antipsychotic
bipolar affective disorder
depression
dopamine
electroconvulsive therapy
extrapyramidal effects
mania
monoamine oxidase inhibitors
neuroleptic
neurosis
noradrenaline
phenothiazine
psychosis
psychotropic
schizophrenia
selective serotonin reuptake inhibitors
serotonin (5-HT)
tardive dyskinesia
tranquilliser
tricyclic antidepressants
tyramine reaction

KEY ABBREVIATIONS

ADHD	attention deficit hyperactivity disorder
AMH	*Australian Medicines Handbook*
BAD	bipolar affective disorder
CBT	cognitive behaviour therapy
CNS	central nervous system
DA	dopamine
ECT	electroconvulsive therapy
5-HT	5-hydroxytryptamine (serotonin)
MAO	monoamine oxidase
MAOI	monoamine oxidase inhibitor
NA	noradrenaline
RIMA	reversible inhibitor of MAO-A
SSRI	selective serotonin reuptake inhibitor
TCA	tricyclic antidepressant

PSYCHIATRY is the branch of medicine dealing with treatment of disorders of the mind. Traditionally in psychiatry disorders were classified into the major conditions, the **psychoses**, which affect a person's whole mind and mental state, and the more minor, less pervasive conditions, the **neuroses**, in which a person's mental state is only partly changed. There are two major types of psychosis: **schizophrenia** and the mood disorders (**depression**, **mania** and **bipolar affective disorder**). The neurotic disorders include conditions such as anxiety, obsessive–compulsive disorder and phobias; in these disorders, responses to stress are considered to be at the extreme of the normal range rather than abnormal. Psychiatrists also see patients with organic mental disorders (dementias, delirium and drug-related disorders), developmental disorders (autism, mental retardation and specific disorders of speech, attention etc) and personality disorders involving maladaptive responses to circumstances and unusual behaviour patterns.

These conditions are not static but are defined in terms of relationships and the person's responses to the environment. There is often a high risk of suicide, hence the importance of early effective treatment. The general clinical features are of disordered thought, perception, emotion, behaviour, intellect and personality.

PSYCHOTROPICS AND ANTIPSYCHOTICS

Psychotropic literally means affecting the mind. The term 'psychotropic agents' could thus include all drugs that primarily affect the mind, such as sedatives and hypnotics, antianxiety agents, central nervous system (CNS) stimulants, general anaesthetics and social drugs, including alcohol, marijuana and caffeine, as well as the drugs used to treat the major psychiatric disorders. In this text, however, 'psychotropic' is used in the narrower sense to refer to drugs used to treat the major psychoses. Although the term 'antipsychotic' could apply to drugs used in all psychoses, including affective (mood) disorders, it has come to be used to refer only to drugs used in schizophrenia; the other term used similarly is 'neuroleptic', meaning a drug that can modify abnormal psychotic behaviour.

The main emphasis in this chapter will be on the **antipsychotic** drugs used in the treatment of schizophrenia, and the **antidepressant** and antimanic drugs used in mood disorders. See Clinical Interest Box 19-1 for the historical background to psychiatric treatments.

MODELS USED IN PSYCHIATRY

Various models are used in psychiatry to help describe and manage conditions:
- the biological model, in which genetic, biochemical and physiological factors are considered
- the behavioural model, which emphasises that symptoms are learned habits that can be corrected
- the social model, which considers disruptive circumstances, relationships and family situations
- the psychoanalytical model (based on Sigmund Freud's work), in which inborn drives are considered to conflict with outside demands.

CLINICAL INTEREST BOX 19-1   HISTORICAL BACKGROUND TO PSYCHIATRIC DRUGS

Historically, people perceived as being mad or insane were hidden in cellars or attics in their homes or committed to custodial care in gaols or in lunatic asylums. Physical restraints (stone walls, straitjackets, tranquilliser chairs); shock therapy with water, ice packs, insulin or electricity; or major CNS surgery such as lobotomy were often the only ways to deal with severe mental illness. As sedating medicines became available, sufferers could be drugged into oblivion with narcotics or early hypnotics (bromides, alcohols, paraldehyde, chloral hydrate and the barbiturates).

Psychiatry as a specialist branch of medicine started in the 20th century, and scientific psychiatry in the 1920s, as studies were carried out to define and classify types of mental illness and relate them to inheritance or traumatic events. **Electroconvulsive therapy** (ECT) was discovered as an effective form of treatment of severe depression in 1938.

The first specific drug treatment was discovered in 1949: **lithium** was recognised by Dr John Cade, a Melbourne psychiatrist, as being effective in mania. Reserpine (from the plant *Rauwolfia serpentina*), an Indian drug used to encourage meditation and introspection, was demonstrated to have tranquillising and antihypertensive properties (due to inhibition of storage of monoamines in vesicles, see Figure 19-1) but caused severe depression and parkinsonian effects. The first safe major tranquilliser, or **neuroleptic** drug (**chlorpromazine**), was developed in 1952 and an effective **antidepressant** drug (**imipramine**) was developed soon afterwards.

These drugs revolutionised the treatment of mental illness. People successfully treated could remain in their families, jobs and communities. Even more specific, safe and effective drugs are continually being developed, tested and used clinically, e.g. the new selective serotonin reuptake inhibitors (SSRIs) such as fluoxetine in depression, and the atypical antipsychotics in schizophrenia.

Overall, an eclectic approach that borrows from all models where relevant is perhaps most useful. In the context of pharmacology and attempts to explain the mechanism of a psychoactive drug's actions, we inevitably tend to emphasise the biological model, particularly the imbalances in CNS neurotransmitter levels that can be corrected by drugs.

THE CENTRAL NERVOUS SYSTEM, THE MIND AND EMOTIONS

To understand the actions of drugs in treating the symptoms of mental illness, it is important to have knowledge of the functioning of the nervous system. Refer to Chapter 14 for a review of the physiology and functions of the various components of the CNS, including the CNS functional systems (e.g. reticular activating system [Figure 17-3], limbic system [Figure 14-3] and extrapyramidal system). Understanding of the major CNS neurotransmitter systems (catecholamines, 5-hydroxytryptamine [5-HT, serotonin] and acetylcholine, see Figures 14-5 and 14-6) is also necessary as background to this chapter.

It has become increasingly difficult in practice to separate the functions of the mind from those of the body. The CNS is responsible for consciousness, behaviour, memory, recognition, learning and the more highly developed integrative and creative processes such as imagination, abstract reasoning and creative thought. In addition, it serves to coordinate vital regulatory functions such as blood pressure, heart rate, respiration, salivary and gastric secretions, muscular activity and body temperature. The interrelationships among the various circuits in the brain produce patterns of behaviour that can be modified by conscious choice, by external situations or by internal adjustments. This allows the individual to adapt to changes in both the external and the internal environments.

Neurotransmitter mechanisms

The putative CNS neurotransmitters are discussed briefly in Chapter 14 and their proposed relationships to psychiatric disorders are shown diagrammatically in Figure 14-6. Because the monoamine neurotransmitters are particularly involved in the aetiology, pathogenesis and pharmacological treatment of schizophrenia and depression, these will be described in more detail in this context. Virtually all psychotropic drugs interact with catecholamine-containing neurons by some mechanism. It should be recognised that while there may be evidence that a transmitter is depleted in a condition (e.g. **5-HT** in depression, **dopamine** in Parkinson's disease) and that enhancement of that transmitter improves the patient (e.g. selective serotonin reuptake inhibitor antidepressants, levodopa plus dopa decarboxylase inhibitor in antiparkinson therapy), many links in the cause–effect –cure chain remain to be completed.

Noradrenaline

High concentrations of noradrenaline are located in neurons in the hypothalamus, pons (locus coeruleus), medulla and cranial nerve nuclei; these noradrenergic neurons innervate virtually the entire CNS from the cerebral cortex to all spinal levels. Noradrenergic pathways are thought to have global activating functions in responses to various sensory stimuli, maintaining attention and vigilance.

Dopamine

The relationship of **dopamine** to the major psychoses has received much attention. Dopamine is found in high concentrations in the striatum and caudate nucleus and especially in the basal ganglia and **extrapyramidal tracts**. It is both a neurotransmitter in its own right and a precursor for noradrenaline synthesis. There are various dopamine receptors in the brain, especially in the basal ganglia and limbic areas, but D_1 and D_2 receptors are the primary receptor types influenced by the antipsychotic agents. Although both receptor types are involved with movement disorders in the basal ganglia, **tardive dyskinesia**, a severe adverse effect of chronic treatment with antipsychotic agents, is thought to be due to supersensitivity of D_2 receptors. In schizophrenia, the density of D_2 receptors in the caudate and putamen brain regions is consistently high. Newer antipsychotic agents with low affinity for D_2 receptors but high affinity for D_4 receptors, such as clozapine, are less apt to cause **extrapyramidal effects**. Further research in this area may result in the development of more specific agents with fewer adverse effects.

5-hydroxytryptamine

Areas rich in neurons containing **5-HT** include the hypothalamus, pineal gland and midbrain, with pathways projecting especially to the spinal cord, limbic system and thalamus. In most cells, 5-HT causes a decrease in discharge rate and hence is inhibitory. There are many types of 5-HT receptors (at least 15 distinct types have been cloned), with more than eight types found in brain regions. 5-HT_1 receptors are involved particularly in thermoregulation, hypotension, sexual behaviour and the serotonin syndrome; 5-HT_2 receptors mediate excitation rather than inhibition.

5-HT appears to coordinate complex sensory and motor patterns. Alterations of 5-HT levels in the nervous system are associated with changes in behaviour and mood: 5-HT activity levels are highest during waking arousal and lowest during REM sleep. Clinical conditions that are influenced by 5-HT levels include affective disorders, ageing and neuro-degenerative disorders, anxiety, developmental disorders, eating disorders, vomiting, migraine, obsessive–compulsive disorder, pain sensitivity, sexual disorders, sleep disorders and substance abuse.

Many drugs mimic or block the action of 5-HT on peripheral tissues and produce changes in mood and behaviour, which suggests that they interfere with the action of 5-HT in the brain. For example the Indian drug reserpine, used to treat hypertension, causes severe depression; and many hallucinogenic agents, including lysergic acid diethylamide (LSD), are chemically related to 5-HT (see Figure 22-4). Ecstasy, or 3,4-methylenedioxymethamphetamine (MDMA), a neurotoxic 'party drug', decreases 5-HT turnover in the brain and causes a loss of 5-HT-containing axons. The efficacy of the selective serotonin reuptake inhibitors (SSRIs) in treating major depression is good evidence that 5-HT function is impaired in depressive illness.

Histamine

Histamine, although not a catecholamine, is included in the monoamine transmitters. The fact that systemically administered antihistamines cause CNS effects (sedation, hunger) is evidence for the roles of histamine in the brain. Histamine-containing neurons in the posterior hypothalamus send long projecting fibres to many areas, including the cortex, hippocampus, striatum and thalamus. Histamine is thought to be involved in altering food and water intake, and in thermoregulation, autonomic activity and hormone release; its effects are mediated by histamine H_1, H_2 and H_3 receptors. As many of the psychotropic agents (antipsychotics and antidepressants) have antagonistic activity on histamine receptors, there are frequently adverse effects such as sedation, weight gain and antiemetic actions.

Acetylcholine

Acetylcholine is the neurotransmitter in many short inter-neurons in the CNS, especially in the spinal cord. There are also two major cholinergic tracts in the brain, starting in the basal forebrain and the pons–tegmental areas. Acetylcholine may participate in pain perception, and cholinergic dysfunction has been implicated in degenerative diseases, including Huntington's chorea and Alzheimer's disease (see Chapter 21).

Effects in the peripheral nervous system

These monoamine neurotransmitters and acetylcholine are also neurotransmitters in the peripheral nervous system, particularly in the autonomic and enteric nervous systems. It is highly likely, therefore, that drugs given for their central effects in disorders affecting the mind will have potentially major adverse effects in the periphery. Adverse effects on blood pressure (orthostatic hypotension), gastrointestinal tract functions (dry mouth, constipation, weight gain), sexual function (impotence, decreased libido) and eye functions (blurred vision) are common with antipsychotic and antidepressant drugs.

CLINICAL ASPECTS OF DRUG THERAPY IN PSYCHIATRY

Indications for drug therapy

The impact of mental illness within populations is becoming increasingly apparent; this could include both the milder neuroses (anxiety, phobias and personality disorders) and the more severe psychoses (schizophrenia and bipolar affective disorder). The 1997 National Survey of Mental Health and Wellbeing by the Australian Bureau of Statistics showed that 18% of adults in the community had a mental disorder in the 12 months preceding the survey; mental disorders constitute the leading cause of disability burden in Australia, accounting for 27% of the total years lost due to disability.

Drugs play an important role in contemporary approaches to psychiatric care. Although many people with mild psychological conditions can be treated successfully with psychotherapies, patients with moderate and severe disorders usually require drugs or electroconvulsive therapy. Clinically, drug therapy reduces or alleviates symptoms and allows the patient an opportunity to participate more easily in other forms of treatment that may produce a permanent change in mood and behaviour. The effects of drugs can be additive, potentiating or antagonistic, depending on their structures and mechanisms of actions. The environment can potentiate the effectiveness of the drug treatment or detract from it.

Guidelines for prescribing psychotropic drugs suggest:
- a thorough diagnostic assessment is necessary
- drugs should be used only if essential, not in place of talking to the patient
- the patient's response will guide future drug use
- the patient should be informed of the expected time-course of response and likely adverse effects
- compliance is promoted with simplest and lowest effective dose regimen and regular follow-up
- drug therapy needs to be tailored to the specific patient (young/elderly/pregnant/concurrent disease).

Drug selection

Generally, prescribers select psychotherapeutic agents on the basis of the diagnostic category: schizophrenia, bipolar affective disorder or psychoneurosis. The prescriber will try to match a particular drug's therapeutic advantages to the patient's symptoms, assuming the person's diagnosis warrants the use of a psychotropic agent. Since their introduction, the antipsychotic and antidepressant agents have been widely prescribed, frequently overprescribed and, in many instances in the elderly, inappropriately used. Inappropriate prescribing exposes the older person to an increased risk of adverse reactions and drug interactions that are often detrimental to the person's cognitive and functional health status.

Informed consent

Informed consent is usually taken to imply that the patient has agreed to participate in particular treatment after being given adequate information to assist in making the decision.

In the context of mental illness, however, the concept of informed consent can be difficult. A person suffering severe anxiety may be in no state to weigh up potential benefits or adverse effects of treatment; a person in acute mania or drug-induced delirium may need restraint before long-term clinical plans can be instituted; and the disordered thought patterns of schizophrenia may make it difficult for the person to make reasoned judgements about possible therapies. Patients need to be assisted to make wise and balanced decisions about their treatment—the patient's involvement in and 'owning' of the treatment plan will improve compliance with it.

Adverse drug reactions

The adverse effect profile of a drug is a useful tool to help a prescriber select an appropriate antipsychotic agent. Drugs

TABLE 19-1 Selected antipsychotic agents: potency and major effects

CHEMICAL, GENERIC NAME	DAILY ORAL DOSE (mg)	FREQUENCY OF EFFECTS AND ADVERSE EFFECTS*				
		Antiemetic	Sedation	Hypotension†	Anticholinergic	Extrapyramidal**
Phenothiazines						
Chlorpromazine	75–800	3	3	3	2	2
Thioridazine	50–600	1	3	3	3	2
Fluphenazine	2.5–10	1	2	1	1	2
Prochlorperazine	10–40	3	2	1	1	3
Trifluoperazine	2–20	3	2	1	1	2
Thioxanthines						
Flupenthixol	20–40 every 2 to 4 weeks (depot injection, not oral)	—	1	1	1	3
Other compounds						
Haloperidol	0.5–20	2	1	1	1	3
Pimozide	2–12	—	1	1	1	3
Atypical agents						
Amisulpride	100–1000	—	1	1	0	2
Aripiprazole	10–30	—	2	1	0	1
Clozapine	100–600	1	3	3	3	1
Olanzapine	5–20	—	2	1	1	1
Quetiapine	400–800	—	1	2	1	1
Risperidone	0.5–6	—	1	2	0	1

Source: Psychotropic Expert Group 2003; *Australian Medicines Handbook* 2005.
Grading: 1, low; 2, moderate; 3 high.
†Orthostatic hypotension.
****Extrapyramidal** side-effects include akathisia, dystonia, parkinsonism and tardive dyskinesia.

TABLE 19-2 Antipsychotic medications: adverse reactions

RELATIVELY FREQUENT ADVERSE REACTIONS

Sleepiness, dizziness, dry mouth, constipation and nasal congestion reported with phenothiazines and thioxanthines

Weight gain commonly reported with most antipsychotics

GENERAL ADVERSE REACTIONS

Visual changes and hypotensive episodes (more common with phenothiazines and thioxanthines)

Dystonia and/or parkinsonian effects, including shuffle in walk, arm or leg stiffness, tremors, mask-like facial expression, dysphagia, imbalance and muscle spasms or unusual twisting effects of face, neck or back (more common with phenothiazines, thioxanthines, risperidone and haloperidol)

Akathisia (abnormal motor restlessness and agitation), increased pacing, and insomnia (more often reported with haloperidol and thioxanthines). This may be misinterpreted as worsening of agitation associated with the psychosis

Tardive dyskinesia, a late-developing serious adverse reaction in about 20% of patients, especially older women, who show involuntary repetitive hyperkinetic movements, usually of the mouth and face; possibly due to supersensitivity to dopamine following upregulation of receptors. There is no effective treatment

Neuroleptic malignant syndrome, a rare but potentially fatal adverse effect; features include high temperature, muscle rigidity and altered consciousness

Hyperkinesia, agitation and aggressive behaviour

---

that antagonise neurotransmitter receptors in both central and peripheral nervous systems are liable to have wide-ranging effects. This problem is compounded in the case of antipsychotic drugs by the fact that many of the drug groups act at receptors for several transmitters; for example the classic antischizophrenic agents, the phenothiazines, are notoriously 'dirty' drugs as they antagonise receptors for dopamine (D_2), acetylcholine (muscarinic), noradrenaline (α-), 5-HT and histamine (H_1).

As can be seen from Tables 19-1 and 19-2, the adverse effect profiles of various antipsychotic agents can be compared and tabulated to aid in choice of drug. If a drug with a strong sedative property is desired, chlorpromazine or thioridazine might be prescribed, whereas haloperidol is less likely to cause daytime drowsiness. An important group of common adverse effects from antipsychotics are the **extrapyramidal effects**, i.e. those involving marked motor stimulation mediated via pathways in the extrapyramidal tract (see Chapter 14 and Clinical Interest Box 19-2). If extrapyramidal effects are troublesome, thioridazine, which has less potential for inducing extrapyramidal effects but the greatest anticholinergic effect, might be chosen. If **anticholinergic effects** (such as dry mouth, blurred vision, constipation and urinary retention) continue and are disturbing to the patient, the prescriber could select an agent with less potential for inducing such effects, such as fluphenazine, thiothixene or haloperidol.

Similar rationales can be used in choosing among antidepressants (see Table 19-3). In this case, anticholinergic effects, orthostatic hypotension and gastrointestinal distress are the likely adverse effects. Once stabilised on a drug, the patient is then closely monitored for continued drug effectiveness and the development of adverse reactions.

Some antipsychotic agents, especially those with sedative effects, impair psychomotor performance and thus can impair driving skills, ability to operate machinery and reaction times to dangerous stimuli. Sedative effects of other CNS depressants taken concurrently, including alcohol, will be increased. New drugs, and old drugs being used for new indications, require post-marketing monitoring for adverse effects (see Clinical Interest Box 19-3).

Neuroleptic malignant syndrome is a rare but potentially fatal adverse effect occurring in 0.5%–1% of patients on typical antipsychotics. It involves high temperature, muscle rigidity, altered consciousness and impaired autonomic homeostasis. Treatment requires withdrawal of the drug, hydration and sometimes bromocriptine (a dopamine agonist) and dantrolene to control muscle spasms.

Treatment of adverse drug reactions

In some cases, adverse effects are sufficiently severe to require treatment if administration of the antipsychotic or antidepressant drug is to continue. Specific drugs are used where possible, e.g. diazepam or propranolol to decrease severe agitation and benztropine to treat anticholinergic or parkinsonian effects.

CLINICAL INTEREST BOX 19-2
NEUROLEPTIC EXTRAPYRAMIDAL ADVERSE EFFECTS

AKATHISIA

Description   Motor restlessness; person unable to sit or stand still, feels urgent need to move, pace, rock, or tap foot. Can also present as apprehension, irritability and general uneasiness, and may be mistaken for worsened agitation. More common in females than males; usually occurs within a few weeks of starting drug therapy.

Treatment   Lower dose of neuroleptic agent, switch to an atypical antipsychotic, or administer an antiparkinson drug such as benztropine, or diazepam.

DYSTONIA

Description   Acute reaction requiring immediate intervention. Patient exhibits muscle spasms of face, tongue, neck, jaw and/or hands. Hyperextension of neck and trunk and arching of back. Oculogyric crisis may occur (fixed upward gaze and/or eye muscle spasms); laryngeal spasm is potentially fatal. Commonly occurs after large doses of neuroleptics, usually within a week of drug therapy. Occurs more often in males than females.

Treatment   Depending on the severity of reaction, lower neuroleptic dose, administer benztropine IM or IV.

DRUG-INDUCED PARKINSONISM

Description   Symptoms similar to Parkinson's disease: shuffling gait, drooling, tremors, increased rigidity (cogwheel). Bradykinesia (slow movements) and akinesia (immobility) also reported.

Treatment   Add antiparkinson drug, such as benztropine or benzhexol. Physician may switch to a neuroleptic less likely to induce this effect, such as a newer atypical agent.

TARDIVE DYSKINESIA

Description   Oral or facial dyskinesias, i.e. abnormal involuntary muscle movements around the mouth, lip smacking, tongue darting, constant chewing movements, or tics. Patient might also have involuntary movements of arms or legs. More common in older women but has been reported in younger people.

Treatment   Prevention is vital, as it may be irreversible. Monitor for early signs, and reduce or cease neuroleptic agent as soon as possible. No effective treatment.

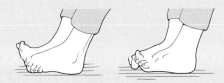
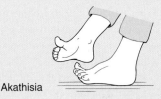

Akathisia

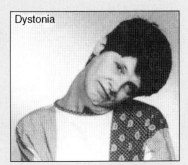

Dystonia

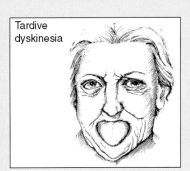

Tardive dyskinesia

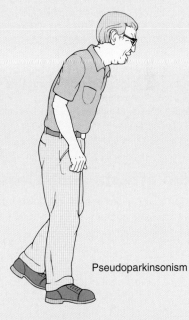

Pseudoparkinsonism

CLINICAL INTEREST BOX 19-3
THIORIDAZINE AND ARRHYTHMIA;
MOCLOBEMIDE AND HYPERTENSION

THIORIDAZINE AND ARRHYTHMIA: PRESCRIBING CHANGES

Thioridazine, a phenothiazine tranquilliser, increases the risk of arrhythmias from QT prolongation. After reviewing international and New Zealand data, the NZ Medicines Adverse Reactions Committee has recommended that thioridazine should not be prescribed if there are interacting medicines or predisposing conditions:

- a history of QT prolongation
- abnormal serum potassium levels
- concomitant use of medicines that inhibit CYP2D6 (e.g. cimetidine, many antidepressants) or inhibit thioridazine metabolism by another mechanism (e.g. fluvoxamine, pindolol, propranolol)
- concomitant use of medicines that might prolong the QT interval (e.g. antiarrhythmic agents, cisapride, tricyclic antidepressants, other tranquillisers)

Source: NZ Prescriber Update No. 21, pp 4–7; June 2001.

MOCLOBEMIDE CAN PUT THE PRESSURE UP

A reduction in blood pressure associated with postural hypotension, as well as spontaneous hypertension, are considered to be typical side-effects of conventional, irreversible and non-selective MAO (A+B) inhibitor antidepressants. The new-generation of reversible MAO-A inhibitors is, however, expected to have negligible cardiovascular effects and low propensity to induce either blood pressure increases or decreases. However, the true incidence of such changes is largely unknown since observation studies assessing the frequency of blood pressure changes in selected populations of patients treated in practice, are lacking. The frequency of hypertension in patients treated with moclobemide was reported to be 0.5/100, whereas there were no reports of hypertension associated with the SSRI antidepressant fluoxetine.[1]

1. Delini-Stula A, Baier D, Kohnen R, Laux G, Philipp M, Scholz HJ. *Pharmacopsychiatry.* 32(2): 61–7, 1999 Mar.

Rebound effects and relapses

After discontinuation of therapy, there are often withdrawal effects that may be related more to rebound phenomena than to any dependence on the drug. For example, after discontinuation of use of antipsychotics, there may be nausea, vomiting, restlessness and excessive cholinergic stimulation effects; after cessation of antidepressant therapy, agitation and insomnia; and after abrupt withdrawal of lithium, relapse of mania. These effects can often be avoided by slow tapering off of the drug. Many patients eventually relapse and require renewed medication.

Compliance

Ongoing compliance with long-term antipsychotic therapy is often a problem; many of these medications have unpleasant and disabling adverse effects and the treatment might seem to the patient to be worse than the disease. It is noteworthy in this context that animals in the laboratory situation will self-administer many drugs (for reward), including alcohol, cocaine, opioids, nicotine and amphetamines, but will not self-administer antipsychotic agents such as phenothiazines. In addition, patients may not have sufficient insight into their own condition to recognise the need for medication. Compliance can be improved by:

- patients and physicians agreeing on management plans
- discussions about the goals, advantages and disadvantages of treatments
- simple once-daily drug regimens
- use of reminders and involvement of family and friends in therapy
- written information and instructions
- regular monitoring of compliance by means of tablet counts or assay of drug levels in plasma
- administration of long-acting depot preparations (e.g. IM injections of oily preparations of antipsychotics every 2–4 weeks).

Adverse drug interactions

There are long lists of potential interactions with psychotropic drugs (e.g. see Tables 14M, N in *Therapeutic Guidelines: Psychotropic* and *Australian Medicines Handbook*, Appendix A). Elderly patients are particularly at risk, because of the likelihood of renal impairment leading to prolonged half-lives of drugs and because of polypharmacy to treat multiple pathologies. In general, because of their mechanisms of action in altering the levels of CNS neurotransmitters, psychotropic agents are likely to interact with other drugs affecting the central or autonomic nervous systems. These include opioids, anxiolytics, cardiovascular drugs, antihistamines, anaesthetics, sedatives, antiepileptics, endocrine drugs, stimulants, antiemetics, sympathomimetic amines, muscle relaxants, anticholinergics and alcohol. Lithium, because of its effects on the kidney, has specific interactions with other drugs affecting the kidneys, such as diuretics, sodium salts and non-steroidal anti-inflammatory agents.

It is impossible for anyone—health-care professional or student—to learn all these potential drug interactions. It is more sensible and safer to understand the general principles and look up reference texts for specific interactions of drugs prescribed concurrently.

TABLE 19-3 Adverse effect profiles of some antidepressant medications

DRUG	ADVERSE EFFECTS					
	Anticholinergic	Sedation	Insomnia or agitation	Orthostatic hypotension	Gastro-intestinal distress	Weight gain (over 6 kg)
TRICYCLIC/TETRACYCLIC ANTIDEPRESSANTS						
Amitriptyline Doxepin Imipramine	3+	4+	0	3/4+	0	3+
Nortriptyline	1+	2	0	1	0	1+
Clomipramine	3+	2	0	2+	0	2+
Mianserin	1+	3+	1	1+	1	0
SELECTIVE SEROTONIN REUPTAKE INHIBITORS						
Citalopram	0	1	2	0	2	1
Fluoxetine Paroxetine Sertraline	0	0	2+	0	3+	1
MONOAMINE OXIDASE INHIBITORS						
Phenelzine Tranylcypromine	1	1+	2+	2+	1+	2+
Moclobemide	2+	—	2+	—	2+	0
OTHERS						
Nefazodone Venlafaxine	—	—	2+	—	3+	0

Adapted from: Psychotropic Expert Group 2003; *Australian Medicines Handbook* 2005,
0 = absent or rare; 1+ = least common; 2+ = uncommon; 3+ relatively common; 4+ = most common; — indicates not relevant.

PAEDIATRIC IMPLICATIONS OF PSYCHOTROPIC AGENTS

Children are at a greater risk of developing neuromuscular or extrapyramidal adverse effects, especially dystonias. Monitor closely if antipsychotic agents are administered.

Paediatric patients with chickenpox, CNS infections, measles, dehydration, gastroenteritis or other acute illnesses will be at special risk of developing adverse reactions and possibly Reye's syndrome. Extrapyramidal effects may be confused with CNS signs of encephalopathy or Reye's syndrome. Avoid use of phenothiazine antiemetic therapy in such patients.

The tricyclic antidepressants are usually not recommended for the treatment of depression in children younger than 12 years. Children are very sensitive to an acute overdose, which should always be considered very serious and potentially fatal. Adolescents often require a lower dose because of their sensitivity to this drug group.

Adverse effects reported in children receiving tricyclic antidepressants include changes in electrocardiogram patterns, increased nervousness, sleep disorders, complaints of tiredness, hypertension and mild stomach distress.

Lithium may decrease the bone density or bone formation in children. If it must be used, closely monitor serum levels and for signs of toxicity.

GERIATRIC IMPLICATIONS PSYCHOTROPIC AGENTS

The elderly tend to have higher serum levels of antipsychotic and antidepressant drugs because of changes in drug distribution resulting from a decrease in lean body mass, less total body water, less serum albumin and usually a relative increase in body fat. Therefore these patients often require a lower drug dose and a more gradual drug dose titration than younger adult patients.

Geriatric patients are more prone to have orthostatic hypotension, anticholinergic effects, extrapyramidal effects and sedation. They should be carefully evaluated before starting such potent medications, and if the antipsychotic agents are necessary, the elderly person generally should receive only half the recommended adult dose. When clinical improvement is noted, attempts at tapering the dose and discontinuing the drug should be instituted.

The tricyclic antidepressants may cause increased anxiety in geriatric patients. If the patient has cardiovascular disease, the use of tricyclic antidepressants increases the risk of inducing arrhythmias, tachycardia, stroke, congestive heart failure and myocardial infarction.

Lithium is more toxic in geriatric patients so lower lithium dosages, a lower lithium serum level and very close monitoring are critical in this age group. Generally, excessive thirst and polyuria may be early adverse effects of lithium toxicity, and CNS toxicity, lithium-induced goitre and clinical hypothyroidism may develop.

PREGNANCY SAFETY

ADEC Category	Drug
B1	Pimozide, reboxetine
B2	Fluvoxamine, mianserin, tranylcypromine, venlafaxine
B3	Amisulpride, aripiprazole, citalopram, mirtazapine, moclobemide, nefazodone, olanzapine, phenelzine, quetiapine, risperidone, sertraline
C	Amitriptyline, chlorpromazine, citalopram, clomipramine, clozapine, dothiepin, doxepin, droperidol, escitalopram, fluoxetine, flupenthixol, fluphenazine, fluvoxamine, haloperidol, imipramine, nortriptyline, paroxetine, pericyazine, prochlorperazine, sertraline, thioridazine, trifluoperazine, trimipramine, zuclopenthixol
D	Lithium

Note: The phenothiazines (although not recommended during pregnancy) are generally classified C (including prochlorperazine, which is mainly indicated as an antiemetic).

Psychotropic therapy in special groups
Psychiatric disorders in childhood

It is estimated that 15% of children show symptoms leading to psychosocial impairment and requiring treatment. Common conditions are anxiety disorders, depressive disorders, attention deficit hyperactivity disorder (ADHD) and conduct disorders. In general, girls are more likely to have emotion-type problems and boys to have behaviour-type problems. Contributing factors are thought to include genetic factors, socioeconomic problems, family disruption, child abuse and stressful life experiences. The prevalence of some disorders decreases with age (e.g. ADHD), whereas for others it increases with age (e.g. depression, schizophrenia, substance abuse).

The increasing use of psychotropic medications in children and adolescents is of concern (see Paediatric Implications box and discussion of ADHD in Chapter 20). Compliance with long-term medication regimens can be a problem, particularly with teenagers, who usually do not like feeling different.

Children and young adolescents may suffer depression, however antidepressants are not recommended for children.

Psychiatric disorders in the elderly

Although most elderly people are healthy, fit and active, many very old people have physical or mental limitations on their independence. Multiple pathologies and polypharmacy can confound diagnosis of mental illness, as can gradually increasing neurodegenerative or endocrine disorders, anxiety, dementia or depression. Psychotropic drugs need to be used with caution, because of the likelihood of impaired renal function, prolonged half-lives and possible drug toxicity (see Geriatric Implications box).

Psychiatric disorders specific to women

It is now recognised that there are gender issues in mental health. Some are psychosocial: e.g. in certain societies girls and women may have inferior status and roles, less opportunity for education, paid employment or health care, and may be more at risk of violence and abuse. Biological differences in hormones and stresses due to menstruation, pregnancies, breastfeeding, child care and menopause can all precipitate mental illness. Syndromes specific to women include:

- premenstrual syndrome: anxiety, depression and insomnia are more frequent in the premenstrual period, and retained fluid can alter pharmacokinetic parameters of drugs being taken
- a major postpartum psychosis occurs within 1–4 weeks of childbirth with an incidence of 1–2 per 1000 births; mood disorders are more common than schizophrenia
- postpartum depression, with persistent severe lowering of mood, has a prevalence of 15%–25% in the first post-natal year; milder postpartum blues affect 60%–70% of new mothers but do not require drug treatment
- stillbirth, habitual miscarriage or infertility will affect a woman's self-image and can cause grief and psychological symptoms
- menopausal changes, including vasomotor symptoms and insomnia, can trigger perimenopausal depression
- the ageing population and longer lifespan of women mean that in Western societies about two-thirds of people over 80 years old are women, so most mentally ill people in nursing homes for the aged are women; depression, anxiety and dementia (usually from Alzheimer's disease)

are the main diagnoses. Older women with continuing social links, interests and support are least at risk of psychiatric symptoms.

Drugs should be avoided during pregnancy if possible. Some drugs pose a teratogenic risk (see Pregnancy Safety box); however, the health of the mother and baby are paramount, so if the mother's psychiatric condition is so serious as to warrant medication during pregnancy or breastfeeding, then the safest drugs should be used at the lowest effective doses. Sertraline is the recommended antidepressant if one is required during pregnancy or breastfeeding.

Psychiatric disorders in indigenous populations

Indigenous communities have suffered major disruption after colonisation of their lands, with subsequent discrimination, dispossession, poverty, poor health, suppression of traditional cultures and family supports, and lack of educational and employment opportunities. These are all established risk factors for psychological distress and mental illness, particularly for depression, anxiety and substance abuse (see Clinical Interest Box 19-4).

Non-drug therapy

Detailed discussion of non-drug therapeutic modalities is beyond the scope of this pharmacology text. Because the psychotropic drugs are generally used only after other therapies have been unsuccessful, most patients taking psychotropics have already experienced non-drug therapies, possibly on an ongoing basis, so these therapies are described briefly here.

Psychotherapies

Psychotherapies include various types of treatment based on a relationship between a person needing help for psychological distress or disturbed behaviour or relationships and a trained health-care professional (e.g. psychologist, psychiatrist, social worker, occupational therapist) who systematically uses psychological principles in therapy (see Clinical Interest Box 19-5).

Electroconvulsive therapy

Electroconvulsive therapy (ECT) is used mainly as a safe, highly effective treatment for severe depression. It was originally introduced (in the 1930s) for schizophrenia, on the rationale that inducing a series of epileptic-type fits would help the disordered CNS functions. Early techniques were primitive; in current practice anaesthetics and muscle relaxants are used, dosage of the electrical current is more accurately determined and applied, and EEG is routinely monitored. The convulsion induced by the current is essential; ECT is thought to act by causing consistent readjustment in monoamine levels in the brain.

There is a higher positive response from ECT (80%) than from antidepressants (60%) in severe depression, especially when associated with psychotic features, suicidal ideas, psychomotor slowing and weight loss. ECT is relatively contraindicated in severe cardiovascular and respiratory disorders, or in conditions with raised intracranial pressure. The main adverse effect is memory impairment.

Psychosurgery

In the early 20th century, the technique of prefrontal lobotomy was used to treat severe schizophrenia by severing the connections between the frontal lobes and the rest of the brain. The much more specific technique currently used, limbic system surgery, targets the connections between the frontal lobes and particular components of the limbic system (see Chapter 14 and Figure 14-3). It is sometimes used in severe cases of depression and obsessive–compulsive disorder that are unresponsive to other treatments.

ANTIPSYCHOTIC AGENTS

Antipsychotic, or **neuroleptic**, **agents** are the mainstay of treatment of schizophrenia. They are also used in acutely disturbed patients in the manic phase of bipolar disorder or in acute agitation or delirium. The first antipsychotic agent, which is also the prototype **phenothiazine**, was chlorpromazine, well known by its trade name Largactil. This was the first effective **tranquilliser** (a drug prescribed to calm an agitated or anxious individual) without serious sedating actions. It was released in the early 1950s, and revolutionised treatment of 'madness'. Hundreds of analogues were developed as me-too drugs, of which a few are still in use (see Table 19-1).

Schizophrenia

Schizophrenia (sometimes erroneously referred to as split personality) is manifested by disordered mood, thought, perception and volition, leading to delusions, withdrawal and loss of insight (see Clinical Interest Box 19-6). It is thought to be due to abnormal brain circuitry or disturbed neurotransmission, especially overactivity of the mesolimbic dopaminergic pathways. It has an insidious onset in young adults (aged 15–35 years) and a prevalence in virtually all societies of about 1%. It causes considerable morbidity, lost work time and mortality (from suicide).

Aetiological factors have been studied at length: there is a strong biological basis and genetic vulnerability, and

---

CLINICAL INTEREST BOX 19-6
SIGNS AND SYMPTOMS OF SCHIZOPHRENIA

Patients with schizophrenia have a wide variety of symptoms and signs, sometimes described as positive (those which appear excessive, or hyper-behaviours), negative (reduced, or hypo-behaviours) and impaired cognitive powers. A deficit of willed action can explain many of the negative symptoms, and many of the bizarre positive symptoms may be due to a deficit in self-monitoring systems.

Most antipsychotic agents produce useful effects on the following positive symptoms: hallucinations, delusions (paranoia, bizarre, religious), disorganised thinking, communication and behaviour (agitation, anxiety, hyperactivity and hostility). The negative symptoms — flat affect (mood), withdrawal, lack of motivation, poor hygiene and dress, social inadequacy, and diminished speech patterns — are usually less responsive to drug therapy, as are the cognitive aspects — impaired memory, planning and mental flexibility.

The target symptoms are used as monitoring parameters to evaluate the individual's response to the medication. The newer, atypical antipsychotic drugs, such as clozapine and risperidone, appear to be more effective than other neuroleptic agents against the negative symptoms.
See: publications by the Schizophrenia Fellowship of New Zealand and the Schizophrenia Fellowship of Victoria, Inc, and www.sfv.org.au.

environmental associations with perinatal complications (i.e. first few days of the patient's life) or stressful relationships or life events. The current view is that many cases of schizophrenia are caused by a defect in early brain development. A related condition, schizophreniform psychosis, has an acute onset related to drugs or trauma (physical or emotional). There is now a strong association between use of cannabis (marijuana) in adolescence and increased risk of developing schizophrenia.

DRUG MONOGRAPH 19-1 CHLORPROMAZINE

INDICATIONS Phenothiazine derivatives are used in the treatment of schizophrenia, nausea and vomiting, intractable hiccups and severe behavioural disorders in children, and as adjuncts to the treatment of acute mania, dementias, depression, pain, tetanus and alcohol-induced hallucinations.

PHARMACOKINETICS Phenothiazines are lipid-soluble so are well absorbed orally and concentrate in the CNS. **Chlorpromazine** is subject to first-pass metabolism and oral bioavailability ranges from 10% to 80%. Peak plasma levels are reached in 1–4 hours after oral administration or in 15–30 minutes after IM injection. The onset of antipsychotic effect is achieved gradually, usually requiring several weeks, and peak therapeutic effect occurs between 6 weeks and 6 months. Duration of action ranges from 6 to 24 hours or more depending on dosage and frequency of drug administration. Chlorpromazine is metabolised in the liver via many pathways to various metabolites, which are generally inactive and are excreted primarily by the kidneys.

ADVERSE EFFECTS See the earlier discussion on adverse effects of psychotropic agents and Tables 19-1 and 19-2. Common adverse effects include orthostatic hypotension, sedation, **anticholinergic** and **extrapyramidal effects** (akathisia, dystonia, drug-induced parkinsonism and **tardive dyskinesia**: see Clinical Interest Box 19-2) and phototoxic skin reactions. IM injections are painful and can cause muscle necrosis. Note that tardive dyskinesia has no known effective treatment so early assessment and diagnosis are crucial to prevent progression.

DRUG INTERACTIONS Many interactions are possible; reference texts should be consulted for specific interactions. Some of the more common effects that can occur when chlorpromazine is given with other drugs are listed below:

Alcohol and CNS depressants, including anaesthetics, benzodiazepines, lithium and opioids — can result in enhanced CNS depression, respiratory depression and increased hypotensive effects. The drug dosage should be reduced.

Anticholinergic drugs — concurrent drug use may result in an increase in anticholinergic adverse effects.

Antihypertensive agents — concurrent drug use with the phenothiazines may result in an exacerbation of hypotensive effects.

Adrenaline — phenothiazines block α-adrenoceptors, thus administration of adrenaline to treat phenothiazine-induced hypotension can result in severe hypotension. (This is an example of the classic vasomotor reversal effect of adrenaline, discovered by Dale in 1913: when α receptors are blocked, adrenaline's effects on β receptors are unmasked, resulting in lowering of blood pressure and in tachycardia.) Avoid or a potentially serious drug interaction may occur.

Levodopa (L-dopa) — concurrent use with the antipsychotic agents can render levodopa ineffective in controlling Parkinson's disease and antipsychotics ineffective in schizophrenia.

Lithium — variable effects: can decrease gastrointestinal absorption of chlorpromazine, or increase clearance, or increase extrapyramidal symptoms and neurotoxicity.

Quinidine — when given concurrently with chlorpromazine, an increase in cardiac depression can occur.

Tricyclic antidepressants — metabolism of the phenothiazines and the antidepressants can be inhibited, leading to raised plasma levels and toxicity.

WARNINGS AND CONTRAINDICATIONS Use with caution in patients with breast cancer, cardiovascular disease, severe liver impairment, hyperthyroidism, Parkinson's disease, chronic respiratory disease or epilepsy, in glaucoma and other conditions involving problems of parasympathetic control, in children (see Paediatric Implications box) and in the elderly (see Geriatric Implications box).

Avoid use in patients with phenothiazine hypersensitivity, phaeochromocytoma, profound CNS depression, in alcohol abusers, in pregnant women (see Pregnancy Safety box), during lactation and in people often exposed to sunlight.

DOSAGE AND ADMINISTRATION The dosage of antipsychotic agents varies according to the individual, the indication for treatment and the patient's response to the medication. It is best to titrate from a low dose, increasing when necessary to produce a therapeutic response. When stopping antipsychotic therapy, the dosage should be reduced gradually over 2 or 3 weeks, otherwise rebound nausea, vomiting, dizziness, tremors and dyskinesias may occur.

Actions and mechanisms of antipsychotics

Antipsychotics are particularly effective against the positive symptoms of schizophrenia. They decrease hallucinations, delusions, initiative, emotion, aggression, responses to external stimuli and thought disorder, and can prevent relapses. The patient may become drowsy but is readily arousable without confusion. There is good evidence that the mechanism of action of antipsychotics is by antagonism of **dopamine** receptors, especially the D_2 subclass, which mediate the main inhibitory effects of dopamine in the CNS, particularly in the nigrostriatal, mesolimbic and tuberoinfundibular systems. This action leads to useful therapeutic effects (slower thinking and movements and antiemetic actions), and to common adverse reactions (**extrapyramidal effects** [see Clinical Interest Box 19-2] and hyperprolactinaemia, which infrequently results in swelling of the breast and milk secretion).

Clinically, it is known that many antipsychotic drugs (and antidepressants) take many weeks before their actions are most effective, even though their biochemical actions may be immediate. It is thought that the delay for antipsychotics may be due to a transient increase in dopaminergic activity, which changes after about 3 weeks to inhibition, when the antipsychotic effects 'kick in'.

As discussed earlier, the phenothiazines also block receptors for acetylcholine, noradrenaline (α receptors), histamine, and 5-HT, so there are wide-ranging adverse effects, including sedation, **anticholinergic** and gastrointestinal effects, hypotension and movement disorders. Partly because of the adverse effects, there is often poor compliance with antipsychotics and they have no abuse potential. Long-acting depot IM injections of oily solutions of some of the agents help overcome compliance problems.

Classification of antipsychotics

Antipsychotic medications (**neuroleptics**, major **tranquillisers**) have been classified based on average dose required as low-potency, intermediate-potency and high-potency drugs. The basis for the classification is the quantity of medication necessary to produce an equivalent effect when compared with other agents in the same category. For example, 100 mg chlorpromazine or thioridazine (low-potency agents) is considered to be about equivalent to 5 mg trifluoperazine or 2 mg haloperidol (high-potency agents) (see Table 19-1 for antipsychotic dosages).

On the basis of chronology, antipsychotics are also classified as being first-generation agents (i.e. the older agents), such as the phenothiazines, thioxanthines and haloperidol-type drugs, which came to be considered typical, and second-generation agents, such as clozapine, olanzapine and risperidone, which appear to have rather different profiles of actions (see Tables 19-1 and 19-2) and are known as the **atypical antipsychotics**; they are less likely to induce extrapyramidal side-effects.

Phenothiazines are also sometimes classified chemically into subgroups depending on the type of side-chain in the molecule, e.g. the piperidine compounds (such as thioridazine and pericyazine) and the piperazine compounds (such as fluphenazine, perphenazine, prochlorperazine and trifluoperazine).

Phenothiazine derivatives

Chlorpromazine will be considered in detail as the prototype **phenothiazine** antipsychotic drug (see Drug Monograph 19-1) and brief information will be given on other phenothiazines.

Other phenothiazines

Tables 19-1 and 19-2 show the properties of various phenothiazines. Fluphenazine and trifluoperazine cause extrapyramidal reactions relatively frequently. Fluphenazine is available as an oral liquid formulation and as a depot IM injectable for chronic use. Pericyazine is a low-potency drug and is recommended in low doses for behavioural disturbances in the elderly and in dementias. Thioridazine is less likely to produce extrapyramidal reactions; however, it can cause other potentially dangerous effects: pigmentary changes in the skin and eyes leading to retinopathy and impaired vision, cardiotoxicity in overdose, and endocrine disturbances.

Prochlorperazine is a phenothiazine that is mainly used for its antiemetic actions: it is usually more effective than simple antihistamines in severe vomiting, especially in vertigo and migraine. It is available as tablets, injections and suppositories.

Thioxanthines

The thioxanthines flupenthixol and zuclopenthixol resemble the piperazine phenothiazines (such as fluphenazine) in their antipsychotic effects, including the high incidence of extrapyramidal effects (see Table 19-1). Their antipsychotic indications, adverse effects, precautions and drug interactions are similar to those for the phenothiazines. Zuclopenthixol is available in three different chemical and pharmaceutical forms: as tablets, as a short-acting depot injectable preparation (for initial use, for 2–3 days only), and in a long-acting depot form.

Other 'typical' antipsychotics
Butyrophenone derivatives: haloperidol, droperidol

Haloperidol and droperidol, although structurally different from the other antipsychotic agents, have similar properties in terms of antipsychotic efficacy, adverse effects and drug interactions.

Haloperidol appears to have a selective CNS effect. It competitively blocks D_2 receptors in the mesolimbic system and causes an increased turnover of brain **dopamine** to produce its antipsychotic effect. It is associated with a significant degree of extrapyramidal effects but has less effect on noradrenergic receptors. It is a useful antipsychotic and antiemetic and is used to treat severe behavioural problems in children, in acute mania, and in Tourette's syndrome, a rare CNS disorder that presents as involuntary, rapid and repetitive motor movements, tics (facial grimaces and blinking) and vocal noises.

Droperidol is used as an adjunct in anaesthesia and in short-term management of disturbed behaviour and severe anxiety. It is available only as an injection.

Pimozide

Pimozide antagonises dopamine receptors in the CNS and increases dopamine turnover. It has very weak α-blocking and hypotensive actions. It is indicated for treating psychoses and for treating severe motor and vocal tics in people with Tourette's syndrome who have failed to respond to haloperidol. Extrapyramidal effects are common and there is a risk of arrhythmias when used in combination with drugs that affect heart rate or if the pimozide plasma level becomes high, so ECG should be monitored regularly.

'Atypical' antipsychotic agents

The second-generation 'atypical' antipsychotics have much less potential than earlier neuroleptics to cause extrapyramidal effects or sedation but are more likely to cause weight gain (see Tables 19-1 and 19-2). They may be better at treating the negative symptoms of schizophrenia. These drugs are still relatively new and efficacy and safety in children, pregnancy or lactation are not yet established. They are much more expensive than older drugs.

Clozapine

Clozapine differs from the other neuroleptics by antagonising D_1, D_2 and D_4 dopamine receptors, with less affinity for D_2 receptors, so it is less apt to induce extrapyramidal effects. It also antagonises 5-HT_2, α_1-adrenoceptors and histamine H_1 receptors. Because it has the potential for causing agranulocytosis and cardiomyopathies, this drug is reserved for treatment-resistant schizophrenia or for when the adverse effects of other drugs preclude their continued use. Treatment with clozapine is closely monitored. The manufacturer recommends dispensing only weekly supplies and performing weekly white blood cell counts. Other common adverse effects include drowsiness and seizures, and orthostatic hypotension when treatment is started. In Australia, there is a national distribution system requiring registration of doctors, pharmacists and patients involved with the clinical use of clozapine.

Olanzapine and risperidone

Olanzapine and risperidone also block both 5-HT_2 and dopamine D_2 receptors. Compared with clozapine, they are less sedating, cause fewer anticholinergic effects and do not have the same potential to cause serious agranulocytosis. There are clinically significant drug interactions with CNS depressants, antihypertensives, dopamine agonists, the new antidepressants and drugs that inhibit or enhance drug-metabolising enzymes. Olanzapine has also been approved for IM use in treatment of acute manic episodes associated with bipolar disorder, agitation, and behavioural symptoms in dementia.

Others

Quetiapine is an antagonist at many CNS neurotransmitter receptors, such as 5-HT (5-HT_{1A} and 5-HT_2), dopamine (D_1 and D_2), histamine (H_1) and adrenergic (α_1 and α_2) receptors. It is indicated for the treatment of psychotic disorders. It has low potency and has a short half-life, so twice-daily doses are required. Other new 'atypicals' include amisulpride and aripiprazole; their places in the range of antipsychotic drugs are not yet established.

TREATMENT OF AFFECTIVE DISORDERS

Affective disorders, or mood disturbances, include **depression** (which is the most common affective disorder) and **mania**.

Aetiology of affective disorders

No single factor has been identified as the cause of affective disorders. Psychiatrists who emphasise psychosocial therapies will probe to identify stressful events or mental conflicts (divorce, death of a parent or partner, inadequate parenting, physiological stressors, illness, infection or childbirth) that preceded the onset of depression. Others adhering to the biological theory tend to explain affective disorders by reference to the monoamine theory, i.e. reduced levels of catecholamine (noradrenaline, **dopamine**, adrenaline) and indoleamine (**5-HT**) transmitters in the CNS, or to changes in hormone or sodium levels, or to familial predisposition to pessimism. Functional polymorphisms in the promoter region of the serotonin transporter gene have been found to moderate the influences of stressful life events on a person's liability to suffer depression or tendency to suicide. Many practitioners today believe that genetic, psychosocial and biological factors lead to a common pathway that results in an affective disorder.

Many drugs themselves can evoke depression, probably by altering amine neurotransmitter levels in the CNS. Drug groups implicated include sedatives (alcohol, benzodiazepines, barbiturates), antipsychotics, antihypertensives (reserpine, β-blockers), hormones (corticosteroids, oral contraceptives), opioids and hallucinogens.

The monoamine theory in affective disorders

Imbalances in the centrally acting monoamine neurotransmitters, especially noradrenaline and 5-HT, have been theorised to be the cause of depression and mania. A deficiency in central noradrenaline or **5-HT** has been associated with depression, whereas an excess of **noradrenaline** is believed to be related to mania (see Figure 14-6).

Mechanisms of action of antidepressants

The storage, release, action on receptors and inactivation of CNS amine neurotransmitters are shown in Figures 14-7 and 19-1. Although the exact mechanism of action of the **antidepressant** drugs is not yet known and there are inconsistencies in some of the theories (e.g. why is cocaine not an effective antidepressant, and why and how is mianserin effective?), it is generally accepted that:
- many antidepressants (including the **tricyclics**) act by inhibiting the reuptake of noradrenaline or 5-HT, which

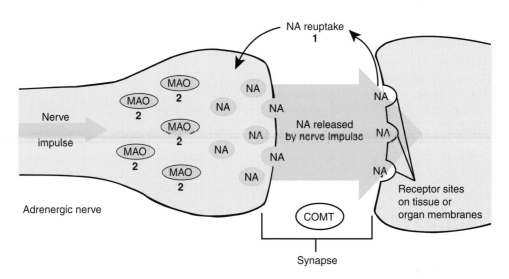

FIGURE 19-1 Proposed mechanisms of action of antidepressant drugs. Normally, **noradrenaline** (NA) is released from storage sites in vesicles within the noradrenergic nerve ending by the arrival of a nerve impulse. The released NA traverses the synaptic cleft and acts on adrenoceptors on the postsynaptic nerve or other cell. Released NA is inactivated mainly by reuptake back into the nerve ending (uptake 1 process) and then stored again in vesicles. Released NA may also be metabolised by catechol-O-methyltransferase (COMT) enzymes located in the synaptic cleft or by the enzyme monoamine oxidase (MAO) within the nerve terminal.
Antidepressant drug therapy: **1. tricyclic antidepressants** block the reuptake of released NA and prevent it from re-entering the adrenergic nerve, thus there is more NA available to act on receptors. **2. MAO inhibitors** block MAO located on the surface of the mitochondria within the cell, leaving more NA available for release. **Selective serotonin reuptake inhibitors** (SSRIs) selectively block the reuptake process for 5-hydroxytryptamine (**5-HT, serotonin**), analogous to mechanism 1 for NA, thus allowing more 5-HT to act on postsynaptic 5-HT receptors.
Other drugs acting on monoamine transmission in the CNS include reserpine, which blocks storage of catecholamines and hence inhibits aminergic transmission; cocaine, which is a powerful inhibitor of the NA reuptake process; amphetamine and tyramine, which are accumulated by uptake 1 and stored in vesicles, displacing NA, which is free to act; and entacapone, a COMT inhibitor used in Parkinson's disease.

increases the amount of neurotransmitter available to act and reverses the relative deficiency of monoamine
- other antidepressants (**monoamine oxidase inhibitors**, MAOIs) act by inhibiting the monoamine oxidase enzymes found in the mitochondria of nerve cells and responsible for metabolising noradrenaline, thus allowing a build-up of neurotransmitter available for release from the nerve terminal.

Depression

Over the years many classifications of **depression** have been used, such as the time during life at which depression occurred (childhood, adolescent, postnatal or senile depression), or the reason for the depression, such as exogenous (reactive or secondary) depression or endogenous depression.

Exogenous (from outside) depression may be a person's response to a loss, such as the loss of a loved one or loss of a job, or the presence of a debilitating illness, or disappointment. The response may manifest as lack of pleasure or interest in activities and everyday living. This is usually referred to as normal depression or 'the blues' and generally improves within a few months without the use of antidepressant medications. The mobilisation of support systems and, if necessary, psychotherapy are useful in exogenous depression, and benzodiazepines can help with associated anxiety.

Endogenous (from within) depression is characterised by the absence of external causes for depression. This type of depression may be caused by genetic determination and biochemical alterations and can be relieved by antidepressant medications.

The current classification of depressive disorders has eliminated the use of the terms 'exogenous' and 'endogenous'. Instead, major affective disorders are defined as **bipolar affective disorders** (BAD; manic–depressive psychosis, including one or more manic or hypomanic episodes) or major unipolar depressive disorders (single major depressive episode or recurrent episodes). There are also atypical affective disorders, and **depression** can occur along with neurotic and personality disorders.

Criteria for major depression include the presence of:
- mood changes (sadness, despondency, guilt feelings, self-pity, pessimism and loss of interest in life and social activities)
- psychological symptoms (low self-esteem, poor concentration, hopeless or helpless feelings and suicidal tendencies or increased focus on death)
- physiological manifestations (sleep disturbances, decreased interest in sex, fatigue, loss of energy, menstrual dysfunction, headaches, palpitations, constipation, loss of appetite and weight loss or weight gain)
- thought alterations (a decrease in ability to concentrate, poor memory, confusion, delusions relating to health, persecution or religion).

Mood variations are usually diurnal and often worse in the morning.

Mania, the opposite pole of bipolar depressive illness, is characterised by wild mood swings, excessive energy, high pressure of speech, extravagant gestures and gifts and seeming lack of need for sleep.

It is estimated that in Australia at any time one in five people has depressive symptoms, many of which are transient and normal. Clinical BAD has a prevalence of about 10% and is being recognised as a serious public health issue as there is a high risk of suicide—10%–19% in people with BAD.

Measures to treat depression include reduction of environmental stressors, ECT, psychotherapy and drug therapy. In some patients, antidepressant drug therapy in combination with one or more adjunct measures is more effective than drug therapy alone. A herbal remedy, St John's wort, is becoming popular (see Clinical Interest Box 19-7). Referral to a specialist psychiatrist is advisable in cases of severe depression when the patient has not responded to antidepressants or other measures.

Antidepressant therapy
Antidepressant drugs: clinical aspects
INDICATIONS FOR ANTIDEPRESSANTS

As well as for mood disorders, **antidepressants** are indicated for neuroses (some anxiety disorders, panic disorder, obsessive–compulsive disorder and eating disorders), in the management of enuresis and incontinence, premenstrual dysphoric disorder, and as adjunctive therapy in neuropathic pain, migraine and ADHD in children.

ANTIDEPRESSANT DRUG GROUPS

The first antidepressant drugs were discovered by serendipity (sheer good luck): iproniazide, an antitubercular agent, and imipramine, a drug being tested as an antischizophrenic, were found to elevate mood in subjects taking the drugs. This led to studies of the actions and mechanisms of similar drugs, which came to be called the tricyclic antidepressants (TCAs, imipramine-like drugs) and MAO inhibitors (iproniazide-like drugs). The main groups of antidepressant agents are:

- the **tricyclic antidepressants**: these prevent the reuptake of monoamines (**noradrenaline, 5-HT**) and hence have sympathetic nervous system effects; they also have significant **anticholinergic** actions, are characterised by a long delay in onset, and can cause sleepiness, weakness, and impaired cognition
- **selective serotonin reuptake inhibitors** (SSRIs; e.g. fluoxetine): a relatively new group of drugs, these have a more potent effect on 5-HT uptake than on noradrenaline uptake; they have fewer cardiovascular effects and are

less lethal in overdose than the TCAs; these drugs now dominate antidepressant prescribing in Australia
- **monoamine oxidase (MAO) inhibitors**: the early examples (e.g. tranylcypromine) are irreversible and non-selective for MAO isoenzymes (see Clinical Interest Box 19-8), but the newer one, moclobemide, is a reversible inhibitor of MAO-A (RIMA).

SELECTION OF AN ANTIDEPRESSANT

Overall, the antidepressants appear to have similar efficacies, although there is a wide variability in patient responses to particular drugs. *Therapeutic Guidelines: Psychotropic* recommends as first-line therapy the SSRIs, RIMA (moclobemide), nefazodone and venlafaxine. Only after unsuccessful trials of several of these agents are the second-line agents indicated: the TCAs and mianserin, then the non-selective MAOIs, which have a large number of potentially serious drug and food interactions.

Selection of an antidepressant is empirical, taking into consideration the adverse effect potential of each antidepressant compared with the medical problems of the individual patient. For example, a prescriber might select a sedating antidepressant (amitriptyline, doxepin or mianserin) for an agitated depressed person, or a drug less likely to cause sedation or hypotension (nortriptyline) for an elderly patient. SSRIs are relatively activating, so best administered early in the day. Toxicity in overdose is also important, especially if the patient is at risk of attempting a deliberate overdose—SSRIs are safer than TCAs.

PLASMA LEVELS AND COMPLIANCE

Plasma levels of the tricyclic antidepressants can vary widely between individuals and, with the possible exceptions of nortriptyline and imipramine, they often do not correlate with dose or therapeutic response. Prescribers may order plasma concentration measurements to monitor and help identify non-compliant patients. A lower than expected plasma level should initially indicate the need to interview the person to verify adherence to the prescribed schedule. The reason for the patient's ineffective management of the therapeutic medication regimen (intolerable adverse effects, misunderstanding of directions, potential drug interaction or inadequate finances to purchase prescriptions) can then be identified and perhaps resolved.

If compliance is verified and plasma concentration remains low, dosage adjustments may be necessary or the prescriber might consider switching to a different antidepressant. If the person is non-responsive to a predominantly noradrenaline-potentiating medication, a 5-HT-potentiating agent might be indicated.

SPECIAL GROUPS

The elderly often have reduced levels of liver drug metabolising enzymes, and thus higher plasma drug concentration and a greater potential for adverse effects exist. Many prescribers start geriatric patients at one-third to one-half the usual adult dosage, adjusting as necessary according to therapeutic response or presence of undesirable effects.

In children, antidepressants should be reserved for those with severe conditions not manageable with psychotherapy, and supervised by a specialist child psychiatrist—SSRIs are considered the first-line drugs. In the context of safety in pregnancy (see Pregnancy Safety box), most antidepressants are classified as C; however, some are considered safer, e.g. mianserin, moclobemide and venlafaxine. Postnatal depression affects about 10%–20% of mothers, who may need drug treatment. The SSRIs (except fluoxetine) appear to be safest with respect to transfer into breast milk.

As antidepressants generally elevate the mood and raise levels of 'stimulating' CNS neurotransmitters, they can cause unwanted effects in patients with other conditions. For example, TCAs and mianserin lower the seizure threshold and can precipitate epileptic seizures, provoke manic episodes in patients with bipolar disorder, and cause arrhythmias or angina in those with cardiac disease.

DELAYED ONSET OF ACTION
These drugs tend to have a long-delayed onset of antidepressant action, due to their long half-lives and mechanism of action (alteration of neurotransmission in CNS pathways and subsequent elevation of mood). A trend towards improvement in clinical symptoms may be apparent in 2–3 weeks and full effects may not appear for 6–8 weeks; this time corresponds with an inhibition rather than facilitation of monoaminergic transmission. During this period, patients are at great risk of deepening depression ('nothing is ever going to help') and might need adjunct treatment with psychotherapy or ECT. The initial drug tried should be given in adequate doses for an adequate period, and compliance checked, before changing to another class of antidepressant. After symptoms improve, therapy should be continued for at least 6 months.

ADVERSE EFFECTS
Many of the antidepressant drugs affect levels of several neurotransmitters, so they have effects in both the central and peripheral nervous systems. Common adverse effects are **anticholinergic** actions, sedation or insomnia, hypotension, gastrointestinal distress and weight gain (see Table 19-3).

An adverse effect due to excessive stimulation of 5-HT$_{1A}$ receptors is the **serotonin syndrome**. This is characterised by mental state changes (confusion, delirium, hypomania), GI tract effects (diarrhoea), motor effects (hyperreflexia, incoordination, tremor), autonomic instability, sweating, fever and shivering. Other drugs that interfere with 5-HT transmission, including drugs used in migraine, analgesics and St John's wort, can also cause or exacerbate the syndrome.

Tricyclic antidepressants
All the **TCAs** act by the same mechanism and appear to have similar efficacies. Although they were the first major group of drugs successful in treating depression, they have been largely overtaken by newer, safer drugs (e.g. the SSRIs such as fluoxetine) so they are currently used as second-line agents if the newer agents do not bring benefit.

Typical characteristics of the tricyclics such as **imipramine** are as follows:
* mechanism of action: inhibition of reuptake of monoamine neurotransmitters into nerve terminals, leading to improved mood
* other actions: antagonism of receptors for other transmitters, acetylcholine (muscarinic), histamine H$_1$, **noradrenaline** α$_1$ and **5-HT**, leading to adverse reactions in many body systems
* many drug interactions, with drugs affecting all the neurotransmitters mentioned above, including other antidepressants and antipsychotics, also all CNS depressants, and drugs inhibiting or inducing drug metabolism

Precautions need to be taken in people with many other conditions, including other psychoses, seizure disorders, urinary retention, cardiac, liver, renal or thyroid disease, glaucoma, and during pregnancy or breastfeeding. Dosage is started low, and gradually increased while monitoring therapeutic and adverse effects. Therapeutic effects may not become apparent for some weeks after commencement of therapy.

OTHER TRICYCLIC ANTIDEPRESSANTS
Imipramine and trimipramine are fairly typical TCAs. Nortriptyline is less likely than others to cause sedation, hypotension or anticholinergic effects, so is safer in the elderly. Dothiepin is thought to be the most toxic in overdose and doxepin is the most sedating.

Clomipramine, an analogue of imipramine, is a more selective inhibitor of 5-HT reuptake (over noradrenaline) than are the other TCAs, hence it may have fewer autonomic effects but is more likely to provoke the serotonin syndrome. It is indicated for the treatment of obsessive–compulsive disorders and premenstrual tension.

Selective serotonin reuptake inhibitors
SSRIs are as effective as other **antidepressants** and considerably safer because they increase levels of 5-HT but have much less effect on NA levels, hence fewer autonomic effects. The first, **fluoxetine** (see Drug Monograph 19-2), was so successful that soon after its release it took over the market for antidepressants (see Clinical Interest Box 19-9). Fluoxetine was soon followed by sertraline, fluvoxamine, paroxetine and citalopram then the latter's active isomer escitalopram.

DRUG MONOGRAPH 19-2 FLUOXETINE

Fluoxetine (better known by its original trade name, Prozac) is a selective serotonin reuptake inhibitor (SSRI) antidepressant; it is much more potent at inhibiting reuptake of serotonin than of noradrenaline. It is much less effective at antagonism of acetylcholine, histamine and α-adrenergic receptors than are the tricyclic antidepressants. It helps elevate mood, relieve other symptoms and reduce social impairment.

INDICATIONS Fluoxetine is indicated for treatment of major depression, obsessive–compulsive disorder and premenstrual dysphoric disorder. It can also be used for bulimia nervosa, panic disorder and post-traumatic stress disorder.

PHARMACOKINETICS Fluoxetine is readily absorbed after oral administration and reaches peak plasma levels after about 6–8 hours. It is highly protein-bound, and has a very high volume of distribution. It has non-linear kinetics as it inhibits its own metabolism. It is extensively metabolised in the liver; one metabolite (norfluoxetine) is active as an antidepressant. Metabolites are excreted via the kidneys. With chronic administration, the half-lives of fluoxetine and norfluoxetine are respectively 4–6 and 9–16 days, hence it takes some weeks for the concentration at steady state to stabilise.

DRUG INTERACTIONS Fluoxetine inhibits metabolism by the CYP2D6 isoenzymes, hence it raises plasma levels of drugs metabolised by that enzyme, including many antiepileptic drugs, antipsychotics, benzodiazepines, tricyclic antidepressants and St John's wort. There are protein-binding interactions with warfarin.

ADVERSE REACTIONS Common reactions include rashes, anxiety, dizziness, weight loss, nausea and headaches; seizures are rare. There is some debate as to whether antidepressants may increase the risk of suicide in depression, or whether this and worsening symptoms occur in the interval between dosing and when the drug's effects begin to occur.

WARNINGS AND CONTRAINDICTIONS Patients need to be warned of possible adverse effects, of the delay before therapeutic effects, and of caution required if driving or operating machinery. Withdrawal reactions can occur after cessation of the drug, due to its long half-life. The dose needs to be reduced in severe liver disease. Fluoxetine is in pregnancy category C as it crosses the placenta and can lead to withdrawal reactions in the neonate. It is not recommended during lactation due to its lipid solubility and long half-life. Antidepressants are not generally indicated for treatment of childhood depression.

DOSAGE AND ADMINISTRATION The usual starting does in depression is 20 mg/day in adults, which may be increased after several weeks' trial gradually to a maximum of 80 mg/day in divided doses. It is available in tablet, capsule and oral liquid formulations.

The SSRIs are generally indicated to treat depression, obsessive–compulsive disorder and panic disorder; fluoxetine is also indicated for treating bulimia nervosa. They have similar efficacies to the TCAs and the same delayed onset of action. Unlike the TCAs, which often cause weight gain, the SSRIs (except paroxetine) can cause anorexia and weight loss. They have little affinity for receptors for DA, acetylcholine, histamine or NA and are the least toxic antidepressants in overdose. There are numerous potential drug interactions, especially with other antidepressants and with drugs implicated in the serotonin syndrome, and they can inhibit the metabolism of many drugs.

Adverse effects are as shown for fluoxetine. Early suggestions that use of fluoxetine is associated with enhanced suicidal behaviour have not been supported by longer studies.

As well as being a marketing phenomenon, fluoxetine is interesting from a pharmacokinetic viewpoint. While most SSRIs have half-lives of about 24 hours, fluoxetine has an active metabolite with a half-life of up to 16 days. Consequently, it takes weeks to achieve steady-state concentrations or to eliminate the active metabolite after discontinuation of the drug, and there is an extended period for drug interactions.

Monoamine oxidase inhibitor antidepressants
MONOAMINE OXIDASE

MAO, an enzyme found in mitochondrial membranes in nerve terminals, the liver and the brain, is involved in the inactivation and degradation of various monoamines. Tyramine, catecholamines (**noradrenaline** [NA], adrenaline and **dopamine** [DA]), **5-HT** and several amine drugs are all substrates for the enzyme. Compounds that inhibit the enzyme thus interfere with the inactivation of amine neurotransmitters and may potentiate their actions, particularly the vasopressor effects.

Two types of MAO enzymes have been identified: MAO-A and MAO-B. MAO-A appears to have a preference for 5-HT, NA and DA and is located throughout the body (high concentrations are present in the human placenta). MAO-B is contained mainly in human platelets but about equal amounts of both types are found in the liver and brain. DA and tyramine, a monoamine with sympathomimetic effects found in many foodstuffs, are inactivated by both MAO-A and MAO-B. Hence an inhibitor that selects for the MAO-A form is likely to be better clinically as an **antidepressant**, as it will raise

BOX 19-1 MANAGEMENT OF DRUG OVERDOSE: TRICYCLIC ANTIDEPRESSANTS

Tricyclic antidepressant (TCA) overdose can be life-threatening, resulting in serious adverse reactions such as cardiac arrhythmias, heart block, hypotension, seizures, coma and, in many instances, death. TCAs are relatively more toxic than most other drugs taken for self-poisoning; 70%–80% of people who take overdoses of TCAs do not reach the hospital alive. Therefore, it is important that safer antidepressants be prescribed whenever possible, especially for patients with suicidal ideas.

SIGNS AND SYMPTOMS
The signs and symptoms of a TCA overdose vary in severity depending on numerous factors, including the amount ingested and absorbed, other drugs taken, the age of the individual and the interval between ingestion and initiation of treatment. Any acute overdose or unwarranted ingestion of a TCA in children or adults must be considered serious and potentially fatal.

CNS abnormalities include agitation, ataxia, choreoathetoid movements, drowsiness, hyperactive reflexes, muscle rigidity, seizures and coma. Cardiac abnormalities include arrhythmias, signs of congestive heart failure and tachycardia. Vomiting, dilated pupils and hyperpyrexia can occur.

TREATMENT
Patients suspected of having taken an overdose of a TCA should be admitted to hospital immediately. Symptomatic and supportive measures are instituted according to the individual patient's requirements. These may include:

- emesis or use of gastric lavage to empty the stomach followed by administration of activated charcoal to absorb any remaining drug in the gastrointestinal tract
- close monitoring of cardiovascular functioning for at least 5 days; cardiac arrhythmias have occurred up to 6 days after massive TCA doses and may require treatment with digitalis or propranolol
- maintenance of body temperature and respiratory and cardiac functions
- administration of anticonvulsants or an inhalation anaesthetic to control seizures.

Haemodialysis, peritoneal dialysis, forced diuresis and exchange transfusions are not successful for treating a TCA overdose because of the low plasma levels of the drug.

CLINICAL INTEREST BOX 19-8 TYRAMINE-CONTAINING SUBSTANCES

Patients taking old-style non-selective MAOIs are at risk of the **tyramine reaction** if they eat or drink tyramine-containing preparations, as the tyramine (usually inactivated by MAO-B) can build up to high levels and raise the blood pressure by a sympathomimetic action (see 'MAOI Advice Card' in *Australian Medicines Handbook* 2005, Appendix E).

The tyramine content of foods varies because of different conditions or preparation of the foods, different food samples or different producers or manufacturers. The major goal should be to advise the patient to avoid foods and drinks with reported moderate to high tyramine contents as follows:

- cheeses: especially mature and aged (e.g. blue, Brie, Emmenthaler, Gruyère, Parmesan, Roquefort, Stilton)
- aged, cured and pickled meats and fish: game, caviar, herring, sausages (kabana, pepperoni, salami), bacon, hot-dogs
- vegetables: overripe avocado, broad bean pods, pickled vegetables
- fruit: overripe figs, bananas and raisins
- meat or yeast extracts (Vegemite, Bonox) and stock cubes or packet soups
- alcoholic beverages: red wines, especially Chianti; sherry, beer, liqueurs
- coffee substitutes, soy products.

Some foods that contain tyramine or other pressor amines, if eaten in moderation when fresh, are less apt to cause a serious reaction. Such foods include yoghurt, sour cream, cream cheese, cottage cheese, chocolate and soy sauce.

(As a colleague who was taking tranylcypromine once complained: "I'm going to a cocktail party, and I won't be able to eat or drink *anything*!")

---

the levels of neurotransmitter amines (see Figure 19-1) while allowing inactivation of tyramine and other potentially toxic monoamines.

MAO INHIBITORS (MAOIs)
The early **MAOIs** were irreversible and non-selective in their inhibitory effects, i.e. they inhibited both MAO-A and

MAO-B, for 2–3 weeks. Current research indicates that the MAOIs also desensitise the α_2- or β-adrenoceptors and 5-HT receptors (downregulation). Examples are the drugs phenelzine and tranylcypromine. They raise the level of monoamines and elevate the mood, but there is a long delay in mood improvement. There are many serious adverse reactions, including autonomic and sexual dysfunction, severe hypertension and insomnia.

MAOIs impair the metabolism of many other drugs, including adrenaline and sympathomimetic amines, DA (including that formed after administration of levodopa), methyldopa and pethidine, and enhance the activity of drugs that cause release of amine transmitters. Interactions can occur with prescription-only and over-the-counter medications, caffeine and tyramine-containing foods and beverages (the **tyramine reaction**: see Clinical Interest Box 19-8). The major adverse reaction with these agents is the occurrence of sudden and possibly very severe hypertension that if untreated can

CLINICAL INTEREST BOX 19-9 PROZAC BEATS THE BLUES

Fluoxetine (Prozac) was released in the USA in 1987. By 1990 it had made the covers of both *Newsweek* and *The New Yorker* as the new wonder drug for depression, and by 1993 sales had reached US$1.2 billion worldwide. It was so widely prescribed in the USA that in some towns most of the population were said to be taking the 'happy pill'.

In Australia, prescriptions for antidepressants surged by 35% in the 1990s, from 5.1 million in 1990 to 6.9 million in 1996. There was a rapid market uptake of SSRIs with only a small decrease in prescribing of TCAs.

Specialist physicians were unsure whether the prevalence of depression had risen or whether people were more aware of the condition, more prepared to consult their doctors about it or more aware that there are drugs to treat it. A depression institute (*beyondblue*) has been set up to study the disorder.

Antidepressant use in Australia is similar to that in the USA and second only to that in Sweden.
Source: Gray 1997; McManus et al 2000; Turkington 1994.

BOX 19-2 FACTORS AFFECTING LITHIUM PLASMA CONCENTRATION

Lithium levels are elevated by:
- renal dysfunction
- diarrhoea or vomiting
- fluid or salt loss, diuretics or dehydration
- low-salt diets
- excess sweating, high fever or strenuous exercise
- non-steroidal anti-inflammatory drugs (NSAIDs) or angiotensin-converting enzyme (ACE) inhibitors.

Lithium levels are lowered by:
- high salt intake
- high intake of sodium bicarbonate
- pregnancy.

Because of the large number of adverse drug reactions and interactions, the old non-selective MAOIs are now indicated only as second- or third-line antidepressants for the treatment of depression that does not respond to other, safer drugs. Some patients, however, respond only to MAOIs.

REVERSIBLE INHIBITORS OF MAO-A

Moclobemide is a reversible inhibitor of MAO-A (RIMA), a new **antidepressant** drug group. It is much less likely to cause tyramine reactions, as tyramine and other amines can still be

progress to vascular collapse and fatality. (Reference texts should be consulted for potential drug interactions whenever another drug is added to a regimen containing an MAOI.)

CLINICAL INTEREST BOX 19-10   VAN GOGH'S AFFECT AND ART

Vincent van Gogh, the great Dutch artist, suffered what would most likely now be classified as severe **bipolar affective disorder**, or manic–depressive pyschosis.

Vincent was born in 1853 into an austere religious and artistic Dutch family. There was a history of mental illness (epilepsy, nervous complaints) on both sides of his family. His childhood was dominated by his mother's grief over the earlier death of her first son. He became an art dealer and preacher but his self-martyrdom and solitude were found to be unacceptable, so he turned to painting.

His four important relationships with women — two of whom were 'mentally unbalanced' — all ended in shame and humiliation. His friendship and collaboration with the painter Gauguin in Arles (Provence, France) was short-lived, with Vincent suffering a severe mental disturbance and cutting off part of his ear and sending it to a prostitute.

There are many references to his self-abasement, misery, moodiness, melancholy, neglect of his appearance and health, excessive drinking and feeling a prisoner. At other times he was remarkably energetic, with strong exalted emotions, swarms of ideas for his work and extravagant gestures. He painted prolifically but was financially dependent on his brother. He suffered many episodes of mental disorder, with confusions, hallucinations, delusions, paranoia and aggression, or anguish, immobility and guilt, identifying with

the suffering and rejection of Christ. He committed himself to a mental asylum for a year and committed suicide a few months after leaving it, aged 37.

Many of the swings in Vincent's moods can be traced in his paintings, which vary between brilliant yellow sunny scenes such as sunflowers and harvests and dark sombre visions of gloomy peasant life, ruined churches or flocks of black birds foreboding evil.

Genetic features played a part in Vincent's illness, as did his unhappy childhood, rejection by women and peers, unhappy events, physical ill-health and heavy drinking of alcohol and absinthe (known to contain the neurotoxins thujone and santonin). There are other theories: that he had epilepsy or Ménière's disease, was poisoned by drinking turpentine, had gonorrhoea or syphilis and glaucoma. He was treated for epilepsy with digitalis and it has been suggested that the bright yellow–green colours and swirling halos around lights in his later paintings are due to the altered colour vision indicative of severe digitalis toxicity. Inevitably, Vincent's affective disorder, of whatever aetiology, influenced his art. Perhaps if effective treatment for bipolar disorder had been available, his art would have been less imaginative and creative?
After: Wolf 1994 and various sources.

inactivated by MAO-B. The fact that it is reversible means that MAO activity is restored within 1–2 days of stopping administration of the drug. Nausea, headache and insomnia are adverse effects and there may be adverse interactions with sympathomimetic amines and pethidine. A tyramine-free diet is not required, although large quantities of tyramine-rich foods should be avoided. Moclobemide is relatively safe in overdose.

Other miscellaneous antidepressants

There are other new atypical **antidepressants**, which act by various mechanisms affecting amine neurotransmitter levels.

MIANSERIN

Mianserin has a tetracyclic chemical structure, rather than tricyclic. It does not inhibit the reuptake of monoamine transmitters but enhances postsynaptic 5-HT$_{1A}$ receptors, hence its antidepressant actions. It shares some of the other properties of the TCAs, as it antagonises α_1-adrenoreceptors and histamine H$_1$ receptors, but has less anticholinergic action so has fewer cardiovascular adverse effects. A rare adverse effect unrelated to the antidepressant actions is reversible neutropenia, which is monitored by blood counts before and during therapy.

NEW ANTIDEPRESSANTS

Two relatively new antidepressants are reboxetine and venlafaxine. Their precise mechanisms of action differ but

---

DRUG MONOGRAPH 19-3 LITHIUM

INDICATIONS Lithium is indicated for prevention of manic or depressive episodes in bipolar affective disorder and in treatment of acute mania. It is also used as adjunctive therapy in schizophrenia and treatment-resistant depression.

PHARMACOKINETICS With the exception of the slow-release dosage form, lithium is rapidly absorbed and reaches peak plasma concentrations in 1–3 hours. It has a long half-life: in adults 24 hours, in adolescents 18 hours, and in geriatric patients up to 36 hours, hence steady-state plasma concentrations are not reached for 5–7 days. Lithium is not metabolised so it is excreted unchanged by the kidneys; it is partly reabsorbed from the proximal tubule along with sodium.

THERAPEUTIC DRUG MONITORING Lithium has a very narrow therapeutic range, with concentrations only 1.5 times therapeutic concentration causing severe toxicity, so plasma levels must be monitored regularly. Samples are taken 12 hours post-dose to measure trough levels. Therapeutic plasma concentrations for the treatment of bipolar disorder are: acute, 0.8–1.2 mmol/L; and maintenance, 0.6–0.8 mmol/L. A clinical response is usually reported in 1–3 weeks. Levels are monitored weekly during dosage adjustment, then every 1–3 months once stabilised (see Box 19-2 for other factors affecting lithium serum levels).

DRUG INTERACTIONS The following effects may occur when lithium is given with the drugs listed below:

Antithyroid drugs or iodides — can enhance the hypothyroid goitrogenic effects of lithium or these medications; monitor closely for lethargy or intolerance to cold.

Non-steroidal anti-inflammatory agents — can decrease excretion of lithium, leading to raised lithium levels and toxicity; monitor closely for blurred vision, confusion and dizziness.

Phenothiazines, fluoxetine, haloperidol — lithium levels may be altered, with risk of neurotoxicity. Monitor physical symptoms and drug serum levels closely.

Diuretics, especially thiazides — decreased lithium excretion results in a raised lithium level and toxicity. A reduction in lithium dosage may be indicated. Monitor closely.

ADVERSE EFFECTS These include tremors of hands, thirst, nausea, increased urination, diarrhoea, weight gain and irregular pulse rate. Long-term effects include acne, psoriasis, hypothyroidism and renal damage. A specific effect is nephrogenic diabetes insipidus, in which lithium inhibits the actions of antidiuretic hormone on the distal tubule cells, leading to polyuria. Early signs of toxicity include confusion, vomiting, tremors, slurred speech and drowsiness. Later signs are blurred vision, convulsions, severe trembling, ataxia, arrhythmias and increased production of urine. Prolonged toxic levels can lead to irreversible brain damage, and even relatively low plasma levels can be fatal. Treatment of toxicity is by gastric lavage, forced diuresis and dialysis.

WARNINGS AND CONTRAINDICATIONS Lithium should be used with caution in patients with diabetes mellitus, hypothyroidism, goitre or psoriasis, and in pregnant or severely debilitated patients or patients on a sodium-restricted diet. Avoid use in people with a history of lithium hypersensitivity or with severe dehydration or renal impairment, and during lactation.

DOSAGE AND ADMINISTRATION Lithium, as the carbonate salt, is available as tablets and controlled-release tablets. The usual adult dose of lithium for acute mania is 250–500 mg, 3 times daily, adjusted according to the patient's response and tolerance up to a maximum dose of 2.5 g/day. The maintenance dose is 1000–2500 mg daily in divided doses. Geriatric patients usually require a much lower dosage (one-third to one-half).

CLINICAL INTEREST BOX 19-11
THERAPEUTIC VALUE OF LITHIUM DISCOVERED IN MELBOURNE

Chemically, lithium (Li) is a simple metal, first isolated in 1817. It is the third lightest element, related in its properties to the other alkaline earth metals sodium and potassium. Lithium salts were once used for gout and as sedatives and a salt substitute. It was known that excess lithium caused cardiac depression, nausea and upset stomach, and mental depression. How lithium came to be used in psychiatric medicine is an interesting story.

In 1948 Dr John Cade, a Melbourne psychiatrist, was doing research into the chemical basis of mania. He established that patients' urine contained a 'manic toxin' that had excitant effects when injected into guinea pigs.

Working on the theory that urea was the neurotoxin and that urates would enhance the toxicity, he tested the lithium salt, lithium urate, but found it caused the animals to become lethargic and unresponsive to stimuli.

To his surprise, Cade found that other lithium salts had similar protective, calming effects, and concluded it was lithium, not urate, that was the pharmacologically important ion.

He tested lithium clinically in 10 patients with mania and showed that lithium salts have specific effects in controlling mania but are ineffective in schizophrenia or acute depression. Cade recognised that the adverse effects (abdominal discomfort, slurred speech, ataxia, depression) could be fatal if the drug administration was not immediately stopped.

Cade speculated "as to the possible aetiological significance of a deficiency in the body of lithium ions in the genesis of this disorder", and reported that lithium treatment was "much preferred to prefrontal leucotomy". He published his work in the *Medical Journal of Australia* (1949), but it met with little interest. Was the journal (then) too obscure? the remedy too simple? the drug not patentable? the cure potentially too toxic?

By the 1960s, lithium had been re-evaluated and its efficacy in reducing the prevalence, severity and duration of recurrent manic episodes proven. There is an 80%–85% response rate when lithium is used prophylactically in manic–depressive psychosis.

---

both show some inhibition of 5-HT and NA reuptake and affect various other neurotransmitters. Adverse effects include autonomic, CNS and sexual dysfunctions.

Mirtazapine is a new antidepressant released for general use in mid-2001. It is chemically related to mianserin and has different mechanisms of action from those of the tricyclics and MAOIs. Mirtazepine, by selective blockade of histamine H_1 receptors, α_2-adrenoceptors and 5-HT_{2A}, 5-IIT_{2C} and 5-HT_3 receptors, appears to enhance noradrenergic activity and 5-HT activity at $5HT_{1A}$ receptors, which gives it better antidepressant efficacy and fewer peripheral and central adverse effects. In particular, it is safer in overdose, has fewer anticholinergic effects, and does not cause nausea or diarrhoea, insomnia or sexual dysfunction.

In bipolar depression, other drugs sometimes useful are the anticonvulsant lamotrigine and antipsychotic olanzapine.

Antimanic therapy
Mania

Bipolar affective disorder involves mood swings between the poles of depression and mania; patients with unipolar mania are rare. Bipolar disorders are much less common than unipolar depression, with bipolar conditions accounting for only about 10% of affective disorders. The peak age of onset of bipolar illness is in the late 20s, about 15 years earlier than that of unipolar depression.

Mania is characterised by the presence of speech and motor hyperactivity, reduced sleep requirements, flights of ideas, grandiose or paranoid thoughts, elated, irritable or angry mood, poor judgement, aggressiveness and hostility, overspending and possibly promiscuity. (The hypomanic state may cause social problems, with overactivity, uncompleted tasks, irritability, excessive untidy bright clothing, poor judgement and increased sexual interest.) Then the person with bipolar disorder may suffer a mood swing to depression, which can persist for several months (see Clinical Interest Box 19-10).

Counselling, psychotherapy and drug therapy are useful for treating bipolar disorders. ECT may be required for severe mood disturbance or for suicidal depression. Antipsychotic drugs (e.g. phenothiazines) are useful for sedation and control of the mania symptoms and antidepressants in the depressive phases for at least 6 months. Olanzapine and quetiapine, both atypical antipsychotic agents, have been approved for use in treatment of acute manic episodes associated with bipolar disorder, in which they help control disruptive behaviour and cause the patient to become more settled and sleep better.

Lithium is the specific treatment for prevention of recurrences of manic episodes (see Clinical Interest Box 19-11). Other mood-stabilising drugs include the antiepileptic agents sodium valproate, lamotrigine and carbamazepine (see Chapter 18), sometimes used in combination with lithium or with olanzapine.

Lithium: the antimanic drug

Lithium's mechanism of action has still not been established. Sodium in the cells has been reported to increase by as much as 200% in manic patients. Lithium and sodium are both actively transported across cell membranes but lithium cannot be pumped out of the cell as effectively as sodium can. Lithium can impair sodium actions in many physiological processes. It inhibits or slows down G-protein coupling with receptors, adenylate cyclase activity, phosphoinositol cycling and various phosphokinase activities, and affects neuro-

protective proteins. Overall, it inhibits transmitter release at synapses, increases the turnover of NA and 5-HT in the brain and decreases postsynaptic receptor sensitivity, with the result that the presumed overactive catecholamine systems in mania are corrected (see Drug Monograph 19-3).

DRUGS AT A GLANCE 19: Psychotropic agents

Therapeutic group	Pharmacological group	Key examples	Key pages
Antipsychotic agents	Phenothiazines	chlorpromazine	315, 323–4
		fluphenazine	315, 324
	Thioxanthines	flupenthixol	315, 324
	Others	haloperidol	315, 325
		pimozide	315, 325
	Atypical antipsychotics	clozapine	315, 325
		olanzapine	315, 325
Antidepressants	Tricyclic antidepressants	imipramine	319, 329
		nortriptyline	319, 329
	Selective serotonin reuptake inhibitors (SSRIs)	fluoxetine	319, 329, 30
		citalopram	319, 329
	Monoamine oxidase inhibitors	tranylcypromine	319, 331
	• Reversible inhibitors of MAO-A (RIMA)	• moclobemide	319, 332
	Others	mianserin	319, 333
		venlafaxine	319, 333–4
Antimanic agents		lithium	333–5

Note: See also Tables 19-1, 19-2 (antipsychotics); Table 19-3, Figure 19-1 (antidepressants).

KEY POINTS

● To treat mental illness, the health-care professional needs some understanding of the pathogenesis and clinical manifestations of the major psychoses schizophrenia and bipolar affective disorder, and the relevance of imbalances in brain neurotransmitters, especially the monoamines noradrenaline, dopamine and 5-HT.

● Important clinical aspects include the importance of informed consent and compliance with therapy; the frequency of serious adverse drug reactions and interactions; concomitant non-drug therapy with psychotherapy, electroconvulsive therapy and psychosurgery; and the selection of appropriate therapy for patients in special groups: children, elderly, female and indigenous people.

● Since the discovery of antipsychotic tranquillisers in the 1950s, there has been a marked decrease in the length of institutionalisation for psychiatric disorders. Many people are now treated as outpatients at community mental health centres.

● The main antipsychotic (antischizophrenic) agents are the phenothiazine derivatives, thioxanthines and atypical antipsychotics. Although the exact mechanisms of their antipsychotic effect are unknown, a primary effect is dopamine blockade in specific areas of the CNS. Receptors for many other neurotransmitters are also likely to be blocked.

● Major adverse effects occur in the central, autonomic and motor nervous systems, including sedation, hypotension, behaviour changes, dystonias and parkinsonian effects, and akathisia. Serious adverse effects are tardive dyskinesia and neuroleptic malignant syndrome.

- The major affective disorders are depression and bipolar affective disorder. The monoamine theory of affective disorders suggests that during depressive episodes levels of monoamines, especially noradrenaline and 5-HT, are low in parts of the brain related to mood.

- Antidepressant drug groups include the tricyclic antidepressants, the selective serotonin reuptake inhibitors and the monoamine oxidase inhibitors. All appear to act by increasing brain levels of 5-HT and noradrenaline.

- Lithium is usually the drug of choice for prophylaxis and treatment of mania or bipolar affective disorder.

- All psychotherapeutic medications can produce undesirable adverse effects. Therefore patient education and close monitoring are necessary to improve compliance and clinical outcome and to avoid or reduce the potential for unwanted and potentially serious adverse effects and drug interactions.

REVIEW EXERCISES

1. Review Table 19-1 'Selected antipsychotic agents, potency and major effects' and answer the following questions:
   - Name three drugs on this chart that have high antiemetic effects.
   - If the prescriber wants to change therapy from chlorpromazine to an antipsychotic agent with an equivalent antiemetic effect but less sedation, less hypotension and fewer anticholinergic effects, which drug might be selected?
   - Why do the adverse effect profiles for the atypical agents differ from those of the phenothiazines?

2. Discuss the use of antipsychotic and antidepressant drugs in the elderly, considering usual dosages, pharmacokinetics and adverse effects.

3. Explain the warning about the need for caution in using antipsychotic agents in patients with Parkinson's disease.

4. List several reasons why the selective serotonin reuptake inhibitors are preferred over the tricyclic antidepressants for the treatment of depression.

5. Describe the various theories for the mechanism of action of lithium in the treatment of mania.

6. Name one drug from each category (phenothiazines, atypical antipsychotics, the various antidepressant categories and lithium) and discuss indications, actions and adverse effects, mechanisms of action, significant drug interactions, warnings and contraindications.

7. Discuss the signs, symptoms and management of the extrapyramidal adverse effects reported with the antipsychotic agents.

8. Describe and explain the mechanism of the tyramine reaction that can occur in patients taking MAO inhibitor drugs, and name four common tyramine-containing substances.

REFERENCES AND FURTHER READING

Andreason NC. Symptoms, signs and diagnosis of schizophrenia. *Lancet* 1995; 346: 477–81 (and the articles on schizophrenia in each of the subsequent five issues of *The Lancet*).
Anonymous. *NZ Prescriber Update*; June 2001; no. 21: 4–7.
Australian Medicines Handbook 2005. Adelaide: AMH, 2005.
Bloch S, Singh BS. *Understanding Troubled Minds: A Guide to Mental Illness and its Treatment*. Melbourne: Melbourne University Press, 1997.
Bloch S, Singh BS (eds). *Foundations of Clinical Psychiatry*. 2nd edn. Melbourne: Melbourne University Press, 2001.
Braun L, Cohen M. *Herbs and Natural Supplements: An Evidence-Based Guide*. Sydney: Elsevier Mosby, 2005.
Brown TM, Dronsfield AT, Ellis PM. Li-Mg: a life-saving relationship. *Education in Chemistry* 1997; 34: 72–4.
Buckley NA, Whyte IM, Dawson AH et al. Self-poisoning in Newcastle, 1987–1992. *Medical Journal of Australia* 1995; 162: 190–3.
Cade JFJ. *Mending the Mind: A Short History of Twentieth Century Psychiatry*. Melbourne: Sun Books, 1979.
Campbell D. The management of acute dystonic reactions. *Australian Prescriber* 2001; 24: 19–20.
Carr V. Are atypical antipsychotics advantageous?—the case against. *Australian Prescriber* 2004; 27(6): 149–51.
Caspi A, Sugden K, Moffitt TE et al. Influence of life-stress on depression: moderation by a polymorphism in the 5-HT T gene. *Science* 2003; 301(5631): 386–9.
Caswell A (ed.). *MIMS Annual June 2005*. Sydney: CMPMedica Australia, 2005.
Cooper JR, Bloom FE, Roth RH. *The Biochemical Basis of Neuropharmacology*. 8th edn. New York: Oxford University Press, 2003.
Creamer M, McFarlane A. Post-traumatic stress disorder. *Australian Prescriber* 1999: 22: 32–4.
Delini-Stula A, Baier D, Kohnen R et al. Undesirable blood pressure changes under naturalistic treatment with moclobemide, a reversible MAO-A inhibitor—results of the drug utilization observation studies. *Pharmacopsychiatry* 1999; 32(2): 61–7.
Fugh-Berman A, Cott JM. Dietary supplements and natural products as psychotherapeutic agents. *Psychosomatic Medicine* 1999; 61: 712–28.

Gaster B, Holroyd J. St John's wort for depression: a systematic review. *Archives of Internal Medicine* 2000; 160: 152–6.

Gibbons RD, Hur K, Bhaumik DK, Mann JJ. The relationship between antidepressant medication use and rate of suicide. *Archives of General Psychiatry* 2005; 62(2): 165–72.

Gray D. More seek drugs to help beat the blues. *The Age* 16 November 1997.

Hall M. Serotonin syndrome. *Australian Prescriber* 2003; 26(3): 62–3.

Healy D. *Psychiatric Drugs Explained.* 4th edn. Edinburgh: Churchill Livingstone, 2005.

Hegarty K. Management of mild depression in general practice: is self-help the solution? *Australian Prescriber* 2005; 28(1): 8–10.

Jureidini JN. Suicide and antidepressants in children. *Australian Prescriber* 2005; 28(5): 110–1.

Keks NA. Are atypical antipsychotics advantageous?—the case for. *Australian Prescriber* 2004; 27(6): 146–9.

Lampe L. Antidepressants: not just for depression. *Australian Prescriber* 2005; 28(4): 91–3.

McManus P, Mant A, Mitchell PB et al. Recent trends in the use of antidepressant drugs in Australia, 1990–1998. *Medical Journal of Australia* 2000; 173: 458–61.

Mant A, Rendle VA, Hall WD et al. Making new choices about antidepressants in Australia: the long view. *Medical Journal of Australia* 2004; 181(7 Suppl): S21–4.

Mitchell PB. St John's wort: quack medicine or novel antidepressant treatment? *Australian Prescriber* 1999; 22: 112–13.

Mitchell PB, Mahli GS, Ball JR. Major advances in bipolar disorder. *Medical Journal of Australia* 2004; 181(4): 207–10.

National Prescribing Service. St John's wort—drug interactions. *NPS Newsletter* 11, August 2000.

Psychotropic Expert Group. *Therapeutic Guidelines: Psychotropic, version 5.* Melbourne: Therapeutic Guidelines Limited, 2003.

Rang HP, Dale MM, Ritter JM, Moore PK. *Pharmacology.* 5th edn. Edinburgh: Churchill Livingstone, 2003 [chs 37, 38].

Schweitzer I, Maguire K. Stopping antidepressants. *Australian Prescriber* 2001; 24: 13–15.

Snowdon J. Late-life depression: what can be done? *Australian Prescriber* 2001; 24: 65–7.

Spencer JW, Jacobs JJ. *Complementary/Alternative Medicine: An Evidence-Based Approach.* St Louis: Mosby, 1999.

Stahl SM. *Essential Psychopharmacology: Neuroscientific Basis and Practical Applications.* 2nd edn. Cambridge: Cambridge University Press, 2000.

Tiller JWG. The new antidepressants: clinical applications. *Australian Prescriber* 1999; 22: 108–11.

Tiller JWG. Cognitive behaviour therapy in medical practice. *Australian Prescriber* 2001; 24: 33–7.

Turkington CA, Kaplan EF. *Making the Prozac Decision: Your Guide to Antidepressants.* Los Angeles: Lowell House, 1994.

Various authors. Depression and the community. *Medical Journal of Australia* 2002; 176 (10, Suppl.): S60–S101.

Wolf PL. If clinical chemistry had existed then . . . *Clinical Chemistry* 1994; 40: 328–35.

ON-LINE RESOURCES:

beyondblue, the national depression initiative: www.beyondblue.org.au/index.aspx

Mental Illness Fellowship of Victoria (formerly Schizophrenia Fellowship of Victoria): www.mifellowship.org/facts&stats.htm

New Zealand medicines and medical devices safety authority: www.medsafe.govt.nz

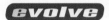 More weblinks at http://evolve.elsevier.com/AU/Bryant/pharmacology/

CHAPTER 20

Central Nervous System Stimulants

CHAPTER FOCUS

The central nervous system (CNS)-stimulant drugs such as amphetamine and caffeine may produce dramatic effects by increasing the activity of CNS neurons; however, their therapeutic usefulness is limited because of their many general effects and adverse reactions in the body. Chronic use and misuse have occurred with these drugs, resulting in patients developing drug tolerance, drug dependence and drug abuse problems. If taken in sufficient doses, all CNS stimulants may cause convulsions. This chapter reviews the CNS-stimulant drugs that are available for clinical use. Their approved indications are for treatment of attention disorders and narcolepsy, and to suppress the appetite. The methylxanthines (caffeine, theophylline and theobromine) are mainly taken in beverages (coffee, tea, cocoa and soft drinks) to increase alertness, while amphetamines have limited clinical applications but are widely abused for their stimulant effects.

OBJECTIVES

- To discuss the main groups of CNS-stimulant drugs (amphetamines and methylxanthines), including their mechanisms of action, pharmacological effects, indications, significant drug interactions, and common adverse effects.

- To describe attention-deficit hyperactivity disorder (ADHD) and its effects in the child and adult, and outline its clinical management.

- To describe narcolepsy and the drugs useful in treating this condition.

- To discuss the use of amphetamines as anorectic agents.

- To describe the multiple effects of caffeine in the body, list its indications, and identify the signs of and treatment for a caffeine overdose.

KEY DRUGS

caffeine
dexamphetamine
methylphenidate

KEY TERMS

amphetamines
analeptics
anorectics
attention deficit hyperactivity
    disorder
narcolepsy

KEY ABBREVIATIONS

ADHD	attention deficit hyperactivity disorder
cAMP	cyclic adenosine monophosphate
CNS	central nervous system
MAO	monoamine oxidase
TCAs	tricyclic antidepressants

THE TWO main groups of CNS stimulants are the **amphetamines** and related drugs, and the methylxanthines, such as **caffeine**.

The CNS stimulants exert their major effects on the cerebrum, medulla, brainstem and the hypothalamic or limbic regions. Amphetamines are mainly stimulants of the cerebral cortex; anorectic agents suppress the appetite, possibly by a direct stimulant effect on the satiety centres in the hypothalamic and limbic regions; **analeptics** (restorative drugs) primarily affect centres in the medulla and the brainstem. CNS stimulants act by increasing the neuronal discharge in excitatory pathways or by blocking inhibitory pathways.

Cerebral stimulants were commonly prescribed in the past for obesity and to counteract CNS-depressant overdosage, but such use today is generally considered obsolete. Although CNS stimulants suppress appetite, tolerance develops to the anorectic effect, usually before the weight reduction goal is reached. The main drugs used to suppress appetite are phentermine and diethylpropion (see later section on anorectic agents). Treating severe CNS depression with stimulants is also discouraged because close monitoring and supportive measures have been found to be quite successful, avoiding undesirable adverse reactions.

These drugs may also affect other parts of the nervous system, including the autonomic nervous system, so side-effects are common. With their narrow therapeutic indicies between effectiveness and toxicity, CNS stimulants may induce cardiac arrhythmias, hypertension, convulsions and violent behaviour. They therefore have limited use in practice today and are primarily used for the treatment of 'alertness disorders' such as **attention-deficit hyperactivity disorder (ADHD)** and narcolepsy and as appetite suppressants. They are also being examined for their effectiveness in improving functional recovery after brain injuries such as stroke.

AMPHETAMINES

Amphetamine itself (α-methylphenethylamine) is closely related chemically to noradrenaline, adrenaline and many other sympathomimetic amines (see Chapter 12). There are also trace amounts of similar amines in the brain, such as octopamine, tyramine and phenylethylamine, which, as well as being chemicals in the biosynthetic pathways for neurotransmitters, may act as neuromodulators. The amphetamine-like analogues have fewer hydroxyl (–OH) groups than do the catecholamines and thus have higher lipid solubilities and CNS activities. The generic term 'phenylethylamines' is sometimes used to refer to all the drugs in this group, including the four drugs described in this section: dexamphetamine, methylphenidate, phentermine and diethylpropion; however, as they are all related chemically to the prototype amphetamine, we will refer to the group as the **amphetamines**.

Amphetamine-like drugs have four main effects on the CNS:
- euphoria ('feel-good' excitement—people become hyperactive and talkative, fatigue is reduced, and sex drive is said to be enhanced; however, overconfidence may mask impaired performance*)
- locomotor stimulation (increased alertness and activity; animals are described as appearing busier rather than brighter)
- anorexia (appetite suppression)
- stereotyped behaviours (repeated inappropriate actions, such as animals gnawing, sniffing, or moving the head; in humans, choreas can develop, with repeated involuntary, purposeless movements).

The proposed mechanism of action for the **amphetamines** includes the release of noradrenaline, dopamine and other monoamines from storage sites in nerve terminals (hence an indirect sympathomimetic effect), direct stimulating effects on α- and β-adrenoceptor sites, and effects on dopamine transmission. The primary action centrally appears to be in the cerebral cortex and possibly the reticular activating system. Stimulation results in an increase in mental alertness and motor function, decreased sense of fatigue and, usually, a euphoric effect. These effects are probably mediated through effects on central adrenoceptors. Amphetamines can also cause stereotyped behaviours in animals (compulsive gnawing and sniffing) and paranoid psychosis in humans, similar to an acute schizophrenic attack. These effects are most likely related to actions on dopaminergic pathways, as they can be reversed by antipsychotic drugs.

Indirect actions at glutamate receptors have also been implicated in the mechanism of action of amphetamines and related CNS stimulants. Many of the actions of amphetamines (which cause convulsive, locomotor, stereotyped and circulatory behaviours) are blocked by antagonists at both types of glutamate receptors, and glutamate-receptor blockers may be useful in treatment of psychostimulant toxicity (Box 20-1). The acute toxicity of amphetamines, which causes cellular necrosis and loss of CNS neurons, is thought to be due to the formation of active free radicals and hence mitochondrial malfunction. In chronic abuse of amphetamines there is a strong association with psychoses and especially schizophrenia; whether this is a causal effect (amphetamines causing psychosis) and/or a 'dual diagnosis' effect (people with schizophrenia more likely to use or abuse drugs) is at present unclear.

---

*Amphetamines may improve performance in endurance sporting events and may increase alertness and reduce fatigue; hence they are prohibited by the World Anti-Doping Agency (see Chapter 57). Pharmacological folklore includes many anecdotes of university students who sat for examinations while 'high' on amphetamines (taken to help their studying), and spent the entire 3-hour exam time writing out their names!

BOX 20-1 MANAGING AMPHETAMINE OVERDOSE

Signs and symptoms of amphetamine overdose include dilated pupils, euphoria, confusion, delirium, convulsions, insomnia, psychosis, fever, sweating, tremors, rapid respiration, arrhythmias, cerebrovascular accidents and death.

There is no specific antidote for an overdose of amphetamines. Institute symptomatic and supportive measures according to the individual patient's requirement.

Generally, emesis and/or gastric lavage is indicated, followed by administration of activated charcoal to adsorb any remaining drug in the gastrointestinal tract; haemodialysis is ineffective. Excessive stimulation and seizures may be counteracted with diazepam or haloperidol (to decrease dopaminergic effects and hyperthermia). Urine acidification and forced diuresis are recommended in patients who do not respond to sedatives.

Vital signs, cardiac and respiratory functions, and hydration and nutrition should be monitored frequently. Medications usually used are: for hypertension, IV phentolamine or nitrites; for arrhythmias, lignocaine IV.

Tolerance develops readily to the peripheral and anorectic effects of amphetamines; indeed, the anorectic effects wear off a few days after taking these drugs, which detracts from their clinical usefulness. Addiction to and dependence on amphetamines can develop, possibly due to users taking more of the drugs to overcome the unpleasant mood swing (depression and tiredness) after the effects of a dose wear off, leading to 'binge' drug-taking behaviour. (These aspects of amphetamine abuse are covered in Chapter 22.) Because of their potential for abuse, amphetamines are no longer readily prescribed for use as appetite suppressants; instead, they are indicated only for the treatment of ADHD and in the treatment of narcolepsy. **Dexamphetamine** and **methylphenidate** fall under the Australian Poisons and Controlled Substances Regulations into the 'Controlled Drug' classification, Schedule 8, for drugs with a high abuse potential. Other proposed clinical uses are in recovery from stroke and from traumatic brain injury.

In the peripheral nervous system, amphetamines and related phenylethylamines have indirect sympathomimetic actions by causing the release of noradrenaline; hence they have vasoconstrictor and hypertensive effects. Drugs such as oxymetazoline and phenylephrine are used topically in the nose and eye for their decongestant effects (see Drug Monograph 32-8).

CNS STIMULANTS IN TREATMENT OF ADHD AND NARCOLEPSY

Attention-deficit hyperactivity disorder

The syndrome of **ADHD** is considered a psychiatric disorder of childhood (previously these children were probably just considered naughty or unmanageable). It is characterised by distractibility, a short attention span, impulsive behaviour, hyperactivity and learning disabilities; and the child may be moody and irritable and have low self-esteem. Improper functioning of the monoamine neurotransmitter systems (noradrenergic, dopaminergic and serotonergic) have been implicated in this syndrome. Paradoxically, CNS-stimulant medications tend to decrease the distractibility and hyperactivity, resulting in a lengthened attention span and improved cognitive performance and social behaviour.

The prevalence of ADHD in the community is about 1% and may be greater in more socially disadvantaged groups. Symptoms may present from infancy and ADHD usually becomes apparent between the ages of 3–7 years, with boys affected more often than girls by a 10:1 ratio. Usually professional intervention is unnecessary until the child enters the

CLINICAL INTEREST BOX 20-1 METHYLPHENIDATE — ITS (MIS)USE IN NEW ZEALAND

Medicines with legitimate medical indications are being increasingly diverted for illicit purposes. **Methylphenidate** is used for the treatment of narcolepsy and for ADHD in children and is regarded as a first choice pharmacological agent in the treatment of ADHD. It is available as an immediate-release (10mg) or sustained-release (20mg) tablet.

Methylphenidate stimulates the central nervous system and has a calming effect on ADHD children and allows them to focus on schoolwork. Patients with ADHD do not get addicted to the stimulant drug. However, when misused as an illicit drug, being snorted like cocaine or injected like heroin, it has powerful stimulant effects and can cause serious health risks. The street names include 'Rits' and 'poor mans coke'. In New Zealand, from February 1 2000, methylphenidate prescriptions were restricted to specialist recommendation, reflecting concerns that parents and children were obtaining methylphenidate too readily and then supplying it to others. Up till March 2002, more than 72 000 prescriptions for methylphenidate had been written, an increase of more than 30% over 2000. The street value of methylphenidate tablets is about $5, considerably less than in the US where the street value is about NZ$20.

school setting. ADHD may persist into adulthood, with higher incidences of substance abuse, antisocial personality disorders, anxiety and depression being observed in comparisons with control groups.

Managing this disorder requires a behavioural modification program (family support, directed activities, special educational programs, and psychotherapy) with use of pharmacological therapy as an adjunct if necessary. Around

DRUG MONOGRAPH 20-1 DEXAMPHETAMINE

Dexamphetamine, the (+) or dextro-isomer of amphetamine, is the prototype drug of this group. It is indicated for use in ADHD in children, and in narcolepsy (see later discussions).

PHARMACOKINETICS Amphetamines are well absorbed from the gut, with peak plasma concentrations reached 2 hours after oral administration. They are widely distributed to body tissues, with especially high concentrations in the brain and cerebrospinal fluid, lungs and kidneys. Some dexamphetamine is metabolised in the liver, and the remainder is excreted unchanged by the kidneys.

Excretion (and therefore half-life) is pH-dependent; excretion is increased in acidic urine and decreased in more alkaline urine. Approximate half-lives are 6–8 hours in acidic urine with pH <5 (e.g. after taking ammonium chloride); 15–30 hours in alkaline urine of pH >7.5 (e.g. after taking sodium or potassium citrate).

DRUG INTERACTIONS

Drug	Possible effect and management
Tricyclic antidepressants; CNS stimulants; sympathomimetics	Effects of these drugs are enhanced, which may result in adverse cardiovascular and CNS effects, such as arrhythmias, tachycardia or severe hypertension. Avoid or a potentially serious drug interaction may occur
MAO inhibitors, including reversible inhibitors of MAO-A (RIMAs)	Avoid concurrent usage because metabolism of amphetamines is inhibited; hence release of catecholamines is increased; headaches, arrhythmias, vomiting, sudden severe hypertension or hyperpyrexia may result. Avoid or a potentially serious adrenergic crisis may occur
β-Adrenergic blocking drugs (systemic and ophthalmic) and other autonomic antihypertensive agents	Amphetamines may overcome adrenoceptor antagonism of α- or β-blockers, causing sympathomimetic effects resulting in loss of blood pressure control, and hypertension

Drug	Possible effect and management
Digitalis glycosides	May result in an increase in cardiac arrhythmias
Thyroid hormones	Concomitant administration may result in enhanced effects of thyroid hormones or amphetamines

ADVERSE REACTIONS Important adverse reactions include:
- CNS: euphoria, increased irritability, insomnia, visual disturbance, dizziness, anorexia, dyskinesia and Tourette's syndrome
- cardiovascular system: tachycardia, angina
- autonomic nervous system: excessive sweating, dry mouth
- gastrointestinal system: nausea or vomiting,
- endocrine system: impotence, alterations in libido.

With high dosage or prolonged consumption, mood changes, including depression, increased agitation, choreas and psychosis may occur. Drug dependence and tolerance may also develop.

Treating amphetamine overdose consists of symptomatic and supportive care and reversal of CNS stimulation with sedatives, as outlined in Box 20-1.

WARNINGS AND CONTRAINDICATIONS Amphetamines have a high liability for abuse. The CNS stimulation and the depression after withdrawal both impair abilities to drive or operate machinery.

Avoid use in persons with amphetamine hypersensitivity, hyperthyroidism, hypertension, glaucoma, history of drug abuse, cardiovascular disease, severe agitation, severe arteriosclerosis and Tourette's syndrome. Amphetamines are contraindicated during pregnancy, as they cause increased risk of malformations, premature delivery and withdrawal symptoms in the infant (Category B3).

DOSAGE AND ADMINISTRATION Dosage depends on the indications for which the drug is prescribed and is adjusted individually to the lowest effective dose, not taken in the evenings because of the CNS excitation effects. Typical doses for school-age children are initially 5–10 mg daily, increasing to a maximum of 40 mg/day in ADHD.

15%–20% of children do not respond or their symptoms increase with the stimulant drugs; in these cases, antidepressant therapy with tricyclic agents or treatment with clonidine is indicated. To promote the child's proper psychosocial development, the distractibility and hyperactivity must be managed during school hours and at other times (e.g. for participation in clubs, music lessons or social events).

The two amphetamine-related drugs approved for treatment of ADHD in Australia are **dexamphetamine** (see Drug Monograph 20-1) and **methylphenidate**, which is more selective at blocking dopamine transporters. Use of these psychostimulants helps improve academic performance, vocational success and social and emotional development. Response is usually rapid and obvious. Doses are started low and gradually increased to a maximum of 30 mg dexamphetamine per day, provided effective responses are obtained. The prescriber needs to work closely with the child, the parents, carers and school staff in evaluating results and planning dosages. There are as yet no clear guidelines as to how long therapy should be continued. Widespread use of the drugs increases their availability for abuse, and diversion of the drugs from the school playground to the black market is becoming a problem, in both Australia and New Zealand (see Clinical Interest Box 20-1). New extended-release, long-acting formulations of methylphenidate are now available; these have many advantages including once-daily dosing, which improves the privacy of patients taking them and minimises the likelihood of the drugs being diverted or abused.

A new non-stimulant drug now available in treatment of ADHD is atomoxetine. This compound inhibits the reuptake of noradrenaline (as do cocaine and amphetamines); however, it appears not to cause CNS stimulation, and does not cause dependence, hence is not a controlled (S8) drug. It is well absorbed but has variable bioavailability; the half-life varies from 5 to 22 hours. Clinical placebo-controlled trials in children showed its efficacy in reducing ADHD symptoms; it was approximately equiactive with (but not better than) methylphenidate. As expected, autonomic side-effects are common, including dry mouth and raised pulse rate and blood pressure. Other recommended non-stimulant therapies include behavioural modification techniques in children, and cognitive behavioural therapy in adolescents and adults; drugs used include antidepressants, α_2-adrenoceptor agonists and cholinergic agents.

Narcolepsy

Narcolepsy is a condition characterised by excessive drowsiness and uncontrollable sleep attacks during the daytime, even during eating, driving or talking.* In addition, the

---

*As a colleague explained the condition to his students: 'If you fall asleep during my lectures, that's normal. If I do, that's narcolepsy.'

patient may exhibit a sleep paralysis (inability to move that occurs immediately on falling asleep or on awakening), cataplexy (stress-induced generalised muscle weakness), and hypnagogic illusions or hallucinations (vivid auditory or visual dreams occurring at onset of sleep). It is a specific, permanent neurological disorder, coming on in early adulthood and causing great distress to the sufferers.

Although narcolepsy is essentially incurable, education about the condition assists the patient to recognise the symptoms and adapt the daily schedule. CNS stimulants such as methylphenidate are useful in controlling the daytime drowsiness and excessive sleep patterns, whereas tricyclic antidepressants are being tested in conjunction with the stimulants for cataplexy and sleep paralysis.

A new non-amphetamine drug, modafinil, has been shown to be clinically effective in treating narcolepsy, with significantly increased scores on tests for maintenance of wakefulness and sleep latency. Modafinil was approved for use in Australia in February 2002. Its mechanism of action is unclear: it does not appear to bind with receptors for any monoamine transmitters. It improves alertness, and opposes the impaired cognitive functioning caused by lack of sleep, while not affecting appetite, behaviour, nocturnal sleep or the autonomic nervous system. A single dose taken in the morning is slowly absorbed, and eliminated mainly by metabolism in the liver to inactive metabolites which are excreted via the kidneys. The elimination half-life is approximately 10–12 hours. There are potential drug interactions with other drugs metabolised by CYP3A4; in women, combined oral contraceptives may be inactivated faster so other contraception should be used. Main adverse effects are central: headache, nausea, nervousness and possibly euphoria, hence the drug might be abused. The standard dose is 200–400 mg each morning. Modafinil may also prove useful in other disorders of sleep/wakefulness such as obstructive sleep apnoea and in shift-work.

CNS STIMULANTS AS ANORECTIC AGENTS

Anorectic (also called anorexiant or appetite-suppressant) drugs include a variety of medications used for the short-term treatment of obesity. They are indirectly acting sympathomimetics and are phenylethylamine-like or amphetamine-like drugs. Their exact mechanism of action is unknown but they appear to reduce hunger by effects in the hypothalamus and limbic areas of the brain. In the past, many such drugs were readily available to treat obesity by decreasing appetite; however, the amphetamines are liable to be abused because of their dependence potential, and tolerance develops rapidly, so amphetamine and dexamphetamine are no longer prescribed for obesity. Two other amphetamine analogues, fenfluramine and dexfenfluramine, were withdrawn in Australia because of their tendency to cause adverse cardiovascular effects (particularly pulmonary hypertension).

The only two remaining amphetamine-related compounds indicated as **anorectics** are diethylpropion and phentermine. These act mainly on adrenergic pathways and, while they do cause some CNS stimulation and mild euphoria, they are less liable to lead to dependence than are other amphetamines. Actions, adverse effects and drug interactions are generally similar to those of dexamphetamine.

Anorectic agents have several limitations, so careful selection and dosing are necessary to minimise the unwanted effects. As appetite suppressants they are recommended only for the short term because tolerance to the anorectic effect may occur within a few weeks. They are used as adjuncts to other obesity treatment regimens such as reducing absorption of fats, reducing energy intake, modifying diet, increasing physical activity, behavioural therapy and surgery (see Chapter 58 for pharmacological aspects of obesity).

Sibutramine, newly released in Australia, is a serotonin and noradrenaline reuptake inhibitor (SNRI) used to treat obesity. Other selective serotonin reuptake inhibitors (SSRIs, e.g. fluoxetine) used as antidepressants have also been shown to reduce appetite (see Table 19-3 and Clinical Interest Box 19-9 on Prozac).

METHYLXANTHINES CAFFEINE

The methylxanthines—**caffeine** (Drug Monograph 20-2), theophylline, theobromine and the herbal medicine *Paullinia cupana* (commonly known as guarana)—are naturally occurring chemicals found in beverages such as coffee, tea, cocoa and cola drinks. Caffeine is also present in many foods, over-the-counter drugs and prescription drugs; it is probably the most commonly used stimulant worldwide. A large daily intake of caffeine-containing products may increase alertness but may also induce insomnia and heart arrhythmias in some persons, especially the elderly. (Aspects of caffeine related to the social use of, and dependence on, caffeine-containing products are discussed in Chapter 22. The clinical use of methylxanthines as bronchodilators is considered in Chapter 32, including Figures 32-3 and 32-4 [showing their mechanisms of action], Drug Monograph 32-3 on theophylline and Box 32-1 on managing theophylline overdose.)

Mechanism of action

The mechanism of action of **caffeine** was initially postulated to involve raising of cyclic adenosine monophosphate (cAMP) levels through blocking of the enzyme phosphodiesterase (Figure 32-4), leading to smooth muscle relaxation and other

effects. However, it is now recognised that the concentrations required for this action are probably not reached in clinical (or social) doses.

Recent studies indicate that caffeine's effects are primarily due to antagonism of adenosine receptors (adenosine is an endogenous nucleoside and a neuromodulator that is structurally similar to caffeine). Adenosine mediates CNS depression, has cardiac depressant and bronchoconstrictor effects, inhibits platelet aggregation and is an important regulator of blood flow (vasodilator in most regions, including the coronary circulation, but vasoconstrictor in the renal and cerebral circulations). Adenosine is used clinically in supraventricular tachycardias: rapid IV injection decreases atrioventricular conduction and effectively converts the arrhythmia to sinus rhythm.

By antagonising adenosine A_1 and A_{2A} receptors, methylxanthines oppose these effects and indirectly lead to increased cAMP levels. This 'second messenger' is involved in activating many protein kinases, which may cause variations in energy metabolism, cell division and differentiation, changes in ion transport and ion channel functions, and contraction of cardiac and smooth muscle—hence the pharmacological effects described.

Some of the behavioural effects of caffeine are thought to be mediated by dopamine. By antagonising inhibitory effects of adenosine on dopamine receptors, caffeine may indirectly stimulate dopamine activity. This mechanism could explain the similarities between the behavioural effects of caffeine, amphetamines and cocaine; antagonists at A_{2A} receptors are being trialled in Parkinson's disease.

Pharmacological effects of caffeine

Because caffeine has effects on many body functions and is so widely used, both its short-term and possible long-term effects are important. Overall, moderate habitual coffee intake is not a health hazard.

CENTRAL NERVOUS SYSTEM

Although all levels of the CNS may be affected, regular doses of caffeine (100–150 mg) will stimulate the cortex and produce increased alertness but decreased motor reaction time to both visual and auditory events (see Clinical Interest Box 20-2). Drowsiness and fatigue generally disappear. Larger doses may affect the medullary, vagus, vasomotor and respiratory centres, resulting in slowing of the heart rate, vasoconstriction and increased respiratory rate.

Caffeine is thus useful for counteracting fatigue in shift-workers (and students) and as a cognitive enhancer, but can cause anxiety. The mechanism is thought to be via antagonism of adenosine receptors and consequent enhancement of dopamine activity. Caffeine also lifts the mood and may have antidepressant effects; it has been shown to reduce the risk of suicide. Caffeine withdrawal leads to headaches, fatigue, decreased alertness, and irritability;* it has therefore been used clinically to relieve postoperative withdrawal symptoms, and for post-dural-puncture headaches.

RESPIRATORY EFFECTS

Although the mechanism of action is not clearly defined, caffeine appears to stimulate the medullary respiratory centre and normalise autonomic function. Thus it may be useful for treating apnoea in preterm infants and Cheyne–Stokes respiration in adults, as an adjunct to non-drug measures and as an alternative to theophylline. The methylxanthines are an important group of bronchodilator agents; in particular, aminophylline, a derivative of theophylline, is used in childhood asthma.

CARDIOVASCULAR SYSTEM

In low doses caffeine is thought to enhance vagal stimulation and thus slow the heart. In higher doses, caffeine stimulates the myocardium, increasing both heart rate and cardiac output. Overstimulation may cause tachycardia and cardiac irregularities.

Depending on the dose, caffeine may cause either vasodilation, or a reflex increase in systemic vascular resistance, which can cause a rise in blood pressure. This latter effect

may be secondary to stimulation of the sympathetic nervous system and blockade of adenosine-induced vasodilation. Overall, caffeine has a weak vasodilator action, with little effect on blood pressure.

ANALGESIC ADJUNCT AND VASCULAR EFFECTS

Caffeine is used in analgesic products and in combination with ergotamine for treating migraine and other headaches, to enhance pain relief. The enhanced effect of ergotamine may be a result of better absorption of the ergotamine in the presence of caffeine; caffeine itself may also have some direct antimigraine action. Caffeine and theophylline cause potent cerebral vasoconstriction; the latter has been trialled in ischaemic stroke, on the rationale that a decrease in blood flow in perfused areas in the brain may enhance development of collateral vessels in ischaemic areas after stroke. Clinical evidence for benefit is not yet convincing.

MUSCULOSKELETAL SYSTEM

Caffeine affects voluntary skeletal muscles to increase the force of contraction and decrease muscle fatigue. These effects are via activation of the 'ryanodine receptor' family, activation of which opens calcium channels in the sarcoplasmic reticulum of skeletal muscle cells, causing calcium release and contraction of the muscle (see Clinical Interest Box 20-3, and Chapter 15, under Adverse effects of general anaesthetics). Caffeine also has a general thermogenic action, increasing heat production,

---

*This contributes to the morning 'hangover' in people who insist they are not fit to be spoken to until they have had their morning 'hit' of coffee.

DRUG MONOGRAPH 20-2 CAFFEINE

INDICATIONS Caffeine is used in the treatment of fatigue or drowsiness and as an adjunct to analgesics to enhance relief of pain; it is sometimes used as a respiratory stimulant in infants with respiratory difficulties.

PHARMACOKINETICS Caffeine is rapidly and totally absorbed after oral administration. It is only 35%–40% protein-bound and is distributed to all body compartments. It crosses the blood–brain barrier and enters the CNS, and passes readily through the placenta. The peak plasma level is achieved within 50–75 minutes, with therapeutic plasma levels at 5–25 mg/mL.

Caffeine is metabolised in the liver. In adults it is metabolised to theophylline and theobromine whereas in the neonate only a small portion is metabolised to theophylline. Caffeine's half-life is 3–10 hours (average 4 hours) in adults and 65–130 hours in neonates. In adults, caffeine is excreted by the kidneys, with only 1%–2% excreted unchanged; in neonates it is excreted by the kidneys, with about 85% excreted unchanged.

DRUG INTERACTIONS The following effects may occur when caffeine is taken with the drugs listed below:

Drug	Possible effect and management
Other CNS-stimulating drugs, other caffeine-containing medications or drinks	May result in increased CNS stimulation and undesirable side-effects such as increased nervousness, and arrhythmias
Adenosine	Caffeine and theophylline decrease the sensitivity of the myocardium to adenosine; larger doses of adenosine may be needed

ADVERSE REACTIONS Common adverse reactions include increased nervousness or anxiety and irritation of the gastrointestinal tract, resulting in dyspepsia and nausea. More frequent adverse reactions in neonates include abdominal swelling or distension, vomiting, body tremors, tachycardia or nervousness.

Signs of overdose include raised temperature, headache, confusion, increased irritability and sensitivity to pain or touch, tinnitus, insomnia, palpitations, fine tremor, increased urination, dehydration, nausea and vomiting, abdominal pain and convulsions.

A withdrawal syndrome of irritability, headache and increased weakness has been reported when users of more than 600 mg/day (about six cups of coffee) decrease or eliminate this intake.

WARNINGS AND CONTRAINDICATIONS Use with caution in persons with insomnia, nervousness and tachycardia.

Avoid use in patients with caffeine or xanthine hypersensitivity; severe anxiety, including agoraphobia or panic attacks; severe cardiac disease; liver function impairment; or hypertension.

DOSAGE AND ADMINISTRATION The adult dose is 100–200 mg orally, repeated in 3–4 hours if necessary to a maximum of 500 mg daily. (A standard cup of coffee contains 50–150 mg caffeine.) Caffeine is not recommended for use in children up to 12 years of age. It is present in combination with ergotamine in several formulations for treatment of migraine (see Chapter 21), in caffeinated beverages, and in some 'tonic' preparations in combination with vitamins and glucose; the usual dose of caffeine in these formulations is 100 mg.

---

possibly via the hypothalamus or by enhancing catecholamine effects.

Recently, interesting effects of methylxanthines have been demonstrated in bone. In animals some abnormalities of fetal bone and joint development have been shown. In humans there is some evidence that high caffeine intake may increase urinary excretion of calcium, decreasing bone mineral density. This could have important implications for the development of osteoporosis, especially in postmenopausal women.

GASTROINTESTINAL TRACT

Caffeine increases secretion of pepsin and hydrochloric acid from the parietal cells; hence coffee may cause dyspepsia, and intake is restricted in patients who have a gastric or duodenal ulcer.

RENAL SYSTEM

The methylxanthines produce a mild diuretic effect by increasing renal blood flow and glomerular filtration rate and by decreasing the tubular reabsorption of sodium and water. Theophylline is the only xanthine still used for this diuretic effect; however, the effect is well known to coffee drinkers and is additive with the diuretic effects of alcohol (see Figure 20-1).

ADDITIONAL EFFECTS

Caffeine also increases metabolic activity, inhibits uterine contractions, transiently raises glucose levels by stimulating glycolysis, and raises catecholamine levels in plasma and urine.

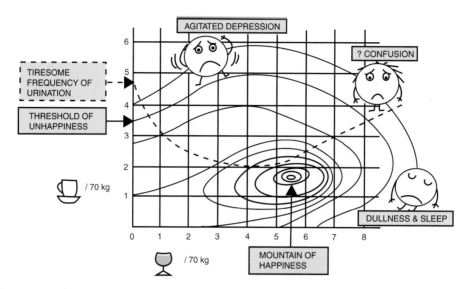

FIGURE 20-1 Drug interactions between caffeine and alcohol. The scenario is a dinner party or nightclub: alcohol is consumed during the evening, and coffee before leaving. Doses of alcohol (measured in glasses of wine per 70 kg adult) are plotted along the X-axis, and doses of caffeine (measured in cups of coffee per 70 kg adult) up the Y-axis. The CNS-depressant effect of alcohol taken alone leads to dullness and sleep, whereas the CNS-stimulant effect of caffeine alone causes agitation and depression. These effects are antagonistic, causing CNS confusion at high doses of both taken together. Unfortunately, the diuretic effects of the two drugs compound, leading to a tiresome frequency of urination.
Figure courtesy of Dr Andrew Herxheimer, in Laurence 1973; used with permission.

PREGNANCY SAFETY	
ADEC Category	**Drug**
A	Caffeine
B2	Diethylpropion, methylphenidate, phentermine
B3	Dexamphetamine, methylphenidate

DRUGS AT A GLANCE 20: Central nervous system stimulants

Therapeutic group	Pharmacological group	Key examples	Key pages
CNS stimulants	Amphetamines	dexamphetamine	339–2
	Others	methylphenidate	340–2
		modafinil	342
	Anorectics	diethylpropion phentermine }	342–3
	(Methyl)xanthines	caffeine	343–5

KEY POINTS

- The CNS-stimulant drugs have limited use in clinical practice today, as mild stimulants, appetite suppressants and in treating 'alertness disorders'.

- The amphetamines and related drugs have sympathomimetic actions (indirect and direct) and may also act through effects on dopamine and glutamate receptors.

● The main actions of the amphetamines are to cause euphoria, locomotor stimulation, anorexia and stereotyped movements. In overdose or chronic use they may lead to the development of tolerance, dependence and psychoses.

● The amphetamine-related stimulants dexamphetamine and methylphenidate are approved for use in treatment of attention deficit hyperactivity disorder (ADHD) and narcolepsy.

● When used as appetite suppressants, diethylpropion and phentermine are usually recommended as adjuncts to other regimens that include physical exercise, behaviour modification, diet and exercise.

● Caffeine and other methylxanthine alkaloids are CNS stimulants that are present in many beverages and medications. They have diverse pharmacological effects, and are used as mild CNS stimulants, bronchodilators and social drugs.

REVIEW EXERCISES

1. Differentiate between the proposed mechanisms of action for amphetamines and methylxanthines. Compare their main pharmacological effects and clinical uses.

2. Diethylpropion and phentermine have been promoted as being advantageous over the previous anorectic drugs that were removed from the market. Why?

3. List three contraindications for amphetamines and explain why CNS stimulants should not be used in these conditions.

4. Explain why CNS-stimulant drugs should not be used to treat patients who are currently taking (a) timolol ophthalmic drops, or (b) antidepressants (tricyclics or MAO inhibitors).

5. Describe the epidemiology and pathology of attention deficit hyperactivity disorder and outline its management.

6. When taking a medication history, why is the amount of caffeine consumed daily by the patient a concern? Name three illnesses or conditions that may be induced or exacerbated by the chronic consumption of large amounts of caffeine.

REFERENCES AND FURTHER READING

Australian Medicines Handbook 2005. Adelaide: AMH, 2005.
Banerjee D, Vitiello MV, Grunstein RR. Pharmacotherapy for excessive daytime sleepiness. *Sleep Medicine Reviews* 2004; 8(5): 339–54.
Bowman WC, Rand MJ. *Textbook of Pharmacology.* 2nd edn. Oxford: Blackwell, 1980 (chs 11, 24, 43).
Cauli O, Morelli M. Caffeine and the dopaminergic system. *Behavioural Pharmacology* 2005; 16(2): 63–77.
Guilleminault C, Pelayo R. Narcolepsy in children: a practical guide to its diagnosis, treatment and follow-up. *Paediatric Drugs* 2000; 2(1): 1–9.
Hazell P. Review of new compounds available in Australia for the treatment of attention-deficit hyperactivity disorder. *Australasian Psychiatry* 2004; 12(4): 369–75.
Juliano LM, Griffiths RR. A critical review of caffeine withdrawal: empirical validation of symptoms and signs, incidence, severity, and associated features. *Psychopharmacology* 2004; 176(1): 1–29.
Laurence DR. *Clinical Pharmacology.* 4th edn. Edinburgh: Churchill Livingstone, 1973.
Pockley P. Memory drugs flood the classroom. *Australasian Science* 2000; Nov/Dec: 28.
Psychotropic Expert Group. *Therapeutic Guidelines: Psychotropic, version 5.* Melbourne: Therapeutic Guidelines Limited, 2003.
Rang HP, Dale MM, Ritter JM, Moore PK. *Pharmacology.* 5th edn. Edinburgh: Churchill Livingstone, 2003.
Selikowitz M. *ADHD: The Facts.* Oxford: Oxford University Press, 2004.
Smith N, Temple W. Dosis facit venenum: raves that can kill with speed. *Australian Pharmacist* 2000; 19(8): 483.
Sulzer D, Sonders MS, Poulsen NW, Galli A. Mechanisms of neurotransmitter release by amphetamines: a review. *Progress in Neurobiology* 2005; 75(6): 406–33.
Waxmonsky JG. Nonstimulant therapies for attention-deficit hyperactivity disorder (ADHD) in children and adults. *Essential Pharmacology* 2005; 6(5): 262–76.

ON-LINE RESOURCES

New Zealand medicines and medical devices safety authority: www.medsafe.govt.nz

evolve More weblinks at http://evolve.elsevier.com/AU/Bryant/pharmacology/

CHAPTER 21

Drugs for Neurodegenerative Disorders and Migraine

CHAPTER FOCUS

This chapter covers the drugs used in treating various neurodegenerative disorders and dementias. Drugs with centrally mediated actions on skeletal muscle are also discussed, and the pharmacological treatment of headaches, especially migraine, is considered. These conditions are often progressive and incapacitating, and will become more common as our population ages. Hence an understanding of the disease processes and appropriate interventions is important for health-care professionals.

OBJECTIVES

- To explain the neurotransmitter balance theory in Parkinson's disease and describe the involvement of dopamine and acetylcholine in motor function and balance.

- To discuss the primary agents (dopaminergic, anticholinergic) used to treat Parkinson's disease, including their mechanisms of action, pharmacokinetics, drug interactions and primary adverse reactions.

- To review medications used to treat muscle spasm and spasticity, myasthenia gravis and dementias, including Alzheimer's disease.

- To compare the mechanisms of action of centrally acting and directly acting skeletal muscle relaxants and discuss their clinical use.

- To describe the treatment of headache, especially the involvement of 5-hydroxytryptamine (5-HT, serotonin) in the pathogenesis of migraine, and the use of 5-HT agonists and antagonists in treatment and prophylaxis.

KEY DRUGS

amantadine
apomorphine
baclofen
benztropine
botulinum toxin
carbidopa
dantrolene
donepezil
levodopa
methysergide
pergolide
pyridostigmine
rivastigmine
selegiline
sumatriptan

KEY TERMS

akinesia
Alzheimer's disease
anticholinergic
anticholinesterase agents
bradykinesia
dementia
dystonia
headache
migraine
myasthenia gravis
on–off syndrome
Parkinson's disease
skeletal muscle relaxant
spasms
spasticity

KEY ABBREVIATIONS

CNS	central nervous system
COMT	catechol-O-methyltransferase
DA	dopamine
DDC	dopa decarboxylase
DDI	dopa decarboxylase inhibitor
dopa	dihydroxyphenylalanine
GABA	gamma-aminobutyric acid
GIT	gastrointestinal tract
5-HT	5-hydroxytryptamine (serotonin)
MAO	monoamine oxidase
NMDA	N-methyl-D-aspartate
NMJ	neuromuscular junction

THE neurodegenerative disorders include a loose grouping of conditions such as Parkinson's disease, myasthenia gravis, multiple sclerosis and other movement disorders, and the dementias, including Alzheimer's disease and stroke-related cognitive impairments. The pathological processes occurring in these nervous system dysfunctions are not completely understood, and good animal models of the diseases and specific drug therapies are not always available.

The need to develop and monitor rational pharmacological interventions for these progressively deteriorating conditions is apparent. Currently there are no cures; therefore drug therapies are the primary methods used to minimise the symptoms of these illnesses. In some of the conditions, novel techniques involving transplantation of neurons and gene therapy are being trialled.

Spasticity of the skeletal muscles can also be debilitating; these muscles are affected by many pharmacological substances. Agents with effects at different levels in the central nervous system (CNS), i.e. in the brain or the spinal cord, or at the neuromuscular junction, are also discussed in this chapter, as are drugs used in treating migraine and other headaches.

DRUG TREATMENT OF PARKINSON'S DISEASE

Parkinson's Disease

Parkinson's disease is a progressively debilitating disorder of the basal ganglia, characterised by tremors at rest, bradykinesia (abnormal slowing of all voluntary movements and speech), forward flexion of the trunk, muscle rigidity, loss of postural reflexes and weakness. It occurs usually between the ages of 50 and 80 years, affecting both sexes equally. The prevalence is about 110 per 100,000 in the Australian population; however, about 1% of the population over the age of 55, and 1.5% of people in the 70–79 age group, have Parkinson's disease. Although the cause is unknown, genetic factors, viral influences and environmental contaminants have been suspected. Parkinsonism is classified as idiopathic (no known cause), postencephalitic (particularly after viral encephalitis), degenerative (e.g. due to arteriosclerosis), or drug-induced (especially by chronic administration of the antidopamine neuroleptic agents for schizophrenia).

The signs and symptoms are caused by a dopamine-deficiency state of the extrapyramidal motor system (see Figure 14-5), particularly in the nigrostriatal tracts. In affected patients, the levels of dopamine (DA, an inhibitory transmitter) in the basal ganglia fall to as low as 20% of normal levels. This produces a dopamine/acetylcholine imbalance, with a relative increase in acetylcholine (excitatory neurotransmitter). The correct balance of DA and acetyl-choline is important in regulating posture, muscle tone and voluntary movement (Figure 14-6 and Figure 21-1). The amounts of other monoamine neurotransmitters (e.g. noradrenaline and 5-hydroxytryptamine [5-HT, serotonin]) and of other transmitters (e.g. somatostatin, substance P and enkephalins) are also decreased in the brain of a person with Parkinson's disease. The condition has even been induced by designer drugs (Clinical Interest Box 21-1).

The CNS has two major types of DA receptors: D_1 and D_2 receptors. The exact role of the D_1 receptor is not currently known (although D_1 receptor activation is necessary for maximal expression of D_2 receptor activity), but D_2 and especially D_{2A} receptors are particularly involved with the motor effects of levodopa and the other dopamine agonists effective in Parkinson's disease.

Drug therapy is focused on correcting the DA/acetylcholine imbalance by raising DA levels or blocking acetylcholine effects. The classes of drugs used in treatment include (1) drugs that raise brain DA levels or stimulate DA receptors to enhance dopaminergic mechanisms, and (2) drugs with central **anticholinergic** activity (anticholinergics and antihistamines). No agents have yet been found that cure the condition or slow its progression. Drug treatment is usually not started until the symptoms have become disturbing to the patient. Non-drug therapies that have been tried include physiotherapy, surgery to specific tracts in the CNS and transplantation of dopaminergic neuronal tissue from fetal CNS. This is an exciting and busy area of pharmacological research, with a wide range of new molecules undergoing clinical trials: esterified forms of levodopa, MAO-B inhibitors, dopamine agonists and reuptake inhibitors, and new formulations of some older drugs. In addition, efforts are being made to treat dyskinesias with drugs acting at various receptors, and to halt or reverse disease progression with neuroprotective agents.

Drugs affecting brain dopamine

Three classifications of drugs mimic brain DA: those that raise brain levels of DA, those that release DA, and directly acting dopaminergic agonists. The drugs of choice in the treatment of Parkinson's disease are those that raise the brain levels of DA. The other two groups are used as adjuncts or when normal therapy is contraindicated.

The drugs enhancing brain DA have their major effect on the bradykinesia (slowed movements), **akinesia** (difficulty in initiating or the lack of ability to initiate muscle movement) and rigidity caused in Parkinson's disease by lowered levels of brain DA. The person with akinesia exhibits a mask-like facial expression, impairment of postural reflexes and eventually an inability for self-care. Dopamine enhancers are less effective in relieving the tremor associated with the condition.

Levodopa

In the biosynthetic pathways for the formation of the catecholamine neurotransmitters (see Figure 10-9), the starting point is the absorption of the essential amino acids phenylalanine and tyrosine from proteins in the diet. These are converted in adrenergic nerves to dopa (dihydroxyphenylalanine), the immediate precursor for DA. Dopamine itself cannot be given as a drug to 'top up' the stores in dopaminergic pathways, as it would be metabolised too rapidly, and would not pass the blood–brain barrier, so its precursor, levodopa, is administered. Levodopa is the first-line treatment for most patients. A large proportion (99%) of administered **levodopa** is metabolised in the liver and other cells by the enzyme dopa decarboxylase (DDC, also known as L-aromatic amino acid decarboxylase). Hence only a small proportion (1%) survives to cross the blood–brain barrier and be converted in dopaminergic neurons to DA (see Figure 21-2). For this reason large doses of levodopa used to be given, leading to

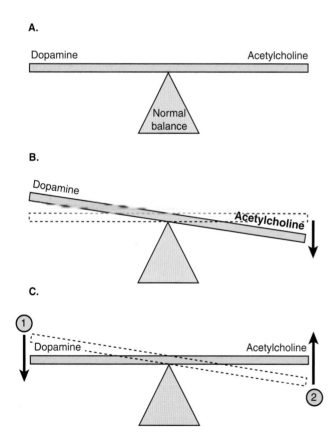

FIGURE 21-1 Central acetylcholine/dopamine balance. **A.** Normal 'balance' of acetylcholine and dopamine. **B.** In Parkinson's disease, a decrease in dopamine results in an acetylcholine/dopamine imbalance. **C.** Drug therapy for Parkinson's disease focuses on (1) increasing the dopamine level, which restores the acetylcholine/dopamine balance towards normal by increasing the supply of dopamine or stimulating dopamine receptors, and/or (2) blocking acetylcholine receptors or reducing acetylcholine levels.

**CLINICAL INTEREST BOX 21-1
PARKINSONISM INDUCED BY DRUGS**

'Designer drugs' (i.e. chemical variations of illegal or controlled substances) are an increasing problem in many societies. Such products are usually not yet illegal but are produced to mimic the psychoactive effects of various illegal products. Often the user consumes an unknown substance that may or may not be the desired product.

1-methyl-4-phenyl-1,2,3,6-tetrahydropyridine (MPTP), initially a contaminant of a preparation produced as an analogue of pethidine in clandestine laboratories, has been sold on the streets as heroin, cocaine or a contaminant of other 'street drugs'. MPTP in some users induces a severe degenerative CNS disorder characterised by tremors and muscle paralysis similar to the symptoms of Parkinson's disease. In some patients the paralysis has been permanent.

MPTP causes irreversible destruction selectively of the nigrostriatal dopaminergic pathways in various species, and has been used to induce in primates a parkinsonian syndrome. This is a very useful animal model in which to study the actions of drugs potentially useful in treating Parkinson's disease.

Not surprisingly, parkinsonian symptoms can also be induced by chronic administration of dopamine receptor antagonists. Thus antischizophrenic (neuroleptic) agents such as the phenothiazines (chlorpromazine, prochlorperazine) have been implicated in drug-induced parkinsonism.

---

major peripheral adverse reactions, including constipation, difficult urination, orthostatic hypotension, irregular heart rate and severe nausea or vomiting.

In a fine piece of pharmacological detective work and synthetic organic chemistry research, compounds were developed that inhibit the DDC enzyme in the peripheral nervous system, thus allowing a greater proportion of the levodopa dose to enter the CNS. Because the DDC inhibitors themselves were designed so as not to pass the blood–brain barrier, the enzyme is not inhibited in the CNS, where DA can still be synthesised from dopa. Thus the stores in the remaining functional CNS dopaminergic pathways are replenished, DA release is facilitated, and the remaining functional receptors are 'flooded' with DA. The dose of levodopa required is only 1/5 to 1/4 of that previously needed. The doses are taken orally immediately after meals.

The DDC inhibitor drugs used clinically, administered orally in conjunction with levodopa, are **carbidopa** (see Drug Monograph 21-1) and benserazide; both are structural analogues of DA and competitive inhibitors of the decarboxylase enzyme. So successful has this strategy been in reducing the dose of levodopa required and the peripheral adverse reactions, that levodopa is no longer available in Australia for use without a DDC inhibitor. The CNS effects of levodopa (confusion, especially in the elderly, nightmares, mood changes, and choreiform and involuntary movements of the body) are a greater risk with this combination because more levodopa reaches the brain to be converted to DA. The effectiveness of the combination often declines over years of chronic administration, resulting in the 'on–off syndrome', with increasing fluctuations in motor control (see Clinical Interest Box 21-2). Doses of levodopa and the frequency of administration eventually need to be increased to maintain therapeutic effect, and taking the dose without food can increase the rapidity of onset of action.

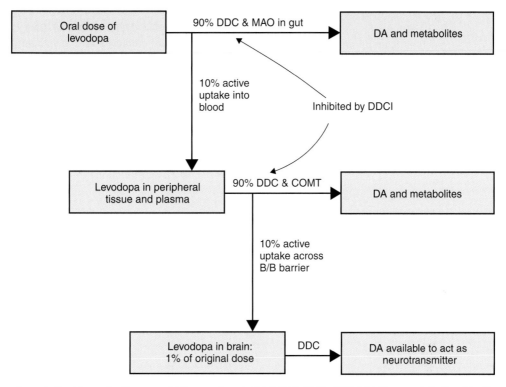

FIGURE 21-2 Levodopa in Parkinson's disease. Of the orally administered dose, about 99% is metabolised in the periphery by the enzymes dopa decarboxylase (DDC), monoamine oxidase (MAO) and catechol-*O*-methyltransferase (COMT), allowing only 1% to cross the blood–brain barrier (B/B barrier) and be converted to dopamine (DA). In the presence of a DDC inhibitor (DDCI), the enzyme in the periphery is inhibited, thus allowing a much greater proportion of administered dose to reach the CNS and be converted to active dopamine.

DRUG MONOGRAPH 21-1 LEVODOPA–CARBIDOPA

This combination formulation consists of **levodopa** plus **carbidopa** in a 4:1 or 10:1 ratio.

INDICATIONS Levodopa–carbidopa is indicated for the treatment of idiopathic, postencephalitic and symptomatic Parkinson's disease. The combination is particularly effective against rigidity and bradykinesia; tremor is less well treated.

PHARMACOKINETICS Levodopa is absorbed by active transport; much is metabolised in the gut by monoamine oxidase (MAO) and dopa decarboxylase (DDC), so only about 30%–50% reaches the systemic circulation. The drug is distributed to most body tissues; the CNS receives less than 1% of the dose. Levodopa has a half-life of

1–3 hours. The duration of action is up to 5 hours per dose. Metabolites, principally homovanillic acid, are excreted by the kidneys.

After an oral dose of carbidopa, 40%–70% of the carbidopa dose is absorbed. Carbidopa is distributed widely to many body tissues, with the exception of the CNS. Peak plasma levels of carbidopa appear in 2–5 hours. The drug's metabolism is insignificant; it is excreted by the kidneys.

Usually, improvement is seen within 2–3 weeks, although some patients require levodopa for up to 6 months to obtain a therapeutic effect.

DRUG INTERACTIONS The following effects can occur when levodopa plus a DDI is given with the drugs listed:

DRUG MONOGRAPH 21-1 LEVODOPA–CARBIDOPA

Drug	Possible effect and management
Anticonvulsants, neuroleptics, including phenothiazines and metoclopramide	Can result in decreased levodopa effects, because hydantoin anticonvulsants increase levodopa metabolism, and metoclopramide and antipsychotic neuroleptic agents such as phenothiazines block dopamine receptors in the brain. If possible, avoid the combination of neuroleptics with levodopa
Antihypertensives	Increased risk of postural hypotension; decrease dose
Monoamine oxidase (MAO) inhibitors (type A)	This combination can result in a hypertensive crisis. MAO inhibitors should be discontinued 2–4 weeks before starting levodopa therapy
Monoamine oxidase (MAO) inhibitors (type B) (selegiline)	This combination may be used (see later), but can result in increased levodopa-induced nausea and CNS effects. Levodopa dose should be reduced

ADVERSE REACTIONS Adverse reactions due to levodopa include anxiety, dyskinesias, confusion (especially in the elderly), difficult urination, depression, orthostatic hypotension, mood changes, irregular heart rate, severe nausea or vomiting and sudden loss of mobility. The effectiveness of levodopa appears to wear off after chronic administration (see Clinical Interest Box 21-2 for more information on the on–off syndrome).

A withdrawal syndrome can occur, resembling the 'neuroleptic malignant syndrome' related to decreased dopaminergic transmission.

Adverse reactions due to levodopa–carbidopa are similar to those for levodopa. Eyelid spasms or closing (blepharospasm) may be an early sign of drug overdose.

WARNINGS AND CONTRAINDICATIONS Caution is required in severe cardiovascular, pulmonary, renal, hepatic, psychiatric and endocrine diseases, in glaucoma and peptic ulcer, and during pregnancy (Category B3). The combination is contraindicated in wide-angle glaucoma. Levodopa can activate melanomas. Monitoring should be carried out for mental, behavioural and intraocular pressure changes, and for arrhythmias.

Dopamine agonists are contraindicated during lactation, as dopamine inhibits secretion of prolactin (see Clinical Interest Box 39-3), and during treatment with typical antipsychotic agents.

DOSAGE AND ADMINISTRATION Levodopa dosage for adults is initiated with 50 mg twice daily, increasing by 100–125 mg until a therapeutic response is achieved, to a maximum of 2 g/day. The tablets should always be taken before food.

The available levodopa–carbidopa combination dosage forms include 100/25 (100 mg levodopa and 25 mg carbidopa), 250/25 (250 mg levodopa and 25 mg carbidopa), and a controlled-release formulation 200/50 (200 mg levodopa and 50 mg carbidopa). These three combination dosage forms are available to permit greater flexibility in prescribing sufficient amounts of both levodopa and carbidopa, and in titrating the dose–response relationship for the individual. The controlled-release formulations can minimise the on–off swings, but they have lower oral bioavailability, so higher levodopa doses may be required.

CLINICAL INTEREST BOX 21-2 LEVODOPA 'ON–OFF' SYNDROME

On–off syndrome refers to a complication following prolonged levodopa therapy (2 years or more). The patient fluctuates from being symptom-free ('on') to demonstrating full-blown Parkinson's symptoms ('off') during therapy. These effects can last from minutes to hours, and might be due to a decrease in delivery of dopamine centrally, an alteration in sensitivity of the dopamine receptors, a variation in the amount and rate of drug absorption, a dopamine metabolite interference or a combination of effects.

Treatment may require more frequent administration of levodopa or levodopa–DDC inhibitor, and perhaps the addition of a direct-acting dopamine agonist, bromocriptine. Concurrent administration of a COMT inhibitor (entacapone) helps reduce 'off' times. After a drug holiday (drug withdrawal) of several days to a week, some people demonstrate an improved response to the drug therapy. This might be because of the re-establishment of dopamine receptor sensitivity to levodopa, which is usually only temporary. Because symptoms can worsen during the drug-free period, this approach should be instituted in a hospital setting.

Ergot derivatives

The ergot alkaloids are derivatives of a fungus, *Claviceps purpurea*, which grows on damp rye grains and can cause outbreaks of poisoning (ergotism). These compounds are renowned for having different effects on a variety of receptors, and thus can cause intense vasoconstriction, ischaemia and hypertension (sympathomimetic effects), or vasodilation and flushing (by blocking α-adrenoceptors), uterine contractions (an oxytocic effect on uterine smooth muscle) and agonistic or antagonistic actions on 5-HT receptors. Derivatives include ergometrine (used as an oxytocic agent: see Drug Monograph 45-1); ergotamine, dihydroergotamine and methysergide (used in migraine); bromocriptine (a central DA agonist, used to inhibit lactation); and lysergic acid diethylamide (LSD, the classic hallucinogenic agent, discussed in Chapter 22).

The ergot derivatives used in Parkinson's disease are bromocriptine, **pergolide** and cabergoline. They stimulate central DA receptors, and thus improve bradykinesia and rigidity, but are less effective than levodopa. The ergot derivatives, however, used together with a levodopa–DDC inhibitor combination allow lower doses of levodopa, and hence can delay the onset of motor fluctuations (on–off syndrome) and dyskinesias. A peripheral DA antagonist (domperidone, an antiemetic) is sometimes given concurrently to minimise peripheral dopamine effects (nausea, hypotension).

Pergolide is more potent and longer-acting (for 4–6 hours) than bromocriptine and directly stimulates both D_1 and D_2 receptors. Many patients who did not respond to levodopa have improved with the addition of pergolide to levodopa therapy.

Drug interactions can be expected with DA antagonists, such as the phenothiazines, thioxanthines, haloperidol and metoclopramide. In addition, drugs that produce hypotension can have an additive hypotensive effect when administered concurrently with ergot alkaloids.

Adverse reactions are similar to those for levodopa, and include effects in the GIT and CNS. The drugs should be used with caution in patients with arrhythmias and psychosis. Because of their DA agonist actions, these ergot derivatives inhibit lactation, so are contraindicated in breastfeeding women. Cabergoline is used as a lactation inhibitor and to treat hyperprolactinaemia.

Other dopaminergic agonists

Apomorphine is a DA agonist not related chemically to ergot derivatives; it is, as its name implies, a morphine derivative but has very little analgesic activity (see Clinical Interest Box 21-3).

In Parkinson's disease, apomorphine is used in people severely disabled by motor fluctuations in levodopa response that are non-responsive to other treatment. Adverse reactions are similar to dopaminergic effects of levodopa or the ergot alkaloids, especially vomiting, hypotension and psychiatric disturbances. Apomorphine is contraindicated in many conditions, including cardiovascular diseases, respiratory or CNS depression, dyskinesias and psychiatric disorders. Because of its low therapeutic index and the need to determine an effective dose range during an 'off' motor period, the drug is best administered in a hospital setting under specialist supervision.

CLINICAL INTEREST BOX 21-3 APOMORPHINE, THE ARCHETYPAL EMETIC AGENT

Apomorphine is a morphine derivative with a four-ring structure that can be imagined to contain the dopamine backbone. It acts as a dopamine (DA) analogue and stimulates central DA receptors. Its pharmacology is interesting:

- It stimulates the medullary chemoreceptor trigger zone and is a powerful emetic in animals that can vomit (including dogs and humans).
- In animals that cannot vomit (e.g. rats, rabbits), it causes excitation, agitation and stereotyped behaviours, similar to the effects of amphetamines.
- Its actions are antagonised by chlorpromazine, the classic antidopamine phenothiazine neuroleptic agent.
- It has been used as an emetic in medicine, to treat poisoning by orally ingested (non-corrosive) substances.
- It has been used in aversion therapy to break the pattern of drug use in dependent people; for example given with a dose of the addictive drug, it induces vomiting, and the response becomes conditioned such that eventually the drug without apomorphine induces vomiting.
- In Parkinson's disease, apomorphine is useful for relief of tremor and corrects the sudden loss of levodopa efficacy in late-stage disease.
- It is administered parenterally (SC) or sublingually, as it has little effect if taken orally.
- To prevent its powerful emetic actions, the antiemetic domperidone is given prophylactically before apomorphine; domperidone is a DA antagonist that does not cross the blood–brain barrier, so does not antagonise the actions of apomorphine or DA in the CNS.
- The cocktail of domperidone (peripheral DA antagonist), apomorphine (central DA agonist), carbidopa (peripheral dopa-decarboxylase inhibitor) plus levodopa (central DA precursor) is a powerful combination.

Other non-ergot dopaminergic agonists include ropinirole and pramipexole; however the latter drug is not marketed in Australia.

Drugs raising brain dopamine levels
Amantadine, a dopamine-releasing drug

Amantadine is a synthetic antiviral compound used occasionally to treat influenza (see Chapter 32). Although its mechanism of action is not completely known, it is postulated that amantadine releases DA and other catecholamines from neuronal storage sites. It also blocks the uptake of DA into presynaptic neurons, thus permitting peripheral and central accumulation of DA. It has useful antimuscarinic activity, and may give the person a sense of wellbeing and elevation of mood. It is less effective than levodopa but produces more rapid clinical improvement and causes fewer untoward reactions.

Amantadine is indicated for use as an antidyskinetic agent in treatment of mild Parkinson's disease, and as an antiviral drug used in treatment of influenza. It is well absorbed orally and is excreted by the kidneys unchanged, so doses need to be reduced in patients with kidney impairment. There are clinically significant drug interactions with dopamine antagonists (which oppose its effects) and other drugs with anticholinergic actions (which are additive).

Adverse reactions are typical anticholinergic (atropinic) effects and effects of DA agonists (GIT, mood and cardiovascular changes). In addition, amantadine can cause unusual purple-red skin spots (livedo reticularis, usually seen with chronic therapy).

Selegiline, a monoamine oxidase inhibitor

There are two types of monoamine oxidase (MAO) in the body: monoamine oxidase A is relatively specific to metabolism of noradrenaline and 5-HT; monoamine oxidase B metabolises mainly DA. (Reversible inhibitors of MAO-A are used as antidepressants: see moclobemide in Chapter 19.) Selegiline irreversibly inhibits MAO-B, thus preventing the breakdown of DA, and blocks DA reuptake (see Drug Monograph 21-2). As a result it will enhance or prolong levodopa's antiparkinson effect, which might result in a lowering of the daily dose of levodopa. Another MAO-B inhibitor, rasagiline, has been approved but is not marketed in Australia.

Entacapone, a catechol-*O*-methyltransferase inhibitor

The other main enzyme involved in metabolism of the catecholamines, including noradrenaline and DA, is catechol-O-methyltransferase (COMT). Thus a COMT inhibitor, analogous to an MAO inhibitor (MAOI), will also inhibit

---

DRUG MONOGRAPH 21-2 SELEGILINE

Selegiline is used as adjunctive therapy in late-stage Parkinson's disease, in combination with levodopa or levodopa–carbidopa.

PHARMACOKINETICS Selegiline, a phenylethylamine derivative, is well absorbed orally, reaching its peak plasma level in 30 minutes to 2 hours. It is rapidly metabolised and has three active metabolites, including L-amphetamine and methamphetamine (with half-lives of 2–20 hours), so has low bioavailability. It readily crosses the blood–brain barrier; metabolites are excreted slowly via the kidneys.

DRUG INTERACTIONS The following effects can occur when selegiline is given with the drugs listed below:

Drug	Possible effect and management
Other MAO inhibitors, selective serotonin reuptake inhibitors (SSRIs) (including fluoxetine and sertraline), sumatriptan and pethidine	Concurrent use with selegiline can result in mania and a reaction similar to the serotonin syndrome (confusion, restlessness, hyperreflexia, sweating, shivering, tremors, diarrhoea, ataxia and fever). Avoid or a potentially serious drug interaction could occur. These drugs should not be initiated until 2–5 weeks after selegiline is discontinued

Drug	Possible effect and management
Levodopa	Although selegiline is indicated to be given concurrently with levodopa, this combination can increase levodopa-induced adverse reactions such as dyskinesias, nausea, hypotension, confusion and hallucinations. To reduce this potential, the dose of levodopa should be lowered
Tyramine-rich foods	The 'tyramine reaction' is less severe than with MAO-A inhibitors; however, hypertension can occur

ADVERSE REACTIONS These are typical dopaminergic effects, including nausea, vomiting, insomnia, dizziness, stomach distress or pain, dyskinesias and mood alterations.

WARNINGS Use with caution in patients with movement or cardiovascular disorders, psychoses, history of peptic ulcer disease, or selegiline hypersensitivity.

DOSAGE AND ADMINISTRATION The usual adult dose of selegiline is 2.5–5 mg twice daily.

the inactivation of DA and prolong the clinical response to levodopa, increasing the 'on' time for motor response. The only COMT inhibitor currently available for use in Parkinson's disease is a relatively new drug, entacapone, a reversible and specific inhibitor. It is always used with a levodopa–DDC inhibitor combination.

As entacapone increases both clinical effects of and adverse reactions to levodopa, the dose of levodopa needs to be decreased by 10%–30%. Drug interactions are similar to those for other drugs that increase dopaminergic activity, i.e. with MAOIs, catecholamines and tricyclic antidepressants. Currently drug trials are underway to test whether addition of entacapone to levodopa–DDCI therapy early in the course of treatment will delay development of motor complications. Entacapone is contraindicated in hepatic impairment, and liver functions are monitored, as a similar drug was withdrawn from use due to severe hepatic reactions.

Drugs with central anticholinergic activity

Symptoms of Parkinson's disease caused by an excess of cholinergic activity include muscle rigidity and muscle tremor (see Figure 21-1). The muscle rigidity or increased tone appears as ratchet resistance, or cogwheel rigidity, in which the affected muscle moves easily, then meets resistance or remains fixed in the new position. The muscle tremors appear to have a to-and-fro movement caused by the sequence of contractions of agonistic and antagonistic muscles involved. The tremors are usually worse at rest and are commonly manifested as a pill rolling motion of the hands and a bobbing of the head. Anticholinergics are more useful early in the course of the disease because the adverse reactions to DA depletion are not prominent at this stage.

The **anticholinergics**, which readily cross the blood–brain barrier, can block central cholinergic excitatory pathways, returning the DA–acetylcholine balance in the brain (especially in the basal ganglia) to normal and producing some improvement in functional capacity and relief of tremor. There is less effect on the rigidity and akinesia.

The belladonna alkaloids atropine (see Drug Monograph 11-2) and hyoscine were the first centrally active (i.e. crossing the blood–brain barrier) anticholinergic agents used to treat parkinsonism; for many years they were the only drugs available for such treatment. These drugs have been supplanted by synthetic anticholinergics, which were developed in an effort to produce drugs as effective as the belladonna drugs but with fewer adverse reactions. In this group **benztropine** is the key drug; there is little to choose between the various anticholinergics, but benztropine and orphenadrine have more pronounced antihistaminic actions than do others, such as benzhexol and biperiden. The usefulness of these drugs is limited because of their anticholinergic (atropinic)

adverse reactions and their tendency to be less effective with continued use. Some anticholinergics are also used to control extrapyramidal reactions, such as rigidity, akinesia (difficulty in or lack of ability to initiate muscle movement), tremor and akathisia, which are caused by antipsychotic drugs such as the phenothiazines.

DRUGS AFFECTING SKELETAL MUSCLES

The physiology of the motor nervous system is reviewed in Chapter 13, and drugs that affect transmission at the neuromuscular junction (NMJ) are discussed there. These drugs are used in many different clinical contexts, e.g. as **skeletal muscle relaxants** during surgical operations, to stimulate acetylcholine receptors in muscle weakness, to relieve spasticity and spasms in skeletal muscle and to treat ocular disorders such as glaucoma. These clinical uses are discussed in the relevant chapters. Here we discuss drugs affecting central control of skeletal muscle and some drugs that affect skeletal muscle actions in movement disorders with a central component, such as cerebral palsy and multiple sclerosis.

Thus the drugs considered here are those that affect central control of motor activity via gamma-aminobutyric acid (GABA) receptors, or affect neurotransmission at the NMJ via acetylcholine receptors. Drugs that have motor effects via actions on central DA receptors have been covered in the previous section on Parkinson's disease, and in Chapter 19 (on psychotropic agents).

Anticholinesterases

The **anticholinesterase agents** (cholinesterase inhibitors) enhance cholinergic actions by inhibiting the effect of the cholinesterase enzymes that inactivate acetylcholine at cholinergic nerve terminals (see Figures 10-8 and 13-4; and Drug Monograph 13-3 on neostigmine). This permits the accumulation of acetylcholine and enhanced effects at autonomic ganglia, parasympathetic neuroeffector junctions, and neuromuscular junctions. In **myasthenia gravis** (see Clinical Interest Box 21-4 and Figure 21-3), the increased amount of acetylcholine (ACh) at the NMJ competes more successfully with antibodies against the ACh receptors for receptor binding sites and thus reduces fatigue in muscle. Anticholinesterases that are lipid-soluble and thus cross the blood–brain barrier are used for their central effects on cholinergic transmission, especially in dementias (see later section).

The anticholinesterase agents are generally divided into three groups based on their duration of action, which is determined largely by the type of binding to the enzyme. Of the medium-acting agents, **pyridostigmine** has better oral bioavailability than neostigmine, a longer half-life and fewer GIT adverse reactions, so it is the first-line drug for myasthenia gravis.

Skeletal muscle relaxants

Most muscle strains and spasms are self-limited and respond to rest and physiotherapy and short-term skeletal muscle relaxants. Spasticity (a form of muscular hypertonicity with increased resistance to stretch) as the result of stroke, closed head injuries, cerebral palsy, multiple sclerosis, spinal cord trauma and other neurological disorders may require long-term use of these agents.

Skeletal muscle spasm and spasticity

Skeletal muscle **spasms**, or cramps, result when there is an involuntary contraction of a muscle or group of muscles, accompanied by pain or limited function. Most skeletal muscle spasms are caused by local injuries, but some result from low calcium or sodium levels or epileptic myoclonic seizures. Each type of spasm is treated according to its cause. Skeletal muscle injuries are usually self-limiting and can be treated with rest, physiotherapy, or immobilisation by use of casts, neck collars, crutches or arm slings. When tissue damage and oedema are present, however, anti-inflammatory drugs may be used.

Central skeletal muscle relaxants are used mainly for conditions in which muscle spasms do not quickly respond to other forms of therapy. Such conditions include musculoskeletal strains and sprains, trauma, and cervical or lumbar radiculopathy (disease of the spinal nerves and their roots) as a result of degenerative osteoarthritis, herniated disc, spondylosis or laminectomy. Diazepam is useful in the treatment of muscle spasms.

Skeletal muscle **spasticity**, characterised by skeletal muscle hyperactivity, occurs when gamma motor neurons (which tonically control muscle spindle contractile activity) become hyperactive. There are two primary types of muscle spasticity: spinal and cerebral.

Spinal spasticity can be identified by a marked loss of inhibitory influences with hyperactive tendon stretch reflexes, clonus (alternate contraction and relaxation of muscles), primitive flexion withdrawal reflexes, and a flexed posture. Varying degrees of spasticity of the bladder and bowel can also occur.

Cerebral spasticity has less reflex excitability, increased or impaired muscle tone, and no primitive flexion withdrawal reflexes or flexed posture.

Muscle spasticity is most commonly seen in patients with CNS injuries and strokes. Moderate to severe spasticity occurs in two-thirds of patients with multiple sclerosis. Individuals with cerebral palsy and rare neurological disorders can also have muscle spasticity.

Centrally acting and directly acting skeletal muscle

CLINICAL INTEREST BOX 21-4 MYASTHENIA GRAVIS

Although this condition is very rare — occurring with a world-wide prevalence of about 7.5–10 per 100,000 population — it has long been of great interest to pharmacologists, because of the interesting pharmacological concepts that it exemplifies.

Myasthenia gravis is a progressive, incurable disease characterised by the loss of or decrease in acetylcholine receptors, which is caused by an autoimmune process and results in skeletal muscle weakness and fatigue. The thymus gland is believed to be involved in the causation of myasthenia gravis, through the production of antibodies directed against the acetylcholine receptor proteins. Nearly 15% of all myasthenia gravis patients have a thymoma, or tumour of the thymus gland. Clinical signs and symptoms, and implications, are shown in Figure 21-3.

The most common early reported symptoms are ptosis and diplopia. The person might complain of shoulder fatigue after shaving or combing the hair, or of hand weakness, finding it difficult to open doors or kitchen jars or to perform repetitive tasks, such as playing the piano. The most serious consequences of myasthenia gravis are dysphagia and respiratory muscle weakness, since these can result in aspiration pneumonia or respiratory failure.

Treatment of this disease state may include thymectomy, which brings partial or complete remission in two-thirds of patients, plasmapheresis to remove antibodies, and drug therapy, including cholinesterase inhibitors, corticosteroids and azathioprine. Anticholinesterases allow increased levels of ACh at cholinergic nerve endings, thus competing with antibodies for binding sites on remaining receptors.

---

relaxants are the drugs of choice in treating muscle spasticity. These drugs include baclofen, diazepam and dantrolene. They are more effective in the treatment of spinal spasticity than cerebral spasticity; concurrent physiotherapy is always required for optimal treatment. Excessive muscle relaxation can cause the serious adverse reactions of dysphagia (difficulty in swallowing) and choking.

Centrally acting skeletal muscle relaxants

The exact mechanism of action of the central skeletal muscle relaxants is not known. The drugs cause CNS depression in the brain (brainstem, thalamus and basal ganglia) and spinal cord that results in relaxation of striated muscle spasm; thus CNS depression accompanies the muscle relaxation. Consequently, these drugs create the adverse reactions of drowsiness, blurred vision, light-headedness, headache and feelings of weakness, lassitude and lethargy that make their long-term use undesirable. The main centrally acting drugs used primarily as antispastic agents are **baclofen** (see Drug

CLINICAL SIGNS

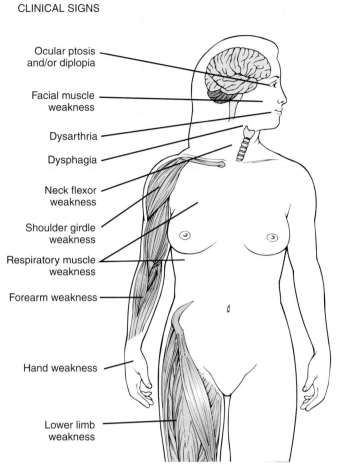

Ocular ptosis and/or diplopia

Facial muscle weakness

Dysarthria

Dysphagia

Neck flexor weakness

Shoulder girdle weakness

Respiratory muscle weakness

Forearm weakness

Hand weakness

Lower limb weakness

SYMPTOMS

- Drooping of upper eyelids
- Double vision
- Diminished expression
- Slurred speech
- Difficulty swallowing
- Shoulder tiredness
- Exhaustion, decrease in respirations
- Arm fatigue and/or weakness

IMPLICATIONS

- Symptoms become worse with exertion but will improve with rest.
- Stress, menstruation, infections, surgery and vigorous physical exercise may worsen symptoms.
- Symptom severity may fluctuate from morning to night and from day to day.
- Muscle weakness common; sensory loss and coordination difficulties not reported in myasthenia gravis patients.

FIGURE 21-3 Signs, symptoms and implications of myasthenia gravis.

Monograph 21-3) and diazepam, both of which act via effects on gamma-aminobutyric acid (GABA) transmission. A related compound, gamma-hydroxybutyric acid, previously used as an anaesthetic agent, has been subject to abuse as a street drug (see Clinical Interest Box 21-5).

DIAZEPAM

The clinical uses of diazepam as an antianxiety and anti-epileptic agent are discussed in detail in Chapters 17 and 18, under the benzodiazepines (see Drug Monograph 17-1). It appears to act primarily by modulation of GABA transmission, leading to hyperpolarisation of cells and postsynaptic inhibition, in brain and spinal pathways, and thus reduces muscle tone and coordination. It can also directly suppress muscle function at the neuromuscular synapse.

Diazepam is used in the treatment of skeletal muscle spasm caused by reflex spasm to local pathological conditions, such as inflammation of muscle and joints or secondary to trauma. It is also used to treat spasticity caused by upper motor neuron disorders (cerebral palsy and paraplegia), athetosis, tetanus and stiff-man syndrome (to overcome the widespread chronic muscular rigidity, pain and skeletal muscle spasms).

TETRABENAZINE

Tetrabenazine is a centrally acting skeletal muscle relaxant that acts via effects on dopamine pathways. It releases monoamine neurotransmitters and depletes brain DA levels, and thus causes sedation and muscle relaxation. It was formerly used as a neuroleptic agent, but causes parkinsonism, extrapyramidal effects and depression, so is now used only occasionally in treatment of movement disorders.

Peripherally acting skeletal muscle relaxants

NEUROMUSCULAR BLOCKING AGENTS

Perhaps the most important skeletal muscle relaxants are those classified as the neuromuscular blocking agents. The two groups are:

- the non-depolarising drugs, which compete with ACh at the NMJ end-plate and antagonise nicotinic receptors and thus cause flaccid paralysis (exemplified by curare and pancuronium, Drug Monograph 13-1)
- the depolarising blockers (suxamethonium, Drug Monograph 13-2), which activate the nicotinic receptors,

CLINICAL INTEREST BOX 21-5
GRIEVOUS BODILY HARM
AND FANTASY

Since 2002 it has been illegal for people to possess and supply the drug Fantasy (Misuse of Drugs Act 1975). Fantasy and Grievous Bodily Harm are misnomers for the sedative drug gamma-hydroxybutyric acid (GHB, also known as sodium oxybate), which is an analogue of the inhibitory neurotransmitter GABA. GHB is a naturally occurring metabolite of GABA. Muscimol, a natural hallucinogenic ingredient of some mushrooms, is also an analogue of GHB that has psychotomimetic effects.

The structures of GHB and GABA are very similar:

GHB $CH_2OH-(CH_2)_2-COOH$

GABA $CH_2NH_2-(CH_2)_2-COOH$

GHB injected IV causes a long-lasting unconsciousness (90 min) after a delay of 8–15 min, and has been used as an induction anaesthetic. It has weak analgesic actions, but en¬hances the actions of narcotic analgesics and neuro¬muscular blocking agents. It causes little depression of the cardiovascular or respiratory systems, but can cause hallucinations, hence is no longer used medically. The drug comes in a clear liquid form (although food colourant can be added) and is often mixed with drinks. It is becoming known as a 'date rape' drug. Particular risks for these substances include the following:

- There is a very fine line between the dose required to give the desired effect and that causing an overdose;
- There is delayed onset of effect, which causes people to use too much of the drug; the unpredictability, effects and drug interactions;
- There is a likelihood of people becoming dependent; and
- It increases the risks associated with driving while intoxicated, or of drug-assisted sexual assaults.

In October 1996, Australian Police in Victoria issued a warning after several people in a Gold Coast night club suffered respiratory depression and hallucinations. It is thought that their drinks were spiked with Grievous Bodily Harm, which is used in the rave dance music scene in Europe and the United States as an alternative to ecstasy or speed.

In New Zealand, the number of people admitted to accident and emergency departments after taking life-threatening overdoses of Fantasy/Grievous Bodily Harm has been increasing over the past few years. In 2001, the Ministry of Health repeated its warning to the public about products containing butanediol, GHB, or fantasy. Three people became unconscious in 2000 as a result of taking 1,4 butanediol. In 2002, the *Dominion Post* reported the second fatal Fantasy overdose in New Zealand, although final blod tests confirming the presence of the drug were pending. Fantasy overdoses are becoming more common, with doctors in Auckland and Wellington emergency departments treating cases on most weekends.
Adapted from: www.moh.govt.nz and www.ndp.govt.nz

DRUG MONOGRAPH 21-3 BACLOFEN

The effects of baclofen are mediated via gamma-aminobutyric acid (GABA), an inhibitory neurotransmitter in many pathways especially in the grey matter in the brain, and at about 30% of CNS synapses. Baclofen is a GABA agonist, stimulating GABA receptors and thus inhibiting release of transmitters from many types of nerve terminals; it depresses the CNS and has an antispastic action in the spinal cord, inhibiting activation of motor neurons.

INDICATIONS It is used orally in the treatment of spasticity resulting from multiple sclerosis or from injuries to the spinal cord or head injury; it may be effective in the chronic spasticity associated with cerebral palsy, but not in epilepsy. Baclofen may also reduce pain in spastic patients by inhibiting substance P release in the spinal cord.

PHARMACOKINETICS Absorption after oral administration (with meals) is generally good, but can vary among individuals. Baclofen crosses the blood–brain barrier and acts centrally. The time to peak plasma concentration is 2–3 hours. The onset of action is variable and can occur in hours or may take weeks. Baclofen has a half-life of 2.5–6 hours. Intrathecal administration minimises GIT adverse effects. Baclofen is partly metabolised in the liver, and is excreted in the kidneys 70% unchanged.

DRUG INTERACTIONS Enhanced CNS-depressant and hypotensive effects can occur when baclofen is given concurrently with other CNS-depressant medications, antihypertensive agents, or with MAO inhibitors or tricyclic antidepressants. With levodopa, there is increased risk of psychotic reactions.

ADVERSE REACTIONS These include transient drowsiness, headache, vertigo, confusion, muscle weakness, nausea, hallucinations, depression, urinary disorders, tinnitus and GI upset.

WARNINGS AND CONTRAINDICATIONS Use with caution in patients with cerebral lesions, cerebrovascular accident, diabetes mellitus, seizure disorders, kidney impairment, respiratory disease or a history of psychiatric problems, and in the elderly. Not recommended for cerebral palsy. Use with extreme caution in children <16 years. Avoid use in people with peptic ulcer or known baclofen hypersensitivity.

DOSAGE AND ADMINISTRATION Dosage begins low to minimise adverse effects. The adult dose is 5 mg orally three times daily, increased by 5 mg per dose every 3 days until the desired response is achieved, not to exceed 80 mg/day.

leading to loss of excitability, and cause muscle twitching followed by short-duration paralysis.

These are mainly used during surgical operations, so are discussed in more detail in Chapter 15, under Adjuncts to anaesthesia: muscle relaxants.

BOTULINUM TOXIN A

The type A toxin from the bacteria *Clostridium botulinum* has long been known to be poisonous, and is implicated in food poisoning in which the anaerobic organism multiplies in poorly preserved or refrigerated food. The toxin blocks release of ACh from cholinergic nerves and thus causes a chemical denervation. It has a permanent toxic effect, decreasing muscle tone and contractility, leading to flaccid paralysis and atrophy of the affected muscles. It is a protein toxin and

---

**CLINICAL INTEREST BOX 21-6
BULGARIAN SNOWDROPS FOR
ALZHEIMER'S DISEASE**

Dementia is a global disorder developing over months to years, with cognitive, emotional and behavioural abnormalities leading to a decline in social and occupational functioning. The only drugs currently approved by the TGA in Australia for use in dementias are the cholinesterase inhibitors. These drugs do not cure Alzheimer's disease; but may slow the progression and improve alertness and cognition for 1–4 years. Examples are donepezil, rivastigmine and, more recently, galantamine; the latter drug has been used for hundreds of years in a traditional European herbal remedy from snowdrops (*Galanthus nivalis*).

There are reports that in the 1950s a Bulgarian pharmacologist noticed people rubbing the common snowdrop on their foreheads to ease nerve pain, and giving an infusion of the bulbs to relieve poliomyelitis-associated paralysis. Russian pharmacologists identified the anticholinesterase activity of extracts of *Galanthus* species in 1951, and determined the chemical structure of the active ingredient galantamine in 1952; it is a complex polycyclic alkaloid. It was soon introduced into Russian medicine as an antidote to neuromuscular blockade and for many neurological conditions, such as myasthenia gravis.

Perhaps because its pharmacology was originally studied in Russia during the Cold War period, it was some decades before galantamine made its appearance in the West. In Australia, it is now marketed in tablets and capsules (4–24 mg), and is subsidised for use in mild-to-moderate dementia. Galantamine has dual mechanisms of action: both by inhibition of acetylcholinesterase and enhancement of the binding of acetylcholine to nicotinic receptors. Clinically, galantamine improves cognitive performance (memory, attention, reasoning and language) and performance in activities of daily living. Its adverse reactions, as with other cholinomimetic agents, include gastrointestinal stimulation, depression and weakness.
Sources: Neurology Expert Group 2002; Caswell 2005; The Pharmaceutical Journal Online: www.pjonline.com/Editorial/20041218/christmas/p905alzheimers.html, accessed 4 October 2006.

---

extraordinarily potent: it is estimated that less than a 10^{-12} g dose will kill a mouse.

These effects have been put to good clinical use in the parenteral administration of the toxin to specific muscle groups undergoing involuntary spasm, e.g. in blepharospasm (uncontrollable winking or sustained tight closure of the eyes due to spasm of the eyelid muscles; see Drug Monograph 35-3), equinus foot deformity or other focal muscle **dystonias**. **Botulinum toxin** is also used to paralyse superficial facial muscles to (apparently) reduce wrinkles (see Clinical Interest Box 13-1). The toxin is injected SC to the muscle and relieves muscle spasm for several months until new motor end-plates sprout and reinnervation occurs.

Botulinum toxin A is contraindicated in myasthenia gravis, which it exacerbates, and has adverse interactions with aminoglycoside antibiotics and other drugs that impair ACh release and cause neuromuscular blockade. Adverse reactions include muscle weakness in muscle groups adjacent to the site of injection.

DANTROLENE

Dantrolene acts directly on skeletal muscles to produce skeletal muscle relaxation by inhibiting the release of calcium from the sarcoplasmic reticulum to the myoplasm. This results in a decreased muscle response to the action potential and decreased muscle contraction. As an antispastic agent, dantrolene's direct effect on skeletal muscle dissociates the excitation–contraction coupling. This effect is probably induced by the interference with calcium ion release from the sarcoplasmic reticulum. Dantrolene reduces both mono-synaptic- and polysynaptic-induced muscle contractions (see Drug Monograph 21-4).

DRUG TREATMENT OF OTHER MOVEMENT DISORDERS

Drug treatment of other movement disorders (myopathies, neuropathies and palsies) involves selection from a wide range of drugs, depending on the aetiology and clinical manifestations of the disorder. Frequently there is a suspected immunological cause, so immunosuppressants are administered rather than drugs directly affecting skeletal muscle control or function.

Multiple sclerosis

Multiple sclerosis is the most common cause of progressive neurological disability in the 20–50 age group. Its incidence varies with latitude, being higher further from the equator. Thus the incidence in Tasmania is about seven times that in north Queensland. There is widespread demyelination of neurons in the brain (white matter) and spinal cord, leading to muscle weakness and sensory and visual disturbances. Environmental and genetic factors have been implicated in triggering the autoimmune reaction against CNS myelin. There is a relapsing–remitting course of progressive disability over a period of about 30 years.

Centrally acting antispasticity drugs such as baclofen and diazepam are used, as well as dantrolene, corticosteroids and other immunosuppressants, beta-interferon (antiviral and immunomodulatory), anticonvulsants and antidepressants (for sensory disturbances, pain and depression) and autonomic drugs (for relief of urinary problems). Glatiramer is a new unusual drug specifically for use in multiple sclerosis, to reduce the frequency of relapses. A simple synthetic tetrapeptide, it appears to block T-lymphocyte action against myelin antigens. As a peptide, it must be injected daily, and reactions at the injection site are common. Other adverse effects include chest pain, dyspnoea, anxiety, oedema, tremor and delayed development of antibodies to the drug.

Amyotrophic lateral sclerosis

This is a motor neuron disease in which degeneration of neurons progressively leads to bulbar palsy and atrophy of skeletal muscles, and eventually to respiratory failure and/or choking. It is possibly due to accumulation of glutamate in affected neurons.

Riluzole, a new drug that specifically inhibits the release of glutamate, has been trialled as a neuroprotective agent in this condition. It significantly slows the deterioration in muscle strength, and prolongs life by a few months. Common adverse

effects are weakness, nausea and decreased lung function, and liver function requires monitoring.

DRUG TREATMENT OF DEMENTIAS

Dementia

Dementia is described as a progressive mental disorder characterised by chronic personality disintegration, confusion and deterioration of intellectual capacity and impulse control. Confusional states affect about 1% of the general population, but the incidence is about 16% in hospital admissions and up to 80% in geriatric or aged care units. **Alzheimer's disease** accounts for about 50%–60% of dementia, while vascular dementia (including multi-infarct dementia, formerly known as cerebrovascular arteriosclerosis), Pick's disease, Parkinson's disease dementia and other forms comprise the balance. In Australia, dementia is the sixth leading cause of disease burden in the community, accounting for 3.5% of total disability-adjusted life years; it ranks ahead of diabetes and asthma in terms of disease burden.

Reversible dementias can be caused by drugs, emotion, metabolic or endocrine alterations, poor nutrition, trauma, infection, alcoholism and systemic illness. The medications most associated with this type of dementia include anticholinergic agents, cardiac drugs, antihypertensives, anti-inflammatories, anticonvulsants and psychotropics. Clinical Interest Box 21-7 lists potentially reversible causes of dementia.

The syndrome of dementia usually develops slowly; the phases of cognitive decline occurring in Alzheimer's disease

---

DRUG MONOGRAPH 21-4 DANTROLENE

INDICATIONS Dantrolene is used in the treatment of spasticity, especially upper motor neuron disorders such as multiple sclerosis, cerebral palsy, spinal cord injury and cerebrovascular accident, and in prophylaxis and treatment of malignant hyperthermia that occurs during surgery.

PHARMACOKINETICS Dantrolene is available orally and parenterally. Oral absorption is incomplete and slow; the onset of action when dantrolene is used to treat the spasticity of upper motor neurons can take 1 week or more. The drug has a half-life (orally) of about 9 hours. It is metabolised in the liver and excreted in the kidneys and bile.

DRUG INTERACTIONS When dantrolene is given concurrently with other CNS depressants, an increase in CNS-depressant effects can result. Monitor closely, as dosage reduction of one or both drugs may be necessary. When dantrolene is used chronically, concurrent use of hepatotoxic medications (e.g. oestrogens) increases the

potential risk for hepatotoxicity.

ADVERSE REACTIONS These include diarrhoea, dizziness, sleepiness, unusual fatigue, muscle weakness, nausea, vomiting, respiratory depression, and cardiovascular, haematological and CNS changes.

WARNINGS AND CONTRAINDICATIONS Potentially fatal hepatitis can occur, so liver function should be monitored. Use with caution in patients with myopathy, liver or pulmonary function impairment, or neuromuscular diseases and in individuals older than 35 years (especially women), as they have an increased potential for hepatotoxicity. Patients should be cautioned against driving or other hazardous occupations.

Avoid use in people with dantrolene hypersensitivity and active liver diseases, such as hepatitis or cirrhosis.

Dosage begins low (25 mg orally daily), with gradual increases to a limit of 50 mg 4 times daily to monitor effects and minimise toxicity.

are described in Table 21-1. Early signs include depression, loss of ability to concentrate and increased anxiety, irritability and agitation. Intellectual ability is usually the first to decline and then recent memory (such as names of acquaintances or recent events), followed by the loss of orientation to time, place and person. Personal habits change. The person may become loud or obscene, or some personality characteristics that were present might become magnified. Helplessness, total dependency and loss of manual skills may occur next. In the final stages, the person may be bedridden, with loss of sphincter control, and eventually will die, usually of bronchopneumonia.

CLINICAL INTEREST BOX 21-7
POTENTIALLY REVERSIBLE CAUSES OF DEMENTIA

- Drugs, chemicals or toxins: bromides, mercury; CNS depressant drugs such as butyrophenones, phenothiazines, sedatives and alcohol; diuretics
- Emotional problems: depression, chronic alcoholism
- Metabolic disorders: hyperglycaemia, hypothyroidism, hypopituitarism
- Sensory deprivation: blindness, deafness
- Nutritional deficits: deficiency of vitamin B_{12}, folic acid, niacin
- Tumours: brain tumours or metastases
- Acute trauma: subdural haematoma
- Infections or fever: viral infections, bacterial (tuberculosis)
- Arteriosclerotic events: vascular occlusion, stroke

In management, all the possible reversible causes of dementia should be considered first. Then treatment should be instituted to try to prevent or reduce the ongoing damage and to support the patient and family in managing this disease process. Drug treatment is indicated only for symptom control, i.e. the use of low-dose antipsychotic agents for treating severe agitation, delusions and hallucinations, or antidepressants for severe depression. Supportive care should include proper nutrition, moderate exercise if permitted, vitamins if indicated and the use of environmental aids in a consistent fashion, such as night lights and daily calendar reminders.

Alzheimer's disease

Alzheimer's disease is a dementia of insidious onset and gradually progressive course, characterised by confusion, memory failure, disorientation, restlessness, speech disturbances and impaired cognitive abilities. It is currently incurable, and accounts for more than half the people with dementia. There is a linear incidence with age, so that about 50% of the population over 85 years shows some evidence of Alzheimer's disease. It has been estimated to be the major underlying reason for over 50% of all nursing home admissions. Clinically, a progressive decline in intellectual functions is noted (see Table 21-1).

While researchers are still searching for the cause of Alzheimer's disease, many theories have been proposed. The theories currently under study include:

- a deficiency in the neurotransmitter acetylcholine, and perhaps other neurotransmitters in the brain
- a slow viral or other infection that attacks selected brain cells

---

TABLE 21-1 Staging of cognitive decline in Alzheimer's disease

STAGE	CLINICAL PHASE	SYMPTOMS
1	Normal	No change in cognition
2	Very mild	Forgets object location, some deficit in word finding
3	Mild (early confusion)	Early cognitive decline in one or more areas: memory loss, decreased ability to function in work situations, name-finding deficit, some decrease in social functioning, recall difficulties, and anxiety
4	Moderate	Unable to perform complex tasks such as managing personal finances, planning a dinner party, concentrating, and recalling knowledge of current events
5	Moderately severe (early dementia)	Usually needs assistance for survival: reminders to bathe, help in selecting clothes, and other daily functions; may be disoriented; may become tearful
6	Severe (dementia)	Needs assistance with dressing, bathing and toilet functions; may forget names and details of personal life, and be unaware of surroundings; may have incontinence of urine and faeces; shows an increase in CNS disturbances such as agitation, delusions, paranoia, obsessive anxiety, and violent behaviour
7	Very severe (late dementia)	Unable to speak (speech limited to 5 words or less); may scream or make other sounds; unable to ambulate, sit up, smile or feed self; unable to hold head erect, will ultimately slip into stupor or coma

- a genetic predisposition
- an autoimmune theory (that the body fails to recognise host tissue and attacks itself)
- beta-amyloid protein accumulation in the CNS
- excess glutamate in central pathways, leading to neuronal degeneration.

The best hypothesis to date is that Alzheimer's disease results from the loss of cholinergic neurons in the CNS, particularly the cholinergic input from the basal forebrain to the hippocampus and cerebral cortex, hence the impairment in memory and learning. There is also reactive gliosis (glial scarring), and formation of dendritic plaques and tangles, especially in the grey matter.

Current pharmacotherapy is focused on improving cognitive functioning or limiting disease progression and symptom control. Unfortunately, no known medication cures or prevents Alzheimer's disease. The medications currently approved in Australia for cognitive improvement are centrally acting reversible cholinesterase inhibitors (**donepezil**, galantamine and **rivastigmine**), which act to raise and prolong ACh levels in cholinergic pathways and have been demonstrated to enhance cognitive functioning and slow the decline in functions. Other drugs may be tried to relieve behavioural disturbances and mood changes, especially antipsychotics. New therapies currently under trial include muscarinic M_1 agonists, nicotinic agonists, molecules that mimic nitric oxide, metal chelators and factors influencing amyloid beta-precursor protein, including antioxidants, vitamin E, and the curry spice curcumin.

Centrally acting anticholinesterases

These drugs such as **donepezil** act to enhance neurotransmitter actions of acetylcholine in CNS pathways; the mechanism is discussed in the previous section on drugs affecting skeletal muscle. As ACh is also the neurotransmitter at neuroeffector junctions in the parasympathetic nervous system, these drugs can be expected to have many adverse reactions, especially in the GIT and heart (see Drug Monograph 13-3). The clinical benefits have proven to be small, and are considered not cost-effective. Currently in Australia there are strict guidelines as to provision of authority for a doctor to prescribe the drugs subsidised by the PBS.

Memantine, an NMDA antagonist

Memantine, a new drug that antagonises receptors for *N*-methyl-D-aspartate (NMDA), is thought to reduce neuronal degradation due to excess glutamate present in Alzheimer's disease. It is approved for use in moderate-to-severe dementia; adverse CNS effects are common. Functional status should be reviewed regularly and the drug discontinued unless deterioration is slowed.

Symptom management

The benefits from anticholinesterases have been limited; therefore, many other drugs are under clinical investigation, including:

- newer anticholinesterases, e.g. velnacrine maleate
- non-steroidal anti-inflammatory drugs (NSAIDs) such as indomethacin, on the rationale that some mediators of inflammation are increased in cognitive decline conditions
- nimodipine, a calcium channel blocker, can improve functions via its vasodilator effects
- selegiline an MAO-B inhibitor that may have antioxidant effects and increase 5-HT and noradrenaline concentrations, can improve monoaminergic functions
- oestrogens (it has been reported that postmenopausal women treated with oestrogen are less likely to get Alzheimer's disease than those who were untreated)
- 5-HT antagonists and angiotensin-converting enzyme inhibitors
- antipsychotic agents, such as haloperidol and risperidone, for management of behavioural disturbances, including delusions and hallucinations; adverse reactions should be monitored, and antipsychotic agents or any medications with anticholinergic effects could worsen the cognitive functioning of the patient
- antidepressants might be required, as 20%–40% of Alzheimer's patients experience depression; low doses of antidepressants with a low anticholinergic profile, such as desipramine or nortriptyline, are preferred
- antianxiety agents, especially those with short-to-intermediate half-lives such as lorazepam, oxazepam or alprazolam, are selected for patients who exhibit severe anxiety or agitation, the potential for inducing a paradoxical reaction (increase in activity, restlessness, and agitation), which might be confused with increasing dementia, is present
- other compounds that have shown some effect as cognitive enhancers, including glycine agonists, vitamins (pyridoxine) and phospholipids.

Treatment of stroke

Ischaemic brain damage can lead to the commonest type of secondary dementias, i.e. multi-infarct or arteriopathic dementia. There are about 40,000 strokes per year in Australia; hypertension and atheroma are important aetiological factors. Treatment is for the underlying conditions; for example recent research has shown that in patients who have had a stroke, aggressive lowering of blood pressure with an angiotensin-converting enzyme inhibitor and a diuretic significantly reduces the risk of another stroke. Other drugs tried include aspirin and other antiplatelet drugs, warfarin, thrombolytics and calcium channel blockers, and various complementary and alternative therapies (see Clinical Interest Box 21-8).

CLINICAL INTEREST BOX 21-8 COMPLEMENTARY AND ALTERNATIVE THERAPIES IN NEUROLOGICAL DISORDERS

Many CAM methods have been tried in neurological disorders (stroke, brain injury, multiple sclerosis, Parkinson's disease, dementias, epilepsy and spinal cord injury), possibly reflecting the inadequate success of conventional medicine in treating these distressing chronic/degenerative conditions. The best validated research is on acupuncture and *Ginkgo biloba*.

- Acupuncture, in varied techniques, has provided some improvement in stroke patients.
- Extracts of the herb *Ginkgo biloba* have been used for 5000 years in traditional Chinese medicine; there is evidence for efficacy in producing cognitive improvements in patients with stroke, Alzheimer's disease and cerebral ischaemia. In experimental studies, *Gingko biloba* extracts have demonstrated antiplatelet, anticoagulant and free-radical scavenger activities and 'vascular regulatory activity'.
- The herb feverfew (*Tanacetum parthenium*), which is

proposed to have actions inhibiting serotonin release from platelets, has a long history of use in migraine patients.
- Fish oil supplementation has been shown to alleviate dementia, and a diet high in fish reduces the risk of Alzheimer's disease.
- Galantamine, an alkaloid from the bulbs of the Russian snowdrop *Galanthus woronowii*, has anticholinesterase activity, with actions similar to those of neostigmine; it has been used effectively in neuromuscular disorders and is now available in tablet form.
- Other CAM therapies shown to be useful are phyto-oestrogens, hypnotherapy and music therapy in improving mood and motivation, and massage therapy in improving circulation.

From: Spencer & Jacobs 1999; *Australian Prescriber* 24 (4): 100–101, 2001; Braun & Cohen 2005.

DRUGS USED IN MIGRAINE AND OTHER HEADACHES

Drugs used in migraine
Migraine

Migraine is a severe intermittent **headache** sometimes preceded or accompanied by flashing lights or other disturbances of brain function. More specifically, migraine attacks have been defined as headache with at least two of the following four features: pain affecting one side of the head only, pulsating in quality, moderate or severe in intensity, aggravated by exertion; plus nausea with or without vomiting, and sensitivity to light and sound. The nature of the attacks varies between patients, and within a patient at different times.

Migraine has been known and described for thousands of years. At various times, it has been considered a bad headache, a spontaneous 'concussion', an inflammatory disorder, a vascular disorder, a form of epilepsy or a platelet disorder. The fact that dilation of cerebral blood vessels is involved was proved by showing that if patients are (gently) centrifuged feet-outwards, the head pain is relieved, by taking the blood to the periphery. It is now generally considered that migraine is a syndrome of unstable cerebral blood vessels, probably mediated by 5-HT, with the first, prodromal, stage involving vasoconstriction of intracranial vessels, followed by reflex vasodilation with severe unilateral pulsating pain.

The prevalence of migraine is the community is about 7% in males and 16% in females (during reproductive non-

pregnant years). Migraine can occur in young children, and prevalence rises from about 3% in 7-year-olds to 9% in 15-year-olds. In Australia, it is estimated that a quarter of people suffering migraines require medical attention, and about 70% have some positive family history of migraines. While the exact aetiology is unknown, many factors are known to trigger a migraine attack; these are summarised in Clinical Interest Box 21-9.

The course and pathogenesis of a typical migraine attack begins with the prodrome or aura phase, during which

CLINICAL INTEREST BOX 21-9 TRIGGERING FACTORS IN MIGRAINES

While the specific factor(s) causing migraines are not known, many patients come to realise that particular events or factors seem to trigger off an attack. Some of the common 'triggers' are:

- mechanical: a blow to the head or pressure on the head
- environmental changes: hot winds (the sirocco of the Mediterranean, the sharav in Israel, and hot north winds in Melbourne), changes in barometric pressure or the weather
- stress (emotions, glare, noise) or relaxation after stress
- hormone level changes, e.g. at puberty, pre- and during menstruation (the declining oestrogen phase)
- drugs: oestrogens, vasodilators, including nitrates
- foods (those implicated include chocolate, cheese, oranges, preservatives) and alcohol, especially red wines; however, placebos (inactive substances) have also triggered attacks
- deydration
- changes in sleep patterns, especially in REM sleep.

there is vasoconstriction of the intracranial vessels. This is thought to lead to impairment of blood flow to the brain, starting in the visual cortex and causing the sensation of flashing lights, pin-pricking, impaired speech and weakness. Blood flow is reduced in the parts of the brain subject to the symptoms.

The second phase of the attack is that of headache, thought to be due to a protective reflex vasodilation, during which blood flow to the brain, face and head is increased by about 20%. The nervous system is overreactive, responding rapidly to intense stimuli. There are sensations of flashing lights, spectra, double vision, and increased sensitivity to light (photophobia), smells and noise. Autonomic effects include nausea and vomiting, diarrhoea, fluid retention and afterwards diuresis, and CNS effects of vertigo, ataxia, incoordination and impaired consciousness.

During the early phase, platelet levels of 5-HT drop due to release of 5-HT, which causes the vasoconstriction, aura and pain. Later, 5-HT levels are low, allowing vasodilation. GIT symptoms are due to effects of 5-HT on receptors in the gut. The headache is thought to be due partly to arterial dilation and sensitisation to pain by released 5-HT and bradykinin. Spontaneous discharge along trigeminal nerve pathways releases other neurotransmitters (substance P, calcitonin gene-related peptide), which contribute to pain, vasodilation and visual and GIT disturbances.

Thus the main neurotransmitter involved in migraine appears to be 5-HT, and the specific drugs involved in treatment are 5-HT agonists in the acute attack and, apparently paradoxically, 5-HT antagonists in prophylaxis against attacks.

Treatment of migraine
NON-PHARMACOLOGICAL TREATMENT
Before pharmacological treatment of migraine is commenced, it is important that the diagnosis be confirmed and other causes of severe headache excluded. Trigger factors need to be managed; often attacks can be pre-empted if the person can remove to a quiet dark room, take mild analgesics, and sleep off the attack. Behavioural therapies such as attention to sleep and rest habits, relaxation and assertiveness training, and avoidance of stress are useful.

TREATMENT OF THE ACUTE ATTACK
Mild analgesics should be tried first, with stronger drugs tried as necessary, moving up the analgesic ladder (see Figure 16-7). Suitable analgesics are paracetamol in children, and in adults aspirin (600–900 mg every 4 hours) or paracetamol (1–1.5 g every 4 hours, to a maximum of 4 g/day).

An antiemetic (metoclopramide, prochlorperazine or domperidone) can be used if nausea is severe.

If stronger analgesia is required, compound analgesics should be tried: aspirin or paracetamol, plus codeine or dextropropoxyphene, or a stronger non-steroidal anti-inflammatory drug (naproxen or ibuprofen). Opioids are avoided due to potential problems with dependence and adverse GIT effects.

Ergotamine, a powerful vasoconstrictor, acts both as an α-adrenoceptor agonist and 5-HT agonist. A dose of 1–2 mg can be given at the onset of the attack, either orally or rectally. Caffeine or diphenhydramine is sometimes given concurrently with ergotamine (with doubtful pharmacological rationale). If parenteral administration is necessary due to nausea, then the dihydroergotamine derivative can be given SC or IM. Ergot alkaloids have many adverse reactions so are used cautiously, and rebound headaches can occur after cessation of administration.

If the above therapies have been ineffective in relieving previous attacks, one of the new 'triptan' drugs may be prescribed: **sumatriptan** (see Drug Monograph 21-5), zolmitriptan or naratriptan. These are structural analogues of 5-HT and are selective agonists at 5-HT$_1$ receptors and effective vasoconstrictors especially on cerebral arteries, relieving migraine headache in 50%–75% of cases within 2–4 hours of oral administration. They can be administered orally, parenterally or as a nasal spray. They are relatively new drugs that came into use in the 1990s and revolutionised treatment of migraine for many patients.

PREVENTION OF MIGRAINE ATTACKS
Triggering factors need to be identified and avoided if possible, and any underlying conditions, such as hypertension or anxiety, treated first. Increasing frequency of attacks can be due to overuse of ergotamine, as the withdrawal effect causes rebound headache.

If the patient suffers more than one severe attack per month, prophylactic agents are tried, in the following order:
- antidepressants (amitriptyline, MAO inhibitors)
- anticonvulsants (phenytoin, topiramate, valproate)
- calcium channel blocker
- β-blockers (propranolol, metoprolol)—their clinical efficacy may be due to effects at 5-HT receptors rather than β-blocking actions
- antiserotonin/antihistamine agents (pizotifen)
- methysergide, a potent 5-HT antagonist (see below).

Methysergide is an ergot derivative that is a potent 5-HT$_2$ antagonist. It suppresses migraine headache in about 25% of patients, but is ineffective in treatment of acute attacks. An initial dose of 1 mg/day orally is given, increasing gradually to 3–4 times/day, then reducing over 2–3 weeks. The drug must be discontinued after 4 months due to the risk of fibrosis (retroperitoneal, or in the heart valves or pleura). The drug may be reintroduced after a drug holiday of 1–2 months if no fibrosis has occurred.

There is a high incidence of adverse reactions, especially in the CNS, GIT and cardiovascular system, with behavioural changes and peripheral vascular disease. Methysergide is

DRUG MONOGRAPH 21-5   SUMATRIPTAN

Sumatriptan selectively constricts cranial vessels by agonist actions at 5-HT receptors.

INDICATIONS It is indicated for treatment of an acute migraine attack, in patients unresponsive to or intolerant of other therapies. It is also indicted by injection for acute relief of cluster headache pain.

PHARMACOKINETICS After oral administration, absorption of sumatriptan is rapid but incomplete; a high first-pass metabolism means low bioavailability. After SC administration, the peak plasma concentration is reached in about 30 minutes, and there is much higher bioavailability, so doses are considerably lower (6 mg compared with 50–100 mg orally). Intranasal administration as a spray has a quicker onset of action than orally (hence it is useful to relieve pain and retard development of the migraine attack, especially in people with severe nausea and vomiting) but shorter duration of action.

DRUG INTERACTIONS The triptan drugs interact significantly with the following agents administered concomitantly:

Drug	Possible effect and management
Monoamine oxidase inhibitors including moclobemide	Increased risk of ischaemia; contraindicated

Drug	Possible effect and management
Selective serotonin reuptake inhibitors	Increased risk of adverse drug reactions; monitor effects

ADVERSE REACTIONS Minor reactions include dizziness, fatigue, drowsiness, chest pain, nausea and vomiting, feelings of heaviness and rash. Rarely, there have been reports of arrhythmias, stroke, anaphylactic reactions, seizures, and even acute myocardial infarction and death.

WARNINGS AND CONTRAINDICATIONS Sumatriptan should be taken as monotherapy, i.e. other antimigraine preparations should be avoided. It should not be taken within 24 hours of ergotamine preparations. Caution is advised in the elderly and during pregnancy. The drug is contraindicated in ischaemic diseases (ischaemic heart disease, myocardial infarction, coronary vasospasm), hypertension, and in a history of cerebro- or peripheral vascular disease. It should not be used during lactation or in severe liver disease, and is not licensed for use in children.

DOSAGE AND ADMINISTRATION The oral dose is 50–100 mg as soon as possible in the attack, repeating after 2 hours if necessary to a maximum of 300 mg/day. The SC dose regimen is 6 mg, repeating after 1 hour to maximum of 12 mg/day. For intranasal administration the dose is 10–20 mg into one nostril, repeating after 2 hours to a maximum of 40 mg/day. Note: Sumatriptan must not be taken less than 24 hours after ergot, and ergot not for 6 hours after sumatriptan.

---

contraindicated in many conditions: CVS disease, hyperthyroidism, collagen disease, urinary tract disorders, renal or liver disease, and in children, pregnancy or lactation.

The herb feverfew (*Tanacetum parthenium*), which is proposed to have actions inhibiting 5-HT release from platelets, has a long history of use in migraine patients. Recent clinical trials have confirmed that it has some prophylactic efficacy; however, the content of active ingredients varies widely among plants and at different times.

Drugs used in other headaches
Normal headaches

There is a wide variety of conditions in which **headaches** can occur, with accompanying triggering factors:
- excess stimulation of the nerves of the scalp (tight hat or goggles)
- 'ice-cream headache', from eating ice-cream or other very cold food or drinks
- 'hot-dog' headache, from the nitrite preservatives in cured meats
- 'Chinese restaurant syndrome', from monosodium glutamate
- hangover headache, from dehydration, aldehydes and acetate after excessive alcohol consumption
- fasting, from low blood sugar levels
- rebound or medication overuse headache, after withdrawal from drugs such as analgesics, caffeine, nicotine, ergotamine and β-blockers
- mountain sickness, from changes in fluid balance and low oxygen levels
- drug-induced headache, from vasodilators, oral contraceptives, tetracyclines, indomethacin, amphetamines, pethidine, histamine H_2-antagonists or epidural anaesthesia
- exertional vascular headaches, from strenuous exercise,

coughing, straining or sexual intercourse (due to increased blood pressure, vasodilation, muscle contractions)

• other pain conditions, including neuralgias, sinusitis, neck pain and toothache.

In most of these types of headache, simple analgesics provide adequate pain relief. Appropriate doses are aspirin 600 mg orally every 4 hours or paracetamol 0.5–1 g orally every 3–6 hours, with a maximum of 4 g/day. In medication overuse headache, the causative drug must be withdrawn.

Tension headache

Tension headache is a chronic headache without aura or vomiting, affecting both sides of the head, often with depression or anxiety. It affects women more frequently than men. It has been suggested that it is a syndrome of low 5-HT levels.

Physical management includes relaxation, exercises and massage, and avoidance or reduction of caffeine intake. Drug treatments tried (after simple analgesics) are amitriptyline (an antidepressant) and diazepam (an antianxiety agent).

Cluster headache

Cluster headache is a severe one-sided pain, centred on one eye, often with one blocked or runny nostril, which recurs within 24 hours. There is decreased sympathetic function on the affected side; it has been called 'migrainous neuralgia'. Men are affected more frequently than women; it is triggered particularly by vasodilators, including alcohol.

Treatment is with inhaled oxygen, and sumatriptan is effective. Prevention is with prophylactic use of ergotamine, methysergide, corticosteroids, lithium or calcium channel blockers.

More serious causes of headache

Although most headaches are mild and self-limiting, there are potentially serious causes of headaches that need to be checked: cerebral oedema, a space-occupying lesion (e.g. intracranial haemorrhage, meningitis or encephalitis, or tumour), vascular insufficiency, temporal arteritis, or headache after head injury.

PREGNANCY SAFETY	
ADEC Category	**Drug**
A	Bromocriptine
B1	Benzhexol, cabergoline, galantamine, pizotifen
B2	Benztropine, biperiden, dantrolene, memantine, neostigmine, orphenadrine, rivastigmine, selegiline
B3	Amantadine, apomorphine, baclofen, benserazide, botulinum toxin A, carbidopa, donepezil, entacapone, levodopa, levodopa carbidopa, naratriptan, riluzole, ropinirole, sumatriptan, zolmitriptan
C	Diazepam, dihydroergotamine, ergotamine, methysergide, pergolide, pyridostigmine

GERIATRIC IMPLICATIONS ANTICHOLINERGICS

• The elderly are highly susceptible to adverse effects of anticholinergic drugs, especially constipation, dry mouth and urinary retention (usually in men).
• Avoid use of these agents in people with narrow-angle glaucoma or a history of urinary retention.
• Memory impairment has been reported with continuous administration of these agents, especially in older people.
• When usual adult doses are administered, some elderly people may have a paradoxical reaction: hyperexcitability, agitation, confusion and sedation.
• Chronic use decreases or inhibits the flow of saliva, which can contribute to oral discomfort, periodontal disease and candidiasis.
• Overheating resulting in heat stroke has been reported in people receiving anticholinergic drugs during vigorous exercise or periods of hot weather.
• Blurred vision and/or increased sensitivity to light can occur.
• Anticholinergic dosing in the elderly should begin at the lowest dose, with gradual increases until maximum improvement is noted or intolerable adverse effects occur.

DRUGS AT A GLANCE 21: Drugs for neurodegenerative disorders and migraine

Therapeutic group	Pharmacological group	Key examples	Key pages
Antiparkinson agents	Dopaminergic agents		
	• Drugs increasing brain DA levels + dopa-decarboxylase inhibitor:	levodopa + carbidopa or benserazide	350–2
	• DA releasers	amantadine	353–4
	• MAO-B inhibitors	selegeline	354
	• COMT inhibitors	entacapone	354–5
	DA agonists		
	• Ergot derivatives	bromocriptine, pergolide, cabergoline }	352–3
	• Others	apomorphine	353
	Anticholinergics (central)	benztropine	355
Drugs affecting skeletal muscle Centrally acting	Anticholinesterases	pyridostigmine	355–6
	Skeletal muscle relaxants: GABA agonists	baclofen diazepam	356–8 357
Peripherally acting	Inhibitors of acetylcholine release	Botulinum toxin	359
	Inhibitors of calcium release	dantrolene	359–60
Drugs used in dementias	Centrally acting anticholinesterases	donepezil rivastigmine }	362
	NMDA antagonists	memantine	362
Antimigraine drugs Acute treatment	Analgesics/NSAIDs	aspirin paracetamol naproxen	364
	5-HT agonists		
	• Ergot alkaloids	ergotamine	353, 64
	• Triptans	sumatriptan	364–5
Prophylaxis	5-HT antagonists	methysergide	364–5

5-HT = 5-hydroxytryptamine; DA = dopamine; MAO = monoamine oxidase; COMT = catechol-O-methyltransferase; GABA = gamma-aminobutyric acid; NMDA = N-methyl-D-aspartate; NSAIDs = non-steroidal anti-inflammatory drugs.

KEY POINTS

● This chapter reviews the pathology and treatment of Parkinson's disease, myasthenia gravis, movement disorders and muscle spasticity, dementia and Alzheimer's disease, and migraine and other headaches. These neurological disorders often incapacitate the individual. Use of pharmacological agents is essential for symptom control, which allows the patient to function as independently as possible for as long as possible.

● People with Parkinson's disease usually require correction of the disorder's imbalance of dopamine/acetylcholine neurotransmitters. They are therefore treated with dopaminergic agents, to raise brain levels of dopamine, and/or with drugs that have central anticholinergic effects.

- The main dopaminergic agents are levodopa with a decarboxylase inhibitor, the ergot derivatives, and apomorphine, amantadine and selegiline. These all tend to have adverse reactions on dopamine receptors in the CNS and GIT.

- Centrally acting anticholinergic drugs (such as benztropine) inhibit acetylcholine-mediated motor activity but have adverse reactions on other ACh receptors in the motor and autonomic nervous systems.

- Myasthenia gravis, which is characterised by skeletal muscle weakness and fatigue, is a debilitating disease. The drugs of choice in treatment are the anticholinesterase drugs acting at the neuromuscular junction, such as pyridostigmine; these increase ACh activity at the motor end-plate.

- Drugs that act as skeletal muscle relaxants can have central actions (e.g. baclofen, diazepam) or peripheral actions (botulinum toxin A, dantrolene). They are usually the drugs of choice in the treatment of muscle spasticity. The neuromuscular blocking agents used in surgery (such as curare and suxamethonium) also act at the neuromuscular junction.

- There is no current medication to cure or prevent Alzheimer's disease and dementia. Centrally acting anticholinesterases (e.g. donepezil) slow cognitive decline by enhancing ACh functions. Other pharmacotherapy is used for symptom control and to manage agitation, delusions and hallucinations.

- Migraine is a severe unilateral headache; it is thought to be due to fluctuating levels of 5-HT in the brain, causing vasoconstriction then vasodilation of cerebral blood vessels. For treatment of acute attacks, analgesics and 5-HT agonists (ergotamine, sumatriptan) are used. To prevent attacks, 5-HT antagonists (methysergide) and various other drugs are used prophylactically. It is also important for patients to identify and avoid triggering factors.

- Other headaches ('normal', tension and cluster headaches) are treated with simple analgesics, and antidepressants, antianxiety agents or antimigraine drugs as required.

REVIEW EXERCISES

1. Describe the classifications of drugs that affect brain dopamine levels. Name one drug from each category, and explain its mechanism of action in Parkinson's disease.

2. Discuss the rationale for the combined administration of levodopa with carbidopa in patients with Parkinson's disease.

3. Outline the common adverse reactions that occur with drugs that enhance central dopamine transmission, and describe three potentially serious drug interactions with dopaminergic agonists.

4. Discuss the theory of dopamine/acetylcholine imbalance in Parkinson's disease, and describe the pharmacology of centrally acting anticholinergic agents (actions, mechanism of action, adverse reactions).

5. What is myasthenia gravis? Describe the action, adverse reactions and overdose effects of the anticholinesterase drugs.

6. Discuss the mechanisms of action and clinical uses of the skeletal muscle relaxants baclofen, diazepam, botulinum toxin A and dantrolene.

7. Describe the pathogenesis of Alzheimer's disease and the rationale and use of anticholinesterases in its management.

8. Describe the involvement of 5-HT and triggering factors in the pathogenesis of migraine, and discuss the use of drugs in treatment of the acute attack, and prophylaxis of recurrent attacks.

9. Outline the use of drugs in treatment of other headaches (normal, tension and cluster).

REFERENCES AND FURTHER READING

Arulmozhi DK, Veeranjaneyulu A, Bodhankar SL. Migraine: current concepts and emerging therapies. *Vascular Pharmacology* 2005; 43(3): 176–87.

Attia J, Schofield P. What now for Alzheimer's disease? An epidemiological evaluation of the AD2000 trial. *Australian Prescriber* 2005; 28(6): 134–5.

Australian Medicines Handbook 2005. Adelaide: AMH, 2005.

Beal MF, Lang AE, Ludolph AC (eds). *Neurodegenerative Diseases: Neurobiology, Pathogenesis and Therapeutics*. Cambridge: Cambridge University Press, 2005.

Bloch S, Singh BS. *Foundations of Clinical Psychiatry*. 2nd edn. Carlton: Melbourne University Press, 2001.

Bowman WC, Rand MJ. *Textbook of Pharmacology*. 2nd edn. Oxford: Blackwell, 1980 [chs 18, 19, 25].

Bradberry JC, Fagan SC, Gray DR, Moon YS. New perspectives on the pharmacotherapy of ischemic stroke. *Journal of the American Pharmacists Association* 2004; 44(2 Suppl. 1): S46–56.

Braun L, Cohen M. *Herbs and Natural Supplements: An Evidence-Based Guide*. Sydney: Elsevier Mosby 2005.

Byrne GJ. Pharmacological treatment of behavioural problems in dementia. *Australian Prescriber* 2005; 28(3): 67–70.

Caswell A (ed.). *MIMS Annual June 2005*. Sydney: CMPMedica Australia, 2005.

Cooper JR, Bloom FE, Roth RH. *The Biochemical Basis of Neuropharmacology.* 8th edn. New York: Oxford University Press, 2003.

Coughlan CM, Breen KC. Factors influencing the processing and function of the amyloid beta precursor protein—a potential target in Alzheimer's disease? *Pharmacology & Therapeutics* 2000; 86: 111–45.

Fung VSC, Hely MA, de Moore G, Morris JGL. Drugs for Parkinson's disease. *Australian Prescriber* 2001; 24: 92–95.

GlaxoWellcome. *The 'Not Another Headache' Handbook.* Melbourne: GlaxoWellcome Australia, 1999.

Goldney RD, Stoffell BF. Ethical issues in placebo-controlled trials in Alzheimer's disease. *Medical Journal of Australia* 2000; 173: 147–8.

Johnston TH, Brotchie JM. Drugs in development for Parkinson's disease. *Current Opinion in Investigational Drugs* 2004; 5(7): 720–6.

Lance JW. *Migraine and Other Headaches.* Sydney: Compass, 1993.

Lance JW. Headache and face pain. *Medical Journal of Australia* 2000; 172: 450–5.

Lindley RI, Landau PB. Early management of acute stroke. *Australian Prescriber* 2004; 27(5): 120–3.

Mann J. *Murder, Magic and Medicine.* Oxford: Oxford University Press, 1992.

Neurology Expert Group. *Therapeutic Guidelines: Neurology, version 2.* Melbourne: Therapeutic Guidelines Limited, 2002.

Poewe W, Wenning GK. Apomorphine: an underutilized therapy for Parkinson's disease. *Movement Disorders* 2000; 15: 789–94.

Pender MP. Multiple sclerosis. *Medical Journal of Australia* 2000; 172: 556–62.

Psychotropic Expert Group. *Therapeutic Guidelines: Psychotropic, version 5.* Melbourne: Therapeutic Guidelines Limited, 2003.

Sacks O. *Migraine.* Berkeley: University of California Press, 1992.

Schrag A. Entacapone in the treatment of Parkinson's disease. *Lancet Neurology* 2005; 4(6): 366–70.

Smith N, Temple W. Dosis facit venenum. Date rape drugs. *Australian Pharmacist* 2000; 19: 357.

Spencer JW, Jacobs JJ. *Complementary/Alternative Medicine: An Evidence-Based Approach.* St Louis: Mosby, 1999.

Thomas T. Monoamine oxidase-B inhibitors in the treatment of Alzheimer's disease. *Neurobiology of Aging* 2000; 21: 343–8.

Williams D. Medication overuse headache. *Australian Prescriber* 2005; 28(6): 143–5.

ON-LINE RESOURCE

Alzheimer's Australia website: www.alzheimers.org.au

New Zealand medicines and medical devices safety authority: www.medsafe.govt.nz

evolve   More weblinks at http://evolve.elsevier.com/AU/Bryant/pharmacology/

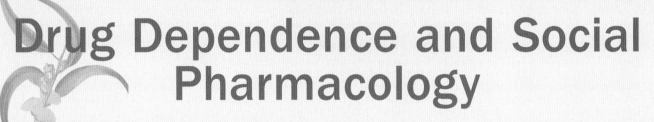

CHAPTER 22

Drug Dependence and Social Pharmacology

CHAPTER FOCUS

Substance and drug misuse is one of the top public health issues in societies today. It is widespread despite legislation, enforcement, and educational efforts to curb drug abuse. This chapter addresses drug misuse and abuse by identifying the problem and its effects on the individual and society, the issues that affect drug abuse in professionals, problems in drug testing, and the aetiological factors and pharmacological basis of dependence and tolerance. The drugs most commonly abused are identified and discussed, especially opioids (heroin, morphine); CNS depressants (including alcohol, the benzodiazepines and inhalants); CNS stimulants (cocaine, amphetamines, caffeine and nicotine); psychotomimetics (cannabis); and hallucinogens (LSD, MDMA). Health-care professionals may need to be able to recognise the signs and symptoms of abuse of various drugs. They must also be informed about the proper interventions (pharmacological and non-pharmacological) used for treatment in clinical practice.

OBJECTIVES

● To describe the difference between drug misuse and drug abuse.

● To discuss the scope and impact of substance and drug abuse in Australia and New Zealand.

● To identify the pharmacological basis of physical drug dependence and tolerance.

● To describe the general methods of treatment of drug dependence (treatment of acute overdose, detoxification, substitution, withdrawal and maintenance).

● To discuss the pharmacology of the drugs that are commonly abused, describe how the drugs are abused and explain related problems, toxic effects, withdrawal syndromes and methods of treatment.

● To describe the pathophysiological changes and effects on individuals and society resulting from chronic drug abuse.

KEY DRUGS

acamprosate
alcohol
amphetamines
caffeine
cannabis
cocaine
ecstasy
ethanol
heroin
lysergide
marijuana
methadone
naltrexone
nicotine
Δ⁹-tetrahydrocannabinol

KEY TERMS

addiction
alcoholism
dependence
designer drugs
drug abuse
drug misuse
euphoria
flashback phenomena
hallucinogen
illicit drugs
physical dependence
psychological dependence
reinforcement
reward
tolerance
withdrawal syndrome

KEY ABBREVIATIONS

ANS	autonomic nervous system
BP	*British Pharmacopoeia*
cAMP	cyclic adenosine monophosphate
CNS	central nervous system
DTs	delirium tremens
ETS	environmental tobacco smoke
GABA	gamma (γ)-aminobutyric acid
HIV–AIDS	human immunodeficiency virus–acquired immune deficiency syndrome
5-HT	5-hydroxytryptamine (serotonin)
IDUs	intravenous drug users
LSD	lysergic acid diethylamide
MDMA	3,4-methylenedioxymethamphetamine
PCP	phencyclidine
THC	tetrahydrocannabinol

DRUG DEPENDENCE, MISUSE AND ABUSE

Drug misuse or abuse

ALL drugs prescribed or self-administered have the potential to be misused or abused. The prescribing of drugs without adequate exploration of the patient's presenting complaint represents **drug misuse** by a prescriber. Prolonged and unsupervised administration of drugs for symptomatic relief, such as over-the-counter (OTC) analgesics for pain relief, is another example. In general, drug misuse refers to inappropriate or indiscriminate use of drugs.

Drug abuse refers to self-administration of a drug in chronically excessive quantities, in a manner that deviates from approved medical or social patterns in a given culture, resulting in physical or psychological harm. There are three important aspects to this definition:

- abuse is defined by what is accepted in the society, which may depend on its laws, history, religion and ethos
- it is a legal definition, implying that what deviates from the approved norm is illegal
- it involves knowing what is accepted medical practice; for example opiates are approved on medical prescription for pain but not for relief of anxiety or to constrict the pupil; β-blockers are approved in cardiovascular disease but restricted in some sporting events.

The drugs that are most commonly abused in Western societies are caffeine, nicotine and ethanol (alcohol). There are double standards prevalent in this area in terms of what is considered acceptable; for example, most governments condemn abuse of alcohol and tobacco products but do not ban them, as they receive enormous amounts of revenue from taxes on the products. However, the revenue received falls far short of the amount required in health care for treatment of adverse reactions and chronic health and social problems arising from abuse of these drugs.

Drug abuse is neither a new nor a recent phenomenon. It has been known throughout history as one expression of an individual's search for relief of physical, psychological, social or financial problems. Contemporary drug abuse has attained prominence as an issue with moral, legal, religious, social, psychological and medical implications. Drug abuse is not a problem confined to any particular socioeconomic, cultural or ethnic group.

Drug abuse may take a variety of forms:

- Experimental abuse occurs when people use drugs in an exploratory way, after which they accept or reject continuing use of the drugs.
- Social or recreational drug abuse may occur in social contexts, e.g. with alcohol, nicotine, caffeine, marijuana, 'ecstasy' and cocaine.
- Compulsive drug abuse is characterised by irrational, irresistible abuse of a drug.

- Ritualistic drug abuse may be related to religious practices, e.g. with psychotomimetic or hallucinogenic drugs.
- Polydrug or multiple drug abuse is common. Marijuana, alcohol and other depressants are often used together and in conjunction with central nervous system (CNS) stimulants. Many people in Western societies are dependent on both alcohol and caffeine, taking alcohol in the afternoons and evenings, and requiring caffeine in the mornings to overcome their hangovers from the night before.
- Drug abuse also occurs in sport: many drugs (anabolic steroids and sympathomimetics, stimulants, narcotic analgesics, diuretics, some hormones) are banned or restricted in sporting competitions, as they are seen as being dangerous or offering unfair advantages to the users. (This topic is covered in Chapter 57.)

Apart from caffeine, nicotine and ethanol, drugs that are commonly abused are:

- opioid analgesics ('narcotic analgesics', e.g. morphine and heroin)
- other CNS depressants (benzodiazepines, barbiturates, inhaled solvents)
- other CNS stimulants (cocaine, amphetamines)
- psychotomimetics or hallucinogens (cannabis, lysergic acid diethylamide [LSD], phencyclidine [PCP]).

Aspects of these drug groups relevant to drug abuse or dependence will be considered in detail in this chapter; many of the drugs with therapeutic uses are discussed in other chapters of the text.

Drug dependence

Note that drug abuse does not always entail dependence on the drug: people may abuse simple analgesics or megadoses of vitamins or asthma puffers. Generally, however, the stimulus to keep taking the drug is dependence on it. Drug **dependence** is the condition in which administration of a drug is compulsively sought in the absence of a therapeutic indication and despite adverse psychological, social or physical effects; dependence may lead to disturbed behaviour to ensure further supplies of the drug. Dependence does not always cause problems; thus a person may be dependent on caffeine, which is safe and cheap, without breaking laws or suffering serious adverse effects or withdrawal reactions.

There are two main types of dependence:

- **psychological dependence**: a behavioural pattern characterised by out-of-control craving for the pleasure of the drug's effects, denial of excessive drug use, and continuing abuse of the drug despite personal, social or legal difficulties; the use of the drug does not improve the person's quality of life
- **physical dependence**, which is manifest by intense

disturbances when administration of the drug ceases (the **withdrawal syndrome**).

Note that patients may well be in a state of medical dependence on a drug required for effective therapy; for example patients with type 1 diabetes are said to be 'insulin-dependent' and those with chronic asthma may be dependent on regular use of inhaled corticosteroids to control their symptoms.

Two other aspects of drug dependence also need to be defined. **Addiction** (a term sometimes used synonymously with dependence) is a behavioural pattern of drug use characterised by an overwhelming involvement with the procurement and use of the drug and a high tendency to relapse back into drug dependence. **Tolerance** is a physical state in which repeated doses of the drug cause decreasing effects, or doses must be increased to maintain the same effects. Not all drugs of dependence induce tolerance; for example tolerance develops rapidly to most of the effects of morphine (but not to the constipating or miotic effects), whereas there is little tolerance to marijuana.

Governments worldwide have regulated and restricted the use of most drugs of dependence (see Chapter 4); some, however (alcohol, nicotine, caffeine), are considered differently, and are readily available in most countries. In Australia drugs of dependence are generally listed in Schedule 8: CONTROLLED DRUGS, and thus are subject to the strictest controls in terms of availability, storage, labelling and prescribing. (An exception is low-dose codeine, which is readily available in cough mixtures and compound analgesics.) Thus most drugs of dependence are illegal other than on prescription and so if available outside approved medical use, they are considered **illicit**.

AETIOLOGICAL FACTORS LEADING TO DRUG ABUSE AND DEPENDENCE

Sociocultural factors

Different societies use and accept certain drugs as legal, while they may restrict or ban the use of other drugs. Such patterns of usage may depend on the particular society's religious rules, ethos (aggressive or meditative), history, traditional medicine practices, and experiences with the drugs. As Rang et al (1999) pointed out: "… drug-taking is clearly seen by society in a quite different light from other forms of addictive self-gratification, such as opera-going, football or sex". In smaller units of society, whether or not a drug is 'popular' may depend on its availability, ease of sharing, and peer-group pressures. In areas where particular drugs are illegal and are in short supply, the non-law-abiding people in society may be

motivated to obtain and sell the banned substances, which is usually a very profitable criminal venture.

In Japan amphetamines are major drugs of abuse, used to boost personal productivity and achievement. In Middle Eastern societies cannabis is considered a legal drug, encouraging introspection and meditation and decreasing sex drive, whereas alcohol is usually a forbidden substance. By contrast, in most Western cultures use of alcohol is encouraged despite its adverse effects on individuals, families and societies, while cannabis is illegal and may be considered an aphrodisiac! In high-altitude regions such as the South American Andes and Peru, coca leaves (the source of cocaine) are brewed as a tea or chewed to decrease hunger sensations, improve work performance, and increase a feeling of wellbeing.

Personality factors

The usual reason for a person to initially take an illicit drug is because of belief that a desirable pharmacological effect will result. The drug generally is used as a maladaptive coping mechanism to provide relief from anxiety or from personal problems, to achieve pleasure or gratification, or to alter the state of mind. Clinical Interest Box 22-1 summarises some theories on why people abuse drugs.

Psychological studies on people dependent on or abusing drugs have shown the three most important predictors to be rebelliousness, tolerance of deviance, and low school performance. Other factors include curiosity; impulsiveness; a low threshold of frustration; boredom; peer pressure; alienation; hedonism (pleasure-seeking behaviour); affluence; feelings of fear, inadequacy, shame or failure; personal conflicts; a predisposition to depression, which may result in emotional and behavioural problems; aggressiveness in childhood; the need to escape; and the widely publicised attention to drug abuse in the mass media. In particular, the 'alcoholic personality' has a higher than average incidence of depression and antisocial tendencies plus a genetic predisposition to dependence on the drug. Organisations such as Alcoholics Anonymous have been developed to help individuals overcome their dependence in a supportive, non-judgemental environment.

Pharmacological factors
Drugs of abuse

Although many drugs have some abuse potential, few drugs without CNS effects are misused or abused. The most frequently abused substances are those that have short onset of action and alter the mind, producing **euphoria**, enhanced alertness, relief from anxiety or pain, or hallucinations. Tolerance and/or physical dependence and a withdrawal syndrome may develop. Table 22-1 summarises several aspects of the main drugs of abuse. Other drugs that may induce altered states of perception, thought and feelings, and drug-induced psychoses as a result of prolonged use or

CLINICAL INTEREST BOX 22-1
WHY DO PEOPLE ABUSE DRUGS?

Many theories have been proposed as to why some people abuse drugs. Theories that see drug abusers as deviants include:

- the sinner (the moralistic model): the person lacks moral willpower to 'just say no'
- the sick person (the disease model): the patient suffers a psychopathology or is genetically predisposed to dependence
- the social victim (the poor environment model): poor home, schooling or role models, or unemployment, racism or other disadvantage.

Psychological theories to explain drug abuse include:

- cognitive–behavioural theory: dependence is due to a learned (reinforced) set of dysfunctional behaviours, which can be unlearned
- psychoanalytical theory: behaviours are determined by unconscious forces, so drugs are used in self-medication to improve mood or perception
- poor self-care theory: people struggling to cope abuse drugs, leading to 'suicide by degrees'
- the dual-diagnosis theory: the person concurrently suffers both psychiatric difficulties and substance dependence.

Note that there are different patterns of drug misuse or abuse in various sections of society, e.g. between men and women, indigenous and non-indigenous people, and adolescents and adults. Theories (and management programs) need to be sensitive to these patterns of drug abuse.

Adapted from: Hamilton et al 1998.

abuse include the methylxanthines (caffeine and theophylline, found in coffee, tea, chocolate and colas), anticholinergics, corticosteroids, psychotropic agents and levodopa. The pharmacological effects of some of these mind-altering drugs are graphically illustrated in Figure 22-1, showing the webs woven by spiders sprayed with amphetamine, caffeine, chloral hydrate or marijuana (NASA 1995).

Reinforcement and reward

The various drugs that have dependence potential have very little in common in terms of their chemical structures or effects on particular receptors. The one property they share is that of producing **reinforcement** or **reward** in animals or humans: that is, once familiar with the drug's effects, subjects will carry out work to obtain further doses of the drug as a reward. Drugs may be strong or weak reinforcers. Strong reinforcers include cocaine and morphine. Animals trained to self-administer cocaine will press a bar many thousands of times to obtain a dose, to the point of toxicity and self-mutilation. Animals trained with morphine will administer

doses that avoid either toxicity or withdrawal syndrome. Weak reinforcers include nicotine and caffeine; however, some drug addicts have been recorded as finding it easier to give up heroin than quit smoking. Non-reinforcers include cannabis: animals will not bother to self-administer this drug.

Some drugs are in fact negative reinforcers, i.e. animals will learn to avoid them; phenothiazines such as chlorpromazine are examples, which helps explain the poor compliance of patients prescribed these drugs chronically. The withdrawal syndrome that occurs after stopping drugs that cause physical

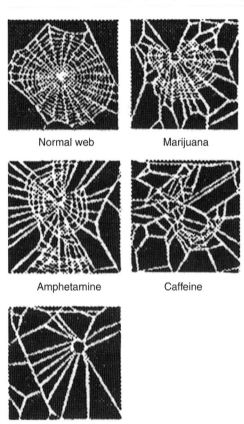

Normal web   Marijuana

Amphetamine   Caffeine

Chloral hydrate

FIGURE 22-1 Effects of mind-altering drugs on spiders. In a technique developed to test the toxicity of chemicals, household spiders were sprayed with solutions of the chemicals and the shapes of the webs subsequently spun were analysed using techniques of statistical crystallography. The figure shows the effects on web-spinning prowess of marijuana (a drug causing relaxation and impairment of motor coordination and memory), amphetamine and caffeine (CNS stimulants), and chloral hydrate (a sedative drug). The technique was developed as an alternative to toxicity testing in higher animals, which is expensive, time-consuming and subject to ethical concerns. The head of the research team, Dr David Noever, was quoted as saying that he did not expect complaints from animal rights groups. "We're all concerned about tests on warm and fuzzy creatures, but in this case they are only fuzzy." (quoted in *The Sunday Age*, 7 July 1995). Reproduced from *NASA Tech Briefs* 1995; 19(4): 82, with permission.

TABLE 22-1 Selected drugs commonly abused and symptoms of abuse

DRUG CATEGORY	STREET NAMES	METHODS OF USE	SYMPTOMS OF USE	HAZARDS OF USE
Marijuana/hashish	Pot, grass, dope, hooch, reefer, weed, gunga, Columbian, green, skunk, hash, hash oil, sinsemilla, joint, bhang, ganja, charas, kif, dagga	Most often smoked; can also be swallowed in solid form	Sweet, burnt odour; neglect of appearance; loss of interest and motivation; possible weight loss; red eyes	Impaired memory and perception; interference with psychological maturation; possible damage to lungs, heart, reproductive and immune systems; psychological dependence; increased risk of schizophrenia
Alcohol	Booze, hooch, juice, brew, grog, piss, turps	Swallowed in liquid form	Impaired muscle coordination and judgement	Heart and liver damage, death from overdose, death from car accidents, addiction, unsafe sex
Stimulants *Amphetamines** Amphetamine Dextroamphetamine Methamphetamine	Speed, uppers, pep pills, Bennies, Dexies, Moth, crystal, black beauties	Swallowed in pill or capsule form, injected into veins, dissolved in drinks	Excess activity, irritability; nervousness, mood swings, needle marks, violence	Arrhythmias, loss of appetite, hallucinations, paranoia, convulsions, coma, brain damage, death from overdose
Ecstasy	E, XTC, eccies, love drug	Taken as tablets	Increased confidence, paranoia, dry mouth, hangover, 'burnout'	High blood pressure, heart rate and temperature; thirst and overhydration
Cocaine	Coke, snow, toot, white lady, crack, ready rock, Charlie, blow	Most often inhaled (snorted); also injected or swallowed in powder form, smoked	Restlessness, anxiety, intense short-term high followed by dysphoria	Intense psychological dependence, sleeplessness, anxiety, nasal passage damage, lung damage, death from overdose (highly addictive)
Nicotine/tobacco	Smoke, cancer stick, ciggie, durry, death stick, fag, gasper, coffin nail, butt	Smoked in cigarettes, cigars and pipes; snuff; chewing tobacco	Smell of tobacco, high carbon monoxide blood levels, stained teeth	Cancers of the lung, throat, mouth and oesophagus; cardiovascular disease; emphysema
Depressants *Barbiturates* Pentobarbitone	Barbs, downers Yellow jackets Blue devils	Swallowed in pill form or injected into veins	Drowsiness, confusion, impaired judgement, slurred speech, needle marks, constricted pupils	Infection after parenteral use, addiction with severe life-threatening withdrawal symptoms, loss of appetite, death from overdose, nausea
Opioids Methadone, pethidine Morphine	Dreamer, junk	Swallowed in pill or liquid form, injected, smoked	Drowsiness, lethargy; miosis	Addiction with severe withdrawal symptoms, loss of appetite, constipation, tolerance, death from overdose

*Includes lookalike drugs resembling amphetamines that contain caffeine, phenylpropanolamine (PPA), and ephedrine.

TABLE 22-1 Selected drugs commonly abused and symptoms of abuse—cont'd

DRUG CATEGORY	STREET NAMES	METHODS OF USE	SYMPTOMS OF USE	HAZARDS OF USE
Heroin	Smack, hammer, horse	Injected into veins, smoked	Needle marks, intense high	As for other opioids
Codeine	School boy	Swallowed in pill or liquid form		
Hallucinogens				
PCP (phencyclidine)	Angel dust, killer weed, supergrass, hog, peace pill	Most often smoked; can also be inhaled (snorted); injected or swallowed in tablets	Distorted sensations, slurred speech; blurred vision, incoordination, confusion, agitation, aggression	Anxiety, depression, impaired memory and perception, psychological dependence, death from accidents, death from overdose
LSD	Acid, trip, cubes, purple haze	Injected or swallowed in tablets	Dilated pupils, delusions; hallucinations, mood swings	Breaks from reality, emotional breakdown, flashback
Mescaline	Mesc, cactus	Usually ingested in their natural form		
Psilocybin	Magic mushrooms			
Inhalants				
Solvents				
Gasoline, glue, paint thinner, lighter fluid	Chroming, glue sniffing	Inhaled or sniffed, often with use of paper or plastic bag or rag	Initial high, then CNS depression; poor motor coordination; impaired vision, memory and thought processes; abusive, violent behaviour; slowed thought; headache	High risk of sudden death; drastic weight loss; brain, liver and bone marrow damage; anaemia; death by anoxia
Nitrites				
Amyl, butyl	Poppers, locker room, rush, snappers	Inhaled or sniffed from gauze or ampoules		

dependence can act as a type of negative reinforcement, such that addicts learn rapidly to try to avoid the withdrawal syndrome by taking another dose.

Pharmacological bases of dependence and tolerance

DEPENDENCE

Much research has gone into the mechanisms of drug dependence. Currently the best accepted theory involves central dopaminergic pathways, in particular the mesolimbic pathway from the substantia nigra through the nucleus accumbens to the frontal cortex. All dependence-producing drugs have been shown to increase the release of dopamine in this pathway and to cause increased cyclic AMP (cAMP) activity. In addition, the dopamine transporter (uptake mechanism) plays a key role in mediating the actions of cocaine and amphetamines.

Further evidence is that interruption of this pathway, e.g. with neuroleptic (antidopamine) drugs, leads to a decrease in drug-seeking behaviours. Drugs that increase dopamine turnover cause decreased ethanol consumption in ethanol-preferring mice, and dopamine-transporter 'knockout' mice

(i.e. mice with their dopamine-activator genes inactivated) can be used as models for long-term drug abuse of cocaine and amphetamines. In addition, variants in the dopamine-receptor gene are associated with the 'reward deficiency syndrome', which involves such varied pathologies as drug dependence, smoking, alcoholism, obesity, pathological gambling and attention-deficit hyperactivity disorder.

This explanation is oversimplified, however, and other mediators and transmitters may also be involved, including 5-hydroxytryptamine (5-HT, serotonin), glutamate and corticosteroids.

TOLERANCE

Tolerance, the tendency for successive doses to have lesser effects, may exist with either psychological or physical dependence and may be viewed in two ways. Receptor-site (pharmacodynamic) tolerance is a form of adaptation in which the effect produced depends on both the concentration of the drug and the duration of the exposure. In this type of tolerance the clinical effect of the drug is reduced as the duration of exposure continues. Receptor synthesis may be downregulated or receptors may be lost or desensitised, or there may be exhaustion of chemical mediators or transmitters.

The second type of tolerance is metabolic (pharmaco-kinetic) tolerance, which refers to aspects of drug disposition or elimination. Prolonged exposure to a drug can change the body's handling of the drug, increasing drug clearance with repeated ingestion. With prolonged exposure to barbiturates, for example, the steady-state blood concentrations will fall progressively because of barbiturates' inducing effect on hepatic microsomal enzymes, which increases barbiturate metabolism and inactivation.

PROBLEMS ASSOCIATED WITH DRUG ABUSE

The scale of trafficking in drugs

It is estimated that worldwide the trade in drugs amounts to 10% of all international trade. Many studies have shown that law enforcement agencies cannot prevent the supply of illicit drugs, despite enormous operating budgets, which leads to the conclusion that prohibition is simply not working.

In the USA, alcohol was generally estimated to play a role in 40% of assaults reported, 50% of crimes, 50% of all traffic accidents, 35% of suicides and 50% of unintentional injury fatalities. Over 70% of all prison inmates are imprisoned for drug-related crimes.

Overall, the economic cost of drug misuse and abuse in Australia, including tangible and intangible costs, was estimated at more than A$34.5 billion in 1998/99. Of this, about 60% was due to tobacco, 22% due to alcohol, and only 17% due to illicit drugs. Thus it is the licit drugs (alcohol and tobacco) that cause the most medical and economic harm in our community.

Individual, family and society problems

Substance abuse is a major medical, social, economic and interpersonal problem, affecting people from all economic backgrounds and across the lifespan. The craving for further doses of the drug may come to dominate the individual's life, even leading to an unacceptable lifestyle or a life of crime to support the drug dependence.

While deaths from overdose of heroin or other illicit drugs are tragic and newsworthy, the vast majority of non-prescription drug-related deaths in Australia are due to tobacco (72%) or alcohol (25%). It has been estimated that in

1992 about 23,000 Australians died from drug-related causes. Another relevant statistic is that in Victoria, around 10% of hospital bed-days are used to treat conditions associated with the use of alcohol, tobacco or illicit drugs. Of clients attending specialist drug treatment services, about 50% of problems were related to alcohol, 25% to opioid abuse and 7% each to amphetamines or cannabis. Over 12% of clients reported multiple drug use and 38% reported injecting drugs.

The harm done may be directly to the individual, from adverse drug reactions or interactions such as liver cirrhosis from chronic alcoholism, psychosis from amphetamines or lung cancer and cardiovascular disease from smoking. The signs and symptoms of acute drug intoxication are summarised in Table 22-2.

There are indirect effects as well; for example IV drug abuse may lead a person into the subculture of 'shooting up', with the risk of sharing of non-sterile needles and hence HIV–AIDS and hepatitis, or into a life of crime and possible imprisonment. As a consequence of all the above factors, the life-expectancy of people who are dependent on drugs is generally lower than the life-expectancy of non-dependent individuals. Clinical Interest Box 22-2 describes some of the myths related to drug abuse.

Families of drug-dependent persons may have to cope with reduced earnings and resources, aggressive behaviour, increased medical expenses, destructive relationships and increased dependence on state welfare for support. Drug abuse during pregnancy poses major problems for both mother and fetus (see the Pregnancy Safety box at the end of this chapter).

At the society level there may be escalating crime in the community, with the attendant requirements for increased policing, court procedures and prisons to deal with offences related to production, supply and possession of illicit drugs; and alcohol-related intoxication, violence and drink-driving, with increased risk-taking and deaths. Abuse of injectable drugs (opioids, amphetamines and cocaine) leads to spread of infections such as viral hepatitis and HIV–AIDS.

Withdrawal syndromes

As well as acute adverse pharmacological effects and toxicity, there are longer-term problems of withdrawal after chronic administration. In many cases, the **withdrawal syndrome** is due to or manifests as a rebound in the systems affected by the drug. Withdrawal from chronic use of benzodiazepines (antianxiety agents and CNS depressants), for example, is likely to lead to feelings of anxiety and agitation, while withdrawal from amphetamines (CNS stimulants) leads to depressed mood and drowsiness. Characteristics of individual withdrawal syndromes will be discussed in later sections under specific drug groups.

TABLE 22-2 Signs and symptoms of acute drug intoxication

DRUG(S) ABUSED	SIGNS AND SYMPTOMS
Cannabis drugs	Tachycardia and postural hypotension, conjunctival vascular congestion (red eyes), distortions of perception, dryness of mouth and throat, possible panic
Cocaine	Increased stimulation, euphoria, raised blood pressure and heart rate, anorexia, insomnia, agitation; in overdose: elevated body temperature, hallucinations, seizures, death
Opioids	Depressed blood pressure and respiration, fixed pinpoint pupils, coma, pulmonary oedema
Barbiturates and other general CNS depressants	Depressed blood pressure and respiration; ataxia, slurred speech, confusion, depressed tendon reflexes, coma, shock
Amphetamines	Elevated blood pressure, tachycardia, other cardiac arrhythmias, hyperactive tendon reflexes, pupils dilated and reactive to light, hyperpyrexia, perspiration, shallow respirations, circulatory collapse, possible hallucinations, paranoid feelings
Hallucinogenic agents	Elevated blood pressure, hyperactive tendon reflexes, piloerection, perspiration, pupils dilated and reactive to light, anxiety, distortion of body image and perception, delusions, hallucinations

CLINICAL INTEREST BOX 22-2 MYTHS RELATED TO DRUG ABUSE

Many myths circulate in the community related to drug misuse and abuse. Some examples of misinformation are:

- 'Medicines you can buy in the supermarket or health shop aren't real drugs, so they can't harm you.' (*Wrong*: vitamins, minerals, aspirin, paracetamol, cough mixtures, herbal preparations etc can and do have adverse effects.)
- 'Recreational use of drugs is not harmful.' (*Wrong*: all drugs can have adverse effects; tobacco and alcohol cause by far the greatest harm to the Australian community.)
- 'Only weak individuals become addicts — I can control my drug-taking.' (*Wrong*: people take drugs for a variety of reasons and anyone can become addicted, depending on the drug and dose.)
- 'My mate lined his stomach with milk before we started drinking, so he'll be OK to drive us all home.' (*Wrong*: milk is quickly absorbed and does not delay the absorption of alcohol.)
- 'I stopped using heroin for a while, but I'm going back onto it — it's OK because I'm used to it.' (*Wrong*: tolerance is quickly lost and the strength and purity of preparations can vary widely, so doses at levels previously taken may be toxic.)
- 'All street drugs are so addictive that one dose will make you an addict.' (*Wrong*: several doses over a period of time may be required before dependence develops.)
- 'My friends told me that marijuana is not dangerous but one of them went mad — it might make me crazy too.' (It may, but occasional use is unlikely to cause

psychosis; however, it can precipitate mental illness in people predisposed to it.)
- 'My drug taking is hurting only me.' (*Wrong*: drug abuse can harm friends, family and society. No individual has the right to damaging or destructive behaviour.)
- 'You can't stop me taking drugs.' (*True*: only the drug user can stop the drug abuse; but first you must admit you have a problem.)
- 'The doctor prescribed these drugs, so they must be OK; I won't get hooked on them.' (*Wrong*: prescription drugs such as pethidine, codeine, amphetamines, benzodiazepines [Valium] and phenobarbitone can cause dependence.)
- 'If I take "speed" pills, they will pep me up and burn up the booze, so I can drink as much alcohol as I like.' (*Wrong*: even though the stimulant effects of amphetamines may partly counteract the depressant effects of alcohol, the blood alcohol level will continue to rise, and may go higher than expected because of the dehydrating effects of the combination.)
- 'All drug addicts should be imprisoned.' (*Wrong*: what about those dependent on caffeine, alcohol or nicotine? Treatment and rehabilitation are more effective than imprisonment.)
- 'Growing and pushing drugs is one way poor people can make money.' (Maybe, but it is illegal, takes the trafficker into the criminal world, increases crime, and is dangerous.)

Adapted from: Hamilton et al 1998; Walters 1996.

Problems among health professionals

Career pressures and easy accessibility to drugs place health-care professionals, particularly doctors, pharmacists, nurses, anaesthetists and dentists, at greater risk of drug abuse. Studies among health professionals in the USA have shown that the combination of alcohol and other drugs was quite prevalent, especially with physicians and nurses. Health-care professionals who abused medications generally used more than four substances, including prescription drugs (opioid analgesics and benzodiazepines), alcohol, tobacco and nitrous oxide.

POLICIES RELATED TO DRUG ABUSE AND ITS MANAGEMENT

History of legislation against drugs of abuse

Opium, as a source of active alkaloids with analgesic, sedative (narcotic) and antidiarrhoeal activities, has been used in various cultures for thousands of years. An international Opium Convention was set up in 1912 to curb the trade; this was ratified after World War I. Other drugs of addiction were added to the charter, including cannabis in 1925.

The responsibility for worldwide control of narcotics (by then defined to include cocaine and cannabis) was handed over to the United Nations after World War II (1946). Most countries now attempt to keep their official drug regulation legislation in line with that of the UN but this can be problematic if a country wishes to trial an alternative policy (e.g. supervised injecting facilities).

Extent of drug abuse in Australia

To estimate the extent of drug abuse in Australia, large-scale population surveys on household drug use patterns, attitudes and behaviours have been carried out regularly every 3–4 years since 1985. The data collected from these surveys have formed the basis for the development of policies for Australia's response to drug-related issues. The first results from the 2004 survey of almost 30,000 Australians aged from 12 years up are available from the Australian Institute of Health and Welfare, Drug Statistics Series no. 13. Some interesting facts and trends since the previous survey in 2001 are:

- almost half the respondents aged over 14 years had smoked more than 100 cigarettes in their lives; however, the proportion who smoked daily declined to 17.4%

- the proportion of people drinking alcohol daily remained stable at 8.9%
- almost 2 out of every 5 Australians had used an illicit drug at some time in their lives; recent marijuana use dropped significantly from 12.9% to 11.3%
- tobacco, alcohol and illicit drug use contributes to significant disease, injury, workplace problems, violence, crime and family breakdown in Australia
- economic costs associated with both licit and illicit drug use in 1998/99 amounted to $34.5 billion, of which tobacco accounted for 60%, alcohol 22% and illicit drugs 17%
- however, when people are asked to nominate which drugs they consider cause drug problems in Australia, the first nominated is generally heroin (39.4%), then marijuana, well before alcohol, cocaine, amphetamines, then tobacco
- data on the proportion of the population that had recently used drugs are as follows: alcohol: 83.6%, tobacco: 20.7%, any illicit drug: 15.3%
- the only illicit drug whose use is increasing is ecstasy, up from 2.9% in 2001 to 3.4% in 2004
- when drugs were ranked in order of 'acceptability' for regular use, the order was alcohol > tobacco > marijuana, then non-medical use of analgesics and CNS depressants, before ecstasy, amphetamines and hallucinogens
- support for the legalisation of illicit drugs has declined slightly
- public support has grown for measures to reduce the problems associated with tobacco use, such as banning smoking in public places and increasing tax on tobacco products.

Tobacco and alcohol

The extent of the problem of drug abuse in Australia is not easy to define. As discussed in the previous section, the most commonly abused drugs are in fact legal: alcohol and tobacco. Overall, tobacco use has been dropping since the 1940s, when about 75% of Australian men smoked, to about 30% of men smoking in the mid-1990s and 20% in 2004. The proportion of young women smoking, however, has risen, and this group is particularly vulnerable to advertising and to the use of tobacco to decrease appetite.

With respect to alcohol, Australians rank about 15th highest as per capita consumers (on average, 7.65 litres of pure alcohol per person per year). About 12% of men drink alcohol daily, and 5.8% of women. About 27% of teenagers aged 14–19 years drink at least weekly. Over the 200-odd years since alcohol was introduced into Australia, patterns of drinking have changed, from rum to beer to wines. Surveys attempting to estimate the extent of problem drinking (drinking to above the accepted safe limits of four standard drinks per day for men, or two for women) suggest that overall about

CLINICAL INTEREST BOX 22-3
DRUG MISUSE IN NEW ZEALAND

ALCOHOL

Alcohol is the most commonly consumed drug in New Zealand. It is estimated that alcohol-related conditions account for 3.1% of male deaths and 1.41% of female deaths.

Alcohol affects the road toll, street crime and petty dishonesty. It is related to:
- 60 per cent of all incidents reported to the Police
- 41 per cent of all fatal motor accidents
- 77 per cent of street disorder and fighting offences
- 40 per cent of serious assaults

The Sale of Liquor Amendment Act 1999 introduced a number of major changes. The legal minimum drinking age was lowered from 20 to 18 years, and minors under 18 years are not allowed to purchase alcohol or consume it on licensed premises or in public places unless accompanied by a parent or guardian.

The upper legal limit of alcohol for licensed drivers aged over 20 years is 80 mgs of alcohol per 100 mls of blood or 400 microgrammes per litre of breath on a breathalyser. For all licensed drivers aged under 20 years, the upper legal limit is 30 mgs of alcohol per 100 mls of blood or 150 microgrammes per litre of breath

To stay under the limit:
- Male drivers should have no more than one 375 ml can of beer (4.5% alcohol) or two cans of low alcohol beer (2% alcohol).
- An average-size woman could go over the limit even after a double nip of spirits or a small glass of wine, or a can of beer.
- Under 20-year-olds are best advised not to drink and drive.

SMOKING

Tobacco is the second most commonly used recreational drug after alcohol. It is estimated to kill approximately 4700 New Zealanders each year. Many people in New Zealand suffer from a wide range of chronic illnesses associated with smoking. On 3 December 2003, an amendment to the Smoke-free Environments Act 1990 was passed. Premises became smoke free and the display of tobacco products became restricted, as was the sale to under 18's. Herbal smoking products were included in the ban. The aim was to reduce the effects of second-hand smoke which was reported to kill 350 New Zealanders annually.

The 1996–97 Health Survey showed that nearly half of all Maori adults reported that they were current smokers, compared with 23.2% of European/Pakeha, 27.7% of Pacific Island and 10.1% of 'other' adults. Maori adults reported starting to smoke at an earlier age and were more likely to have smoked for more than 20 years. A smoking cessation shceme introduced in 1999 offering nicotine-containing smoking cessation patches and gum from pharmacies and clinics in exchange for vouchers and a small fee has been taken up by New Zealanders in large numbers. In July 2003 the Maori Tobacco Control Strategy was launched. The culturally appropriate Aukati Kai Paipa programmes have a quit rate of 29%. The next Health Survey is due to be conducted during 2006/7.

CANNABIS

Marijuana is the third most popular recreational drug in New Zealand after alcohol and tobacco (excluding caffeine)

Cannabis was the main illicit drug used in 1999, with only a small percentage reporting current or regular use and associated drug-related problems. It is used disproportionately by young males, Maori and some rural communities, particularly in Northland and on the East Coast where cannabis is widely grown for economic purposes. It is these demographic areas which report the most cannabis-related harm.

New Zealand debated whether or not the possession or use of marijuana should be decriminalised; about 70% of the 18,720 prosecutions for offences involving cannabis resulted in a conviction in 1998. The National Organisation for the Reform of Marijuana Laws (NORML) works to end cannabis prohibition, but their campaign was opposed by the select committee of the Youth Parliament in 2000. In July 2005, the Labour Governement reported that it would not introduce legislation to legalise marijuana.

METHAMPHETAMINE

Methamphetamine can be produced easily in a clandestine home laboratory using pseudoephedrine tablets (available without prescription in New Zealand), using simple extraction techniques, common household equipment and readily available chemicals to do the 'bake', following recipes available on the Internet. Police are observing the trend of 'shoppers' who move from pharmacy to pharmacy purchasing cold/flu products containing pseudoephedrine. There has been a marked increase in the number of clandestine laboratories for the manufacture of 'P', with a peak in 2003 of nearly 200 labs detected.

If it is contained in a cold/flu preparation containing less than 1.8grams it will be a partially exempt drug, as will controlled release formulations containing no more than 240mg. This allows the sale of these medicines from pharmacies. In many pharmacies, identification is required for the purchase of pseudoephedrine containing medicines. This is in accordance with the pharmacist's Code of Ethics (Principle 3) of non-maleficence, which requires that the pharmacist plays an active role in preventing the sale of medicines for illegal purposes.

Pseudoephedrine and pseudoephedrine-containing products became controlled drugs from 15 October 2004. There was a steady increase in the size of parcels of pseudoephedrine products seized by Customs officials, with examples of parcels containing 1800, 2400, and 20,000 tablets in single imports. Such imports were often arranged through internet pharmacy sites.

Pseudoephedrine is used as a precursor substance in the manufacture of methamphetamine or 'P', an addictive drug misused for its stimulant potential. Methamphetamine sells on the street for between $180 to $1000 for one gram. Known also as 'speed', 'pure', 'burn' and 'ice', the name 'P' is used only in New Zealand. 'Ice' is the name of the most pure form, which is highly addictive.

Adapted from: www.moh.govt.nz, www.crime.co.nz, www.ndp.govt.nz, accessed 19 January 2006

76% of men are responsible drinkers, 6.7% at-risk drinkers and 3.5% high-risk drinkers; the analogous figures for women are 70% responsible, 7.2% at-risk and 2.2% high-risk. Female teenagers are twice as likely as males to consume alcohol at risky levels.

Illicit drugs

The abuse of **illicit drugs** (especially cannabis, heroin and cocaine) is decreasing in Australia. Generally, men are more likely to use illicit drugs than women, and young people (<35 years) more so than older adults. There is a huge jump in use of drugs during the teenage years, especially between Year 7 at school (11–12-year-olds) and Year 11 (16–17-year-olds); alcohol and marijuana are most commonly used.

Cannabis is the most widely used illicit drug, with about 33% of the Australian population (in large-scale surveys) admitting to having tried it and 10%–13% having used it in the previous 12 months. Young people are more likely to use cannabis: 55% of 20–29-year-olds have used it. Cannabis use has been decriminalised in some states (South Australia, ACT) so that private use is no longer a crime. There is no evidence that this has led to an increase in use or abuse, and it has allowed police and courts to concentrate on more dangerous illicit drugs.

With respect to use of other illicit drugs in Australia:

- about 9% of the population claim to have tried amphetamines, and 6% have tried ecstasy; this use is increasing, mainly for recreational use and abuse in the 20–39 age group
- 6%–10% have tried hallucinogens, such as LSD or psilocybin; these drugs came to prominence in the 1960s and are now mainly used in the 'rave' party scene
- 5% use barbiturates for non-medical purposes
- 3% use cocaine or inhalants, and 2% ecstasy or heroin; these illicit drugs tend to be abused by particular subcultures of society
- generally, illicit drugs are most commonly obtained from friends or acquaintances (70%); heroin, however, is most commonly obtained from dealers (64%), and steroids from gyms and sports clubs (65%).

Therapeutic drugs

Therapeutic drugs (prescribed and OTC) can also be misused or abused for non-medical purposes; the extent of this is difficult to determine. Drug regulations have become increasingly tight since the early 1900s, when narcotics were banned. Amphetamines were readily available in the 1950s and 1960s but are now indicated only for narcolepsy and attention-deficit hyperactivity disorder (ADHD). They are, however, frequently abused by people wanting the CNS-stimulant effects (e.g. long-distance drivers), and children prescribed stimulants for ADHD have been known to sell

them on to schoolmates and adults. Pseudoephedrine, another amphetamine-type stimulant, is readily available in cough and cold medicines (see Clinical Interest Box 22-3). Codeine and other mild narcotic analgesics used in pain relievers and as cough suppressants are frequently abused; naive young hospital pharmacists are sometimes surprised at the number of patients turning up regularly at respiratory clinics for their bottle of Pholcodine Linctus! The benzodiazepine antianxiety drugs are renowned for causing dependence, which can be difficult to break.

Doctors and pharmacists need to be aware that patients become very persuasive in faking symptoms to get certain drugs prescribed, and often 'shop around' to augment their supply.

Policy approaches
Australian drug policies

Many possible policy approaches can be adopted by governments in response to problems of drug abuse in the community. The current policies in Australia are based on the American prohibition model of 'zero tolerance' for illicit drug abuse, as well as on demand reduction and harm minimisation (see www.nationaldrugstrategy.gov.au, and Clinical Interest Box 22-4). Worldwide, prevention policies have been proven to be enormously expensive and ineffective and the extent of drug abuse has changed little over several decades.

Other possible drug policies

In the Netherlands and some other European countries, policies are based on normalisation and destigmatisation, whereby less harmful drugs ('soft drugs') are less tightly controlled and may be ignored by police (e.g. cannabis can be ordered in a coffee shop). Supervised injecting facilities have been demonstrated to operate well in some German cities, leading to decreased public nuisance, fewer heroin overdose deaths and decreased frequency of drug-related infections.

TREATING DRUG DEPENDENCE
General aspects of treatment

Many treatment modalities are possible in the area of drug abuse and the choice is determined by whether it is a case of acute toxicity, chronic abuse or long-term management. Drug dependence is a chronic relapsing–remitting disorder and the person must first acknowledge that the drug use has become a problem. As stated previously, the only person who can stop drug abuse is the drug user himself or herself. In this section, general aspects of treatment will be discussed; specific treatments for particular drug-related problems will be considered

CLINICAL INTEREST BOX 22-4 'TURNING THE TIDE' ON DRUGS

The Victorian state government drug program 'Turning the Tide' was set up in response to community concern about the perceived rising drug problem. It emphasised education (school, tertiary, professional and community); improved services, especially to at-risk young people and adult offenders; and improved research, data collection, monitoring and testing procedures. About A$60 million was approved for the program over 1996–99, and a Premier's Drug Advisory Council was instituted. Unfortunately, many of its recommendations were considered 'too hot to handle' politically.

The following harm minimisation advice was promulgated, in recognition that people will continue to abuse drugs and need some protection:

- Use only one drug at a time.
- If injecting, use clean syringes, needles and water; inhaling is safer.
- If using ecstasy in the 'rave' scene, take frequent rest and water breaks.
- Don't use drugs when alone.
- Practise safe sex.

- Dispose of used needles and syringes safely.
- If someone collapses, put him or her in the recovery position, call an ambulance immediately and stay with the person.

The Victorian Premier's Drug Advisory Council's Report concluded in 2000 that maintaining the status quo (prohibition of all currently illicit drugs) is not an option: it will only lead to increased abuse and more heroin deaths. With respect to marijuana, the Council acknowledged that school children (rightly) see cannabis as less dangerous than alcohol or tobacco and can obtain it as easily as getting a pizza! Cannabis is widely used but is not highly addictive, only one in 10 users having problems. Decriminalisation of marijuana was recommended on the basis that in other places this has not led to increased use (except by 'drug tourists'). Decriminalisation breaks the nexus between cannabis and more dangerous illicit drugs, allows redirection of police and court time to control of trafficking in more serious drugs and diverts scarce funds to treatment and rehabilitation of drug abusers.

in the section on the drug of abuse. Some general points relevant to treatment are:

- multiple drug abuse is common so a full drug screen should be carried out
- for many patients, counselling about the drug-related problems is helpful, with respect to reducing intoxication, risks and consumption
- psychiatric problems often occur concurrently with drug abuse, especially depression, psychoses, anxiety disorders and personality disorders; likewise, people with psychiatric disorders often abuse drugs. This is known as 'dual diagnosis'. Long-term use of benzodiazepines may thus be an addiction requiring treatment, or it may be appropriate medication for chronic medical or psychiatric conditions
- intravenous drug users (IDUs) run extra risks of contracting blood-borne virus diseases, such as hepatitis B or C or HIV infection through sharing of equipment (syringes, needles); needle exchange programs and supervised injecting rooms may be advised
- drug abusers become very skilled at conning doctors into prescribing more of the drugs they crave
- other treatment modalities include education and information, self-help strategies, psychological therapies and complementary and alternative medicine (CAM) methods (see Clinical Interest Box 22-5).

The guiding principle should be to consider a combination of therapeutic approaches, depending on the individual's needs.

Treating acute overdose

The first aim of treatment is resuscitation of the patient, if necessary, then elimination of the drug taken, if possible, and treatment of toxic effects and complications. Specific

CLINICAL INTEREST BOX 22-5 COMPLEMENTARY AND ALTERNATIVE THERAPIES IN MANAGEMENT OF DRUG DEPENDENCE

Patients with problems related to drug abuse frequently turn to CAM methods for relief. Methods tried include prayer, removal to a sanatorium (with fresh air, controlled diet and healthy lifestyle), hypnosis, acupuncture, and mutual support programs such as the famous 12-step program of Alcoholics Anonymous.

Few clinical trials have been done to test the efficacy of CAM methods and there is a high drop-out rate, with return to the abused drug (recidivism). Some evidence exists for the effectiveness of biofeedback in treatment of misuse of alcohol and opioids; transcendental meditation in opioid, nicotine, cocaine or alcohol abuse; rest and yoga in alcohol or nicotine abuse; acupuncture for cocaine abuse; and various herbs for detoxification and 'liver cleansing' in alcohol abuse.

Overall, combinations of Western and CAM therapies are common and often effective, e.g. specific replacement or antagonist drugs, along with behavioural psychotherapy, nutritional therapy and acupuncture.

Adapted from: Spencer & Jacobs 1999.

DRUG MONOGRAPH 22-1 NALTREXONE

Naltrexone is an opioid antagonist with no agonist actions. It competitively binds to opioid receptors and reversibly blocks the effects of all opioids, including the physical dependence produced. In alcohol-dependent people, naltrexone reduces alcohol craving, alcohol consumption and relapse rates, presumably by antagonism of endogenous opioids involved in alcohol-dependence mechanisms. Naltrexone can precipitate a withdrawal syndrome in opioid-dependent people.

INDICATIONS This drug is indicated for adjuvant treatment in the detoxified opioid-dependent or alcohol-dependent person, in conjunction with a comprehensive psychological and social rehabilitation program.

PHARMACOKINETICS Absorption is rapid but naltrexone undergoes an extensive first-pass metabolism in the liver to the major metabolite 6 β naltrexol, which also has opioid antagonist effects. Oral bioavailability is only 5%–40%. The peak serum concentration is reached in 1 hour. Elimination half-life for naltrexone is 4 hours and, for its major metabolite, about 13 hours. Its duration of action is dose-dependent and ranges from 24 to 72 hours. Excretion of the drug and its metabolites is via the kidneys.

ADVERSE DRUG REACTIONS Serious adverse effects are uncommon, as naltrexone has little intrinsic activity. Mild adverse effects are also the symptoms of opioid withdrawal and include anxiety, GI and sleep disturbances and headache.

DRUG INTERACTIONS There have been few studies of drug interactions. In opioid-dependent people not yet adequately detoxified a serious withdrawal reaction is precipitated. The opioids present in other opioid-containing

medications (such as narcotic analgesics and cough suppressants) will be antagonised, leading to decreased effectiveness. In alcohol-dependent people the combination with disulfiram can lead to additive hepatotoxicity.

WARNINGS AND CONTRAINDICATIONS Naltrexone is contraindicated in patients receiving opioids, those dependent on them or those in acute withdrawal. Patients must be opioid free for 7–10 days before starting naltrexone therapy. If necessary this status should be confirmed with a naloxone challenge test (low-dose naloxone is given under close supervision and the patient observed for signs of acute withdrawal reaction). Naltrexone is also contraindicated in severe liver disease.

There are dangers if a patient resumes opioid administration while on naltrexone or after stopping naltrexone therapy, as previous tolerance may have waned and there is risk of a potentially fatal overdose. If patients on naltrexone therapy suddenly require opioids for analgesia in an emergency, there are difficulties in overcoming the receptor blockade caused by naltrexone.

Naltrexone is classified B3 with respect to pregnancy warnings, as there has been limited use to establish safety. Similarly, safety in children or during breastfeeding has not been established.

DOSAGE AND ADMINISTRATION Treatment with naltrexone is started cautiously, usually at a dose of 25 mg orally, with close monitoring for withdrawal signs and symptoms for about 1 hour. If no withdrawal effects occur, the balance of the daily dose is given. Maintenance is usually 50 mg orally daily. Compliance with therapy is improved if a trusted adult supervises administration of the drug.

---

antagonist drugs may be used to block the toxic effects of the drug of dependence, e.g. the opioid antagonists naloxone or nalorphine for opioid overdose, or flumazenil for benzodiazepine overdose. Antidepressants such as fluoxetine or bupropion may be useful, particularly for withdrawal syndromes and quitting smoking. Drugs that may potentiate toxicity, particularly in the CNS or cardiovascular system, should be avoided.

Treating chronic abuse

Initially, a comprehensive assessment of the person is required, for organic diseases, drug screening and a full history—medical, drug, social, family, psychological and psychiatric. The goals of treatment are to achieve withdrawal from the drug, detoxification and treatment of any withdrawal reactions. A milder substitute drug helps maintain effects while reducing harms, e.g. oxazepam for diazepam, or methadone

for morphine or heroin. Dopamine agonists may help reduce craving for the pleasure reinforcement. Naltrexone has effects in treating more than one type of drug dependence (see Drug Monograph 22-1). A multidisciplinary approach to treatment is required and may be best carried out in a hospital or 'detox' facility.

Long-term maintenance

The preferred scenario is to achieve abstinence from any drug abuse; however, this is recognised as being very difficult and perhaps unrealistic. A more reachable goal is harm minimisation, without reliance on pharmacological agents for support. An exception is the use of methadone in maintenance programs for opioid addicts; methadone prescribed by authorised physicians and dispensed in authorised clinics or pharmacies reduces the withdrawal symptoms and craving for opioids.

Responses to drug-seeking behaviour

Health-care professionals have to remain alert to drug-seeking behaviours. Many patients 'shop around' among doctors to obtain prescriptions for drugs on which they are dependent, particularly seeking codeine, pethidine, oxycodone, amphetamines and benzodiazepines. A recent study in Australia revealed over 850 people who had seen more than 50 different doctors in one year, and over 20,000 people who had seen 15 or more doctors.

While it is important that patients with genuine need of a drug are not denied it, drug seekers need to be identified and referred to an appropriate treatment facility. Signs of drug-seeking behaviours include:

* requests for a specific drug (of dependence) and refusing other suggestions
* reporting inconsistent symptoms
* reporting a recent move into the area, with a (forged?) letter of support
* signs of drug intoxication or withdrawal, especially impaired cognitive functions, injection-site marks and constricted or dilated pupils.

OPIOIDS (HEROIN, MORPHINE AND OTHER AGONIST OPIOIDS)

Opiates are the narcotic drugs from natural sources and include the opium alkaloids morphine and codeine. Related drugs are the semisynthetic compounds heroin and hydromorphone and the synthetic drugs pethidine, methadone and fentanyl. The term opioid is preferred because it refers to both natural and synthetic products that have morphine-like effects on enkephalin (opioid) receptors. The pharmacology of these drugs when used clinically as analgesics is discussed in depth in Chapter 16. Because opioids can rapidly relieve pain, change or elevate mood, relieve tension, fear and anxiety, and produce feelings of peace, euphoria, and tranquillity, they are particularly likely to lead to physical and psychological dependence. Tolerance develops to most of the effects, especially to analgesia, euphoria, sedation and respiratory depression, but not to the constipation or miosis. Heroin, morphine, pethidine, methadone and pholcodine are the most frequently abused; as described earlier, health-care professionals who have ready access to opioids are at particular risk.

Opioid abuse
Heroin abuse

Diacetylmorphine (**heroin**, diamorphine) is a synthetic morphine derivative with no accepted medical use in Australia. It was initially introduced into medicine as a cough suppressant and to treat morphine addiction. It was banned in most countries because of its high potential for abuse and the increasing number of heroin addicts.

Heroin abuse and dependence is not an easy lifestyle: the drug has a short half-life, requiring frequent doses, and the practice is illegal and expensive, estimated at costing A\$50–200 per day. Recent studies estimate that in 1997/98 there were about 75,000 dependent heroin users in Australia, i.e. about seven per thousand adults. The mortality rate is 1%–2% of users per annum; in 1998 there were 737 reported deaths from heroin overdose. In New Zealand a 1998 survey found that about 1% of the population reported using any opiate drug, with 0.6% as current users. These prevalence figures are similar to those in Britain and the European Union. The purity of heroin supplies varies widely—from 25% pure to 90% pure—and users can never be sure of the strength of the sample they procure or what it is adulterated with (often sugar, sedatives or amphetamines). It is therefore fatally easy for addicts to overdose. Impurities injected along with the opioid can cause collapsed veins, infections and organ damage.

Pharmacologically, heroin is a prodrug. When it is administered it is rapidly converted in the liver to morphine. Heroin is highly lipid-soluble and quickly passes the blood–brain barrier, producing a rapid intense 'rush'. It is highly addictive and tolerance develops rapidly to most effects. Controlled studies comparing heroin and morphine in terms of effects achieved when abused do not support the generally held belief that heroin is 'better'.

MODE OF ADMINISTRATION. The opioids generally have low oral bioavailability and so are administered percutaneously (absorbed through the mucous membranes) by sniffing (snorting), by subcutaneous injection (skin popping) or by direct IV injection (mainlining, 'shooting up'). The rate of absorption is increased by injection, with mainlining producing almost immediate drug effects.

ACUTE OVERDOSAGE. Acute overdosage of opioids may result in severe pulmonary oedema and respiratory depression. These outcomes are dose-dependent, and what constitutes a lethal dose also depends on the individual's tolerance for the drug. Symptoms occur rapidly in most patients. Opioid toxicity is manifested as slow, shallow breathing, severe hypoxia, cold clammy skin, miosis, bradycardia, hypotension, muscle spasm and lethargy; urinary retention may also occur. The presence of thrombophlebitis, scarred veins and puckered scars from subcutaneous injections may help identify the patient with opioid dependence. The treatment of choice for acute overdosage is administration of an antagonist (e.g. naloxone) and respiratory and cardiovascular support.

WITHDRAWAL SYNDROME. In a patient who is physically dependent on opioids, sudden withdrawal of the substance of abuse, or an abrupt reversal of opioid effects with an opioid antagonist, may precipitate an acute abstinence or withdrawal syndrome, with excitation and diarrhoea.

While unpleasant, the withdrawal symptoms are not particularly dangerous. Milder symptoms (craving and sleep disturbances) may continue for many months, and some authorities claim that psychological dependence continues for the rest of the person's life.

Treating opioid dependence

The main aim of treatment is to keep users alive and help them 'mature out' of their condition. Treatment programs concentrate on either withdrawal and continuing total abstinence, including 'rapid detoxification' programs with an opioid antagonist such as naltrexone; or (more realistically) withdrawal then substitution and ongoing maintenance with another less dangerous opioid such as methadone. Chilling statistics report that on average after 10 years' treatment, 30%–40% of former users remain abstinent, 40%–50% are active users or imprisoned, and 10%–20% have died.

Withdrawal and detoxification programs

Generally, opioid withdrawal is difficult and repeated relapses may be expected. Abrupt and complete withdrawal (cold turkey) can be accomplished but is dangerous (especially in patients with a coexisting medical illness) and inhumane. Therapeutic withdrawal by successively tapering the drug's dosage over a period of several days may be accomplished in a hospital or clinic with close medical supervision.

Therapeutic community programs (such as Odyssey House in Melbourne) and halfway houses have been established; they offer group psychotherapy and support and self-help approaches.

METHADONE SUBSTITUTION AND WITHDRAWAL

One method of withdrawal is substitution of **methadone** for heroin or morphine, then withdrawal of methadone over a 6-week period. Methadone is a synthetic opioid analgesic that is effective orally (see Drug Monograph 22-2). By virtue of cross-tolerance, methadone dependence can be substituted for heroin dependence. Methadone can forestall the euphoriant effects of heroin and the craving for the drug without producing heroin's deleterious physical and mental effects, and without the requirement for parenteral administration and the attendant risks of infections. When properly administered, methadone allows the individual to function adequately without intellectual or emotional impairment.

Methadone withdrawal programs are not always successful, however: relapse is common and the person may need to go onto a methadone maintenance program.

During the opioid withdrawal phases, other pharmacological agents may be required to treat the withdrawal symptoms: antidiarrhoeal agents, antispasmodics, nonsteroidal anti-inflammatory drugs and sedatives such as diazepam are used. Clonidine is specifically useful in treating the sympathetic nervous system symptoms and is helpful in lessening discomfort of the withdrawal syndrome. It is also under investigation for relieving the symptoms of acute withdrawal from other drugs, including nicotine and alcohol.

NALTREXONE RAPID DETOX PROGRAMS

Naltrexone is a specific opioid antagonist used to prevent relapse in alcohol and opioid withdrawal and detoxification programs (and also to treat acute overdose with opioids, see Drug Monograph 22-1). Administration to an opioid-dependent person precipitates an acute withdrawal syndrome within a few minutes, as the naltrexone binds to opioid receptors in the CNS and competitively inhibits their activation by endogenous enkephalins/endorphins or by administered opioids. Naltrexone is also being used in 'rapid-detox' procedures, in which the antagonist is administered under close medical supervision while the opioid-dependent person is under anaesthesia or sedation. In addition, naltrexone may be used in long-term abstinence programs, a daily dose being given to continuously block the effects of any opioids taken. Counselling and support are usually necessary to help the person remain committed to the opioid abstinence and ongoing naltrexone treatment.

OPIOID SUBSTITUTION AND MAINTENANCE PROGRAMS

METHADONE OR BUPRENORPHINE MAINTENANCE. Methadone or buprenorphine maintenance is the long-term substitution of prescribed, supervised oral opioid for injected illicit opioids.

In Australia, methadone or buprenorphine programs must comply with the requirements of the state Department of Health or Human Services. The patient attends the pharmacy for a supervised oral dosing of methadone (daily) or buprenorphine (daily or alternate days). Occasional take-away doses are allowed to enable patients to go away for 1–2 days; take-away doses are dispensed in large volumes of cordial to obviate the risks of injection of the dose or inadvertent toxicity. Buprenorphine is a partial agonist at μ-opioid receptors (see Ch 16) and, due to its long half-life, is proving a useful alternative to methadone in maintenance therapy or detoxification programs.

A similar program operates in New Zealand (see Clinical Interest Box 22-6).

CLINICAL INTEREST BOX 22-6
THE METHADONE MAINTENANCE PROGRAM

The objectives of the **methadone** maintenance programme in New Zealand are in line with the national Drug Policy: the aim is to minimise the harms associated with the misuse of opioid drugs, a strategy referred to as 'harm reduction'.

The Opioid Substitution Treatment New Zealand Practice Guidelines were published by the Ministry of Health in 2003. They replace the National Protocol for Methadone Treatment (1996), and emphasise the importance of the continuity of care ranging from intensive intervention and stabilisation management, to treatment through the GP primary-care network.

Each methadone client receives an individualised treatment plan that should be reviewed every six months. The first dose of methadone is usually in the range 10–40 mg and should not exceed 40mg. The dose should be maintained for the first 3 to 4 days of treatment so as to reach steady state. Maximum daily doses are in the range 60-120mg, and some individuals require 'split doses'. The aim is to achieve effective management of withdrawal symptoms. Treatment should be started early in the week to allow monitoring during the working week; steady state blood levels are often not achieved before five days' treatment.

Methadone doses should be sufficient to provide clinical stability and minimisation of withdrawal symptoms. Clients should be able continue their role in society, and remain in the programme.

Adapted from: www.moh.govt.nz and www.mhc.govt.nz

DRUG MONOGRAPH 22-2 METHADONE ORAL SYRUP

Methadone is an orally active opioid agonist that helps reduce illicit drug use and the associated crime and social problems, while maintaining the addict's dependence on a relatively safe opioid drug. Methadone is available as a syrup, the formulation usually used for treating opioid dependence, or as tablets or parenteral solution for pain relief as an alternative to morphine. Oral administration reduces IV administration requirements, removes the opioid-taking from the 'street drug' scene and can be readily supervised by the authorised physician, pharmacist or other health professional.

INDICATIONS Methadone is indicated either for short term treatment and management of withdrawal symptoms during opioid detoxification programs, or in long-term use for maintenance of opioid dependence in methadone maintenance programs.

PHARMACOKINETICS Methadone is well absorbed orally and has good bioavailability but its pharmaco-kinetic handling by the body is very variable. Peak plasma levels are reached in 1–5 hours, it is widely distributed via the bloodstream, and protein binding ranges from 60% to 90%. Metabolism occurs in the liver, to at least two inactive metabolites; however, autoinduction of metabolising enzymes occurs, leading to a shorter half-life and pharmacokinetic tolerance. Methadone and its metabolites are excreted in urine and faeces. The half-life is variable (15–60 hours), so several days may be required before steady-state levels are reached, and careful dose adjustment is required; some people may require more than one dose per day.

ADVERSE DRUG REACTIONS The adverse-reaction profile of methadone is similar to that of all opioids, i.e. euphoria, CNS and respiratory depression, GI and cardiovascular disturbances, and spasm of biliary and renal-tract smooth muscle. Because methadone may be taken daily for many months or years, long-term effects need to be considered. Tolerance develops in a few weeks to most of the effects, so people on methadone maintenance can usually resume normal lifestyle and work patterns. In men, fertility may be impaired and gynaecomastia may develop.

DRUG INTERACTIONS Any other CNS depressant, when combined with methadone, will have additive depressant effects; this includes alcohol, antihistamines, sedatives and many psychotropic agents. Typical enzyme inducers will speed up the metabolism of methadone, which can precipitate a withdrawal syndrome, thus requiring higher or more frequent methadone doses, while other drugs may inhibit the metabolism of methadone, so doses may need to be reduced.

WARNINGS AND CONTRAINDICATIONS Methadone is contraindicated in respiratory depression, acute alcoholism or head injury and in severe hepatic or GI diseases. Precautions are required in elderly patients (because of the prolonged half-life), and in patients with diabetes mellitus or other endocrine disorders. Prolonged use leads to dependence, but it is generally considered that it is easier to wean an addict off methadone than off heroin or morphine. Deaths have occurred in patients in poor physical health, so medical examination including liver function tests and tests for blood-borne viral diseases should be carried out before starting treatment.

Because of the CNS depression caused, there are cautions against driving or operating machinery while taking methadone. Methadone is in Category C with respect to pregnancy safety classification, with the warning that higher doses may be required in pregnancy because of faster metabolism.

DRUG MONOGRAPH 22-2 METHADONE ORAL SYRUP

DOSAGE AND ADMINISTRATION Methadone syrup is classified as Schedule 8 and there are strict regulations as to its prescribing, dispensing and administration. The strength of the formulation is 5 mg/mL. Because of its long half-life, it may take several days for effects to stabilise.

The initial dose is 10–20 mg, with the dosage increased gradually to the minimum required maintenance dosage, usually 30–50 mg/day, with a maximum of 80 mg/day. Many patients eventually choose to come off methadone by gradually reducing daily dosage.

CENTRAL NERVOUS SYSTEM DEPRESSANTS

Alcohols

The term 'alcohol', defined chemically, simply refers to a hydrocarbon derivative in which one or more of the hydrogen atoms (–H) has been replaced by a hydroxyl group (–OH). Although there are many different kinds of alcohol, the term alcohol in the medical or social context usually refers to ethanol (ethyl alcohol—see Clinical Interest Box 22-7). Methyl, propyl, butyl and amyl alcohols are examples of other alcohols; these are very toxic when taken orally.

Ethanol (ethyl alcohol, 'alcohol')

sources

Alcohols are naturally produced from the fermentation of cereals and fruits. Most wines are produced from fermentation of grapes from the plant species *Vitis vinifera*, while beer has been traditionally brewed from grains with hops added for flavouring. Rum is distilled after fermentation of sugar cane, and other spirits from grains, fruits or vegetables (e.g. whisky from barley or rye).

USES

Ethanol is the only alcohol used extensively in medicine and in alcoholic beverages. Therapeutically, ethanol administered orally has been used as an appetite stimulant and as a mild hypnotic. Ethanol denatures proteins by precipitation and dehydration, which may be the basis for its germicidal, irritant and astringent effects. For local or *in-vitro* effects, ethanol has been used as a skin antiseptic and disinfectant, in topical pharmaceutical preparations, as a preservative in many formulations, in sclerotherapy (e.g. to cause hardening and closure of varicose veins), and to cause lesions to sensory nerves in neuralgias.

Alcohol is found in many oral pharmaceuticals, as a solvent or as a component of flavoured vehicles. (Table 22-3 lists the ethanol contents of various Australian OTC preparations.)

Ethanol is used in alcoholic drinks, and a low level of alcohol intake (e.g. two glasses of red wine daily for men, one glass for women) has been shown to be protective against some cardiac conditions. While ethanol is not usually taken for therapeutic purposes, it is a very commonly taken drug so it is discussed in the usual format (Drug Monograph 22-3).

PHARMACOLOGICAL EFFECTS

CNS-DEPRESSANT ACTIONS. Contrary to popular belief, alcohol is not a stimulant but a CNS depressant, causing progressive and continuous depression in sequence of the

CLINICAL INTEREST BOX 22-7 ALCOHOLS — WHAT'S YOUR POISON?

The strengths of alcoholic solutions could scientifically (and logically) be expressed in SI units, e.g. in g/L, mg/mL or even molar terms; however, the unit % v/v is most commonly used (i.e. the number of millilitres of pure ethanol per 100 mL solution), and other archaic traditional units and terms are still in current use. In the *British Pharmacopoeia*, absolute alcohol, or dehydrated alcohol, refers to 100% pure ethanol, whereas Alcohol BP is a mixture of ethyl alcohol (approximately 96%) and water.

'Proof spirit' is an old term originally defined as 'a solution of alcohol of such strength that it will ignite when mixed with gunpowder' (an important concept in the early days of naval warfare) and more recently as 'the alcoholic solution that weighs 12/13 of an equal measure of distilled water'. Proof spirit contains about 57% v/v ethanol in the UK. The strengths of alcoholic spirits are still sometimes stated in terms of proof spirit, thus '60 over proof' refers to spirit of a strength such that 100 volumes contain as much alcohol as 160 volumes of proof spirit.

There are several forms of 'methylated spirits', all consisting largely of ethyl alcohol that has been purposely contaminated with other solvents including methanol, acetone and pyridine to render it unfit for human consumption. It is used clinically for skin disinfection. The toxicity is mainly due to acute poisoning with methanol, which can cause severe abdominal pain, metabolic acidosis, blindness, coma and respiratory failure.

Alcoholic beverages contain varying amounts of ethanol, ranging from about 1% v/v for low-alcohol beer to 40%–50% v/v for spirits such as brandy, rum and whisky (see Table 22-4).

TABLE 22-3 Content of ethyl alcohol in some OTC products

PRODUCT NAME	OTHER ACTIVE INGREDIENTS	AMOUNT OF ALCOHOL	COMPANY/MANUFACTURER
Benadryl For The Family – Chesty	Guaifenesin, pseudoephedrine HCl	4.26% w/v	Pfizer
Benadryl For The Family – Dry	Dextromethorphan HBr, pseudoephedrine HCl, diphenhydramine HCl	Alcohol-free	Pfizer
Brondecon Elixir	Choline theophyllinate	8.5% v/v (0.85 ml/L)	Pfizer
Brondecon Expectorant	Choline theophyllinate, guaifenesin	8.5% v/v	Pfizer
Dimetapp Chest Congestion Paediatric Drops	Guaifenesin	4.8%	Wyeth
Dimetapp DM Elixir and Paediatric Drops	Brompheniramine maleate, phenylephrine HCl, dextromethorphan HBr	2.3% v/v	Wyeth
Duro-Tuss Decongestant	Pholcodine, pseudoephedrine HCl	Alcohol-free	3M Pharmaceuticals
Paedamin Elixir	Diphenhydramine HCl, phenylephrine HCl	7.2% v/v	Paedpharm
Robitussin DM	Guaifenesin, dextromethorphan HBr	4.8% v/v	Wyeth
Robitussin DM-P Extra Strength	Dextromethorphan HBr, pseudoephedrine	Alcohol-free	Wyeth

cerebrum, cerebellum, spinal cord and medulla. What sometimes appears to be stimulation results from depression of the higher faculties of the brain and represents the loss of inhibitions acquired by socialisation. Alcohol is thought to interfere with the transmission of nerve impulses at synaptic connections but the precise mechanism is not known. It inhibits calcium entry into nerve cells, possibly by enhancing γ-aminobutyric acid (GABA)-mediated inhibition and/or antagonising excitatory amino acid transmitters (e.g. glutamate).

The action of alcohol varies with the blood alcohol level, the individual's tolerance, the presence or absence of extraneous stimuli, the rate of ingestion, and gastric contents. Small or moderate quantities produce a feeling of wellbeing (euphoria) and increased confidence. Then finer powers of concentration, judgement and memory are lost, visual acuity is diminished, and sensorimotor functions (including driving) are impaired. Many drivers will take chances when under the influence of alcohol that they would never take ordinarily, as accident statistics reveal (see Figure 22-2). Table 22-5 compares the blood alcohol level with clinical observations of behaviour and pharmacological effects.

EFFECTS ON OTHER SYSTEMS. The effects of alcohol on other body systems are as follows:
- cardiovascular: depression of the vasomotor neurons in

TABLE 22-4 Content of ethyl alcohol in various beverages

BEVERAGES	ETHANOL CONTENT (%)	ETHANOL PER STANDARD MEASURE (g)
Beer	1–5	5–20
Wine (red/white)	9–15	5–18
Fortified wines (sherry)	16–23	8
Spirits (brandy, whisky, vodka)	35–55	8–10

Adapted from: Bowman & Rand 1980; Whelan 2002.

the medulla, causing vasodilation, especially in the skin, and rapid heat loss; chronic alcoholism may result in hypertension, arrhythmias and cardiomyopathy
- gastrointestinal: stimulation of secretion of gastric juice rich in acid, and of salivary secretions (hence the use of alcoholic drinks as 'tonics' and aperitifs); chronic alcohol ingestion causes nutritional deficiencies, gastritis, pancreatitis and hepatic cellular damage, which results in fatty liver, hepatitis, fibrosis and scarring (cirrhosis)

DRUG MONOGRAPH 22-3 ALCOHOL (ETHANOL)

Taken orally, **alcohol** is a sedative and euphoriant; it is usually taken in the form of alcoholic drinks.

PHARMACOKINETICS Being a very small molecule (molecular weight 46), **ethanol** does not require digestion before absorption. It is very water-soluble but because of its small molecular size it readily diffuses through lipid membranes and hence rapidly enters cells. A small amount is absorbed from the stomach, while most is absorbed from the small intestine. Peak blood alcohol levels are reached about 30–60 minutes after administration. After absorption, alcohol is distributed in every tissue of the body in about the same ratio as its water content. Therefore a rough estimate of the quantity consumed and of the levels in the brain may be obtained from an analysis of the blood (see Table 22-5). The volume of distribution is about 35 L for a 70 kg adult.

About 90% of the alcohol absorbed is metabolised in the liver. The liver enzyme alcohol dehydrogenase oxidises ethanol to acetaldehyde, then acetaldehyde is oxidised to acetic acid and eventually to carbon dioxide and water. The remainder of the ethanol is primarily excreted by way of the lungs, sweat and kidneys. The amount of alcohol excreted in expired air — as measured by 'breathalyzers' — is very small: the amount in 2 L expired air is equivalent to that in 1 mL blood; however, this small amount may have considerable forensic importance if it indicates greater than 0.05% blood levels.

As plasma ethanol levels rise, the hepatic alcohol dehydrogenase pathway becomes saturated, resulting in an increase in the unmetabolised alcohol proportion. The maximum rate of metabolism is about 120 mg/kg/h, and the clearance and half-life are dose-dependent. This explains why blood alcohol levels remain high if the person keeps drinking steadily. The plasma levels tend to be higher in women than in men after the same amount of alcohol is consumed, both because women have lower levels of dehydrogenase enzymes and because their higher proportion of fat to lean tissue means that they have a smaller volume of distribution for water-soluble drugs. Heavy exercise may slightly increase the rate of elimination of alcohol. Chronic administration (i.e. in alcoholics) initially increases the rate of metabolism by the liver enzyme pathway, but as liver damage and cirrhosis develop, metabolism becomes impaired.

ADVERSE DRUG REACTIONS Alcohol affects many body systems (see Pharmacological effects in text above). In particular, it causes euphoria and reduces inhibitions, causes sensorimotor impairment, increases gastric acidity and has a diuretic effect. The therapeutic index is estimated at about 4; i.e. while one or two drinks may make you the life of the party, 4–8 may make you raging drunk, comatose or incapable of driving safely.

Chronic alcohol use may result in hyperlipidaemia, fatty deposits in the liver and, ultimately, alcoholic cirrhosis. Alcohol has a diuretic effect both because of the increase in fluid intake (although this may be small with wines and spirits) and through inhibition of antidiuretic hormone (ADH) release. If an individual has pre-existing renal disease, the kidney may be further damaged.

DRUG INTERACTIONS Alcohol is the most commonly used and abused drug in Australia. It interacts with many prescription and OTC drugs, in particular with any other CNS depressant, resulting in frequent adverse drug interactions (see Table 22-6).

WARNINGS AND CONTRAINDICATIONS Because of the increased risk of fetal alcohol syndrome (mental retardation, craniofacial dysgenesis and growth retardation), pregnant women are advised not to drink more than two standard drinks per day; there is a 10% risk of fetal malformations if consumption exceeds 2 g ethanol/kg/day during the first trimester. During breastfeeding, ethanol partitions into milk to about the same level as in maternal plasma; the time to maximum level in milk is about 1 hour. Drinking alcohol is not recommended for lactating women because of the possible depressant effects on the infant's CNS and respiration.

Generally, alcohol is not recommended for people with liver disease or psychiatric problems, or patients taking any of the many drugs with which alcohol interacts.

DOSAGE AND ADMINISTRATION As can be seen from Table 22-4, the standard 'measures' of alcoholic drinks have developed such that the average drink contains in the range 5–20 grams of ethanol: the stronger the drink, the smaller is the typical container. Thus a beer stein is larger than a wine glass, and a sherry glass larger than a 'shot' glass for spirits. It is generally recommended that men drink no more than four standard drinks per day, and women no more than two.

- endocrine: levels of adrenocorticotrophic hormone may be raised; levels of many other hormones are lowered: low antidiuretic hormone (ADH) causes diuresis, leading to dehydration; low oxytocin causes delayed labour during parturition; and low testosterone causes feminisation and impotence
- lipid metabolism: a low daily alcohol intake may raise plasma levels of high-density lipoproteins (HDLs, the 'good' lipids), and thus reduce the incidence of ischaemic heart disease and stroke
- effects on the fetus: there is a 19% incidence of fetal alcohol syndrome (mental retardation, craniofacial

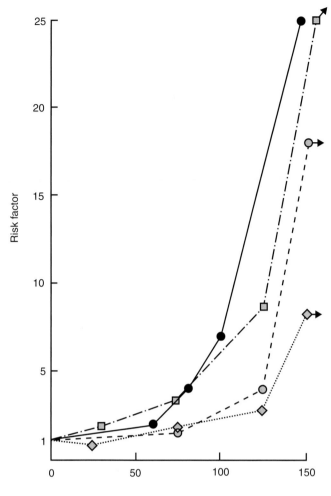

Risk factor

Blood ethanol concentration (mg/dL)

FIGURE 22-2 Results of four surveys on the relation between traffic accidents and blood ethanol concentration. The risk factor is the ratio of traffic accidents in subjects with a given blood ethanol concentration to all traffic accidents in the population from which the subjects are drawn. Note that 50 mg/dL equates to 0.05%.
From data reviewed in Wallgren H, Berry M. *Actions of Alcohol.* Amsterdam: Elsevier, 1970; as shown in Bowman & Rand 1980; used with permission.

dysgenesis and growth retardation) in infants born to women who consumed four or more drinks per day during the first trimester of pregnancy.

METHANOL (METHYL ALCOHOL, WOOD ALCOHOL)

If taken orally, methanol is a CNS toxin: the fatal dose is in the range 100–200 mL and as little as 10 mL has been known to cause permanent blindness. The reason for this severe toxicity compared with the very similar alcohol, ethanol, is that whereas ethanol is metabolised to acetaldehyde and then acetate, methanol is metabolised to formaldehyde

(formalin) and formate, which are more toxic. Formic acid is slowly metabolised, with maximum concentrations in the blood 2–3 days after ingestion of methanol, and is the cause of severe metabolic acidosis. The specific ocular toxicity of formaldehyde is because it is a potent inhibitor of respiration and glycolysis in the retina.

Alcohol abuse
ALCOHOL MISUSE AND ABUSE, AND ALCOHOLISM

Alcohol abuse has been defined simply as any form of drinking that is more than customary, traditional or dietary use. **Alcoholism** is a physical or psychological dependence on alcohol, with a compulsion to consume despite adverse effects.

Alcohol use and misuse have been classified as:
* social drinking: no regular excessive drinking, no problems or symptoms
* heavy drinking: habitual excessive drinking, but no problems or symptoms
* problem drinking: problems for self, family or work, but no symptoms of addiction leading to physical or mental impairment
* alcoholic addiction: strokes, blackouts, loss of control, with impairment to health and intellect.

PREVALENCE OF ALCOHOL ABUSE

Compared with 31 other countries (in 1987), Australians ranked 15th highest in total alcohol consumption (European countries were highest): 10th highest for beer (Germany highest), 18th for wines (Italy and France highest), and 30th for spirits (Eastern European countries highest). Australian men in the age range 35–55 averaged about 15 drinks per week, and women about 7 per week. Since that survey, the rate of consumption of beer has been decreasing and that of wine increasing.

In Australia, it is estimated that about:
* 9.3% of the population over 13 years old are abstainers from alcohol (teetotallers)
* 73% are safe or responsible drinkers
* 10% drink in a risky manner
* 10.6% of young women and 14% of young men are at risk of harm at least weekly from drinking
* 3700 people die each year due to complications of alcohol abuse.

PROBLEMS WITH ALCOHOL ABUSE

Problem drinking is considered to occur when people drink to escape or to the level of intoxication, or when people work or drive while intoxicated, suffer injury or come into conflict with the law while intoxicated or indulge in behaviour while intoxicated which they would not do when sober. Such problems include: social isolation ranging from family breakdowns to 'skid-row' lifestyle; increase in self-destructive

TABLE 22-5 Concentration of alcohol in blood, and related clinical observations

STAGE	BLOOD ALCOHOL (mg/dL)*	CLINICAL OBSERVATIONS
Subclinical	30–100	Slight evidence of performance deterioration possible, such as in motor function, coordination, personality or mood and mental acuity
Emotional instability	100–200	Decreased inhibitions, emotional instability, slight muscular incoordination, slowing of responses to stimuli, signs of intoxication
Confusion	200–300	Disturbance of sensation, decreased pain sense, staggering gait, slurred speech
Stupor	300–400	Marked decrease in response to stimuli, muscular incoordination approaching paralysis, impaired intelligence
Coma, death	400	Complete unconsciousness, depressed reflexes and respiration, subnormal temperature, anaesthesia, impairment of circulation, coma, possible death

*Note: a blood alcohol level of 0.05% (the legally safe limit in most states of Australia), i.e. 0.05 g/100 mL, equates to 50 mg/dL.

behaviours, suicide and motor vehicle accidents; neuropathies (peripheral and central) and myopathies (skeletal, cardiac); chronic hepatotoxicity and cirrhosis, with associated possible death from oesophageal varices; gastrointestinal (GI) or haematological toxicity; Korsakoff's psychosis, alcohol dementia and cerebellar degeneration; and fetal abnormalities. It is estimated that 15%–25% of all male hospital admissions are due to alcohol-related causes (injuries, accidents, chronic disorders).

Tolerance develops to most of the effects of low doses of ethanol, particularly while blood alcohol levels are rising. There is both pharmacokinetic tolerance, due to induction of drug-metabolising enzymes in chronically alcoholic persons, and pharmacodynamic tolerance, due to some adaptation to the depressant effects.

There is increasing evidence that ethanol increases opioid neurotransmission, and that this interaction accounts for some of the reinforcing effects of alcohol and also for the tolerance that develops to some actions of alcohol. Humans with a family history of alcohol dependence show increased release of endorphins in response to an alcohol challenge, compared to those with no family history of alcohol abuse. Clinical trials of naltrexone in patients with alcohol dependence show a modest therapeutic effect of the opioid antagonist in reducing alcohol consumption.

HANGOVER AND ALCOHOL WITHDRAWAL SYNDROME

A 'hangover' is a mild withdrawal syndrome after acute intoxication. The symptoms (usually suffered on 'the morning after the night before') are headache, nausea, vertigo, pallor, sweating, tachycardia and nystagmus (rapid jerky eye movements). Various mechanisms have been suggested as the cause of hangover symptoms, including hypoglycaemia, dehydration (due to the diuretic effect of alcohol, possibly compounded by

lack of other fluid intake, and vomiting), electrolyte imbalances and persistence of lactic acid and acetaldehyde in the bloodstream. A hangover is a withdrawal reaction, hence it can be 'cured' by another dose of the drug of dependence, i.e. alcohol, which is the basis for the old custom of treating it with another drink, 'the hair of the dog that bit you'.

Treating alcohol abuse

Long-term treatment of ethanol withdrawal and abuse includes monitoring health status, symptom relief, preventing or treating complications, and developing long-term rehabilitation plans. Supportive care includes fluid and electrolyte replacement, adequate nutrition, thiamine to prevent development of Wernicke's encephalopathy, psychotropic agents, psychotherapy to improve coping skills and prevent relapses, and anticonvulsant medications if necessary. Treatment needs to be continued for many months or years; hospitalisation may be necessary for the acute phase during which the patient is on high doses of sedatives to protect against convulsions.

There are also alcohol-sensitising drugs, in particular disulfiram, which when coadministered with alcohol make the person suffer such a severe drug interaction that this deters the person from drinking alcohol. Disulfiram inhibits the enzyme aldehyde dehydrogenase, which converts acetaldehyde to acetate. This permits acetaldehyde to accumulate and cause the unpleasant toxic effects: vasodilation, hyperventilation and raised pulse rate, pounding headache, and copious vomiting. (Table 22-6 lists some drugs that interact with alcohol.)

The drug of choice in treating chronic alcohol abuse is now **acamprosate** (Drug Monograph 22-4), which is used in combination with counselling and lifestyle changes to maintain abstinence from alcohol. Acamprosate is chemically related

DRUG MONOGRAPH 22-4 ACAMPROSATE

Acamprosate is a relatively new drug that reduces neuronal hyperexcitability and sometimes decreases alcohol craving and consumption; there is no abuse risk.

INDICATIONS Acamprosate is indicated to help maintain abstinence from alcohol and reduce relapse rates in alcohol-dependent people. It is used as an adjunct to psychological and social therapies.

PHARMACOKINETICS Absorption after oral administration is moderate, but slow and variable. Absorption and oral bioavailability are decreased by food in the GI tract. Acamprosate is not metabolised and is excreted unchanged in the urine; thus renal impairment reduces drug elimination. The half-life is 13–28 hours, with steady state reached in about 7 days.

ADVERSE DRUG REACTIONS The main adverse effects are in the GI tract (nausea and vomiting, diarrhoea, abdominal pain), and skin rashes.

DRUG INTERACTIONS Few large-scale studies have been carried out. Acamprosate does not alter the CNS effects or metabolism of alcohol.

WARNINGS AND CONTRAINDICATIONS Acamprosate is contraindicated in impaired hepatic or renal functions and is not indicated for treatment of acute alcohol withdrawal.

DOSAGE AND ADMINISTRATION Administration is started about 1 week after drinking has stopped and is recommended for 1 year's duration. Dose depends on body weight; average dose for an adult heavier than 60 kg is 666 mg three times daily.

TABLE 22-6 Selected significant alcohol–drug interactions

SUBSTANCES INTERACTING WITH ALCOHOL	MECHANISM	POSSIBLE EFFECTS
Antihistamines, antidepressants, opioid analgesics, hypnotics, antianxiety agents, antipsychotic drugs	Additive	Enhanced CNS-depressant effects
Disulfiram, some cephalosporins, oral antidiabetic agents, griseofulvin, metronidazole, procarbazine, tinidazde	Inhibition of aldehyde dehydrogenase in metabolism of alcohol, leading to acetaldehyde accumulation (a 'disulfiram-type reaction')	Most severe effects seen with disulfiram and alcohol: flushing, stomach pain, head throbbing, raised heart rate, hypotension, sweating, nausea and vomiting; with antidiabetic agents, mild to severe hypoglycaemia
Phenytoin, warfarin	Increase or decrease in liver metabolism	In chronic alcohol abuse or anticoagulation: possible decrease in anticonvulsant or anticoagulant effect caused by increased metabolism (enzyme induction). In acute alcohol use: a possible decrease in metabolism, causing raised serum level of phenytoin or warfarin, and toxicity
Salicylates	Additive	Increased GI irritability and bleeding
Nitrates, glyceryl trinitrate	Additive	Vasodilation leading to hypotension, syncope
Anticholinergics, antispasmodics	Slowed GI functions	Slowed absorption of alcohol
Prokinetic drugs (metoclopramide)	Accelerated GI functions	Faster absorption of alcohol
Paracetamol	Additive	Enhanced hepatic toxicity of paracetamol

to the neurotransmitters GABA, glutamate and taurine, and may restore inhibitory neurotransmission in these pathways. In rats it decreases alcohol-seeking behaviour. Acamprosate reduces the symptoms of alcohol withdrawal (craving, anxiety, irritability and insomnia), but does not affect the metabolism of alcohol.

Benzodiazepines and barbiturates

Misuse and abuse of other CNS depressants (benzodiaze-pines, barbiturates and chloral hydrate-type sedatives) have declined greatly in recent years, probably as a result of the availability of newer agents with greater safety and effectiveness profiles. (General information about these agents is summarised in Tables 22-1 and 22-2; their pharmacological and clinical aspects are discussed in Chapters 17 and 18.) The general effects are similar to dependence on ethanol but the social setting is different: whereas men tend more to abuse alcohol, women are more likely to become dependent on benzodiazepines ('mother's little helpers').

Benzodiazepines (diazepam, alprazolam, lorazepam)

Benzodiazepines are commonly prescribed medications for anxiety, insomnia and convulsive disorders. Benzodiazepines initially prescribed for medical purposes can cause depend-ence and patients may 'shop around' among doctors and pharmacists to obtain supplies. Tolerance develops to the sedating and intoxicating effects but not to the respiratory depression. Managing benzodiazepine dependence should include gradual drug withdrawal. Flumazenil is a specific benzodiazepine-receptor antagonist that is administered intra-venously for the treatment of benzodiazepine toxicity. As flumazenil has a short half-life (50 minutes), several doses may be required to treat the patient who has overdosed with a long-acting benzodiazepine.

Temazepam, a short-acting benzodiazepine, was formerly available in Australia in gel capsules containing temazepam in solution. Unfortunately these came to be abused, as injecting drug users injected the contents of the gelcaps, particularly at times of heroin shortage, in order to replace the depressant effects of the opioid or alcohol, to deal with stress, or to offset the effects of CNS-stimulant drugs. Common complications included abscesses, skin ulcers, deep venous thromboses, aneurysm and haemorrhage, ischaemia, gangrene and subsequent amputation. The gelcaps have now been withdrawn from the market, which has led to a decrease in their misuse and consequent harm.

Kava

Kava is an intoxicating drink made by fermenting the grated (or chewed) roots of *Piper methysticum*, a plant native to Polynesia, used at religious and welcoming ceremonies. The effects are similar to those of benzodiazepines or alcohol, and include muscle relaxation, anticonvulsant effects, analgesia, reduced anxiety, mild stimulation, then sedation. Chronic use has been associated with skin disorders. Kava has fewer detrimental effects than alcohol on cognitive functions and information processing.

Inhalants

Other CNS-depressant substances of abuse are the volatile hydrocarbons and solvents such as toluene, xylene, benzene, petrol, acetone, paint thinner, correction fluid, lighter fluid, glues and nitrous oxide. Chemically, the substances are hydrocarbons (halogenated, aliphatic or aromatic), ketones, esters or ethers. They are general CNS depressants with pharmacological properties similar to those of the halogenated hydrocarbon general anaesthetics such as chloroform and halothane (see Chapter 15).

When abused, they are sniffed (inhaled); this procedure is referred to as 'chroming' or 'glue sniffing'. This type of sub-stance abuse is most common among children and teenagers (6–15 years of age). In economically depressed populations inhalants are often the first drug of abuse used.

On inhalation these agents may produce a rapid general CNS depression with marked inebriation, dizziness, exhila-ration, disinhibition and aggressiveness—similar to effects seen with alcohol intoxication. Inhalation may also result in bronchial and laryngeal irritation, cardiac arrhythmias, ven-tricular fibrillation and renal tubular acidosis, especially with glue sniffing. At high doses, confusion and coma occur as well as blood dyscrasias. A serious risk is that the person may pass out while inhaling from a plastic bag and suffocate. Generally, treatment is with removal of the inhaled agent and bed-rest. Recovery from lower doses may be seen in 15 minutes to a few hours. Chronic inhalant abuse will lead to neurotoxicity, and hepatic and renal toxicity; deaths from cardiac arrhythmia and respiratory failure have been reported. Habituation and dependence can occur and tolerance also develops with inhalants.

CNS STIMULANTS

The primary CNS stimulants abused are the **amphetamines** and related 'designer drugs' (such as ecstasy) and nicotine, cocaine and caffeine. The pharmacological aspects and clin-ical uses of these drugs are discussed in Chapter 20 and also in Chapter 32 under Respiratory stimulants.

Amphetamines
Actions and mechanisms

Chemically, amphetamines are similar to the natural catecholamines adrenaline, noradrenaline and dopamine. They have weak agonist actions on adrenoreceptor sites and have therefore been classified as sympathomimetic agents. They increase the release of natural catecholamines and block their reuptake into neurons, which causes a 'fight or flight' response; they may also have mild monoamine oxidase inhibitory effects, which contributes to their sympathomimetic and CNS stimulant actions. There are three types of amphetamines: salts of racemic (±) amphetamines, dextroamphetamines and methamphetamines, all of which vary in degree of potency and peripheral effects. Dexamphetamine is said to have fewest peripheral effects, such as hypertension and tachycardia. Central effects include increases in mood, energy, alertness and mental and physical capacities, and decreased appetite and sleep; euphoria and stereotyped behaviours also occur (see Drug Monograph 20-1).

Oral amphetamine is absorbed from the GI tract and concentrates in the brain, kidneys and lungs. It is metabolised in the liver and excreted via the kidneys. Amphetamine is a basic drug with a pK_a (the pH at which half the drug amount in the body is ionised and half un-ionised) of 9.9; therefore alkaline urine with pH >7 reduces excretion of amphetamine and extends its half-life to about 20 hours. Acidic urine at pH 5, by contrast, increases excretion and reduces the half-life to 5–6 hours. People who abuse this drug are usually aware of the prolonged effect they can achieve by alkalinising their urine, whereas prescribers are aware that acidifying the urine to a pH of 4.5–5.5 will enhance amphetamine excretion and help treatment of amphetamine overdose.

Abuse of amphetamines

Amphetamines were widely used during World War II to enhance alertness and reduce battle fatigue and quickly became popular drugs of abuse, amphetamine as 'benzedrine', and methamphetamine or methedrine as 'speed'. Results from the 2004 National Drug Survey in Australia showed that approximately 10% of persons aged 20–29 years had used amphetamines in the previous 12 months, and 12% had used ecstasy; the use of ecstasy has increased steadily since 1995. Most amphetamines are produced in illegal backyard laboratories, with no controls over the manufacturing practices or the purity or strength of the product, and sold illegally. Due to the unknown strength of street supplies, overdose is common and potentially fatal; parenteral use carries the risks of IV drug abuse and infections. Amphetamines are generally taken orally, but can also be inhaled after vaporisation, inhaled as fine powders ('snorted'), or injected.

Intravenous amphetamine injection results in marked euphoria—a rush accompanied by a sense of great physical strength and clear thinking, and engagement in vigorous activity that may actually be inefficient and repetitious.

The sympathetic stimulant properties of amphetamines can cause dramatic effects such as tachycardia, dyspnoea, chest pain and hypertension; infarcts, hyperpyrexia, hepatotoxicity, seizures and circulatory collapse have been reported. Severe anxiety, paranoia, schizophrenia-like symptoms ('snow lights'), insomnia and weight loss also occur. Amphetamine users often use depressants or 'downers', such as large amounts of alcohol, marijuana, benzodiazepines, barbiturates or heroin to offset the overstimulation effects. Detoxification and use of conventional therapies for medical complications, including anticonvulsants and antihypertensive agents, are necessary in treating acute toxicity.

There is a rapid fall-off in drug effects, which enhances the intense craving for the drug and rapidly leads to addiction. Drug withdrawal is followed by long periods of sleep, and on waking the individual often feels hungry, extremely lethargic and profoundly depressed (anhedonia). This phenomenon is known as 'crashing', and is typical of the rebound swings after withdrawal of drugs of dependence. Suicide risk is quite possible during this period.

Amphetamine (especially methamphetamine) use is on the rise. Crystal methamphetamine (known as 'ice' or 'crystal meth') is gaining popularity because a high occurs usually in less than a minute when these crystals are heated and the vapour is inhaled. In some instances, oral amphetamine users are also inhaling or smoking methamphetamine concurrently, which vastly increases the intensity and toxicity of the effect, and its duration (a high can persist for 12 hours).

Amphetamine-like agents
'DESIGNER DRUGS'

These are drugs designed and synthesised to be amphetamine look-alikes and mimic the CNS-stimulant effects of amphetamines and cocaine. The classic **designer drug** is 3,4-methylenedioxymethamphetamine (MDMA, better known as 'ecstasy', see Figure 22-4 later), originally synthesised in 1914 as an appetite suppressant but which has recently found popularity as a stimulant. Related compounds have varying chemical substituents (methoxy-, methyl-, halogen or sulfur) on the phenyl ring of the amphetamine or methamphetamine. They have similar mechanisms of action to amphetamine, interfering with uptake processes (transporters) in CNS neurons to raise levels of monoamine neurotransmitters and cause CNS stimulation.

The typical scene for abuse of ecstasy and other such drugs is at dance parties (the rave scene), where the drugs are taken to produce euphoria, feelings of closeness and confidence; hence the street names ecstasy and 'love drug'. It is estimated that about 7.5% of Australians aged over 14 have tried ecstasy (see Clinical Interest Box 22-8). Unwanted effects include jaw clenching and teeth grinding, anxiety, paranoia and confusion, mild hallucinations, impaired cognition, bizarre behaviour and possibly psychosis. Overdose can result in hypertension, tachycardia and hyperthermia; deaths have occurred from excess CNS and autonomic stimulation. Users of ecstasy in the dance scene are advised to take frequent rest breaks and sip water regularly to rehydrate.

Nicotine and tobacco smoking

As discussed in Chapter 10, the major neurotransmitter at all autonomic ganglia is acetylcholine. Its effects at ganglia are mediated at receptors described as nicotinic because the early physiologists found that the effects of stimulating autonomic ganglia were most closely mimicked by the compound nicotine. As stimulation of postganglionic fibres produces effects on smooth muscle, cardiac muscle, and glands (see Figure 10-7), non-selective ganglionic stimulants that stimulate both parasympathetic and sympathetic pathways can result in a broad range of pharmacological effects. Nicotinic-type acetylcholine receptors are also present at the end-plate in neuromuscular junctions, and acetylcholine is a CNS neurotransmitter as well, so nicotine also has effects on skeletal muscle and on neurotransmission in the brain and spinal cord.

Nicotine

Nicotine is an oily liquid alkaloid, freely soluble in both organic solvents and water. It turns brown on exposure to air and is the chief alkaloid in the tobacco plant *Nicotiana tabacum*. Nicotine has no therapeutic use (other than in nicotine replacement therapy for smokers trying to quit), but is of great pharmacological interest and toxicological importance. Nicotine is readily absorbed from the GI tract, respiratory mucous membrane, and skin. It is most commonly self-administered by smoking cigarettes (which contain about 1 g nicotine each), or cigars or pipes. Tobacco smoking was introduced into European societies from Central America in the 16th century.

PHARMACOLOGICAL EFFECTS

Nicotine may produce a variety of complex and often unpredictable effects in the body. Many actions are dose-related, with small doses generally inducing activation or stimulation at receptors, and larger doses producing a decreased or depressed response.

At autonomic ganglia nicotine temporarily stimulates all sympathetic and parasympathetic ganglia. This is followed by depression, which tends to last longer than the period of stimulation. Its effects on skeletal muscle are similar: stimulation then a depressant phase during which nicotine exerts a curare-like action on skeletal muscle.

Nicotine stimulates the CNS, especially the medullary centres (respiratory, emetic and vasomotor). Large doses may cause tremor and convulsions. Stimulation is followed by depression. Death may result from respiratory failure, caused mainly by the curare-like action of nicotine on nerve endings in the diaphragm. Central effects commonly reported by humans are increased alertness and concentration and reduced boredom and anxiety; learning and performance have been shown to improve, and dependence occurs.

The actions and effects of nicotine on the cardiovascular system are complex. Heart rate is frequently slowed at first but later may be accelerated. The small blood vessels in peripheral parts of the body constrict but later may dilate, and the blood pressure rises then falls; this occurs in nicotine poisoning. Nicotine also has an antidiuretic action and decreases GI motility. Repeated administration of nicotine causes development of tolerance to some of its effects, particularly to the nausea, sweating, antidiuretic effects and feelings of unease, so that habitual smokers find smoking pleasurable and relaxing, whereas first-time smokers become anxious and nauseated. (It is an indication of the strong 'rewarding' effect and addictive potential of nicotine—and of the aggressive advertising practices and peer pressures encouraging smoking—that anyone goes on to smoke a second cigarette.)

BENEFICIAL EFFECTS

Chronic smokers have a lower than average prevalence of both Alzheimer's disease and Parkinson's disease; the rationale is that nicotine may enhance dopaminergic and cholinergic activity in central pathways. Nicotinic agonists have been tried in treatment of both conditions but, because of their slowly progressive course, clearcut effects are difficult to prove, and further long-term prospective studies are required.

TOXICITY

Nicotine has both short- and long-term toxic effects that are extremely important in public health terms. Nicotine toxicity has resulted from percutaneous absorption after misuse of insecticides containing nicotine, which at times has led to the deaths of farm workers. Because nicotine is a major ingredient in tobacco products, both acute toxicity (with ingestion of such products by small children) and chronic toxicity are well documented.

Tobacco smoking and nicotine

Tobacco smoke is an aerosol containing about 4×10^9 particles per mL, i.e. in the range 10–80 mg per cigarette; nicotine accounts for about 0.14–1.21 mg (30 Australian brands; 1996). Burning of tobacco also generates around 4000 compounds in the gaseous and particulate phases, including 60 known carcinogens such as tars, formaldehyde, hydrogen cyanide, benzene and nitrosamines, implicated as aetiological factors in cancers of the bladder, lung, buccal cavity, oesophagus and pancreas. Other smoking-related illnesses include pulmonary emphysema, chronic bronchitis, coronary heart disease, strokes, myocardial infarction and chronic dyspepsia. Male smokers have about one-third the sperm count of non-smokers. Cigarette smoking is thought to be responsible for more than 50% of all domestic fires. Smoking is also a considerable financial outlay: it has been estimated that someone who has smoked 10 cigarettes a day since the age of 20 and has the good luck to live to be 50 will be A$250,000 poorer than a non-smoker of the same age.

Smokers absorb sufficient nicotine to exert a variety of effects on the autonomic nervous system. In people with peripheral vascular disease such as thromboangiitis obliterans (Buerger's disease), nicotine is generally believed to be a contributing factor by causing spasms of the peripheral blood vessels. Vasospasm in the retinal blood vessels of the eye, associated with smoking of tobacco, is thought to cause serious disturbance of vision. Most male smokers of 20 years duration are impotent by the age of 50, owing to microvascular damage. Mothers who smoke usually deliver infants with low birth weights and a higher incidence of congenital abnormalities; prematurity and stillbirth are more common.

Passive smoking

Passive smoking (inhalation of environmental tobacco smoke) refers to the inhalation of cigarette smoke by non-smokers.

Reports from studies in Australia, the USA and UK all indicate that:

- environmental tobacco smoke can cause lung cancer and other cancers in healthy non-smokers (non-smoking partners of smokers have a 20%–30% greater risk of lung cancer than partners of non-smokers)
- children of parents who smoke have a greater incidence of asthma, respiratory tract symptoms and infections and middle ear disease than children from a non-smoking family and have a greatly increased likelihood of becoming smokers
- environmental tobacco smoke is a risk factor for cardiac disease (24% increase in risk of dying from coronary artery disease)
- environmental smoke exposure is causally linked to sudden infant death syndrome.

Dependence on nicotine

Tobacco is Australia's worst 'killer' drug, the most abused and the most harmful, killing "more people than alcohol, drugs, murder, suicide, road, rail and air crashes, poisoning, HIV, drowning, fires, falls, lightning, electrocution, snakes, spiders and sharks put together" (Jamrozik & Le 2001). A 2004 national survey of drug use found that about 19% of Australians aged 14 years and over smoked regularly at least weekly.

The addictive component of tobacco is nicotine. Monkeys trained to press a bar to receive an IV injection of nicotine will self-administer up to a point, at which the adverse effects presumably outweigh the rewarding effects. Nicotine is also postulated to have an antidepressant action, and ex-smokers who successfully abstain often suffer clinical depression.

The dose of nicotine absorbed from one cigarette is estimated to amount to about 10–40 mcg/kg body weight, and smokers tend to maintain their plasma nicotine concentration at about 10–50 ng/mL. By comparison, nicotine is absorbed more slowly from cigars and pipes but the doses of nicotine achieved are in the same order, about 20–40 mcg/kg (see Figure 22-3).

Treating nicotine dependence
NICOTINE BY OTHER ROUTES

Smoking is notoriously hard to quit; the withdrawal syndrome, consisting of irritability, impatience, anxiety, restlessness and headaches, continues for several days; the craving persists for weeks or months. As with other drug-dependent states, treatment may be by replacement of the drug with a less harmful related drug or, in this case, nicotine delivered in a less harmful formulation such as a gum (Drug Monograph 22-5) or patch. Unfortunately there does not appear to be a nicotinic antagonist agent effective in treating dependence analogous to the use of naltrexone in opioid dependence.

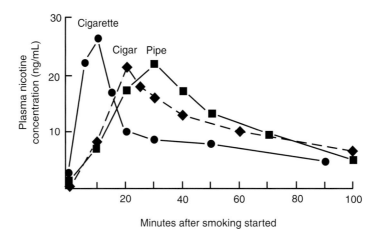

FIGURE 22-3 Plasma concentration of nicotine after smoking. Habitual smokers used a cigarette, pipe or cigar; blood samples were taken and plasma levels of nicotine measured. The mean dose of nicotine over the period of smoking was estimated at, for a cigarette, 21 mcg/kg over 8–10 minutes; pipe, 45 mcg/kg over 20–30 minutes; cigar, 41 mcg/kg over 22 minutes. *Source*: Bowman & Rand 1980, used with permission; data obtained by Dr M.P. Giles, Department of Pharmacology, University of Melbourne.

Physician advice and follow-up can lead to maintained cessation rates of about 10%, and behavioural therapy has about a 20% success rate. Doctors in general practice are recommended to follow the '5As framework' (see Litt 2005) when encouraging patients to quit smoking:

Ask: about smoking status and habits

Assess: interest in quitting, barriers to quitting

Advise: on nicotine dependence and health hazards of smoking

Assist: enrolment in quit program, plus drug therapies and support

Arrange: follow-up reviews and support.

This program, together with follow-up by QuitLine, advice offered by the nurse and pharmacist, and combination pharmacotherapy, can significantly enhance quit rates.

Nicotine replacement therapy (patches, gum, lozenges, sublingual tablets, spray or inhaler) doubles the cessation rate of advice or behavioural therapy alone. Patches are formulated in a range of doses providing from 21 mg/24 h to 7 mg/24 h; the dose is tapered off over several weeks. The patches and gum are available OTC (Schedule 2) but it has been suggested that until nicotine replacement therapy is more available and cheaper than cigarettes, there are financial reasons why nicotine-dependent persons continue smoking.

Bupropion, previously used as an antidepressant, enhances cessation rates to 10%–24%; it is thought that the antidepressant effects contribute to helping smokers give up smoking, as nicotine itself has antidepressant and antianxiety actions. When the cost of the drug was partly subsidised after its introduction into the Pharmaceutical Benefits Scheme (PBS), there was an unexpectedly high demand for the new therapy, with an estimated 200,000 Australians believed to have started using the drug within 4 months.

Cocaine

Cocaine is an alkaloid related to the belladonna alkaloids atropine and hyoscine; it is an ester-type local anaesthetic (see Clinical Interest Box 15-6). Its central and autonomic effects are largely due to its ability to inhibit the reuptake of catecholamines back into nerve terminals. Thus it potentiates the actions of noradrenaline, adrenaline and dopamine in the peripheral and central nervous systems, and has sympathomimetic effects. It is classified as a controlled substance (Schedule 8).

Cocaine has central stimulant properties, causing excitement, talkativeness, tremors, vomiting and increased respiration and blood pressure. It is a powerful reinforcer, rapidly producing sensations of reward and exhilaration, thus it rapidly causes dependence. There is no typical withdrawal syndrome, but rebound effects after withdrawal may manifest as fatigue and depression. Topically it has local anaesthetic and vasoconstrictor therapeutic effects; thus it has a limited use in a few selected surgical procedures, such as nasal and ophthalmic surgery (Clinical Interest Box 22-9).

Orally administered cocaine is readily absorbed but subject to an extensive first-pass effect; thus there is low oral bioavailability (as for all local anaesthetics) and short half-life (about 1 hour); cocaine abusers may need to use the drug every half hour or less to maintain the high. Cocaine is given parenterally for its local anaesthetic effects. When abused, cocaine is taken as a snuff ('snorted') or by injection; when coca leaves are chewed, the cocaine is probably absorbed via the buccal mucosa. The free-base form ('rock' or 'crack') is smoked for a rapid, intense effect.

DRUG MONOGRAPH 22-5 NICOTINE GUM

Nicotine is an autonomic ganglion-stimulant agent with widespread effects in the body. When used medically in nicotine replacement therapy by smokers trying to quit, it decreases the severity of the tobacco withdrawal syndrome and increases the likelihood of smoking cessation. Nicotine is available in gum (resin), inhaler formulations and transdermal systems (patches) for use in smoking cessation programs. The most effective treatment currently is a combination of patch (providing steady nicotine replacement) with gum or spray (to provide the 'hit' when a boost of euphoriant effect is required). Dependence on nicotine replacement therapy is considered easier to break than is the smoking habit.

INDICATIONS The nicotine resin is in the form of chewing gum for the nicotine-dependent patient who is undergoing acute cigarette withdrawal or who is trying to sustain abstinence from smoking. It is most effective in moderate to heavy smokers who are well motivated to quit and who have good counselling and social support. When the person has a strong urge to smoke, a stick of gum is chewed instead, which relieves the physical symptoms of nicotine withdrawal. The number of pieces of gum chewed is gradually reduced over a 2- to 3-month period. Nicotine replacement therapy is of little benefit to light smokers, for whom behavioural techniques to support quitting are recommended.

PHARMACOKINETICS Pure nicotine is a colourless–pale yellow oily liquid. It is very lipid-soluble and rapidly absorbed across lipid membranes of the mouth, skin, airways and GI tract. When chewed as a gum (or from tobacco) it is absorbed through the buccal mucosa, more slowly than if inhaled while smoking. When saliva containing nicotine is swallowed, the drug is absorbed through the GI tract and inactivated in the liver.

It is metabolised primarily in the liver, with smaller amounts metabolised in the kidney and lung. Most of the metabolites are inactive, although cotinine, the main oxidation product, is said to have antidepressant and psychomotor stimulant properties. The half-life is 1–2 hours. Elimination is primarily renal, with 10% excreted unchanged and the remainder as metabolites; the drug is excreted in breast milk.

DRUG INTERACTIONS The effects in the table below may occur when nicotine is taken with the drugs listed.

Drug	Possible effect and management
Paracetamol, caffeine, oxazepam, propranolol and theophylline	Smoking increases metabolism of these drugs, which may result in lower blood concentrations, so higher or more frequent drug dosing may be required

Drug	Possible effect and management
Adrenergic agonists or blocking agents, catecholamines, corticosteroids	Smoking and nicotine raise catecholamine and cortisone levels; therefore therapy with adrenoceptor agonists or antagonists or corticosteroids may require dosage adjustment based on the individual's response
Insulin	Smoking cessation may result in an increased insulin effect; dosage reduction may be necessary. Monitor closely for symptoms of hypoglycaemia
Autonomic drugs	The effects of nicotine on autonomic ganglia are complicated and dose-dependent. Doses of other autonomic drugs may need adjusting
Vasoconstrictors	Nicotine decreases myocardial oxygen supply and increases demand; these effects are compounded by other vasoconstrictors
Acidic beverages (coffee, soft drinks)	May decrease buccal absorption of nicotine
Nicotine (in other forms, e.g. cigarettes, patches)	Additive effects, leading to chest pains and palpitations

ADVERSE REACTIONS Adverse effects of nicotine include fast heart beat, mild headache, increased appetite, increased watering of mouth or dry mouth, sore mouth or throat, coughing, dizziness or light-headedness, hiccups, irritability, indigestion and difficulty in sleeping. Adverse reactions with nicotine gum include local injury to mouth, teeth or dental work. Transdermal patches may also cause pruritus and/or erythema under the patch. Some of the signs and symptoms may in fact be due to stopping smoking, rather than to nicotine gum.

Early signs of overdose are nausea and vomiting, severe increased watering of the mouth, severe abdominal pain, diarrhoea, cold sweat, severe headache, severe dizziness, disturbed hearing and vision, confusion and severe weakness; while signs of toxicity include fainting, hypotension, difficulty breathing and fast, weak or irregular pulse, and convulsions.

WARNINGS AND CONTRAINDICATIONS Use with caution in people with cardiovascular disease, insulin-

DRUG MONOGRAPH 22-5   NICOTINE GUM

dependent diabetes mellitus, hyperthyroidism, peptic ulcer disease or phaeochromocytoma. Avoid use in patients with nicotine hypersensitivity, severe angina pectoris or life-threatening cardiac arrhythmias, and after myocardial infarction.

Use is not recommended in pregnancy or breastfeeding; however, nicotine replacement therapy is preferable to smoking.

DOSAGE AND ADMINISTRATION Nicotine gum comes in two strengths, either 2 mg or 4 mg nicotine per piece. The

patient should be instructed to stop smoking before using nicotine replacements (gum, patches or inhaler) and not to use any other nicotine products.

The gum is chewed intermittently and very slowly when the individual has the urge to smoke. The user controls the dose, by biting the gum to release nicotine. The oral dosage is 2 or 4 mg as a chewing gum, repeated as needed to curb the person's urge to smoke, with 10–12 pieces of gum per day, tapering off over 8–12 weeks. Most patients require about 10 pieces of gum per day during the first month of treatment.

CLINICAL INTEREST BOX 22-9 COCAINE AND COCA-COLA

Cocaine is the active ingredient of the leaves of the plant *Erythroxylon coca* and has been used for thousands of years in Central and South American countries, particularly in the Andes, where its stimulating properties suppressed hunger, alleviated misery, and enhanced endurance at high altitudes.

It was introduced into Europe in the 16th century by returning Spanish conquistadors and rapidly achieved popularity. It was soon incorporated into wines, lozenges and tonic mixtures, most famously Coca-Cola, advertised as a 'temperance drink' that would aid digestion and stimulate the nervous system. Cocaine was removed from Coca-Cola only in 1908 because of fears about its addictive effects; after a lawsuit, the name was allowed to retain the word 'coca'.

The potential medical usefulness of the new agent was recognised by European physicians, including Sigmund Freud, who experimented with the drug and described its CNS-stimulant effects, as well as the 'fuzziness on the lips and palate' (due to local anaesthesia). Freud's assistant Carl Köller demonstrated the efficacy of cocaine as a local anaesthetic, particularly in eye surgery.

The acute toxicity of cocaine was quickly recognised, and studies of its chemical structure and pharmacological properties led to the synthesis of many analogues with lower toxicity, including benzocaine, procaine and lignocaine (see Chapter 15 and Drug Monograph 15-4).

Caffeine

The xanthine alkaloids **caffeine**, theophylline and theobromine are found naturally in plants used for the stimulating beverages coffee, tea and cocoa. The xanthines have legitimate medical uses, as CNS stimulants (see Chapter 20) and as bronchodilators (Chapter 32); they also have mild diuretic and cardiac-stimulant effects and have been used to treat respiratory failure in premature infants. Caffeine (Drug Monograph 20-2) is the most powerful CNS stimulant of the

three xanthine alkaloids, hence it is most used and abused in drinks. Theophylline (Drug Monograph 32-3) is the most powerful smooth muscle relaxant, hence is used in asthma. Caffeine is also present in maté (an infusion of the leaves of the shrub *Ilex paraguayensis*), cola and guarana preparations.

Chemically, the xanthines are closely related to the purine bases adenine and guanine (building blocks for DNA and RNA, see Figure 49-1), and caffeine is thought to act through effects on adenosine receptors. At higher concentrations, the xanthines also inhibit the enzyme phosphodiesterase (PDE), which leads to raised intracellular levels of cAMP and may contribute to some of caffeine's actions.

Social use of caffeine

Caffeine is the most widely used psychoactive substance. About half the world's annual coffee production is consumed in the USA, where the average daily caffeine dose is over 250 mg. By comparison, tea accounts for about 43% of all caffeine consumption; the British tend to drink more tea than coffee, and average over 300 mg caffeine daily (see Clinical Interest Box 22-10). Two to three cups of strong coffee are sufficient to raise the caffeine levels in the plasma or brain to approximately 100 μM, a concentration at which adenosine-receptor blockade and some PDE inhibition occur.

Caffeine reduces fatigue, improves concentration (leading to decreased reaction times and increased speed of calculations in tests) and improves motor tasks. In contrast to the amphetamines, caffeine does not cause euphoria, stereotyped behaviours or psychoses. Some tolerance and dependence may develop to caffeine but there is little evidence of an acute withdrawal syndrome (possibly a mild irritability and headache). Animals cannot be trained to self-administer caffeine, which implies that it does not produce reward or dependence; and caffeine does not act on the dopaminergic structures related to reward, motivation and addiction.

In large doses, caffeine can be mutagenic and teratogenic in animals but these effects have not been seen in humans. Large doses (300–600 mg) can cause insomnia, anxiety, palpitations, tremor, headache, increased gastric secretions, and seizures.

CLINICAL INTEREST BOX 22-10 COFFEE, TEA OR COCOA?

The plant from which coffee is extracted, *Coffea arabica*, is thought to have originated in Ethiopia; the technique for preparing the seeds to produce the stimulant beverage was developed in the 9th century in Yemen near the town Mocha.

Coffee was introduced into Western Europe in the 16th century and rapidly became popular in coffee houses; coffee plantations were started in many colonies of the European powers, including in Africa, Brazil and New Guinea.

Tea is a beverage made by infusing dried leaves of the plant *Camellia sinensis* in boiling water; this has been done in China and Japan for over 1600 years. Tea also reached Europe in the 16th century and plantations were established in many colonies (India, Sri Lanka, Indonesia).

Cocoa and chocolate come from the seed of *Theobroma cacao*, discovered in the Aztec court in Mexico by Cortes in the early 16th century. The bitter beverage made from cacao beans, peppers and other herbs was called chocolatl, and was thought to have aphrodisiac properties. It was only when the beans were steeped in hot water, and vanilla and sugar added, that the drink became palatable and popular, as chocolate and cocoa.

All of these beverages rely for their popularity and stimulant qualities on the content of the xanthine alkaloids caffeine, theophylline and theobromine. The caffeine content depends on how the drinks are brewed, with coffee containing about 50–150 mg caffeine per cup, tea 50–100 mg, and cocoa 50 mg. While caffeine can induce a mild dependence, those who claim to be 'chocoholics' are most likely addicted to the sugar and flavours in chocolate rather than the caffeine content. The average consumption from beverages by regular tea- or coffee-drinkers is about 200 mg caffeine/day.
Adapted from: Bowman & Rand 1980; Mann 1992.

There have been suggestions that high regular intakes of caffeine are associated with increased incidence of cancers (breast, pancreatic, urogenital) but this association could be due to carcinogens from the roasted coffee beans (which contain more than 1000 different chemicals) rather than related to caffeine intake. Habitual moderate coffee intake does not represent a health hazard. Caffeine has also been implicated in female infertility and in low-birth-weight infants. Diterpenes (present in unfiltered coffee brews, e.g. from Turkish or Greek methods of making coffee) have been shown to raise cholesterol levels in the blood. Caffeine is also present in many other OTC medications, in some prescribed medicines and in soft-drinks (see Clinical Interest Box 22-11)

Tea, on the other hand, may be protective, as the tannins and flavonoids, especially in green teas, are antiatherosclerotic. Polyphenols in tea have been shown to have inhibitory effects on carcinogenesis in animals, delay cancer onset in humans and have antioxidant (protective) properties.

Overall, social use of caffeine is generally not problematic and any dependence is mild. Caffeine abuse is not considered sufficiently severe to warrant treatment and is usually self-limiting because of the negative adverse effects (diuresis, insomnia and dyspepsia) and lack of positive effects on reward pathways.

PSYCHOTOMIMETICS

The term psychotomimetics literally means drugs that are powerful in producing or mimicking psychotic reactions, and could thus refer to a wide range of drugs, including cocaine, amphetamines, antidepressants, centrally acting antimuscarinics and even some antimicrobial agents. It has, however, come to be used in a more restricted sense to refer to drugs with a history of religious, social and/or paramedical use in producing changes in perception or hallucinations. The main groups are the cannabinoids, and hallucinogens such as lysergic acid diethylamide (LSD) and mescaline.

Cannabis drugs (marijuana, hashish)

The **cannabis** drugs are derived from the leaves, stems, fruiting tops and resin of both female and male hemp plants (*Cannabis sativa*), which were probably originally native to Central Asia. The plants have historically been used for the very strong fibres in the stems, which are fast-growing and can be up to 5 m in length. The fibres are used for weaving into fabric (hence the term canvas), for twisting into ropes (hemp), and for making paper. Hempseed is a source of oil similar to linseed oil and is used as birdseed. There are also dermatological preparations (oils, soaps, lotions etc), and foods and fabrics based on cannabis. The resin provides compounds that are used for mental relaxation and euphoria.

The active drugs (cannabinoids) are from the resin of the plant, exuded from the leaves, tops of the stems and the flowering tops of the plants. The potency of the active ingredient (Δ^9-tetrahydrocannabinol [Δ^9-THC]), is greatest in the flowering tops and varies according to the climatic conditions under which the plant is grown, with the typical leaf containing 3% THC. Imported **marijuana**, when carefully cultivated, may contain 6%–10% THC. Marijuana grown under scientifically controlled conditions as a THC source may contain up to 15% THC, and is much more potent than the domestic variety smoked or grown for production of fibres or seeds.

CLINICAL INTEREST BOX 22-11 CAFFEINE CONTENT IN SELECTED PRODUCTS

Gaining prominence in the soft-drink market are 'formulated caffeinated beverages'. Marketed as 'energy- or performance-enhancing drinks', these products promise to 'sustain energy levels' and 'improve mental acuity'. These drinks may also contain guarana, which consumers are often unaware is a natural source of caffeine. Until recently in Australia, manufacture of these products was prohibited, although importation of products from New Zealand and other countries was allowed. There has been insufficient regulation of these products in regard to both caffeine levels and labelling.

Safety concerns have been accentuated in the community by various media reports of caffeine intoxication. Examples have been the death of a 25-year-old woman from ventricular arrhythmias after ingesting energy drinks; her blood caffeine level was equivalent to that of ingesting 15–20 cups of coffee. Also, the possibility of caffeine-induced psychosis or

'caffeinism' was discussed in a court case where an armed robbery occurred after the assailant consumed eleven cans of an energy drink.

An expert working group under the auspices of the Australia New Zealand Food Authority (ANZFA) has, since 1999, examined safety aspects of dietary caffeine. The effects on high-risk groups — children, pregnant or lactating women or those with hypersensitivity to caffeine — are under consideration, as is the potential for low-dose behavioural changes and caffeine addiction.

In August 2001, it was proposed to develop an Australian standard for these caffeinated beverages and to limit caffeine levels to a range of 145–320 mg/L. Mandatory nutritional information is required on these drinks and it is proposed that there be an advised daily limit and warning to those at risk. The table below shows the caffeine contents of a range of commercial products.

CAFFEINE CONTENTS OF SELECTED BEVERAGES AND FOODS

Substance	Amount of caffeine	Conditions
Instant coffee[1]	30–120 mg per cup	
Brewed coffee	40–180 mg per cup	Dependent on type of beans and method of brewing
Decaffeinated coffee	2–5 mg per cup	
Tea[2]	30–110 mg per cup	Dependent on strength of brew
Yerba maté[3]	25–150 mg per cup	
Cocoa (derived from *cacao* beans)[4]	4–70 mg per cup	
Chocolate bars	30–75 mg per 100 g bar	

CAFFEINE CONTENTS OF SELECTED OTC MEDICATIONS

OTC medication	Caffeine per tablet/capsule	Other active ingredients
No-Doz	100 mg	
No-Doz Plus	100 mg	Thiamine, nicotinic acid
Travacalm Original	20 mg	Hyoscine HBr, dimenhydrinate
Dynamo	100 mg	Thiamine HCl, nicotinic acid

CAFFEINE CONTENTS OF SELECTED PRESCRIPTION MEDICATIONS

Prescription medication	Amount of caffeine	Other active ingredients
Cafergot	100 mg per tablet or suppository	Ergotamine tartrate

CAFFEINE CONTENTS OF SOFT-DRINKS

Trade name	Approximate amount of caffeine	Other additives
Professor Head's Smart Drink 'Energy'	80 mg per 250 mL	Ginseng, yerba maté,[3] taurine, guarana,[5] other (choline, leucine, valine, arginine, inositol)
Red Bull	80 mg per 250 mL	Taurine, inositol
Diet Coke	32 mg per 250 mL	Unspecified
Coca-cola	32 mg per 250 mL	Unspecified
Pepsi-cola	27 mg per 250 mL	Unspecified

1. Coffee beans; *Coffea arabica, Coffea robusta* or various blends (1.2%–1.4%).
2. Tea leaves; *Camellia sinensis* (1%–5% caffeine).
3. Yerba maté; leaves of *Ilex paraguayensis* (0.2%–2% caffeine).
4. Cacao beans; *Theobroma cacao* (0.25%–1.7% caffeine).
5. Guarana, from the 'beans' of the South American plant *Paullina cupana* (1%–5% caffeine).
1 cup = about 150–200 mL; 'demi-tasse' = about 75 mL; one teacup = about 150 mL; one coffee mug = about 250–350 mL.

Preparations and active constituents

Marijuana (cannabis prepared for smoking) and hashish are the most common forms of cannabis in use. Hashish refers to the powdered form of the plant's resin, which contains 7%–12% THC. Other forms of cannabis, used in such countries as Jamaica, Mexico, Africa, India and the Middle East, include bhang, ganja and charas. In Morocco kif is used and in South America a cannabis form called dagga.

Marijuana plants contain hundreds of different chemicals, generally termed cannabinoids; they have complex 3-ring structures. Of these, Δ^9-THC and closely related compounds, and cannabidiol (CBD) have been most studied in humans to identify their pharmacological effects. While many questions are still unanswered, it is believed that the major psychoactive ingredient in cannabis is THC. Marijuana cigarettes contain about 0.5–2 g marijuana, of which only 0.5%–1% is THC.

Mode of administration and pharmacokinetics

Tetrahydrocannabinols are highly lipid-soluble, so are readily absorbed when administered by oral, subcutaneous or pulmonary routes, but they are most potent when inhaled. Either the pure resin or the dried leaves of the cannabis plant may be smoked in pipes or cigarettes. The smoke is inhaled deeply and retained in the lungs as long as possible to achieve maximal saturation of the absorbing surface; about 15%–50% of the THC present in preparations is actually absorbed after smoking.

The peak plasma level of THC after smoking one marijuana cigarette is reported to occur within minutes. THC is highly protein-bound, so only a small proportion enters the CNS; it persists in the body in adipose tissue depots (for over 4 weeks) and in the lungs and liver, with a long half-life. It is metabolised in the liver to various hydroxylation products, some of which are pharmacologically active. The metabolites are excreted in the urine, bile and faeces. Only trace amounts of the unchanged THC are detected in the urine. Note that the long half-life of marijuana and the consequent prolonged period for detection of cannabinoids in the urine have made it difficult for accurate correlations to be made between blood cannabinoid concentrations and impaired driving performance, whereas with alcohol the correlation between alcohol in expired air (breath-testing) and impaired psychomotor performance is clear.

Pharmacological effects

Marijuana cigarettes ('joints') are illegal in Australia but in some states there is a more lenient attitude to marijuana use than to 'harder' illicit drugs such as opioids, amphetamines and cocaine, and a few plants may be grown for personal use. The main effects are in the CNS, where the drug has intoxi-cating and mind-altering properties. The drug experience is highly subjective, with a high placebo reaction.

Cannabinoids can affect most systems and organs of the body, as shown below:
- CNS: euphoric effect, anxiety-free state, perceptions of time and space distorted—time is perceived to pass slowly; loss of concentration, disconnected thoughts, impaired decision making, floating sensations, weakness, tremors, incoordination and ataxia; stimulation of appetite and antiemetic effects; anticonvulsant and antiepileptic activities; analgesic effects; hypothermia; hallucinations can occur with high doses, also lethargy and sedation; anxiety and acute toxic psychoses are possible
- cardiovascular system: palpitations, tachycardia and delayed bradycardia, postural hypotension and possible vasovagal syncope, conjunctival vascular congestion (red eyes)
- GI tract: dry mouth and throat, decreased GI motility, delayed GI disturbances and enhanced appetite and flavour appreciation
- respiratory tract: bronchodilation; smoking-related problems, including sore throat, bronchitis and emphysema, and increased risk of lung cancer
- ocular effects: reddening of the eyes; ptosis (drooping of eyelids); decreased intraocular pressure (useful antiglaucoma effect)
- endocrine system: diuretic effect (decreased antidiuretic hormone release); oestrogenic effects (reduced fertility and libido in male chronic users)
- other actions: reported antibacterial, immunosuppressant and antineoplastic effects
- toxic effects: marijuana has a low acute toxicity, with few if any human deaths ever attributed solely to its use; its therapeutic index is estimated to be greater than 1000.

Mechanism of action

The cannabinoids exert various distinct actions: they seem to act as CNS depressants, similar to ethanol, and also as mild hallucinogens like mescaline; THC has effects on lipid membranes similar to those of general anaesthetics. As dosage increases, their effects proceed from relief of anxiety, disinhibition and excitement, to anaesthesia. If dosage is high enough, respiratory and vasomotor depression may occur.

Much research work has gone into attempting to identify the mechanism of action of cannabinoids and the possible natural neurotransmitters or receptors involved. Cannabinoid receptors have been isolated and studied, and the search for a 'natural' endogenous cannabinoid has shown up the compound anandamide, an arachidonic acid derivative related to the eicosanoids and prostaglandins. Much active research work is focused on this substance and its possible use or exploitation in development of new classes of drugs.

Medical use of cannabinoids

Synthetic cannabinoids (dronabinol, a pure preparation of Δ^9-THC, and nabilone) have been prepared and tested for the treatment of nausea and vomiting induced by cancer chemotherapy and not responsive to standard therapies. Both products have a high potential for abuse and so are closely regulated; neither is available in Australia. Other potential uses of cannabinoids are as an adjunct in treating patients with wasting conditions such as HIV–AIDS, and in chronic pain syndromes, insomnia, epilepsy, opioid withdrawal, glaucoma, asthma, and neurological diseases with spasticity. Problems that can be envisaged related to medical use of cannabis are the issues of placebo reactions; consistency of dosing and bioavailability after administration by smoking; and the long half-life and potential prolonged adverse effects on concentration and driving.

Marijuana abuse

Traditionally, marijuana was used in Eastern and African countries in religious ceremonies to enhance meditation and as a mild intoxicant (especially in times when and countries where alcohol was prohibited). In Australia, 50%–60% of the adult population admit to having used marijuana at some stage and in 1998, 18% used marijuana regularly, a much higher figure than in the USA, UK, Canada or Spain. The prohibitions on the use of cannabis are much debated, with valid arguments both for and against prohibition.

TOLERANCE, DEPENDENCE AND WITHDRAWAL

With regular doses at low levels, no tolerance develops to the effects of cannabis; on the contrary, there appears to be a type of 'reverse tolerance', in which users become more familiar with the administration techniques and effects and less anxious about the use of an illicit substance. There is no marked dependence, and withdrawal causes only mild 'rebound' effects such as anxiety, sleep disturbances and muscle weakness and tremor, which may persist for weeks. Craving for the drug can recur intermittently for months after the drug is stopped. If treatment for withdrawal is required, non-pharmacological interventions and an exercise program are preferred to substitution of another drug product.

PROBLEMS WITH CHRONIC USE

Heavy daily use over many years has been shown to be associated with the following major probable adverse reactions:
- respiratory diseases associated with smoking
- cannabis dependence
- cognitive impairment, especially of attention and memory, possibly reversible by long abstinence (secondary school teachers report that they can identify which students are regular users).

Serious possible adverse reactions include:
- increased risk of developing cancers (respiratory tract, GI tract)
- impaired occupational performance
- higher risk of birth defects and leukaemia in offspring exposed in utero
- increased risk of developing schizophrenia.

High-risk groups are adolescents, especially those who are poor performers at school, who are at risk of moving on to more dangerous illicit drugs; pregnant women and their offspring; people with pre-existing diseases, especially cardiovascular, respiratory or psychotic conditions; and drug-dependent people.

Overall, the health risks from regular use of cannabinoids are less dangerous than those from some legal drugs of dependence, particularly alcohol and tobacco.

Hallucinogens

A **hallucinogen** is a drug that produces auditory or visual hallucinations. The most common hallucinogenic agents include LSD and its variants, mescaline, psilocybin and PCP; drugs based on amphetamine are also hallucinogenic (see earlier discussion). Various psychoactive hallucinogenic drugs have been used as adjuncts to religious ceremonies or were used experimentally by young people in the hippie scene in the 1960s and are now experiencing a resurgence in popularity. LSD (Clinical Interest Box 45-3), dimethyltryptamine (DMT), PCP, mescaline, psilocybin and ecstasy (Clinical Interest Box 22-12) are examples of drugs that can produce distortions in perception or thinking at very low doses.

Many of the hallucinogenic agents have chemical structures related to central neurotransmitters or are methylated derivatives of the transmitters (see Figure 22-4). This raises the fascinating possibility that some neurological and psychiatric disturbances may be due to altered metabolic pathways producing endogenous methylated transmitters in CNS pathways, or to higher than normal levels of transmitters being shunted down unusual metabolic paths.

LSD (lysergic acid diethylamide; lysergide)

Lysergide is a very potent hallucinogenic drug that is usually available illicitly in doses of around 200 mcg. LSD is related to the ergot alkaloids (see Drug Monograph 45-1) and thus can affect many body systems and neurotransmitters. After oral administration, it will cause a central sympathomimetic effect within 20 minutes: hypertension, dilated pupils, hyperthermia, tachycardia and enhanced alertness. Effects on mood are unpredictable, ranging from euphoria to severe depression and panic. The psychoactive effects occur in about 1–2 hours and have been described as heightened perceptions, distortions of the body and visual hallucinations.

CLINICAL INTEREST BOX 22-12 OTHER HALLUCINOGENS

MDMA (ecstasy, Adam, XTC) is a stimulant–hallucinogenic used largely by students and other young adults. Evidence indicates that it can destroy brain dopamine neurons. High-dose or chronic use may lead to parkinsonian symptoms and eventually paralysis.

MDA, methylenedioxyamphetamine, is an amphetamine-type drug, similar in structure to MDMA. It destroys serotonin-producing neurons in the brain.

MPPP (a pethidine analogue used as a heroin substitute) synthesis usually produces a toxic byproduct, MPTP, which has caused permanent, irreversible Parkinson's disease in users by selectively destroying nigrostriatal dopaminergic neurons.

DOM, dimethoxymethamphetamine, is a hallucinogenic agent with about 50 times the potency of mescaline.

GHB (γ-hydroxybutyric acid, 'grevious bodily harm', 'fantasy'), originally an anaesthetic, has CNS-depressant and mild hallucinogenic effects (see Clinical Interest Box 21-5).

Bufotenine, a plant alkaloid also present in the skin of toads, and dimethyltryptamine (DMT) are weak hallucinogens and interfere with monoamine transmitters.

Hallucinogenic properties have been reported for many other natural compounds:

- betel (used in India and Asia, chewed with lime; the psychoactive agent is arecoline, a parasympathomimetic drug)
- nutmeg and mace (producing intoxication similar to that produced by cannabis)
- banana skins (containing tryptamine derivatives, which are weak hallucinogens)
- *Amanita muscaria* (the classic white-spotted orange mushroom, containing muscarine, bufotenine and related alkaloids)
- pituri (a preparation used by indigenous Australians in ceremonies and to reduce hunger)
- the old English plants belladonna, thornapple, mandrake, henbane and monkshood, most of which contain centrally acting antimuscarinic agents similar to atropine.

Unpleasant experiences with LSD (a 'bad trip') are rather frequent. Clinically, evidence of impaired judgement in the toxic state is common, and altered states of consciousness may cause psychosis to develop or trigger a latent psychosis into activity. Feelings of acute panic and paranoia during a toxic LSD psychosis can result in homicidal or suicidal thoughts and actions. Long-term effects include **flashback phenomena**, in which unfavourable reactions induced by LSD, such as depression and long-term schizophrenic or psychotic reactions, recur weeks or even years after using the drug. Flashbacks occur in most LSD users.

Mescaline

Mescaline is the chief alkaloid extracted from mescal buttons (flowering heads) of the peyote cactus. It produces subjective hallucinogenic effects similar to those produced by LSD but has only about 0.02% of the potency of LSD. The trimethoxy- and dimethoxy- derivatives of mescaline are also hallucinogenic. It is usually ingested in the form of a soluble crystalline powder that is either dissolved into teas or encapsulated. The usual dose of mescaline is 300–500 mg, which produces GI disturbances, then vivid and colourful visual hallucinations, plus a syndrome of sympathomimetic effects. The half-life of mescaline is about 6 hours and it is excreted in the urine.

Psilocybin

Psilocybin and psilocyn are drugs derived from Mexican mushrooms. They produce subjective hallucinogenic effects similar to those produced by mescaline but of shorter duration.

Within 0.5–1 hour after ingestion of 5–15 mg psilocybin, a hallucinogenic dysphoric state begins. A dose of 20–60 mg may produce effects lasting 5–6 hours. The mood is pleasant to some users, while others experience apprehension. The user has poor critical judgement capacities and impaired performance ability. Also seen are hyperkinetic compulsive movements, laughter, mydriasis, vertigo, ataxia, paraesthesia, muscle weakness, drowsiness and sleep.

Ketamine and phencyclidine (PCP)

Ketamine ('K', 'special K') is a dissociative anaesthetic with hallucinogenic properties; overdose can cause CNS stimulation and delirium. Dependence and flashbacks can occur.

PCP (phencyclidine, also known as 'angel dust') was originally introduced into medicine as an anaesthetic similar to ketamine, but its use was discontinued because of its hallucinogenic effects. PCP has a history of serious adverse outcomes, including many suicides, assaults and murders. Common peripheral signs include flushing, profuse sweating, nystagmus, diplopia, ptosis, analgesia and sedation. PCP produces a state similar to alcohol intoxication, with other perceptual distortions (visual or auditory) that can recur unpredictably, and symptoms that mimic schizophrenia. Toxic pressor effects may cause hypertensive crisis, intracerebral haemorrhage, convulsions, coma and death.

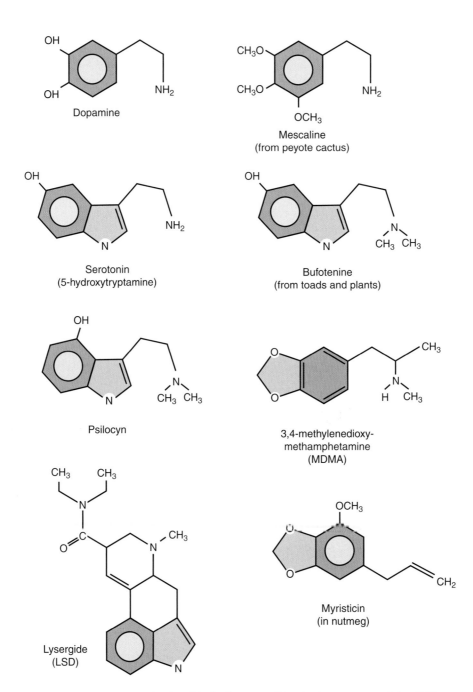

FIGURE 22-4 Monoamine neurotransmitters and related hallucinogens. Chemical structures of the CNS neurotransmitters dopamine and 5-hydroxytryptamine (5-HT, serotonin) are shown, as well as various natural and synthetic hallucinogenic agents — all are methylated compounds in which a backbone structure similar to that of dopamine or serotonin can be traced.

OTHER DRUGS OF ABUSE

Non-opioid analgesics (paracetamol, aspirin, ibuprofen)

Paracetamol, aspirin, ibuprofen and other non-steroidal anti-inflammatory drugs (NSAIDs—see Chapters 16 and 55) are OTC drugs that are readily available in many outlets such as pharmacies and supermarkets. These same ingredients may also be contained in combination formulations and sold with or without a prescription. Thus the potential for intentional and unintentional drug overdose exists with this category of drugs, although they do not cause dependence. They are particularly risky when combined with CNS depressants such as alcohol or benzodiazepines.

Overdoses from non-opioid analgesics are commonly seen in emergency departments; paracetamol is especially dangerous when taken in massive overdoses, owing to its toxic effects on the liver. In Australia, young teenage girls (aged 10–14) overdose on 'headache tablets' at 14 times the rate of boys of the same age. It is thought that the girls are beginning to self-medicate at a turbulent time in their lives and that, whereas boys tend to use more violent means to harm themselves, girls are more likely to use drugs. About one in 100 females admitted to hospital for analgesic poisoning dies from the toxic effects.

Drugs restricted in sport

Many drugs are restricted or prohibited in particular sports, such as anabolic steroids, opioid analgesics, β-blockers, alcohol and even caffeine. This is a specific type of drug abuse, which is considered in Chapter 57.

PREGNANCY SAFETY

As usual, it is recommended that drug use be minimised during pregnancy to only what is essential to the health of the mother (and fetus). Most drugs of dependence, being lipid-soluble, are likely to cross the placental barrier and consequently adversely affect the fetus. Illicit drugs such as heroin, cannabis and ecstasy do not have pregnancy safety classifications, nor do non-scheduled substances such as caffeine, alcohol and tobacco. There are difficulties in gaining data on the safety of these drugs, particularly as drug-abusers often use many different drugs, and lifestyle factors may lead to poor antenatal care.

ADEC Category	Drug
B1	Naloxone
B2	Acamprosate, bupropion, disulfiram
B3	Dexamphetamine, naltrexone
C	Methadone
D	Nicotine (gum, patches, inhaler, lozenges, sublingual tablets)

With respect to other drugs of dependence, the following should be noted:
• alcohol: a moderate to high intake during pregnancy leads to risk of fetal alcohol syndrome (discussed earlier)
• tobacco use leads to poor pregnancy outcomes (increased risk of spontaneous abortion, preterm delivery, low birth weight); note that nicotine is in category D but nicotine substitution is considered safer than smoking
• cocaine: use leads to poor outcomes and is teratogenic (genitourinary tract malformations)
• opioids: use during pregnancy can cause opioid withdrawal in the neonate, with CNS excitability; for heroin-dependent women, methadone maintenance is the preferred treatment
• cannabis and the hallucinogens: have not been shown to be teratogenic
• caffeine: appears to be safe in moderate amounts, but caffeine clearance decreases during pregnancy, so lower amounts should be consumed.
   With respect to breastfeeding, it is generally considered that the benefits outweigh any potential risks from drugs that a mother may take, so moderate amounts of caffeine, alcohol, amphetamines and tobacco may be preferable to withdrawal syndromes or to weaning the infant. However, the 'hard' illicit drugs are considered of such risk to the infant that breastfeeding is not advised; cocaine in particular is contraindicated owing to the risk of toxicity to the infant.

DRUGS AT A GLANCE 22: Drug dependence and social pharmacology

Therapeutic group	Pharmacological group	Key examples	Key pages
Analgesics	Opioids	heroin	375, 7, 83, 4
		morphine	374, 83, 4
		methadone	374, 84–6
		buprenorphine	384
CNS depressants	Alcohols	ethanol (= 'alcohol')	374, 8, 86–91
	Benzodiazepines	diazepam	392
	Barbiturates	phenobarbitone	374, 7
	Inhaled hydrocarbons	petrol, xylene	392
CNS stimulants	Amphetamines	methamphetamine } dexamphetamine	374, 7, 92, 3
	'Designer drugs'	MDMA (= 'ecstasy')	374, 93, 4
	Nicotinic agonists	nicotine, tobacco	374, 8, 94–8
	Local anaesthetics; catecholamine reuptake inhibitor	cocaine	374, 7, 96–8
	(Methyl)xanthines	caffeine, } theophylline	398–400
Psychotomimetics	Cannabinoids	marijuana, Δ^9-THC (cannabis)	374, 7, 99, 401, 2
	Hallucinogens	lysergide (= lysergic acid diethylamide)	375, 7, 402–4
		ketamine	403
Antidotes for toxicity or abuse			
Opioid dependence	Opioid antagonists	naltrexone	382
Alcohol dependence	Alcohol deterrents	acamprosate	390–2
Benzodiazepine dependence	Benzodiazepine antagonists	flumazenil	382, 392
Nicotine dependence	Antidepressants	bupropion	396

Note: See also summary Tables 22-1, 22-2.
MDMA = 3,4-methylenedioxymethamphetamine; THC = tetrahydrocannabinol.

KEY POINTS

- Drug dependence may be psychological and/or physical; related problems are addiction, tolerance and withdrawal syndromes. Trafficking in illicit drugs leads to problems in individuals, families and society, and government policies attempt to reduce supply and demand and minimise harm arising from drug dependence.
- Aetiological factors leading to drug abuse may be based on sociocultural aspects that dictate which drugs are prohibited, personality factors that predispose to drug dependence, and pharmacological factors that cause some drugs to be reinforcing or rewarding. Drugs of dependence may be legal and even prescribed, such as alcohol, caffeine, morphine and benzodiazepines or illicit, such as heroin, marijuana and cocaine.

- The drugs most commonly abused are opioids (heroin); CNS depressants, including alcohol, the benzodiazepines and inhalants; CNS stimulants (cocaine, amphetamines, caffeine and nicotine); psychotomimetics (cannabis) and hallucinogens (LSD, MDMA).

- Treating drug dependence involves managing the acute overdose situation or withdrawal reaction, attempts to detoxify, reduce dependence and maintain abstinence, or maintenance of dependence with the least harmful substitute drug.

- In the case of opioid dependence, naloxone is used as an opioid antagonist to treat acute toxicity, naltrexone is used for detoxification, and methadone as an opioid substitute for long-term maintenance.

- Alcohol abuse is very common in Australian society and ranges from occasional problem drinking through to chronic alcoholism; treatment is with naltrexone or acamprosate. Other CNS depressants abused are the prescription sedatives, such as benzodiazepines, and solvents, which are inhaled.

- CNS stimulants including amphetamines, ecstasy and similar designer drugs, cocaine and caffeine are commonly abused for their euphoriant effects.

- The most problematic drug of dependence in Australia is nicotine, taken by smoking; smoking-related cardiovascular disease and cancers are a major public health problem. Nicotine dependence is treated by substituting nicotine by less dangerous routes, such as gum, patches or inhalers. Bupropion, an antidepressant, improves the rate of smoking cessation in smokers who are well motivated to quit.

- The illicit drug most frequently abused is cannabis and its derivative marijuana; it is used to produce euphoria, distorted perceptions and freedom from anxiety and has been used clinically for treating severe vomiting, pain and glaucoma.

- Hallucinogens include lysergide (LSD), mescaline and various designer drugs, amphetamines and natural products; these can produce 'bad trips', flashback phenomena and psychoses.

- As everyone is likely to be affected in some way by drug abuse, professionals must be informed about the current drug abuse issues, the reported signs and symptoms of drug abuse with each agent, and the recommended interventions and treatment approaches.

REVIEW EXERCISES

1. Ethanol abuse is a common problem in society today. Review the pharmacological effects of ethanol systemically on the central nervous system, cardiovascular system and the gastrointestinal organs, both in short-term use and in chronic alcohol consumption. Name at least three major drug interactions with alcohol and other drugs.

2. What are the differences between cocaine hydrochloride, free-base cocaine, and crack or rock cocaine? What are cocaine's effects on the body initially and with chronic use? What are some medical complications associated with cocaine abuse?

3. Explain why the opioid drug methadone was selected as a substitute drug for heroin and withdrawal maintenance. Name the advantages and disadvantages of methadone use.

4. Discuss the major problems caused to individuals, families and society by chronic drug abuse.

5. Describe the signs, symptoms and treatment for overdose of heroin, amphetamine and alcohol.

6. Discuss types of policies that governments might consider in attempting to curb problems arising from drug abuse.

7. Describe the factors that cause some drugs to be abused, and some people to abuse drugs.

8. Why is clonidine, an antihypertensive drug, used to treat acute opioid, nicotine and alcohol withdrawal and detoxification? Explain its pharmacological effects and the main adverse effects associated with its use.

9. Discuss the general treatment methods available for managing drug abuse and give examples.

10. Describe the pharmacological actions of nicotine and problems related to tobacco abuse.

11. Outline the extent of drug abuse in Australian or New Zealand society, discussing the main groups of drugs liable to be abused.

12. Debate the statement 'Cannabis is much safer than tobacco, so smoking marijuana should be allowed and cigarettes banned'.

REFERENCES AND FURTHER READING

Adverse Drug Reactions Advisory Committee. Update on bupropion (Zyban SR). *Australian Adverse Drug Reactions Bulletin* 2001; 20(2): 6–7.

Analgesic Expert Group. *Therapeutic Guidelines: Analgesic, version 4*. Melbourne: Therapeutic Guidelines Limited, 2002.

Australian Institute of Health and Welfare. 2004 national drug strategy household survey: detailed findings. Canberra: Australian Institute of Health and Welfare, 2005.

Australian Medicines Handbook 2005. Adelaide: AMH, 2005.

Bloch S, Singh BS. *Understanding Troubled Minds: A Guide to Mental Illness and its Treatment*. Melbourne: Melbourne University Press, 1997 [ch. 13].

Bowman WC, Rand MJ. *Textbook of Pharmacology*. 2nd edn. Oxford: Blackwell, 1980 [ch. 42].

Brailowsky S, Garcia O. Ethanol, GABA and epilepsy. *Archives of Medical Research* 1999; 30(1): 3–9.

British Pharmacopoeia Commission. *British Pharmacopoeia 2000*. Vol 1. London: The Stationery Office, 2000.

Cannon ME, Cooke CT, McCarthy JS. Caffeine-induced cardiac arrhythmia: an unrecognised danger of healthfood products. *Medical Journal of Australia* 2001; 174: 520–1.

Caswell A (ed.). *MIMS Annual June 2005*. Sydney: CMPMedica Australia, 2005.

Christopherson AS. Amphetamine designer drugs—an overview and epidemiology. *Toxicology Letters* 2000; 112–13: 127–31.

Cooper JR, Bloom FE, Roth RH. *The Biochemical Basis of Neuropharmacology*. 8th edn. New York: Oxford University Press, 2003.

Gonzalez G, Oliveto A, Kosten TR. Combating opioid dependence: a comparison among the available pharmacological options. *Expert Opinion on Pharmacotherapy* 2004; 5(4): 713–25.

Guy GW, Whittle BA, Robson PJ. *The Medicinal Uses of Cannabis and Cannabinoids*. London: Pharmaceutical Press, 2004.

Hall W, Solowij N, Lemon J. The health and psychological effects of cannabis. *National Drug Strategy Monograph Number 25*. Canberra: AGPS, 1994.

Hall WD, Ross JE, Lynskey MT et al. How many dependent heroin users are there in Australia? *Medical Journal of Australia* 2000; 173: 528–31.

Hamilton M, Kellehear A, Rumbold G. *Drug Use in Australia: A Harm Minimisation Approach*. Melbourne: Oxford University Press, 1998.

Hollister LE. Marijuana (cannabis) as medicine. *Journal of Cannabis Therapeutics* 2001; 1(1): 5–27.

Intergovernmental Committee on Drugs, and the Australian National Council on Drugs. *The National Drug Strategy: Australia's Integrated Framework 2004–2009*. Canberra: Commonwealth of Australia, 2004.

Iversen L. Neurotransmitter transporters: fruitful targets for CNS drug discovery. *Molecular Psychiatry* 2000; 5(4): 357–62.

Jamrozik K, Le M. Tobacco's uncounted victims. *Medical Journal of Australia* 2001; 174: 490–1.

Kritz H, Sinzinger H. Tea consumption, lipid metabolism, and atherosclerosis. *Wiener Klinische Wochenschrift* 1997; 109(24): 944–8.

Litt J. What's new in smoking cessation? *Australian Prescriber* 2005; 28(3): 73–5.

Lucas G. How to detect the alcoholic in your practice. *Modern Medicine of Australia* 1981; October: 36–9.

Mann J. *Murder, Magic and Medicine*. Oxford: Oxford University Press, 1992.

Morland J. Toxicity of drug abuse—amphetamine designer drugs (ecstasy): mental effects and consequences of single dose use. *Toxicology Letters* 2000; 112–13: 147–52.

Mundell M. Ecstasy con: it's the unreal thing. *The Age* 2001; Feb 3, News: 15.

NASA. Using spider-web patterns to determine toxicity. *NASA Tech Briefs* 1995; 19(4): 82.

Nawrot P, Jordan S, Eastwood J, Rotstein J, Hugenholtz A, Feeley M. Effects of caffeine on human health. *Food Additives and Contaminants* 2003; 20(1): 1–30.

Norton SA. Betel: consumption and consequences. *Journal of American Academy of Dermatology* 1998; 38(1): 81–8.

Odyssey House. *About Us. Odyssey House*. Melbourne: Odyssey House, 2001.

Oswald LM, Wand GS. Opioids and alcoholism. *Physiology and Behavior* 2004; 81(2): 339–58.

Paton A, Touquet R. *ABC of Alcohol* 4th edn. Malden, MA: Blackwell, BMJ Books, 2005.

Penington D. *Drugs In Our Community—Taking Stock*. Discussion Paper no. 3, 1999. Melbourne: Trust for Young Australians, 1999.

Penington D. *Illicit Drugs, Community Perception and Public Policy Imperatives*. Melbourne: University of Melbourne Centre for Public Policy, 1996.

Psychotropic Expert Group. *Therapeutic Guidelines: Psychotropic, version 5*. Melbourne: Therapeutic Guidelines Limited, 2003.

Public Health Division, Department of Human Services. *Methadone Treatment in Victoria: User Information Booklet*. Melbourne: Victorian Government Department of Human Services, 2001.

Rang HP, Dale MM, Ritter JM, Moore PK. *Pharmacology*. 5th edn. Edinburgh: Churchill Livingstone, 2003.

Reynolds JEF (ed.). *Martindale: the Extra Pharmacopoeia*. 31st edn. London: Royal Pharmaceutical Society, 1996.

Robinson SE. Buprenorphine: an analgesic with an expanding role in the treatment of opioid addiction. *CNS Drug Reviews* 2002; 8(4): 377–90.

Robson P. Therapeutic aspects of cannabis and cannabinoids. *British Journal of Psychiatry* 2001; 178: 107–15.

Scott T, Grice T. The great brain robbery: what everyone should know about teenagers and drugs. Sydney: Allen & Unwin, 2005.

Silagy C, Mant D, Fowler G, Lancaster T. *Nicotine Replacement Therapy for Smoking Cessation*. (Cochrane Review.) The Cochrane Library, Issue 2, 2001. Oxford: Update Software, 2001.

Singh YN (ed.). *Kava: From Ethnology to Pharmacology*. Boca Raton: CRC Press, 2004.

Smith PF, Smith A, Miners J et al. *Report from the Expert Working Group on the Safety Aspects of Dietary Caffeine*. Canberra: Australian New Zealand Food Authority, 2000.

Speight TM, Holford NHG (eds). *Avery's Drug Treatment*. 4th edn. Auckland: Adis International, 1997.

Spencer JW, Jacobs JJ. *Complementary/Alternative Medicine: An Evidence-Based Approach*. St. Louis: Mosby, 1999.

Stahl SM. *Essential Psychopharmacology: Neuroscientific Basis and Practical Applications*. 2nd edn. Cambridge: Cambridge University Press, 2000 [ch. 13].

State Government of Victoria. *Drugs, the Facts: A Practical Guide to Reducing the Harm From Drugs*. Melbourne: State Government of Victoria, Department of Human Services, 'Turning the Tide' program, 1997.

Stick S. Environmental tobacco smoke—physicians must avoid fanning the flames. *Australian and New Zealand Journal of Medicine* 2000; 30: 436–8.

Sudano I, Binggeli C, Spieker L, Luscher TF, Ruschitzka F, Noll G, Corti R. Cardiovascular effects of coffee: is it a risk factor? *Progress in Cardiovascular Nursing* 2005; 20(2): 65–9.

Twist C. *Facts on the Crack and Cocaine Epidemic*. London: Gloucester Press, 1989.

Walters E. *The Cruel Hoax: Street Drugs in Australia*. Melbourne: Shield, 1996.

Whelan G. The management of the heavy drinker in primary care. *Australian Prescriber* 2002; 25(3): 70–3.

White J, Taverner D. Drug-seeking behaviour. *Australian Prescriber* 1997; 20(3): 68–70.

Wilce H. Temazepam capsules: what was the problem? *Australian Prescriber* 2004; 27(3): 58–9.

Williamson EM, Evans FJ. Cannabinoids in clinical practice. *Drugs* 2000; 60(6): 1303–14.

Wills S. *Drugs of Abuse*. 2nd edn. London: Pharmaceutical Press, 2005.

Wodak A. Drug treatment for opioid dependence. *Australian Prescriber* 2001; 24(1): 4–6.

Zevin S, Benowitz NL. Drug interactions with tobacco smoking: an update. *Clinical Pharmacokinetics* 1999; 36(6): 425–38.

ON-LINE RESOURCES

Australian Drug Foundation (2001): www.adf.org.au

Australian Institute of Health and Welfare. *2004 National Drug Strategy Household Survey: First results*. AIHW cat. no. PHE57 (Drug Statistics Series no. 13). Canberra: AIHW, 2005: www.aihw.gov.au

DirectLine, Turning Point Alcohol and Drug Centre: www.turningpoint.org.au

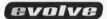 More weblinks at http://evolve.elsevier.com/AU/Bryant/pharmacology/

UNIT V
Drugs Affecting the Heart and Vascular System

CHAPTER 23

Overview of the Heart and Vascular System

CHAPTER FOCUS

Cardiovascular disease is a major health problem in Australia and annually accounts for approximately 40% of all deaths. During 2002/03 hypertension accounted for 6.1% of all problems managed by general practitioners (AIHW: Britt et al 2003). As life expectancy increases, it is anticipated that more people will be diagnosed with acute and chronic cardiovascular conditions, and they will rely increasingly on care provided by health professionals. An understanding of the anatomy and physiology of the heart and vascular system is essential to understanding the action and use of drugs in the treatment of hypertension, cardiac failure, angina, atherosclerosis and thromboembolic disorders.

OBJECTIVES

● To describe the structure and function of the atria, ventricles, valves and major blood vessels of the heart.

● To describe the vascular supply of the heart and explain the relationship between myocardial demand and supply.

● To explain the functional characteristics of the cardiac conduction system.

● To describe the phases of a cardiac action potential.

● To describe the electrical, mechanical and contractile aspects of myocardial function.

● To describe the electrical basis of the P, QRS and T waves of an electrocardiogram (ECG).

● To explain the relationship between cardiac output, stroke volume and heart rate.

● To describe the effects of the autonomic nervous system on the heart.

● To describe the structure and function of the various blood vessels and explain their contribution to total peripheral vascular resistance.

KEY TERMS

action potential
afterload
atria
automaticity
AV node
capacitance vessels
cardiac output
conductivity
depolarisation
diastole
electrocardiogram
Frank–Starling relation

myocardium
preload
refractoriness
resistance vessels
repolarisation
rhythmicity
SA node
sarcolemma
sarcomere
stroke volume
systole
ventricles

KEY ABBREVIATIONS

ATP	adenosine triphosphate
AV	atrioventricular
CO	cardiac output
ECG	electrocardiogram
HR	heart rate
mV	millivolts
SA	sinoatrial
SV	stroke volume
SVR	systemic vascular resistance
TPR	total peripheral resistance

ADVANCES in science and technology have resulted in greater understanding of, and new treatments for, cardiac disease. With these advances has come the increased use of electrocardiographic monitoring of persons with known or suspected cardiovascular disorders. Microelectrode techniques have grown increasingly sophisticated and have helped provide greater understanding of the electrical properties of cardiac fibres and the causes of various cardiac disorders. This expansion in knowledge of cardiac anatomy, electrophysiology and pharmacology has resulted in improvements in the diagnosing and treatment of cardiac arrhythmias, heart failure and coronary vascular disease. This chapter reviews our current understanding of the physiological properties of the heart and blood vessels which comprise the cardiovascular system.

THE HEART

The heart is a hollow muscular organ that consists of four chambers — the upper right and left **atria** and the lower right and left **ventricles**. The main pumping chambers are the right ventricle, which pumps deoxygenated blood through the pulmonary circulation, and the left ventricle, which pumps oxygenated blood through the systemic circulation. The pericardium is a bag-shaped membrane that surrounds the heart and confines it to its position in the chest. Between the pericardium and the wall of the heart is the pericardial cavity, which contains pericardial fluid, a slippery substance that reduces friction between the pericardium and the heart wall when the heart contracts. The heart wall consists of the external smooth epicardium, the middle layer of myocardium, or muscle tissue, and the inner endocardium which lines the chambers of the heart and the valves. The valves open, enabling blood to flow in the forward direction, and close, preventing backflow into the chambers. The tricuspid valve lies between the right atrium and right ventricle, the mitral (bicuspid) valve between the left atrium and left ventricle, the semilunar valves between the right ventricle and the pulmonary trunk (pulmonary valve) and between the left ventricle and the aorta (aortic valve) (Figure 23-1).

Cardiac muscle

The pumping action of the heart depends on the ability of the cardiac muscle to contract. The **myocardium**, the thick, contractile middle layer of the heart wall, is composed of many interconnected branching muscle fibres,

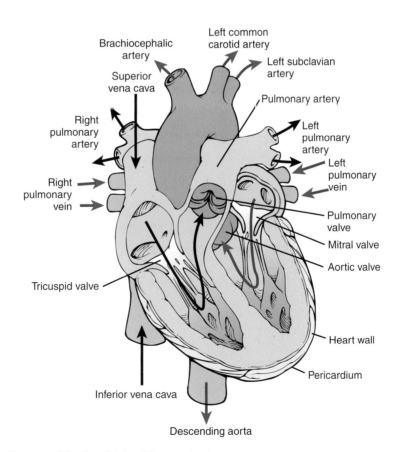

FIGURE 23-1 A schematic diagram of the heart, blood flow and valves.

or cells, that form the walls of the atria and the ventricles. Each individual cardiac muscle cell contains a nucleus in the middle and a plasma membrane (cell membrane), the **sarcolemma** (Figure 23-2A). By joining end to end, the cells form a long fibre, with each cell contacting its neighbour through a thickening of the sarcolemma called the intercalated disc. These discs contain desmosomes that hold the fibres together, and gap junctions, which provide sites of low electrical resistance, permitting the spread of muscle action potentials throughout the cardiac muscle.

Each individual muscle fibre (cell) comprises a group of multiple parallel myofibrils, the end unit of which is the myofilament. The myofibrils are arranged end to end in a series of repeating units called **sarcomeres** (Figure 23-2B, 2C). At the point of separation of the sarcomeres, known as the Z line, the sarcolemma of the muscle fibre interlocks (invaginates) at its end with the sarcomere to form the transverse sarcotubule, or T system, which penetrates deeply into the cell. An extensive network of internal membranes, the sarcoplasmic reticulum, encircles groups of myofibrils and makes contact with the sarcotubules.

The sarcomere, which is the basic unit of contraction in the heart, lies between two successive Z lines and is part of the myofibril. Examination by light microscope reveals the most characteristic feature of the muscle fibre, alternating light (I) bands and dark (A) bands (Figure 23-2C). The darkness of the A bands results from the thicker myosin filaments, while the lightness of the I bands reflects the thinner actin filaments. In the middle of the darker A band is a less dense portion called the H zone; the myosin filaments run the entire length of the A band, passing through the H zone. The lighter I band, by contrast, is divided by a darker appearing region called the Z line, where actin filaments from neighbouring sarcomeres join each other; actin filaments run through the whole I band and terminate at the edge of the H zone, which accounts for the lighter appearance of this zone (Figure 23-2D, 2E). Cross-bridges, which are small projections that extend from the sides of the myosin filament, appear along the entire length of the filament. The interaction between these cross-bridges of myosin and the active sites of actin produces contraction by sliding the A bands and I bands with respect to each other.

The tremendous energy requirements for cardiac muscle contraction can be seen by the great numbers of mitochondria lined up in long chains between the myofibrils (Figure 23-2B). The heart derives most of its energy from oxidative metabolism of fatty acids and lactate, which occurs in mitochondria and cardiac muscle cells.

Coronary vascular supply of the heart

The entire blood supply to the myocardium is provided by the right and left coronary arteries, which arise from the base

of the aorta (Figure 23-3). The right atrium and ventricle are supplied with blood from the right coronary artery. The left coronary artery divides into the anterior (descending) branch and the circumflex branch and supplies blood to the left atrium and ventricle. These main coronary vessels continue to divide, forming numerous branches, resulting in a profuse network of coronary vessels. The major arterial vessels supplying the heart are located on the external surface of the ventricles. Branches penetrate the myocardium towards the endocardial (inner) surface. Venous coronary blood drains via the coronary sinus into the right atrium. Coronary perfusion occurs as a result of the high pressure of blood in the aorta and occurs primarily when the ventricles have relaxed and the coronary vessels are no longer compressed. Ventricular contraction compresses the coronary vascular bed but increases coronary outflow. Increased oxygen delivery to the myocardium is supported almost exclusively by increased coronary blood flow.

When the demand for oxygen and nutrients by body tissues increases, cardiac output must increase. At the same time, the heart muscle itself must be supplied with enough oxygen and nutrients to replace the energy it expends. In other words, a balance must be maintained between energy expenditure and energy restoration. The increase in heart rate increases the metabolic needs of the heart and, normally, coronary dilation occurs in an attempt to meet the higher metabolic demand and to overcome restricted blood inflow. Whenever the delivery of oxygen to the myocardium is inadequate to meet the increased oxygen consumption by the heart, myocardial ischaemia occurs. In many instances atheroma formation is one of the major causes of ischaemia, which manifests in the signs and symptoms of angina (Chapter 25).

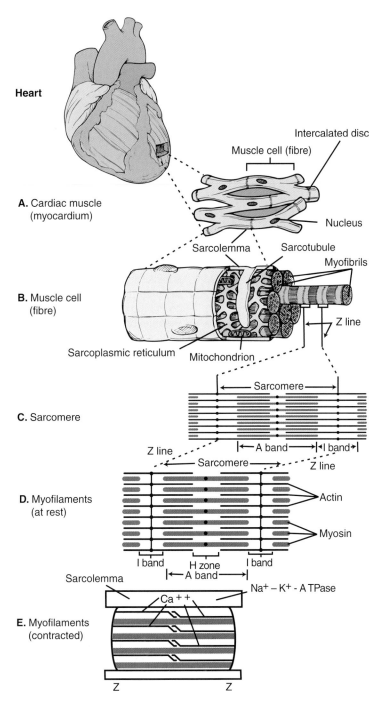

FIGURE 23-2 Structure of heart and cardiac muscle cell fibres. The enlargement of the square illustrates a portion of the cardiac muscle (myocardium) (**A**), which is composed of myocardial cells. Each cell contains a centrally located nucleus and a limiting plasma membrane (sarcolemma), which forms the intercalated disc at the termination of each cell. An individual muscle cell (fibre) (**B**) consists of multiple parallel myofibrils. Each myofibril is arranged longitudinally in a series of light and dark repeating units. Each unit is called a sarcomere. At the Z line, the sarcolemma invaginates to form the transverse sarcotubules, or T system. An extensive network, called the sarcoplasmic reticulum, encircles groups of myofibrils and makes contact with the sarcotubules. The sarcoplasmic reticulum contains a high concentration of calcium ions. The mitochondria appear in long chains between the myofibrils. The sarcomere (**C**) is the unit of muscle contraction. It is composed of two types of bands, the A band and the I band. The Z line divides the latter. Myofilaments (**D**) of the sarcomere include the thin filament, actin, and the thick filament, myosin. The dark appearance of the A band is caused by the myosins and the lighter appearance of the I band by the actin. When contracted (**E**), the sarcomere shortens so that the thick filaments approach the Z line and the width of the H zone between the thin filaments narrows. Calcium ions are required for contraction.

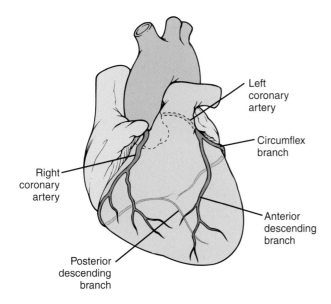

FIGURE 23-3 Coronary blood supply to the heart. Dark shaded vessels are those located on the external surface of the ventricles; light shaded vessels show penetration of arterial branches towards the endocardial surface.

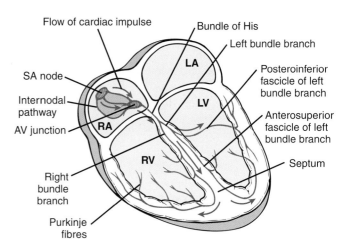

FIGURE 23-4 Conduction system of the heart. The cardiac impulse is initiated at the SA node and is transmitted through the internodal pathways to the two atria, resulting in atrial contraction. At the AV node, the electrical impulse is delayed. Conduction then speeds up at the bundle of His, with the impulse travelling through the right bundle branch and the left bundle branch and continuing through the posteroinferior fascicle and anterosuperior fascicle of the latter bundle branch. Finally, the arrival of impulses at the Purkinje fibres results in their distribution to all parts of both ventricles, where, on excitation, ventricular contraction is produced. RA = right atrium; RV = right ventricle; LA = left atrium; LV = left ventricle.

The cardiac conduction system

The effective pumping action of the heart depends on the regularity of events occurring in the cardiac cycle. Each cycle consists of a period of relaxation, **diastole**, followed by a period of contraction, **systole**. The rhythm and rate of the cardiac cycle are regulated by the conduction system, specialised cardiac cells that have the ability to initiate and transmit the electrical impulses needed to stimulate contraction of the cardiac muscle.

The conduction system (Figure 23-4) is made up of:
• the sinoatrial (SA) **node**
• internodal pathways
• the atrioventricular (AV) **node**
• the bundle of His
• right and left bundle branches
• Purkinje fibres.

In the normal heart, the SA node, located in the right atrium, initiates the heartbeat. The impulses generated are then conducted through the interatrial and internodal pathways to both atria, producing atrial contraction. Having travelled through the atria the impulses arrive at the AV node, which links the conducting pathways of the atria to the ventricles. Electrical conduction is delayed at the AV node, allowing time for the atria to contract fully and the ventricles to finish filling before contraction. At the bundle of His, conduction speeds up and the impulses travel through the right and left bundle branches, then through the posteroinferior and anterosuperior fascicles of the left bundle branch. The

transmission of impulses at the Purkinje fibres, which consist of tiny fibrils that spread around the ventricles and connect directly with the myocardial cells, is very rapid. Finally, the synchronised depolarisation of both ventricles produces ventricular contraction, resulting in the ejection of blood through both the pulmonary artery and the aorta by the ventricles.

Electrophysiological properties

The coordinated pumping action of the heart is initiated and regulated by the specialised fibres of the conduction system. The individual fibres of this system possess three basic electrophysiological properties: automaticity, conductivity, and refractoriness.

AUTOMATICITY

The specialised fibres of the conduction system have the inherent ability to spontaneously initiate an electrical impulse without any external stimuli. This is the most fundamental mechanism of impulse formation, and the cells that possess this property of **automaticity**, the ability to initiate an impulse, are called pacemaker cells. They are found in specialised conducting tissues such as the SA and AV nodes and the His–Purkinje system.

Normally, the impulse of the heart is spontaneously and regularly initiated at the pacemaker cells of the SA node. During the resting phase the membrane of the cell depolarises itself, spontaneously and gradually, until it reaches the threshold and generates an action potential (see later section, Electrical excitation). Thus the membrane of pacemaker cells is never truly at rest. The slow depolarisation of the membrane in the resting state is called spontaneous diastolic depolarisation, or phase 4 depolarisation, and defines automaticity. This property is attributed to the continuous influx of sodium ions into the interior of the cells, which readily drives the membrane towards the threshold potential. The resting potential of automatic pacemaker cells differs from that of contractile myocardial cells. After full repolarisation, the membrane of myocardial cells maintains a steady resting potential until an external stimulus causes it to depolarise. Automaticity is thus a property of fibres of the conduction system that normally controls heart rhythm — it is not a feature of 'working' muscle (atria and ventricles); however, in some circumstances (e.g. cardiac disease, use of certain drugs), myocardial cells have the potential to exhibit spontaneous depolarisation.

The spontaneous excitation of pacemaker cells establishes the normal rhythm of the heart. The regularity of such pacemaking activity is termed **rhythmicity**. Under normal circumstances, only one functional pacemaker, the SA node, predominates because it has the highest frequency of depolarisation. The normal rate of impulse formation is about 72 beats/min. If the SA node substantially slows its rate of impulse formation, then the AV node becomes the primary pacemaker of the heart and will drive the heart at about 40 beats/min.

CONDUCTIVITY

Conductivity refers to the ability of a cell (e.g. cardiac muscle, nerve) to transmit an action potential along its plasma membrane. The property of conductivity therefore exists not only in the cells of the conduction system but also in the cardiac musculature. The speed with which electrical activity is spread within the SA node is quite slow — about 0.05 m/s. The impulse then spreads out rapidly over the atrial musculature at a rate of about 1 m/s. When the impulse reaches the AV node, there is a delay of about 0.01 seconds, then atrial systole occurs, allowing the atria to contract fully and the ventricles to fill. The impulse then spreads rapidly at about 2–4 m/s, along the right and left bundle branches and Purkinje fibres. This rapid activation of contractile elements evokes a synchronous contraction of the ventricles. The conduction velocity is determined by the threshold size of the resting potential of the cell membrane and by membrane responsiveness.

REFRACTORINESS

Cardiac tissue is non-responsive to stimulation during the initial phase of systole (contraction). This is known as refractoriness, and it determines how closely together two action potentials can occur. Throughout most of the repolarisation phase, the cell cannot respond to a stimulus. The effective refractory period represents that period in the cardiac cycle during which a stimulus, no matter how strong, fails to produce an action potential. After the effective refractory period and as repolarisation nears completion, a relative refractory period occurs. This is defined as that period during which a propagated action potential can be elicited, provided that the stimulus is stronger than normally required in diastole. When this happens, the fibre is stimulated to contract prematurely, giving rise to an ectopic (extra) beat. Drugs such as digoxin, caffeine and nicotine can trigger ectopic activity.

Myocardial contraction

Throughout the past decade, our understanding of the fundamental mechanisms governing contraction of cardiac muscle in both normal and disease states has improved tremendously. Yet some aspects of this complicated process are still unknown. Cardiac muscle contraction begins with a rapid change in the resting membrane potential of the cell. This electrical current spreads to the interior of the cell, where it causes the release of calcium ions from the sarcoplasmic reticulum. The calcium ions then initiate the chemical events of contraction. The overall process for controlling cardiac muscle contraction, called excitation–contraction coupling, involves electrical excitation, mechanical activation and contractile mechanisms.

Electrical excitation
THE VENTRICLES

Cardiac muscle contraction begins with an action potential initiated by the SA node. The **action potential**, the difference in conductance, which produces rapid changes in concentrations of sodium, potassium and calcium ions, occurs in the membrane of the myocardial cell. The resting state of a muscle cell in the ventricle is created by the difference in electrical charge across the sarcolemma. In this case, the inside of the cell is negative with respect to the outside, which is positively charged. Because the sarcolemma separates these opposite charges, the membrane is in effect polarised. At rest, the extracellular environment is rich in sodium ions (Na^+) and the intracellular environment in potassium ions (K^+), with a rich calcium ion (Ca^{2+}) concentration in the region of the sarcolemma and where it invaginates on the sarcotubule (Figure 23-2).

The cardiac action potential is divided into two stages, **depolarisation** and **repolarisation**. These stages are further subdivided into five phases, 0–4. The resting potential of a myocardial cell is called **phase 4**; in this phase the membrane is polarised with a charge of around –90 **millivolts** (mV). At this voltage the interior of the cell is negative with respect to the exterior and the membrane is relatively impermeable to ions. Any stimulus that changes the resting membrane potential to a critical value, called the threshold, can generate an action potential. See Figure 23-5 for steps of the action potential.

The critical threshold for depolarisation (around −60 mV) may be reached as a result of normal pacemaker activity or of propagation of an electrical impulse from a nearby cell, which opens voltage-dependent sodium channels. The fast inward current of sodium ions (fast channel) results in a membrane that is positively charged to 20 mV. This difference in membrane po-tential results in depolarisation and is designated as phase 0 of the action potential. Within a few milliseconds, the sodium channels close and are unavailable for initiation of another action potential until repolarisation has occurred. Soon after, repolarisation occurs in three phases. The beginning of phase 1 is a partial repolarisation due to inactivation of the sodium current. Phase 2 is the plateau phase that results from a slow inward current of calcium ions via L-type voltage-sensitive calcium channels and a small outward flow

of potassium ions. Calcium ion entry into the cell is essential for the excitation–contraction coupling mechanism.

Phase 3 results from rapid potassium ion efflux from the cell via voltage-gated potassium channels. As more potassium leaves the cell and less calcium enters during this phase, the membrane potential reverts to −90 mV. After repolarisation, phase 4, a resting period, ensues, during which the cell membrane actively transports sodium ions out and potassium ions in, against their concentration gradients. These cation exchanges during recovery require an adenosine triphosphate (ATP)-dependent transport mechanism, the Na+–K+ pump located in the sarcolemma. Binding to the sarcolemma, Na+–K+-ATPase contributes to the pharmacological effects of digoxin on myocardial contraction (Chapter 24).

THE SA AND AV NODES

In the cells of the **SA and AV nodes**, the action potential consists of only phases 0, 3 and 4 (Figure 23-6). The principal distinguishing feature of the pacemaker fibre resides in phase 4. A slow spontaneous depolarisation occurs that requires no external stimulus and is termed diastolic depolarisation.

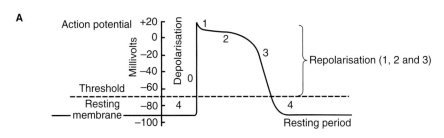

Depolarisation

Phase 0 — membrane becomes permeable to Na+
    which rapidly flows into the cell

Repolarisation

Phase 1 — membrane potential becomes slightly positive because of
    the rapid influx of Na+
Phase 2 — slow inward flow of Ca2+ and outward flow of K+
Phase 3 — rapid outward flow of K+

Resting period

Phase 4 — cell membrane actively transports Na+
    outside and K+ inside, returning cell membrane
    to state of polarisation

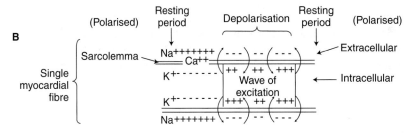

FIGURE 23-5 A. Action potential of a single myocardial cell. **B.** Ion movements across the myocardial cell membrane during an action potential.

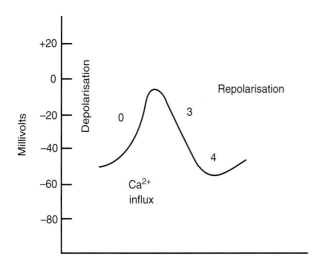

FIGURE 23-6 Three-phase action potential of a slow-channel fibre, the SA node. Unlike the case in the fast fibres of myocardial cells, the depolarisation (phase 0) is attributed primarily to Ca^{2+} influx through slow calcium channels of the cell membrane. Repolarisation involves only phase 3, which is followed by phase 4.

This is responsible for automaticity. Unlike the fast sodium channels of the myocardium, depolarisation (or phase 0) is achieved predominantly by the slower current carried by calcium ions (to a minor extent by sodium ions) through the slow Ca^{2+} channels of nodal cells. Thus, phase 0 results in a slower conduction velocity in nodal cells than in myocardial cells. Calcium channel blockers inhibit these slow channels. Repolarisation is more gradual and involves only phase 3. The membrane then finally returns to phase 4.

VASCULAR SMOOTH MUSCLE

The smooth muscle of blood vessels depends primarily on the presence of calcium ions to initiate and sustain contraction. It is believed that the onset of depolarisation (phase 0) in smooth muscle is caused mainly by calcium ions rather than by sodium ions. Calcium ions enter the smooth muscle cell through voltage-gated and receptor-operated calcium channels. The rise in free calcium ion concentration is considered to be the primary event in excitation–contraction coupling, which increases smooth muscle tone, causing vasoconstriction. Activation of smooth muscle can reduce the calibre of small vessels markedly, as is apparent from the 'spasm' that may occur in coronary vessels. Calcium channel-blocking drugs are capable of blocking the slow calcium ion influx in smooth muscle of blood vessels, thereby producing relaxation (Chapter 25).

MECHANICAL ACTIVATION

As previously stated, the muscle unit that contracts is the sarcomere. It consists of two contractile proteins, actin and myosin. Myosin, the thicker filament, contains the **adenosine** triphosphate (ATP) enzyme system (ATPase) needed to hydrolyse ATP. Hydrolysis is required to provide the energy for contraction. ATP is synthesised in the mitochondria, which are normally abundant in cardiac muscle. Actin, the thin filament, is involved with calcium ion activity. These two filaments combine to help effect cardiac contraction.

Contraction is initiated when the impulse reaches the myocardial cell and travels along the sarcolemma of the muscle fibre. As the depolarisation wave spreads along the sarcotubules, calcium enters through 'L-type' (long-lasting and large) voltage-sensitive calcium channels, causing a secondary release of calcium from the sarcoplasmic reticulum. Hence the plateau, which is phase 2 of the action potential, is maintained through this slow inward calcium current. Calcium ion movement is the chief component that couples electrical excitation of the sarcolemma with muscle activation of the myofilaments in the sarcomere. Normally, interaction between actin and myosin is prevented by tropomyosin, which is bound to the actin filament. Binding of calcium ions to troponin C, a component of the troponin complex, results in a conformational change that moves tropomyosin out of the way and allows binding of the myosin cross-bridges to the actin filaments. These changes initiate the contractile mechanism.

THE CONTRACTILE MECHANISM

Activation of the actin filaments by calcium ions allows formation of the myosin cross-bridges. This interaction pulls the actin along the immobile myosin filaments towards the centre of the A band, shortening the sarcomere and producing muscle contraction. In this process, the lengths of individual filaments remain unchanged. The I band narrows as the thick filaments approach the Z line, and the H zone narrows between the ends of the thin filaments when they meet at the centre of the sarcomere (Figure 23-2D, 2E). The greater the quantity of calcium ions delivered to troponin, the greater the rate and numbers of interactions between actin and myosin. As a result of this response, the development of tension and contractility is increased.

When magnesium is present, ATP is cleaved by myosin ATPase. This reaction provides the energy necessary for the actin filaments to move along the myosin and produce muscle contraction. Muscle relaxation depends on removing calcium ions from the sarcomere, thereby allowing the actin–myosin filaments of the sarcomere to return to their resting positions. This is achieved by a calcium ATPase (located in the walls of the sarcoplasmic reticulum), which actively returns some calcium ions to the sarcoplasmic reticulum while the remainder are removed from the cell by a Na^+–Ca^{2+} exchange protein that exchanges three Na^+ ions for every Ca^{2+} ion.

Electrocardiograms

An **electrocardiogram** (ECG) is a graphic representation of electrical currents produced by the heart. It is a useful tool in determining abnormalities of cardiac rhythm, the heart's response to exercise and the effectiveness of certain drugs. An electrode is placed on each limb and a single electrode placed independently in six different positions on the chest. Combinations of limb and chest leads provides 12 different recordings that, when compared, provide information on the functioning of the heart.

Electrical activity typified by three distinct waves on the ECG (P, QRS and T) always precedes mechanical contraction. The P wave represents atrial depolarisation and follows the firing of the SA node. Immediately after, a wave of electrical activity moves through atrial muscle, the muscle contracts and blood flows from the atria into the ventricles. After the P wave, a short pause or interval (P–R interval) occurs while the electrical activity is transmitted to the AV node, conduction tissue and ventricles. The second wave, the QRS complex, represents ventricular depolarisation and the ventricles contract shortly after it begins. Repolarisation, or recovery, of the ventricles is indicated by the third and smaller T wave. Atrial recovery or repolarisation does not show on the ECG because it is hidden in the QRS complex (Figure 23-7).

CARDIAC FUNCTION
Cardiac output

The primary function of the heart is the supply of oxygenated blood to the rest of the body, both during periods of rest and during increased physical activity. When the body's requirement for oxygen increases, heart rate and cardiac output increase to meet the demand. **Cardiac output** (CO) is a function of both the **stroke volume** (SV) and **heart rate** (HR); that is:

$$CO = SV \times HR$$

SV of the heart depends on the volume of blood remaining in the heart at the end of diastole and the volume that remains after ventricular contraction. For example, in a healthy resting adult, if SV was about 70 mL and HR 72 beats/min, CO would equal 5040 mL/min.

The factors that regulate SV include the degree of stretch of heart fibres before contraction (**preload**), the force of contraction of the ventricles and the pressure that must be overcome before the ventricles can eject the

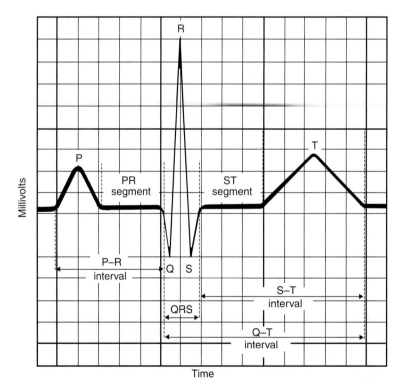

FIGURE 23-7 Graphic representation of the normal electrocardiogram. Vertical lines represent time, each square represents 0.04 s, and every five squares (set off by heavy black lines) represents 0.20 s. The normal P–R interval is less than 0.20 s; the average is 0.16 s. The average P wave lasts 0.08 s, the QRS complex is 0.08 s, the ST segment is 0.12 s, the T wave is 0.16 s, and the Q–T interval is 0.32–0.40 s if heart rate is 65–95 beats/min. Each horizontal line represents voltage; every five squares equals 0.5 mV.

blood (**afterload**). The greater the preload, the greater the stretch and the greater the contraction. This relation means that the longer the muscle fibres are at the end of **diastole** (period of heart relaxation), the more forceful the contraction will be during **systole** (the period of contraction). This mechanism applies only when the muscle fibre is lengthened within physiological limits and is known as the **Frank–Starling relation** (or the Frank–Starling law of the heart). This relation ensures that outputs from the right and left ventricles are the same.

If a diseased heart is dilated and the fibres are stretched to a critical point beyond their limit of extensibility, the forces of contraction and cardiac output are both diminished and ineffective. If the right ventricle fails, blood pools in systemic vessels, causing peripheral oedema, while failure of the left ventricle results in pulmonary oedema because of the backing up of blood in the lungs. Thus the functional significance of the Frank–Starling relation is that effective cardiac output can be brought about only by adequate relaxation and refilling of cardiac chambers after each myocardial contraction.

Control of the heart by the autonomic nervous system

Although the conduction system possesses the inherent ability for spontaneous rhythmic initiation of the cardiac impulse, the autonomic nervous system has an important role in the regulation of the rate, rhythm and force of myocardial contraction of the heart. Both the parasympathetic and sympathetic nerves innervate the heart. Vagal nerve fibres of the parasympathetic branch are found primarily in the SA and AV nodes and atrial muscles, whereas the sympathetic fibres innervate both nodes and the atrial and ventricular muscles.

Vagal stimulation to the heart is mediated by the release of acetylcholine. This acts on muscarinic (M_2) receptors of the SA node to decrease heart rate, on the AV node to decrease conduction velocity, and on the atria to decrease force of contraction. Control by the vagus nerve ensures that the heart rate is slowed to about 75 beats per minute. In the absence of any regulation from the parasympathetic nervous system the heart would contract at about 90–100 beats per minute, which is the normal automatic firing rate of the SA node. The ventricles are relatively unaffected because of a lack of vagal innervation. By contrast, sympathetic stimulation is mediated by the release of noradrenaline, which acts specifically on the β_1 receptors (located in both nodes and atrial and ventricular muscles) to increase heart rate, automaticity, conduction velocity and force of contraction. Circulating adrenaline from the adrenal medulla also elicits cardiac responses. High doses of administered adrenaline may exert a direct effect on the electrophysiological properties of cardiac tissue, causing cardiac arrhythmias. Normally the heart rate is under the continuous influence of both parasympathetic and sympathetic nervous systems; the resting heart rate is the result of their opposing influences.

THE PERIPHERAL VASCULAR SYSTEM

The vascular system comprises the arteries and arterioles, and veins and venules that carry blood away from, and back to, the heart, respectively. Arterioles and capillaries are the main resistance vessels and regulate afterload, while the venules and veins are capacitance vessels contributing to preload of the ventricles.

The arterial wall consists of three layers: the inner, *tunica intima*; the middle, *tunica media*; and the outer, *tunica adventitia*. The middle (thickest) layer is composed of elastic and smooth muscle fibres, and the outer of elastic and collagen fibres. The smooth muscle is arranged in a circular layer, and stimulation by the sympathetic nervous system causes contraction of the smooth muscle, which narrows the lumen of the vessel (vasoconstriction). In contrast, a diminution in sympathetic stimulation results in relaxation of the smooth muscle (vasodilation). The elastic properties of the arteries enable distension when the ventricles eject a volume of blood, and the elastic recoil aids in the forward propulsion of the blood. Arteries branch to form arterioles and capillaries, the main **resistance vessels**, which play a key role in blood pressure regulation. Capillaries are the smallest of the arterial vessels and connect the arterioles to the venules. The combined resistance of the systemic blood vessels, but principally the arterioles, capillaries and venules, is referred to as **systemic vascular resistance** (SVR) or **total peripheral resistance** (TPR).

Venules are the conduits through which blood flows from the capillaries to the veins. Veins consist of the same three layers as arteries but these differ in terms of their relative thickness, with the tunica adventitia forming the thickest layer. Unlike arteries, veins have a system of valves that ensure blood flows in a forward direction towards the heart. About 60% of the blood volume is contained within the systemic veins and venules; hence they are referred to as **capacitance vessels**.

Numerous drugs affect the vascular system and are used in the treatment of hypertension, cardiac failure and angina (Chapter 25), migraine (Chapter 21), atherosclerosis (Chapter 26) and thromboembolic disorders (Chapter 30).

KEY POINTS

- The heart comprises four chambers, two upper atria and two lower ventricles, with the left atrium and ventricle separated from the right by the septum, and the atria from the ventricles by the atrioventricular (tricuspid and mitral) valves.

- The myocardium is composed of cardiac muscle tissue that comprises sarcomeres, the basic contractile units of the heart.

- The heart is supplied with blood and nutrients by the right and left coronary arteries.

- The cardiac conduction system comprises the sinoatrial (SA) and atrioventricular (AV) nodes, internodal pathways, the bundle of His, right and left bundle branches and the Purkinje fibres.

- The cardiac conduction system involves automaticity, conductivity and refractoriness, attributes required for the initiation and transmission of electrical impulses necessary for myocardial contraction.

- The overall process of controlling cardiac muscle contractions involves electrical excitation, mechanical activation and contractile mechanisms.

- The cardiac action potential is divided into two stages, depolarisation and repolarisation, which are further subdivided into five phases (0–4) on the basis of ion movement.

- Electrocardiograms are graphic representations of electrical currents produced by the heart, and consist of a P wave (atrial depolarisation), the QRS complex (ventricular depolarisation) and the T wave (ventricular repolarisation).

- Cardiac output (CO) is a function of stroke volume (SV) and heart rate (HR): CO = SV × HR.

- Factors regulating stroke volume include the degree of stretch of heart fibres before contraction (preload), the force of contraction of the ventricles, and the pressure that must be overcome before the ventricles can eject the blood (afterload).

- The Frank–Starling law of the heart defines the relationship between the force of ejection and the length of cardiac muscle fibres.

- The sympathetic and parasympathetic nervous systems increase the rate and force of contraction and decrease heart rate respectively.

- The walls of arteries and veins consist of the tunica intima, tunica media and tunica adventitia, in differing proportions.

- Constriction and dilation principally of arterioles, capillaries and venules play a key role in determining total peripheral vascular resistance.

REVIEW EXERCISES

1. Discuss myocardial contraction by addressing the electrical excitation, mechanical activation and contractile mechanisms.
2. Describe the cardiac conduction system, including heart structures and electrophysiological properties of the heart.
3. Describe the cardiac effects of the parasympathetic and sympathetic nervous systems.
4. Explain the relationship between cardiac output, stroke volume and heart rate. What are the determinants of stroke volume?
5. Discuss the Frank–Starling relation in a normal heart.

REFERENCES AND FURTHER READING

AIHW: Britt H, Miller GC, Knox S et al. General practice activity in Australia 2002–03. General Practice Series No. 14. AIHW Cat. No. GEP 14. Canberra: AIHW, 2003.

Australian Institute of Health and Welfare. *Australia's Health 2004*. Canberra: AIHW, 2004.

Ministry of Health. *A Portrait of Health: Key Results of the 2002/03 New Zealand Health Survey*. Wellington: Ministry of Health, 2004.

Roden DM. Antiarrhythmic drugs. Ch. 35 in: Hardman JG, Limbird LE, Gilman AG (eds). *Goodman & Gilman's The Pharmacological Basis of Therapeutics*. 10th edn. New York: McGraw-Hill, 2001.

Seeley RR, Stephens TD, Tate P. *Anatomy and Physiology*. 3rd edn. New York: McGraw-Hill, 1995.

Thibodeau GA, Patton KT. *Anatomy and Physiology*. 4th edn. St Louis: Mosby, 1999.

Tortora GJ, Grabowski SR. *Principles of Anatomy and Physiology*. 9th edn. New York: HarperCollins, 2000 [chs 20, 21].

Van Wynsberghe D, Noback CR, Carola R. *Human Anatomy and Physiology*. 3rd edn. New York: McGraw-Hill, 1995.

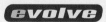 More weblinks at http://evolve.elsevier.com/AU/Bryant/pharmacology/

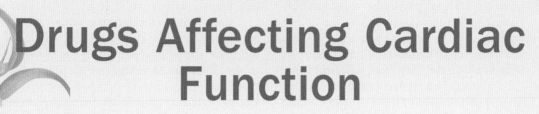

CHAPTER 24

Drugs Affecting Cardiac Function

CHAPTER FOCUS

Numerous drugs affect the heart and vascular system both directly and indirectly. The digitalis glycosides were discovered more than 400 years ago and are still used today for the treatment of heart failure. Over the past decade, other drugs have proved to be more beneficial in treating heart failure, and digoxin is no longer considered the single first-line drug of choice. Digoxin has a narrow therapeutic index and there is a need to be aware of both its tendency to cause arrhythmias and its range of adverse effects. The drugs used to treat arrhythmias are very potent, with as great a potential to cause sudden cardiac death as to save lives. Careful drug selection, along with close monitoring of a person's clinical condition, is crucial to achieving the goal of safe and effective antiarrhythmic therapy.

OBJECTIVES

- To describe the primary actions of digoxin on the heart.

- To describe two potentially serious drug interactions with digoxin.

- To discuss predisposing factors that may increase the risk of digoxin toxicity.

- To review the role of digoxin immune Fab in digoxin poisoning.

- To describe two mechanisms by which cardiac arrhythmias may arise.

- To discuss the mechanism of action of each of the four classes of antiarrhythmic drugs currently available.

- To describe in general terms the main effects of the class I, II, III and IV antiarrhythmic drugs on the electrophysiology of the heart.

- To name one drug from each of the four antiarrhythmic classes.

KEY DRUGS

amiodarone
digoxin
lignocaine
quinidine
sotalol

KEY TERMS

arrhythmia
automaticity
chronotropic
conductivity
dromotropic
heart failure
inotropic
negative inotropic effect
positive inotropic effect
proarrhythmogenic
sinus bradycardia
sinus tachycardia

NUMEROUS drugs affect the heart and vascular system and provide the mainstay for treating diseases such as **heart failure**, arrhythmias, hypertension, ischaemic heart disease and shock and hypotensive states. (The authors acknowledge that the prefix 'a' means 'without', and in that regard the only arrhythmia is asystole [a flat line on the ECG]. The correct term is 'dysrhythmia', the prefix 'dys' meaning 'difficulty with'. However, as the terms **'arrhythmia'** and 'antiarrhythmic drugs' are in common usage, they have been retained.) Many of these drugs exert a direct effect on the heart or vasculature, while others indirectly affect cardiac function as a consequence of actions on vascular tissue.

Drugs acting directly on the heart include:

- the autonomic neurotransmitters adrenaline, noradrenaline and acetylcholine, and the related drugs that were discussed in Chapters 11 and 12 (e.g. muscarinic and adrenergic receptor agonists and antagonists)
- cardiac glycosides
- antiarrhythmic drugs.

Drugs with a **positive inotropic effect** increase the force of myocardial contraction (e.g. digoxin, dobutamine, adrenaline and isoprenaline), whereas drugs with a **negative inotropic effect** decrease the force of myocardial contraction (e.g. propranolol).

Drugs with a **chronotropic** action affect heart rate. A positive chronotropic effect is produced if the drug accelerates the heart rate by increasing the rate of impulse formation in the sinoatrial (SA) node (e.g. adrenaline). A negative chronotropic drug has the opposite effect and slows the heart rate by decreasing impulse formation (e.g. digoxin).

A **dromotropic** effect refers to drugs that affect conduction velocity through specialised conducting tissues. A drug with a positive dromotropic effect increases conduction (e.g. phenytoin), and one with a negative dromotropic effect delays conduction (e.g. verapamil).

Drugs in the digitalis group are among the oldest drugs known to affect both cardiac contractility and rhythm. They increase the force of contraction (positive inotropism) and alter the electrophysiological properties of the heart by

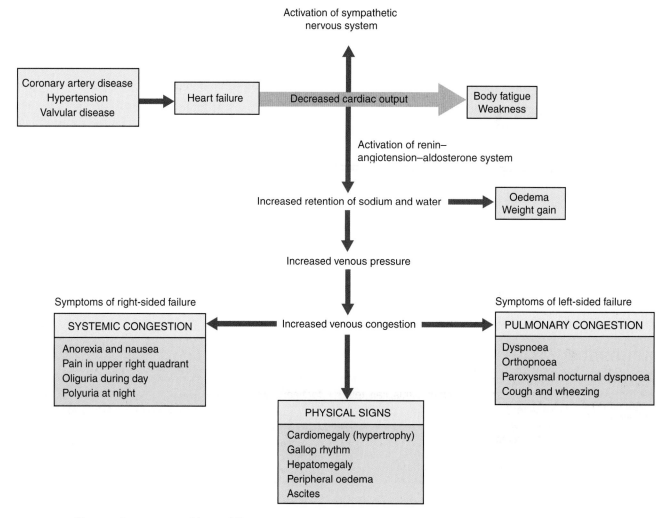

FIGURE 24-1 Signs and symptoms of heart failure.

slowing the heart rate (negative chronotropism) and slowing conduction velocity (negative dromotropism).

CARDIAC GLYCOSIDES

The story of the origin of digitalis demonstrates a herbal remedy (it was called 'housewife's recipe') that was used for hundreds of years by 'common' people (farmers and housewives) for dropsy (fluid accumulation). More than 400 years ago, Dr Leonhard Fuchs recommended that physicians use it "to scatter the dropsy, to relieve swelling of the liver, and even to bring on menstrual flow" (Silverman 1942). Dr Fuchs was a botanist–physician, and at that time the medical profession paid little attention to a 'mere flower picker'.

In the mid-1700s, a female patient shared an old family recipe for curing dropsy with Dr William Withering, which he then used for his dropsy patients. After studying digitalis for 10 years, he published his conclusions in *An Account of the Foxglove*. This remarkable publication stressed instructions that are still valid today—for example, the necessity of individualising dosage according to response. Digitalis was listed in the *London Pharmacopoeia* in 1722.

The term digitalis glycoside refers specifically to cardiac glycosides derived from the *Digitalis* species and includes digoxin and digitoxin. The mechanisms of action of the cardiac glycosides (digoxin, digitoxin and oubain) are fundamentally the same, with minor differences occurring among the pharmacokinetic parameters of the individual agents. Digoxin is the most widely used cardiac glycoside and was previously considered first-line therapy for heart failure. Its use in that setting has declined in the face of more effective drugs, such as the angiotensin-converting enzyme inhibitors (see Clinical Interest Box 24-1).

Digoxin

The main effects produced by digoxin on the heart are:
- increased contractile force (positive inotropism)
- decreased conduction through the AV node (negative dromotropism)
- decreased heart rate (negative chronotropism)
- disturbance of rhythm.

Digoxin also causes adverse effects that include disturbances of the gastrointestinal tract and the central nervous system.

Positive inotropic action

Digoxin inhibits the active transport of Na^+ and K^+ across the myocardial cell membrane by inhibiting the action of the membrane-bound enzyme Na^+–K^+-ATPase. Normally, this enzyme hydrolyses ATP to provide the energy for the Na^+–K^+

CLINICAL INTEREST BOX 24-1   HEART FAILURE

In 2002, 2729 people died of heart failure; 90% of these deaths occurred in people over the age of 75 years (AIHW 2004). In general, heart failure is a disease of the elderly population, with most hospital admissions occurring in people over the age of 65. Risk factors predisposing to heart failure include high blood pressure and coronary heart disease. The cost of treating Australians with heart failure exceeds that of any other medical condition for persons aged 65 years or over (AIHW 2004).

Heart failure is a complex problem and the symptoms (fatigue, shortness of breath and congestion) are related to inadequate cardiac output (and hence inadequate tissue perfusion) during exertion, and to the retention of fluid (Figure 24-1). As a consequence of inadequate performance of the myocardium, compensatory mechanisms are activated, and incomplete emptying of the heart during ventricular systole eventually allows blood to accumulate, causing dilation or enlargement of the heart. In the left atrium, this can lead to pulmonary congestion; in the right atrium, systemic congestion, including ascites, may occur. During the interim, the heart attempts to pump blood out to the systemic circulation, but instead the increased fluid in the left ventricle produces stretching of the myocardial fibres and dilation of the ventricles. The ventricles start to fail and cardiac output is reduced.

Mechanisms to compensate, involving adrenergic (sympathetic) stimulation, occur as the body attempts to maintain an adequate cardiac output. The increased heart rate and peripheral vascular resistance also elevate the heart's demand for oxygen, further contributing to myocardial dysfunction. The decrease in cardiac output leads to decreased tissue perfusion and, following activation of the renin–angiotensin system, the kidneys respond by retaining more sodium and water. The increase in circulatory blood volume increases the demands on the heart.

The short-term goals of therapy are the relief of symptoms and improvement in the quality of life. Long-term management is aimed at retarding disease progression and prolonging survival. Non-pharmacological approaches include modifying risk factors (diet, smoking and alcohol intake), encouraging exercise, often through rehabilitation programs, and providing home support.

Although digoxin was previously the mainstay of therapy for heart failure, the first-line agents are now the angiotensin-converting enzyme (ACE) inhibitors, diuretics and β-blockers. Recent studies have shown that β-blockers may have favourable effects in some cases of heart failure but, because of adverse effects on left ventricular function, these drugs are started in low doses and titrated upwards. Digoxin is now a second-line drug that provides valuable therapy in people with chronic heart failure accompanied by atrial fibrillation (National Heart Foundation 2001).

pump that expels intracellular Na$^+$ and transports K$^+$ into the cardiac cell during repolarisation. Digoxin binds specifically to the Na$^+$–K$^+$-ATPase and inhibits its action (Figure 24-2). Intracellular Na$^+$ accumulates, which inhibits the extrusion of calcium ions, so more calcium is taken up by the sarcoplasmic reticulum. Free calcium ions are essential for linking the electrical excitation of the cell membrane to the mechanical contraction of the myocardial cell, a mechanism known as excitation–contraction coupling.

The increased availability of calcium ions released from the sarcoplasmic reticulum increases the coupling of actin and myosin, which results in more forceful myocardial contraction with a concomitant increase in cardiac output. Inhibition of Na$^+$–K$^+$-ATPase activity is proposed to be the mechanism by which the cardiac glycosides increase myocardial contraction without causing increased oxygen consumption.

Negative chronotropic and negative dromotropic actions

Digoxin has negative chronotropic (decreased heart rate) and dromotropic (slowed conduction velocity) effects because it can alter the electrophysiological properties of cardiac tissues.

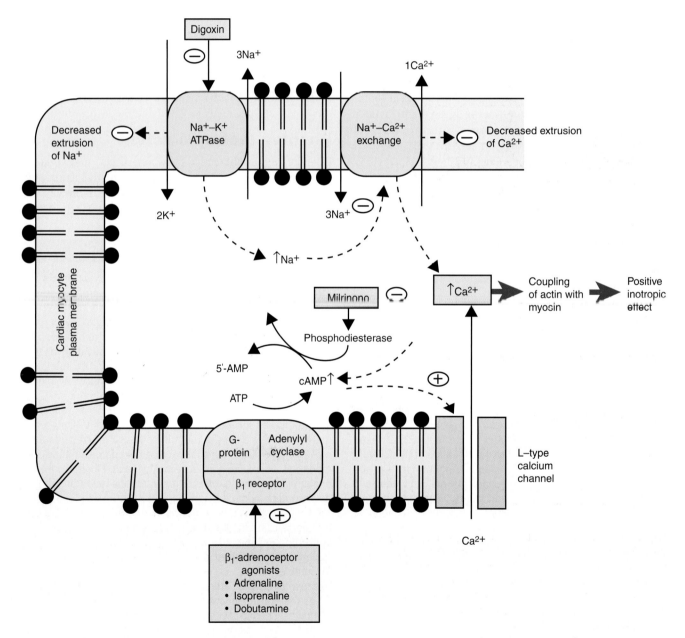

FIGURE 24-2 Schematic representation of cardiac myocyte indicating sites of action of digoxin, milrinone and β-adrenoceptor agonists. – = inhibitory effect; + = positive effect.

AUTOMATICITY

Cardiac tissue has the inherent ability to initiate and propagate an impulse without external stimulation, called **automaticity**. This property affects the rate and rhythm of the heart. At therapeutic plasma concentration, digoxin decreases automaticity and increases the resting membrane potential of atrial tissue and the AV node. These actions occur as a result of augmentation of vagal activity (slowing of heart rate) by a direct effect on the central vagal nuclei, which modifies the excitability of efferent vagal fibres, and by a decrease in the sensitivity of the SA and AV nodes to catecholamines and sympathetic impulses. With increasing plasma concentration of digoxin, severe bradycardia and heart block can occur. On the other hand, toxic concentrations of digoxin can increase sympathetic nervous system activity and directly increase automaticity. This increases the rate of spontaneous depolarisation and is one of the mechanisms responsible for digitalis-induced ectopic pacemakers. Toxic doses of digitalis can significantly increase impulse formation in latent or potential pacemaker tissue, causing arrhythmias.

CONDUCTION VELOCITY

All concentrations of digoxin decrease conduction velocity. The atrioventricular (AV) conduction velocity is slowed both by the direct action of digoxin, which increases the effective refractory period of the AV node, and by increased vagal action. The electrocardiogram (ECG) shows a prolonged P–R interval (Figure 24-3A) and in toxic doses the drug can lead to increased heart block.

REFRACTORY PERIOD

The effect of digoxin on the refractory period varies in different parts of the heart. A prolonged refractory period occurs because of decreased conduction velocity and an increase in the effective refractory period of the AV conduction system, which is very sensitive to digoxin. This action is partly direct and partly caused by increased vagal tone. Toxic doses of digoxin can prolong the refractory period and depress conduction in the AV conduction system until complete heart block occurs.

Indications

Digoxin is used for treating heart failure and cardiac arrhythmias, especially atrial fibrillation, atrial flutter and paroxysmal atrial tachycardia. During atrial fibrillation, several hundred impulses originate from the atria, but only few of them are transmitted through the AV junction. (Figure 24-3B shows the electrocardiographic pattern of atrial fibrillation.) Digoxin slows the ventricular rate because it increases the refractory period of the AV junction and slows conduction at this site, thereby reducing the possibility of inducing ventricular tachycardia.

Pharmacokinetics

The absorption of digoxin varies, depending on the formulation. The drug is 60%–80% absorbed from tablets, and 70%–85% from the elixir. Absorption is delayed after food and about 20% is bound to plasma proteins. The plasma half-life of digoxin is 20–50 hours in people with normal renal function, thus permitting once-daily dosing. Steady-state plasma concentration is reached after about 5 days in people with normal renal function. Digoxin is widely distributed to all body tissues and is excreted predominantly as unchanged drug (about 70%–80%) in the urine. The concentration of digoxin in tissues such as the heart, liver and skeletal muscle tends to be higher than that in plasma.

A.

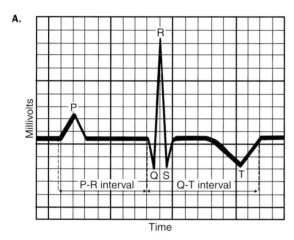

B.

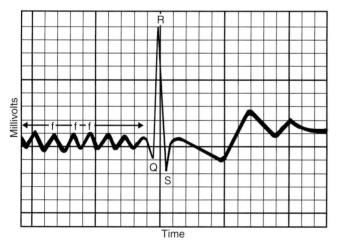

FIGURE 24-3 A. Representation of typical effects of digoxin on the electrical activity of the heart as shown on the electrocardiogram (ECG). Note the prolonged P–R interval, the shortened Q–T interval, and the T wave inversion.
B. Representation of atrial fibrillation as seen on the ECG. No true P waves are noted, but fibrillation waves (indicated on the figure by 'f') consisting of rapid, small, irregular waves are noted. The QRS complex is normal in configuration and duration but occurs irregularly.

DRUG INTERACTIONS 24-1 Digoxin

Drug	Possible effect	Management
Amiodarone	Marked increase in plasma concentration of digoxin, with increased risk of toxicity	Reduce dosage of digoxin and monitor plasma digoxin concentration and clinical status
Antacids (esp. aluminium and magnesium types), antidiarrhoeals (kaolin–pectin type), bile acid-binding resins (cholestyramine, colestipol) and sucralfate	Decreased bioavailability of digoxin	Give these drugs 6–8 hours after digoxin dosage
Calcium channel-blocking drugs (verapamil and diltiazem)	Increased plasma digoxin concentration, enhanced negative effect on atrioventricular conduction and heart rate	Monitor plasma digoxin concentration and anticipate need to reduce dose
Potassium-depleting drugs, such as amphotericin B (parenteral), corticosteroids, or loop or thiazide diuretics	The potential for inducing hypokalaemia with these drugs, if used concurrently with digoxin, increases the possibility of digoxin toxicity	Ensure adequate intake of potassium, monitor potassium levels closely and watch for clinical signs and symptoms of hypokalaemia
Quinidine	Possibly a marked increase in plasma concentration of digoxin	Monitor plasma concentration and clinical response closely; dosage reduction may be necessary
Spironolactone	Increased plasma digoxin concentration	Monitor plasma digoxin concentration and anticipate need to reduce dose
St John's wort	Possibly decreases plasma digoxin concentration and clinical effect	Avoid combination

DRUG INTERACTIONS 24-1 Digoxin

Drug	Possible effect	Management
Suxamethonium	Risk of dangerous arrhythmias (e.g. bradyarrhythmia)	Avoid or potentially serious drug interaction may occur

Sources: AMH 2006; Speight & Holford 1997.

Drug interactions

See Drug Interactions table 24-1 for digoxin.

Adverse reactions

Adverse reactions include anorexia and gastrointestinal disturbances such as nausea, vomiting and diarrhoea. Central nervous system effects such as visual disturbances, confusion, nightmares, agitation and drowsiness are less frequent, as are arrhythmias. The arrhythmias seen with digitalis toxicity are premature ventricular beats, paroxysmal atrial tachycardia with AV block, progressing AV block, and ventricular arrhythmias such as ventricular tachycardia or fibrillation. Loss of appetite, nausea, vomiting and abdominal distress may indicate digoxin toxicity. Hypokalaemia and hypomagnesaemia increase the risk of digoxin toxicity, whereas hypocalcaemia may reduce the effectiveness of digoxin. See Box 24-1 for information on digitalis toxicity.

Warnings and contraindications

Use with caution in people with renal impairment (decreased elimination), hypothyroidism (increased sensitivity), hyperthyroidism (digoxin resistance), electrolyte abnormalities (e.g. hypokalaemia, hypomagnesaemia or hypercalcaemia) or acute myocardial infarction.

Digoxin is contraindicated in people with digoxin hypersensitivity, Wolff–Parkinson–White syndrome, constrictive pericarditis, cor pulmonale, complete heart block, ventricular arrhythmias or obstructive cardiomyopathy.

Dosage and administration

Digoxin has a narrow therapeutic range and people can display toxic effects when the drug is in the normal range. Dosage should be individualised depending on assessment of renal function, clinical response and plasma drug concentration monitoring. See Box 24-2 for information on the therapeutic drug monitoring of digoxin. Elderly people may have age-related, renal or hepatic impairment and a decreased volume of distribution for digoxin; thus lower doses are necessary to avoid toxicity. See the Geriatric Implications box for more information about cardiac glycosides.

BOX 24-1 DIGOXIN TOXICITY

Almost every type of arrhythmia can be produced by digoxin. The type of arrhythmia produced varies with age and other factors. Premature ventricular contractions and bigeminal rhythm (two beats and a pause) are common signs of digoxin toxicity in adults, whereas children tend to develop ectopic nodal or atrial beats. Other digoxin-induced arrhythmias are caused by depression of the SA and AV nodes of the heart. This results in various conduction disturbances (first- or second-degree heart block or complete heart block). Digoxin can also cause increased myocardial automaticity, producing extrasystoles or tachycardia.

Health-care professionals need to be aware of the predisposing factors for digoxin toxicity. The presence of any of these factors indicates the need for close observation for signs and symptoms of toxicity:

Hypokalaemia	Low potassium levels can increase digoxin cardiotoxicity. Because potassium competes with digoxin for binding to the Na^+–K^+-ATPase pump, a depletion of potassium increases cardiac excitability. Low extracellular potassium is synergistic with digoxin and enhances ectopic pacemaker activity. Potassium loss can occur as a result of vomiting, diarrhoea or gastric suctioning. Poor dietary intake or severe dietary restrictions that decrease electrolyte intake can also

alter potassium levels. The use of corticosteroids and various diuretic agents (e.g. frusemide and thiazide preparations) can induce potassium loss.

Corticosteroids cause potassium loss and sodium retention. Surgical procedures associated with severe electrolyte disturbances such as abdominoperineal resection, colostomy, ileostomy and colectomy cause loss of potassium.

Use of potassium-free intravenous fluids can cause hypokalaemia.

Hypercalcaemia	Excess calcium in the presence of digoxin may cause sinus bradycardia, atrioventricular conduction block, and ectopic arrhythmia.
Hypomagnesaemia	Low magnesium concentration increases the risk of digoxin toxicity.
Coexisting conditions	About 70% of digoxin is excreted by the kidneys and, in cases of diminished renal function, the plasma half-life of digoxin increases, necessitating dosage reduction. If the individual should develop digoxin toxicity, management becomes an issue, as the plasma half-life of digoxin may be in the order of 120 hours.

For situations of atrial fibrillation, an initial loading dose (oral/IV) of 250–500 mcg is given, with further dosing every 4–6 hours to a maximum of 1.5 mg. In the elderly or in the presence of chronic renal failure, an initial loading dose of 125–250 mcg is given, with further dosing every 4–6 hours to a maximum of 500 mcg. The usual adult oral maintenance dose is 125–250 mcg once daily, or 62.5–125 mcg in the elderly. The paediatric loading dose is 30–40 mcg/kg in three or four divided doses, and an oral maintenance dose of 5–10 mcg/kg daily in one or two divided doses (see Paediatric Implications box).

Treatment of digoxin poisoning

Digoxin-specific immune antigen-binding fragment (Fab)

The antidote used for life-threatening digoxin poisoning is an ovine digoxin-specific immune antigen-binding fragment (Fab). These fragments, which are derived from antidigoxin antibodies, bind the digoxin molecules, preventing them

from interacting at their site of action. The digoxin–fragment complex accumulates in blood and is excreted by the kidneys. As more tissue digoxin is released into the blood to maintain equilibrium, it is bound by the antigen fragments and removed, which results in lower levels of digoxin in tissues, thereby reversing its effects.

After IV administration the onset of action is rapid and initial signs of improvement in digoxin toxicity may be seen within 15–30 minutes. The half-life of digoxin immune Fab appears to be in the order of 15–20 hours, but data on use in humans are limited. The complex is excreted by the kidneys.

Close monitoring is necessary, as withdrawal of digoxin can result in a decrease in cardiac output, congestive heart failure and hypokalaemia. An increase in ventricular rate may be seen in people with atrial fibrillation. Safety of digoxin immune Fab has not been completely defined because of its limited use. There are no known contraindications to use, but caution should be exercised in people with kidney function impairment; a history of allergies, particularly to sheep proteins; and in those previously treated with digoxin immune Fab.

The adult dose varies according to the amount of digoxin that is required to be complexed. One vial of antibody

BOX 24-2 THERAPEUTIC DRUG MONITORING OF PLASMA DIGOXIN CONCENTRATION

Digoxin has a narrow therapeutic range of 0.5–2 mcg/L. In situations of chronic heart failure, studies suggest that a plasma concentration of 0.5–1 mcg/L should be the target range. Although adverse effects are in general related to plasma digoxin concentration, often the plasma concentration does not clearly delineate patients with toxic levels from those with non-toxic levels. It has been reported that 38% of individuals with actual digoxin toxicity had a digoxin plasma concentration of 2 mcg/L while some with hypokalaemia exhibited toxic signs with plasma levels of 1.5 mcg/L (Kradjan 1995). Plasma digoxin concentration should be used as a guide in conjunction with clinical observations.

Criteria for determining plasma digoxin concentration
- Suspected toxicity
- Individual's compliance questionable or unreliable
- Failure to respond appropriately to therapy
- Presence of impaired renal function
- Use of drugs with documented interactions (e.g. quinidine, calcium channel-blocking drugs)
- Confirmation of unusual or abnormal digoxin concentration

The time that a blood sample is drawn for determination of plasma digoxin concentration is critical. Blood should be taken at least 6–8 hours after the last oral dose or immediately before the next dose (trough concentration).

GERIATRIC IMPLICATIONS DIGOXIN

Digoxin is a commonly prescribed drug, particularly in the elderly, who are often more sensitive to it. Some degree of renal impairment generally exists and hence elderly people require lower doses to reduce the potential for toxicity. As the volume of distribution can also be lower in the elderly, smaller loading doses are used. Early toxic signs often include anorexia, nausea and vomiting; difficulty with reading, which may appear as visual alterations such as green and yellow vision, double vision or seeing spots or haloes; headaches; dizziness; fatigue; weakness; confusion; depression; increased nervousness; and diarrhoea.

PAEDIATRIC IMPLICATIONS DIGOXIN

A fall in plasma potassium concentration enhances the effect of digoxin and increases the risk of toxicity. Individualise dosing with very close monitoring, especially in infants. Monitor plasma potassium levels closely. In contrast to adults, the early signs of toxicity in infants and children are cardiac arrhythmias, including sinus bradycardia, which suggest digoxin intoxication. In children, digoxin can produce any type of arrhythmia, including atrial tachycardia, supraventricular tachycardia and nodal tachycardia. Be extremely careful in calculating digoxin dosages and double-check all calculations with another health-care professional (nurse, pharmacist or physician).

binds about 0.5 mg digoxin. The dose required can be calculated from the number of tablets ingested or from the plasma digoxin concentration. The full product information should be consulted for calculation of the dosage of digoxin antibodies (Box 24-3), and the shelf expiration date of the product checked before use.

PHOSPHODIESTERASE INHIBITORS

Milrinone

Milrinone is a selective inhibitor of phosphodiesterase, the enzyme that metabolises cAMP in cardiac and vascular tissue (Figure 24-2). Inhibition of the breakdown of cAMP results in elevated levels of cAMP within those tissues. This then results in increased calcium influx and uptake by the sarcoplasmic reticulum, causing improvement in myocardial contractility and vasodilation without increasing myocardial oxygen consumption and heart rate. Milrinone is a positive inotrope and vasodilator with very little chronotropic activity.

It is indicated for short-term treatment (about 48 hours) of severe heart failure refractory to other drugs, and for low-cardiac-output states (e.g. following cardiac surgery). It is principally used in coronary and intensive care units, and prolonged use is associated with increased mortality.

Administered intravenously, milrinone has a half-life of 2.5 hours and a duration of action of 3–6 hours. It is excreted by the kidneys, and a reduction in dose is necessary in people with severe renal impairment. Common adverse reactions include ventricular arrhythmias, angina and hypotension.

ANTIARRHYTHMIC DRUGS

Disorders in cardiac electrophysiology

Antiarrhythmic drugs are used for the treatment and prevention of disorders of cardiac rhythm. A cardiac **arrhythmia** is defined as any deviation from the normal rhythm of the

---

BOX 24-3 FORMULAE FOR DIGOXIN IMMUNE FAB (OVINE) (DIGIBIND)

Estimate of total body load of digoxin

Oral ingestion:

   body load (mg) = dose ingested (mg) × 0.8*

Plasma digoxin concentration:

$$\text{body load (mg)} = \frac{\text{digoxin concentration (ng/mL)} \times 5 \text{ L/kg}^{**} \times \text{body weight (kg)}}{1000}$$

Calculation of dose of antibody

$$\text{Dose (number of vials)} = \frac{\text{body load (mg)}}{0.5 \text{ (mg/vial)}}$$

---

*0.8 is used to correct for incomplete absorption.
**Assumed volume of distribution of digoxin.

---

heartbeat. Disorders of cardiac rhythm arise because of abnormality in spontaneous initiation of an impulse, i.e. in automaticity; or abnormality in impulse conduction, i.e. in **conductivity**. In some circumstances a combination of both processes occurs.

Abnormality in automaticity

A disturbance in automaticity can alter the heart's rate, rhythm or site of origin of impulse formation. When the rate of pacemaker activity is affected, a decrease in automaticity of the sinoatrial (SA) node produces **sinus bradycardia** (an abnormal condition in which the myocardium contracts steadily but at less than 60 contractions per minute). An increase in automaticity of the SA node results in **sinus tachycardia** (an abnormal condition in which the myocardium contracts regularly but at more than 100 beats per minute). A shift in the site of origin of impulse formation can generate an abnormal pacemaker or an ectopic focus, resulting in activation of a part of the heart other than the SA node. This is called an ectopic pacemaker, and it may discharge at either a regular or an irregular rhythm. It occurs because the cardiac fibres depolarise more frequently than the SA node.

Abnormal automaticity can develop in cells that usually do not initiate impulses (e.g. atrial or ventricular cells). Clinical disorders such as hypoxia or ischaemia can cause impulse disturbances in automaticity and in conductivity, and both manifestations are responsible for ectopic beats. Ectopic beats are classified as escape beats, premature beats or extrasystoles, and ectopic tachyarrhythmia.

Abnormality in conductivity

Altered conduction of the cardiac impulse probably accounts for more arrhythmias than changes in automaticity. A disturbance in conductivity may be caused by a delay or block of impulse conduction or by the re-entry phenomenon.

DELAY OR BLOCK OF IMPULSE CONDUCTION

In abnormal circumstances, conduction of an atrial impulse to the ventricles can be delayed or blocked in the AV node or structures beyond this region in the conduction pathway. In first-degree AV block, the impulses from the SA node pass through to the ventricles very slowly; this is shown by a prolonged P–R interval on the electrocardiogram (ECG). In second-degree block, some atrial beats fail to pass into the ventricles through the AV node. In third-degree block, or complete heart block, no impulses reach the ventricle, in which case the Purkinje fibres initiate their own spontaneous depolarisation at a very slow rate. This results in independent ventricular and atrial rhythms referred to as ventricular 'escape'.

RE-ENTRY PHENOMENON

The re-entry phenomenon is the mechanism responsible for initiating ectopic beats. For example, when an impulse travels down the Purkinje fibre, it normally spreads along two branches, and when it enters the connecting branch impulses are extinguished at the point of collision in the centre (Figure 24-4A). At the same time, other impulses that begin laterally from the Purkinje fibres activate ventricular muscle tissue. In an abnormal situation, the impulse descending from the central Purkinje fibre travels down one branch normally but encounters a block in the other branch due to ischaemia or injury (Figure 24-4B). This is a unidirectional block, because the impulse can pass in one direction only. In the injured branch, where the impulse is blocked in the forward direction at the site of injury, a retrograde (reverse) impulse from the ventricular tissue re-enters the depressed region from the other direction, provided the pathway proximal to the block is no longer refractory. When the effective refractory period of the blocked area is over, re-entry of the impulse from the ventricular muscle into this site causes the impulse to circulate or recycle repetitively through the loop, resulting in a circus-type movement that produces arrhythmia.

TABLE 24-1 Pharmacokinetics of selected antiarrhythmic drugs

DRUG	ONSET OF ACTION (h)	HALF-LIFE (h)	THERAPEUTIC RANGE* (mg/L)
Class Ia drugs			
Disopyramide	0.5–3	4–10	2–4
Procainamide	0.25–1	2.5–5	4–10
Quinidine	1–4	6	2.5–5
Class Ib drugs			
Lignocaine	IV: 1 min	1.6	–
	IM: 3–15 min		
Mexiletine	2–4	Varies (10–20)	0.5–2
Class Ic drugs			
Flecainide	1–6	Varies (12–27)	0.2–0.9
Class II drugs			
β-blockers (see Chapter 12)			
Class III drugs			
Amiodarone	3–7	14–59 days (metabolite 60–90 days)	1–2.5
Sotalol	2–3	12–14	
Class IV drugs			
Calcium antagonists (see Chapter 25)			

Sources: USP DI 1998; AMH 2006.
*Local or regional laboratories should be consulted.

Drugs that decrease or slow conduction velocity can convert unidirectional block to a two-way or bidirectional block (Figure 24-4C). As the impulses travelling in the antegrade (forward) direction and those moving in a retrograde (reverse) direction are blocked at the injured site, the re-entry pathway is interrupted, abolishing the ectopic beats. In Figure 24-4D, the conditions required for preventing re-entry by another mechanism are also illustrated.

Antiarrhythmic drugs were classified into categories based on their fundamental effects on cardiac electrophysiology by Vaughan Williams in 1970. This grouping is of value in predicting the drug's therapeutic efficacy, although not all drugs belonging to a particular class necessarily possess identical actions. The currently available antiarrhythmic drugs are grouped into four classes (Table 24-1) according to their mechanisms of action (Figure 24-5) but there are a number of drugs that are not classified in the Vaughan Williams system.

Classification of antiarrhythmic drugs

Class I drugs block sodium channels interfering with sodium influx during phase 0 of the action potential. These are further divided into:
- Class Ia drugs: disopyramide, procainamide and quinidine
- Class Ib drugs: lignocaine and mexiletine
- Class Ic drugs: flecainide.

Class II drugs are the β-adrenoceptor antagonists and include atenolol, esmolol and metoprolol.

Class III drugs in general increase the duration of the action potential and the effective refractory period; they include amiodarone and sotalol.

Class IV drugs are the calcium channel blockers verapamil and diltiazem.

Drugs not classified under this scheme include adenosine, atropine (Chapter 11), adrenaline (Chapter 12) and digoxin.

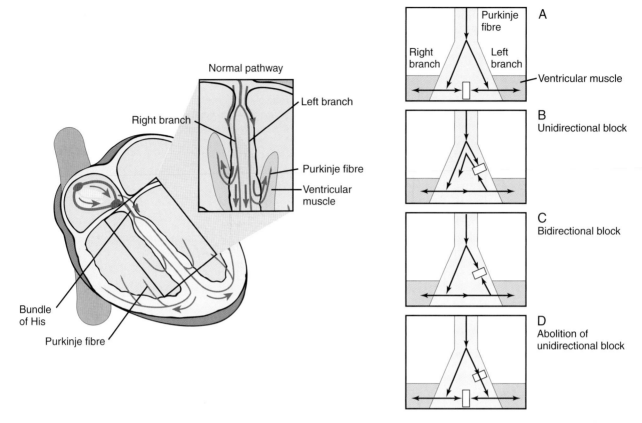

FIGURE 24-4 Re-entry phenomenon. Illustration of a branched Purkinje fibre that activates ventricular muscle.

The rationale for use of antiarrhythmic drugs includes restoration of haemodynamic stability, prevention of life-threatening arrhythmias, prevention of sudden cardiac death, controlling ventricular rate and preventing thromboembolism in atrial fibrillation (AMH 2006). Despite their use for the treatment of arrhythmias, these drugs all possess proarrhythmic potential, and can worsen the arrhythmia and cause sudden death. Use of these drugs requires careful consideration of other treatment options and, following institution of therapy, careful monitoring of the clinical condition of the patient.

Class Ia drugs

The use of class Ia drugs such as quinidine has declined because of evidence of increased mortality with chronic use (Ninio 2000).

Quinidine

Quinidine prevents movement of sodium and potassium across cell membranes. This inhibition of cation exchange results in a decrease in the rate of diastolic depolarisation from resting potential during phase 4 and an increase in the threshold potential (the voltage shifts towards 0 mV). Therefore quinidine decreases impulse conduction and delays repolarisation in the atria, ventricles and Purkinje fibres. By decreasing impulse generation at ectopic sites, quinidine suppresses or abolishes arrhythmias. Abnormal or ectopic pacemaker tissue appears to be more sensitive to quinidine than the SA node, thus permitting the SA node to re-establish control over impulse formation in the heart. Changes observed in the ECG when quinidine is used include widening of the QRS complex, which indicates a decrease in intraventricular conduction, and lengthening of the P–R interval, which represents slower conduction through the AV junction.

The most significant action of quinidine is its ability to prolong the effective refractory period of atrial and ventricular fibres. A delay in completion of repolarisation probably exerts an important antiarrhythmic action. The tissue remains refractory for a period after full restoration of the resting membrane potential. This property is believed to influence the conversion of unidirectional block to bidirectional block, thereby abolishing the re-entry type of arrhythmia (Figure 24-4C).

Quinidine exerts an anticholinergic effect, resulting in inhibition of vagal action on the SA node and AV junction. This effect permits the sinus node to accelerate and can often provoke a dangerous sinus tachycardia. The main non-cardiac action of quinidine is peripheral vasodilation, which results from quinidine's α-adrenergic blocking effect on vascular

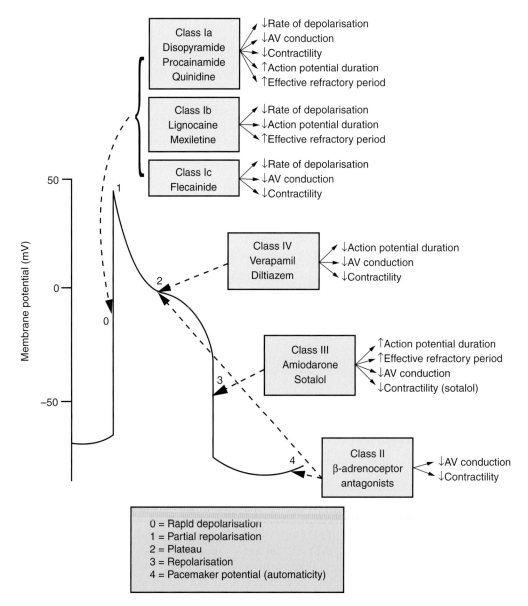

FIGURE 24-5 Phases of the cardiac action potential and the effects produced by the various classes of antiarrhythmic drugs.

smooth muscle. The combined effect of a decrease in peripheral vascular resistance and a reduced cardiac output caused by depressed myocardial contractility contributes to the development of hypotension, a condition that may become a serious problem during quinidine therapy. Quinidine is used for the management of ventricular tachyarrhythmias unresponsive to other treatment.

The pharmacokinetics of quinidine are detailed in Table 24-1. Quinidine is well absorbed and undergoes extensive oxidative metabolism in the liver. Around 20% of unchanged drug is excreted by the kidneys. The usual adult quinidine dose is 0.75 g twice daily, which is adjusted depending on the results of plasma drug concentration monitoring. The therapeutic range for quinidine is 2.5–5.0 mg/L. Slow-

release formulations of quinidine should be taken whole and preferably with food.

Adverse reactions include anorexia, diarrhoea (dose-related), bitter taste, nausea, vomiting, abdominal distress, flushing, rash, tinnitus, confusion and blurred vision. Quinidine should be used with caution in people with asthma, emphysema, hyperthyroidism, hypokalaemia, infection or psoriasis. In people with renal failure, a reduction in dosage may be necessary. Avoid use in people with quinidine hypersensitivity, incomplete or complete AV block, digoxin toxicity with AV conduction alterations, severe conduction defects, myasthenia gravis or thrombocytopenia. Quinidine is a potent inhibitor of CYP2D6 and is subject to many drug interactions. See Drug Interactions table 24-2 for quinidine.

DRUG INTERACTIONS 24-2 Quinidine

Drug	Possible effect and management
Amiodarone	Quinidine clearance is reduced. Reduce dose by 30%–40% when adding amiodarone
Antiarrhythmic drugs	Additive effects are observed. Monitor ECG closely
β-blockers	Potentiation of β-blocker effect due to inhibition of metabolism (metroprolol and propranolol). Monitor closely
Digoxin	Increased risk of toxicity due to decreased clearance of digoxin. Decrease digoxin dose and monitor plasma drug concentrations
Diuretics	Hypokalaemia can increase risk of arrhythmias. Correct hypokalaemia
Urinary alkalisers and antacids	Can result in increased reabsorption of quinidine and elevated plasma concentration. Monitor plasma quinidine concentration if toxicity is suspected
Verapamil	Quinidine clearance reduced. Due to increased risk of toxicity, use combination when no other alternative is an option
Warfarin	Inhibition of warfarin metabolism can potentiate anticoagulant effect. Monitor INR when adding or stopping quinidine and for signs of additional anticoagulant effects, such as excessive bruising, bleeding gums, black stools, haematuria and haematemesis

DRUG INTERACTIONS 24-3 Disopyramide

Drug	Possible effect and management
Azole antifungals	Increase disopyramide plasma concentration. Avoid combined use
Erythromycin	Increases disopyramide plasma concentration. Avoid combined use
Other anti-arrhythmic agents, such as diltiazem, flecainide, lignocaine, procainamide, quinidine, verapamil and β-adrenergic blocking agents	Monitor closely for evidence of negative chronotropic (bradyarrhythmia) and inotropic effects (heart failure). β-adrenergic blocking agents may exacerbate heart failure, especially in individuals with compromised ventricular function. Avoid combined use or potentially serious drug interactions may occur
Phenytoin	Induction of hepatic enzymes reduces disopyramide plasma concentration. Monitor plasma concentration and increase dose if required
Tricyclic and tetracyclic antidepressants	Avoid combined use as prolongation of the Q–T interval increases the risk of proarrhythmic effect

Disopyramide

The effects of disopyramide are similar to those of quinidine with the exception that disopyramide does not possess α-adrenergic receptor antagonist properties and its anticholinergic effects are more prominent. The latter is the reason why a drug that slows AV conduction may be administered with disopyramide when it is used in the treatment of atrial flutter or atrial fibrillation (see Box 24-4 for definitions). Disopyramide is indicated for treatment of ventricular arrhythmias, and re-entrant arrhythmias are abolished by converting a unidirectional block into a bidirectional block (Figure 24-4C).

Disopyramide is well absorbed and has a weakly active metabolite with both antiarrhythmic and anticholinergic effects. The therapeutic plasma concentration range for disopyramide is 3–8 mg/L (see Table 24-1).

See the Drug Interactions table 24-3 for disopyramide.

Common adverse reactions include blurred vision, constipation and dry mouth. In addition, disopyramide can cause urinary retention, hypersensitivity reactions, severe disturbances of cardiac rhythm and exacerbation of heart failure. Disopyramide should be used with caution in people with diabetes mellitus, glaucoma (closed-angle), hypokalaemia, myasthenia gravis, enlarged prostate or renal impairment. Avoid use in people with disopyramide hypersensitivity, AV block, cardiogenic shock, cardiac conduction abnormality, cardiomyopathy or heart failure.

Dosage and administration are individualised according to response and tolerance, to a maximum of 800 mg per day. The usual adult oral loading dose is 200–300 mg, with a maintenance dose of 100–150 mg every 6 hours (400–600 mg daily). A dose of 100 mg is administered every 8 hours in people with mild renal impairment, every 12 hours in people with moderate impairment, and once daily in people with severe renal impairment.

Procainamide

Procainamide is an analogue of the local anaesthetic procaine, and its electrophysiological effects are similar to those of quinidine except that it lacks α-adrenergic receptor antagonism and exerts weak anticholinergic effects via a reduction in acetylcholine release. The result is that the direct depressant effect of procainamide on the SA and AV nodes

DRUG INTERACTIONS 24-4 Procainamide	
Drug	**Possible effect and management**
Amiodarone, cimetidine and trimethoprim	Coadministration increases plasma concentration of procainamide, increasing the risk of toxicity. Monitor plasma drug concentration of procainamide or avoid combination
Anticholinesterases (e.g. neostigmine)	Reduction of acetylcholine release by procainamide may cause increased muscle weakness in persons with myasthenia gravis. Increased dose of anticholinesterase drug may be required
Antihypertensive drugs	Increased hypotension has been reported, especially when parenteral (intravenous) procainamide is given. Monitor closely, as dosage adjustments may be necessary
Neuromuscular blocking agents	Concurrent use may result in enhanced neuromuscular blockade. Use reduced dose of neuromuscular blocking drug
Other antiarrhythmic drugs	Monitor for enhanced or additive proarrhythmic effects. Avoid combined use

may not be as effectively balanced by vagal blockade as it is with quinidine. In people with a pre-existing ventricular dysfunction, procainamide can also cause severe congestive heart failure. The primary indications for procainamide are to treat atrial and ventricular arrhythmias, such as premature ventricular contractions, ventricular tachycardia, atrial fibrillation and paroxysmal atrial tachycardia.

Procainamide is rapidly eliminated by hepatic metabolism and by renal excretion (50%–60% unchanged drug). It has a half-life of 2.5–4.5 hours and its active metabolite N-acetylprocainamide has a half-life of 6 hours. See Table 24-1. See the Drug Interactions table 24-4 for procainamide.

Adverse reactions are similar to those of quinidine except for tinnitus and visual changes, which are specific to quinidine. In addition, a systemic lupus erythematosus-type reaction can occur (i.e. fever, chills, painful joints, and rash). Procainamide can cause an exacerbation of heart failure, severe rhythm disturbances, a worsening of muscle weakness in people with myasthenia gravis, and an exacerbation of lupus erythematosus. Avoid use in people with procainamide hypersensitivity, heart block (second- and third-degree) or signs of digoxin toxicity.

Class Ib drugs

The class Ib drugs lignocaine and mexiletine differ from class Ia drugs because in general they do not affect conduction velocity. Lignocaine and mexiletine are structurally very similar and are particularly useful for acute ventricular arrhythmias. A high incidence of adverse effects has limited the usefulness of mexiletine. Like the class Ia drugs, these drugs are can worsen arrhythmias.

Lignocaine

Lignocaine, an agent used extensively as a local and topical anaesthetic agent, is also an antiarrhythmic agent, especially for ventricular arrhythmias seen after cardiac surgery or an acute myocardial infarction. Lignocaine appears to act primarily on the sodium channel, blocking both the activated and inactivated sodium channels, although its greater effect is in depolarised or ischaemic tissues. These effects are indicative of the efficacy of lignocaine for suppressing arrhythmias associated with depolarisation (such as ischaemia and digoxin-induced toxicity) and its lack of effectiveness in arrhythmias that occur in normal polarised tissues (atrial fibrillation and atrial flutter). Lignocaine has few electrophysiological effects in normal cardiac tissue.

Lignocaine does not inhibit vagal activity, nor does it influence cardiac output and arterial pressure. In addition, it does not depress myocardial contractility, thereby reducing the potential for development of heart failure. Because it exerts a limited effect, if any, on the SA node and atrial myocardium, the drug has no use in the treatment of supraventricular tachycardia. The major use of lignocaine is in the treatment of severe ventricular arrhythmias.

Lignocaine is administered only intravenously and is metabolised by the liver to active metabolites, which, after a 24-hour infusion, also contribute to the therapeutic and toxic effects (see Table 24-1). Concurrent drug administration with β-blockers or cimetidine can inhibit metabolism of lignocaine and increase the risk of toxicity. Additive toxicity may also occur with other antiarrhythmic drugs.

Adverse reactions include dizziness, anorexia, nausea, vomiting, tinnitus, tremor and visual disturbances. Of a more serious nature are bradycardia, convulsions, respiratory depression and cardiac arrest. Use lignocaine with caution in people with liver or kidney function impairment, as lignocaine and its active metabolites can accumulate. Avoid use in people with lignocaine hypersensitivity, complete heart block, sinus bradycardia or Stokes–Adams syndrome (see Box 24-4 for definitions).

The lignocaine adult dose of 1 mg/kg is given IV over 1–2 minutes and is repeated after 5 minutes if necessary. Children receive the same 1 mg/kg dose initially, but repeat dosages in 5 minutes should not exceed a total dose of 3 mg/kg. By IV infusion, the maintenance dose is usually 10–50 mcg/kg/min.

Mexiletine

Mexiletine is structurally similar to lignocaine, but because it has been modified to reduce hepatic first-pass metabolism, it may be administered orally (see Table 24-1 for pharmacokinetics). Ventricular arrhythmias that respond to parenteral lignocaine are usually responsive to mexiletine.

Drug interactions occur with mexiletine and other antiarrhythmic drugs, resulting in additive depressant effects on conduction of the AV node and myocardium. Mexiletine inhibits the metabolism of theophylline and increases the risk of theophylline toxicity.

Adverse reactions are similar to those for lignocaine. In addition, paraesthesia of fingers and toes, rash, tremors and indigestion can occur. Rarely, pulmonary fibrosis, Stevens–Johnson syndrome (erythema multiforme presenting with macules, papules and vesicles on the mucous membranes of the lips, mouth, genitalia and conjunctiva), hepatotoxicity and cardiac arrest have been reported. Use mexiletine with caution in people with severe heart failure, an acute myocardial infarction, convulsive disorders, hypotension, sinus node or intraventricular conduction dysfunction, or liver function impairment. Avoid use of mexiletine in people with drug hypersensitivity, AV block or cardiac shock.

The mexiletine adult oral loading dose is usually 400 mg, with an oral maintenance dose of 100–250 mg three times daily.

Class Ic drugs

The class Ic drug available in Australia is flecainide, which is used to treat atrial fibrillation and flutter, and serious ventricular arrhythmias. The potential for proarrhythmic effect is of special concern, especially in people with poor left ventricular function or sustained ventricular arrhythmias. The class Ic drugs can also aggravate congestive heart failure.

Flecainide

Flecainide is a sodium channel-blocking agent used to treat ventricular arrhythmias; it has minimal effects on repolarisation and no anticholinergic properties. It suppresses premature ventricular contractions, and in high doses can exacerbate arrhythmias in people with a pre-existing ventricular tachyarrhythmia or in people with a previous myocardial infarction.

Flecainide is well absorbed after oral administration. It is metabolised by the polymorphic hepatic CYP2D6 and can accumulate to toxic levels in people deficient in this enzyme. The therapeutic range for flecainide is 0.2–0.9 mg/L (see Table 24-1). The administration of flecainide with other antiarrhythmic drugs (digoxin, β-blockers, verapamil) can result in enhanced adverse cardiac effects. In people with diuretic-induced hypokalaemia, there is an increased risk of arrhythmias.

BOX 24-4 CARDIAC TERMS AND DEFINITIONS	
Atrial flutter	Atrial tachycardia with heart rates between 230 and 380 beats/min. Two types have been identified.
Atrial fibrillation	An arrhythmia caused by disorganised electrical activity in the atria, resulting in a fast, irregular ventricular response.
Cardiomyopathy	Illness/disease that affects heart structure and function.
Cardiogenic shock	A low cardiac output that occurs with myocardial infarctions and congestive heart failure. If not corrected it can be fatal.
Heart block	Interference with the conduction of electrical impulses in heart muscle. This is often further defined, e.g. as a first-degree AV block (atrial impulses reach the ventricles but are delayed) or the delay that occurs in a specific area, such as bundle branch block or intraventricular block.
Sick sinus syndrome	Sinus node dysfunction that is characterised by severe sinus bradycardia and symptoms of weakness, dizziness, lethargy and syncope. Treatment usually requires a pacemaker.
Stokes–Adams syndrome	Incomplete heart block that causes episodes of loss of consciousness.
Supraventricular tachycardia	A heart rate exceeding 100 beats/min that originates above the ventricles, such as in the atria, SA node or AV junction.
Torsade de pointes	A ventricular tachycardia with a prolonged repolarisation. It can be drug-induced (usually by the antiarrhythmic agents, tricyclic antidepressants, and other drugs). Contributing factors include hypokalaemia, hypomagnesaemia and bradycardia.
Wolff–Parkinson–White syndrome	A disorder in AV conduction that is often seen as two AV conduction pathways.

Adverse reactions include blurred vision, dizziness, headaches, constipation, nausea, weakness, chest pain, irregular heartbeats and arrhythmias. Use flecainide with caution in people with heart failure, hypokalaemia or hyperkalaemia, and renal impairment. Flecainide is contraindicated post-myocardial infarction, in people with heart block, or in situations of cardiogenic shock.

The flecainide adult oral dose is 50–100 mg every 12 hours, increasing by 50 mg every four days to a maximum of 400 mg daily.

Class II drugs

The class II drugs include atenolol, esmolol and metoprolol. All three drugs are β-adrenoceptor antagonists that are used to control cardiac arrhythmias caused by excessive sympathetic nerve activity. These drugs are the only class of antiarrhythmics to show a reduction in mortality post-myocardial infarction.

Drugs such as atenolol are used to treat atrial tachy-arrhythmias and ventricular arrhythmias, whereas esmolol is indicated for short-term treatment of supraventricular tachy-cardia induced by atrial fibrillation or atrial flutter (these drugs are discussed extensively in Chapter 12).

Class III drugs

The electrophysiological properties of drugs in this group differ markedly from those of the other classes. Drugs in this group prolong the effective refractory period by prolonging the action potential duration.

Amiodarone

Amiodarone increases the refractory period in all cardiac tissues through a direct effect on the tissues. It decreases automaticity, prolongs AV conduction and decreases the automaticity of fibres in the Purkinje system. It can block potassium, sodium (class I effect) and calcium channels (class IV effect) and β receptors (class II effect). It has the potential to cause a variety of complex effects on the heart and has serious adverse effects. Amiodarone is reserved for the prevention and treatment of serious atrial and ventricular arrhythmias in people not responding to or tolerating other drug therapies.

Amiodarone is a structural analogue of thyroid hormone and is highly lipophilic. It is poorly absorbed and has a bioavailability of about 30%. It is widely distributed in the body (e.g. in adipose tissues, liver and lung), and reaches steady-state plasma concentration after several weeks. Its onset of action varies from several days to weeks, even if loading doses are administered. It has a biphasic elimination half-life: the initial half-life is 2.5–10 days, and the terminal half-life is 26–107 days. It has one active metabolite (desethylamiodarone), which has a terminal half-life of about 60 days (see Table 24-1).

See the Drug Interactions table 24-5 for amiodarone.

Adverse reactions include dizziness, bitter taste, headache, flushing, nausea, vomiting, constipation, ataxia, weight loss, tremors, paraesthesias of fingers and toes, photosensitivity, blue–grey skin discoloration, pulmonary fibrosis or pneumonitis, cough, fever, allergic reaction and blurred vision.

DRUG INTERACTIONS 24-5 Amiodarone

Drug	Possible effect and management
Digoxin	Can increase the plasma concentration of digoxin, causing toxicity. Monitor plasma digoxin concentration and reduce dose of digoxin as necessary. Can also see additive effects of both drugs on the SA node and AV junction
Other antiarrhythmic agents	Can increase cardiac effects and the risk of inducing tachyarrhythmias. It also raises plasma levels of quinidine, procainamide and flecainide. If amiodarone must be given with class I antiarrhythmic agents, reduce the dose of the class I drug by 30%–50% several days after starting amiodarone
Phenytoin	Can result in increased plasma concentration of phenytoin, possibly resulting in toxicity. Monitor plasma concentration of phenytoin and decrease dosage if necessary
Warfarin	Can increase anticoagulant effect by inhibiting metabolism of warfarin. Decrease warfarin dose as necessary and monitor INR

Use amiodarone with caution in people with heart failure, liver or thyroid function impairment. Avoid use in people with amiodarone hypersensitivity, second- or third-degree AV block and bradycardia.

The usual adult dose for chronic atrial or ventricular tachyarrhythmias is 200–400 mg 8 hourly for 1 week, then 200–400 mg twice daily for one week. The maintenance dose is 100–400 mg (or less if indicated) once daily. For children, the oral maintenance dose is 4 mg/kg once daily.

Sotalol

Sotalol is a β-adrenoceptor antagonist that also blocks cardiac K^+ channels, prolonging the action potential duration and increasing the effective refractory period in atrial and ventricular tissue and AV node. It is indicated for treatment and prevention of atrial and serious ventricular arrhythmias. Sotalol is predominantly cleared renally (around 90%) and therefore accumulates in people with renal impairment (Table 24-1). Additive depressant effects occur with other antiarrhythmic drugs, including verapamil and diltiazem, producing bradyarrhythmia, atrioventricular block and an increased risk of heart failure. Increased risk of arrhythmias also occurs in the presence of diuretic-induced hypokalaemia.

Common adverse effects include hypotension, dyspnoea, fatigue, dizziness, impotence, nausea, vomiting and diarrhoea.

Similar to the other classes of antiarrhythmic drugs, sotalol is **proarrhythmogenic**, potentially producing new or worsening arrhythmias. Care should be exercised in people with heart failure, airways disease, diabetes or peripheral vascular disease. Sotalol is contraindicated in the presence of heart block, sinus bradycardia, severe heart failure and hypotensive states. See Chapter 12 for further information.

Sotalol is available as both an IV and an oral formulation. The adult oral dose range is 40–160 mg twice daily.

Class IV drugs

Drugs in this class include verapamil and diltiazem, which are reviewed in Chapter 25.

Unclassified antiarrhythmic agents

This group includes digoxin (discussed previously) and adenosine.

Adenosine

Adenosine is produced endogenously. Via an action on A_1 receptors on the AV node, it slows AV node conduction. It is indicated for the acute treatment of supraventricular tachycardia. Administered by intravenous bolus, it has an immediate onset and its action is terminated rapidly (20–30 s) by uptake into red blood cells and vascular endothelial cells. It is metabolised to inosine (which is processed to uric acid) and adenosine monophosphate (AMP). Caffeine and theophylline can antagonise the effect of adenosine, whereas dipyridamole increases the effects of adenosine because it inhibits metabolism of adenosine and blocks adenosine reuptake.

Adverse reactions include dyspnoea, flushing, cough, dizziness, tingling in arms, nausea, headache, and transient arrhythmias such as premature ventricular contractions, sinus bradycardia, sinus tachycardia, skipped beats and chest pain/pressure. These all resolve rapidly because of the short duration of action of adenosine. Use adenosine with caution in people with asthma as it may cause bronchospasm. Avoid use in people with adenosine hypersensitivity, AV block or sick sinus syndrome.

The usual dose is 3 mg administered rapidly in an IV bolus over 1–2 s, followed by 6 mg as a second dose if the arrhythmia has not resolved. If the arrhythmia is still present 1–2 min after the second injection, a third dose of 12 mg may be administered.

ADEC Category	Drug
A	Digoxin, lignocaine
B1	Mexiletine
B2	Adenosine, digoxin immune Fab (ovine), disopyramide, procainamide
B3	Flecainide
C	Amiodarone, quinidine, sotalol

PREGNANCY SAFETY

DRUGS AT A GLANCE 24: Drugs affecting Cardiac Function

Therapeutic group	Pharmacological group	Key examples	Key Pages
Drugs affecting cardiac function	Cardiac glycoside	digoxin	423–8
	Phosphodiesterase inhibitor	milrinone	428
	Antiarrhythmic drugs	amiodarone	436
		flecainide	435
		lignocaine	434
		mexiletine	435
		quinidine	431–3

KEY POINTS

- Numerous drugs that affect the heart and vascular system provide the mainstay for the treatment of diseases such as heart failure, arrhythmias, hypertension and ischaemic heart disease.
- Many drugs exert a direct effect on the heart or vasculature; others indirectly affect cardiac function as a consequence of actions on vascular tissue.
- Drugs acting directly on the heart include catecholamines (Chapter 12), cardiac glycosides (typified by digoxin) and antiarrhythmic drugs.
- Drugs may exert inotropic, chronotropic or dromotropic actions.
- Digoxin decreases heart rate and slows conduction. It is used in the treatment of cardiac arrhythmias, especially atrial flutter and fibrillation, and heart failure.
- Digoxin has a narrow therapeutic index, can exacerbate or worsen arrhythmias, and is subject to many serious drug interactions.
- Several factors such as hypokalaemia, hypercalcaemia and hypomagnesaemia, may predispose to digoxin toxicity.
- Ovine digoxin-specific immune antigen binding fragments (Fab) are used to treat digoxin poisoning.
- The antiarrhythmic drugs are used to treat and prevent cardiac rhythm disorders.
- Cardiac rhythm disorders are usually the result of an abnormality in the electrophysiology of the cells in the cardiac conduction system or cardiac muscle cells.
- The antiarrhythmic drugs are subdivided into four classes (I–IV) according to their mechanism of action.
- Class Ia, Ib and Ic drugs suppress automaticity. Class Ia includes disopyramide, procainamide and quinidine, which decrease conduction velocity and prolong the action potential.
- Class Ib drugs (lignocaine and mexiletine) may increase or have no effect on conduction velocity.
- The class Ic drug flecainide is indicated for the treatment or prevention of supraventricular tachyarrhythmias.
- Class II drugs have β-adrenergic-blocking action and are discussed in Chapter 12.
- The class III drugs are amiodarone and sotalol.
- The class IV drugs have calcium channel-blocking activity and are discussed in Chapter 25.
- All antiarrhythmic drugs are potent medications that require careful patient selection and close monitoring to avoid drug-induced adverse effects or toxicity.

REVIEW EXERCISES

1   Explain why digoxin itself can produce cardiac arrhythmias.
2   Describe the use of digoxin immune Fab (ovine) in digoxin toxicity. How is the dose calculated?
3   Why is the plasma concentration of digoxin routinely monitored?
4   Describe the pharmacological effects of quinidine.
5   Why are quinidine and disopyramide contraindicated for use in people with myasthenia gravis?
6   What are the differences in the electrophysiological effects of procainamide and quinidine?
7   Discuss the primary therapeutic effects and adverse effects of amiodarone. Why is it contraindicated for use in people with AV block?

REFERENCES AND FURTHER READING

Australian Institute of Health and Welfare. *Australia's Health 2004*. Canberra: AIHW, 2004.
Australian Institute of Health and Welfare (AIHW). *Heart, Stroke and Vascular Diseases—Australian Facts 2001*. AIHW cat. no. CVD 13. Cardiovascular Disease Series No. 14. Canberra: AIHW, National Heart Foundation of Australia, National Stroke Foundation of Australia, 2001.
Australian Medicines Handbook 2006. Adelaide: AMH, 2006.
Cardiovascular Expert Group. *Therapeutic Guidelines: Cardiovascular, version 4*. Melbourne: Therapeutic Guidelines Limited, 2003.
Kradjan WA. Congestive heart failure. In: Young LY, Koda-Kimble MA (eds). *Applied Therapeutics: the clinical use of drugs*. 6th edn. Vancouver: Applied therapeutics Inc, 1995.

Krum H. Recent advances in the management of chronic heart failure. *Australian and New Zealand Journal of Medicine* 2000; 30: 475–82.

National Heart Foundation of Australia and Cardiac Society of Australia and New Zealand Chronic Heart Failure Clinical Practice Guidelines Writing Panel. Guidelines for management of patients with chronic heart failure in Australia. *Medical Journal of Australia* 2001; 174: 459–66.

Ninio DM. Contemporary management of atrial fibrillation. *Australian Prescriber* 2000; 23: 100–2.

Ooi H, Colucci W. Pharmacological treatment of heart failure. In: Hardman JG, Limbird LE, Goodman AG (eds). *Goodman & Gilman's The Pharmacological Basis of Therapeutics.* 10th edn. New York: McGraw-Hill, 2001 [ch. 34].

Quinn DI, Day RO. Guide to clinically more important drug interactions. In: Speight TM, Holford NHG (eds). *Avery's Drug Treatment.* 4th edn. Auckland: Adis International, 1997 [Appendix B].

Rang HP, Dale MM, Ritter JM, Moore PK. *Pharmacology.* 5th edn. Edinburgh: Churchill Livingstone, 2003 [ch. 17].

Roden DM. Antiarrhythmic drugs. In: Hardman JG, Limbird LE, Goodman AG (eds). *Goodman & Gilman's The Pharmacological Basis of Therapeutics.* 10th edn. New York: McGraw-Hill, 2001 [ch. 35].

Silverman M. *Magic in a Bottle.* New York: Macmillan, 1942.

Speight T, Holford N (eds). *Avery's Drug Treament.* 4th edn. Auckland: Adis Inernational, 1997.

United States Pharmacopeial Convention. *USP DI: Drug Information for the Health Care Professional.* 18th edn. Rockville: United States Pharmacopeial Convention, 1998.

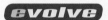 More weblinks at http://evolve.elsevier.com/AU/Bryant/pharmacology/

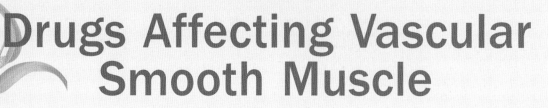

CHAPTER 25

Drugs Affecting Vascular Smooth Muscle

CHAPTER FOCUS

The focus of this chapter is the vasodilator drugs that produce vasodilation by relaxing smooth muscle in the blood vessel walls by either direct or indirect action. Some drugs act primarily on veins or arterioles, while others dilate both types of blood vessels. The principal uses of these drugs, which include the organic nitrates, calcium channel blockers, potassium channel activators, angiotensin-converting enzyme inhibitors and angiotensin-II-receptor antagonists, are in the treatment of angina, hypertension and heart failure. These drugs are frequently prescribed, either alone or in combination therapy, so it is important that health-care professionals are knowledgeable about all of these drug classes.

OBJECTIVES

- To discuss the mechanism of action of nitrates.

- To describe the therapeutic effects of glyceryl trinitrate in the treatment of angina pectoris.

- To compare the effects of nitrates, β-blockers and calcium channel-blocking agents on ventricular volume, heart rate, coronary blood flow and collateral blood flow.

- To describe the effects of calcium channel blockers on cardiac muscle, the cardiac conduction system and vascular smooth muscle.

- To compare and contrast the effects and primary indications of the different calcium channel-blocking drugs.

- To describe three potentially serious drug interactions reported with the calcium channel blockers.

- To explain the mechanism of action of the angiotensin-converting enzyme inhibitors and the angiotensin-II-receptor antagonists.

- To explain why diuretics, β-blockers, vasodilators, ACE inhibitors, angiotensin-II-receptor antagonists and calcium channel blockers are effective antihypertensive drugs.

KEY DRUGS

captopril
clonidine
diltiazem
glyceryl trinitrate
losartan
nicorandil
nifedipine
oxpentifylline
verapamil

KEY TERMS

angina pectoris
angiotensin II
angiotensin-II-receptor antagonists
angiotensin-converting enzyme
calcium channel blockers
centrally acting adrenergic inhibitors

hypertension
nitrates
peripheral vascular disease
potassium channel activators
renin–angiotensin–aldosterone system
vasodilator

THE vascular system comprises the arteries and arterioles, and venules and veins that carry blood away from, and back to, the heart, respectively. Arterioles and capillaries are the main resistance vessels and regulate afterload, while the venules and veins are capacitance vessels, contributing to preload of the ventricles. Contraction of vascular smooth muscle is effected by an increase in intracellular calcium concentration. Modulation of calcium concentration forms the basis for the actions of a range of drugs that affect the vascular system. Drugs causing vasoconstriction by acting on α-adrenoceptors (e.g. α-adrenoceptor agonists such as adrenaline) and vasodilation (α_1-adrenoceptor antagonists such as prazosin) are discussed in Chapter 12.

This chapter describes the drugs that directly and indirectly affect vascular smooth muscle contraction. Emphasis is on **vasodilator drugs** used for the treatment of a variety of disorders, including hypertension, angina, shock, cardiac failure and peripheral vascular conditions. These drugs produce vasodilation by relaxing smooth muscle in the blood vessel walls. The main groups of drugs to be discussed are:

* direct-acting vasodilators
  — nitrates
  — calcium channel blockers
  — potassium channel activators
* indirect-acting vasodilators
  — centrally acting adrenergic inhibitors
  — angiotensin-converting enzyme (ACE) inhibitors
  — angiotensin-II-receptor antagonists.

ANGINA

The term **angina pectoris** refers to temporary interference with blood flow that reduces oxygen and nutrient supply to heart muscle, resulting in intermittent myocardial ischaemia, typically characterised by pain (see Box 25-1 for types of angina pectoris). Angina may occur at rest or can be precipitated by exertion or excitement. When coronary blood flow is inadequate, hypoxia causes an accumulation of pain-producing substances such as lactic acid (anaerobic metabolite) and other chemical factors such as potassium ions, kinins and adenosine. Stimulation of cardiac sensory nerve endings, which transmit impulses to the central nervous system, results in the typical anginal pain response. Coronary atherosclerosis or vasomotor spasm of the coronary vessels may cause inadequate oxygenation. Other causes of anginal pain may be pulmonary hypertension and valvular heart disease. Individuals with severe anaemia, even with minimal coronary artery disease, may suffer from anginal attacks because of inadequate oxygen supply.

Drug therapy of angina is aimed at either relaxing coronary artery smooth muscle, thus improving perfusion, or reducing the metabolic demand of the heart, or both. An ideal antianginal drug would:

* establish a balance between coronary blood flow and the metabolic demands of the heart
* have a local rather than a systemic effect, acting directly on coronary vessels to promote coronary vasodilation with little or no effect on other organ systems
* promote oxygen extraction by the heart
* be effective when taken orally and have a sustained action
* be devoid of tolerance.

Currently no one drug meets all these criteria and the drugs now available provide only temporary relief.

VASODILATOR DRUGS —DIRECT-ACTING

Organic nitrates

The **nitrates** glyceryl trinitrate (also called nitroglycerine), isosorbide dinitrate and isosorbide mononitrate are very effective drugs for the treatment of angina pectoris because of their dilating effects on veins and arteries (Drug Monograph 25-1; Figure 25-1). The resulting pooling of blood in the veins (capacitance blood vessels) decreases the amount of blood returned to the heart (preload), which reduces left ventricular end-diastolic volume. This decrease in blood return helps reduce the myocardial oxygen demand (chest pain caused by angina pectoris largely results from an inadequate supply of oxygen to the heart).

BOX 25-1 TYPES OF ANGINA PECTORIS

Stable angina
Stable angina is usually associated with coronary arteriosclerosis and the pain predictably occurs with exertion or stress (e.g. cold, fear, emotion) and after eating.

Unstable angina
Unstable angina is a progressive form of angina in which pain occurs more frequently and becomes more severe with time. The pain may appear during rest and may last longer, with less relief by antianginal drugs. People with this condition eventually show signs and symptoms of impending myocardial infarction or coronary failure.

Variant angina (Prinzmetal angina)
This form of angina is uncommon and is caused by focal spasm of coronary arteries. In about 75% of people, the spasm occurs near an area of atherosclerosis. The pain often occurs during rest or without any cause.

Nitrate dosage forms

See Table 25-1 for pharmacokinetics of nitrates. Sublingual tablets and the sublingual spray are used to abort an acute attack or during an episode of angina. The person should sit or lie down first and then place the sublingual tablet under the tongue or in the buccal pouch allowing it to dissolve fully, or spray the aerosol under the tongue. Patients should not swallow, eat, drink or smoke while the tablet is in the mouth. If necessary, the sublingual tablet dosage is repeated at 5-minute intervals for a total of three doses. If chest pain is not relieved within a 15-minute period, an ambulance should be called and the person transported immediately to a hospital. A maximum of two sublingual sprays 5 minutes apart is used and if no relief occurs after 5 minutes an ambulance should be called. After use of sublingual preparations, a transient headache lasting 15–20 minutes and flushing may occur.

The sublingual tablets should be stored in a tightly closed dark container and the bottle dated when first opened. The

CLINICAL INTEREST BOX 25-1 MANAGEMENT OF ANGINA

Guidelines for the management of unstable angina were published jointly by the National Heart Foundation of Australia and the Cardiac Society of Australia and New Zealand in 2000. Drug therapies recommended (in the absence of contraindications) included the use of aspirin in all patients and, in low-risk patients, glyceryl trinitrate and β-blockers.

Use of the latter is based on evidence of a decrease in progression to myocardial infarction. If β-blockers were contraindicated because of pre-existing asthma, then in the absence of heart failure or heart block, a calcium channel blocker could be used. If used alone, verapamil and diltiazem were recommended because of their beneficial effects in reducing heart rate.

Recommendations for long-term management included the use of an HMG-CoA reductase inhibitor (statin) in persons with a cholesterol level >4 mmol/L, and an angiotensin-converting enzyme inhibitor in persons with hypertension or diabetes. Subsequent addenda to the guidelines have been published in August 2001, October 2001 and July 2002.

Amendments to these guidelines can be found at: www.heartfoundation.com.au/index.cfm?page=45

DRUG MONOGRAPH 25-1 GLYCERYL TRINITRATE

Glyceryl trinitrate is the key drug in the nitrate category. It is available as a sublingual tablet, sublingual spray, transdermal patch or IV infusion. The other drugs in this category include isosorbide dinitrate, which is available as a sublingual or oral tablet, and isosorbide mononitrate, available as a slow-release formulation.

MECHANISM OF ACTION After interacting with tissue sulfhydryl groups all of the nitrates release the free radical nitric oxide (NO). The release of NO activates guanylate cyclase in vascular smooth muscle, thereby increasing formation of cyclic guanosine monophosphate (cGMP). This in turn leads to changes in the degree of phosphorylation of smooth muscle proteins. Ultimately, dephosphorylation of the myosin light chain leads to relaxation. The biochemical steps for the metabolism of nitrates to the active NO and the ultimate therapeutic effect of vasodilation are illustrated in Figure 25-1.

Glyceryl trinitrate at low doses causes venodilation, with little effect on arterial resistance vessels. This causes a reduction in preload and stroke volume. With higher doses, dilation of arteries occurs, resulting in a reduction in arterial pressure which, coupled with venous pooling when standing, often results in postural hypotension and dizziness. As both cardiac output and arterial pressure are reduced, the oxygen demand by the myocardium is also reduced. Nitrates also dilate normal coronary and coronary collateral vessels. The resultant increased coronary perfusion and hence oxygen

delivery ensures more efficient distribution of blood to ischaemic areas of the myocardium.

INDICATIONS Glyceryl trinitrate is used to prevent or treat stable angina, and to treat unstable angina and heart failure associated with acute myocardial infarction.

PHARMACOKINETICS (Table 25-1) Glyceryl trinitrate is rapidly metabolised by the liver to dinitrates that have about 10% of the biological activity of the parent drug.

DRUG INTERACTIONS The concurrent use of nitrates with alcohol, antihypertensives, other drugs causing hypotension, and vasodilators (including sildenafil, tadalafil and vardenafil) may result in enhanced orthostatic hypotensive effects.

ADVERSE REACTIONS These include dizziness, headaches, nausea or vomiting, agitation, facial flushing, increased pulse rate, dry mouth, rash, prolonged headaches and blurred vision.

WARNINGS AND CONTRAINDICATIONS Nitrates are contraindicated in persons with cardiomyopathy, hypotension, hypovolaemia, aortic or mitral stenosis, severe anaemia, raised intracranial pressure and glaucoma, and with concurrent use of sildenafil.

DOSAGE AND ADMINISTRATION See Table 25-1.

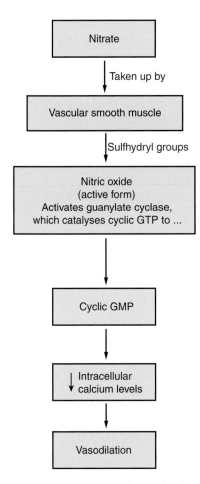

FIGURE 25-1 Mechanism of action of organic nitrates.

container should not be left opened or exposed to heat or moisture. To maintain potency the unused tablets should be discarded 3 months after opening the container.

The lingual spray should not be inhaled and the mouth should be closed immediately after delivery of the dose. If using a pump delivery system the pump may need to be primed to ensure an even spray.

Oral sustained-release tablets should not be crushed or chewed but swallowed whole with a full glass of water.

Transdermal glyceryl trinitrate is a patch system that contains a drug reservoir from which the drug is slowly released (passive diffusion). The drug is absorbed through the skin and transported by blood to the site of action to produce its beneficial effects. This system is applied daily to a hairless skin area, usually on the chest (preferred site), shoulder or inside upper arm. The site should be changed to avoid skin irritation but avoid applying the patch to extremities, especially below the knee or elbow.

Transdermal systems with different release rates are available (releasing 0.2–0.6 mg/h), and each has a different mechanism for drug delivery. The systems should not be considered to be interchangeable. (See Figure 25-2 for an

illustration of transdermal systems.) As tolerance develops to glyceryl trinitrate, it is recommended that the patch be applied for 12–14 hours and removed for 10–12 hours each day. This drug-free interval helps maintain the efficacy of the product.

Calcium channel blockers

The **calcium channel blockers**, while having diverse chemical structures, all block the inward movement of calcium through the slow channels of the cell membranes of cardiac and smooth muscle cells. (See Chapter 23 for a discussion of vascular smooth muscle contraction.) This activity, however, varies according to the specific type of cardiovascular cells involved. The three types of tissues or cells are cardiac muscle, or myocardium; the cardiac conduction system (SA and AV nodes); and vascular smooth muscle.

Pharmacological effects
MYOCARDIUM
Calcium channel blockers decrease the force of myocardial contraction by blocking the inward flow of calcium ions through the slow channels of the cell membrane during phase 2 (plateau phase) of the action potential (see Figure 23-5). The diminished entry of calcium ions into the cells fails to trigger the release of large amounts of calcium from the sarcoplasmic reticulum within the cell. This free calcium is needed for excitation–contraction coupling, an event that activates contraction by allowing cross-bridges to form between the actin and myosin filaments of muscle. The force of contraction by the heart is determined by the number of actin–myosin cross-bridges formed within the sarcomere. Decreasing the amount of calcium ions released from the sarcoplasmic reticulum results in fewer actin–myosin cross-bridges being formed, thus decreasing the force of contraction and resulting in a negative inotropic effect.

CARDIAC CONDUCTION SYSTEM (SA NODE AND AV JUNCTION)
In these tissues, calcium channel blockers decrease automaticity in the SA node and decrease conduction in the AV junction. Depolarisation (phase 0) of the action potential is normally generated by the inward calcium ion current through the slow channels. These drugs block the inward calcium ion current across the cell membrane of the SA node, decreasing the rate of depolarisation and depressing automaticity. The result is a decrease in heart rate (negative chronotropic effect). Similarly, decreasing calcium ion influx across the cell membrane of the AV junction slows AV conduction (negative dromotropic effect) and prolongs AV refractory time. When AV conduction is prolonged, fewer atrial impulses reach the ventricles, thus slowing the rate of ventricular contractions.

VASCULAR SMOOTH MUSCLE

The effect of calcium channel blockers on smooth muscle of the coronary and peripheral vessels has a significant influence on cardiovascular haemodynamics. Coronary artery dilation occurs, which lowers coronary resistance and improves blood flow through collateral vessels, as well as improving oxygen delivery to ischaemic areas of the heart.

These agents also inhibit the contraction of smooth muscle of the peripheral arterioles. This results in widespread reduction in resistance to blood flow through the body (determined by the tone of the vascular musculature and the diameter of the blood vessels) and blood pressure. The haemodynamic change reduces afterload, which also decreases oxygen demand of the heart.

TABLE 25-1 Pharmacokinetics and dosages of nitrates

DRUG	ONSET OF ACTION	DURATION OF ACTION (h)	METABOLISM	EXCRETION	USUAL ADULT DOSE
Glyceryl trinitrate			Liver	Kidneys	
Sublingual tablet	1–3 min	0.5–1			300–600 mcg repeated every 3–4 min to a maximum of 1200–1800 mcg
Lingual aerosol	2–4 min	<1			400–800 mcg
IV infusion	Immediate	Variable*			5–10 mcg/min increased by 5 mcg/min every 3–5 minutes until desired response
Transdermal patch	>4 h	8–24			Relates to amount of drug released/24 hours
Isosorbide dinitrate			Liver	Kidneys	
Oral tablet	15–40 min	4–6			3–30 mg up to 4 times daily
Sublingual tablet	2–5 min	1–2			5–10 mg every 2–3 hours
Isosorbide mononitrate			Liver/kidneys	Kidneys	
Controlled-release tablet	1–2 h	24			30–60 mg once daily to a maximum of 120 mg daily

*Depends on duration of infusion.

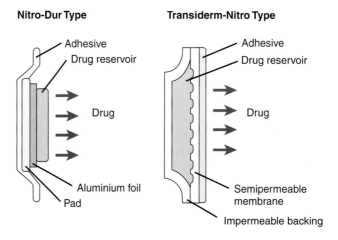

FIGURE 25-2 Transdermal systems. Nitro-Dur is a gel-like matrix surrounded by fluid. Transiderm-Nitro contains a semipermeable membrane between the drug reservoir and the skin that controls the drug delivery.

The calcium-channel blockers include the:

- phenylalkylamine type (verapamil)
- benzothiazepine type (diltiazem)
- dihydropyridine type (amlodipine, felodipine, nifedipine, nimodipine and lercanidipine).

Verapamil was the first calcium channel blocker released and is the key drug for this category. It has greater effects on the heart, reducing AV conduction and blocking the SA node, resulting in a decrease in heart rate and contractility. It is considered a moderate peripheral vasodilator. **Diltiazem** has similar pharmacological effects on vascular tissue but has less effect on the heart than verapamil. These agents dilate coronary arteries and arterioles, inhibit coronary artery spasm and dilate peripheral arterioles, reducing total peripheral resistance (afterload), thus lowering arterial blood pressure at rest and during exercise.

The dihydropyridine drugs, exemplified by **nifedipine**, have minimal effect on cardiac tissue at therapeutic doses. They act principally on vascular smooth muscle, reducing peripheral vascular resistance. In some circumstances the reflex sympathetic response to vasodilation results in tachycardia, which may be deleterious. Table 25-2 shows a comparison of the effects of the different types of calcium channel blockers.

Indications

Therapeutically, the calcium channel blockers have been used to treat angina, supraventricular tachyarrhythmias (verapamil), hypertension and cerebral vasospasm after subarachnoid haemorrhage (nimodipine).

BOX 25-2 IMPLICATIONS OF THE USE OF CALCIUM CHANNEL BLOCKERS IN THE ELDERLY

The elderly are more susceptible to these agents and the adverse effects of increased weakness, dizziness, fainting episodes and falls. Although glyceryl trinitrate (or other nitrates) may be taken concurrently with these agents, the person should be advised to report any increase in frequency or intensity of angina attacks to the physician. Alcohol consumption may result in hypotensive episodes in some people. Whenever possible, the use of alcohol should be avoided. In the elderly, treatment should be started at a lower dose because a reduction in hepatic metabolism may result in increased plasma concentration. Plasma half-life increases in the elderly with amlodipine, diltiazem, felodipine and verapamil. These agents should not be discontinued abruptly, as severe rebound angina attacks may result (gradual drug withdrawal is recommended).

Pharmacokinetics

See Table 25-3 for pharmacokinetics of the calcium channel-blocking agents. Diltiazem is metabolised to a major metabolite, desacetyldiltiazem, which may be responsible for up to 50% of its coronary dilation effect. Verapamil's active metabolite, norverapamil, accounts for about 20% of the antihypertensive effect of verapamil. Nifedipine has no known active metabolite, while the other agents have metabolites that may or may not have significant therapeutic effects. Nimodipine is highly lipophilic and crosses the blood–brain barrier, having a greater effect on cerebral arteries than other arteries in the body.

Drug interactions

Drug interactions are quite extensive and vary for each of the calcium channel-blocking drugs (see Table 25-4). Relevant drug information sources should be consulted.

Adverse reactions

These include headache, nausea, hypotension, dizziness, skin flushing or rash, oedema of the ankles and feet, dry mouth and tachycardia. (See Box 25-2 for implications of the use of the calcium channel blockers in the elderly.) Gingival hyperplasia is a rare adverse effect reported with amlodipine, diltiazem, felodipine, verapamil and, most often, nifedipine. It starts as an inflammation of the gums, usually in the first 9 months of therapy. When the drug is discontinued, this effect usually improves within 1–4 weeks. Good dental hygiene, along with professional teeth cleaning, is necessary to reduce the potential for this adverse effect.

Warnings and contraindications

Use with caution in persons with severe bradycardia, congestive heart failure (caution with felodipine, nifedipine and nimodipine, as they have a slight negative inotropic effect), hypotension, acute myocardial infarction or liver or kidney impairment. Avoid use in persons with hypersensitivity to calcium-blocking agents, cardiac shock, severe bradycardia or congestive heart failure (use extreme caution with diltiazem and verapamil).

Potassium channel activators

Drugs of this class include **nicorandil**, which may be used as an alternative to long-acting nitrates to reduce the frequency of anginal attacks, and diazoxide and minoxidil, which have limited use in treating hypertension. These drugs relax smooth muscle by acting on ATP-sensitive potassium channels. Normally, intracellular ATP closes the channel, causing the smooth muscle cells to depolarise. Drugs that activate the potassium channel antagonise the action of ATP, preventing

TABLE 25–2 Comparison of effects of calcium channel-blocking agents

EFFECTS	AMLODIPINE	DILTIAZEM	FELODIPINE	NIFEDIPINE	VERAPAMIL
Contractility	↑	↓	↑	0/↓	↓↓
Vasodilation					
Coronary	↑	↑↑↑	↑	↑↑↑	↑↑
Peripheral	↑↑↑	↑	↑↑↑	↑↑↑	↑↑
Heart rate	+/–	0/↓	↑	↑	↑↓
Cardiac output	↑	0/↑	↑	↑↑	↑↓

↑ = slight increase; ↓ = slight decrease; ↑↑ = intermediate increase; ↓↓ = intermediate decrease; ↑↑↑ = significant increase; ↓↓↓ = significant decrease; +/– = minimal effect; ↑↓ = slight effect; 0 = no effect.

TABLE 25-3 Pharmacokinetics and dosages of calcium channel-blocking drugs

DRUG	ONSET OF ACTION (min)	TIME TO PEAK CONCENTRATION (h)	DURATION OF ACTION (h)	METABOLISM	EXCRETION	USUAL ADULT DAILY DOSE
Amlodipine	2–5 (IV)	6–12	No data	Liver	Kidneys	2.5–5 mg daily, maximum 10 mg/daily
Diltiazem	30	2–3	4–8	Liver	Kidneys and bile	30 mg 3–4 times daily to a maximum of 180–240 mg/day
Controlled-release	30–60	6–11	12	Liver	Kidneys and bile	180 mg once daily to a maximum of 360 mg once daily
Felodipine (controlled-release)	120–300	2.5–5	24	Liver	Kidneys	5 mg once daily to a maximum of 20 mg once daily
Lercanidipine	No data	1.5–3	24	Liver	Kidneys	10 mg once daily increasing to 20 mg (maximum) once daily. Use low dose for at least 2 weeks before increasing dose
Nifedipine	20	0.5–1	4–8	Liver	Kidneys	10–20 mg twice daily to a max of 20–40 mg twice daily
Verapamil	Oral: 60–120 IV: 1–5	1–2	IV: 2 Oral: 8–10 Controlled-release: 24	Liver	Kidneys and faeces	80 mg 2–3 times daily to a max of 160 mg 2–3 times daily (conventional product)

closure of the channel. This results in hyperpolarisation and relaxation of the vascular smooth muscle.

Nicorandil

In addition to its action as an activator of potassium channels, which leads to arterial vasodilation and a reduction in after-load, **nicorandil** relaxes the venous vascular system. This is due to an increase in cGMP brought about by the nitrate moiety of the drug (a similar effect to that of glyceryl trinitrate). Nicorandil's use in chronic stable angina is as a result of evidence that it exerts a direct effect on normal and stenotic coronary arteries.

All the antianginal drugs discussed in preceding

TABLE 25-4 Drug interactions of calcium channel-blocking drugs

DRUG	POSSIBLE EFFECT AND MANAGEMENT
β-adrenergic-blocking agents	An increased risk of bradycardia occurs with co-administration with diltiazem, and monitoring of cardiac function is necessary. This combination with verapamil is not recommended because of the risk of heart block
Carbamazepine and cyclosporin	Diltiazem and verapamil increase plasma concentrations of carbamazepine and cyclosporin. Monitor such combinations closely, as dosage adjustments may be necessary
Digoxin	Increased plasma concentration of digoxin has been reported with coadministration of verapamil or diltiazem. Monitor digoxin plasma concentration closely whenever a calcium channel-blocking agent is started or discontinued or when dosage is changed. Monitor for prolonged AV conduction, bradycardia or AV blocks, especially during the initial week of therapy, as digoxin dose may need to be changed
Hepatic enzyme-inducing drugs (phenytoin, barbiturates)	May increase metabolism of dihydropyridines and verapamil. Monitor clinically and increase dose if necessary

sections (nitrates, calcium channel blockers and β-blockers [Chapter 12]) provide symptomatic relief in persons with angina. These drugs may be used alone or in combination because they improve the balance between myocardial oxygen supply and demand. A comparison of the effects of these drugs on cardiovascular parameters is shown in Table 25-5.

After oral administration nicorandil is absorbed rapidly, with bioavailability in the order of 75%, indicating no extensive first-pass metabolism. Maximal plasma concentrations are reached in 30–60 minutes and the drug has a rapid elimination phase, with a half-life of about 60 minutes. Nicorandil is metabolised by de-nitration, with the metabolites excreted in the urine within 24 hours.

Common adverse reactions include nausea, flushing, headache, dizziness, palpitations and myalgia. At high doses, hypotension may be problematic. Precaution should be exercised in persons with severe hepatic impairment, as lower doses may be required. Nicorandil is contraindicated in individuals with hypotension or left ventricular failure.

The initial dose is 10 mg orally twice daily (less for patients prone to headache or adverse reactions), increasing after 1 week to 10–20 mg twice daily.

Diazoxide

The antihypertensive action results of diazoxide from potassium channel activation and hence relaxation of smooth muscles in the peripheral arterioles, which causes a decrease in peripheral resistance. As blood pressure falls, a reflex increase in heart rate and cardiac output occurs, with resultant maintenance of coronary and cerebral blood flow. This cardiovascular reflex mechanism also inhibits the development of orthostatic hypotension. Concurrent use with other antihypertensives or peripheral vasodilators may result in additive effects.

Diazoxide is administered intravenously to reduce blood pressure promptly in hypertensive emergencies such as malignant hypertension and hypertensive crisis. Intravenous diazoxide is ineffective in reducing elevated blood pressure in persons with MAO-induced hypertension or phaeochromocytoma. Because of its adverse effects, the drug is not used orally for treatment of chronic hypertension. Administered intravenously (intermittently or by infusion) the onset of action is 1 minute, the peak effect occurs within 2–5 minutes, the half-life is about 28 hours, and the duration of effect is 2–12 hours. Diazoxide is metabolised by the liver and excreted by the kidneys.

Adverse reactions include hyperglycaemia, tachycardia, anorexia, headache, flushing, dizziness, constipation, abdominal cramps, changes in taste perception, and oedema (sodium and water retention). With rapid IV injection severe adverse reactions including angina, bradycardia, hypotension, cerebral ischaemia and confusion may occur. Use diazoxide with caution in persons with gout, diabetes and heart failure. Avoid use in persons with diazoxide hypersensitivity, coronary or cerebral insufficiency, or aortic dissection.

The adult dose is 1–3 mg/kg up to a maximum of 150 mg IV, repeated after 5–15 minutes if necessary. Intravenous infusion at a rate of 7.5–30 mg/min is the preferred route and dosage, to minimise the risk of a precipitous fall in blood pressure.

Capsules of diazoxide are available through the Special Access Scheme for the treatment of intractable hypoglycaemia. The oral route is not normally used for the treatment of hypertension because of poor tolerance of oral diazoxide.

Minoxidil

Minoxidil is an orally effective direct-acting peripheral vasodilator. It reduces blood pressure by decreasing peripheral vascular resistance in the arteriolar vessels, with little effect on veins. It does not cause orthostatic hypotension. It

TABLE 25-5 Comparison of effects of nitrates, β-blockers and calcium channel blockers

EFFECT	NITRATES	β-BLOCKERS	CALCIUM CHANNEL BLOCKERS
Systolic blood pressure	(–)	(–)	(–)
Ventricular volume	(–)	(+)	(–) or (0)
Heart rate	(+)	(–)	(–),(+) or (0)
Myocardial contractility	(0)	(–)	(–)
Coronary blood flow	(+)	(+) or (0)	(+)
Coronary vessel resistance	(–)	(+) or (0)	(–)
Coronary spasm	(–)	(+) or (0)	(–)
Collateral blood flow	(+)	(0)	(–)

(–) = decreased; (+) = increased; (0) = no change.

is a potent vasodilator and also causes a reflex increase in cardiac output, induces sodium retention, promotes development of oedema, and increases plasma renin activity. Minoxidil is reserved for severe hypertension unresponsive to traditional agents, i.e. severe hypertension associated with chronic renal failure. Concomitant administration of a β-adrenergic-blocking agent such as propranolol is necessary to prevent severe reflex tachycardia. Administration of a diuretic agent is also essential to counteract sodium and water retention. Its more commonly recognised topical use is for male-pattern baldness in both men and women.

The onset of action of minoxidil is 30 minutes, with the peak effect occurring in 2–3 hours (after a single dose). Although the plasma half-life is about 4 hours, the duration of its hypotensive action may exceed 24 hours. With daily administration steady-state plasma concentration is achieved after 3–7 days. It is metabolised by the liver and excreted by the kidneys.

Adverse reactions occur with oral dosing and include nausea; vomiting; tachycardia; anorexia; headaches; excessive hair growth (hypertrichosis), usually on face, arms and back; red flushing of skin; oedema; angina and pericarditis. Use with caution in persons with heart failure, angina, phaeochromocytoma, cerebrovascular disease and post-myocardial infarction. Avoid use in persons with minoxidil hypersensitivity or pulmonary hypertension secondary to mitral stenosis, and in pregnant or lactating women.

For children 12 years and over and adults, the initial dose is 5 mg orally daily as a single dose. For adults this can be increased every 3 days by 5–10 mg until a maintenance dose of 10–40 mg daily in one or two divided doses is achieved. For children up to 12 years of age the dose is 0.2 mg/kg (maximum 5 mg/day). The maximal daily dose for adults is 100 mg, and for children 50 mg.

Miscellaneous vasodilators

The drugs discussed below include hydralazine and sodium nitroprusside. Both these agents are used during hypertensive emergencies because they are rapid direct-acting vasodilators that produce an immediate fall in arterial pressure.

Hydralazine

Hydralazine hydrochloride is believed to produce its hypotensive effects by direct relaxation of vascular smooth muscle, particularly the arterioles, with little effect on veins, leading to reduction in peripheral resistance. Consequently, renal blood flow is increased, providing an advantage to patients with renal failure. Hydralazine also maintains cerebral blood flow and causes sodium and water retention. The resulting hypotension is thought to stimulate the baroreceptor reflex, causing an increase in heart rate and cardiac output. Unfortunately, this response offsets the antihypertensive effects of the drug. Tolerance to the antihypertensive action may be counteracted by combination with other antihypertensive drugs. Hydralazine also increases plasma renin activity. It is used for the treatment of hypertensive emergencies and in combination with a β-blocker and a diuretic in persons with hypertension refractory to other drugs.

An oral dose of hydralazine has an onset of action of 45 minutes; with IV administration the onset is within 10–20 minutes. The peak effect is within 1 hour (orally) or 15–30 minutes (IV). The plasma half-life is 3–7 hours and duration of action is 3–8 hours. It is metabolised principally by acetylation in the liver, with the metabolites excreted by the kidneys. Identification of slow acetylator phenotype (see Chapter 6) in both Caucasians (about 50%) and Asians (about 20%), which results in significant increases in the plasma concentration of the drug and hence the risk of toxicity, has limited the usefulness of this drug. Concurrent drug administration with monoamine oxidase inhibitors or other antihypertensives may result in severe hypotension.

Adverse reactions include diarrhoea, nausea, vomiting, tachycardia, anorexia, headache, facial flushing, stuffy nose, oedema, angina, rash, peripheral neuritis and a systemic lupus erythematosus (SLE)-like syndrome. The SLE-like syndrome may include myalgia, arthralgia, arthritis, weakness, fever and skin changes. Use with caution in patients with angina, cerebral artery disease, and renal and hepatic impairment. The drug is contraindicated in persons with hydralazine hypersensitivity, aortic dissection, severe tachycardia and heart failure, and SLE.

The adult oral dose is 25 mg twice daily increasing as required to a maintenance dose of 50–200 mg daily. Doses above 100 mg daily increase the risk of the SLE-type adverse reaction, and the acetylator phenotype should be determined in advance. Parenterally, the adult dose is 5–10 mg IV slowly over 20 minutes, repeated if necessary.

BOX 25-3 MANAGING SODIUM NITROPRUSSIDE OVERDOSE

Metabolism and toxicity

Nitroprusside contains five cyanide groups. When the drug is administered IV, one molecule of nitroprusside reacts with one molecule of haemoglobin to form one molecule of cyanmethaemoglobin, four cyanide ions and nitric oxide, the active substance. Nitric oxide then activates the enzyme guanylate cyclase to produce cGMP, and vasodilation. The free cyanide ions react with thiosulfates, catalysed by the mitochondrial enzyme rhodanase, forming the final metabolite thiocyanate, which is excreted by the kidneys.

Processing of cyanide ions from sodium nitroprusside to thiocyanate can proceed normally at a rate of about 2 mcg/kg/min. Infusion rates greater than this can lead to accumulation of cyanide ions. In persons with normal renal function the half-life of thiocyanate is 3 days, but this may double or triple in persons with renal failure.

Cyanide toxicity may manifest as tachycardia, sweating, hyperventilation, metabolic acidosis, hypotension, arrhythmias and death. In contrast, thiocyanate toxicity causes nausea, dyspnoea, blurred vision, confusion, psychosis and tinnitus.

Treatment

Discontinue sodium nitroprusside and administer sodium nitrite (3% solution) at a dose of 4–6 mg/kg IV over 2–4 minutes. After administration of sodium nitrite, administer sodium thiosulfate (150–200 mg/kg) IV to convert the cyanide to thiocyanate. The nitrite/thiosulfate regimen can be repeated using 2–3 mg/kg sodium nitrite and 75–100 mg/kg sodium thiosulfate after two hours (eMIMS 2006).

Thiocyanate is less toxic and rarely a problem, but if thiocyanate toxicity occurs, use haemodialysis. Be aware, however, that haemodialysis does not remove cyanide.

Sodium nitroprusside

Sodium nitroprusside (nitroferricyanide) is a potent and rapid direct-acting vasodilator agent that greatly reduces arterial blood pressure. It relaxes both arterial and venous smooth muscles. The decrease in systemic resistance causes a reduction in preload and afterload, improving cardiac output. It is indicated for rapid reduction of blood pressure in hypertensive emergencies and for controlled hypotension during surgery.

Sodium nitroprusside is useful only for short-term treatment, as it must be given intravenously. Its onset of action and peak effect occur almost immediately (within minutes) after administration by IV infusion. The half-life of nitroprusside is 2 minutes; the half-life of thiocyanate, a toxic metabolite, is 3 days. The duration of effect is 1–10 minutes after discontinuation of the infusion. Metabolism is by erythrocytes (to cyanide) and the liver (cyanide to thiocyanate). The drug is excreted by the kidneys.

The hypotensive effect of sodium nitroprusside is exacerbated by other antihypertensive drugs, volatile anaesthetics and other negative inotropes. Adverse reactions include dizziness, excessive sweating, headaches, anxiety, abdominal cramps, tachycardia, hypothyroidism, flushing, rash and muscle twitching. Ataxia, blurred vision, headache, nausea, vomiting, tinnitus, shortness of breath, delirium and unconsciousness may occur with thiocyanate toxicity. Hypotension, metabolic acidosis, pink coloration, very shallow breathing pattern, decreased reflexes, coma and widely dilated pupils may be observed with cyanide toxicity. (See Box 25-3 for treatment of sodium nitroprusside overdose.) Use with caution in persons with hypothyroidism, hypothermia or lung disease. Avoid use in persons with nitroprusside hypersensitivity, cerebrovascular or coronary artery disease, liver disease, kidney disease or metabolic-induced vitamin B_{12} deficiency.

For hypertensive emergency, the initial dose is 0.3 mcg/kg/min, which is slowly increased as necessary. The maximum dose is 10 mcg/kg/min.

Solution should be freshly prepared using 5% glucose intravenous infusion (no other solution should be used) and protected from light by wrapping the container in the supplied opaque sleeve, aluminium foil or other opaque material. The prepared solution should be discarded within a 24-hour period. A freshly prepared solution has a faint brown tinge; discard if it is highly coloured (e.g. blue, green or dark red).

PERIPHERAL VASCULAR DISEASE

Peripheral vascular disease, which results in coolness or numbness of the extremities, intermittent claudication and leg ulcers, is a common problem in the elderly. The primary risk factors include hyperlipidaemia, diabetes, obesity, high blood pressure and smoking. The use of various direct-acting vasodilators for peripheral occlusive arterial disease has generally been very disappointing. **Oxpentifylline** and hydroxyethylrutosides are used for symptomatic relief but there is a lack of convincing evidence for efficacy of either drug. If no benefit is seen after a short trial of use, the drugs should be stopped. (See Drug Monograph 25-2.)

MANAGEMENT OF HYPERTENSION

Non-pharmacological measures are the first-line approach for managing hypertension and include weight and alcohol reduction, limiting dietary sodium intake and embarking on a program of regular physical activity. When instituting drug therapy the lowest dose of the chosen drug is used, adding a second drug from a different drug class if necessary. The overriding goal of drug therapy is to lower the blood pressure, with minimal adverse effects. Long-acting drugs that allow once-daily dosing are preferable, as they aid compliance.

Effective drug combinations include:
- an ACE inhibitor or angiotensin-II-receptor antagonist plus a calcium channel blocker
- a β-blocker plus an α-blocker
- a β-blocker plus a dihydropyridine calcium channel blocker (amlodipine, felodipine or nifedipine)
- a thiazide diuretic plus a β-blocker
- a thiazide diuretic plus an ACE inhibitor or angiotensin-II-receptor antagonist.

Figure 25-3 summarises the physiological factors controlling blood pressure (the sympathetic nervous system and the renin–angiotensin–aldosterone system) and indicates the sites of action of currently used oral antihypertensive drugs.

VASODILATOR DRUGS —INDIRECT-ACTING

The main groups of drugs in this category include centrally acting drugs that inhibit vasoconstriction through mediation by the sympathetic nervous system, and inhibitors of the renin–angiotensin system. Both groups are used principally for the treatment of hypertension.

Centrally acting adrenergic inhibitors

The centrally acting agents **clonidine** and methyldopa are effective antihypertensive drugs, especially when combined with a diuretic. When given as the sole agent, clonidine and methyldopa usually cause sodium and water retention.

CLINICAL INTEREST BOX 25-2 HYPERTENSION

Hypertension is defined as an elevated systolic blood pressure, diastolic blood pressure, or both. In clinical practice elevated systolic blood pressure is a greater predictor of cardiovascular risk than elevated diastolic pressure. Worldwide definitions of hypertension vary and recently a suggested classification has been developed following a review of systems in the USA and Europe (Heart Foundation 2004).

CATEGORY	SYSTOLIC (MMHG)	DIASTOLIC (MMHG)
Normal	<120	<80
High–normal	120–139	80–89
Grade 1 (mild hypertension)	140–159	90–99
Grade 2 (moderate hypertension)	160–179	100–109
Grade 3 (severe hypertension)	≥180	≥110

This classification has also stratified people based on blood pressure levels, the presence of risk factors and the degree of target-organ damage secondary to hypertension. The major risk factors in hypertensive patients include cigarette smoking, diabetes mellitus, raised total or LDL cholesterol or reduced HDL cholesterol, age (>55 years male, >65 years female), family history of heart disease, male gender (increased risk at any age compared to females), obesity, excessive alcohol intake and a sedentary lifestyle. Psychosocial risk factors include depression, social isolation and lack of quality support. Those populations most at risk include people of Aboriginal, Torres Strait Islander, Maori or Pacific Islander origin and those in lower socioeconomic groups. The target-organ damage or cardiovascular disease in hypertensive patients includes stroke or transient ischaemic attacks (TIA), kidney disease, retinopathy and various cardiac diseases such as angina, heart failure, left ventricular hypertrophy and prior myocardial infarction.

"A therapeutic plan should be implemented in all patients with hypertension (BP ≥140 mmHg systolic and/or ≥90 mmHg diastolic). The plan should be aimed at both blood pressure reduction and reduction of overall cardiovascular risk. The management strategy should be related to the patient's absolute risk category. In all individuals whose blood pressure is ≥120/80 mmHg, modification of lifestyle should also be recommended." (Heart Foundation 2004).

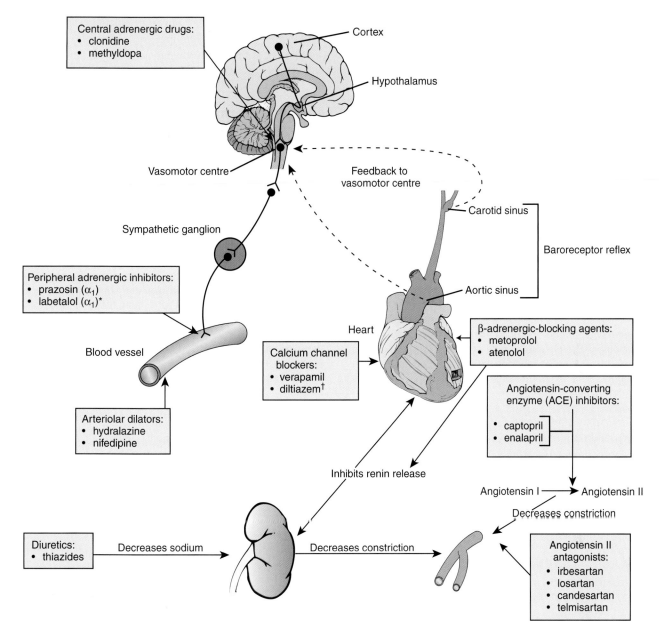

FIGURE 25-3 Physiological control of blood pressure and sites of action of currently used oral antihypertensive drugs. *Labetalol acts on both α_1- and β_1-adrenoceptors. †Diltiazem acts on both the heart and arteriolar vascular smooth muscle.

Clonidine

Clonidine is a centrally acting α_2 agonist. It reduces systolic and diastolic blood pressure by stimulating central α_2 receptors, which *decreases* sympathetic outflow from the brain to the blood vessels and heart. Blood pressure is lowered as a result of decreased cardiac output, heart rate and peripheral vascular resistance. The effect on cardiac output is the result of a reduction in both heart rate and stroke volume, which can lead to bradycardia.

The decreased sympathetic outflow to the kidneys reduces renal vascular resistance, preserving renal blood flow. In some persons, renin activity may be suppressed (Hoffman 2001).

With continued clonidine use, a diuretic is used to correct fluid retention.

Clonidine is marketed for the treatment of hypertension and menopausal flushing but is also used for the diagnosis of phaeochromocytoma, for attention-deficit hyperactivity disorder and for managing the symptoms of opioid withdrawal. At a low dose (100 mcg), clonidine is also used for migraine or recurrent vascular headache prophylaxis in adults unresponsive to other drug therapies.

Clonidine is well absorbed after oral administration, with bioavailability approaching 100%. Oral clonidine has an onset of action within 0.5–1 hour, a peak effect in 2–4

DRUG MONOGRAPH 25-2 OXPENTIFYLLINE

Oxpentifylline is a xanthine derivative that improves haemorrhagic disorders in the microcirculation, which involves the flow of blood through the fine vessels (arterioles, capillaries and venules). Although the mechanism of action of oxpentifylline is not completely understood, current evidence shows the drug possesses several properties that improve microcirculatory blood flow to ischaemic tissues. (It improves red blood cell flexibility and reduces blood viscosity by decreasing fibrinogen concentrations and inhibiting aggregation of red blood cells and platelets.) The result is increased microcirculatory blood flow and oxygenation of tissues.

INDICATIONS Oxpentifylline is indicated for the treatment of intermittent claudication caused by occlusive arterial disease of the limbs.

PHARMACOKINETICS Oxpentifylline is administered orally as a controlled-release tablet. The drug is almost completely absorbed and undergoes extensive first-pass metabolism. The plasma half-life of the parent drug ranges from 0.4 to 0.8 hours, and for the metabolites, from 1 to 1.6 hours. Peak plasma concentration occurs in 2–4 hours

and the onset of action with chronic dosing is between 2 and 4 weeks. It is metabolised in the liver and excreted by the kidneys.

DRUG INTERACTIONS Concurrent use with antiplatelet and thrombolytic medications may prolong prothrombin time and bleeding. Use with sympathomimetics and xanthines may result in an increase in central nervous system stimulation.

WARNINGS AND CONTRAINDICATIONS Avoid use in persons with bleeding problems (e.g. peptic ulcers), cerebrovascular or coronary artery disease or acute myocardial infarction. In severe renal impairment dosage reduction may be required.

ADVERSE REACTIONS These include dizziness, headaches, abdominal distress, nausea and vomiting. Rarely, chest pain, an irregular heart rate, rash, bleeding and hallucinations are encountered.

DOSAGE AND ADMINISTRATION For adults, the oral dose is 400 mg 2–3 times daily. Treatment should be stopped after 6–12 weeks if unsuccessful.

---

hours and a duration of action of up to 8 hours. Clonidine is excreted predominantly as unchanged drug in urine (60%), with the remainder excreted as hydroxylated metabolites.

See the Drug Interactions table 25-1 for clonidine. Adverse reactions include dry mouth, headaches, constipation, weakness, postural hypotension, impotency or decreased sexual drive, insomnia, anxiety, anorexia, nausea, vomiting and pruritus.

Use with caution in the elderly and in persons with impaired atrioventricular (AV) node or sinus node function, coronary insufficiency, depression or a history of depression, Raynaud's syndrome, or a recent myocardial infarction. Clonidine is contraindicated in sick sinus syndrome and heart block.

The adult dose for the treatment of hypertension is 0.05–0.1 mg twice daily initially, increased every 2–3 days by 0.1 or 0.2 mg. For maintenance, the dose is 0.15–0.3 mg daily in two divided doses.

Methyldopa

Although the exact hypotensive mechanism of methlydopa is unknown, the theory is that a metabolite of methyldopa (α-methylnoradrenaline) stimulates the central α_2 receptors, which results in a reduction in noradrenaline (sympathetic) outflow to the heart, kidneys and peripheral vasculature.

Methyldopa's peak effect occurs in 4–6 hours after a single dose or in 48–72 hours with multiple dosing. The duration of

action is 12–24 hours (after a single oral dose), 1–2 days (after multiple oral doses) or 10–16 hours (after IV administration). Methyldopa is metabolised centrally to α-methylnoradrenaline within adrenergic nerve endings and in the liver to a sulfate conjugate (30–60%). Excretion is primarily by the kidneys.

See the Drug Interactions table 25-2 for methyldopa.

Adverse reactions include drowsiness, dry mouth, headaches, oedema of the feet and legs, fever, postural hypotension,

DRUG INTERACTIONS 25-1 Clondine

Drug	Possible effect and management
β-adrenergic-blocking agents	Concurrent administration with clonidine may lead to loss of blood pressure control. Bradycardia may be exacerbated. Monitor pulse rate closely. If discontinuing both drugs, the β-blocking agent should be stopped first. Discontinuing clonidine first may increase the risk of inducing a withdrawal hypertensive crisis
Tricyclic antidepressants	The antihypertensive effectiveness of clonidine may be reduced. This usually occurs in the first or second week of therapy. Monitor closely, as dosage adjustments and/or an alternative drug may need to be considered

DRUG INTERACTIONS 25-2 Methyldopa

Drug	Possible effect and management
Iron	Ferrous sulfate or gluconate may reduce bioavailability, interfering with blood pressure control
Monoamine oxidase (MAO) inhibitors	Excessive sympathetic stimulation may occur, causing hallucinations, headache and hypertension. Avoid or a serious drug interaction may occur
Sympathomimetics (cocaine, adrenaline and others)	A decrease in methyldopa's antihypertensive effect and a possible increase in the pressor effects of these medications may result. Avoid or a serious drug interaction may occur

impotency, insomnia, depression, anxiety and nightmares. Use with caution in persons with sulfite sensitivity or kidney impairment. Avoid use in persons with methyldopa hypersensitivity, hepatitis, cirrhosis, haemolytic anaemia or phaeochromocytoma.

The initial adult oral dose is 125–250 mg twice daily for 2 days, adjusted by 250–500 mg daily at 2-day intervals as necessary. The maintenance dose is 250–2000 mg/day, divided into 2–4 individual doses.

The renin–angiotensin–aldosterone system

The **renin–angiotensin–aldosterone system** regulates blood pressure by increasing or decreasing blood volume through modulation of renal function (Figure 25-4). The initiating factor is renin, an enzyme secreted from the juxtaglomerular cells located in the afferent arteriolar walls of the nephron. When blood flow through the kidneys is reduced, renal arterial pressure is reduced, which causes the release of renin into the circulation. Renin catalyses the cleavage of angiotensinogen (a plasma globulin) to form angiotensin I, a weak vasoconstrictor. Subsequently, in the small vessels of the lung, angiotensin I is converted by **angiotensin-converting enzyme** (ACE) to angiotensin II.

Angiotensin II is one of the most potent vasoconstrictors known. It is particularly effective in constricting arterioles, which increases peripheral resistance and raises blood pressure. In addition, angiotensin II acts on the adrenal cortex to stimulate the secretion of aldosterone, a hormone that promotes reabsorption of sodium by the kidneys. The increased sodium elevates the osmotic pressure in the

CLINICAL INTEREST BOX 25-3 NEW ZEALAND HEALTH INFORMATION

Population health surveys and record linkage studies are managed by Public Health Intelligence. The findings are integrated into New Zealand Health Monitor, which compiles social statistics, and operates under strict ethical standards. The surveys are conducted nationwide at different intervals, as shown below:

Survey	Frequency (Years)	Next survey
NZ Health Survey	3	2006/7
NZ Adult Nutrition Survey	10	2007/8
NZ Child Nutrition Survey	10	2012
NZ Tobacco Use Survey	2 out of every 3	2006/8
NZ Alcohol and Drug Use Survey	3	2007
NZ Sexual and Reproductive Health Survey	5	2006
NZ Mental Health and Wellbeing Survey	10	2012

Key findings on chronic disease from the 2002/3 survey include:
- One in four adults had been diagnosed with chronic neck or back problems.
- One in five adults aged 15–44 years had been diagnosed with asthma.
- One in six adults had been diagnosed with arthritis.
- One in 10 adults had been diagnosed with heart disease.
- One in 17 adults had been diagnosed with migraine headaches
- One in 18 adults aged over 45 years had been diagnosed with chronic obstructive pulmonary disease.
- One in 20 adults had been diagnosed with cancer.
- One in 40 adults had been diagnosed with a serious mental disorder
- One in 42 adults had been diagnosed with osteoporosis.

Adapted from: www.moh.govt.nz Ministry of Health. 2004. A Portrait of Health: Key results of the 2002/03 New Zealand Health Survey. Wellington: Ministry of Health.

plasma, causing a release of antidiuretic hormone from the hypothalamus, leading to increased reabsorption of water from the renal tubules, which adds to the rise in blood pressure. Angiotensin II itself also acts on the kidney tubules to promote reabsorption of water.

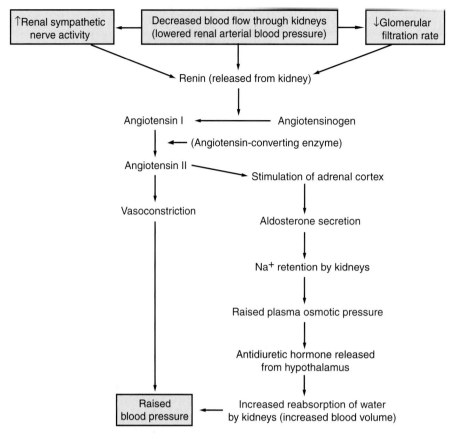

FIGURE 25-4 The renin–angiotensin–aldosterone system.

Excessive fluid retention is controlled by negative feedback mechanisms operating within this system so that fluid balance is restored to a normal level. Thus the renin–angiotensin–aldosterone system involves slow adjustments to changes in fluid volume. The kidneys are by far the most important organs in the body for long-term regulation of blood pressure. When the operation of the system fails, increased peripheral resistance and retention of fluid volume produce a combination of hypertensive effects, which keep blood pressure constantly elevated.

Knowledge of the normal mechanisms for blood pressure control has led to the development of drugs inhibiting the conversion of angiotensin I to angiotensin II, commonly known as ACE inhibitors, and drugs that block the action of angiotensin II on AT$_1$ (angiotensin II type I) receptors, the angiotensin-II-receptor antagonists.

Angiotensin-converting enzyme (ACE) inhibitors

ACE inhibitors competitively block the angiotensin-converting enzyme necessary for the conversion of angiotensin I to angiotensin II. Angiotensin II is a powerful vasoconstrictor that raises blood pressure and also causes aldosterone release,

DRUG INTERACTIONS 25-3 ACE inhibitors	
Drug	**Possible effect and management**
Diuretics	Concurrent administration with an ACE inhibitor may result in first-dose hypotension. Withhold diuretic for 24 hours before initiating ACE inhibitor therapy
General anaesthetics	Additive hypotensive effect. Monitor blood pressure
Lithium	Reduced excretion of lithium, with increased risk of toxicity. Monitor plasma lithium concentration and renal function
NSAIDs, including COX-2 inhibitors	Increased risk of hyperkalaemia and reduced hypotensive effect of ACE inhibitor. Avoid combined use
Potassium-sparing diuretics, potassium supplements	Closely monitor plasma electrolytes, especially potassium, because of the high risk of hyperkalaemia

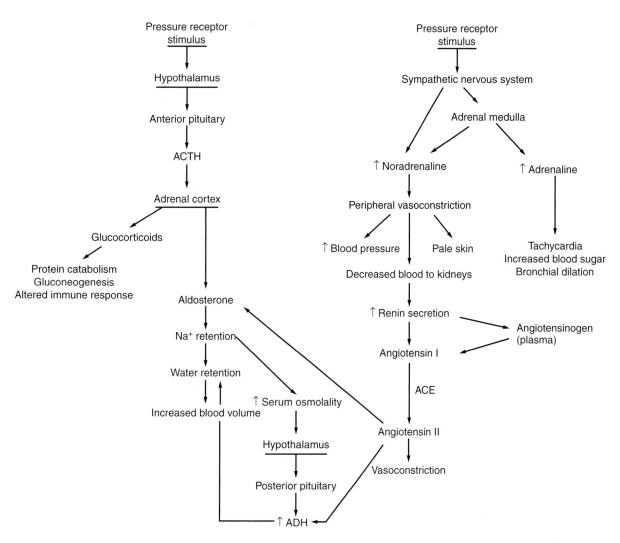

FIGURE 25-5 Control of blood pressure. Activation of the sympathetic nervous system causes increased release of noradrenaline, resulting in peripheral vasoconstriction and raised blood pressure. Increased release of adrenaline increases heart rate and the force of myocardial contractions, also resulting in elevation of blood pressure. Vasoconstriction results in increased blood supply to the kidneys, which activates the angiotensin system. Ultimately, the release of angiotensin II (a potent vasoconstrictor) results in an increase in aldosterone release from the adrenal cortex, an increase in release of antidiuretic hormone (ADH), and increased blood volume. (See the text for a description of mechanisms.)

TABLE 25-6 Pharmacokinetics and adult dosing of ACE inhibitors in hypertension

DRUG	ONSET OF ACTION (h)	DURATION OF EFFECT (h)	ACTIVE METABOLITE	ADULT DOSE RANGE (mg/day)*
Captopril	0.25–1	6–12	—	50–100
Enalapril	1	24	Enalaprilat	10–40
Fosinopril	≤1	24	Fosinpril diacid	10–40
Lisinopril	1	24	—	20–40
Perindopril	3–6	24	perindoprilat	2–8
Quinapril	≤1	≤24	Quinaprilat	10–40
Ramipril	1–2	24	Ramiprilat	2.5–10

*Oral doses titrated as needed and tolerated (AMH 2006).

DRUG MONOGRAPH 25–3 LOSARTAN

PHARMACOKINETICS (TABLE 25-7) Losartan is orally administered, with peak concentration occurring within 1 hour, while that of the active carboxylic acid metabolite occurs in 3–4 hours. The drug undergoes substantial first-pass metabolism in the liver and is metabolised by hepatic CYP2C9 and CYP3A4 (see Chapter 6) to at least six metabolites. The active carboxylic acid metabolite is 10–40 times more potent than the parent drug. The half-life of losartan is 2 hours, and for the carboxylic acid metabolite, between 6 and 9 hours. The duration of action is at least 24 hours, with metabolism in the liver and excretion in bile (around 60%) and urine (35%).

DRUG INTERACTIONS When losartan is administered with a diuretic, potentiation of the hypotensive effect may result. Usually, a lower losartan dose is necessary, with close monitoring. Drug interactions are similar to those of the ACE inhibitors.

ADVERSE REACTIONS These include headache, tiredness, back or muscle pain, diarrhoea, nasal congestion, dizziness and upper respiratory infection. Dry cough and insomnia are considered rare effects.

WARNINGS AND CONTRAINDICATIONS Use with caution in persons with kidney impairment. Use extreme caution if administering losartan to volume- or sodium-depleted individuals, as severe hypotension may result. Correct the deficiency first or start with a smaller drug dose. Avoid use in persons with losartan hypersensitivity, liver impairment or stenosis of the renal arteries, and in women contemplating pregnancy.

DOSAGE AND ADMINISTRATION The initial adult dose is 50 mg orally daily; the maintenance dose is 25–100 mg daily. With concurrent administration of diuretics, start at a dose of 25 mg once daily.

resulting in sodium and water retention (Figure 25-4). Inhibition of ACE results in:

- a decrease in vascular tone, thereby directly lowering blood pressure.
- inhibition of aldosterone release, reducing sodium and water reabsorption; the resultant excretion of fluid is thought to cause only a secondary reduction in blood pressure (decrease in aldosterone secretion does lead to a slight elevation in serum potassium)
- increase in plasma renin activity, caused by a loss of negative feedback on renin release.

Figure 25-5 illustrates the physiological control of blood pressure.

Captopril is the prototype drug of this class, which now also includes perindopril, enalapril, quinapril, fosinopril, ramipril, lisinopril and trandolapril.

INDICATIONS

ACE inhibitors are indicated for the treatment of hypertension, heart failure, diabetic nephropathy and left ventricular dysfunction, and after myocardial infarction. All drugs of this class demonstrate similar antihypertensive efficacies, and adverse reactions do not differ significantly among the individual ACE inhibitors. With the exception of captopril, most of these drugs maintain an antihypertensive effect for up to 24 hours, allowing once-daily dosing.

PHARMACOKINETICS (SEE TABLE 25-6)

DRUG INTERACTIONS

See the Drug Interactions table 25-3 for ACE inhibitors.

ADVERSE REACTIONS

These include headaches, diarrhoea, loss of taste, weakness, nausea, dizziness, hypotension, rash, fever and joint pain. The cough associated with ACE inhibitor use occurs in a significant number of people and is thought to be due to the inhibition by the ACE inhibitor of the enzyme that degrades bradykinin (see Clinical Interest Box 25-4).

WARNINGS AND CONTRAINDICATIONS

Use with caution in persons with SLE, scleroderma, bone marrow depression, cerebrovascular insufficiency, coronary

CLINICAL INTEREST BOX 25-4 ACE INHIBITOR COUGH

A well-known adverse effect of ACE inhibitors is a dry persistent cough that has been reported to occur in 5%–35% of individuals prescribed ACE inhibitors. Interestingly, this cough occurs more often in women, non-smokers and Chinese persons. The cough is not dose-dependent, can occur within hours of the first dose, may take weeks to months to develop, and normally resolves within 1–4 weeks of cessation of therapy. In a small number of individuals the cough may persist for 3 months after stopping the ACE inhibitor.

In general, it has been considered that the cough occurs as a consequence of inhibition of ACE, which is normally responsible for the metabolism of bradykinin (a vasodilator peptide) to inactive fragments. Inhibition of ACE results in accumulation of bradykinin and substance P, protussive mediators that sensitise airway nerves that produce a cough as a result of a tickling or scratching sensation in the throat (Dicpinigaitis 2006).

insufficiency, type 1 diabetes or liver function impairment (the last of these warnings is for all ACE inhibitors except for lisinopril and quinapril). Avoid use in persons with ACE inhibitor hypersensitivity, angio-oedema or hyperkalaemia and in renal artery stenosis, transplant or impairment. ACE inhibitors should be avoided in pregnancy because of their potential to produce a range of abnormalities (see Pregnancy Safety box at the end of this chapter).

Angiotensin-II-receptor antagonists

After the discovery of two subtypes of angiotensin II receptors, it was found that stimulation of the type 1 receptor (AT_1) mediated all the actions of angiotensin II. This meant a more precise target was available for blocking the vasoconstrictor effects of angiotensin II, rather than the broader effects (and possibly adverse effects) resulting from inhibition of ACE. The AT_1 receptor quickly became the target for the development of the new antihypertensive drugs called **angiotensin-II-receptor antagonists**. These agents, which include candesartan, eprosartan, irbesartan, losartan and telmisartan (see Table 25-7), block the receptors for angiotensin II; thus they inhibit vasoconstriction and the increase in aldosterone release but they have very little effect on plasma potassium concentration. In addition, they do not inhibit the breakdown of cough-producing bradykinin. Losartan is indicated for the treatment of hypertension and is considered the key drug in this category.

TABLE 25-7 Pharmacokinetics and adult dosing of angiotensin-II-receptor antagonists in hypertension

DRUG	BIOAVAILABILITY	TIME TO PEAK EFFECT (h)	HALF-LIFE (h)	ADULT DOSE RANGE (mg/day)*
Candesartan	15%	6–8	5–10	8–16
Irbesartan	60%	3–6	11–15	150–300
Losartan	14%	6	1.5–2 (parent) 4–9 (metabolite)	25–100
Telmisartan	40%	0.5–1	24	20–80

Adapted from: Robinson 2001.
*Once-daily dosing (AMH 2006).

PREGNANCY SAFETY

ADEC Category	Drug
A	Methyldopa
B1	Isosorbide dinitrate, oxpentifylline
B2	Glyceryl trinitrate, isosorbide mononitrate
B3	Clonidine, nicorandil
C	Amlodipine, diazoxide, diltiazem, felodipine, hydralazine, minoxidil, nifedipine, nimodipine, nitroprusside, verapamil
D	Candesartan, captopril, enalapril, fosinopril, irbesartan, lisinopril, losartan, perindopril, quinapril, ramipril, telmisartan, trandolapril
Unclassified	Hydroxyethylrutosides

DRUGS AT A GLANCE 25: Drugs affecting vascular smooth muscle

Therapeutic group	Pharmacological group	Key examples	Key pages
Antianginal drugs	Nitrates	glyceryl trinitrate	441–4
		isosorbide dinitrate	441
Antihypertensives	Calcium channel blockers	amlodipine	443–6
		diltiazem	443–6
		lercanidipine	446
		nifedipine	443–6
		verapamil	443–6
	Potassium-channel activators	diazoxide	447
		minoxidil	447–8
		nicorandil	446
	Vasodilators	hydralazine	439–49
		sodium nitroprusside	449
	Centrally acting antihypertensives	clonidine	451–2
		methyldopa	452
	ACE Inhibitors	captopril	454–7
		enalapril	455
		lisinopril	455
		ramipril	455
	Angiotensin II antagonists	candesartan	457
		irbesartan	457
		losartan	456

KEY POINTS

- Vasodilator drugs are used for the treatment of a range of disorders, including hypertension, angina, shock, cardiac failure and peripheral vascular conditions.
- Vasodilator drugs work by relaxing smooth muscle in the blood vessel walls. Some drugs act primarily on veins or arterioles, while others dilate both types of blood vessels.
- The main groups of direct-acting vasodilator drugs are the organic nitrates, calcium channel blockers and potassium channel activators.
- The indirect-acting vasodilators include the centrally acting adrenergic inhibitors, ACE inhibitors and angiotensin-II-receptor antagonists.
- The organic nitrates produce vasodilation through the production of nitric oxide and an increase in cGMP.
- At low doses, glyceryl trinitrate causes venodilation, reducing preload and stroke volume. Higher doses dilate arteries and the overall effect is a reduction in myocardial work and oxygen demand, hence their beneficial effect in angina.
- Calcium channel-blocking drugs block the inward movement of calcium ions through the slow channels of the cell membrane of cardiac and vascular smooth muscle cells.
- These drugs decrease the force of myocardial contraction (negative inotropic effect), decrease automaticity in the SA node and decrease conduction in the AV junction (negative chronotropic and negative dromotropic effects), and inhibit calcium ion influx in smooth muscle cells (reduction in peripheral vascular resistance).
- These drugs are very effective for the treatment of angina, hypertension and cardiac arrhythmias.
- Not all calcium channel blockers have equivalent therapeutic effects. Nifedipine is a potent peripheral vasodilator with minimal cardiac effects; therefore it is an effective antihypertensive agent. Nimodipine is indicated for the treatment of subarachnoid haemorrhage while the other calcium channel-blocking agents are used for their cardiovascular effects (antianginal, antiarrhythmic and antihypertensive).

- Drugs such as diazoxide, nicorandil and minoxidil relax smooth muscle by activating ATP-dependent potassium channels. They activate the potassium channel, antagonising the action of ATP and preventing closure of the channel. This results in hyperpolarisation and relaxation of the vascular smooth muscle.

- Diazoxide and minoxidil have limited use in the treatment of hypertension, while nicorandil is used for the treatment of angina.

- The main indirect-acting vasodilator drugs are the centrally acting drugs that inhibit sympathetic outflow, and inhibitors of the renin–angiotensin–aldosterone system.

- The centrally acting agents clonidine and methyldopa are effective antihypertensives, especially when combined with a diuretic. When given as the sole agent, clonidine and methyldopa usually cause sodium and water retention.

- ACE inhibitors such as captopril competitively block the angiotensin-converting enzyme necessary for the conversion of angiotensin I to angiotensin II. Angiotensin II is a powerful vasoconstrictor that raises blood pressure and also causes aldosterone release, resulting in sodium and water retention.

- ACE inhibitors are indicated for the treatment of hypertension, heart failure, diabetic nephropathy, left ventricular dysfunction, and after myocardial infarction. All drugs of this class demonstrate similar antihypertensive efficacy, and adverse reactions do not differ significantly among the individual ACE inhibitors.

- Angiotensin-II-receptor antagonists inhibit the action of angiotensin II, thereby preventing vasoconstriction, and are indicated for the treatment of hypertension.

- Five drug classes are used to treat hypertension. These include diuretics, β-blockers, ACE inhibitors, angiotensin-II-receptor antagonists and calcium channel blockers.

- Depending on an individual's response to therapy, combination drug therapies are often required for good control of hypertension. Such combinations are based on an understanding of the physiological control of blood pressure and the sites of action of the drugs used.

- Non-pharmacological management of hypertension includes lifestyle changes or modifications such as weight reduction, sodium restriction, elimination or limited consumption of alcohol and tobacco, reduction of dietary saturated fats and exercise.

REVIEW EXERCISES

1 Name and describe the three types of angina pectoris.

2 Glyceryl trinitrate sublingual tablets were prescribed for Mr Jones, with instructions to place one tablet under the tongue and repeat at 5-minute intervals if necessary, for a total of three doses. What additional instructions should be given to Mr Jones about the use of this product?

3 Why are calcium channel-blocking drugs effective antihypertensive agents?

4 What advice would you give an elderly person with a prescription for a calcium channel-blocking drug to reduce the potential for adverse reactions?

5 Discuss the action, metabolism and the main toxicity associated with the use of nitroprusside.

6 Why were drugs developed to target the renin–angiotensin–aldosterone system?

7 Why do about 20% of persons prescribed ACE inhibitors develop a cough?

8 Describe the pharmacological effects of two antihypertensives from different drug classes (e.g. a diuretic and a β-blocking agent, or a diuretic and a calcium antagonist). What is the purpose of combining antihypertensive drugs?

REFERENCES AND FURTHER READING

Australian Institute of Health and Welfare. *Australia's Health 2004*. Canberra: AIHW, 2004.

Australian Medicines Handbook 2006. Adelaide: AMH, 2006.

Dicpinigaitis PV. Angiotensin-converting enzyme inhibitor-induced cough. *Chest* 2006; 129(1): Suppl 169S–173S.

Hoffman BB. Catecholamines, sympathomimetic drugs, and adrenergic receptor antagonists. Ch. 10 in: Hardman JG, Limbird E, Gilman AG (eds). *Goodman & Gilman's The Pharmacological Basis of Therapeutics*. 10th edn. New York: McGraw Hill, 2001.

Johnson CI. Angiotensin receptor antagonists for the treatment of hypertension. *Australian Prescriber* 1998; 21: 95–7.

Kerins DH, Robertson RM, Robertson D. Drugs used for the treatment of myocardial ischaemia. Ch. 32 in: Hardman JG, Limbird E, Gilman AG (eds). *Goodman & Gilman's The Pharmacological Basis of Therapeutics*. 10th edn. New York: McGraw Hill, 2001.

Oates JA, Brown NJ. Antihypertensive agents and the drug therapy of hypertension. Ch. 33 in: Hardman JG, Limbird E, Gilman AG (eds). *Goodman & Gilman's The Pharmacological Basis of Therapeutics*. 10th edn. New York: McGraw-Hill, 2001.

Quinn DI, Day RO. Guide to clinically more important drug interactions. Ch. 1 Appendix B in: Speight TM, Holford NHG (eds). *Avery's Drug Treatment*. 4th edn. Auckland: Adis International, 1997.

Rang HP, Dale MM, Ritter JM, Moore PK. *Pharmacology*. 5th edn. Edinburgh: Churchill Livingstone, 2003 [ch. 8].

Robinson M. Angiotensin receptor antagonists for hypertension. *Australian Pharmacy Trade* 2001; 14 June: 14–18.

Unstable Angina Writing Group. Management of Unstable Angina Guidelines–2000. *Medical Journal of Australia* 2000; 173: Suppl. S65–S88.

ON-LINE RESOURCES

Hypertension Management Guide for Doctors 2004. Heart Foundation Website [Online]. Available: http://www.heartfoundation.com.au/index.cfm?page=36

The assessment and management of cardiovascular risk 2003. New Zealand Guidelines Group (NZGG), 2003. New Zealand Guidelines Group Website [Online]. Available: http://www.nzgg.org.nz

National Heart Foundation of Australia: www.heartfoundation.com.au

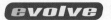 More weblinks at http://evolve.elsevier.com/AU/Bryant/pharmacology/

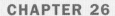

CHAPTER 26

Lipid-lowering Drugs

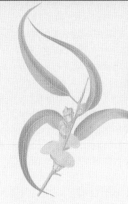

CHAPTER FOCUS

Dyslipidaemia, or increased plasma concentrations
of cholesterol and triglycerides in the body, has
been clinically associated with atherosclerosis.
Atherosclerosis is a disorder of the arteries that is
characterised by cholesterol deposits in the lining
of the blood vessels, which eventually produce
degenerative changes and obstruct blood flow.
Atherosclerosis can result in angina, heart failure,
myocardial infarction, cerebral artery disease and renal
artery insufficiency. It is also a factor in hypertension.
The treatment guidelines for the management of
dyslipidaemia include dietary and lifestyle modifications
and drug treatment. The main classes of lipid-lowering
drugs are the 'statins', bile acid-binding resins and
fibrates.

OBJECTIVES

- To describe the three main classes of lipoproteins (VLDL, LDL and HDL) and discuss their functions.

- To discuss the current management strategies for treating dyslipidaemia.

- To name the three main classes of lipid-lowering drugs and describe their principal indications.

- To explain why the HMG-CoA reductase inhibitors are the most effective drugs for lowering plasma LDL-cholesterol concentration.

- To explain why HMG-CoA reductase inhibitors and bile acid-binding resins are subject to numerous drug interactions.

KEY DRUGS

simvastatin
cholestyramine
gemfibrozil

KEY TERMS

apolipoproteins
atherosclerosis
chylomicrons
dyslipidaemia
high-density lipoproteins
HMG-CoA reductase
lipoprotein lipase
lipoproteins
low-density lipoproteins
very-low-density lipoproteins

KEY ABBREVIATIONS

CAD	coronary artery disease
HDL	high-density lipoproteins
HMG-CoA	3-hydroxy-3-methylglutaryl coenzyme A
IDL	intermediate-density lipoproteins
LDL	low-density lipoproteins
VLDL	very-low-density lipoproteins

DYSLIPIDAEMIA

DYSLIPIDAEMIA is a metabolic disorder characterised by increased concentrations of lipids and lipoproteins. Lipid-lowering drugs are used along with dietary modifications to treat dyslipidaemia. Clinical and experimental studies have provided evidence of an important relation between high levels of circulating triglycerides and cholesterol and **atherosclerosis**. Atherosclerosis, a disorder that involves large- and medium-sized arteries, is characterised by cholesterol deposits in the arterial wall, which eventually produce degenerative changes and obstruct blood flow.

Atherosclerosis is a causative factor in coronary artery disease (CAD), which can result in angina, heart failure and myocardial infarction; cerebral arterial disease that results in senility or cerebrovascular accidents; peripheral arterial occlusive disease, which can cause gangrene and loss of limb; and renal arterial insufficiency. It is also a factor in hypertension. Intensive research to develop effective and safer lipid-lowering drugs is ongoing.

Lipids do not circulate freely in the bloodstream. Instead, they are transported as complexes called **lipoproteins**. Lipoproteins are composed of an interior core, consisting of cholesteryl esters and triglycerides, that is covered by a layer of phospholipids, free cholesterol and apolipoproteins. Hyperlipoproteinaemias are always associated with an increased concentration of one or more lipoproteins.

Classification of lipoproteins

The three primary lipoproteins found in the blood of fasting individuals are **very-low-density lipoproteins** (VLDLs), **low-density lipoproteins** (LDLs), and **high-density lipoproteins** (HDLs). The intermediate-density lipoproteins (IDLs) have short half-lives (minutes to a few hours) and their concentrations in plasma tend to be very low (Table 26-1).

VLDLs contain a large amount of triglyceride (50%–65%) and 20%–30% cholesterol, and are formed in the liver from endogenously synthesised triglycerides, cholesterol and phospholipid. These lipoproteins contain 15%–20% of the total blood cholesterol and most of the triglyceride found in the body (McKenney 1995). Because these particles are quite large, they are not thought to be involved in atherosclerosis.

After VLDL particles are secreted from the liver into the circulation, their triglyceride content is released as a result of the action of the enzyme **lipoprotein lipase**, which is located in the endothelium of adipose and muscle tissue capillaries. Drugs that enhance the action of lipoprotein lipase will lower plasma triglyceride levels. VLDL minus its triglyceride content becomes IDL, which is either returned to the liver or converted to the cholesterol-rich lipoprotein LDL, which contains 60%–70% of total blood cholesterol. The quantity and density of systemic LDL particles correlates with the risk of atherosclerosis, and elevated LDL levels suggest that an individual has a greater potential for developing atherosclerosis.

HDLs are the smallest and most dense lipoproteins. Their function is to transfer cholesterol from peripheral cells to the liver either directly or after transferring to LDL and VLDL. The LDL particles are cleared from plasma by LDL receptors principally in the liver, and the level of hepatic LDL receptors generally controls the level of circulating LDL in humans. High levels of HDL are considered beneficial and they counteract the atherogenic effects of LDL. This transport mechanism prevents the accumulation of cholesterol in the arterial walls, thereby providing protection against the development of atherosclerosis.

Chylomicrons are large particles that transport dietary cholesterol and fatty acids absorbed from the gastrointestinal tract to the liver. This is known as the exogenous pathway of lipid transport, whereas the lipoproteins transporting cholesterol between the liver and peripheral cells are part of the endogenous pathway. Chylomicrons consist mainly of triglycerides (85%–95%), and are produced in the small intestine during absorption of a fatty meal. They are cleared from the bloodstream by lipoprotein lipase after 12–14 hours. The chylomicron that remains following the removal of the triglyceride content is cleared rapidly by the liver and is not converted into LDL.

TABLE 26-1 Lipoproteins: core lipids and lipid transported

LIPOPROTEINS	CORE LIPID	LIPID TRANSPORTED
Chylomicrons/chylomicron remnants	Dietary triglycerides	Dietary triglyceride
VLDL	Endogenous triglyceride	Endogenous triglyceride
IDL	Endogenous cholesteryl esters and triglycerides	Endogenous cholesterol
LDL	Endogenous cholesteryl esters	Endogenous cholesterol
HDL	Endogenous cholesteryl esters	Endogenous cholesterol from periphery

Apolipoproteins

Lipoproteins contain proteins on their surface called **apolipoproteins**. These proteins have a variety of functions: they serve as ligands for cell receptors, activate enzymes involved in lipoprotein metabolism and provide structure for the lipoprotein. If apolipoprotein metabolism is impaired, an increased risk of atherosclerosis exists; thus blood levels of apolipoproteins are important in evaluating lipid disorders. The clinically important apolipoproteins are A-I, A-II, B-100, C-II and E. Apolipoprotein A-I is thought to confer

the beneficial effect of HDL; HDL particles containing A-I alone correlate with a lower risk of coronary heart disease than HDL particles that have both A-I and A-II (McKenney 1995). In contrast, a deficiency of the C-II apolipoprotein in VLDL particles results in impaired triglyceride metabolism and hypertriglyceridaemia.

Figure 26-1 illustrates the normal lipid transport system and indicates the sites of action of the lipid-lowering drugs discussed in the following sections. Dietary fats and cholesterol consumed are transported into the system as

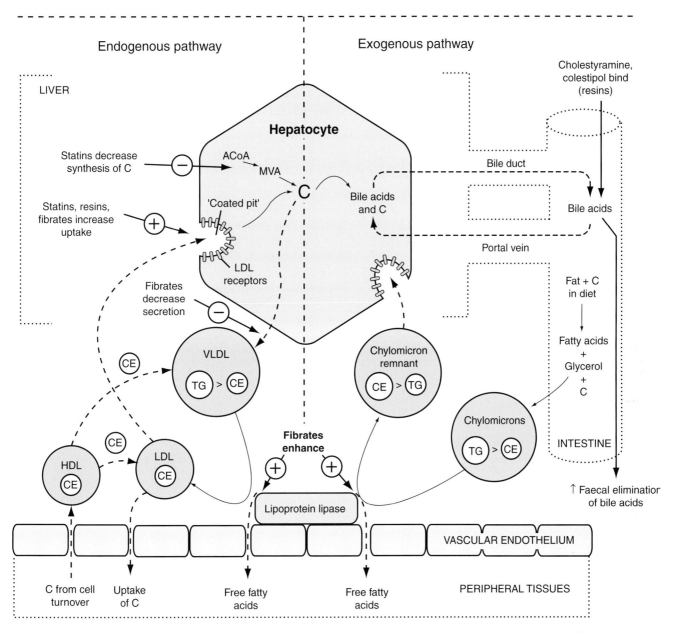

FIGURE 26-1 Schematic diagram of cholesterol transport in the tissues, with sites of action of the main drugs affecting lipoprotein metabolism. C = cholesterol; CE = cholesteryl ester; TG = triglyceride; MVA = mevalonate; HMG-CoA reductase = 3-hydroxy-3-methyl-glutaryl-CoA reductase; VLDL = very-low-density lipoprotein; LDL = low-density lipoprotein; HDL = high-density lipoprotein. *Source*: Rang, Dale, Ritter & Moore 2003. Reproduced with permission.

chylomicrons via the exogenous pathway. In the endogenous pathway the liver synthesises cholesterol and triglycerides, which are transported from the liver to peripheral tissues as VLDL particles. The function of HDL is to carry about 25% of plasma cholesterol from the periphery back to the liver, where it is processed into bile acids. Because the cholesterol HDL carries is ultimately for excretion, it is known as 'good' cholesterol. In contrast, LDL carries more than 50% by weight of cholesterol and its relation with the development of atherosclerosis has resulted in its label of 'bad' cholesterol.

Plasma lipoproteins are usually in a state of dynamic equilibrium. When the liver and tissues outside the liver need cholesterol they increase the synthesis of LDL receptors on their respective cell surfaces (Figure 26-1). These receptors are necessary for the binding of LDL, thus enabling the release of free fatty acids. When the cellular need for cholesterol is met, the synthesis of LDL receptors decreases, and so controls the plasma level of LDL. Modulation of the number of hepatic LDL receptors is an integral part of the therapeutic approach to the management of hypercholesterolaemia.

Hyperlipoproteinaemias

Dyslipidaemias can be classed as primary or secondary. The primary, or genetically determined, hyperlipoproteinaemia forms are classified into six phenotypes, depending on

TABLE 26-2 Frederickson/World Health Organization (WHO) classification of hyperlipoproteinaemia

PHENOTYPE	DISORDER	LIPOPROTEIN ELEVATED	LIPIDS ELEVATED
I	Familial lipoprotein lipase deficiency	Chylomicrons	Triglycerides
IIa	Familial hypercholesterolaemia	LDL	Cholesterol
IIb	Familial combined hyperlipidaemia	LDL + VLDL	Triglycerides + Cholesterol
III	Familial dysbetalipoproteinaemia	Chylomicron remnants + IDL	Triglycerides + Cholesterol
IV	Familial hypertriglyceridaemia	VLDL	Triglycerides
V	Severe hypertriglyceridaemia	Chylomicron remnants + VLDL	Triglycerides

TABLE 23-3 Effects of drugs on plasma lipid profile

DRUG	EFFECT ON LIPIDS*		
	LDL-cholesterol	HDL-cholesterol	Triglycerides
Alcohol	No change	–	↑
β-blockers			
Non-selective	No change	↓	↑
Selective	No change	↓	↑
Corticosteroids	↑	–	↑
Cyclosporin	↑	–	↑
Diuretics			
Thiazides	↑	↑	↑
Loop	No change	↓	No change
Oral contraceptives			
Monophasics	↑	↑/↓	↑
Triphasics	↑	↑	↑

Source: McKenny 1995.
*↑ = increased; ↓ = decreased; – = unknown.

the lipoprotein particle elevated (Table 26-2). Factors such as diabetes mellitus, obesity, hypothyroidism, nephrotic syndrome, excess alcohol consumption and drug treatment (Table 26-3) constitute the secondary causes of dyslipidaemia. In these cases, investigation of underlying disease pathology or current drug treatment is necessary before instituting lipid-lowering drug therapy.

MANAGEMENT STRATEGIES FOR DYSLIPIDAEMIA
Dietary modification

Dietary modification is important in the treatment of high LDL-cholesterol levels. The Heart Foundation's Lipid Management Guidelines 2001 recommend a dietary model based on the consumption of "cereals, vegetables and fruit, with regular intake of fish, legumes and nuts, margarine spreads, a combination of oils, lean meat and skinless chicken and low-fat milk and yoghurt. Intakes of full-fat dairy products such as cheese and ice cream should be limited to twice a week, and takeaways, snacks and cakes each limited to once a week". Currently in Australia, a 6-week period of dietary modification is required before a person is eligible for subsidised drugs available through the Pharmaceutical Benefits Scheme (PBS). If dietary changes are ineffective, drug therapy is usually instituted.

Treatment guidelines

Treatment recommendations are based on a person's cholesterol level and the presence of pre-existing ischaemic heart disease or two other risk factors, such as current cigarette smoking, hypertension, a family history of myocardial infarction or sudden death before age 55 in father or other male first-degree relatives or before age 65 in mother or other female first-degree relatives, and diabetes mellitus. Identification of higher-risk individuals can be aided by tools such as the Sheffield tables (Moulds 1998) and the Australian Pharmaceutical Benefits Scheme (PBS) guidelines (Table 26-4). The Australian PBS guidelines have been developed from data on levels of risk and controlled clinical trials.

In the absence of satisfactory reduction of high plasma lipid levels through exercise, diet and lifestyle modification, lipid-lowering drugs offer health-care professionals a management strategy for the treatment of dyslipidaemia. This is of proven benefit in individuals with high cardiovascular risk factors. The main classes of drugs used are:

- inhibitors of **3-hydroxy-3-methylglutaryl coenzyme A** (HMG-CoA) **reductase** (commonly referred to as 'statins')
- bile acid-binding resins
- fibrates
- additional agents, including nicotinic acid and fish oil (see Clinical Interest Box 26-2) and the new drug ezetimibe.

The choice of drug depends on the individual's plasma lipid profile and whether the aim is to reduce the level of LDL-cholesterol (hypercholesterolaemia) or triglyceride (hypertriglyceridaemia), or both LDL-cholesterol and triglyceride (hyperlipidaemia). Table 26-5 provides an indication of the current drug treatment of dyslipidaemia.

TABLE 26-4 Australian PBS Guidelines for subsidy of lipid-lowering drugs	
CRITERIA	**LIPID CONCENTRATION**
Existing coronary heart disease	Total cholesterol >4 mmol/L
Others at high risk plus one or more of the following additional risk factors: diabetes mellitus, familial hypercholesterolaemia, family history of coronary heart disease, hypertension, peripheral vascular disease	Total cholesterol >6.5 mmol/L or Total cholesterol >5.5 mmol/L and HDL <1 mmol/L
People with HDL <1 mmol/L	Total cholesterol >6.5 mmol/L
Men aged 35–75 years	Total cholesterol >7.5 mmol/L or Triglyceride >4 mmol/L
Others not eligible in categories above	Total cholesterol >9 mmol/L or Triglyceride >8 mmol/L

Source: Schedule of Pharmaceutical Benefits 2005.

There is substantial interest in the use of plant sterols as a component of dietary management of people with hyper-lipidaemia. Plant sterols such as sitosterol are similar in structure to cholesterol and, although minimally absorbed, they compete with cholesterol for incorporation into micelles in the gastrointestinal tract. This results in less absorption of cholesterol. In turn, this stimulates hepatic LDL receptor formation, increasing uptake of LDL and so lowering the plasma cholesterol level. Plant sterols have been incorporated into margarine and mayonnaise. A daily intake of 2–3 g reduces LDL cholesterol by 5%–10%, but there is evidence that absorption of dietary carotenoids might be impaired. Toxicity appears not to be an issue in the short term, but long-term safety studies have yet to be undertaken.
Source: Heart Foundation of Australia, Guidelines & Publications: www.heartfoundation.com.au/

Evidence exists that consumption of omega-3 fatty acids found in fish and fish oil reduces the incidence of ischaemic heart disease and sudden death from myocardial infarction, and prolongs the life of myocardial infarction survivors. The consumption of omega-3 fatty acids by humans has decreased as a result of the increased consumption of commercial livestock, which have lower levels of omega-3 fatty acids than their wild or free-range counterparts (Horrocks & Yeo 1999). One of the active components of fish oil is docosahexaenoic acid (DHA), which is present in oily fish such as mackerel, salmon and tuna. Consumption of a fish-rich diet is thought to account for the lower incidence of coronary heart disease in the Japanese and in Greenland Eskimos. In a recent trial, subjects treated with simvastatin but with persistent hypertriglyceridaemia were additionally prescribed fish oil (2 g twice daily) for 1 year. A significant reduction was observed in plasma triglycerides (20%–30%) and VLDL-cholesterol (30%–40%) (Durrington et al 2001). Fish oil can be added to a lipid-lowering drug regimen but a daily dose of at least 2 g is required (Table 26-5). As the content of fatty acids varies among formulations, the dosage of omega-3 fatty acids must be calculated for each individual product. Common products include Blackmores Fish Oil, Maxepa and Nature's Way Omega 3.

HMG-CoA reductase inhibitors

These agents, also known as 'statins', include atorvastatin, fluvastatin, pravastatin and simvastatin. They are competitive inhibitors of **HMG-CoA reductase**, the rate-limiting enzyme necessary for cholesterol biosynthesis (Figure 26-1), and were introduced into clinical practice in the 1980s. **Simvastatin** and pravastatin are fungal metabolites; the others are produced synthetically. These drugs are particularly effective, lowering total cholesterol by 10%–45% and raising HDL by 2%–13%. The decrease in cholesterol production in the liver leads to increased expression of hepatic LDL receptors, resulting in a greater clearance of LDL-cholesterol from the circulation. A modest increase also occurs in HDL and a slight reduction in plasma triglycerides. The widespread use of these drugs world-wide is attributable to their proven efficacy in randomised clinical trials in reducing CAD, angina, strokes and the need for angioplasty and coronary artery bypass grafts.

In addition to beneficial effects on lipid profiles, the statins have a number of other 'antiatherosclerotic' properties (Corsini et al 1999). These include:

- beneficial effects on endothelial function
- modification of inflammatory responses
- reduced platelet aggregability
- modification of thrombus formation
- stabilisation of atherosclerotic plaques
- decreased smooth muscle cell migration and proliferation
- increased fibrinolytic activity.

Clearly these antiatheromatous actions may contribute to the overall beneficial effects observed with statin therapy.

HMG-CoA reductase inhibitors are indicated for the treatment of primary hypercholesterolaemia (types IIa and IIb) caused by an elevated LDL-cholesterol level that is not controlled by diet or other treatment measures. Atorvastatin, fluvastatin and pravastatin are administered as the active drug, whereas simvastatin is administered as a prodrug that requires metabolic activation by the liver. With the exception of fluvastatin, which is metabolised by CYP2C9, the drugs are metabolised by CYP3A4. The predominant route of excretion is via the faeces, with renal excretion accounting for <2% with atorvastatin, 6% with fluvastatin and 47% with pravastatin. An initial response is seen within 1–2 weeks, and the maximum therapeutic response occurs within 4–6 weeks of chronic drug administration. Bile acid-binding resins can impede absorption, so statins should be administered either 1 hour before or 4 hours after administration of the resin.

Significant drug interactions occur with antibiotics, antifungal drugs, HIV-protease inhibitors and cyclosporin (see Drug Monograph 26-1). An increased risk of rhabdomyolysis (necrosis of skeletal muscle with the release of myoglobulin) and acute renal failure may occur. Grapefruit juice should be avoided if taking atorvastatin or simvastatin because grapefruit juice inhibits metabolism of both of these statins. Inhibition of metabolism leads to an increased plasma drug concentration and the likelihood of adverse effects.

Although the agents are well tolerated, adverse reactions include stomach cramps or pain, rash, constipation or diarrhoea, nausea, headaches, myalgia and, rarely, myopathy,

TABLE 26-5 Current drug treatment of dyslipidaemia

DISORDER	LIPID-LOWERING DRUGS
Hypercholesterolaemia	Statin, bile acid-binding resin, nicotinic acid, ezetimibe, fibrate
Hypertriglyceridaemia	Fibrate, fish oil, nicotinic acid
Combined hyperlipidaemia	Statin, fibrate, nicotinic acid

Source: AMH 2006.

DRUG MONOGRAPH 26-1 SIMVASTATIN

Simvastatin is a semisynthetic analogue of lovastatin (not available in Australia). It was originally isolated from cultures of *Aspergillus terreus*. Administered as a prodrug, simvastatin is metabolised in vivo to a hydroxy acid known as simvastatin acid, which is the active form of the drug that inhibits HMG-CoA reductase.

INDICATIONS Simvastatin is indicated for the treatment of hypercholesterolaemia and mixed hyperlipidaemia.

PHARMACOKINETICS Simvastatin is well absorbed and undergoes extensive first-pass metabolism in the liver by cytochrome P450 3A4 (CYP3A4). Availability of the active drug to the general circulation is low and the metabolites are excreted in the bile. The plasma half-life is 1–2 hours. Renal excretion accounts for about 13% of the absorbed dose.

DRUG INTERACTIONS Inhibitors of CYP3A4, such as antibiotics (clarithromycin, erythromycin), antifungal drugs (fluconazole, itraconazole, ketoconazole), cyclosporin, verapamil and grapefruit juice, all elevate the plasma drug concentration. In contrast, inducers of CYP3A4, which include barbiturates, carbamazepine, phenytoin and griseofulvin, all lower the plasma drug concentration.

WARNINGS AND CONTRAINDICATIONS Use of simvastatin is contraindicated in conditions of pre-existing liver or renal impairment, in women of childbearing age unless adequate contraceptive cover is assured (ADEC Category C), in people with severe intercurrent illness (infection, trauma), or prior to major surgery.

ADVERSE REACTIONS Common adverse reactions include gastrointestinal discomfort, headaches, insomnia and dizziness. An elevation of hepatic transaminase levels can occur within the first few weeks of treatment. Of a more serious nature is the potential for the development of myopathy (muscle pain with elevated creatine kinase concentration), which can progress to rhabdomyolysis (muscle breakdown) and renal failure. The latter is more likely when the statins are combined with inhibitors of CYP3A4, but an increased incidence has also been observed in combination with the fibrate class of lipid-lowering drugs and nicotinic acid.

DOSAGE AND ADMINISTRATION As cholesterol synthesis is highest at night, simvastatin is best administered in the evening or at bedtime. The initial dose is 10 mg, increasing to a maximum of 80 mg daily. Effectiveness of the dose is determined by monitoring plasma lipids.

rhabdomyolysis, alopecia, impotence, gynaecomastia, anaphylaxis and angio-oedema. Muscle pain or weakness, severe tiredness or flu-like symptoms should be reported to the treating physician. Overall, long-term safety data with these drugs are limited. Use with caution in situations of impaired hepatic and renal function. Avoid use in people with hypersensitivity to any HMG-CoA reductase inhibitor, organ transplant recipients receiving immunosuppressant drugs, and people with any disease state or condition that may predispose them to renal failure.

The recommended adult dose for atorvastatin is 10 mg daily, titrated monthly as needed (range 10–80 mg/day), and for fluvastatin 20 mg daily in the evening with or after food, titrated monthly as necessary (range 20–40 mg/day). The pravastatin adult dose is 10–20 mg at bedtime, with dosage

adjustments at monthly intervals as needed (to a maximum of 80 mg daily). The simvastatin adult dose is 10 mg in the evening, titrated monthly as necessary to a maximum dose of 80 mg/day.

Bile acid-binding resins

Cholestyramine and colestipol are non-absorbable anion-exchange resins, also called bile acid sequestrants. These drugs are used for their cholesterol-lowering effects. Cholesterol is the major precursor of bile acids, which are secreted from the gallbladder into the small intestine. Bile acids perform two functions in the small intestine: they emulsify fat from food to facilitate chemical digestion, and they are required for absorption of lipids (including fat-soluble vitamins, A, D, E

DRUG INTERACTIONS 26-1
Bile acid-binding resins

Drug	Possible effect and management
Warfarin, or phenindione	Concurrent use significantly decreases absorption of oral anticoagulants and vitamin K; thus the anticoagulant effect might be reduced or enhanced, respectively. It is suggested that oral anticoagulants be given 6 hours before these drugs. Also, monitor international normalised ratio (INR) of prothrombin time and adjust dose as necessary
Digoxin	Reduced absorption occurs. It is recommended that drugs be administered at least 1 hour before or 4–6 hours after administration of resin
Thiazides, frusemide, phenobarbitone, propranolol, benzylpenicillin or tetracyclines	Decreased absorption of these orally administered drugs has been reported. Give several hours before or at least 4 hours after cholestyramine or colestipol
Thyroxine	Decreased absorption of thyroxine. Give thyroxine first and then give cholestyramine or colestipol several hours later

and K). Bile acids are returned to the liver via enterohepatic recirculation.

The anion-exchange resins bind bile acids in the intestine, thereby decreasing absorption of exogenous cholesterol. To compensate for the loss of bile acids removed by the resins and excreted in the faeces, the liver increases the rate of endogenous metabolism of cholesterol into bile acids and increases the expression of hepatic LDL receptors, and hence uptake of LDL-cholesterol from plasma. Long-term increased faecal loss of bile acids causes a reduction of plasma cholesterol concentration that is blunted by the increased synthesis of cholesterol by the liver. An increase in plasma triglycerides limits the use of bile acid-binding resins in people with hypertriglyceridaemia. These drugs used to be the mainstay of lipid-lowering therapy but are now principally used as adjunct therapy to the statins.

Both cholestyramine and colestipol are used in treatment of hypercholesterolaemia and mixed hyperlipidaemia. They are also used to treat pruritus induced by bile acid deposits in dermal tissues (from partial biliary obstruction) and for diarrhoea following ileal resection.

Plasma cholesterol levels usually decrease within 1–2 weeks but in some individuals may increase or exceed previous levels with continued therapy. With cholestyramine, plasma cholesterol levels may continue to fall for up to 1 year. After withdrawal of colestipol and cholestyramine, plasma cholesterol levels tend to rise in around 2–4 weeks. Pruritus will return in about 1–2 weeks after discontinuation of the drugs. Close monitoring for effectiveness is necessary.

The bile acid-binding resins are not absorbed from the gastrointestinal tract and hence there are no major systemic effects. They bind bile acids in the intestine and are excreted via the faeces. See the Drug Interactions table 26-1 for bile acid-binding resins.

Adverse reactions include constipation, indigestion, abdominal pain, nausea, vomiting, flatulence, dizziness, headache and, rarely, gallstones, pancreatitis, bleeding ulcers, and malabsorption syndrome. Use bile acid-binding resins with caution in people with gallstones, hypothyroidism, haemorrhoids, kidney disease or bleeding disorders. Avoid use in people with cholestyramine or colestipol hypersensitivity, biliary obstruction or constipation. Cholestyramine is contraindicated in the presence of phenylketonuria because of the presence of aspartame in the product (aspartame is metabolised to phenylalanine). Safety in pregnancy has not been established.

The adult dose of cholestyramine is 4 g once or twice daily before meals; the maintenance dose is 12–16 g daily in 2–3 divided doses. The colestipol adult dose is 15–30 g daily before meals in 2–4 divided doses. When used in combination with other lipid-lowering drugs, the doses are 4 g for cholestyramine and 5 g for colestipol, once or twice daily.

Additional lipid-lowering drugs

Several additional drugs are discussed below, and a comparison of their lipid-lowering effects is shown in Table 26-6.

Fibrates

Although several fibric acid derivatives are available overseas (e.g. bezafibrate, ciprofibrate, clofibrate, fenofibrate and gemfibrozil), only fenofibrate and **gemfibrozil** are available in Australia (see Drug Monograph 26-2). The results of several large studies have raised specific concerns regarding the use of clofibrate. First, there is the possibility of an increased risk of inducing malignancy and cholelithiasis in humans with the use of this product. Individuals taking clofibrate had twice the risk for cholelithiasis and cholecystitis requiring surgery of non-users. Second, there is no evidence of reduced cardiovascular mortality with its use. In fact, studies reported an increase in cardiac arrhythmias, angina and thromboembolic episodes. The clinical use of clofibrate has consequently declined tremendously.

Gemfibrozil and fenofibrate are more effective in reducing VLDL that is rich in triglycerides than in lowering LDL that is high in cholesterol.

One study (Rubins et al 1999) has suggested that the increase in HDL observed with gemfibrozil reduces the incidence of coronary disease and stroke. In a follow-up period of 5 years, a reduction of 22% was observed in cardiac events (either fatal or non-fatal myocardial infarction). In contrast, the FIELD study (2005) found that fenofibrate did not reduce the risk of coronary events in people with type 2 diabetes. The mechanism of action is not completely understood, but fibrates enhance the action of lipoprotein lipase (increasing hydrolysis of triglycerides), upregulate the expression of LDL-cholesterol genes and cause variable effects on the expression of apolipoprotein genes. These drugs are indicated principally for the treatment of severe hypertriglyceridaemia, mixed hyperlipidaemia and as second-line treatment for hypercholesterolaemia.

TABLE 26-6 Comparison of lipid-lowering effects

DRUG	EFFECT ON LIPIDS*		EFFECT ON LIPOPROTEINS			TYPICAL RESPONSE
	Cholesterol	Triglycerides	VLDL	LDL	HDL	
Cholestyramine	↓	0 or slight ↑	0 or ↑	↓	0 or ↑	Decreases cholesterol 20%–40%
Colestipol	↓	0 or slight ↑	↑	↓	0 or ↑	Decreases cholesterol 20%–40%
Ezetimibe	↓	↓	–	↓	0 or ↑	Decreases cholesterol 10%–18%
Fenofibrate	↓	↓	↓	↓ or ↑	↑	Significantly lowers triglycerides 20%–50%
Gemfibrozi	↓	↓	↓	↓ or ↑	↑	Decreases triglycerides; only slight decrease in cholesterol; increases HDL
Nicotinic acid	↓	↓	↓	↓	↑	Decreases triglycerides (40%–80%) and cholesterol 10%–20%
Simvastatin	↓	↓	↓	↓	↑	Decreases cholesterol 30%–50%

* ↑ = increase; ↓ = decrease; 0 = no change

DRUG MONOGRAPH 26-2 GEMFIBROZIL

Gemfibrozil primarily decreases plasma triglycerides found in VLDL and moderately increases HDL. The mechanism of this action has not been established, but it may involve an inhibition of peripheral lipolysis and a decrease in hepatic extraction of free fatty acids, resulting in reduction of triglyceride production. In addition, the drug may accelerate turnover and removal of cholesterol from the liver, to be excreted in the faeces.

PHARMACOKINETICS Gemfibrozil is well absorbed from the gastrointestinal tract and reaches peak levels in 1–2 hours. Its onset of action in reducing plasma VLDL levels occurs within 2–5 days, with the peak effect seen in 4 weeks. It is metabolised in the liver with glucuronide conjugates, accounting for around 70% of the metabolites excreted by the kidneys. A small proportion (2%) is excreted as unchanged drug and 6% is eliminated via the faeces.

DRUG INTERACTIONS When gemfibrozil is administered with warfarin or phenindione, an increased anticoagulant effect is reported. Monitor INR closely because the anticoagulant dose may need to be decreased significantly. If administered with HMG-CoA reductase inhibitors, an increased risk of rhabdomyolysis, myoglobinuria and acute renal failure can occur. This has been reported within 3 weeks to several months of combined drug therapy, and concurrent drug administration should be avoided.

ADVERSE REACTIONS These include muscle aches and cramps, nausea, vomiting, rash, diarrhoea, flatulence and abdominal distress.

WARNINGS AND CONTRAINDICATIONS Use with caution in people with gallstones or gallbladder disease. Avoid use in people with gemfibrozil hypersensitivity, liver or kidney disease, and especially primary biliary cirrhosis.

DOSAGE AND ADMINISTRATION The adult dose is 1.2 g daily in two divided doses, preferably 30 minutes before food.

Nicotinic acid

The lipid-lowering effect of nicotinic acid (niacin) has been known since 1955. Nicotinic acid is a water-soluble vitamin that inhibits mobilisation of free fatty acids from peripheral tissue. This results in a reduction in the hepatic synthesis of triglycerides and the secretion of VLDL. Nicotinic acid also increases plasma HDL concentration markedly (20%–30%). It is used principally as an adjunct to other therapies such as the fibrates and bile acid-binding resins in the treatment of severe and mixed hypertriglyceridaemia. It is also used to treat niacin (vitamin B_3) deficiency and, because it increases blood flow through skin and muscle, it is used to treat peripheral vascular disease.

Nicotinic acid is well absorbed orally and has a plasma half-life of about 45 minutes. Extensive metabolism occurs in the liver and about 35% of the dose is excreted unchanged in urine. Reduction in plasma triglyceride concentration occurs within several hours of the start of dosing.

Combination with HMG-CoA reductase inhibitors can result in myopathy and rhabdomyolysis. Potentiation of the effect of antihypertensive drugs has also been reported. Adverse reactions include increased feelings of warmth, and flushing of the face and neck. Flushing can be very intense and can be reduced in severity by taking aspirin 30–60 minutes before each dose of nicotinic acid. Other common adverse effects include hypotension, nasal stuffiness, diarrhoea, vomiting and dyspepsia. Less frequently encountered are pruritus, skin rash, dry skin or eyes, hyperglycaemia, hyperuricaemia and jaundice. Liver toxicity has been reported with doses of 2 g per day and higher doses. Use with caution in people with gout, diabetes mellitus, peptic ulcer, liver disease and CAD.

A reduction in dose may be necessary in situations of renal impairment. Nicotinic acid is contraindicated in people with a recent myocardial infarction or symptomatic hypotension.

The adult maintenance dose for hyperlipidaemia is 500 mg–1 g three times daily. The initial dose of 250 mg three times daily is increased by 250 mg every 4 days until the maintenance dose is achieved, to a maximum of 4.5 g daily.

Ezetimibe

Ezetimibe is a novel lipid-lowering drug released in Australia in 2004. It is the first of a new group of drugs that inhibits intestinal absorption of both cholesterol and phytosterols. Not only is it effective in inhibiting intestinal absorption of dietary cholesterol, it also inhibits reabsorption of cholesterol excreted in bile (see Figure 26-1). The exact mechanism of action is unknown but ezetimibe localises at the brush border of the small intestine and is thought to inhibit absorption of cholesterol by binding to a specific transport protein in the small intestine wall. Despite inhibiting cholesterol absorption, ezetimibe does not alter absorption of fat-soluble vitamins and nutrients (Kosoglou et al 2005). The average reduction in LDL-cholesterol with ezetimibe is about 18% and it has minimal effect on HDL-cholesterol and triglycerides. It is primarily used as an adjunct to diet for the treatment of hypercholesterolaemia and homozygous phytosterolaemia.

Ezetimibe is conjugated in the intestine, forming an active glucuronide, which accounts for approximately 90% of the drug in plasma after 30 minutes. Ezetimibe and ezetimibe glucuronide are then transported to the liver and subsequently secreted in bile back into the intestine (enterohepatic recycling). The half-life of both is approximately 22 hours and about 80% of the administered dose is excreted in faeces and about 11% in urine. As ezetimibe is not metabolised to any major extent in the liver, significant interactions with the majority of drugs used to treat dyslipidaemia are not a major issue. However, coadministration with cholestyramine reduces bioavailability, and hence these drugs should be administered several hours apart.

Ezetimibe is administered once daily as a 10 mg dose. As it is a relatively new drug, the full range of adverse effects may not yet be known. Commonly, ezetimibe causes headache

---

GERIATRIC IMPLICATIONS
LIPID-LOWERING DRUGS

Dietary modifications and recommendations are vital to a successful lipid reduction program. When goals are not obtainable by diet alone, drug therapy should be considered.

The elderly often take multiple medications for their illnesses. Health-care professionals should take a thorough drug history to determine whether the person is taking medications that can elevate lipid levels; for example, triglycerides can be increased by 30%–50% by thiazides, 20%–50% by non-selective β-blockers, and up to 50% by ethanol (McKenney 1995).

A common adverse effect, constipation (sometimes severe), has been reported in geriatric patients taking cholestyramine and colestipol. Encourage an increase in daily fluid intake to help reduce the constipating effects of these drugs.

Be aware that long-term use of cholestyramine or colestipol can lead to deficiencies of vitamins A, D, E and K, folic acid and calcium.

PREGNANCY SAFETY

ADEC Category	Drug
B2	Cholestyramine, colestipol, niacin
B3	Ezetimibe, fenofibrate, gemfibrozil
D	Atorvastatin, fluvastatin, pravastatin, simvastatin

and diarrhoea and, as with the statins, muscle disorders (e.g. myalgia, muscle cramps, weakness and pain) have been reported. Recently, a combination of ezetimibe (10 mg) and simvastatin (40–80 mg) has been listed on the Australian Pharmaceutical Benefits Scheme. This combination increases the lipid-lowering effect of the statin by up to 20% and is a valuable combination for individuals who are unable to tolerate a higher dose of a statin.

DRUGS AT A GLANCE 26: Lipid-lowering drugs

Therapeutic group	Pharmacological group	Key examples	Key pages
Lipid-lowering drugs	Statins (HMG-CoA reductase inhibitors)	atorvastatin fluvastatin pravastartin simvastatin	466, 7
	Bile acid binding resins	cholestyramine colestipol	467, 8
	Fibrates	fenofibrate gemfibrozil	468, 9
	Other drugs for dyslipidaemia	ezetimibe nicotinic acid	470

KEY POINTS

- Dyslipidaemia is a metabolic disorder characterised by increased concentrations of plasma cholesterol and triglycerides, two of the major lipids in the body. High circulating levels of these lipids have been associated with atherosclerosis, a disorder in which lipids are deposited in the linings of medium- and large-sized arteries, eventually producing degenerative changes and obstruction of blood flow.
- Atherosclerosis is a causative factor in CAD, which in turn can result in angina, heart failure, myocardial infarction, cerebral artery disease, peripheral artery occlusive disease and renal arterial insufficiency.
- Although there are many contributing causes to and risk factors for atherosclerosis, it is believed that if plasma lipid levels can be controlled, the progression of atherosclerosis may be controlled.
- Treatment recommendations are based on a person's cholesterol level and the presence of pre-existing ischaemic heart disease or two other risk factors, such as cigarette smoking or hypertension.
- Management strategies for the treatment of dysipidaemia include diet and lifestyle modification. If these are ineffective in decreasing plasma lipid concentrations, drug therapy is usually instituted.
- The main classes of lipid-lowering drugs are the HMG-CoA reductase inhibitors ('statins'), bile acid-binding resins and fibrates. These agents may be used either individually or in combination if not contraindicated.
- Effectiveness varies depending on the specific type of dyslipidaemia. See Tables 26-2, 26-5 and 26-6 for classifications of hyperlipoproteinaemia, drug treatment approaches and a comparison of lipid-lowering effects.
- The HMG-CoA reductase inhibitors and bile acid-binding resins are subject to numerous drug interactions. Current drug use should be established before commencing a lipid-lowering drug.

REVIEW EXERCISES

1 Explain the differences between the exogenous and endogenous pathways of lipid transport and indicate the site(s) of action of each of the three main lipid-lowering drug classes.
2 Name five major considerations with the administration of lipid-lowering drugs to the elderly.
3 What effects do thiazide diuretics, corticosteroids and alcohol have on plasma lipids?
4 What is the mechanism of action of simvastatin, and explain why this class of drugs is subject to numerous drug interactions.
5 Name three drugs that increase and three drugs that decrease the plasma concentration of simvastatin.

REFERENCES AND FURTHER READING

Australian Medicines Handbook 2006. Adelaide: AMH, 2006.

Beaumont JL, Carlson LA, Cooper GR, Fejfar Z, Fredrickson DS, Strasser T. Classification of hyperlipidaemias and hyperlipoproteinaemias. *Bulletin of the World Health Organization* 1970; 43: 891–915.

Blumenthal RS. Statins: effective antiatherosclerotic therapy. *American Heart Journal* 2000; 139: 577–83.

Corsini A, Bellosta S, Baetta R et al. New insights into the pharmacodynamic and pharmacokinetic properties of statins. *Pharmacology & Therapeutics* 1999; 84: 413–28.

Durrington PN, Bhatnagar D, Mackness MI, Morgan J, Julier K, Khan MA, France M. An omega-3 polyunsaturated fatty acid concentrate administered for one year decreased triglycerides in simvastatin treated patients with coronary heart disease and persisting hypertriglyceridaemia. *Heart* 2001; 85: 544–8.

FIELD study investigators. Effects of long-term fenofibrate therapy on cardiovascular events in 9795 people with type 2 diabetes mellitus (the FIELD study): randomised controlled trial. *Lancet* 2005; 366(9500): 1849–61.

Horrocks LA, Yeo YK. Health benefits of docosahexaenoic acid (DHA). *Pharmacological Research* 1999; 40: 211–25.

Knopp RH. Drug treatment of lipid disorders. *New England Journal of Medicine* 1999; 341: 498–511.

Kosoglou T, Statkevich P, Johnson-Levonas AO, Paolini JF et al. Ezetimibe: a review of its metabolism, pharmacokinetics and drug interactions. *Clinical Pharmacokinetics* 2005; 44: 467–94.

Lipid Management Guidelines 2001. National Heart Foundation of Australia and The Cardiac Society of Australia and New Zealand. *Medical Journal of Australia* 2001; 175: Suppl S57–S88.

McKenney JM. Dyslipidemias. In Young LY, Koda-Kimble MA (eds). *Applied Therapeutics: The Clinical Use of Drugs.* 6th edn. Vancouver: Applied Therapeutics, 1995.

Mahley RW, Bersot TP. Drug therapy for hypercholesterolaemia and dyslipidaemia. In: Hardman JG, Limbird LE, Gilman AG (eds). *Goodman & Gilman's The Pharmacological Basis of Therapeutics.* 10th edn. New York, 2001 [ch. 36].

Moulds RFW. Sheffield tables for primary prevention of coronary heart disease—an alternative approach. *Australian Prescriber* 1998; 21: 98–9.

Rang HP, Dale MM, Ritter JM, Moore PK. *Pharmacology.* 5th edn. Edinburgh: Churchill Livingstone, 2003 [ch. 19].

Rubins HB, Robins SJ, Collins D, Fye CL et al. Gemfibrozil for the secondary prevention of coronary heart disease in men with low levels of high-density lipoprotein cholesterol [VA-HIT]. *New England Journal of Medicine* 1999; 341: 410–18.

Schedule of Pharmaceutical Benefits for Approved Pharmacists and Medical Practitioners, Commonwealth of Australia, December 2005.

ON-LINE RESOURCES

American Heart Association: www.americanheart.org

National Heart Foundation of Australia: www.heartfoundation.com.au

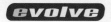 More weblinks at http://evolve.elsevier.com/AU/Bryant/pharmacology/

CHAPTER 27

Overview of the Kidney and Urinary Tract

CHAPTER FOCUS

The kidneys play an important role in maintaining homeostasis by regulating the composition and volume of the extracellular fluid. In addition to this role, the kidneys are essential for eliminating metabolic byproducts such as creatinine, uric acid and urea, and they play a central role in acid–base balance. An important group of drugs that modify the excretion of salt and water by the kidneys is diuretics; these will be discussed in Chapter 28.

OBJECTIVES

- To describe the anatomy and physiology of the urinary system.

- To discuss how the structure of the nephron contributes to regulating the composition of the urine.

- To discuss the role of glomerular filtration, tubular reabsorption and tubular secretion in determining the concentration of electrolytes in urine.

- To describe the sites of action and major effects of antidiuretic hormone and aldosterone on the nephron.

KEY TERMS

aldosterone
antidiuretic hormone
antiporters
glomerular filtration
glomerulus
hypertonic
hypotonic
incontinence

isotonic
nephron
symporters
threshold concentration
tubular reabsorption
tubular secretion
tubular transport maximum
vasa recta

KEY ABBREVIATIONS

ADH   antidiuretic hormone
ESRD   end stage renal disease
GFR   glomerular filtration rate
H^+ hydrogen ion
HCO_3^- bicarbonate ion
T_M tubular transport maximum

THE urinary system is composed of organs that manufacture and excrete urine from the body: two kidneys, two ureters, the bladder and the urethra (Figure 27-1). Urine formed in the kidneys flows through the ureters to the bladder, where it is stored.

When about 250 mL urine is collected, the expansion of the bladder results in a feeling of distension and a desire to void. When voluntary control of the muscles preventing voiding is removed, urine flows from the bladder into the urethra and is expelled from the body.

In males, the urethra is surrounded by the prostate gland; it then passes through fibrous tissue connected to the pubic bones and terminates at the urinary meatus, or tip of the penis (Figure 27-2). The male urethra serves a dual purpose: the elimination of urine from the body, and semen transport. In the female, the only function of the urethra is as the final vehicle for urination (Figure 27-2).

The kidneys are essential for maintaining homeostasis. By processing salts and water and balancing excretion they control the volume and ionic composition of the extracellular fluid, regulate blood pH by excreting hydrogen ions (H^+), excrete waste products such as urea, uric acid and creatinine, and modulate blood pressure via the release of renin and activation of the renin–angiotensin–aldosterone system. In addition to these roles, the kidneys synthesise calcitriol,

an active vitamin D metabolite (see Chapter 42), and the growth factor erythropoietin, which stimulates red blood cell production (see Chapter 29).

ANATOMY AND PHYSIOLOGY OF THE KIDNEY

The kidneys are reddish-brown organs about the size of an individual's closed fist. A cross-section of the kidney shows three distinct regions: the outer cortex, the inner deep reddish-brown medulla and the central hollow pelvis, which is continuous with the ureter (Figure 27-1). The functional units of the kidney are the **nephrons**, the number of which (about 1 million) is determined at birth. Each nephron consists of a **glomerulus** (the glomerular capillaries and the Bowman's capsule) and the renal tubular network comprising, in order of the flow through them, the proximal convoluted tubule, the loop of Henle, the distal convoluted tubule and, finally, the collecting duct. Most nephrons (around 80%) have short loops of Henle that penetrate superficially into the medulla and are termed cortical nephrons. The remaining nephrons

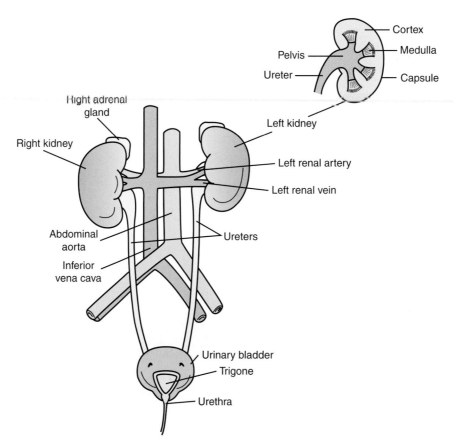

FIGURE 27-1 Urinary system and schematic cross-section of a human kidney.

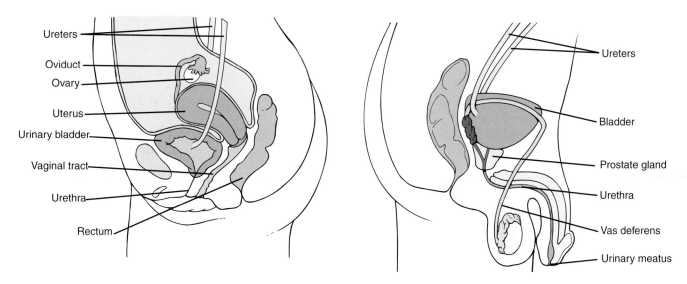

FIGURE 27-2 Sagittal sections of the female and male pelvis.

CLINICAL INTEREST BOX 27-1
RENAL DISEASE IN INDIGENOUS POPULATIONS

The Australian Aboriginal and New Zealand Maori populations have been subject to rapid cultural changes and erosion of traditional lifestyles. One of the most concerning impacts of this on indigenous health is the rise in prevalence of end-stage renal disease (ESRD), now particularly prevalent in Australian Aboriginal people. The crude incidence of ESRD was reported as six times higher for Aboriginals than non-Aboriginals in 1994, but by 1998 the incidence was 21 times that of non-Aboriginal Australians and doubling every four years (Hoy 1996; Hoy et al 1998).

The commonest conditions leading to ESRD are diabetes, hypertension and glomerulonephritis.

Haemodialysis is the most common in-hospital treatment for indigenous people; of the total number of persons registered in 2001 with the Australian and New Zealand Dialysis Transplant Registry, 6.2% were indigenous and of those 66% were under 55 years of age. Of the new cases (~1800) commencing haemodialysis for ESRD in 2001, 9% were indigenous, and within this patient group indigenous females outnumbered males (AIHW 2004).

---

with long loops of Henle that almost traverse the medullary region are called juxtamedullary nephrons and provide the kidney with the ability to concentrate the urine.

The kidneys are highly vascularised and the complex network of arterioles, capillaries and venules gives rise to the glomerular capillaries, the peritubular capillaries that form a dense plexus surrounding the cortical aspects of the renal tubule and the **vasa recta**, the long hairpin loop-shaped capillaries that supply the renal medulla. The peritubular capillaries reunite to form the peritubular venules and blood finally leaves the kidney through a single renal vein. The interface between the unique vascular network and the renal tubular system provides the basis for the three major renal processes: glomerular filtration, tubular reabsorption and tubular secretion.

Glomerular filtration

Glomerular filtration, the initial step in urine formation, occurs as a result of ultrafiltration of water and small solutes through pores of the glomerular capillaries into the capsular space of the Bowman's capsule. In the absence of disease, the glomerular membrane does not filter molecules larger than 6–7 nm in diameter, including plasma proteins such as haemoglobin and albumin. The heart works to create pressure in the blood vessels, which in turn provides the force necessary to accomplish glomerular filtration. Blood flow to the kidney is normally around 1200 mL/min, which is 20%–25% of cardiac output, and the **glomerular filtration rate** (GFR) is about 125 mL/min. This amounts to around 180 litres of filtrate formed per day in a healthy individual, of which 99% is ultimately reabsorbed throughout the nephron tubule.

Maintenance of glomerular hydrostatic pressure depends on systemic blood pressure and is aided by the ability of the afferent and efferent arterioles to alter vessel resistance effectively. Systemic blood pressure has to be significantly reduced before glomerular filtration is greatly altered. Usually, some degree of filtration will exist if the pressure in the glomerular capillaries remains above 50 mmHg.

Tubular reabsorption

Of the 180 L glomerular filtrate delivered to the nephrons per day, about 99% is reabsorbed from the lumen of the proximal convoluted tubule into the peritubular capillaries, with the remainder excreted as urine. This **tubular reabsorption** is a selective process, and the main transport mechanisms that prevail throughout the nephron are:

- simple diffusion and facilitated diffusion; the latter involves carrier-mediated passive transport from a region of high concentration to a region of lower concentration
- primary active transport, principally by the Na^+–K^+-ATPase pump, which transports Na^+ against an electrochemical gradient
- carrier-mediated (secondary active) transport, in which the transport of Na^+ down its concentration gradient provides the energy for the active transport of solutes such as glucose against its concentration gradient. Secondary active-transport membrane proteins that move two substrates in the same direction are called **symporters**, while those that transport two substances in opposite directions are called **antiporters**. Reabsorption of Na^+ and nutrients leads to the reabsorption of water by osmosis.

For almost every substance that is actively transported across the membrane, there is a maximum rate at which the transport mechanism can function. This is called the **tubular transport maximum** (T_M). For example, the T_M for glucose averages 320 mg/min for most adults. If the tubular concentration (mg) of glucose is very high the T_M of 320 mg/min will be reached and the excess glucose remaining will not be reabsorbed but will appear in the urine. Every substance that has a tubular transport maximum also has a renal **threshold concentration**, which is the plasma concentration at which a substance begins to appear in the urine because of saturation of transporters, that is, the exceeding of T_M.

Tubular secretion

The third major renal process is **tubular secretion**, which is the movement of substances from peritubular or interstitial capillaries into the lumen. The proximal convoluted tubule plays an important role in the secretion of hydrogen ions (H^+) which, coupled with preferential absorption of bicarbonate (HCO_3^-), regulates acid–base balance; and in the secretion of metabolic byproducts (e.g. ammonium ions, creatinine) and certain drugs (e.g. penicillin and radio-contrast agents). All of these secretory processes are saturable and exhibit a T_M, just as the reabsorptive processes do.

The roles of various segments of the renal tubule in the movement of water and solutes are summarised in the following sections and in Figure 27-3. The final urinary excretion of a substance, which is influenced by glomerular filtration, tubular reabsorption and tubular filtration, can be summarised as:

$$\begin{array}{l}\text{Amount of} \\ \text{substance} \\ \text{filtered}\end{array} - \begin{array}{l}\text{Amount of} \\ \text{substance} \\ \text{reabsorbed}\end{array} + \begin{array}{l}\text{Amount of} \\ \text{substance} \\ \text{secreted}\end{array} = \begin{array}{l}\text{Amount of} \\ \text{substance} \\ \text{excreted in urine}\end{array}$$

The proximal convoluted tubule

Most of the glomerular filtrate is reabsorbed in the proximal convoluted tubule and returned to the bloodstream. About 70% of the salt and water in the filtrate is reabsorbed rapidly, maintaining nearly the same osmolality between the tubular fluid and the interstitial fluid at the end of the proximal tubule (i.e. the solutions are **isotonic**). The secretion of H^+ that occurs in the proximal tubule is linked to the reabsorption of HCO_3^- in the tubular filtrate. This process involves intracellular formation of carbonic acid (H_2CO_3) from carbon dioxide and water. The carbonic acid formed dissociates to give HCO_3^- and H^+. This reversible reaction is catalysed by carbonic anhydrase. The hydrogen ions formed are secreted into the lumen and combine with bicarbonate in the glomerular filtrate to form carbonic acid in the lumen. This in turn dissociates into water and carbon dioxide, which diffuses into tubule cells and reforms H_2CO_3. Dissociation releases bicarbonate, which is then reabsorbed into the blood.

Acid–base balance is maintained in healthy humans by the action of the body's buffer systems, changes in the rate and depth of breathing, and excretion of H^+ by the kidneys. As the blood becomes more acidic (decreasing pH), the kidneys will respond by increasing the renal tubule excretion of hydrogen and ammonia, which results in an increase in blood bicarbonate and an increase in pH (towards normal).

The loop of Henle

The loop of Henle portion of the nephron is important in regulating urine osmolarity* and osmolality† of body fluids. The descending limb is highly permeable to water, and movement of water out of the tubule produces a hypertonic (more concentrated) filtrate at the tip of the loop of Henle (the papilla). Permeability to urea and sodium is low in this segment of the loop. In contrast, in the ascending limb of the loop of Henle water permeability is almost nil whereas sodium and chloride permeability is high. About 20%–25% of the sodium chloride in the filtrate is reabsorbed and is not accompanied by water. Consequently, two very important situations occur. The tubular filtrates becomes very dilute,

---

*Osmolarity is defined as the total number of dissolved particles per litre of solution. Unit: milliosmoles/L (mOsm/L).

†Plasma osmolality is determined by the total solute content in plasma and the total plasma water mass. Unit: mOsmol/kg H_2O.

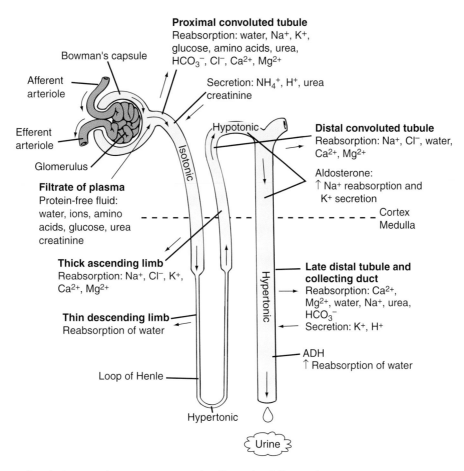

FIGURE 27-3 Summary of main transport processes occurring throughout the nephron.

or **hypotonic** (this is often termed 'free water production'), and the medullary interstitium becomes **hypertonic**, which is necessary for the concentrating capacity of the countercurrent between the renal tubules and the vasa recta. The concentration gradient established across the tubular epithelium becomes multiplied in a longitudinal direction, resulting in a large osmotic gradient between the isosmotic renal cortex and the hyperosmotic medulla and papilla. Potassium is also reabsorbed from the proximal tubules and loop of Henle in percentages equivalent to those for sodium; around 8% of the filtered potassium reaches the distal tubules.

The distal convoluted tubule

Between 5% and 10% of sodium reabsorption takes place actively in the distal convoluted tubule. The net loss of sodium from the filtrate is greater than the reabsorption of water; coupled with reabsorption of chloride, this makes the urine progressively more dilute. Uptake of sodium is largely determined by the presence of the mineralocorticoid **aldosterone**, produced by the adrenal cortex. When the extracellular fluid volume is decreased, the renin–angiotensin–aldosterone system is activated (see Chapter 25), stimulating

the release of aldosterone, which acts to increase the active reabsorption of sodium and secretion of potassium. Parathyroid hormone and calcitriol also act on this segment of the nephron to increase reabsorption of calcium (see Chapter 42).

The collecting duct

Composition of the hypotonic fluid entering the collecting duct may be altered in the medullary portion by the action of **antidiuretic hormone** (ADH) (also called vasopressin) or aldosterone. ADH is a water-conserving hormone synthesised in the hypothalamus and stored in the posterior pituitary gland. When plasma osmolality increases as a result of dehydration or water deprivation, osmoreceptors in the supraoptic area of the hypothalamus stimulate the release of ADH.

The released ADH increases the permeability of the distal tubule and collecting duct to water, which is passively reabsorbed and increases plasma volume, thus lowering plasma osmolality. When ADH concentration is low, a large volume of dilute urine is excreted. In the complete absence of ADH, a condition known as diabetes insipidus occurs and the individual affected can excrete as much as 20 L dilute urine daily.

CLINICAL INTEREST BOX 27-2 URINARY INCONTINENCE

Urinary incontinence is not normal in adults, and of the elderly population it is estimated that urinary incontinence is a significant problem for about 15% of those living in the community and 50% of those living in residential care (Chutka & Takahashi 1998). Within the population of Australian veterans, war widows and war widowers, approximately 15% suffer from incontinence (AIHW 2004).

Reports of incontinence vary from simply reporting a sensation of urgency (urge incontinence), to complaints of leakage of urine when laughing, coughing, sneezing,

exercising etc (stress incontinence), to overflow incontinence (when the bladder fails to empty completely, often as a result of an obstruction) and functional incontinence arising as a result of either the inability to recognise the need to urinate (e.g. as a result of loss of memory) or a physical inability to get to the toilet.

Successful treatment may involve changes to lifestyle (e.g. weight loss and exercising), behavioural therapy and, in some cases, drug or surgical therapy.

MICTURITION

Once formed, urine is carried from the kidneys by the ureters to the urinary bladder, a hollow muscular organ the shape of which is determined by the volume of urine contained at the time. The ureters enter the bladder through the detrusor muscle in the floor of the bladder (the trigone area). The normal tone of the detrusor muscle prevents backflow of urine from the bladder to the ureters. The urethra exits from the bladder at the tip of the trigone, with the detrusor muscle forming the internal sphincter, and passes through the floor of the pelvis (Figure 27-2). In this region, the outer wall of the urethra contains a circular muscle band that forms the external urethral sphincter, which is under voluntary control and prevents urination until socially acceptable circumstances are achieved.

The micturition reflex

The average capacity of the urinary bladder is about 500 mL in an adult. Volume expansion increases tension in the wall of the bladder, triggering stretch receptors in the detrusor muscle and the transmission of sensory impulses by parasympathetic afferent fibres. Reflex parasympathetic discharge via motor efferent fibres causes contraction of the detrusor muscle and relaxation of the internal urethral sphincter. This reflex arc initiates a conscious desire to urinate and, when impulses from the cerebral cortex of the brain inhibit activity in motor neurons to the external sphincter, voluntary relaxation occurs and the bladder contents are expelled. Micturition may be initiated and stopped voluntarily because of control exerted at the level of the cerebral cortex. A lack of voluntary control is referred to as **incontinence**, while failure to either completely or normally urinate may lead to urine retention.

KEY POINTS

- The urinary system comprises the kidneys, ureters, the bladder and the urethra.
- The kidneys are essential for maintaining homeostasis.
- The kidneys process salts and water, balance excretion, regulate the pH of blood via excretion of hydrogen ions, excrete metabolic waste products such as urea and creatinine, modulate blood pressure via release of renin, and synthesise calcitriol and the growth factor erythropoietin.
- The kidney has three distinct regions: the outer cortex, the inner medulla and the central hollow pelvis.
- The functional unit of the kidney is the nephron.
- The nephron consists of the glomerulus and the renal tubule.
- The renal tubule comprises the proximal convoluted tubule, the descending and ascending limbs of the loop of Henle, the distal convoluted tubule and the collecting duct.
- The three major renal processes are glomerular filtration, tubular reabsorption and tubular secretion.
- The glomerular membrane filters substances less than 6–7 nm in diameter, e.g. water, ions, glucose, amino acids and urea. Plasma proteins are not filtered.
- Glomerular filtration rate (GFR) is 125 mL/min; about 180 L filtrate are formed per day in healthy individuals.
- About 99% of the filtrate is reabsorbed throughout the length of the tubule.
- Tubular transport mechanisms include primary active transport, facilitated diffusion and carrier-mediated (secondary active) transport.

- Reabsorbed substances include glucose, amino acids, water and bicarbonate, sodium, potassium and chloride ions.
- Tubular secretion involves movement of substances such as ammonium ions, creatinine and certain drugs from the blood into the lumen of the nephron.
- Both reabsorptive and secretory transport processes exhibit a transport maximum (T_M).
- Differential reabsorption of water and ions occurs along the length of the renal tubule.
- Antidiuretic hormone (ADH) and aldosterone regulate salt and water reabsorption in the distal convoluted tubule and collecting duct.
- Urine is concentrated by the action of ADH and diluted by the action of aldosterone.
- Urine is stored in the urinary bladder. Micturition can be initiated and stopped voluntarily through conscious control at the level of the cerebral cortex.
- A lack of voluntary control over micturition is referred to as incontinence. Failure to completely or normally urinate leads to urine retention.

REVIEW EXERCISES

1 Describe the processes of glomerular filtration, tubular reabsorption and tubular secretion.
2 How is sodium processed by the proximal tubule, the descending and ascending limbs of the loop of Henle, the distal convoluted tubule and the collecting duct?
3 What effect does the secretion of aldosterone have on sodium transport?
4 Explain the process of micturition.

REFERENCES AND FURTHER READING

Australian Institute of Health and Welfare. *Australia's Health 2004*. Canberra: AIHW, 2004.
Chutka DS, Takahashi PY. Urinary incontinence in the elderly. *Drugs* 1998; 56: 587–95.
Hoy WE. Renal disease in Australian Aboriginals. *Medical Journal of Australia* 1996; 165: 126–7.
Hoy WE, Mathews JD, McCredie DA et al. The multidimensional nature of renal disease: Rates and associations of albuminuria in an Australian Aboriginal community. *Kidney International* 1998; 54(4): 1296–304.
Schafer JA. Functional anatomy of the kidney and micturition. Ch. 23 in: Johnson LR (ed) *Essential Medical Physiology*. 2nd edn. Philadelphia: Lippincott-Raven, 1997.
Schafer JA. Reabsorption and secretion in the proximal tubule. Ch. 26 in: Johnson LR (ed) *Essential Medical Physiology*. 2nd edn. Philadelphia: Lippincott-Raven, 1997.
Tortora GJ, Grabowski SR. *Principles of Anatomy and Physiology*. 9th edn. New York: Harper Collins, 2000 [ch. 26].

ON-LINE RESOURCES

Caring for Australians with Renal Impairment: http://www.cari.org.au
Australian Kidney Foundation: www.kidney.org.au

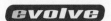 More weblinks at http://evolve.elsevier.com/AU/Bryant/pharmacology/

CHAPTER 28

Diuretics and Drug Treatment of Urinary Incontinence

CHAPTER FOCUS

Diuretics increase urine volume and enhance the excretion of sodium and chloride. They are widely used drugs and are prescribed for treating conditions such as congestive heart failure and hypertension. Electrolyte imbalance is a common adverse effect of diuretic administration. Volume depletion and electrolyte disturbances can be minimised by administering the lowest effective dose and monitoring both clinical response and plasma electrolytes. Urinary incontinence is a common embarrassing problem that afflicts the elderly population in particular. Before starting drug therapy, the health-care professional must eliminate possible contributing factors, such as urinary tract infection, metabolic disorders or certain drugs.

OBJECTIVES

- To name one drug from each of the three major classes of diuretics and identify their primary sites of action in the nephron.

- To compare the efficacy and common adverse reactions associated with each of the three classes of diuretics.

- To name at least five concerns regarding the use of diuretics in the elderly.

- To describe the three main types of urinary incontinence and explain why anticholinergic drugs are effective for treating urge incontinence.

KEY DRUGS

amiloride
frusemide
hydrochlorothiazide
indapamide
oxybutynin
spironolactone

KEY TERMS

diuretics
loop diuretics
osmotic diuretics
potassium-sparing diuretics
thiazide diuretics
urinary incontinence

DIURETICS are among the most extensively used drugs. They are widely prescribed for the treatment of hypertension (see also Chapter 25) and are an integral part of drug therapies in oedematous conditions such as cirrhosis, nephrotic syndrome, chronic renal failure, and acute and chronic congestive heart failure (Chapter 24). Diuretics modify renal function and induce diuresis (increased rate of urine flow) and natriuresis (enhanced excretion of sodium chloride). The increase in urine volume is achieved primarily by inhibiting reabsorption of sodium and chloride in the nephron. The increased excretion of salt leads to an increase in the excretion of water. Understanding the action of diuretics is made easier by having knowledge of the events that take place along the length of the nephron, in particular the loop of Henle and the distal convoluted tubule (see Chapter 27). The three major classes of diuretics are:

• **loop diuretics**, e.g. frusemide
• **thiazide diuretics**, e.g. hydrochlorothiazide
• **potassium-sparing diuretics**, e.g. amiloride.

Although carbonic-anhydrase inhibitors were introduced as diuretics during the 1940s and 1950s, their diuretic effects were very weak and they were found to be ineffective over the long term. Acetazolamide, a carbonic anhydrase inhibitor introduced in 1950, is now reserved for the treatment of

CLINICAL INTEREST BOX 28-1
MERCURIAL DIURETICS

Paracelsus, the 'Grandfather of Pharmacology', was the first to use mercurous chloride as an antisyphilitic agent and as a diuretic in the 16th century. In 1919, while using merbaphen (a mercurial compound) to treat a young female syphilitic patient, Alfred Vogl noticed an increase in urine output from 200 mL to 1200 mL. Also on his ward at that time was a man with syphilitic heart disease. Deciding that this was the ideal patient for the *experimentum crucis*, he injected 2 mL merbaphen intramuscularly and witnessed over the next 24 hours a diuresis of 10 litres (Vogl 1950). Further experimentation confirmed that the diuretic property of merbaphen was independent of its antisyphilitic properties, and for the next 30 years the organic mercurials were the mainstay of diuretic therapy. Severe adverse reactions, including agranulocytosis and thrombocytopenia, and one instance of an immediate fatal reaction, caused mercurial diuretics to be abandoned.

open-angle glaucoma (see Chapter 35) and is used as adjunct treatment with anticonvulsants to manage absence seizures (see Chapter 18).

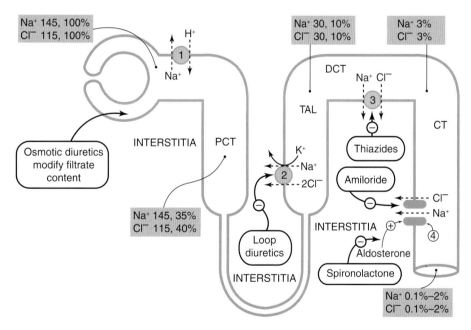

FIGURE 28-1 Schematic summary diagram showing the absorption of sodium and chloride in the nephron and the main sites of action of drugs. The tubule cells are depicted as an orange border around the yellow tubular lumen. Mechanisms of ion absorption at the apical margin of the tubule cell (not of course shown to scale): (1) Na^+/H^+ exchange; (2) $Na^+/K^+/2Cl^-$ co-transport; (3) Na^+/Cl^- co-transport, (4) Na^+ entry through sodium channels. Sodium is pumped out of the cells into the interstitia by the Na^+/K^+-ATPase in the basolateral margin of the tubular cells (not shown). Chloride ions may pass out of the tubule through the paracellular pathway. The numbers in the boxes give the concentrations of ions as millimoles per litre of filtrate and the percentages of ions filtered at the sites specified. No absolute concentrations are given for the DT and CT because they can vary considerably. (PCT, proximal convoluted tubule; TAL, thick ascending loop; DCT, distal convoluted tubule; CT, collecting tubule.) Data from Greger 2000. Reproduced from Rang et al 2003, with permission.

Figure 28-1 shows the various sites of action of current diuretic drugs on the nephron, and highlights the movement of various electrolytes.

DIURETICS

Loop diuretics

The drugs commonly referred to as loop diuretics are bumetanide, ethacrynic acid and **frusemide** (Drug Monograph 28-1). These powerful diuretics are actively secreted into the lumen of the nephron via the organic-base pump in the proximal tubule cells. On reaching the thick ascending limb of the loop of Henle, they inhibit the $Na^+-K^+-2Cl^-$ transporter, thus preventing reabsorption of sodium and chloride. As this site accounts for about 15%–25% of the reabsorption of sodium and chloride, their diuretic effect is greater than that reported with the other diuretics. The mechanism by which they inhibit the transporter is not known, but it is thought they bind to the chloride-binding site on the transporter as these drugs also inhibit the reabsorption of calcium and magnesium.

In addition to diuresis, loop diuretics exert direct vascular effects. In particular, frusemide acutely causes venodilation, but the duration of this effect is too short for frusemide to be used in the treatment of hypertension.

Indications

The indications for loop diuretics include treatment of oedema associated with heart failure, cirrhosis, renal impairment and nephrotic syndrome. In addition, these agents are used as adjunct therapy in patients with acute pulmonary oedema, in people whose conditions are refractory to the other diuretics, and, because they promote excretion of calcium, they are used in people with severe hypercalcaemia.

Drug interactions

Loop diuretics are often included in multiple drug regimens. See the Drug Interactions table 28-1 for loop diuretics.

Warnings and contraindications

Loop diuretics should be used with caution in people with diabetes mellitus, gout, hearing impairment, hepatic and renal impairment, and in those in whom hypokalaemia might precipitate arrhythmias, such as people taking digitalis glycosides. As all loop diuretics are ADEC category C, their use in pregnancy should be avoided.

These drugs should also be avoided in people with known hypersensitivity to loop diuretics, anuria, or severe kidney disease or impairment.

DRUG INTERACTIONS 28-1 Loop diuretics

Drug	Possible effect and management
Amphotericin	Potentiates hypokalaemic effect of frusemide; monitor plasma potassium level and use supplement if indicated
Angiotensin-converting enzyme (ACE) inhibitors	In people on high-dose loop diuretics, increased risk of severe first-dose hypotension. Withhold loop diuretic for 3 days
Aminoglycosides	Increased risk of ototoxicity and renal toxicity. Care required in dosing people with renal impairment. Combination with frusemide is not recommended
Cisplatin	Increased risk of nephrotoxicity and ototoxicity in combination with frusemide
Digoxin	Increased risk of digoxin-induced arrhythmia in people with diuretic-induced hypokalaemia and hypomagnesaemia. Monitor plasma potassium concentration and use supplement if indicated
Lithium	Increased risk of lithium toxicity because of reduced renal clearance. Monitor closely and adjust lithium dose if necessary
NSAIDs	Reduce the effect of loop diuretics; predispose to renal failure in presence of pre-existing hypovolaemia
Sucralfate	Reduces the absorption of frusemide; avoid administration within two hours of each other
Warfarin	Ethacrynic acid displaces warfarin from plasma protein-binding sites and may increase anticoagulant effect. A reduction in warfarin dosage may be required

Thiazide diuretics

The thiazide diuretics were synthesised during the 1950s and were the first real challengers to the use of mercurial diuretics. The current drugs are chemically related to the sulfonamides and include chlorthalidone, **hydrochlorothiazide** (Drug Monograph 28-2), and the thiazide-like drug **indapamide**. All of them inhibit absorption of sodium and chloride in the proximal (diluting) segment of the distal convoluted tubule

DRUG MONOGRAPH 28-1 FRUSEMIDE

Frusemide is one of the most commonly prescribed loop diuretics. The pharmacological effects of all the loop diuretics are similar—all produce a rapid and intense diuresis and in general have a short duration of action (4–6 hours). Lack of response to frusemide is a reasonable indication that a similar non-response will occur with other loop diuretics, and a combination of diuretics should be considered instead.

PHARMACOKINETICS Frusemide is highly protein-bound (>95%) and around 50% of a dose of frusemide is excreted unchanged in urine; the remaining 50% is conjugated with glucuronic acid in the kidney. The oral bioavailability ranges from 10% to 100% (average about 50%) and the elimination half-life in normal subjects is 1.5–2 hours (Brater 1998). The peak effect occurs within 30 minutes when given intravenously and in about 1 hour following oral administration.

DRUG INTERACTIONS See comprehensive listing in the Drug Interactions 28-1 table, which is relevant to all the loop diuretics.

ADVERSE REACTIONS The most common adverse reactions are electrolyte disturbances, including hyponatraemia, hypokalaemia, hypomagnesaemia, hyperuricaemia, and dizziness and postural hypotension (Figure 28–2). Increases in low-density lipoprotein (LDL) cholesterol and triglycerides with a fall in high-density lipoprotein (HDL) cholesterol plasma levels have been reported. High intravenous doses increase the risk of ototoxicity (e.g. tinnitus, vertigo and deafness).

WARNINGS AND CONTRAINDICATIONS Frusemide is contraindicated in states of severe sodium and fluid depletion and where there is an existing history of allergy to frusemide and sulfonamides.

DOSAGE AND ADMINISTRATION This varies according to the condition being treated, and current information sources should be consulted.

DRUG MONOGRAPH 28-2 HYDROCHLOROTHIAZIDE

Of the 697,201 prescriptions for thiazide and thiazide-like diuretics written in Australia in 2004/05, hydrochlorothiazide accounted for 9% of the total. Hydrochlorothiazide is a diuretic used in the treatment of mild to moderate hypertension and oedema associated with hepatic cirrhosis or heart failure.

PHARMACOKINETICS Hydrochlorothiazide is absorbed after oral administration (about 70%) and the maximum plasma concentration occurs 2–4 hours after dosing. The plasma half-life is in the order of 8–12 hours. Hydrochlorothiazide is not metabolised and is excreted almost entirely (>95%) as unchanged drug in urine.

DRUG INTERACTIONS See comprehensive listing in the Drug Interactions 28-2 table.

ADVERSE REACTIONS Common adverse reactions include dizziness, hypotension and electrolyte disturbances (hyponatraemia, hypokalaemia, hyperuricaemia

and hypomagnesaemia). More serious reactions include intrahepatic cholestatic jaundice and a variety of haematological effects (agranulocytosis, aplastic anaemia and thrombocytopenia).

WARNINGS AND CONTRAINDICATIONS
Hydrochlorothiazide is contraindicated in anuria and in people with known hypersensitivity to sulfonamides. The drug should be used with extreme caution in people with renal disease or cirrhosis.

DOSAGE AND ADMINISTRATION This varies according to the condition being treated, and current information sources should be consulted. Hydrochlorothiazide may be administered as a single agent or in combination with a potassium-sparing diuretic (e.g. amiloride or triamterene), an ACE inhibitor (e.g. fosinopril or enalapril) or an angiotensin II antagonist (e.g. candesartan or irbesartan).

Sources: Dollery 1991; AMH 2006.

(Figure 28-1) by binding to the chloride-binding site of the Na^+–Cl^- transporter. Because the maximum portion of the sodium load they can affect at the distal tubule is less than 10%, these drugs are considered moderately potent diuretics in comparison with the loop diuretics. In general, they are well absorbed orally and are usually excreted unchanged by the kidneys. The onset of action is usually within 12 hours,

but the duration of action differs between the drugs. For pharmacokinetics and dosages, see Table 28-1.

The thiazide diuretics promote the renal excretion of water, sodium, chloride, potassium and magnesium, whereas excretion of uric acid and calcium is decreased. When an increased sodium load is presented to the distal tubule, there is a corresponding increase in potassium secretion. In

TABLE 28-1 Selected diuretic pharmacokinetics and dosages*

CLASS	ONSET OF ACTION (hours)	TIME TO PEAK EFFECT (hours)	DURATION OF ACTION (hours)	DOSE RANGE Adults	Infants (6 months–2 years)
Thiazide diuretics					
Chlorthalidone	PO 2	2	48–72	12.5–50 mg/day	0.25–0.85 mg/kg/day
Hydrochlorothiazide	PO 2	4	6–12	25–100 mg/day	12.5–37.5 mg/day in two doses
Loop diuretics					
Bumetanide	PO 0.5–1	1–2	4–6	1–10 mg/day	Not established
	IV within 30 min	0.25–0.5	0.5–1		
Ethacrynic acid	PO 0.5	2	6–8	50–400 mg/day	Not recommended
	IV within 5 min	0.25–0.5	2		
Frusemide	PO 1/3–1	1–2	6–8	20–1000 mg/day	1–6 mg/kg/day
	IV within 5 min	0.5	2		
Potassium-sparing diuretics					
Amiloride	PO 1–2	6–10	24	5–10 mg/day	Not established
Spironolactone	PO 24–48	48–72	48–72	25–200 mg/day	1–3 mg/kg/day

*Use minimum effective dose and monitor clinical response and plasma electrolytes. Data from AMH 2006, Olin 1998.

addition, as the extracellular fluid volume decreases, plasma renin activity and aldosterone levels increase, with resulting potassium loss (Figure 28-2). Potassium is one of the most common electrolytes lost, with loss occurring in 14%–60% of ambulatory hypertensive patients. This loss is dose-related, occurring early in treatment (first month) and more frequently with larger diuretic doses or with the long-acting type of diuretics (e.g. chlorthalidone). Potassium loss can be a serious issue in people who are taking digitalis preparations, as it can precipitate serious arrhythmias as a result of digitalis toxicity. Hypokalaemia may also predispose people with cirrhosis to hepatic encephalopathy or coma. Potassium loss can be minimised by using the lowest possible dose of thiazide, by adding a potassium-sparing diuretic and, if necessary, using potassium supplements. Potassium replacement can be dangerous in the elderly, in patients with renal dysfunction, or when used in combination with potassium-sparing diuretics, because high plasma potassium levels may occur. Dietary modification to include potassium-rich foods may in some circumstances be recommended by practitioners. A cup of dried fruit (e.g. apricots, figs, peaches, pears, prunes or raisins) provides approximately 1000 mg potassium.

Patients receiving thiazide diuretics may have an increase in plasma uric acid. This increase is persistent and probably results from inhibition of tubular secretion of uric acid or increased uric acid reabsorption. This effect is reversible when the drugs are discontinued. In the absence of gout, the hyperuricaemia is usually asymptomatic and requires no treatment; however, in a person with a history of gout, higher doses of thiazides can precipitate an attack that requires treatment (see Chapter 55).

Hyperglycaemia, or impaired glucose tolerance, has been reported with the thiazides and, rarely, with loop diuretics. This effect is reported most often in the elderly, and thiazides can unmask latent diabetes. The mechanism of the thiazide-induced hyperglycaemia is not known but may involve reduced insulin secretion and alterations in glucose metabolism. With the current use of low doses, hyperglycaemia now occurs less often (AMH 2006).

In higher doses the thiazide diuretics have been reported to increase plasma levels of LDL cholesterol, total cholesterol and triglycerides, and to reduce HDL cholesterol (Jackson 1996). The clinical relevance of changes in an individual's lipid profile would need to be considered in the context of the overall health status of the person concerned.

Indications

The indications for the thiazide diuretics include the treatment of mild to moderate hypertension, oedema associated with

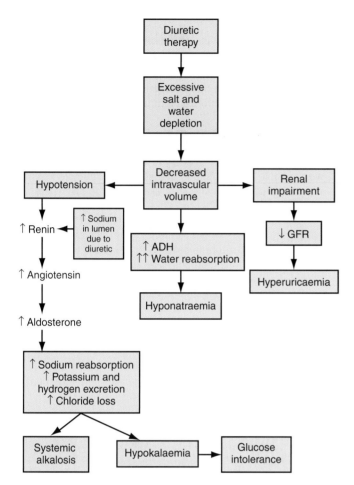

FIGURE 28-2 Interrelationship of thiazide diuretic therapy and unwanted effects.

DRUG INTERACTIONS 28-2 Thiazide diuretics	
Drug	**Possible effect and management**
ACE inhibitors	Increased risk of severe first-dose hypotension. Withhold thiazide diuretic for 24 hours
Cholestyramine and colestipol	Concurrent administration can decrease gastrointestinal absorption of thiazide diuretics. Schedule administration of diuretics at least 1 hour before or 2 hours after administration of these drugs
Digitalis glycosides	Increases risk of digitalis toxicity in presence of hypokalaemia. Monitor potassium and electrocardiogram changes
Lithium	Increased risk of lithium toxicity because of decreased lithium excretion. Monitor plasma lithium concentration and adjust lithium dose if necessary
NSAIDs	Decreased natriuresis and reduced antihypertensive effect. In view of increased potential for nephrotoxicity, avoid concurrent use or adjust dose of diuretic

heart failure or cirrhosis with ascites, the treatment of nephrogenic diabetes insipidus and the prevention of renal calculi formation. Although the initial diuresis produces a fall in blood pressure because of decreased blood volume, during chronic therapy a reduction in total peripheral resistance via an action on blood vessels appears to explain the continued antihypertensive effect.

Drug interactions and adverse reactions

See the Drug Interactions table 28-2 for thiazide diuretics.

In addition to electrolyte imbalances, common adverse reactions include dizziness, weakness, muscle cramps and hypotension. Infrequently rash, blurred vision and male impotence have been reported and, rarely, diarrhoea, photosensitivity, agranulocytosis, cholecystitis, jaundice, and haemolytic anaemia and thrombocytopenia.

Warnings and contraindications

Use with caution in people with type 1 diabetes, gout, renal or hepatic impairment or dyslipidaemias, and in the elderly. Thiazide diuretics are contraindicated in severe renal impairment, anuria and Addison's disease, and in people with known thiazide or sulfonamide hypersensitivity.

See the Geriatric Implications and Pregnancy Safety boxes for more information.

Diuretic combinations

A number of diuretic combination products are available, which are generally used in people whose hypertension is not controlled adequately by a single drug. Fixed-dose combinations, which are commercially available, can provide additional diuretic activity and decrease the potassium depletion characteristic of the thiazide diuretics (e.g. triamterene 50 mg plus hydrochlorothiazide 25 mg, or amiloride 5 mg plus hydrochlorothiazide 50 mg). Additionally, combinations of hydrochlorothiazide with either an ACE inhibitor or an angiotensin II receptor antagonist are available (Table 28-2).

Potassium-sparing diuretics

The potassium-sparing diuretics are **amiloride, spironolactone** and triamterene. Amiloride is also available in combination with hydrochlorothiazide, and triamterene is available only as a combination with hydrochlorothiazide.

TABLE 28-2 Diuretic combinations

ACE inhibitor/diuretic combination

Enalapril (20 mg)/hydrochlorothiazide (6 mg)

Fosinopril (10 or 20 mg)/hydrochlorothiazide (12.5 mg)

Perindopril (4 mg)/indapamide (1.25 mg)

Quinapril (10 or 20 mg)/hydrochlorothiazide (12.5 mg)

Angiotensin II inhibitor/diuretic combination

Candesartan (16 mg)/hydrochlorothiazide (12.5 mg)

Eprosartan (600 mg)/hydrochlorothiazide (12.5 mg)

Irbesartan (150 or 300 mg)/hydrochlorothiazide (12.5 mg)

Telmisartan (40 or 80 mg)/hydrochlorothiazide (12.5 mg)

Combination diuretics

Amiloride (5 mg)/hydrochlorothiazide (50 mg)

Triamterene (50 mg)/ hydrochlorothiazide (25 mg)

Data on the use of potassium-sparing diuretics in Australia 2004/05 indicated that 28,600 prescriptions were written for amiloride alone, 166,559 for the combination of amiloride with hydrochlorothiazide and 53,696 for the combination of triamterene with hydrochlorothiazide. All three are considered to have limited diuretic efficacy and are primarily considered useful when combined with potassium-depleting diuretics such as the thiazides.

Amiloride and triamterene have similar mechanisms of action. They act on the late distal tubules and collecting ducts where they inhibit the reabsorption of sodium and decrease the excretion of potassium. Spironolactone, a synthetic steroidal compound, is a specific antagonist for the mineral-ocorticoid receptor and blocks the action of aldosterone (see Chapter 40). This action results in inhibition of the sodium-retaining property of aldosterone and a concomitant reduction in its potassium-secreting property. The effectiveness of spironolactone is directly related to the circulating level of aldosterone: if the level is high, the effect of spironolactone is greater. It does not interfere with renal tubule transport of sodium and chloride, and does not inhibit carbonic anhydrase. When used alone, all of these drugs have the potential to cause life-threatening hyperkalaemia.

Indications

The potassium-sparing diuretics are indicated for the prevention and treatment of diuretic-induced hypokalaemia. They are also used as adjunct therapy in the treatment of oedema due to heart failure and hepatic cirrhosis. Spironolactone is used

GERIATRIC IMPLICATIONS DIURETICS

As kidneys age, their ability to concentrate and acidify urine and to retain potassium and sodium diminishes. Hence the elderly are more sensitive to diuretic-induced hypotension and electrolyte disturbances than younger adults.

For the elderly patient, start with the lowest dose possible, and titrate slowly to achieve the desired effect.

Diuretics are often referred to as 'water pills', and many people believe fluid intake should be restricted with this drug category. Fluid intake should be discussed with the individual.

Avoid or use *extreme* caution and close monitoring if concurrent potassium supplementation or a potassium chloride salt substitute is ordered for people receiving a potassium-sparing diuretic. Hyperkalaemia and death have been reported with this combination.

Be aware that diuretics can increase urinary incontinence, and be alert to signs and symptoms of diuretic toxicity, such as anorexia, nausea, vomiting, confusion, increased weakness, and paraesthesia of the extremities.

When a diuretic is to be discontinued, reduce the drug gradually to avoid the development of fluid retention and oedema.

**CLINICAL INTEREST BOX 28-2
USE OF SPIRONOLACTONE FOR THE
TREATMENT OF SEVERE HEART FAILURE**

A Randomized Aldactone Evaluation Study (RALES) that was published in 1999 assessed the effectiveness of a combination of spironolactone, an angiotensin-converting enzyme inhibitor (ACE inhibitor), and a loop diuretic in people with severe chronic congestive heart failure. The study was discontinued early because it was evident after 2 years that those patients receiving spironolactone (25 mg daily) had a lower risk of death from progressing heart failure and sudden cardiac death than the placebo group. In addition, the patients receiving spironolactone were hospitalised less frequently and had significant improvement in the symptoms of heart failure (Pitt et al 1999).

The publication of RALES led to a significant increase in the rate of prescription of spironolactone and associated morbidity and mortality from hyperkalaemia (Juurlink et al 2004). Hyperkalaemia is a common adverse effect of spironolactone, and close laboratory monitoring of potassium is necessary on a weekly basis when the drug is first commenced, and then monthly or whenever indicated clinically.

for the treatment of primary hyperaldosteronism, hirsutism in females, for refractory oedema associated with secondary hyperaldosteronism and severe heart failure (Clinical Interest Box 28-2).

Pharmacokinetics

Amiloride has poor oral absorption (15%–25%), whereas triamterene and spironolactone are moderately to well absorbed from the gastrointestinal tract (30%–70%). Spironolactone is metabolised to the active metabolite canrenone, which has a plasma half-life of 16 hours. The onset of action of spironolactone is slow, taking several days to develop. Both spironolactone and triamterene are extensively metabolised in the liver, whereas amiloride is excreted predominantly as unchanged drug by the kidneys. For pharmacokinetic and dosage information, see Table 28-1.

Drug interactions/adverse reactions

See the Drug Interactions table 28-3 for potassium-sparing diuretics.

Common adverse reactions include electrolyte disturbances, particularly hyperkalaemia, hyponatraemia and hypochloraemia (worsened by the combination with hydrochlorothiazide), nausea, vomiting, dizziness, constipation, impotence and headache. Adverse reactions tend to limit the use of spironolactone and, in addition to those already listed, gynaecomastia and decreased libido are a problem.

See Box 28-1 for signs and symptoms of fluid and electrolyte imbalances.

Warnings and contraindications

These drugs are contraindicated in situations of pre-existing hyperkalaemia (plasma potassium >5 mmol/L) and renal failure. Caution should also be exercised in people with type 1 diabetes, renal or hepatic impairment and debilitating

PREGNANCY SAFETY DIURETICS	
ADEC Category	**Drugs**
B1	Oxybutynin
B2	Propantheline
B3	Spironolactone
C	Amiloride, bumetanide, chlorthalidone, ethacrynic acid, frusemide, hydrochlorothiazide, indapamide

cardiopulmonary disease, and in the elderly, who are prone to hyperkalaemia and hypotension. Both amiloride and spironolactone should be avoided in pregnant women; amiloride can cause electrolyte disturbances in the fetus (ADEC Category C) and spironolactone can cause feminisation of the male fetus (ADEC Category B3).

Osmotic diuretics

Osmotic diuretics such as mannitol cause diuresis by adding to the solutes already present in the tubular fluid; they are particularly effective in increasing osmotic pressure because they are not reabsorbed by the tubules. Passive water reabsorption is reduced in their presence; as more fluid remains in the lumen, this alters the electrochemical gradients so less sodium and chloride are reabsorbed in the proximal tubule. Urine volume increases but there is only a small increase in sodium excretion. The availability of other highly effective diuretics has resulted in relegation of these agents for use in non-diuretic indications such as cerebral oedema, reducing intraocular pressure before and after intraocular surgery, and for acute closed-angle glaucoma (see Chapter 35).

DRUGS FOR URINARY INCONTINENCE

Urinary incontinence is a common and embarrassing problem that afflicts in particular the elderly population (see Chapter 27). The storage of urine and the emptying of the bladder involve complex neural integration between the central nervous system (CNS), the spinal cord and peripheral nerves. The bladder has somatic, parasympathetic and sympathetic innervation. Sympathetic innervation controls continence by influencing the function of the internal urinary sphincter. Contraction of the sphincter (closure) ensures that the bladder fills and that leakage of urine does not occur. When the bladder is full (as sensed by stretch receptors in the bladder wall), signals are sent to the brain, the sympathetic system is inhibited and as the internal sphincter relaxes (opens), stimulation from parasympathetic nerves causes contraction

DRUG INTERACTIONS 28-3 Potassium-sparing diuretics	
Drug	**Possible effect and management**
ACE inhibitors, angiotensin II antagonists, potassium supplements	Increased risk of hyperkalaemia. Avoid combined use
Cyclosporin, NSAIDs	Increased risk of hyperkalaemia with both and increased risk of renal failure with NSAIDs. Use with caution and monitor plasma potassium concentration
Lithium	Concurrent use increases the risk of lithium toxicity by reducing renal clearance. Monitor plasma lithium concentration

BOX 28-1 SIGNS AND SYMPTOMS OF FLUID AND ELECTROLYTE IMBALANCES ASSOCIATED WITH DIURETIC THERAPY*

Hypovolaemia	Hypotension, weak pulse, tachycardia, clammy skin, rapid respirations and reduced urinary output
Hyponatraemia	Low plasma sodium levels (reference range 137–143 mmol/L), lethargy, disorientation, muscle tenseness, seizures and coma
Hypokalaemia	Low plasma potassium levels (reference range 2.0–4.5 mmol/L), weakness, abnormal ECG, postural hypotension and flaccid paralysis
Hypocalcaemia	Low plasma calcium levels (reference range 2.10–2.60 mmol/L), irritability, vomiting, diarrhoea, twitching, hyperactive reflexes, cardiac dysrhythmias, tetany and seizures
Hypochloraemia	Low plasma chloride levels (reference range 97–111 mmol/L)
Hypomagnesaemia	Low plasma magnesium levels (reference range 0.70–0.95 mmol/L), nausea and vomiting, lethargy, muscle weakness, tremors and tetany

With potassium-sparing diuretics, be alert for:

Hyperkalaemia	Above the upper limit of the reference range for plasma potassium; nausea, diarrhoea, muscle weakness, postural hypotension and ECG changes

*Consult local/regional laboratories for the equivalent reference ranges.

CLINICAL INTEREST BOX 28-3 RENAL DAMAGE FROM DRUGS, FOODS AND PLANTS

The kidneys are exposed to numerous chemicals every day, forming around 5 million litres of ultrafiltrate over a lifespan of 75 years. Exposure to nephrotoxins occurs from the ingestion of drugs, environmental chemicals, food and plants. Common drugs such as NSAIDs and ACE inhibitors can cause deterioration in renal function, and aminoglycoside antibiotics have been reported to cause an increase in plasma creatinine in about 30% of patients (Saker 2000).

Analgesic abuse was widespread in Australia in the 1970s and was related to widespread advertising and marketing of compound analgesics containing e.g. aspirin combined with phenacetin and caffeine or codeine. Analgesic abusers were typically people with addictive personality traits. The renal function abnormalities included a reduction in glomerular filtration, haematuria and proteinuria, and pathological changes typified by renal papillary necrosis. As a result of legislation introduced in Australia in 1979, restricting the advertising and sale of analgesics, the incidence of analgesic abuse and end-stage renal failure declined (Nanra 1993).

Heavy metals, such as cadmium and lead, and environmental chemicals, such as the pesticides paraquat, chlordane and diquat, all cause renal lesions if ingested, and many of these have been the offending chemical used for suicide. Nephrotoxicity from foods is rare and is more the exception than the rule, although many plants are incredibly toxic to the kidneys. These include the *Amanita phalloides* mushroom, *Datura* species (e.g. angel trumpets), autumn crocus and water hemlock. The damage produced varies enormously and can range from papillary necrosis to acute tubular necrosis to interstitial nephritis and glomerulonephritis.

of the detrusor muscle and urination occurs. When the bladder is empty the nerve signals reverse and the bladder is able to fill with urine again. Defects in these normal pathways lead to incontinence or urinary retention.

Before instituting drug treatment, contributing factors should be eliminated. These include the possibility of a urinary tract infection, excessive fluid intact, high caffeine consumption, metabolic disorders (e.g. hyperglycaemia) and the administration of certain drugs (see Table 28-3). Incontinence can be categorised into three main types: urge incontinence, stress incontinence and overflow incontinence (see Clinical Interest Box 27-2). Anticholinergic drugs are the main group used for the treatment of urinary incontinence.

Anticholinergics

Acetylcholine is the neurotransmitter that controls the detrusor muscle. Overactivity of the detrusor muscle that leads to urge incontinence can be controlled by drugs that block the action of acetylcholine (muscarinic receptor antagonists). This reduces contractility of the bladder muscle, which leads to an increase in bladder capacity. Drugs in this class include **oxybutynin**, propantheline and tolterodine.

Drug interactions and adverse reactions

The main interactions are with other drugs that have

TABLE 28-3 Drug therapy that can contribute to urinary incontinence

DRUG CLASS	SITE OF ACTION	MECHANISM
ACE inhibitors		Chronic cough can worsen stress incontinence
α-adrenergic antagonists	Internal sphincter	Decrease tone
Anticholinergics	Detrusor muscle	Impair contraction
Calcium channel blockers	Detrusor muscle	Decrease contraction
Diuretics		Brisk filling can lead to urgency
Opioids	Detrusor muscle	Impair contraction
Sedatives		Can produce confusion

Adapted from: Chutka & Takahashi 1998; AMH 2006.

DRUGS AT A GLANCE 28: Diuretics and drug treatment of urinary incontinence

Therapeutic group	Pharmacological group	Key examples	Key pages
Diuretics	Loop	frusemide	482, 3
		bumetanide	482
	Thiazide	hydrochlorothiazide	483
		chlorthalidone	484
	Potassium-sparing	amiloride	485–7
		triamterene	485
Urinary antispasmodics	Anticholinergics (genitourinary)	oxybutynin	488
		propantheline	488
		tolterodine	488

anticholinergic properties. These include tricyclic antidepressants, antihistamines, phenothiazines and butyrophenones.

Common adverse reactions related to muscarinic receptor blockade include dry mouth, blurred vision, mydriasis, constipation, urinary hesitancy, orthostatic hypotension and tachycardia.

Warnings and contraindications

These drugs should not be used in people with narrow-angle glaucoma, partial or complete gastrointestinal tract obstruction, severe colitis, urinary obstruction, myasthenia gravis or unstable cardiac rhythms. There is little experience with either drug during pregnancy: ADEC category B1 (oxybutynin) and category B2 (propantheline).

KEY POINTS

- Diuretics are important drugs used for the treatment of hypertension and for other conditions in which fluid volume excess is a problem, such as congestive heart failure, cirrhosis and nephrotic syndrome.
- Diuretics modify renal function and induce diuresis (increased rate of urine flow) and natriuresis (enhanced excretion of sodium chloride).
- There are three major classes of diuretics: the loop diuretics (e.g. frusemide), the thiazide diuretics (e.g. hydrochlorothiazide) and the potassium-sparing diuretics (e.g. amiloride).
- The loop diuretics are potent inhibitors of the reabsorption of sodium and chloride in the thick ascending limb of the loop of Henle.
- A wide variety of drug interactions occur with the loop diuretics.

- Thiazide diuretics inhibit absorption of sodium and chloride in the proximal (diluting) segment of the distal convoluted tubule and are considered less potent than the loop diuretics.
- Thiazide diuretics primarily promote the renal excretion of water, sodium, chloride, potassium and magnesium, whereas excretion of uric acid and calcium is decreased.
- Hyperglycaemia, or impaired glucose tolerance, has been reported with thiazide diuretics but rarely with loop diuretics.
- The potassium-sparing diuretics are amiloride, spironolactone and triamterene. All three are considered to have limited diuretic efficacy and are primarily considered useful when combined with potassium-depleting diuretics such as the thiazides.
- The commonest adverse reactions are electrolyte disturbances (e.g. hyponatraemia, hypokalaemia, hypomagnesaemia).
- Urinary incontinence is a common and embarrassing problem that afflicts in particular the elderly population. Incontinence can be categorised into three main types: urge incontinence, stress incontinence and overflow incontinence. Anticholinergic drugs are the main group used for the treatment of urinary incontinence.

REVIEW EXERCISES

1 Describe the mechanisms and sites of action of the thiazide diuretics. Why are they less potent than the loop diuretics? What effects do they have on glucose, potassium, uric acid, plasma levels of cholesterol and triglycerides?

2 Compare the sites and mechanisms of action of the thiazide diuretics with those of the loop diuretics. Describe three serious drug interactions with the loop diuretics.

3 What are the advantages of combining a thiazide diuretic with a potassium-sparing diuretic?

4 What are the methods of administration for loop diuretics, thiazides and potassium-sparing diuretics?

5 Explain why anticholinergic drugs are effective for the treatment of urinary incontinence.

REFERENCES AND FURTHER READING

Australian Medicines Handbook 2006. Adelaide: AMH Pty Ltd, 2006.
Brater DC. Diuretic therapy. New England Journal of Medicine 1998; 339: 387–95.
Chutka DS, Takahashi PY. Urinary incontinence in the elderly; drug treatment options. Drugs 1998; 56: 587–95.
Dollery C (ed). Therapeutic Drugs. Vols 1 and 2. London: Churchill Livingstone, 1991.
Greger R. Physiology of sodium transport. American Journal of Medical Science 2000; 319: 51–62.
Juurlink DN, Mamdani MM, Lee DS, Kopp A, Austin PC, Laupacis A, Redelmeier DA. Rates of hyperkalemia after publication of the randomized aldactone evaluation study. New England Journal of Medicine 2004; 351: 543–51.
Nanra RS. Analgesic nephropathy in the 1990s—an Australian perspective. Kidney International 1993; 44 Suppl. 42: S86–92.
Olin BR. Facts and Comparisons. Philadelphia: JB Lippincott, 1998.
Pitt B, Zannad F, Remme WJ, Cody R, Castaigne A, Perez A, Palensky J, Wittes J. The effect of spironolactone on morbidity and mortality in patients with severe heart failure. New England Journal of Medicine 1999; 341: 709–17.
Rang HP, Dale MM, Ritter JM, Moore PK. Pharmacology. 5th edn. Edinburgh: Churchill Livingstone, 2003 [Ch. 23].
Saker BM. Everyday drug therapies affecting the kidneys. Australian Prescriber 2000; 23; 17–19.
Vogel A. The discovery of the organic mercurial diuretics. American Heart Journal 1950; 39: 881–3.

evolve More weblinks at http://evolve.elsevier.com/AU/Bryant/pharmacology/

UNIT VII
Drugs Affecting the Blood

CHAPTER 29

Overview of the Haemopoietic System

CHAPTER FOCUS

The haemopoietic system comprises principally blood and bone marrow and the accessory organs: the liver, spleen and kidneys. Blood is the common element that serves every system in the body. It is a multipurpose medium that not only delivers oxygen and nutrients to tissues, removes waste products from cells, regulates pH, adjusts body temperature and affords protection against disease, but also has the capacity to clot, thus preventing haemorrhage. It is crucial for the maintenance of homeostasis—perturbations of the haemopoietic system may manifest in illnesses such as anaemia, haemophilia, thromboembolic disease and leukaemia. Numerous drugs are available that act on the blood, including those that prevent clotting and platelet aggregation, lyse thrombi and treat anaemia. Equally, numerous drugs, notably cancer chemotherapeutic agents, depress bone marrow function as an adverse effect.

OBJECTIVES

- To describe the composition and functions of blood.
- To discuss the structure and function of the three types of blood cells.
- To name and describe the five types of leucocytes found in the blood.
- To discuss the intrinsic and extrinsic pathways for blood clotting.

KEY TERMS

albumin
anaemia
colony-stimulating factors
erythrocytes
erythropoietin
fibrinogen
globulins
haematocrit
haemoglobin
haemopoiesis
haemopoietic system

haemostasis
leucocytes
leucocytosis
leucopenia
phagocytosis
plasma proteins
platelets
thrombocytes
thrombocytopenia
thrombopoietin
thromboxane A_2

KEY ABBREVIATIONS

RBCs red blood cells
WBCs white blood cells
EPO erythropoietin
TPO thrombopoietin
CSFs colony-stimulating factors

THE **haemopoietic system** comprises primarily the blood and bone marrow, complemented by the liver (storage of vitamin B_{12} for erythrocyte production), spleen (removal of expired blood cells and storage of platelets) and kidneys (erythropoietin production). A viscous liquid consisting of plasma and cells, blood is the major transport system in the body and is vitally important for the proper functioning and regulation of the human body. Pumped by the heart, blood carries drugs and nutrients absorbed from the gastrointestinal tract, and oxygen from the lungs to cells throughout the entire body. In addition, it transports waste products from body cells and delivers them to the liver, kidneys and lungs for excretion. Hormones, enzymes, buffers and many other biochemical substances are also transported via the blood to their respective target cells. Blood further helps to regulate body temperature through changes in both its heat-absorbing and cooling properties and by the action of the vascular system in varying its flow through the skin. In addition to its transportation and regulatory roles, blood clots in response to an injury to prevent excessive blood loss and aids in immunity by producing antibodies.

BLOOD COMPOSITION

Blood is composed of two components, cells and plasma—the fluid portion in which the cells are suspended. Although blood volume can vary among individuals and between males and females, the blood volume of an average-sized adult is about 5 L. Of this volume, about 3 L is usually plasma and the remainder is primarily red blood cells. Together, these two components are responsible overall for the viscosity of blood, which is greater than that of water; thus, relative to water, blood tends to flow more slowly. Increased blood viscosity can retard blood flow through blood vessels, resulting in headaches, fatigue, weakness, dyspnoea, and perhaps an enlarged spleen. Buffering is also an important function of blood; the pH of human blood ranges from 7.35 to 7.45.

Plasma

Plasma, a straw-coloured fluid easily seen after centrifuging blood, is about 92% water and 8% plasma proteins (albumin, globulins and fibrinogen). **Plasma proteins** play an important role in maintaining the osmotic pressure of blood, which is important for fluid exchange through capillary walls. **Albumin** is important for the transport of some steroid hormones and fatty acids, and also in the binding of numerous drugs. The **globulins** include the immunoglobulins, also called antibodies, which are important in the body's defence against viruses and bacteria. **Fibrinogen** is essential for blood clotting

and is converted to fibrin by thrombin in the presence of calcium ions. In addition to the proteins, plasma may contain thousands of other substances, such as glucose, electrolytes, vitamins, hormones and waste products. This overview focuses on blood cells, blood proteins and blood groups.

Blood cells

Blood is composed of three types of blood cells:
- red blood cells (RBCs), or erythrocytes, which transport oxygen and carbon dioxide
- white blood cells (WBCs), or leucocytes, which defend the body against bacteria and infections
- platelets, or thrombocytes, which are necessary for blood coagulation.

Changes in various physiological and pathological states may affect blood viscosity; for example, an increase in red blood cells (polycythaemia) increases viscosity. A common laboratory test used is the **haematocrit** (the proportion of packed erythrocytes in blood after centrifugation). The normal range of haematocrit for adult men is 0.4–0.52 and for adult women 0.35–0.47. The higher the haematocrit, the greater the blood viscosity; for example, a person with polycythaemia may have a haematocrit of 0.6 or 0.7, while a person with anaemia may have a significant drop in haematocrit.

BLOOD CELL FORMATION

Haemopoiesis, or blood cell production, occurs within certain parts of bone, principally the red bone marrow. During fetal development, many tissues (e.g. liver, spleen and thymus gland) participate in blood cell production but, after birth, haemopoiesis occurs only in the red bone marrow and, after 20 years of age, principally in the bone marrow of the vertebrae, sternum, ribs and ilia. Differentiation and proliferation of precursor cells into the various types of blood cells is regulated by haemopoietic growth factors such as **erythropoietin** (EPO), **thrombopoietin** (TPO) and the cytokines, which include **colony-stimulating factors** (CSFs) and interleukins (see Chapter 54).

Secretion by the kidneys of EPO, a hormone that regulates production of red blood cells by the bone marrow, is stimulated by hypoxia and/or blood loss. With maximal bone marrow stimulation, red blood cell production can be increased nearly seven times over the normal rate. Thrombopoietin, another hormone, is produced by the liver and substantially increases platelet production, while CSFs and interleukins stimulate formation of leucocytes. A simplified diagram of blood cell differentiation is shown in Figure 29-1.

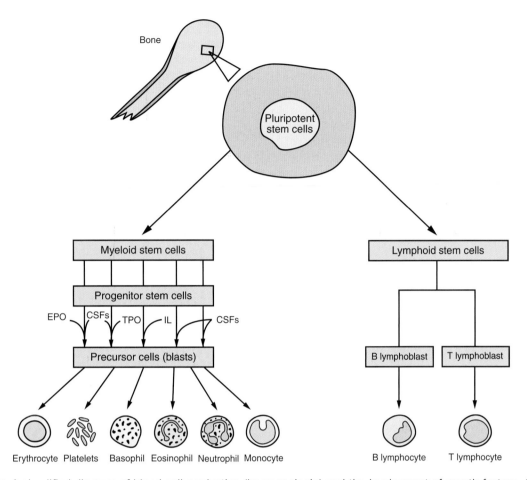

FIGURE 29-1 A simplified diagram of blood cell production (haemopoiesis) and the involvement of growth factors. Cells originating from myeloid stem cells are produced in the bone marrow. Lymphoid stem cells arise in bone marrow but development of lymphocytes is completed in lymphatic tissue. CSFs =colony-stimulating factors; EPO = erythropoietin; IL = interleukin; TPO = thrombopoietin.

RED BLOOD CELLS (ERYTHROCYTES)

RBCs, or **erythrocytes**, are small, non-nucleated, biconcave disc-shaped cells present in large quantities in the blood-stream. Without a nucleus, RBCs have negligible synthetic capacity and hence their lifespan is short, about 120 days. Expired cells are removed from the circulation and destroyed by phagocytes resident in the liver and spleen. It has been estimated that more than 100 million RBCs are produced every minute during adulthood. The normal healthy adult has $4.0–6.0 \times 10^{12}$ cells/L of blood. The body balances production (erythropoiesis) and destruction of these cells to maintain a relatively constant level of RBCs.

Dissolved within the cytosol of RBCs are haemoglobin molecules, the major function of which is the transport of oxygen. Each **haemoglobin** molecule consists of a protein called globin, composed of four polypeptide chains, four non-

protein haem pigment molecules and four iron atoms. Each polypeptide chain is associated with one haem and one iron ion (Fe^{2+}), thus one haemoglobin molecule combines in total with four oxygen molecules. Oxygen is transported from the lungs to the tissues where it is released from the haemoglobin and diffuses through the interstitial fluid into the cells. Haemoglobin can also combine with carbon dioxide that is carried from the cells to the lungs for excretion. More recently, haemoglobin has been reported to be involved in blood pressure regulation by transporting nitric oxide (NO), a gas produced by endothelial cells that line blood vessels and which causes vasodilation. Males tend to have more haemoglobin (range 130–175 g/L) in their blood than females (115–160 g/L).

A condition in which there is a reduced oxygen-carrying capacity of the blood (due to reduced amount or functionality of haemoglobin) is referred to as **anaemia** and often manifests as fatigue. Different types of anaemia exist and are classified on the basis of size and number of functional RBCs and haemoglobin levels. Examples of anaemia include:

- pernicious anaemia, due to a deficiency in absorption of vitamin B$_{12}$ from the small intestine, caused by a lack of intrinsic factor
- iron-deficiency anaemia, due to either inadequate intake or absorption or excessive loss of iron, e.g. during menstruation or as a result of gastric ulceration
- haemorrhagic anaemia, which occurs as a consequence of excessive bleeding and haemolytic anaemia due to premature loss of red cell membrane integrity (e.g. incompatible blood transfusion)
- anaemia induced by increased rate of red cell destruction, which may occur with infections, cancer, or from bone marrow suppression caused by radiation therapy or many cancer chemotherapeutic agents.

WHITE BLOOD CELLS (LEUCOCYTES)

There are five types of nucleated **leucocytes** found in the blood. They are produced primarily in the bone marrow and are classified according to the presence or absence of granules in the cell cytoplasm (see Figure 29-1). There are three types of granular leucocytes: neutrophils, eosinophils and basophils; aged cells that have different-shaped nuclear lobes and an increased number of nuclei (>2, >3 or >5) are referred to as polymorphonuclear leucocytes, or polymorphs. The other two types of leucocytes are lymphocytes and monocytes, which are produced mainly in lymph tissues and organs such as the spleen, thymus, tonsils and various other lymphoid tissue in the bone marrow, gastrointestinal tract, and elsewhere. Blood of a healthy person usually contains $4.0–11.0 \times 10^9$ leucocytes/L. As each type of leucocyte plays a specific role, a differential white blood cell count may be used to detect infections or inflammatory conditions; for example, in acute appendicitis, the percentage of neutrophils increases, as does the total leucocyte count. **Leucopenia** refers to an abnormally low number of leucocytes; **leucocytosis** refers to an increase in WBCs, e.g. in response to infection.

Neutrophils, basophils, monocytes and lymphocytes are very mobile; they leave the capillaries and migrate to sites of infection. The neutrophils and monocytes ingest and destroy the pathogens, a process known as **phagocytosis**, while the lymphocytes defend the body against bacteria, fungi and viruses (see Chapter 54 for an overview of the immune system). In contrast, eosinophils play a dominant role during allergic reactions and parasitic infections.

The lifespan of granulocytes is estimated to be 4–8 hours in the bloodstream and 3–5 days in body tissues. If involved in phagocytosis of pathogens, this lifespan can be reduced to a few hours, because they can also be destroyed. Monocytes also have a short lifespan in the blood, but in body tissues they can increase in size and differentiate to become tissue macrophages (the major phagocytic cells of the immune system that ingest foreign antigens and cell debris), providing a first line of defence against tissue infections. The agranular T and B lymphocytes may live for several years.

PLATELETS

Unlike RBCs and WBCs, **platelets**, or **thrombocytes**, are small, disc-shaped, non-nucleated colourless cell fragments that split off from the megakaryocytes produced by the bone marrow (see Figure 29-1). They have a short lifespan of about 5–8 days. Time-expired platelets are engulfed by resident macrophages in the spleen and liver. Platelets are key substances for blood clotting in the body. If a blood vessel is injured, platelets will congregate at the site and clump together to form a plug to stop the bleeding (see below).

The normal platelet level in the blood is $150–450 \times 10^9$/L. People with a low quantity of platelets have **thrombocytopenia**. Such people tend to bleed and their skin usually displays small purple spots (hence the name thrombocytopenia purpura). Thrombocytopenia is often induced by irradiation injury to the bone marrow, or results from aplasia of the bone marrow induced by specific drugs.

COAGULATION
The haemostatic mechanism

Haemostasis is a process that spontaneously stops bleeding from damaged blood vessels. Blood is normally fluid while circulating in the vessels but with vessel injury it rapidly clots at the site of injury. After any injury to a blood vessel, haemostasis is achieved by three sequential steps:

- blood vessels constrict to retard blood flow from the injured area
- platelet plugs form to temporarily seal the leaking small arteries and veins
- blood coagulates to plug openings in the damaged vessels and wounds to prevent further bleeding.

Blood vessel constriction

Immediately after a blood vessel is injured, vascular constriction occurs, possibly as a reflex response from pain receptors. This response instantly slows the flow of blood from and through the ruptured vessel.

Platelet plug formation

After injury to a blood vessel, interruption of the continuity of its endothelial lining exposes collagen (a fibrous protein) in the underlying connective tissue. Platelets immediately adhere to the exposed collagen to form a dense aggregate, a process known as platelet adhesion. This attachment triggers the release of adenosine diphosphate (ADP) and **thromboxane A$_2$** from the dense granules in the platelet cytoplasm. Liberation of these factors causes further activation of nearby platelets and vasoconstriction through the action of thromboxane A$_2$, which further limits blood flow through the damaged vessel. The outer surfaces of the platelets become extremely sticky and adjacent platelets adhere to one another and the damaged site. This process of recruitment of platelets is called platelet aggregation and eventually the mass forms the platelet plug. Because this plug is relatively unstable, it can stop the bleeding quickly as long as the damage to the vessel is minute. However, for long-term effectiveness the platelet plug must be reinforced with fibrin. This involves a series of chemical reactions called blood coagulation or clotting.

Blood coagulation

Blood coagulation is the final stage of a complex series of events in haemostasis. The process ultimately results in the formation of a stable fibrin clot, which comprises a meshwork of fibrin threads that entraps platelets, blood cells and plasma. Thus the physical formation of a blood clot or thrombus plays a key role in haemostasis by permanently closing the hole in the injured vessel, preventing further bleeding. The chemical events in the blood coagulation mechanism involve two distinct pathways: the intrinsic pathway and the extrinsic pathway.

THE INTRINSIC PATHWAY

As all the chemical substances involved in coagulation are normally found in the circulating blood, this pathway is referred to as the intrinsic system of coagulation. In this complex pathway, activation by proteolysis of the first inactive blood coagulation factors causes activation of the next factor, and this cascading process continues through the whole pathway. The process occurs over several minutes and is initiated by injury to the endothelial lining of the blood vessel wall.

When blood contacts the exposed underlying collagen, factor XII (Hageman factor) is activated by proteolysis to the active 'a' form (factor XIIa). The simultaneous damage of platelets also causes the release of platelet phospholipid (platelet factor III), which is required later in the coagulation process. Factor XIIa then activates factor XI, converting it to factor XIa. The reaction of factor XIa with factor IX requires calcium ions to form activated factor IXa. In the presence of calcium ions and platelet phospholipid, factor IXa interacts with factor VIII and thrombin to form a complex. This combination then speeds up the activation of factor X. Factor Xa combines with factor V, calcium ions and platelet phospholipid to form a complex known as the prothrombin activator (factor IIa). Factor IIa initiates the cleavage of prothrombin to form thrombin, which then converts fibrinogen into fibrin, forming an unstable clot. The final step involves the action of factor XIII (a fibrin-stabilising factor), thrombin and calcium ions, which catalyse the formation of a stronger, stable fibrin clot. See Figure 29-2 for a summary of the main events of the intrinsic pathway, and Table 29-1 for a list of the blood coagulation factors.

THE EXTRINSIC PATHWAY

The extrinsic pathway is activated within seconds by trauma to the vascular wall or to tissue external to the blood vessels. In this pathway, clotting occurs when the tissue protein thromboplastin is released from the damaged tissue, leaks into the bloodstream (hence the name extrinsic) and becomes part of a complex with factor VII and calcium ions. This combination of components activates factor X, which is the step at which the extrinsic pathway converges with the intrinsic pathway; coagulation then continues through a common route with the resultant formation of a stable clot. See Figure 29-2 for the extrinsic pathway.

The final pathway common to both the intrinsic and the extrinsic coagulation systems begins with the activation of factor X and ends in the formation of fibrin. Both systems function simultaneously in the body, and lack of a normal factor in either system will usually result in a blood coagulation disorder.

TABLE 29-1 Blood coagulation factors and synonyms			
FACTOR	**NAME OR SYNONYM**	**FACTOR**	**NAME OR SYNONYM**
I	Fibrinogen	VIII	Antihaemophilic factor (AHF)
II	Prothrombin	IX	Plasma thromboplastin component, Christmas factor
III	Tissue thromboplastin	X	Thrombokinase
IV	Calcium ions (Ca^{2+})	XI	Plasma thromboplastin antecedent (PTA)
V	Proaccelerin (labile factor, accelerator globulin)	XII	Hageman factor
VII	Proconvertin (serum prothrombin conversion accelerator [SPCA])	XIII	Fibrin-stabilising factor

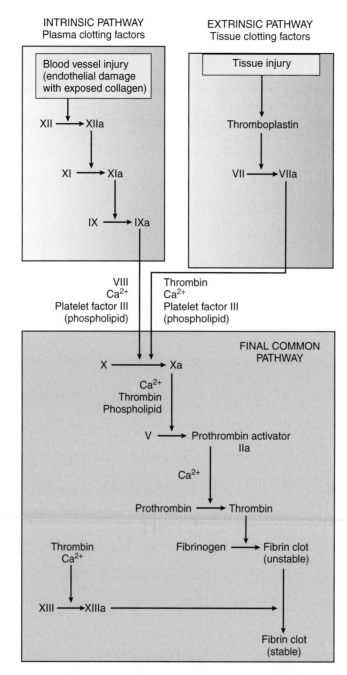

FIGURE 29-2 Coagulation mechanisms for intrinsic and extrinsic pathways for blood clotting. Final pathway (activation of factor X) is common to both the intrinsic and extrinsic coagulation systems.

Blood coagulation abnormalities

Diseases caused by intravascular clotting include some of the major causes of death from cardiovascular sources—coronary occlusion and cerebrovascular accidents. It is estimated that each year over 40,000 Australians have a stroke because of a clot or haemorrhage (Australian Institute of Health and Welfare 2004). Local trauma, vascular stasis and systemic alterations in the coagulability of blood are considered the main factors in the initiation of thrombosis in an unbroken vessel. Basically, coagulation mechanisms are responsible for forming two kinds of thrombi: arterial thrombi and venous thrombi. Arterial thrombi are most frequently associated with atherosclerotic plaques, high blood pressure, and turbulent blood flow that damages the endothelial lining of the blood vessel and causes platelets to stick and aggregate in the arterial system. Venous thrombi occur most often in areas where blood flow is reduced or static. This appears to initiate clotting and produces a thrombus in the venous system.

Thrombi that break away and move in the blood stream are called emboli.

BLOOD GROUPS AND TYPES

The major blood groups are the ABO and Rhesus (Rh) groups, which are based on the A and B type antigens and the Rh antigens (Rh+ and Rh-), respectively, located on red blood cell membranes. Although many erythrocyte antigens have been identified, antigens A, B and Rh are the most important blood antigens involved in blood transfusions and newborn survival. Every person belongs to one of the four ABO blood groups and their RBCs are either Rh+ or Rh-. In addition, the plasma of an individual may carry isoantibodies (agglutinins) (anti-A antibody, anti-B antibody) that react if transfused with the incorrect blood group. The ABO blood groups are as follows:

- type A: A antigen on RBCs and plasma contains anti-B isoantibody
- type B: B antigen on RBCs and plasma contains anti-A isoantibody
- type AB: A antigen and B antigen on RBCs but plasma contains no anti-A or anti-B isoantibodies
- type O: neither A nor B antigens on RBCs but plasma contains both anti-A and anti-B isoantibodies.

People with type A blood can safely receive blood from A and O donors, while people with type B blood can safely receive blood from type B and O donors. (With a type O donor, the donor's anti-A or anti-B antibodies become sufficiently dilute in the recipient's plasma that significant haemolysis is usually not an issue.) Type O persons can receive only type O blood because of the presence of both isoantibodies in their blood. Theoretically people with AB blood can receive all four blood types because their blood is compatible with types AB, A, B and O, hence type AB is known as the universal recipient. Similarly, people of type A, B or AB can receive type O blood, which is therefore referred to as the universal donor. Before transfusion, however, cross-matching of the blood is necessary because other isoantibodies may be present.

A person who is Rh+ carries Rh antigen on their RBCs. One who is Rh- does not have any Rh antigens on the RBCs. About 85% of the population is Rh+. Rh factor is particularly important when an Rh+ man impregnates an Rh- woman. The woman may have antibodies against the Rh antigen, which can cross the placenta and cause haemolysis of fetal blood if the fetus is Rh+. If this occurs, the infant may develop jaundice or be stillborn.

An Rh- woman can acquire Rh antibodies via blood transfusions. It is also possible to develop them if fetal blood enters the maternal bloodstream during childbirth or miscarriage. Because the fetal blood is separate from the maternal circulation until either of these events occurs, the first pregnancy usually has less risk associated with it than subsequent pregnancies. The potential problem with subsequent pregnancies can be reduced by administering human immunoglobulin [anti-Rh(D)] to Rh- women after each pregnancy. This prevents their immune systems from making antibodies to Rh+ blood. Rh- women who have a spontaneous or induced abortion or a termination of an ectopic pregnancy of up to and including 12 weeks' gestation are given a smaller dose of immunoglobulin if their partner is Rh+.

KEY POINTS

- The haemopoietic system comprises primarily the blood and bone marrow, complemented by the liver (storage of vitamin B_{12} for erythrocyte production), spleen (removal of expired blood cells and storage of platelets) and kidneys (erythropoietin production).
- Blood consists of plasma and cells; it transports oxygen, drugs, nutrients, waste products and numerous other substances such as electrolytes and hormones.
- Blood is composed of red blood cells (erythrocytes), white blood cells (leucocytes) and platelets.
- Red blood cells are small, non-nucleated, biconcave discs that have negligible synthetic capacity.
- Haemoglobin dissolved in the red cell cytosol transports oxygen.
- A reduced oxygen-carrying capacity of the blood is referred to as anaemia.
- White blood cells are nucleated and the principal types are neutrophils, eosinophils and basophils, and lymphocytes and monocytes.
- Platelets are small, disc-shaped, non-nucleated cell fragments that are essential for blood clotting.
- Haemopoiesis, or blood cell production, occurs within certain parts of bone, principally the red bone marrow.
- Differentiation and proliferation of precursor cells is regulated by haemopoietic growth factors such as erythropoietin (EPO), thrombopoietin (TPO) and the cytokines, which include colony-stimulating factors (CSFs) and interleukins.

- Haemostasis is a process that stops bleeding and involves blood vessel constriction, platelet plug formation and blood coagulation.
- Clotting involves blood chemicals called coagulation factors and is initiated by two pathways, the intrinsic and extrinsic pathways.
- A clot in an unbroken vessel is called a thrombus, but if it moves from the site of formation it is called an embolus.
- The major blood groups are the ABO and Rhesus (Rh) groups, which are based on the A- and B-type antigens and the presence or absence of the Rh antigen on red blood cells.

REVIEW EXERCISES

1 Describe the composition and function of the two major components of blood.
2 What are the functions of haemoglobin?
3 When a blood vessel is injured, how is haemostasis achieved? Outline the three steps.
4 What are the major blood groups? Explain the basis of Rhesus (Rh) incompatibility.

REFERENCES AND FURTHER READING

Australian Institute of Health and Welfare. *Australia's Health 2004*. Canberra: AIHW, 2004.
Guyton AC. *Textbook of Medical Physiology*. 8th edn. Philadelphia: WB Saunders, 1991 [chs 32, 33, 35, 36].
Tortora GJ, Grabowski SR. *Principles of Anatomy and Physiology*. 9th edn. New York: John Wiley, 2000 [ch. 19].

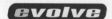 More weblinks at http://evolve.elsevier.com/AU/Bryant/pharmacology/

CHAPTER 30

Drugs Affecting Haemostasis, Thrombosis and the Haemopoietic System

CHAPTER FOCUS

Each year thousands of Australians and New Zealanders die from coronary heart disease and stroke and many more are diagnosed with deep vein thrombosis, pulmonary embolus, transient cerebral ischaemic attacks and other non-fatal thrombotic events. The formation of thrombi or acute thromboembolic disorders requires use of anticoagulant, thrombolytic and antiplatelet agents. By contrast, in some instances excessive bleeding needs to be counterbalanced by the use of specific haemostatic and antifibrinolytic drugs that hasten clot formation and reduce bleeding. All of these drugs are very potent and effective medications requiring a thorough knowledge of their pharmacology for safe usage. Anaemia can occur as a result of a number of factors, many of which are correctable without drug treatment. In some individuals, use of haemopoietics (e.g. erythropoietin) or haematinics (e.g. folic acid) may be necessary.

OBJECTIVES

- To explain the mechanisms of action of heparin and warfarin.

- To discuss common drug interactions that increase the anticoagulant effect of warfarin.

- To describe the use of protamine and vitamin K as anticoagulant antagonists.

- To explain the differences between the effects of thrombolytic and antiplatelet drugs on blood clots.

- To explain the various mechanisms by which haemostatic drugs act.

- To discuss the drug treatment of anaemia.

KEY DRUGS

aprotinin
aspirin
clopidogrel
epoetin alpha
factor VIII
heparin
low-molecular-weight heparin
streptokinase
ticlopidine
warfarin

KEY TERMS

anticoagulant drugs
antifibrinolytic drugs
antiplatelet drugs
embolus
fibrinolytic activity
haemostatic drugs
haemopoietics
haematinics
low-molecular-weight heparin
thrombolytic (fibrinolytic) drugs
thrombus

KEY ABBREVIATIONS

APTT	activated partial thromboplastin time
DIC	disseminated intravascular coagulation
EPO	erythropoietin
HITS	heparin-induced thrombocytopenic syndrome
LMWHs	low-molecular-weight heparins
INR	international normalised ratio

THIS chapter reviews anticoagulant, antiplatelet, fibrinolytic, haemostatic and antifibrinolytic drugs. Although blood clotting is a normal defence mechanism available for protection against excessive haemorrhage, the development of a **thrombus** (an aggregation of platelets, fibrin, clotting factors and the cellular elements of blood) that becomes attached to the inner wall of a blood vessel can obstruct blood flow and cause ischaemia. An **embolus**, a mass of undissolved matter that breaks off from the thrombus, can travel in the vascular system and lodge in a vital area of the body, causing death. In contrast, a defect in the blood coagulation cascade can lead to excessive bleeding or haemorrhage, even after a minor injury.

Arterial or venous thrombus formation is associated with significant morbidity and mortality. Thousands of Australians die each year from coronary heart disease (about 27,000 deaths) and stroke (about 12,000 deaths), and many more are diagnosed with deep vein thrombosis, pulmonary embolus, transient cerebral ischaemic attacks and other non-fatal thrombotic events. In many, cases the first episode of thrombosis can be prevented by prophylactic drug therapy and recurrences prevented by a secondary drug management strategy (Bick 2000). Drugs used for either the prevention or treatment of thrombosis act by modifying:

- coagulation (standard heparin, low-molecular-weight heparins [LMWHs], warfarin and the newer agents bivalirudin, fondaparinux and lepirudin)
- platelet function and aggregation (aspirin, abciximab, clopidogrel, dipyridamole, eptifibatide, ticlopidine and tirofiban)
- fibrinolysis (alteplase, reteplase, streptokinase, tenecteplase and urokinase).

ANTICOAGULANT DRUGS

Anticoagulant drug therapy (Figure 30-1) is primarily prophylactic because these agents act by preventing fibrin deposits, extension of a thrombus and thromboembolic complications. Although long-term anticoagulant therapy remains controversial, there is evidence that anticoagulant therapy reduces the incidence of thrombosis and therefore prolongs life. These drugs have no direct effect on a blood clot that has already formed or on ischaemic tissue injured by an inadequate blood supply because of the clot. The two main groups of **anticoagulant drugs** are parenteral anticoagulant

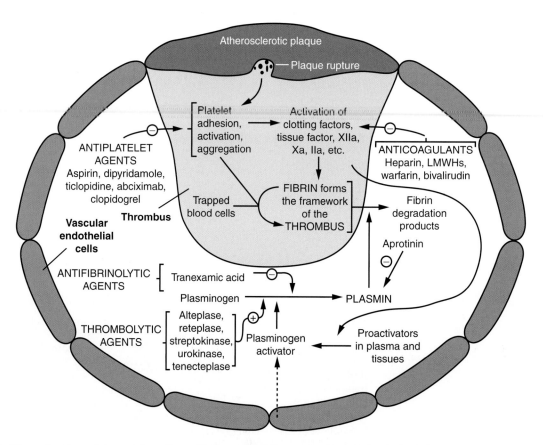

FIGURE 30-1 Sites of action of drugs interacting with the coagulation cascade and the fibrinolytic and platelet activation systems. *Source*: Rang, Dale, Ritter & Moore 2003, with permission.

drugs (e.g. heparin) and oral anticoagulant drugs (e.g. warfarin).

Parenteral anticoagulant drugs
Heparin (unfractionated)

Heparin is a complex substance (a proteoglycan) consisting of repeating disaccharide (sugar) units attached to a core protein. As a consequence, it has a wide range of molecular weights (5000–40,000). This form of heparin is often referred to as 'unfractionated', or 'standard', heparin. It is formed in especially large amounts in the mast cells of the liver, lungs and intestinal mucosa. The source of heparin for injection is bovine (cattle) lung and the mucosal lining of pig intestines. As heparin is obtained from animal tissue, the potency of each preparation varies. Activity is determined biologically, measured against an international standard and reported as units of activity.

Heparin produces its anticoagulant effect by combining with antithrombin III (heparin co-factor), a naturally occurring anticlotting factor in the plasma. The binding of heparin with antithrombin III forms a complex that acts at multiple sites in the normal coagulation system, inactivating factors IXa, Xa, XIa and XIIa. Inactivation of factor Xa of the intrinsic and extrinsic pathways prevents the conversion of prothrombin to thrombin, thereby inhibiting the formation of fibrin from fibrinogen. Furthermore, by preventing the activation of factor XIII (fibrin stabilising factor), heparin prevents the formation of a stable fibrin clot. As fibrin is associated with venous thrombi, heparin is useful in preventing venous thrombosis. The drug does not have **fibrinolytic activity**: it does not dissolve existing clots but can prevent their extension.

INDICATIONS

Heparin is used to prevent and treat all types of venous thromboembolism. It is used prophylactically to prevent blood clotting in surgery of the heart or blood vessels, during blood transfusion, in individuals with disseminated intravascular coagulation (DIC), and in the haemodialysis process. It is considered the drug of choice for acute arterial occlusion because its action is immediate and can be readily reversed if

surgery is necessary. When rapid anticoagulation is necessary, it is used before the oral anticoagulants (Table 30-1).

PHARMACOKINETICS

Heparin is administered parenterally because its large molecular size and polarity prevent any gastrointestinal absorption. Its onset of action is immediate after intravenous injection. Subcutaneous injection usually results in an onset of action within 60–120 minutes. The half-life is dose-dependent but averages 1.5 hours (range 1–6 hours). It is highly protein-bound, and metabolism appears to be principally via the reticuloendothelial system, with only a small amount of unchanged heparin appearing in urine. Heparin dosage is closely monitored with coagulation tests such as the activated partial thromboplastin time (APTT). (See Clinical Interest Box 30-1.)

DRUG INTERACTIONS

The table Drug Interactions 30-1 shows what can occur when heparin is given with the drugs listed.

DRUG INTERACTIONS 30-1 Heparin

Drug	Possible effect and management
Aspirin and other non-steroidal anti-inflammatory drugs (NSAIDs), or other platelet aggregation inhibitors	Increased risk of bleeding is present because of platelet inhibition by these drugs. Also, large doses of aspirin can produce hypoprothrombinaemia. All drugs increase the risk of toxicity because of their potential to produce gastrointestinal ulceration and bleeding. Avoid, or a potentially serious drug interaction could occur
Dextran and dipyridamole	Can increase risk of haemorrhage. Use with caution
Thrombolytics, such as alteplase, reteplase, streptokinase or urokinase	Increased risk of bleeding and haemorrhage is possible with this combination. Avoid, or a potentially serious drug interaction could occur

TABLE 30-1 Anticoagulant drugs: comparison of characteristics

	HEPARIN	WARFARIN
Onset of action	Immediate	Slow (24–48 hours)
Route of administration	Parenteral	Oral
Duration of action	Short (less than 4 hours)	Long (2–5 days)
Laboratory test for dosage control	Activated partial thromboplastin time	International normalised ratio
Antidote	Protamine sulfate	Vitamin K, whole blood, or plasma

ADVERSE REACTIONS

Bleeding, or haemorrhage, is the commonest adverse reaction. Early signs of heparin overdose include increased bruising, nosebleeds or excessive bleeding from minor cuts, wounds, brushing of teeth or menstrual period. Internal signs of bleeding include stomach pain, bloody or black stools, dizziness, persistent headaches, swollen, stiff or painful joints, and vomiting or coughing up of blood. Rarely, asthma-like symptoms, pruritus, urticaria and anaphylaxis have been reported.

At the site of injection, a haematoma or blood accumulation under the skin, pain, or a local skin reaction such as irritation, peeling or sloughing can occur. If observed, immediate discontinuation of therapy is warranted. In 1%–3% of individuals, severe immune-mediated thrombocytopenia (heparin-induced thrombocytopenic syndrome, HITS) can occur, causing complications such as limb ischaemia, stroke, bleeding or death. A substantial drop in the baseline platelet count of 30%–50% indicates the need to withhold heparin.

Heparin should be used with caution in individuals with asthma, a history of allergies, mild to moderate liver impairment or hypertension. Avoid heparin use in people with heparin hypersensitivity, cerebral aneurysm, cerebrovascular bleeding, haemorrhage, severe hypertension, haemophilia, peptic ulcer disease, severe liver or kidney disease, or blood dyscrasias; in women after recent childbirth; and in people who have recently had surgery or anaesthesia.

Low-molecular-weight heparins

The **low-molecular-weight heparins** (LMWHs) are fragments of standard heparin prepared by enzymatic or chemical cleavage. The resulting fragments have a molecular weight range of 4000–6000 and hence are called 'low-molecular-weight' heparins. This difference in molecular weight produces an anticoagulant with properties considerably different

from those of heparin. Both types of heparin can inactivate factor Xa. Heparin (unfractionated) also inactivates thrombin (IIa) because it binds both antithrombin III and thrombin at the same time. In contrast, LMWHs increase the action of antithrombin III on factor Xa, but because of their small size LMWHs can not bind antithrombin III and thrombin at the same time. Hence they have a relatively minor effect on APTT. See Table 30-2 for a comparison of heparin and LMWHs.

LMWHs are considered to be safer, easier to administer (SC), require less monitoring and are now the first choice for thromboembolism associated with pregnancy (Hovanessian 1999). Currently there are two LMWHs on the market, dalteparin and enoxaparin, and one heparinoid, danaparoid. The indications are the same as for standard heparin, with the exception that dalteparin and enoxaparin are used during pregnancy and danaparoid is indicated only for the prevention of venous thromboembolism in surgical patients.

The LMWHs are administered subcutaneously. In comparison with standard heparin, they have a lower affinity for endothelial cells, macrophages and plasma proteins, an increased bioavailability, and a more predictable clearance that is independent of dose. Hepatic clearance plays a minor role and elimination is principally via the kidneys. LMWHs have a longer half-life than heparin (2–4 times greater) when given subcutaneously and their anticoagulant effect also lasts longer. The time to peak plasma concentration is reached in 4 hours with dalteparin and 3–5 hours with enoxaparin. The elimination half-life for dalteparin is 3–5 hours, for enoxaparin 3–6 hours.

Drug interactions for the LMWHs are the same as those for heparin. In addition, if enoxaparin is given concurrently with ticlopidine, inhibition of platelet aggregation resulting in an increased risk of bleeding can result. Monitor closely.

Bleeding is a well-known complication of heparin therapy and the LMWHs have a similar risk. Common adverse

TABLE 30-2 Comparison of regular heparin and low-molecular-weight heparin

PROPERTY	REGULAR HEPARIN	LOW-MOLECULAR-WEIGHT HEPARIN
Molecular weight range	3000–30,000	1000–10,000
Average molecular weight	12,000–15,000	4000–6000
Mechanism of action	Inactivates factor Xa and IIa (thrombin)	Inactivates factor Xa
APTT monitoring required	Yes	No
Inhibits platelet functionç	++++ (high)	++ (medium)
Route of administration	IV, SC	SC only
Protein binding	++++ (high)	+ (low)
Vascular permeability increased	Yes	No
Treatment of bleeding	Protamine	Protamine (partially effective)

reactions include local irritation effects such as erythema, haematomas, urticaria and pain at the injection site. The incidence of thrombocytopenia is less (around 0.6%) and data on osteoporosis also indicate a decreased incidence. Danaparoid

may be used as an alternative to heparin or LMWH in people with heparin-induced thrombocytopenia, as cross-reactivity occurs in fewer than 10% of individuals.

Use LHWH with caution in people undergoing any medical procedure that increases the potential of bleeding. Avoid use in people with LMWH or heparin hypersensitivity, bleeding disorders, severe hypertension, stroke, thrombocytopenia, severe liver or kidney disease, endocarditis or retinopathy, and in those who have recently had surgery. In persons with renal impairment, the risk of bleeding with LMWHs is greater, as they are eliminated by renal excretion. For enoxaparin consider dose reduction in severe renal impairment and avoid completely in end-stage renal disease.

Heparin antagonist
Protamine

Protamine, a protein-like substance derived from the sperm and mature testes of salmon and other fish, is a heparin antagonist and is used in over-anticoagulation. Protamine is a very weak anticoagulant alone, but when the sulfate form is given in conjunction with heparin, a combination is formed that dissociates the heparin–antithrombin III complex, thus reducing the anticoagulant action of heparin. Protamine is a basic protein (containing many free amino groups) and is able to combine with heparin to form an inactive complex.

INDICATIONS

Protamine is indicated for the treatment of an overdose of LMWH or standard heparin that has resulted in haemorrhaging. Blood transfusions may be necessary. It is also used to neutralise the effects of heparin administered during dialysis or cardiac or arterial surgery. It is administered intravenously and has an onset of action within 1 minute. Its duration of action is about 2 hours.

Adverse reactions include back pain, a feeling of warmth or tiredness, flushing, nausea and vomiting. Less often reported are bradycardia, a sudden drop in blood pressure, shock and dyspnoea (all related to the too-rapid administration of protamine), bleeding (caused by protamine overdose or a rebound of heparin activity), hypertension and anaphylaxis.

Use protamine with caution in individuals who have been exposed to protamine in the past, including protamine insulin. Protamine antibodies might have developed, which increases the risk of an allergic reaction. Avoid use in people with protamine hypersensitivity.

Protamine is administered by slow intravenous injection over 10 minutes. One milligram of protamine is necessary to neutralise around 100 units of standard heparin, if injected within 15 minutes of heparin administration. As heparin is cleared quite rapidly, a reduction in the dose of protamine is necessary if it is administered more than 15 minutes after the heparin dose. The standard dose of protamine (1 mg) will partially neutralise 100 units of dalteparin and 1 mg enoxaparin. Close monitoring with blood coagulation tests is required.

Antithrombin-III-dependent and -independent anticoagulants

The antithrombin-III-dependent anticoagulant is fondaparinux, a synthetic and specific inhibitor of factor Xa. Fondaparinux, which binds ATIII, inhibiting both thrombin formation and thrombus development, is as effective and as safe as the LMWHs. It is administered SC and is used in the prevention of venous thromboembolism in high-risk surgery such as hip fracture or replacement, or knee replacement. The

long half-life of 17 hours permits once-daily administration. As with the heparins, this drug is contraindicated in coexisting bleeding disorders and in cases of renal impairment. The latter is important because fondaparinux is excreted unchanged in urine. At present there are no data in pregnancy and breastfeeding, and it is currently listed in ADEC Category C.

The use of medicinal leeches (*Hirudo medicinalis*) has its origins more than 2500 hundred years ago. The discovery in 1884 by John Haycraft that blood in the leech gut did not coagulate finally led to the isolation of the anticoagulant hirudin from leech pharyngeal glands by Markwardt in the late 1950s. The modern anticoagulants are bivalirudin, which is a 20-amino acid synthetic analogue of hirudin, while lepirudin (recombinant hirudin) has been produced using molecular technology. Both drugs bind directly to thrombin

---

DRUG MONOGRAPH 30-1 WARFARIN

Warfarin interferes with hepatic synthesis of the vitamin K-dependent clotting factors, thus depressing the synthesis of factors X, IX, VII and II (prothrombin). Factor VII is depleted quickly; the sequential depletion of factors IX, X and II follows. Warfarin does not affect established clots but prevents further extension of formed clots, thereby diminishing the potential for secondary thromboembolic complications.

INDICATIONS Warfarin is indicated for the prophylaxis and treatment of deep venous thrombosis and pulmonary thromboembolism. It is also used for the prophylaxis of thromboembolism associated with chronic atrial fibrillation, myocardial infarction or in individuals with prosthetic heart valves.

PHARMACOKINETICS The major advantage of this drug is that it is effective orally and can be given once daily after the maintenance dose has been established. Warfarin is well absorbed from the gastrointestinal tract and has a systemic bioavailability of >95%. Peak plasma concentration occurs in 3–9 hours and its duration of action is 2–5 days. The plasma half-life varies from 25 to 60 hours with an average of 40 hours. Warfarin is highly protein-bound (99%). It is metabolised in the liver and eliminated via bile and urine. The elderly are more susceptible to anticoagulant effects (see the Geriatric Implications box).

DRUG INTERACTIONS Many drugs interact with the oral anticoagulant drugs and the international normalised ratio (INR) should be monitored more often when instituting, ceasing or altering other drug therapy. See Box 30-1 for the significant drug interactions.

An increase in the anticoagulant effect of warfarin has been reported with the herbal medicines dong quai, garlic, papaya and St John's wort, and a decrease in anticoagulant effect with ginseng (Campbell et al 2001).

ADVERSE REACTIONS These include bleeding (common), alopecia, anorexia, abdominal cramps or distress, leucopenia, nausea, vomiting, diarrhoea, purple toes syndrome (rare) and kidney damage (rare). Risk of teratogenicity is high and fetal abnormalities and facial anomalies have been reported. If an anticoagulant is necessary during pregnancy, LMWH is usually the drug of choice because it does not cross the placenta.

Risk factors for bleeding include age >70 years, previous history of stroke and falls, liver disease, chronic renal failure, drug interactions and evidence of gastrointestinal bleeding in the previous 18 months (Campbell et al 2001).

WARNINGS AND CONTRAINDICATIONS Use with caution in individuals with a history of severe allergic or anaphylactic reactions, oedema, elevated cholesterol or lipid concentrations or hypothyroidism, in the elderly, and in unsupervised individuals who are alcoholics, psychotic, senile or mentally unstable.

Avoid use in people with known anticoagulant drug hypersensitivity, any medical or surgical condition associated with bleeding (aneurysm, cerebrovascular bleeding, surgery and severe trauma), blood disorders, severe uncontrolled hypertension, pericarditis, severe diabetics, ulcers, visceral cancer, vitamin C or vitamin K deficiencies, endocarditis or severe liver or kidney impairment. Brands of warfarin should not be interchanged due to a lack of bioequivalent data.

DOSAGE AND ADMINISTRATION The usual dose is 5–10 mg daily for 2 days and then adjusted according to the INR. The maintenance dose is in the range 1–10 mg daily and is taken at the same time each day. The INR range varies with specific indications, and local guidelines should be consulted.

independently of ATIII and hence block the thrombogenic activity of thrombin. These drugs are also referred to as direct thrombin inhibitors.

Bivalirudin has a plasma half-life of 25 minutes and lepirudin approximately 1.5 hours; both are administered by IV infusion. Bleeding disorders and significant reduction in renal function are factors for consideration prior to use of either of these drugs. As would be expected, common adverse reactions include bleeding, and in the case of lepirudin a significant number of people (~40%) develop antibodies. Fatal anaphylaxis has been reported on re-exposure to the drug. These are new drugs in the Australasian market, and the full range of adverse drug reactions and drug interactions may not yet be known.

Oral anticoagulant drugs

These drugs were discovered following an outbreak of a haemorrhagic disorder in cattle eating spoiled sweet clover in 1929. The active constituent was later identified as bishydroxycoumarin in 1939. Synthesised analogues, including warfarin (the name comes from the **W**isconsin **A**lumni **R**esearch **F**oundation and **arin** from coumarin), were originally thought to be too toxic and were used as rodenticides. Following survival of a man in 1951 after repeated high doses of the rat poison in an attempt to commit suicide, warfarin was introduced as an anticoagulant for humans in 1959 (see Drug Monograph 30-1). Warfarin is the most widely prescribed oral anticoagulant in Australia (Campbell et al 2001).

Oral anticoagulant antagonist
Vitamin K (phytomenadione)

Vitamin K is essential to the hepatic synthesis of prothrombin (factor II) and factors VII, IX and X. It acts as a co-factor for the carboxylase enzyme, which is necessary for the formation of prothrombin. A deficiency of vitamin K leads to hypoprothrombinaemia and haemorrhage.

BOX 30-1 SIGNIFICANT DRUG INTERACTIONS WITH WARFARIN

Agents that may increase the anticoagulant effect (↑ INR), often necessitating a dosage reduction

Allopurinol	Ciprofloxacin	Ketorolac	Sulfinpyrazone
Amiodarone	Danazol	Leflunomide	Sulfonamides
Anabolic steroids	Dextran	Mefenamic acid	Sulindac
Aspirin	Dextrothyroxine	Metronidazole	SSRIs
Azithromycin	Dipyridamole†	Miconazole	Tamoxifen
Capecitabine	Disulfiram	Phenytoin‡	Thyroid hormone
Cefamandole	Erythromycins	Piperacillin	Ticarcillin
Cefazolin	Fluconazole	Piroxicam	Urokinase
Ceftriaxone	Fluoxetine	Propranolol	Valproate
Celecoxib	Gemcitabine	Propylthiouracil	Zafirlukast
Chloral hydrate*	Gemfibrozil	Quinidine	
Chloramphenicol	Indomethacin	Salicylates	
Cimetidine	Ketoprofen	Streptokinase	

Agents that may decrease the anticoagulant effect (↓ INR), often necessitating an increase in anticoagulant dosage

Aminoglutethimide	Carbamazepine	Haloperidol	Vitamin K
Aprepitant	Colestipol	Primidone	
Azathioprine	Cortisone	Rifampicin	
Barbiturates	Dicloxacillin	Sucralfate	

*Usually occurs during first 2 weeks of therapy. With chronic concurrent therapy, the anticoagulant effect may return to normal or be decreased.
†With doses of dipyridamole >400 mg/day.
‡Increased anticoagulant effect occurs initially. With chronic concurrent therapy, decreased activity may occur. May also see a decrease in metabolism of phenytoin, possibly leading to increased plasma concentrations and toxicity.

INDICATIONS

Vitamin K is used to prevent and treat hypoprothrombinaemia. Prothrombin deficiency can occur because of inadequate absorption of vitamin K from the intestine (usually caused by biliary disease in which bile fails to enter the intestine) or because of destruction of intestinal organisms, which might occur with antibiotic therapy. It is also seen in the newborn, because of a lack of establishment of intestinal organisms. Vitamin K is routinely administered to newborns to help prevent haemorrhage. Although prothrombin levels may be normal at birth, they decline until about day 6–8, when the liver becomes able to form prothrombin.

DRUG INTERACTIONS 30-2 Thrombolytic drugs	
Drugs	**Possible effect and management**
Anticoagulants (oral) or heparin	Concurrent use increases haemorrhage risk, but the combination of heparin and thrombolytic therapy is often prescribed for treatment of an acute coronary arterial occlusion. Monitor closely if concurrent therapies are administered
Antiplatelet drugs	Concurrent use can increase the risk of bleeding episodes. This therapy is not recommended, with the exception of aspirin when indicated for an acute myocardial infarction

Vitamin K is also indicated in the preoperative preparation of individuals with deficient prothrombin, particularly those with obstructive jaundice. In addition, it may be given as an antidote for excessive anticoagulation with warfarin if simple cessation of warfarin therapy is not sufficient. When vitamin K is given concurrently with warfarin, a decrease in the anticoagulant effect is reported.

The onset of action for oral phytomenadione is 6–12 hours, and for the injectable form it is 1–2 hours. Vitamin K is metabolised in the liver and excreted via the kidneys and in the bile. Hence it is used with caution in people with biliary atresia, pancreatic insufficiency or fat malabsorption syndromes. Adverse reactions include facial flushing, taste alterations, and redness or pain at the injection site.

THROMBOLYTIC DRUGS

Thrombolytic (fibrinolytic) drugs are used to treat acute thromboembolic disorders. Unlike anticoagulants, they dissolve clots and are used in a hospital setting by experienced health-care professionals. These agents alter haemostatic capability more profoundly than does anticoagulant therapy. Consequently, when bleeding occurs, it is more severe and very difficult to control. The main drugs in this class include alteplase (also known as recombinant tissue plasminogen activator, rt-PA), reteplase, **streptokinase**, tenecteplase and urokinase. Streptokinase is produced from cultures of β-haemolytic streptococci, urokinase is a product isolated from human urine, and alteplase, reteplase and tenecteplase are produced using recombinant DNA technology.

GERIATRIC IMPLICATIONS   ANTICOAGULANTS

The elderly may be more susceptible to the effects of anticoagulants such as warfarin, so a lower maintenance dose is usually recommended for the geriatric patient, along with very close supervision and monitoring.

The primary adverse effects of excessive drug usage are prolonged bleeding from gums when brushing teeth or from small shaving cuts, excessive or easy skin bruising, blood in urine or stools, and unexplained nosebleeds. These may be early signs of overdose that indicate the need for medical intervention.

Caution individuals to carry an identification card indicating the use of an anticoagulant. Also, remind patients to always consult their prescriber before starting any new drug, including over-the-counter medications and vitamins, or if changing a medication dose or when any drug product is discontinued. Many medications can change the effects of an anticoagulant in the body.

Be aware that administration of concurrent drug therapy that can induce gastric irritation increases the risk of gastrointestinal bleeding. Drugs such as the non-steroidal anti-inflammatory agents (e.g. ibuprofen, indomethacin) that

are commonly prescribed for elderly people often cause gastrointestinal effects.

Alcohol consumption can alter the effect of this medication in the body. Individuals should be instructed to avoid alcohol or at least limit their daily alcohol intake to one alcoholic drink a day. Alcohol may cause liver damage, which increases the individual's sensitivity to anticoagulants. Alcohol intoxication or heavy drinking may predispose to falls, poor compliance and poor nutritional habits, all of which can increase the risk of bleeding (Campbell et al 2001).

Health-care professionals should be aware that diet can interfere with the anticoagulant effect. In a previously stabilised person, vitamin C deficiency, chronic malnutrition, diarrhoea or other illnesses can result in an increased anticoagulant effect, and higher intake of green leafy vegetables (e.g. broccoli, cabbage, silver beet, lettuce and spinach) or consumption of a nutritional supplement or multiple vitamin containing vitamin K can result in decreased anticoagulant effectiveness.

These agents dissolve clots via the endogenous fibrinolytic system. All five drugs have similar biochemical mechanisms of action on the fibrinolytic system, converting plasminogen in the blood to plasmin. Plasmin, a fibrinolytic enzyme, digests or dissolves fibrin clots wherever they exist and can be reached by plasmin. Streptokinase is a key drug because it was the first thrombolytic agent released. Alteplase, reteplase, tenecteplase and streptokinase are indicated for coronary arterial thrombosis associated with an acute myocardial infarction, and alteplase, streptokinase and urokinase for massive pulmonary embolism.

Pharmacokinetics

These agents are administered intravenously. Alteplase, streptokinase and urokinase have elimination half-lives of 35 minutes, 23 minutes and up to 20 minutes, respectively. The time to peak effect after IV injection is from 20 minutes to 2 hours. Duration of the thrombolytic effect is about 4 hours for alteplase, streptokinase and urokinase. Reteplase has an elimination half-life of 13–16 minutes and usually has a peak effect within 2 hours. Tenecteplase shows biphasic elimination kinetics, with an initial half-life of ~25 minutes and a terminal half-life of 130 minutes. The exact mechanisms of elimination for many of these drugs are not fully established.

Drug interactions

See the table Drug Interactions 30-2 for the effects that can occur when a thrombolytic agent is given with the drugs listed.

The commonest adverse reaction is bleeding, including intracerebral haemorrhage. Others occurring less often include fever, headache, nausea, vomiting, hypotension, arrhythmias, allergic reaction, facial flushing, arthralgia and bronchospasm. With streptokinase and urokinase, adverse reactions include stomach pain or swelling, backache, bloody urine and stools, constipation, severe headaches, dizziness, arthralgia, tachycardia, bradycardia and fever.

For all these drugs, the absolute contraindications include:
- active internal bleeding
- recent major trauma or surgery (within 10 days)
- recent cerebrovascular accident (stroke) (within two months)
- bleeding disorder
- intracranial neoplasm or prior intracranial haemorrhage
- bacterial endocarditis, pericarditis
- uncontrolled hypertension (systolic >200 mmHg or diastolic >100 mmHg) (Thomas et al 2000).

Use of streptokinase results in the production of anti-streptokinase antibodies. This drug may be ineffective if given between 5 days and up to 12 months after either a previous streptokinase treatment or an acute streptococcal infection.

CLINICAL INTEREST BOX 30-2   ASPIRIN

Aspirin causes a long-lasting functional deficit in platelets by irreversibly inhibiting cyclo-oxygenase, an enzyme necessary for thromboxane A_2 synthesis. Thromboxane A_2 promotes platelet aggregation and vasoconstriction, and thus aspirin suppresses these actions. Platelets lack the metabolic capacity to synthesise new cyclo-oxygenase, and the deficit induced by aspirin lasts 8–10 days until new platelets are synthesised. This effect on platelet function explains both the effectiveness of aspirin as an antiplatelet agent and why it prolongs bleeding time.

Numerous studies have established the effectiveness of aspirin therapy in people with acute myocardial infarction and demonstrated conclusively a significant reduction in mortality. Follow-up studies in the Second International Study of Infarct Survival (ISIS-2) found that the benefit of early aspirin therapy persisted for several years, and further reductions in the incidence of death, reinfarction and strokes have been reported (Collins et al 1997).

The antiplatelet effect of aspirin is achieved at a dose of 75–300 mg daily and no additional benefit has been observed at higher doses. Low-dose aspirin (100 mg/day) does not cause changes in bleeding time.

In an acute coronary artery thrombosis evolving into a transmural myocardial infarction, thrombolytic therapy is most effective when started as early as possible or within 6–12 hours of the onset of symptoms. In general, bolus administration followed by an intravenous infusion is used. The drug regimens for acute myocardial infarction, pulmonary embolism, deep venous thromboembolism and arterial thromboembolism vary, and local institutional or manufacturer's guidelines should be consulted.

ANTIPLATELET AGENTS

Platelets play a critical role in the production of thrombi following vascular damage. After adhesion of platelets to the thrombogenic surface, they become activated and synthesise mediators such as platelet activating factor and thromboxane A_2, which causes vasoconstriction and platelet aggregation. The latter occurs because the platelets stick to one another via fibrinogen bridges that link between specific receptors, called glycoprotein IIb and IIIa, expressed on the surfaces of the platelets. This is an autocatalytic process, as exposure of certain lipids on the surface of the platelets promotes further thrombin formation, platelet aggregation and fibrin formation. Although this process is desirable when forming a haemostatic plug, it is undesirable when triggered intravascularly. Our knowledge of the role of platelets in thromboembolic disease and our understanding of the pharmacology of aspirin has led to considerable development of drugs with 'antiplatelet activity'.

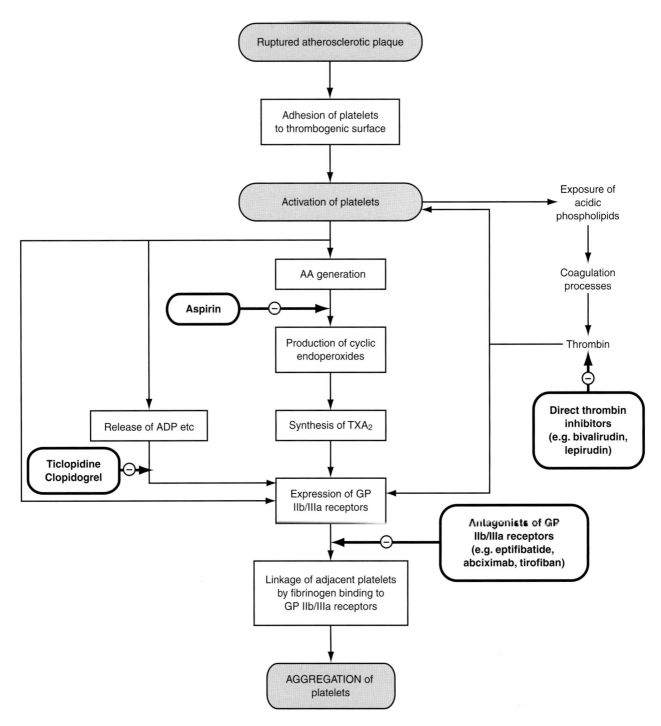

FIGURE 30-2 Platelet activation. Events involved in platelet adhesion and aggregation are shown, with the sites of action of drugs. AA = arachidonic acid; ADP = adenosine diphosphate; GP = glycoprotein; TXA$_2$ = thromboxane A$_2$.
Source: Rang, Dale, Ritter & Moore 2003, with permission.

Antiplatelet drugs are used in the treatment of arterial thrombosis and include aspirin (see Clinical Interest Box 30-2), clopidogrel, dipyridamole, ticlopidine and the glycoprotein IIb/IIIa receptor inhibitors abciximab, eptifibatide and tirofiban (Figure 30-2). (The role of aspirin as an analgesic is discussed in Chapter 16, and as an anti-inflammatory agent in Chapter 55.)

Clopidogrel

Clopidogrel is a thienopyridine derivative structurally related to ticlopidine. It inhibits ADP-induced platelet aggregation through an active metabolite by preventing ADP binding to its platelet receptor. This prevents ADP-mediated activation of the glycoprotein IIb/IIIa complex and hence platelet aggregation. Unlike aspirin it has no effect on prostaglandin synthesis (Figure 30-2). Recent clinical studies have indicated that its effects may be additive with those of aspirin. In individuals with a recent stroke, the risk of bleeding with a combination of aspirin and clopidogrel outweighs any perceived benefit.

Clopidogrel is used widely to prevent thromboebolism in individuals with ischaemic heart disease and those undergoing insertion of an intracoronary stent. As would be anticipated in those with pre-existing bleeding problems, caution should be exercised, and in patients with planned surgery or dental procedures clopidogrel should be halted at least 5 days before the procedure. Bleeding is a common adverse reaction and may be quite severe. Use in pregnancy should be avoided, as there are limited data available.

Dipyridamole

The mechanisms of action for dipyridamole have been proposed to be inhibition of thromboxane A_2 formation; inhibition of phosphodiesterase activity, which results in an increase in platelet cAMP; and inhibition of red blood cell uptake of adenosine, a platelet aggregation inhibitor.

Dipyridamole is used in combination with warfarin for the prevention of postsurgical thromboembolic complications after cardiac valve replacement, and in combination with aspirin for the secondary prevention of ischaemic attacks.

After an oral dose, dipyridamole is rapidly absorbed and reaches peak plasma concentrations within 45–75 minutes. Bioavailability ranges from 40% to 70% and is limited by hepatic first-pass metabolism. It is highly protein-bound, metabolised in the liver, and excreted principally as glucuronides in bile.

Drug interactions

The table Drug Interactions 30-3 shows the effects that can occur when dipyridamole is given with the drugs listed.

Adverse reactions include headache, dizziness, abdominal

DRUG INTERACTIONS 30-3 Dipyridamole	
Drug	**Possible effect and management**
Adenosine	Cellular uptake of adenosine is inhibited and a reduction in dose might be necessary
Aspirin and other antiplatelet drugs	Combined use increases the potential for bleeding episodes. Avoid, or a potentially serious drug interaction could occur. Although the combination of aspirin and dipyridamole has been used commonly for additional therapeutic effects, studies have not proven the combination to be more effective than aspirin alone (United States Pharmacopeial Convention 1998)
Oral anticoagulants, heparin	Concurrent use may increase risk of bleeding. Although the combination of dipyridamole (up to 400 mg/day) and oral anticoagulants has been used without affecting bleeding time, careful monitoring of prothrombin time is recommended
Thrombolytic agents	Concurrent use increases risk of severe bleeding and haemorrhage. Avoid, or a potentially serious drug interaction could occur

upset, rash, allergic reaction, angina pectoris, blood pressure lability (hypertension, hypotension) and tachycardia.

Use dipyridamole cautiously in individuals with unstable angina or recent myocardial infarction and in the presence of aortic stenosis. Avoid use in people with dipyridamole hypersensitivity.

Ticlopidine

Ticlopidine is believed to irreversibly inhibit adenosine diphosphate-induced activation of platelet–platelet aggregation in the same manner as clopidogrel.

This drug is used to decrease the risk of stroke in individuals who have had ischaemic attacks or in those who have had a thrombotic stroke. Recently, it has been used short-term in combination with aspirin to prevent thromboembolic events in people following placement of a coronary stent (see Clinical Interest Box 23-1). Administered orally, the onset of action is slow, taking 3–7 days before a maximal effect is observed. Ticlopidine is metabolised extensively by the liver and no unchanged drug is detected in urine. Binding to plasma proteins occurs for both the parent drug (98%) and metabolites (40%–50%). Coadministration of ticlopidine with aspirin or other anticoagulants increases the risk of bleeding. With theophylline or phenytoin, coadministration increases their respective plasma concentrations, and monitoring of plasma theophylline and phenytoin concentration is recommended.

Adverse reactions include nausea, stomach cramps, bloating, dizziness, skin rash, diarrhoea, tinnitus, bleeding, pruritus, neutropenia and, rarely, agranulocytosis, thrombocytopenia, purpura, hepatitis and Stevens–Johnson syndrome. In people planning dental or elective surgery, the drug should be discontinued 10–14 days before the procedure. Avoid use in people with ticlopidine hypersensitivity, haemophilia, bleeding disorders, current bleeding or severe liver function impairment.

Glycoprotein IIb/IIIa receptor inhibitors

As can be seen in Figure 30-2, inhibition of glycoprotein IIb/IIIa receptors will inhibit all pathways of platelet activation, as they consitute the point at which all the pathways converge. Abciximab is a hybrid murine/human monoclonal antibody while eptifibatide and tirofiban are peptides based on a common sequence that occurs in glycoprotein IIa/IIIb receptors. These drugs are administered parentally and are used in combination with heparin or aspirin (low-dose) to prevent ischaemic cardiac complications in people undergoing percutaneous transluminal coronary angioplasty or intracoronary stenting. To date, development of oral formulations has not been successful.

Abciximab has a longer duration of action than eptifibatide and tirofiban (it remains bound to platelets for about 15 days; platelet function recovers in ~48 hours).

DRUG INTERACTIONS 30-4 Glycoprotein IIb/IIIa receptor inhibitors	
Drug	**Possible effect and management**
Anticoagulants, oral	Administration within a week of the oral anticoagulants is not recommended, because of the increased risk of bleeding
Antiplatelet drugs (dipyridamole, ticlopidine)	Monitor closely if administered concurrently, as the risk of bleeding is increased
Dextran/LMWHs/NSAIDs	Concurrent usage results in increased risk of bleeding and haemorrhage. Avoid, or use cautiously
Thrombolytic drugs	Combined use can result in increased risk of bleeding. Monitor closely if combination or sequential drug therapy is used

The effects that can occur when glycoprotein IIb/IIIa receptor inhibitors are given with the drugs listed are shown in the table Drug Interactions 30-4.

Adverse reactions include bleeding (minor and major), thrombocytopenia, visual changes, confusion, nausea, vomiting and hypotension. Monitor PT, APTT, creatinine clearance, platelet count, haemoglobin and haematocrit before and during treatment.

HAEMOSTATIC AND ANTIFIBRINOLYTIC DRUGS

Haemophilia is a hereditary disorder caused by a deficiency of one or more plasma protein clotting factors. This condition usually leads to persistent and uncontrollable haemorrhage after even minor injury. The symptoms include excessive bleeding from wounds and haemorrhage into joints, the urinary tract and, on occasion, the central nervous system. There are two types of haemophilia: haemophilia A, the classic type in which factor VIII activity is deficient, and haemophilia B, or Christmas disease, in which factor IX complex activity is deficient. In recent years, a correct diagnosis of the coagulation disorder has led to specific factor replacement therapy, and this medical advance has resulted in effective management of patients at home. **Haemostatic** and **antifibrinolytic drugs** are compounds used to hasten clot formation and reduce bleeding. The purpose of these agents is to control rapid loss of blood. Table 30 3 provides a summary of two available drugs. Those not listed are discussed in more detail in following sections.

Factor VIII

Factor VIII, or the antihaemophilic factor, is a glycoprotein necessary for haemostasis and blood clotting. In the intrinsic pathway of the coagulation mechanism, the antihaemophilic factor is required for the transformation of prothrombin to thrombin. In the treatment or prevention of haemophilia A, factor VIII administration is based on replacing the missing plasma clotting factor to control and prevent bleeding.

When administered intravenously, factor VIII has a distribution half-life of 2.4–8 hours and an elimination half-life of 8.4–19.3 hours. The time to peak effect is 1–2 hours after IV administration. No significant drug interactions have been reported with factor VIII, but anticoagulants and antiplatelet drugs should not be administered to haemophiliacs. Mild to severe allergic reactions have been reported, such as bronchospasm, elevated temperature, chills or rash. Other adverse reactions, which might be related to the rate of infusion, include headache, increased heart rate, tingling of fingers, fainting, lethargy, sedation, hypotension, back pain, nausea or vomiting, visual disturbances and chest constriction.

Use factor VIII with caution in individuals with sensitivity to mouse, hamster or bovine proteins. Avoid use in people with antihaemophilic factor hypersensitivity. Individuals who develop antibodies to factor VIII might not respond to factor VIII therapy.

Factor IX complex

Factor IX complex is a purified plasma fraction prepared from pooled units of plasma. It contains factors II, VII, IX and X, which are known as the vitamin K coagulation factors. This agent is used for therapy in individuals with a deficiency of these factors during haemorrhage or before surgery. It is also indicated for patients with haemophilia B in whom factor IX is deficient (Christmas disease). Factor IX complex is used to prevent or control bleeding in individuals with factor IX deficiency. It is also used to treat patients with bleeding problems who have antibodies to factor VIII, and it will reverse haemorrhage induced by warfarin.

Factor IX has an elimination half-life of 18–32 hours and the time to peak effect after IV administration is 10–30 minutes. Interactions with other drugs have not been established.

Adverse reactions include chills and fever, especially when large doses are given. Also, if the intravenous infusion is given too rapidly, headache, flushing, rash, nausea, vomiting, sedation, lethargy, elevated temperature and tingling have been reported. The infusion should be stopped and in most people it can be resumed at a much slower rate.

Thrombosis and DIC have occurred as a result of the administration of factor IX. Myocardial infarction, pulmonary embolism and anaphylaxis have also been reported. It should not be used in individuals undergoing elective surgery, as they are at a greater risk of thrombosis.

Use factor IX with caution in individuals with trauma injuries and severe liver impairment, and in those who have recently had surgery. Avoid use in people with factor IX, hamster protein or mouse protein hypersensitivity, DIC, and those with a history of thromboembolism. Factor IX should be administered slowly by intravenous injection or by intravenous infusion. The dosage is individualised according to the patient's coagulation assay, which is performed before treatment. Check current references for specific dosing recommendations.

Tranexamic acid

Tranexamic acid is a competitive inhibitor of plasminogen activation; at high doses, it is a non-competitive inhibitor of plasmin. It is used after dental surgery in individuals with haemophilia to reduce or prevent bleeding episodes. No significant drug interactions have been reported.

Adverse reactions include nausea, vomiting, diarrhoea, visual disturbances, thrombosis, hypotension, thromboembolism and menstrual discomfort.

Use with caution in women who are breastfeeding. Avoid use in people with tranexamic acid hypersensitivity, colour vision defects, haematuria, subarachnoid haemorrhage, a history of thrombosis, or renal impairment.

Aprotinin

Aprotinin is a proteinase inhibitor obtained from bovine lung. It directly prevents fibrinolysis by inhibiting plasmin and kallikrein, an enzyme of the renal cortex. It is used in cardiopulmonary bypass surgery to reduce blood loss and the need for blood transfusions.

Aprotinin is inactive when given orally and is administered intravenously. It is rapidly distributed in extracellular space, with a terminal half-life of 5–10 hours. It is slowly metabolised by lysosomes in the kidneys and excreted primarily in urine.

Concurrent administration of aprotinin with a thrombolytic agent may result in antagonistic effects.

Adverse reactions are rare but include allergic-type reactions (skin rash, respiratory difficulties, nausea, tachycardia, hypotension and bronchospasm) and anaphylaxis.

Use with caution in individuals with a history of allergies. Avoid use in people who have had previous aprotinin therapy, as re-exposure increases the risk of allergic reactions. Also avoid in patients undergoing surgery of the aortic arch, especially if they are older than 65 years, as instances of renal failure and fatalities have been reported.

A test IV dose is administered at least 10 minutes before the loading dose. If no allergic-type reaction occurs, all other

TABLE 30-3 Haemostatics

DRUG	ACTION	ADMINISTRATION	ADDITIONAL INFORMATION
Eptacog alfa	Recombinant activated factor VII. Activates factors IX and X.	Parenteral	Used both for haemophilia and life-threatening haemorrhage
Prothrombin complex	Normal clotting factors	Parenteral	Purified plasma-derived factors II, IX, and X. Contains heparin (200 units) and ATIII (25 units)

dosages should be administered via a central venous line and no other medication should be given in this line. Consult the manufacturer's instructions for dosing recommendations.

HAEMOPOIETICS AND HAEMATINICS

Darbepoetin alpha and epoetin alpha

The continuous replacement of blood cells is called haemopoiesis and is regulated by growth factors such as erythropoietin (EPO), thrombopoietin (TPO) and the cytokines, which include colony-stimulating factors (CSFs) (see Chapter 29). EPO is not the sole growth factor but it is important, and in its absence severe anaemia is invariably observed. It is produced in the kidney, and production is impaired in chronic renal failure, giving rise to anaemia in that specific condition. In general, anaemia refers to a reduced concentration of haemoglobin in the blood.

Recombinant human erythropoietin (**epoetin alpha**) is almost identical to the human hormone, while darbepoetin alpha, also a recombinant hormone, is a slightly larger version of EPO but nevertheless has the same actions. Epoetin alpha and darbepoetin alpha act specifically through the erythropoietin receptor on erythroid progenitor cells, stimulating erythropoiesis, increasing reticulocyte count and increasing haematocrit and haemoglobin concentration.

The duration of action of darbepoetin alpha is longer, allowing once-weekly dosing, while epoetin alpha is administered three times weekly. These drugs are used to treat anaemia associated with chronic renal failure; surgery with expected blood loss; in cancer chemotherapy; and to stimulate red cell production prior to autologous blood collection in patients with anaemia who are undergoing elective surgery.

Adverse reactions are common and include hypertension (due to a rapid rise in haemoglobin), flu-like symptoms (e.g. headache, bone pain, myalgia and fever) and rash, peripheral oedema, dyspnoea and GI disturbances (e.g. nausea, vomiting and diarrhoea). Administered SC/IV pain at the injection site is more common with darbepoetin alpha, while the development of epoetin antibodies (which may limit usefulness) has been reported.

Iron deficiency anaemia

Iron deficiency anaemia is characterised by small red cells with reduced haemoglobin. Agents commonly used to treat this condition are the **haematinics**: folic acid, iron and vitamin B_{12}. Before commencing therapy, other causes of iron deficiency should be excluded. These include, but are not limited to, blood loss (e.g. chronic NSAID use and GI ulceration), blood donation, pregnancy and lactation (increased iron requirement), malabsorption (e.g. after gastric surgery), inadequate diet (e.g. due to socioeconomic status, vegetarian lifestyle), and previous history of iron deficiency. Iron deficiency not only causes anaemia: iron is also an essential component of myoglobin, enzymes with a haem moiety (e.g. cytochromes and peroxidases) and metalloflavoproteins such as xanthine oxidase, which is involved in purine metabolism (refer to section on hyperuricaemia and gout, Chapter 55).

Iron

The majority of iron (~65%) in the human body circulates as haemoglobin, which contains four haem moieties, each having one iron atom to which one oxygen molecule binds reversibly. In general, iron is obtained through a meat-containing diet, creating a problem for cultures reliant on grain as a major food source. Iron is absorbed from the duodenum and upper jejunum, and carried in plasma bound to transferrin. On average, plasma contains about 4 mg iron and the turnover is about 30 mg per day. The majority of the iron is stored in erythrocytes, with the next highest concentrations occurring in liver, muscle, bone marrow and then small amounts in the spleen and bound in enzymes. Iron concentration is tightly controlled as the body has virtually no mechanism for excreting iron. What iron is lost (~1 mg/day) is via sloughing of mucosal cells containing ferritin and even smaller amounts via bile, sweat and urine.

PREGNANCY SAFETY	
ADEC Category	**Drug**
B1	Alteplase, aprotinin, clopidogrel, dipyridamole, eptacog alfa, ticlopidine, tirofiban, tranexamic acid
B2	Factor VIII, protamine
B3	Lepirudin
C	Abciximab, aspirin, bivalirudin, danaparoid, dalteparin, enoxaparin, eptifibatide, factor IX, fondaparinux, standard heparin, reteplase, streptokinase, tenecteplase
D	Warfarin
Unclassified	Antithrombin III, prothrombin complex†, urokinase, vitamin K_1*

*Use of vitamin K_1 is contraindicated in pregnant women, although it does not readily cross the placenta.
†Contact pregnancy drug information centre.

Iron is administered orally but can also be given parenterally if required. Iron dosage is expressed in terms of elemental iron:

- 1 mg elemental iron = ~9 mg ferrous gluconate
- 1 mg elemental iron = ~ 3 mg ferrous sulfate (dried)
- 1 mg elemental iron = ~0.05 mL iron sucrose (a new product, containing 20 mg iron/mL).

Iron causes most commonly GI disturbances (e.g. abdominal pain, nausea, vomiting, diarrhoea and black-coloured faeces). As acute iron toxicity is serious or even fatal in small children, iron formulations should be kept well out of reach and preferably locked away. In cases of iron overdose, the iron chelator desferrioxamine is administered. This forms water-soluble complexes with the iron, which are then excreted in urine.

Folic acid and vitamin B$_{12}$

In general, folic acid deficiency occurs through poor diet, while vitamin B$_{12}$ deficiency arises from absorptive problems in the terminal ileum (e.g. in Crohn's disease). Folic acid and vitamin B$_{12}$ are both obtained through the diet and both are interrelated in the synthesis of DNA. Folic acid is essential for DNA synthesis, and dietary folic acid is reduced to tetrahydrofolate (FH$_4$). Vitamin B$_{12}$ is required for conversion of methyl-FH$_4$ to FH$_4$, hence a deficiency of either results in defective DNA synthesis.

Folic acid is used to treat folate-deficiency anaemia, to prevent neural tube defects in the growing fetus and to treat or prevent toxicity from methotrexate (Chapter 49). Always exclude vitamin B$_{12}$ deficiency before prescribing folic acid to treat megaloblastic anaemia. In addition, check medications, as some drugs (e.g. antiepileptics, and dihydrofolate reductase inhibitors such as methotrexate [Chapter 49] and trimethoprim [Chapter 51]) cause folic acid deficiency. Except in special circumstances, folic acid is administered orally. Adverse reactions with folic acid are rare.

Vitamin B$_{12}$ (available as hydroxycobalamin and cyanocobalamin) is used principally to treat pernicious anaemia and optic neuropathies (the vitamin is essential to nerve development). Confirm diagnosis before use, as vitamin B$_{12}$ may mask the clinical signs of folic acid deficiency. In cases of malabsorption syndrome, oral formulations are inappropriate and vitamin B$_{12}$ injections will be required. As with folic acid, adverse reactions are rare.

DRUGS AT A GLANCE 30: Drugs affecting haemostasis, thrombosis and the haemopoietic system

Therapeutic group	Pharmacological group	Key examples	Key pages
Anticoagulants	Heparins	enoxaparin heparin	502 501
	Vitamin K antagonist	warfarin	504
	Direct thrombin inhibitor	bivalirudin	504
	Antithrombin-III-dependent anticoagulant	fondaparinux	504
Antifibrinolytic drug	Serine protease inhibitor	aprotinin	511
Antiplatelet drugs	Glycoprotein IIb/IIIa receptor inhibitors	abciximab eptifibatide	510 510
	Other antiplatelet drugs	clopidogrel dipyridamole ticlopidine	509 509 509
Haematinics	Iron preparations	iron	512
	Vitamin B$_{12}$	vitamin B$_{12}$	513
	Folic acid	folic acid	513
Haemopoietics	Recombinant glycoproteins	darbepoetin alpha epoetin alpha	512 512
Haemostatic	Recombinant activated factor VII	eptacog alfa	511
Thrombolytics	Plasminogen activator	streptokinase	506
	Recombinant tissue-type plasminogen activators	alteplase tenecteplase	506 506

KEY POINTS

● Anticoagulant therapy is primarily prophylactic, whereas thrombolytic drugs are used to dissolve already formed clots in the treatment of acute thromboembolic disease states.

● Heparin produces its anticoagulant effect by combining with antithrombin III to form a complex that acts at multiple sites in the normal coagulation system, inactivating factors IXa, Xa, XIa and XIIa. Inactivation of factor Xa of the intrinsic and extrinsic pathways prevents the conversion of prothrombin to thrombin, thereby inhibiting the formation of fibrin from fibrinogen.

● The low-molecular-weight heparins (LMWHs) are fragments of standard heparin prepared by enzymatic or chemical cleavage. They inactivate factor Xa more potently than factor IIa and hence have a relatively minor effect on APTT.

● LMWHs are considered to be safer, easier to administer, require less monitoring than standard heparin and are now the first choice for treatment of thromboembolism associated with pregnancy.

● Bleeding is a well-known complication of heparin therapy, and the LMWHs have a similar risk.

● Warfarin is an orally administered anticoagulant and is indicated for the prophylaxis and treatment of deep venous thrombosis and pulmonary thromboembolism.

● Many drugs interact with warfarin, and the INR should be monitored more often when instituting, ceasing or altering other drug therapy.

● Thrombolytic (fibrinolytic) drugs are used to treat acute thromboembolic disorders. Unlike anticoagulants, they dissolve clots and are used in a hospital setting by experienced health-care professionals.

● Selected antiplatelet drugs inhibit platelet aggregation and can thus be used to reduce the risk of stroke.

● The haemostatic and antifibrinolytic agents are used to promote clot formation and reduce blood loss.

● Haemopoietics and haematinics are used in the treatment of anaemia.

REVIEW EXERCISES

1   Compare the mechanisms of action and indications of the anticoagulant drugs (heparin and warfarin) with those of the thrombolytic agents.

2   What drugs are administered to counteract excessive anticoagulation due to heparin and warfarin? Explain how these drugs work as antidotes.

3   Compare the low-molecular-weight heparins with standard heparin in chemical composition and mechanism of action.

4   Discuss the various biological targets of haemostatic drugs.

REFERENCES

Australian Medicines Handbook 2006. Adelaide: AMH, 2006.

Bick RL. Proficient and cost-effective approaches for the prevention and treatment of venous thrombosis and thromboembolism. *Drugs* 2000; 60: 575–95.

Cambell P, Roberts G, Eaton V, Coghlan D, Gallus A. Managing warfarin therapy in the community. *Australian Prescriber* 2001; 24: 86–9.

Collins R, Peto R, Baigent C, Sleight P. Aspirin, heparin and fibrinolytic therapy in suspected acute myocardial infarction. *New England Journal of Medicine* 1997; 336: 847–60.

Hovanessian HC. New-generation anticoagulants: the low molecular weight heparins. *Annals of Emergency Medicine* 1999; 34: 768–79.

Majerus P, Broze GJ Jr, Miletich JP, Tollenfsen DM. Anticoagulant, thrombolytic, and antiplatelet drugs. In: Hardman JG, Limbird LE, Molinoff PB, Ruddon RW et al (eds). *Goodman & Gilman's The Pharmacological Basis of Therapeutics.* 9th edn. New York, 1996 [ch. 54].

Mannuccio P. Hemostatic drugs. *New England Journal of Medicine* 1998; 339: 245–53.

Rang HP, Dale MM, Ritter JM, Moore PK. *Pharmacology.* 5th edn. Edinburgh: Churchill Livingstone, 2003 [chs 20–21].

Thomas MD, Chauhan A, More RS. Pulmonary embolism: an update on thrombolytic therapy. *Quarterly Journal of Medicine* 2000; 93: 261–7.

Turpie AGG. Management of deep vein thrombosis: prevention and treatment. *Pharmacology and Therapeutics* 1995; 20(6S): 7S–15S.

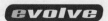   More weblinks at http://evolve.elsevier.com/AU/Bryant/pharmacology/

CHAPTER 31

Overview of the Respiratory System

CHAPTER FOCUS

The respiratory system maintains the exchange of oxygen and carbon dioxide in the lungs and cells and regulates the pH of body fluids. Disorders of other body systems can increase the body's oxygen requirement and therefore increase the work of respiration. Many patients in clinical settings have respiratory problems that require care and interventions by health-care professionals. This chapter provides a review of the relevant anatomy and physiology, and describes how drugs are administered by inhalation, to prepare the student for understanding the drugs affecting the respiratory system.

OBJECTIVES

● To describe the three interrelated respiration processes.

● To name the factors that determine airway efficiency.

● To describe the production and functions of respiratory secretions.

● To describe the autonomic innervation of the airways and explain the β-adrenoceptor mechanism of bronchodilation.

● To discuss the central and peripheral regulation of respiration.

● To describe the administration of drugs in aerosol form to the respiratory tract, via sprays, inhalers and nebulisers.

● To name the objectives of aerosol therapy and explain the relationship of droplet size to therapeutic effectiveness.

KEY TERMS

aerosol
bronchial glands
bronchoconstriction
bronchodilation
carbonic anhydrase
cellular respiration
expiration
gas transport
goblet cells

hypercapnia
hypoxaemia
inspiration
metered dose inhaler
mucociliary blanket
mucociliary transport
nebuliser
pulmonary ventilation
surfactant

KEY ABBREVIATIONS

cAMP	cyclic 3,5-adenosine monophosphate
CFC	chlorofluorocarbon
GMP	guanosine monophosphate
HCO_3^-	bicarbonate ion
M_3	muscarinic type 3 (receptors)
MDI	metered dose inhaler

THE RESPIRATORY SYSTEM

THE respiratory system includes all structures involved in the movement and exchange of oxygen and carbon dioxide: that is, the nose, airway passages, lungs, nasal cavities, pharynx, larynx, trachea, bronchi, bronchioles, pulmonary lobules with their alveoli, the diaphragm, and all muscles concerned with respiration itself (Figure 31-1; see also Figure 32-6).

The most urgent and critical need for maintaining life is an adequate, uninterrupted supply of oxygen. Oxygen is supplied to the body through the process of respiration. 'Respiration' is loosely used to describe three distinct but interrelated processes:

- **pulmonary ventilation** (breathing), which involves the movement of air into and out of the lungs (**inspiration** and **expiration**, respectively)
- **gas transport**, which involves the exchange of gases between the air in the lungs, the blood and the cells
- **cellular respiration**, which involves the utilisation of oxygen in the metabolism of substances to produce energy.

Respiration helps maintain physiological dynamic equilibrium and compensates for rapid adjustment to changes in metabolic states. Parts of the respiratory system also participate in the senses of smell and taste, produce sounds, and assist in control of pH, in removal of foreign bodies and mucus, in immune system defence mechanisms, in inactivation of many biogenic amines and autacoids, and in temperature regulation.

The air passages permit air to flow from the external environment to pulmonary blood, and modify the air taken in by warming, filtering and moistening it. Airway efficiency is determined by the following factors:

- shape and size of each segment of the respiratory tract (nasal cavity, pharynx, larynx, trachea, bronchi, bronchioles and alveolar sacs)
- presence of a ciliated, mucus-secreting, epithelial lining throughout most of the respiratory tract
- character and thickness of respiratory tract secretions
- compliance of the cartilaginous and bony supports
- pressure gradients
- traction on airway walls
- absence of foreign substances in the lumen of the respiratory tract.

Any alteration in these factors affects the ease with

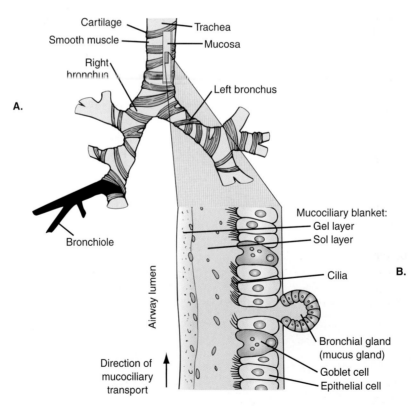

TRACHEOBRONCHIAL TREE

FIGURE 31-1 Tracheobronchial tree and bronchial smooth muscle. **A.** Diagram of tracheobronchial tree. **B.** Longitudinal section of inner lining of airway.

which air flows through the air passages, or effective airway clearance. Congenital anomalies, injuries, allergies or disease cause airflow resistance if these factors are abnormally affected. For example, resistance occurs if there is stenosis, or narrowing, of any portion of the respiratory tract, a loss of cilia that ordinarily sweep out foreign substances, any thick or tenacious secretions, loss of elasticity or the presence of inhaled foreign objects.

Respiratory tract secretions
Mucus

The tracheobronchial tree, made up of repeated branching tubes, is a tubular airway that serves as a conduit for passage of air from the external environment to the alveolar–capillary exchange unit, the respiratory membrane. The inner surface of the tracheobronchial tree is lined with ciliated columnar epithelium interspersed with **goblet cells**. The gelatinous mucus (gel layer) produced by goblet cells is normally discharged into the tubular lumen. In some obstructive pulmonary diseases, mucus secretion is greatly increased, making it difficult for the cilia to transport secretions along the airway.

The **bronchial glands**, which are located in the submucosa of the tracheobronchial tree (Figure 31-1B), secrete a relatively watery fluid (sol layer) through ducts leading to the surface of the ciliated epithelium. Under vagal (parasympathetic) control, the glands can be stimulated by irritant agents or aerosol drugs to release their contents into the lumen of the airway.

The products of the goblet cells and bronchial glands form the sol–gel film that comprises the **mucociliary blanket**. This protective blanket of fluid bathes the ciliated epithelium of the tracheobronchial tree. In addition, the cilia continuously propel the sol–gel film up the respiratory tree towards the larynx. The normal adult produces and swallows about 100 mL respiratory secretions per day. The process of moving mucus along the tracheobronchial tree is called **mucociliary transport** (or mucokinesis). The effectiveness of the mucociliary blanket is a basic concern in chronic obstructive pulmonary disease. The cilia must sustain appropriate function; a dry atmosphere causes the respiratory secretions to become thick and tenacious, which tends to interfere with ciliary movements. Thus adequate humidity should be maintained to prevent thickening in the consistency of the respiratory secretions (see Clinical Interest Box 31-1).

Pulmonary surfactant

Pulmonary **surfactant** (i.e. surface-active agent) is a phospholipid–glycoprotein lipoprotein mixture secreted from alveolar cells and present in the secretions lining the alveoli. Surfactant reduces surface tension in the lung, stabilises the

---

CLINICAL INTEREST BOX 31-1
CYSTIC FIBROSIS AND GENE THERAPY

The disease cystic fibrosis (CF), an inherited autosomal-recessive condition, involves abnormally thick mucus secretions in many organs (including lungs, sweat glands, pancreas and liver) due to abnormal chloride transport. Life expectancy used to be short, but is now more than 30 years.

Most patients suffer from severe respiratory infections due to impaired mucociliary transport. Standard treatment involves use of antibiotics for bacterial infections, enzymes and mucolytics to reduce mucus viscosity, physiotherapy and exercise to clear mucopurulent secretions, bronchodilators, oxygen, anti-inflammatory agents and nutritional support.

The gene for CF was identified in 1989 and its product, the CF transmembrane conductance regulator (CFTR), has been studied intensively. The aim is to develop methods to transfer the gene into cells of the airways of CF patients, so that they can express the CFTR protein and so improve chloride and sodium conductance.

Clinically useful therapy has been carried out in some patients; however, the barrier to effective gene therapy is finding vectors that successfully transfer the gene to the appropriate cells, without inflammatory effects induced by the vector virus.

The respiratory tract is considered particularly feasible as a target for gene therapy because of the ease of access by viral and other vectors. In addition to CF, potential indications for gene therapy include α_1-antitrypsin deficiency, acute transplant rejection and acute lung injury.

Other new methods to improve CFTR protein function include drugs aimed at suppressing premature termination of the synthesis of the protein, stabilising the protein structure, activating the protein or enhancing normal chloride channel functions.
Sources: Flotte & Laube 2001; West & Rodman 2001; Kerem 2005.

---

alveoli and improves lung mechanics. Infants born preterm are at risk of respiratory distress syndrome due to immature mechanisms for producing surfactant, and are likely to suffer rapid shallow breathing, hypoxaemia and acidosis unless treated with synthetic surfactant.

Bronchial smooth muscle
Smooth muscle arrangement

An important component of the tracheobronchial tree is the smooth muscle. The proportion of muscle fibres along the bronchi progressively increases as it extends towards the distal bronchioles (simultaneously, the amount of cartilage decreases). Isolated muscle fibres can be found as far down as the alveolar ducts. The smooth muscle fibres are arranged along the length of the tubular tree in a double helical, or spiral, pattern. Because of this structural feature, the effect of muscle contraction reduces both the diameter and the length of the bronchus or bronchiole.

Efferent nerve supply and receptors

The airway, or tracheobronchial tree, is innervated by the autonomic nervous system. The bronchial smooth muscle tone is influenced by the balance maintained between parasympathetic and sympathetic stimuli during rest. The bronchial smooth muscle tone is normally determined by tonic vagal activity.

Activation of the parasympathetic pathway (vagus nerve) releases acetylcholine (ACh), which stimulates muscarinic type 3 (M_3) receptors in bronchial smooth muscle and glands. Stimulation of the M_3 receptors increases the activity of the enzyme guanylate cyclase in the membrane, thereby increasing the rate of formation of cyclic 3´,5´-guanosine monophosphate (cyclic GMP) from guanosine triphosphate (GTP). This leads to secretion from mucus glands and contraction of bronchial smooth muscle, which result in **bronchoconstriction**, a narrowing of the lumen of the bronchial airway. Cyclic GMP also increases the release of chemical mediators such as histamine from mast cells, which enhances bronchoconstriction.

By contrast, stimulation of the sympathetic pathways releases the catecholamines adrenaline and noradrenaline from the adrenal medulla into the circulation. Their action on the β_2-adrenoceptor sites in the bronchial smooth muscle produces **bronchodilation** by means of smooth muscle relaxation, inhibits mediator release from mast cells and increases mucociliary clearance. All these effects improve ventilation of the lungs. The transduction mechanism whereby catecholamines induce smooth muscle relaxation is via adenylate cyclase, ATP and cyclic AMP (cAMP). Cyclic AMP is inactivated by an enzyme, phosphodiesterase, which catalyses it to the inactive 5´-AMP. This results in a fall in the cAMP level. If the action of phosphodiesterase is inhibited (e.g. by a xanthine drug such as theophylline), the cAMP level remains elevated and the smooth muscle relaxed (see Figures 32-3 and 32-4). Few α-adrenoceptors are present on the bronchial smooth muscle, and their stimulation results in only mild bronchoconstriction.

Thus bronchodilation is induced by circulating catecholamines or by blocking the parasympathetic effects in the airways. Another important natural bronchodilator substance is the mediator nitric oxide, which can be readily formed in the airways by the nitric oxide synthase enzymes. Bronchoconstriction is induced by mimicking the actions of acetylcholine, by blocking β_2-adrenoceptors or by releasing cytokines from mast cells. Excitatory neuropeptides, including substance P and neurokinin A, also cause bronchoconstriction when released during inflammation or chemical irritation.

Control of respiration
Central control

The basic rhythm for respiration is initiated and maintained by the central pattern generator for respiration, in the medullary rhythmicity area located beneath the lower part of the floor of the fourth ventricle in the medial half of the medulla oblongata (see Figure 14-2). Neurons that control inspiration and expiration intermingle and discharge impulses alternately. Signals from the spinal cord, the cerebral cortex and midbrain, the apneustic area of the pons, the pneumotaxic area of the upper pons, and vagal afferents from the lungs can all modify the rhythm of respiration, contribute to the normal pattern of respiration and facilitate 15–20-fold increases in oxygen use during vigorous exercise.

Respiration is normally under involuntary central and autonomic control, and we are unaware of the respiratory process. Voluntary influence and control of breathing, however, are possible via connections between the cerebral cortex and motor neurons that control respiration. This is important when a patient must learn to control breathing patterns voluntarily.

Peripheral control

The medullary rhythmicity area is also influenced by various sensory and peripheral stimuli (via afferent pathways), the vasomotor centre, reflex mechanisms (e.g. the Hering–Breuer reflex), the chemoreceptors in the carotid and aortic bodies (which are highly sensitive to changes in partial pressures of oxygen or carbon dioxide and pH), and the mechanoreceptors in the lungs and airways. Fear, pain, stress, sudden changes in blood pressure or body temperature, irritation of the airways, and blood levels of oxygen and carbon dioxide can all modify the activity of the respiratory centres.

Humoral regulation of respiration is achieved primarily through changes in the concentrations of oxygen, carbon dioxide or hydrogen ions in body fluids. In a healthy individual, carbon dioxide is the chief respiratory stimulant. An increase in the carbon dioxide tension of the blood (**hypercapnia**) directly stimulates the inspiratory and expiratory centres, which increases both the rate and depth of breathing. This results in hyperventilation, which increases loss of carbon dioxide from the lungs to keep the carbon dioxide tension of the blood constant.

Small changes in arterial oxygen concentration usually have little if any direct effect on the respiratory centre, but if the arterial oxygen concentration falls below about 60% of normal (**hypoxaemia**), the chemoreceptors in the carotid and aortic bodies are stimulated and in turn stimulate the respiratory centre to increase alveolar ventilation. This mechanism operates primarily under abnormal conditions such as chronic obstructive pulmonary disease or exposure to high altitude.

Control of pH

The acid–base balance of the body is largely determined by pH homeostatic mechanisms in the kidneys and lungs. Respiration is important in regulating the pH of the blood by controlling the carbon dioxide tension of the blood. Bicarbonate ions (HCO_3^-) and proteins in the blood function as buffer systems, according to the equation:

$$CO_2 + H_2O \rightleftharpoons H_2CO_3 \rightleftharpoons HCO_3^- + H^+$$

This equation shows the combination of carbon dioxide with water to form carbonic acid, which dissociates to bicarbonate and hydrogen ions. This reaction is catalysed by the enzyme **carbonic anhydras**e. The pH of the blood is determined by the ratio of bicarbonate ion (HCO_3^-) to carbon dioxide. When the carbon dioxide content of the blood is increased, there is an increase in the formation of carbonic acid in the blood. This alters the bicarbonate–carbonic acid ratio from the normal value of 20:1 and results in respiratory acidosis. Conversely, a decrease in the carbon dioxide content of the blood results in alkalosis.

AEROSOL THERAPY

Aerosol therapy is a form of inhaled, topical pulmonary treatment. An **aerosol** is a suspension of fine liquid or solid particles dispersed in a gas or in solution. Aerosols can be administered to the skin (as topical sprays) or to body cavities (ear, nose, rectum, vagina), but are most commonly inhaled. After inhalation, some of the particles are deposited in the respiratory tract. Inhalation may be via steam, from a nasal spray or with devices such as **metered dose inhalers**, spacers, face masks and **nebulisers** (see Figures 31-2 and 32-1). Dry powder inhalers are also available. Liquid or solid particles range in size from about 0.005 to 50 μm in diameter. (The terms 'aerosol therapy' and 'nebulisation therapy' are often used interchangeably.)

Aerosol therapy has many advantages:
• drug administration is convenient
• there is minimal irritation or contamination
• lower doses can be given than by systemic administration
• the drug is delivered rapidly to the desired site of action
• systemic adverse effects should be minimised.

Inhaled aerosols can promote bronchodilation and pulmonary decongestion, loosening of secretions, topical application of corticosteroids and other drugs, and moistening, cooling or heating of inspired air.

Metered dose inhalers

Metered dose inhalers (MDIs) are small hand-held 'puffers' containing multiple doses of the active drug in a canister, mixed with a dispersing agent and a propellant. The canister is shaken and then depressed (while inhaling) to deliver an accurate dose of the aerosol along with the inert propellant gas, usually a chlorofluorocarbon (CFC). (These CFC gases, while biologically inert, are infamous for their deleterious effects on the Earth's ozone layer. In countries signatory to the Montreal Protocol of 1987, including Australia, CFCs are being replaced as propellants by less damaging hydrofluoroalkanes, as for example in the 'Ventolin CFC-free inhaler'.)

Effective use of MDIs requires good hand–breath coordination, which may be difficult for young children; breath-activated MDIs, spacers and face masks help improve drug administration (see Clinical Interest Box 31-2).

Dry powder devices

These are similar to MDIs, except that the drug is delivered as finely divided particles rather than in aerosol solution. Examples are the 'Accuhaler', a compact device with a foil strip inside containing doses of finely powdered drug, and the 'Turbuhaler', in which the drug is loaded as a capsule that is broken open when the base is rotated, releasing the active drug. Dry powder inhalers have the advantage that the patient does not need to inhale simultaneously while activating the inhaler device.

Nebulisers

Nebulisers ('pumps') use compressed air or oxygen, or ultrasonic energy, to produce a fine mist of drug in aerosol form from a solution. They are useful for delivering large doses over long periods. Nebulisers are convenient in acute attacks, but otherwise have no sustained advantages over pressurised aerosol or dry powder devices.

Droplet size

The effectiveness of aerosol therapy depends on the number of droplets that can be suspended in an inhaled aerosol. This number is directly related to the size of the droplets. Smaller droplets can be suspended in greater numbers than large droplets. Droplets of more than 40 μm in diameter will be deposited primarily in the upper airway (mouth, pharynx, trachea and main bronchi). This may be useful for keeping large airways (nose and trachea) moist and for loosening secretions. Medium-sized droplets (8–15 μm in diameter) will be deposited primarily in the bronchioles and bronchi. Smaller droplets (2–4 μm in diameter) are more likely to reach the periphery of the lungs—the alveolar ducts and sacs. For comparison, tiny fibres of asbestos dust, which after long-term exposure and inhalation can deposit in the

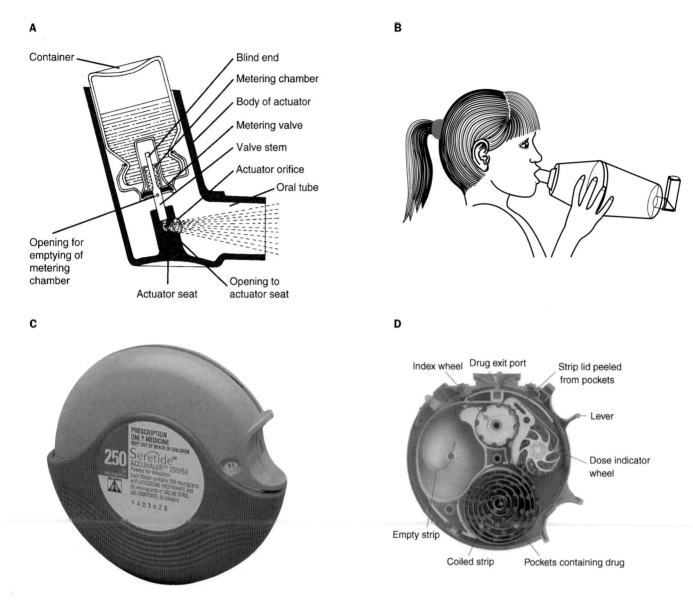

FIGURE 31-2 Devices for drug administration by inhalation. **A.** Metered dose inhaler (MDI, or 'puffer'); cross-section. **B.** MDI in combination with a large-volume spacer. **C.** Accuhaler™. **D.** Accuhaler; cross-section. (A, C and D courtesy GlaxoSmithKline, Australia; used with permission.)

lungs and set up chronic inflammatory responses leading to asbestosis and eventually bronchogenic carcinoma and mesothelioma, are 0.1–1.5 μm in diameter. Particles smaller than about 0.6 μm are unlikely to be deposited, and will be exhaled.

A considerable proportion of an inhaled drug dose is swallowed. This dose can produce systemic effects or may be digested or metabolised rapidly. Other potential problems include oral infections after corticosteroid inhalation, dental caries from acidic drugs, or ocular effects from corneal deposition of drugs if the aerosol mist reaches the eyes.

Rate and depth of breathing are other factors that determine the effectiveness of aerosol therapy. Slow and deep

breathing is required for proper lung aeration and penetration of the mist into peripheral lung areas. The breath should be held for a few seconds after a full inspiration. Rapid or shallow breathing decreases the number of droplets reaching and retained in the periphery of the tracheobronchial tree. Rapid breathing permits escape of significant numbers of fine droplets during expirations; few droplets escape if the breath is held long enough after deep inspiration to permit droplet deposition in the lung periphery. Small droplets are more effective for absorption of bronchodilator drugs.

Droplet size can be controlled in a nebuliser by the pressure used to force oxygen or room air through the solution to produce a mist. The nebuliser tubing diameter, its length

CLINICAL INTEREST BOX 31-2   PUFFERS AND OTHER INHALER DEVICES

Because of the importance of correct use of inhaler devices to maximise drug delivery to the airways, patients need to be shown and reminded of the best way to use inhalers. Patient information sheets are available to demonstrate the correct techniques. With 'puffers', which have been in use for many decades, the technique is as follows:

- Take the cap off the puffer's mouthpiece.
- Hold the puffer upright and shake it well.
- Put the mouthpiece between the teeth and close the lips around it without biting.
- Breathe out slowly and gently without emptying the lungs.
- Tilt the head back slightly and, while breathing in slowly,

press down on the top of the aerosol canister, and continue to breathe in deeply.
- Take the puffer away from the mouth and hold the breath for as long as possible, then breathe out gently.
- Click the cap back onto the puffer.

The technique for handling different styles of inhalers varies, but the inhaling drug–breath holding–exhaling method is similar.

Children sometimes find it easier to use a puffer with a spacer, which reduces the amount of drug deposited in the mouth and throat. With very young children, a small volume spacer or nebuliser and face mask may be useful.

and its number of bends affect the flow and temperature of the mist. With most nebulisers, the maximum density of the inhaled mist is achieved by making the flow of mist as smooth and direct as possible. If a humidity deficit occurs, drug reconcentration can occur with both jet and ultrasonic nebulisers: evaporation of water molecules causes a gradual increase in drug concentration in the droplets, thus increasing the risk of drug toxicity. Control of temperature and humidity can prevent drug reconcentration.

Inhaled aerosols

Aerosol therapy, when used as a method of inhaling drugs such as bronchodilators and anti-inflammatory agents, is intended to minimise systemic absorption and adverse effects. It is important, however, to remember that the lung is an absorptive organ and thus is a route of access for drugs to enter the systemic circulation. Absorption is generally rapid, because of the highly vascular pulmonary capillary system,

but also depends on the drug's lipid solubility, aerosol particle size and pulmonary function. For example, after inhaled general anaesthetic agents enter the airways, they are readily absorbed into the pulmonary capillaries (because they are lipid-soluble). They then circulate rapidly to the brain, readily cross the blood–brain barrier and then act to depress nerve cell functions. Bronchodilator β-agonist aerosols do produce systemic effects such as tremor and tachycardia because the drug stimulates cardiac β-adrenoceptors after absorption into the bloodstream.

When two or more inhalation aerosols are prescribed without specific instructions about the sequence of drug administration, the health-care professional should be aware of the proper recommendations for drug administration. For example, if a corticosteroid or mast-cell stabiliser puffer is prescribed to be administered as well as a bronchodilator puffer, the bronchodilator should be administered 5 minutes before the other drug to promote bronchodilation and maximise inhalation of the second aerosol.

KEY POINTS

- The respiratory system comprises the structures involved in the passage of gases from the nose, via the conducting airways (trachea, bronchi, bronchioles), to the respiratory bronchioles and alveoli in the lungs.
- The primary function of the lungs is gas exchange: oxygen is transported from the air to the blood in pulmonary capillaries and carbon dioxide is removed from the blood and exhaled.
- The main processes involved are pulmonary ventilation (bulk movement of air); gas transport across pulmonary, capillary and red cell membranes; and cellular respiration, providing oxygen for metabolic functions in body tissues and cells.
- Other functions of the respiratory system include regulation of blood pH; defence mechanisms, including removal of foreign particles; participation in speech, taste and smell; and biosynthetic function.
- Respiratory tract secretions, produced by goblet cells and bronchial glands, form a protective mucociliary blanket and provide surfactant functions.
- Bronchial smooth muscle is innervated by the parasympathetic and sympathetic nervous systems, mediating bronchoconstriction (via ACh M_3 receptors) and bronchodilation (via β_2-adrenoceptors), respectively.
- Constriction of the airways can also be produced by neuropeptides and other mediators released during inflammatory responses.

- Respiration is initiated and controlled at the central level (pons and medulla) and influenced at the periphery via sensory receptors, reflexes, oxygen and carbon dioxide partial pressures and blood pH.
- The main buffering capacity of the blood is provided by the bicarbonate–carbonic acid–carbon dioxide equilibrium, which is catalysed by carbonic anhydrase.
- Drugs can be administered locally to the airways as aerosols by means of sprays, inhalers and nebulisers.
- Advantages of inhaled aerosol or fine powder administration include rapid local effect, low dose and few systemic adverse effects.

REVIEW EXERCISES

1 List the functions of the respiratory system and describe how gases are exchanged and blood pH regulated.

2 Describe the central and peripheral control of respiration.

3 Describe the effects of the parasympathetic and sympathetic nervous system on the respiratory system, including the neurotransmitters and receptors involved.

4 Discuss the effects of changes in arterial oxygen or carbon dioxide partial pressures on the respiratory system.

5 Describe how drugs can be administered via the respiratory tract, with examples, and list advantages and potential disadvantages of administration by inhalation.

6 Explain (to an imaginary patient) how to use a 'puffer' inhaler effectively.

REFERENCES AND FURTHER READING

Australian Medicines Handbook 2006. Adelaide: AMH, 2006.

Caswell A (ed.). *MIMS Annual June* 2005. Sydney: CMPMedica Australia, 2005.

Flotte TR, Laube BL. Gene therapy in cystic fibrosis. *Chest* 2001; 120 (3 Suppl): 124S–31S.

Kerem E. Pharmacological induction of CFTR function in patients with cystic fibrosis: mutation-specific therapy. *Pediatric Pulmonology*, 2005; 40(3): 183–96.

Marshall BC, Samuelson WM. Basic therapies in cystic fibrosis: does standard therapy work? *Clinics in Chest Medicine* 1998; 19: 487–504.

Pain MCF. Basic tests of respiratory function. *Australian Prescriber* 2000; 23: 10–12.

Pain MCF. Delivering inhaled asthma therapy. *Australian Prescriber* 2003: 26(1): 5–7.

Powell FL. Part III: Respiratory physiology. In: Johnson LR (ed). *Essential Medical Physiology.* 2nd edn. Philadelphia: Lippincott-Raven, 1999 [chs 18–22].

Respiratory Expert Group. *Therapeutic Guidelines Respiratory, version 3.* Melbourne: Therapeutic Guidelines Limited, 2005.

Shargel L, Mutnick AH, Souney PF, Swanson LN, Block LH. *Comprehensive Pharmacy Review.* 3rd edn. Baltimore: Williams & Wilkins, 1997 [chs 3, 4, 36].

Vaswani SK, Creticos PS. Metered dose inhaler: past, present and future. *Annals of Allergy, Asthma and Immunology* 1998; 80: 11–19.

Virchow JC. Guidelines versus clinical practice—which therapy and which device? *Respiratory Medicine* 2004; 98 Suppl B: S28–34.

West J, Rodman DM. Gene therapy for pulmonary diseases. *Chest* 2001; 119: 613–17.

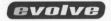 More weblinks at http://evolve.elsevier.com/AU/Bryant/pharmacology/

CHAPTER 32

Drugs Used in Respiratory Disorders

CHAPTER FOCUS

This chapter discusses the various drugs used for effects in the respiratory tract: medical gases (oxygen and carbon dioxide), respiratory stimulants and depressants, drugs affecting mucus and surfactant secretions, antiasthma medications (bronchodilators, symptom controllers and anti-inflammatory agents), and drugs used in respiratory tract infections and conditions affecting the nose. These agents cover a wide range of therapeutic effects on the respiratory system, in many common important conditions.

OBJECTIVES

- To define and describe the key terms in respiratory pharmacology.

- To list the key drugs used in the respiratory tract and describe their actions, clinical uses and adverse effects.

- To discuss the classification of patients with asthma and the stepwise management of asthma.

- To describe the main groups of drugs used in asthma and compare their mechanisms of action, clinical uses and effectiveness.

- To describe the effects of oxygen, oxygen deprivation and oxygen free radicals on the body.

- To explain the differences between a nasal catheter, nasal cannula, oxygen mask and oxygen tent for administration of oxygen.

- To discuss the use and effects of carbon dioxide as a pharmacological agent.

- To describe the drug treatment of respiratory tract infections (viral and bacterial) and of chronic obstructive airways disease.

- To discuss the nasal administration of drugs and describe the treatment of allergic rhinitis.

KEY DRUGS

acetylcysteine
beclomethasone
codeine
cromoglycate
eformoterol
influenza vaccine
ipratropium
oxygen
pseudoephedrine
salbutamol
salmeterol
terbutaline
theophylline
zafirlukast
zanamivir

KEY TERMS

allergic rhinitis
analeptics
asthma
β_2-adrenoceptor
  agonists
bronchodilator
controller
corticosteroids
cough suppressants
cromolyns
decongestants
expectorants
hypercapnia

hypoxaemia
hypoxia
leukotriene-receptor
  antagonists
mast-cell stabilisers
mucoactive agents
mucolytics
oxygen free radicals
preventer
reliever
surfactant
xanthine derivatives

KEY ABBREVIATIONS

COAD	chronic obstructive airways disease
COPD	chronic obstructive pulmonary disease
CR	controlled release
FEV_1	forced expiratory volume
MDI	metered dose inhaler
Pa_{O_2}	partial pressure of oxygen in arterial blood
Pa_{CO_2}	partial pressure of carbon dioxide in arterial blood
P_{O_2}	partial pressure of oxygen
P_{CO_2}	partial pressure of carbon dioxide
ROS	reactive oxygen species
RTI	respiratory tract infection
SRS-A	slow-reacting substance of anaphylaxis

RESPIRATORY GASES
Oxygen

OXYGEN is a gas that is essential for life; it is colourless, odourless and tasteless. It is not itself flammable, but it supports combustion much more vigorously than does air.

Inspired air normally contains 20.9% oxygen, which, at an atmospheric pressure of 760 mmHg, exerts a partial pressure (P_{O_2}) or tension of 159 mmHg. However, as oxygen passes through the bronchial airway, the inspired air becomes saturated with water vapour, which then reduces the P_{O_2} in the alveoli to around 100 mmHg. Finally, the oxygen appears in dissolved form in the arterial blood. The partial pressure of oxygen in arterial blood (Pa_{O_2}) is normally greater than 80 mmHg.

Oxygen must be continuously supplied to tissue cells, as no fibre or cell can remain without oxygen (hypoxic) for very long and survive. Of all the tissues affected by hypoxia (inadequate cellular oxygen), the brain is most susceptible to disruption of normal function and irreversible damage. Whenever any circulatory stress exists, cerebral blood flow tends to be preserved at the expense of other less vital organs. An acute reduction of the Pa_{O_2} level to 50 mmHg decreases mental functioning, emotional stability and fine muscular coordination. Further reduction produces impaired judgement, decreased pain perception, impairment of muscular coordination and, eventually, unconsciousness. Other vital organs in which there must be constancy of blood flow and oxygen supply include the kidneys and heart.

Indications for oxygen therapy

While essential for life, oxygen is also potentially toxic (see below). As with any drug, it should be administered only as required, in specific clinical conditions, in appropriate dosage regimens (% concentration, flow rate and duration) and with careful monitoring of blood gas concentrations. Oxygen is used chiefly to treat **hypoxia** and **hypoxaemia** (an abnormal oxygen deficiency in arterial blood). A Pa_{O_2} of less than 50 mmHg in an acutely ill patient (not adapted to chronic low Pa_{O_2} levels) indicates tissue hypoxia. The four types of hypoxia are:

• hypoxic hypoxia: produced by any condition causing a decrease in P_{O_2}, e.g. high altitude, airway obstruction
• ischaemic hypoxia: inadequate blood flow to an organ or tissue in the presence of a normal P_{O_2} and haemoglobin content, e.g. due to atherosclerosis or thromboembolism
• anaemic hypoxia: inadequate haemoglobin to carry oxygen in the presence of a normal P_{O_2}, e.g. haemorrhage, anaemia, carbon monoxide poisoning
• histotoxic hypoxia: adequate P_{O_2} and haemoglobin but inability of tissues to use oxygen delivered because of the presence of a toxic agent, e.g. cyanide.

Clinically, hypoxic hypoxia is the most common form of hypoxia. A variety of pathological conditions results in hypoxic hypoxia, which necessitates oxygen treatment. Examples are hypoventilation, increased airway resistance, pneumothorax, respiratory centre depression, abnormal ventilation:perfusion ratio, congenital cyanotic heart disease, decreased pulmonary compliance, and breathing oxygen-poor air. The use of oxygen is also indicated in cardiac failure or decompensation, coronary artery occlusion and when administering inhaled general anaesthetics (to increase the safety of general anaesthesia).

The effectiveness of oxygen administration depends on the carbon dioxide content of the blood. High-concentration oxygen therapy (50%–90%) in the hospital situation is used in acute conditions associated with a normal or low Pa_{CO_2}, when there is little risk of CO_2 retention, such as in pulmonary embolism or oedema, myocardial infarction or status asthmaticus (acute severe asthma). People with chronic obstructive pulmonary disease (COPD), however, have difficulty with CO_2–O_2 exchange and are subject to **hypercapnia** (high Pa_{CO_2}) with low Pa_{O_2}. Because of chronic hypercapnia, the medullary centres of these individuals are relatively insensitive to stimulation by carbon dioxide; rather, the low Pa_{O_2} serves as a stimulant to respiration. Oxygen concentration (25%) and flow rates (1–2 L/min) are therefore kept low for patients with COPD; however, the guiding principle is that hypoxaemia will cause death before hypercapnia, so adequate oxygen levels must always be maintained.

Administration

Most of the oxygen administered in hospitals for therapy is provided from a central source, where it is stored as a gas or liquid oxygen. Compressed oxygen is marketed in steel cylinders fitted with reducing valves for the delivery of the gas. The regulators and fittings are non-interchangeable, to minimise the risk of inadvertent administration of the wrong gas (see Clinical Interest Box 32-1); in Australia, oxygen cylinders are black with a white shoulder. Because the gas is under considerable pressure, the tanks must be handled and stored carefully to prevent them from falling or jarring. Oxygen cylinders may also be supplied to the homes (domiciliary oxygen therapy) of patients with severe persistent hypoxaemia, e.g. due to chronic bronchitis and emphysema, pulmonary hypertension or advanced neoplastic disease. Oxygen may also be supplied by an oxygen concentrator, a small mobile floor-standing electrically powered machine that produces oxygen by removing nitrogen from room air.

Oxygen is administered by inhalation via catheters, cannulae or masks (Figure 32-1), each method having advantages and disadvantages. A nasal catheter made of soft plastic is passed through the nose until the tip is just above the epiglottis. The catheter should not be inserted so far that the patient swallows oxygen, as this will cause stomach distension and abdominal discomfort. The catheter is fastened with tape to the forehead and/or nose. Cannulae have either single or double short prongs that are inserted into the lower part of the nostrils. They are much more comfortable for the patient than catheters and are less likely to become obstructed with secretions. Flow rates of 1–3 L/min of a 25%–40% concentration of oxygen are adequate for many patients.

An oxygen mask is the most effective means of delivering high concentrations of oxygen (up to 90%). A simple, lightweight disposable face mask is useful for short-term administration, such as in the early postoperative period or when intermittent oxygen therapy is required. A partial re-breathing mask consisting of a reservoir bag and a partial rebreathing valve conserves roughly one-third of the exhaled air. A non-rebreathing mask is designed to fit tightly over the face; expired air escapes through the one-way flap valve in the mask. The concentration of oxygen in this type of mask is 95%; they are used for short-term therapy such as counteracting smoke inhalation.

The Ventimask (Mix-O-Mask) originated from the Venturi mask and is used for patients with chronic alveolar hypoventilation and CO_2 retention. Exact concentrations of oxygen are delivered to the individual at set flow rates.

HYPERBARIC OXYGEN

Recently, hyperbaric oxygen (oxygen supplied at a pressure of 3–4 times normal) has been used in the treatment of various conditions, such as infections caused by *Clostridium welchii*, the anaerobic bacillus that produces gas gangrene. Increased oxygen pressure in the tissue may exert an inhibitory effect on enzyme systems of anaerobic microorganisms.

Hyperbaric oxygen has also been used in certain circulatory disturbances, such as air or gas embolism, decompression sickness, carbon monoxide and cyanide poisoning, acute traumatic ischaemia, crush injury and compartment syndrome, and also in compromised (ischaemic) grafts and flaps, radiation necrosis, refractory osteomyelitis and to enhance healing in problem wounds.

Oxygen toxicity

While oxygen is essential for life in aerobic organisms including humans, it has also been described as a toxic mutagenic gas; aerobes survive because they have antioxidant defences against oxygen. Exposure of humans to 80%–100% oxygen for a period of 6–10 hours causes an inflammatory response with subsequent destruction of the alveolocapillary membrane of the respiratory tract. Toxicity is often difficult to recognise but the most common symptoms are substernal distress (ache or burning sensation behind the sternum), an increase in respiratory distress with decreased vital capacity, nausea, vomiting, restlessness, tremors, twitching, paraesthesias, convulsions and a dry, hacking cough.

CLINICAL INTEREST BOX 32-1 MEDICAL GASES

Medical gases are supplied in a great range of container sizes, from small portable aluminium cylinders (about 200 L capacity) to steel cylinders of compressed gases (several thousand litres capacity), through to systems of tanks and plumbed-in gas lines servicing hospitals and research institutions. The colour coding adopted in Australia and New Zealand is as follows:

Gas	Colours	Uses
Air, compressed	Green-grey cylinder, black & white shoulder	Breathing apparatus; driving surgical air tools
Carbogen (usually 5% CO_2 in oxygen)	Black cylinder, green-grey & white shoulder	Respiratory stimulant; oxygenation of isolated tissues in physiological and pharmacological research
Carbon dioxide	Green-grey cylinder, green-grey shoulder	Respiratory stimulant; in anaesthesia; in cryosurgery
Helium	Brown cylinder, brown shoulder	Vehicle gas; gaining access to obstructed airways; in balloons
Nitrous oxide	Ultramarine blue cylinder, ultramarine blue shoulder	Analgesia and anaesthesia; vehicle gas in anaesthesia; in cryosurgery
Entonox (50% oxygen, 50% nitrous oxide)	Ultramarine blue cylinder, ultramarine blue & white shoulder	Anaesthetic in obstetrics, first aid, dentistry, ambulances etc
Oxygen, compressed	Black cylinder, white shoulder	Respiratory therapy; carrier gas in anaesthesia; high altitude & underwater breathing; hyperbaric chambers

Equipment used to handle and administer gases includes regulators and flow meters, carry bags, trolleys, oxygen concentrators and conserving devices, pressure gauges, masks, cylinder backpacks, suction units, cannulae, tubing and connectors.

Sources: BOC Gases Group 1999; BOC website: www.boc.com.au, accessed 8 February 2006.
Note: The New Zealand manufacturer refers to green/grey as 'French grey' and ultramarine blue as 'Royal blue'.

OXYGEN FREE RADICALS

Free radicals are chemical species containing one or more unpaired electrons. They tend to be chemically reactive, as the electrons readily participate in oxidation–reduction reactions. Reactive oxygen species (ROS) include the superoxide radical ($O_2\bullet^-$) and hydroxyl radical ($\bullet OH$). These **oxygen free radicals** are formed in many biochemical reactions in the body, e.g. by enzymes such as peroxidases, xanthine oxidase and nitric oxide synthase, and in the electron transport chain.

Oxygen free radicals have been implicated in many pathological processes, in particular in causing oxidative stress, a situation in which there is imbalance between ROS and levels of antioxidant defences. This can lead to adaptation or to cell injury and cell death. Oxygen free radicals are implicated in post-ischaemic reperfusion injury, in many of the processes of ageing, in radiation-induced damage, vitamin E deficiency, atherosclerosis, rheumatoid arthritis, diabetes, inflammatory bowel disease and hypertension, and in some types of cancer and adverse drug reactions.

There is clear evidence that a diet high in antioxidants protects against many of the major diseases of older age, such as ischaemic heart disease and many cancers. The antioxidant vitamins E (tocopherols) and C (ascorbic acid) are protective, and a diet rich in fruit, vegetables, nuts, beans and lentils is encouraged.

Carbon dioxide

Carbon dioxide is a colourless, odourless gas that is heavier than air (normal air contains only 0.04% CO_2). As a pharmacological agent, it affects respiration, circulation and the central nervous system (CNS). Inhalation of 3%–5% CO_2 for a short period increases both rate and depth of respiration unless the respiratory centre is depressed by narcotics or disease.

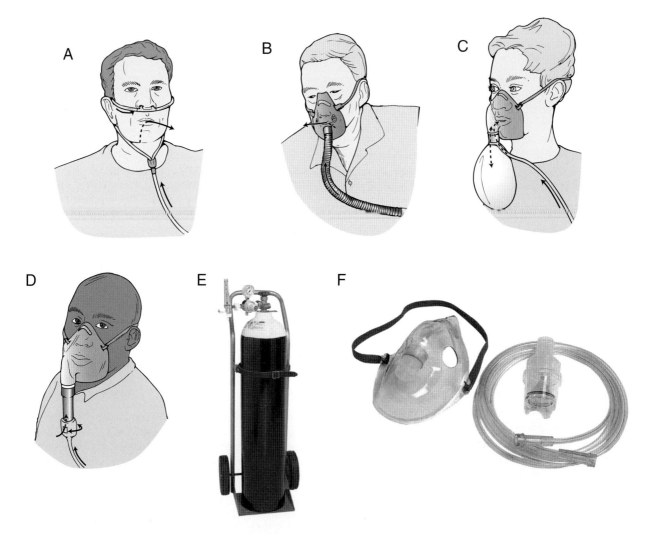

FIGURE 32-1 Various oxygen delivery systems. **A.** Nasal cannula. **B.** Simple face mask. **C.** Partial rebreathing mask. **D.** Venturi mask. **E.** Gas cylinder on trolley, with regulator and flow meter. **F.** Adult nebuliser bowl, tubing and mask. (**E** and **F**: photographs courtesy of BOC Gases Australia Ltd, reproduced with permission.)

Carbon dioxide stimulates cells of the sympathetic nervous system, the respiratory centre and the peripheral chemoreceptors. Inhalation of 5%–7% CO_2 increases cerebral blood flow by around 75%, primarily by dilation of cerebral vessels. When CO_2 increases the rate and force of respiration, venous return to the heart is usually enhanced as a result of decreased peripheral resistance; there is improved rate and force of myocardial contraction and less likelihood of myocardial irritability and arrhythmias.

Too much carbon dioxide in inhaled air (>7%) may cause:
- acidosis
- unresponsiveness of the respiratory centre to the gas
- depression of the cerebral cortex, myocardium and smooth muscle of the peripheral blood vessels
- interference with nerve conduction and transmission
- carbon dioxide narcosis (sleepiness and confusion and, at very high doses, anaesthetic and convulsant effects).

It is therefore important that CO_2 be administered with caution.

Indications

Indications for clinical use of CO_2 are:
- carbon monoxide poisoning: a 5%–7% concentration of CO_2 in oxygen is sometimes used to treat carbon monoxide poisoning. Physiologically, carbon dioxide increases the rate of separation of carbon monoxide from carboxyhaemoglobin
- respiratory depression: when CO_2 is used as a respiratory stimulant, close monitoring by pulse oximetry and Pa_{O_2} is important. Oxygen administration and mechanical assistance of respiration are the usual treatments in respiratory depression
- general anaesthesia and postoperative use: mixtures of O_2 and CO_2 may be used during anaesthesia. Carbon dioxide initially speeds up anaesthesia by increasing pulmonary ventilation; by lessening the sense of asphyxiation, it reduces struggling. In the postanaesthesia period, it hastens the elimination of many anaesthetics
- postoperatively, to increase ventilation and prevent atelectasis; however, deep-breathing exercises, coughing, frequent turning, tracheal suction, and intermittent positive pressure breathing produce better results.

Other uses

Carbon dioxide in solution (as carbonated 'fizzy' drinks) stimulates the absorption of liquids by mucous membranes and hence rapidly relieves thirst (and hastens the absorption of alcohol). Solid CO_2 ('dry ice', at −78°C) has a destructive action on tissues; in cryotherapy it is applied directly to warts to destroy them.

A mixture of CO_2 (usually 5%) in oxygen, known as carbogen (e.g. Carbanox), is used in many pharmacological and physiological experiments to oxygenate isolated tissues (see Clinical Interest Box 32-1).

Carbon dioxide has also been used in the treatment of postoperative hiccups. Relief of hiccups is apparently accomplished by stimulation of the respiratory centre, causing large excursions of the diaphragm, which suppress spasmodic contractions of that muscle, promoting regular contractions.

Carbon dioxide levels are also altered, indirectly, by drugs that inhibit the enzyme carbonic anhydrase (see Chapter 31, under Control of pH). These drugs, such as acetazolamide and dorzolamide, produce a general metabolic acidosis by inhibiting carbonic anhydrase in the kidney, thereby causing loss of bicarbonate and an alkaline diuresis. The acidosis has a stimulatory effect. Carbonic anhydrase inhibitors also have membrane-stabilising and antiepileptic properties, produce drowsiness in high doses, and lower intraocular pressure by inhibiting bicarbonate synthesis; hence they are useful in glaucoma (see Chapter 35).

Administration and toxicity

Carbon dioxide is kept in metal cylinders (coloured grey-green). When it is used for medical purposes it is administered in combination with oxygen. A 5%–10% concentration of CO_2 delivered through a tight-fitting face mask is inhaled by the patient until the depth of respiration is definitely increased. Another way of administering CO_2 is to allow the patient to hyperventilate with a paper bag held over the face. Reinhaling expired air causes the CO_2 content to be continually increased.

Signs of CO_2 overdosage are dyspnoea, breath-holding, markedly increased chest and abdominal movements, nausea and raised systolic blood pressure. Administration should be discontinued when these symptoms appear. Administering 5% CO_2 may produce severe CNS depression if given over 1 hour; a 10% concentration can lead to loss of consciousness within 10 minutes. Administration should be stopped as soon as the desired effects on the patient's respiration have been obtained.

RESPIRATORY STIMULANTS AND DEPRESSANTS

Respiratory stimulants: analeptics

Direct respiratory stimulants come under the broader classification of CNS stimulants and are referred to as **analeptics** (see Chapter 20). These drugs act directly on the respiratory and vasomotor centres in the medulla to increase respiratory rate and tidal exchange and raise the blood pressure. Although these drugs are available for stimulating respiration, they may in large doses cause convulsions, CNS depression and respiratory paralysis; hence airway management and mechanical support of ventilation are more effective in the treatment of respiratory depression. Analeptics have been subject to some controversy: in the past, they were advocated in the treatment of drug-induced respiratory depression and respiratory distress syndrome; however, as these drugs are not specific antagonists to sedatives or narcotics, their use in drug-induced respiratory depression is now considered obsolete.

Reflex respiratory stimulants

Aromatic ammonia spirit and the natural compounds camphor, menthol and thujone (a constituent of absinthe) are given by inhalation for their actions as reflex respiratory stimulants. In cases of fainting, they may be administered by inhaling the vapours ('smelling salts'). Reflex stimulation of the medullary centre occurs through peripheral irritation of sensory nerve receptors in the pharynx, oesophagus and stomach. The rate and depth of respiration are then increased through afferent messages to the respiratory control centres; reflex stimulation of the vasomotor centre results in a rise in blood pressure.

Respiratory depressants

The most important respiratory depressants are the narcotic analgesics, such as opium and its derivatives. These agents depress the sensitivity of the respiratory centre to CO_2, thereby making breathing slower and more shallow and lessening the irritability of the respiratory centre. Respiratory depression, however, is seldom desirable or necessary, although it is sometimes unavoidable. It is also an adverse effect of many otherwise useful CNS depressant drugs, including the benzodiazepines, barbiturates, antihistamines and alcohol.

Occasionally, an opioid such as pholcodine is administered to inhibit the rate and depth of respiration for a painful or harmful cough (see later section on cough suppressants).

DRUGS AFFECTING SECRETIONS AND MUCOCILIARY TRANSPORT

Expectorant and mucoactive drugs

Expectorants are drugs that aid in the removal (and swallowing or spitting out) of sputum from the bronchial passages. **Mucoactive agents** promote the removal of abnormal or excessive respiratory tract secretions by thinning excessively viscous mucus, which allows for more effective ciliary action. These agents prevent sputum retention, which may result from abnormal ciliary activity, defects in air flow or modification of cough effectiveness. Sputum (or phlegm) may be defined as an abnormal viscous secretion of the lower respiratory tree. It consists mainly of mucus, a mucopolysaccharide–glycoprotein material continually produced by the surface cells in the mucous membrane. In addition, sputum contains leucocytes, bacteria, and DNA derived from the breakdown of mucosal cells. These products are responsible for the characteristic thickness and yellow colour of sputum.

People with respiratory disorders such as chronic bronchitis develop disturbances of the mucociliary blanket, resulting in a significant impairment of the mucus clearance process. Consequently, mucus plugging of airways and alveoli (Figure 32-2) and pathogenic colonisation of microorganisms occur in the lower respiratory tract. These changes lead to overproduction of thick, tenacious sputum. The advantage provided by expectorant and mucoactive drugs is that they alter the consistency of the sputum, either by diluting thickened secretions (diluents, irritants) or by chemically breaking down mucus (mucolytics), promoting the eventual expectoration, or spitting out, of these secretions.

Diluents
Water

The agent most commonly used to dilute respiratory secretions is water. People with COPD frequently suffer from dehydration; respiratory secretions become thickened, are retained, and lead to widespread plug formation in the respiratory tree. Water may be administered by ultrasonic nebuliser or, more traditionally, by inhaling steam from a basin of boiling water. Small amounts of water deposited on the gel layer of the respiratory tree appear to reduce the adhesive characteristics and general viscosity of the gelatinous substances found in this layer. Usually large amounts of water are needed to liquefy the respiratory secretions. (For patients receiving restricted fluid intake, water absorbed through the inhalation route must be added to the intake record.)

Saline solutions

Normal saline (0.9% sodium chloride) is an isotonic solution that exerts the same osmotic pressure as plasma fluids. Therapy by nebulisation is well tolerated, resulting in hydration of respiratory secretions. Inhalation of hypotonic solution (e.g. 0.45% sodium chloride) may provide deeper penetration into the more distal airways, whereas inhalation of hypertonic solution (1.8% sodium chloride) stimulates a productive cough.

Irritant expectorants

Older compounds promoted as expectorants are thought to act by an irritant action on the mucous membranes, which increases the secretion of mucus from bronchial secretory cells, facilitating ciliary action and productive coughing and soothing and lubricating dry tissues. Such substances include the natural compounds ipecacuanha, squill, guaifenesin, iodides, liquorice, senega, ammonia and volatile oils (lemon, eucalyptus, tea-tree, pine etc.). While they contribute much to the colour, flavour, smell and placebo effect of many old-fashioned over-the-counter (OTC) cough mixtures (see later section), there is little objective evidence of any pharmacological efficacy. In higher doses, these compounds also have direct and irritant emetic actions.

Mucolytic drugs

Mucolytic drugs exert a disintegrating effect on mucus, facilitating removal of mucus or other exudates from the lung, bronchi or trachea by postural drainage, coughing or spitting. The more commonly used **mucolytics** are **acetylcysteine** (see Drug Monograph 32-1) and bromhexine but there is little hard evidence of clinical efficacy for either compound. They have been proven effective in reducing exacerbations and disability in subjects with chronic obstructive pulmonary disease.

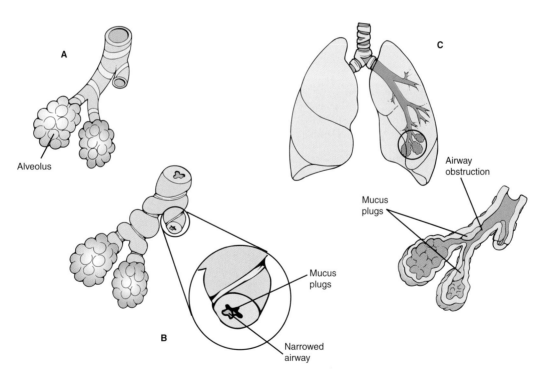

FIGURE 32-2 The airways in asthma. Bronchiole in normal state (**A**) and during an asthma attack (**B** and **C**). An asthma attack is characterised by bronchial muscle spasms, inflammation and excessive mucus, resulting in mucus plugs, oedema and trapped air in the alveoli, which cause airway obstruction (**C**). The total amount of air inhaled and exhaled decreases because of air trapped in the lungs after expiration; wheezing is due to increased airways resistance, especially during expiration.

Bromhexine

This drug is thought to improve mucus flow by enhancing the hydrolysing activity of lysosomal enzymes. It is administered orally as tablets or liquid to reduce mucus viscosity in bronchopulmonary disease.

Dornase alfa

Dornase alfa is a prescribed respiratory inhalant product with some proven mucolytic efficacy. It is used to increase expectoration in cystic fibrosis (see Clinical Interest Box 31-1). It is recombinant human deoxyribonuclease, a DNA-degrading enzyme that digests extracellular DNA released from degenerating neutrophils and cellular debris in purulent sputum, thus improving pulmonary function and reducing the risk of respiratory tract infections common with cystic fibrosis. Its use has resulted in a decrease in the incidence of respiratory infections, hospitalisations and medical costs but it is expensive, so continued treatment needs to be justified by a proven benefit.

The enzyme solution is inhaled via a nebuliser—usually one 2.5 mg ampoule/day regularly for 6–12 months. Inhaled enzyme acts locally in the respiratory tract and does not reach the systemic circulation. Significant improvement in pulmonary function is seen within 3–7 days and a decrease in respiratory infections within weeks to several months.

Adverse reactions include chest pain, sore throat, laryngitis, skin rash and conjunctivitis. No significant drug interaction has been reported.

Muscarinic antagonists (antimuscarinics)

Acetylcholine muscarinic M_3 receptors, present on bronchial smooth muscle cells and gland cells, mediate contraction of smooth muscle (bronchoconstriction) and stimulation of bronchial secretions (see Figures 32-3 and 32-4). Thus, one of the many pharmacological effects of muscarinic-receptor antagonists (antimuscarinic drugs) such as atropine is inhibition of bronchial secretions. Salivary, lacrimal and sweat gland secretions are also inhibited, leading to the common 'atropinic' effect of dry mouth (see Drug Monograph 11-2).

The muscarinic antagonist **ipratropium** is sometimes used in bronchial asthma as a bronchodilator. Potential adverse effects include inhibition of bronchial secretion and mucociliary transport, and accumulation of thickened secretions; however, as there is often excessive mucus production in asthma, the effects tend to cancel out.

Pulmonary surfactants

Surfactant, synthesised in fetal lungs late in fetal life, is a complex mixture of phospholipids, glycoproteins, cholesterol and triglycerides that regulates the surface tension of the fluid on the alveolar surface. Surfactant can be purified from animal lung sources, synthesised in the laboratory or produced by genetic engineering techniques in bacterial cell cultures. Two forms used in Australia are beractant (a modified bovine product) and poractant alfa (derived from pigs' lungs). The products are supplied as solutions for intratracheal administration. These drugs are still relatively new and are normally used only in neonatal intensive care units.

Infant respiratory distress syndrome is a common condition in premature newborn babies (75% prevalence in infants delivered before 28 weeks), with a high mortality rate if not treated rapidly. It is due to a deficiency of surfactant production in the immature lungs, resulting in lung expansion with the risk of alveolar collapse. Treatment of premature infants suffering respiratory distress with exogenous surfactant instilled into the trachea is remarkably effective; surfactant reduces

---

DRUG MONOGRAPH 32-1 ACETYLCYSTEINE

Acetylcysteine reduces the viscosity and stickiness of purulent and non-purulent pulmonary secretions by splitting disulphide bonds in mucoprotein molecules. When administered systemically, it is a specific antidote for paracetamol overdose.

INDICATIONS Acetylcysteine is administered by intratracheal tube or nebuliser to reduce thick or abnormal mucus in bronchopulmonary disease, cystic fibrosis, and atelectasis caused by a mucus obstruction. Note that acetylcysteine is also indicated as an antidote to paracetamol poisoning (see Box 16-2).

PHARMACOKINETICS In inhalation therapy, the primary effects of this agent are local on the mucus in the lungs. When inhaled or instilled directly via an intratracheal

catheter, it produces a rapid effect. The peak response from inhalation occurs within 5–10 minutes. Acetylcysteine is metabolised in the liver.

ADVERSE REACTIONS These include nausea, mouth ulcers and respiratory difficulties, including bronchospasm. No significant drug interaction has been reported.

CONTRAINDICATIONS Avoid use in patients with acetylcysteine hypersensitivity or asthma, and in patients who are unable to cough.

DOSAGE AND ADMINISTRATION The usual adult and paediatric dose by nebulisation using a face mask, mouthpiece, or tracheostomy is 1–10 mL 20% solution 2–6 hourly.

dependence on a ventilator, reduces risk of pneumothorax, increases oxygenation, and has improved survival rates from 30% in the 1970s to 90% today.

If premature birth is anticipated, glucocorticoids given prophylactically to the mother can enhance fetal lung maturation and synthesis of surfactant.

DRUG TREATMENT OF ASTHMA

Pathophysiology of asthma

In **asthma**, the passage of air into and out of the lungs is obstructed because of reversible bronchoconstriction, chronic inflammation of the epithelium of the airways, and increased mucus secretion; there is airway hypersensitivity to a variety of stimuli. The early phase of an acute attack involves bronchoconstriction and excessive secretion of mucus (see Figure 32-2); the late-phase (chronic) response involves inflammation, proliferation of fibroblasts and fibrosis, oedema of the airway mucosa, necrosis of bronchial epithelial cells, and airway wall remodelling, with increased collagen deposition. The principal signs and symptoms are wheezing and cough, dyspnoea (difficult breathing), chest tightness, tachycardia, fatigue, sweating and anxiety. Hypoxaemia and a raised P_{CO_2} may become life-threatening.

The signs and symptoms usually resolve rapidly after administration of bronchodilator drugs, but even during symptom-free periods between attacks, the airway resistance of patients may be 2–3 times normal. In status asthmaticus, the airway obstruction may be irreversible and is potentially fatal.

Extrinsic (atopic, allergic) asthma is triggered by factors not normally in the body, including allergens such as pollens, house dust mites, animal fur, moulds or proteins in foods such as eggs. Other common triggers are drugs, including β-blockers, penicillins and aspirin, chemicals such as sulfites used as preservatives, exercise (breathing cold air is thought to be the stimulus), emotional stress, respiratory infections and environmental pollutants, including cigarette smoke. All people with asthma are hypersensitive to bronchoconstrictor agents, including acetylcholine and $PGF_{2\alpha}$. In 'intrinsic asthma' there is no identified causative agent.

Many mediators are involved in the pathogenesis of an asthma attack, including leukotrienes, histamine, prostaglandins and other cytokines, and neurotransmitters. Not surprisingly, many types of drugs are used to inhibit the pathological effects of these mediators. An overview of the actions of these mediators and the effects of five important drug groups used in treating asthma is given in Figure 32-3. The management of asthma requires assessment and monitoring of severity (by regular checks of FEV_1), and

identification and avoidance if possible of triggering factors. The choice of drugs depends on patient factors, aetiological factors, history and classified severity of asthma, and drug factors such as adverse drug reactions.

Asthma affects more than 10% of Australians (Clinical Interest Box 32-3) and 15% of New Zealanders (Clinical Interest Box 32-4). Patients are classified as mild, moderate or severe, according to the frequency and severity of their asthma attacks during the previous 3 years, because this information is useful when considering pharmacological interventions:

- mild: intermittent attacks (fewer than 1–2 per week), or nocturnal asthma twice or less monthly. Peak expiratory flow (PEF) >80% predicted (i.e. >80% of the expected level); normal after bronchodilator use; PEF variability <20%.
- moderate: attacks more than twice weekly, nocturnal asthma symptoms more than twice per month, and use of a bronchodilator β-agonist inhaler required nearly daily. PEF 60%–80% predicted; normal after bronchodilator use; PEF variability 20%–30%.
- severe: frequent and continuous asthmatic symptoms, including nocturnal asthma and having been hospitalised for asthma in the previous year.

The overall management of asthma is summarised later in this chapter, after discussion of the groups of drugs commonly used in this condition.

CLINICAL INTEREST BOX 32-3   ASTHMA IN THE AUSTRALIAN COMMUNITY

- In Australia, asthma affects:
  — one in four primary-school-aged children
  — one in seven adolescents
  — one in 10 adults.
- The prevalence is increasing, doubling every 15 years.
- In 1997, 730 Australians died from asthma (out of a population of around 17.5 million)—about 14 per week.
- It is believed that 50% of asthma deaths could have been avoided through improved management.
- The estimated total cost of asthma to the Australian community (including medical costs, indirect costs, life-years lost to disability or premature death, and absenteeism) is over $4.3 billion (2000/01 dollars).
- In children, asthma is the most common chronic illness and the most common reason for childhood admissions to hospital and absenteeism from school.
- Over half (54%) of expenditure allocated to asthma in 2000/01 was attributed to drugs used in management.
- Asthma is the ninth leading contributor to disease in Australia.

Sources: National Asthma Campaign: www.nationalasthma.org.au and Asthma Victoria: www.asthma.org.au, accessed 1 September 2006.

The major groups of drugs used in treatment of asthma are:

- reliever medications (bronchodilators: short-acting β₂-receptor agonists, **theophylline**, **ipratropium**)
- symptom controllers (long-acting β₂ agonists)
- preventer medications (inhaled corticosteroids, leukotriene-receptor antagonists, mast-cell stabilisers).

Figure 32-3 gives an overview of the effects of antiasthma medications and the primary sites of action for these drugs. Some of the bronchodilator drugs act by enhancing the production of cyclic 3,5-AMP (cAMP) in bronchial smooth muscle cells to cause bronchodilation (see Figure 32-4). Aerosol therapy and devices used to administer drugs into the airways are described in Chapter 31.

Bronchodilator drugs
History

Bronchodilator drugs are primarily used to treat pulmonary diseases such as asthma, chronic bronchitis and emphysema. They have been used in respiratory medicine for over 5000 years: ephedrine, a sympathomimetic amine closely related structurally to adrenaline, is an alkaloid obtained from the plant *Ephedra sinica* and was introduced from traditional Chinese medicine into Western medicine in 1923. Ephedrine has a predominantly indirect action, via release of noradrenaline from adrenergic nerve terminals; thus it has effects on both α- and β-adrenoceptors. The effects mediated by α-adrenoceptors (especially vasoconstriction and hypertension) and β₁-adrenoceptors (especially cardiac stimulation) count as adverse drug reactions in the context of asthma therapy, so much research effort has gone into development of specific **β₂-adrenoceptor agonist** bronchodilators.

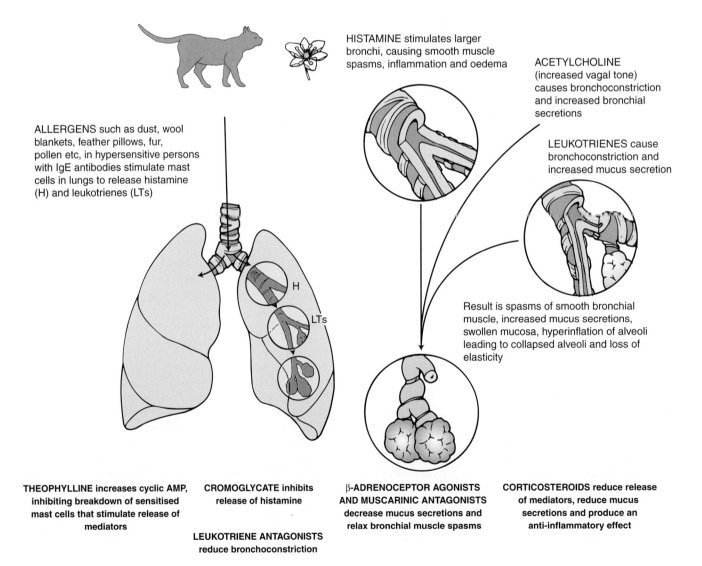

HISTAMINE stimulates larger bronchi, causing smooth muscle spasms, inflammation and oedema

ACETYLCHOLINE (increased vagal tone) causes bronchoconstriction and increased bronchial secretions

LEUKOTRIENES cause bronchoconstriction and increased mucus secretion

ALLERGENS such as dust, wool blankets, feather pillows, fur, pollen etc, in hypersensitive persons with IgE antibodies stimulate mast cells in lungs to release histamine (H) and leukotrienes (LTs)

Result is spasms of smooth bronchial muscle, increased mucus secretions, swollen mucosa, hyperinflation of alveoli leading to collapsed alveoli and loss of elasticity

THEOPHYLLINE increases cyclic AMP, inhibiting breakdown of sensitised mast cells that stimulate release of mediators

CROMOGLYCATE inhibits release of histamine

β-ADRENOCEPTOR AGONISTS AND MUSCARINIC ANTAGONISTS decrease mucus secretions and relax bronchial muscle spasms

CORTICOSTEROIDS reduce release of mediators, reduce mucus secretions and produce an anti-inflammatory effect

LEUKOTRIENE ANTAGONISTS reduce bronchoconstriction

FIGURE 32-3 Overview of the mediators of asthma and the effects of various antiasthma medications.

〰 CLINICAL INTEREST BOX 32-4 ASTHMA IN NEW ZEALAND

The prevalence of asthma in New Zealand is one of the highest in the world. According to the New Zealand Health Survey 2002–2003 one in five adults aged 15–44 years had been diagnosed with asthma. There was no significant difference in prevalence between males and females, but adult males were less likely than females to receive medical treatment. The prevalence of asthma was about four times higher among European/other ethnic groups than among Pacific and Asian ethnic groups, and was highest in the 15–24-year age group. The age of onset in about half of people with asthma is before the age of 10 and most have developed it by the age of 30.

During the 1970s and 1980s, there was an 'epidemic' of asthma-related deaths and hospital admissions in New Zealand, prompting urgent study of possible causes. Since 1989, there has been a decline in these statistics, reflecting changes in management and treatment; however, there is still a high prevalence of reported asthma symptoms in New Zealand, and some evidence that the prevalence may be increasing in New Zealand as in other developed countries.

In 1990, Sears et al reported their findings from a double-blind, placebo-controlled, randomised, crossover 24-week study of regular versus on-demand inhaled bronchodilator therapy: regular inhalation of fenoterol was associated with deterioration of asthma control. They suggested that the trend of using regular, higher doses or longer-acting inhaled bronchodilator β_2 agonists may be an important causal factor in the worldwide increase in morbidity from asthma. Two later case-controlled studies supported the hypothesis that inhaled fenoterol increased the risk of death in patients with severe asthma.

The New Zealand Department of Health issued warnings about the safety of fenoterol and restricted its availability. The asthma death rate fell by half, and time trend data were consistent with fenoterol being the main cause of the New Zealand asthma mortality epidemic. Interestingly, an evaluation of international data on medication sales in countries such as Australia, Belgium, Austria and Germany did not point to a relation between asthma mortality and bronchodilator β_2 agonists in general or fenoterol in particular. Fenoterol is no longer available in New Zealand.

The effectiveness of a 6-month Maori rural community-based asthma self-management program involving a 'credit card' asthma self-management plan was assessed during the 6 years after the formal end of the program. The program participants still had reduced asthma morbidity 6 years after the program had ended but these benefits were less than those measured at 2 years. It appeared that underrecognition and undertreatment of asthma with the appropriate amounts of inhaled steroids were major factors contributing to asthma morbidity. Continued reinforcement of the self-management skills seemed to be an essential component of any follow-up to an asthma self-management program.

To October 1998, the New Zealand Centre for Adverse Reactions Monitoring had received 81 reports of bronchospasm after the ingestion of NSAIDs, and six reports of exacerbation of asthma symptoms, including one fatality after aspirin administration. The reported incidence of 'aspirin-induced asthma' varies from 8% to 20% of adults with asthma and is higher in those who also have chronic rhinitis or a history of nasal polyps. There is marked cross-sensitivity among most NSAIDs, even where they are structurally dissimilar. People with a history of asthma should be warned of the reaction and, as it is difficult to identify those 'at risk', paracetamol should be the antipyretic analgesic of choice unless there are any specific contraindications.
Adapted from: New Zealand Prescriber Update No 18; Sears et al 1990; New Zealand Ministry of Health 1999; D'Souza et al 2000.

β-adrenoceptor agonists

The classification of adrenoceptors and the effects of agents that stimulate or block specific receptors are discussed in Chapter 12; reviewing these will help in understanding the mechanisms and actions of sympathomimetic bronchodilators. While agonists with specific actions on β_2-adrenoceptors are available, it needs to be remembered that any substrate specificity in pharmacology is relative, and such agonists may still stimulate both α and β_1 receptors, so adverse effects in the cardiovascular system (tachycardia), skeletal muscle (tremor) and CNS (anxiety) may occur. The reverse is also true: β_1-adrenoceptor antagonists (β-blockers) used in cardiovascular disease may have potentially life-threatening bronchoconstrictor (β_2) effects in people with asthma (see the case study in Clinical Interest Box 32-5). Agonist actions on uterine β_2-adrenoceptors can cause relaxation of smooth muscle; the drugs are sometimes used to delay threatened miscarriage (see Chapter 45).

The optimal route of administration of β_2 agonists is by inhalation; 'puffers' and 'pumps' deliver low doses of drug directly to the airway smooth muscle and have rapid and relatively specific effects (see Aerosol Therapy in Chapter 31, and Figure 31-2). Some inhaled drug is inevitably deposited in the oropharynx and swallowed; it may be absorbed into the systemic circulation and cause adverse reactions in other tissues. In rare cases, drugs administered by inhalation may cause bronchospasm; propellants may induce cardiac arrhythmias or allergic reactions. 'Epidemics' of deaths from asthma occurred in the 1960s in Britain (attributed to over-the-counter preparations of high-dose isoprenaline) and in the 1980s in New Zealand, attributed to high doses of fenoterol (Clinical Interest Box 32-4). Studies of morbidity have suggested that less selective β agonists may downregulate receptors, leading to the development of tolerance to the bronchoconstrictor effects of these agents, which encourages overuse and exacerbates adverse effects

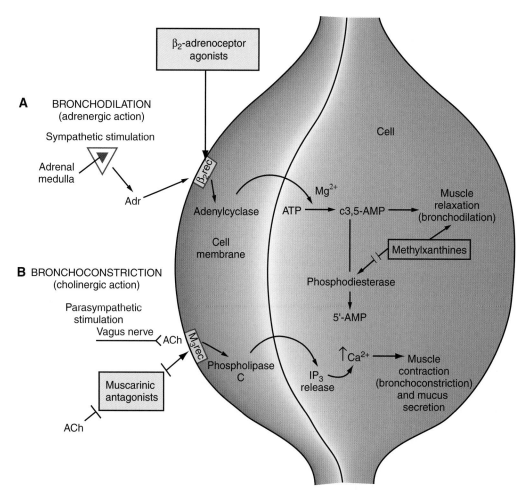

FIGURE 32-4 Proposed mechanisms of action of drugs on bronchial smooth muscle.
A. Bronchodilation pathway. B. Bronchoconstriction pathway. ACh = acetylcholine; Adr = adrenaline; β rec – β₂ receptor;
IP = inositol phosphate; M₃ rec = M₃ muscarinic receptor.

arising from the cardiac and vascular actions (see Abramson
et al 2003).

SHORT-ACTING β₂ AGONISTS

Short-acting β₂ agonists commonly used include salbutamol
(well known as Ventolin) and terbutaline. These are fast-
acting bronchodilators, known as **relievers**, for use in acute
asthma attacks (see Drug Monograph 32-2). Overdependence
on β₂ agonists may indicate that other aspects of asthma
management, including prophylactic use of anti-inflammatory
drugs, and monitoring of FEV₁, are not optimal. Adrenaline,
salbutamol and terbutaline are also available in parenteral
form to be injected in the event of a severe acute asthma
attack.

LONG-ACTING β₂ AGONISTS

Long-acting β₂ agonists commonly used include salmeterol
and eformoterol; they have half-lives in the range 6–12 hours
and are administered once or twice daily. They are known as

symptom **controllers** and are used in conjunction with short-
acting β₂ agonists and inhaled corticosteroids. In addition
to their β₂-agonist actions, these drugs inhibit release of
mast-cell mediators (histamine, leukotrienes, prostaglandins)
from human lung tissue, which helps reduce bronchial hyperreactivity; however, the drugs do not substitute for inhaled
corticosteroids, which should be used concurrently.

XANTHINE DERIVATIVES

The xanthine group of drugs includes caffeine, theophylline
and theobromine. Beverages from the extracts of plants
containing these alkaloids have been used by humans since
ancient times (the social use of the xanthines as coffee, tea,
cocoa and cola drinks is discussed in Chapter 22). **Xanthine
derivatives** relax smooth muscle (particularly bronchial
muscle), stimulate cardiac muscle and the CNS (hence their
social use), and also produce diuresis, probably through
combined actions of increased renal perfusion and increased
sodium and chloride ion excretion. Although caffeine is

CLINICAL INTEREST BOX 32-5 NOT IN THE SCRIPT: A CASE OF DRUG-INDUCED ASTHMA

Mr Bloggs, a busy businessman from Bentleigh, was in a hurry—couldn't wait for an examination, just wanted a prescription for a salbutamol puffer for his asthma. The doctor obliged, against his better judgement, and Bloggs went off.

Three months later Bloggs was back—this time for a repeat prescription for his blood pressure pills. But this time the doctor insisted that Bloggs needed to be examined and it became apparent that he was a red-faced, obese, alcoholic, wheezing smoker. He complained he'd had asthma on and off for 2 years since his blood pressure tablets were changed.

Closer examination of medical records showed that 2 years previously, Bloggs' antihypertensive medication had been changed from methyldopa to metoprolol. When questioned further, Bloggs admitted he had had asthma

when young, but not since adolescence. It became clear that the β-blocker had caused bronchoconstriction, exacerbating his quiescent asthma.

The lessons learned were:
- a β-blocker should be prescribed only after thorough discussion of a patient's past history of respiratory illness
- possible causes of a flare-up of asthma should be investigated before prescribing treatment
- the importance of review consultations should be emphasised, to monitor adverse effects and compliance
- manipulative patients may attempt to rush health professionals in order to hide lifestyle factors such as excessive eating, drinking and smoking.

Adapted from: Murtagh 1992; used with permission.

present in some preparations prescribed for migraine and in some OTC products taken to reduce mental fatigue, the main medical use of these natural products and their synthetic analogues is as bronchodilators.

The drugs in this category are methylated forms of xanthines (i.e. methylxanthines). The most active bronchodilator is theophylline (Drug Monograph 32-3), which is sometimes used as one of its derivatives, either aminophylline (given IV) or choline theophyllinate (as an oral liquid). Note that aminophylline anhydrous contains about 86% theophylline. Optimal clinical use of theophylline compounds can be difficult because of the variable pharmacokinetic parameters, narrow therapeutic index, and many drug interactions, so their use in asthma is declining. However, there is new evidence that low-dose theophylline has useful anti-inflammatory effects and may increase responsiveness to corticosteroids in patients resistant to steroids.

MECHANISMS OF ACTION. Despite their long history and worldwide social and medical use, the mechanism of action of the xanthine derivatives is not well understood. The simple mechanism long held to account for their bronchodilator effect is inhibition of phosphodiesterase (the enzyme that metabolises cAMP), leading to increased intracellular levels of cAMP, smooth muscle relaxation and bronchodilation (see Figures 32-3 and 32-4). The concentrations of theophylline required to inhibit the enzyme in vitro, however, are much greater than therapeutic levels. Other mechanisms proposed include inhibition of cyclic GMP phosphodiesterase, and competitive antagonism of adenosine (which has cardiac-depressant, bronchoconstrictor and platelet-aggregation-suppressant effects) at adenosine receptors. In the treatment of asthma, theophylline derivatives act as bronchodilators, inhibit the late (inflammatory) phase

of asthma and directly stimulate the medullary respiratory centre.

Theophylline is notorious for having very variable pharmacokinetic parameters:
- oral liquids and uncoated tablets of aminophylline and theophylline are rapidly absorbed whereas enteric-coated tablets and sustained-release dosage forms have a delayed and at times an unreliable absorption pattern
- peak level of theophylline is reached in 1–2 hours with the oral solution, immediate-release capsules, or tablets, and in 4–13 hours for sustained-release products
- theophylline's half-life varies with age and with concurrent illness. In premature newborns the half-life is around 30 hours during the first 15 days of life; it is 3.5 hours for children 1–9 years of age, 3–12 hours for the adult non-smoker with uncomplicated asthma, and nearly 10 hours in the elderly
- in patients with acute hepatitis the half-life is 19 hours, with cirrhosis 32 hours, and with hyperthyroidism 4.5 hours
- the theophylline half-life in an adult smoker is only 3–4 hours.

Because of these pharmacokinetic parameters theophylline is a difficult drug clinically and its use is decreasing (see Box 32-1).

Antimuscarinics (Anticholinergics)

Antimuscarinic agents produce bronchodilation by blocking vagal tone and reflexes mediating bronchoconstriction; they may also decrease secretions and make them hard to expectorate. The atropinic drugs ipratropium and tiotropium have useful long-acting bronchodilator actions after inhalation; they are now rarely used in asthma but are useful in COPD.

DRUG MONOGRAPH 32-2
SALBUTAMOL AND TERBUTALINE

INDICATIONS Short-acting β_2-agonist bronchodilators are indicated for symptomatic relief of acute asthma and protection against exercise-induced asthma.

PHARMACOKINETICS Onset of action by inhalation is rapid, within 5–15 minutes, with peak effect within 1–2 hours and duration of action of 3–6 hours. **Salbutamol** is metabolised in the liver and excreted in the kidneys, whereas **terbutaline** is excreted largely unchanged.

DRUG INTERACTIONS Concomitant therapy with other sympathomimetic amines will cause excessive sympathetic stimulation; β-blockers will antagonise the effects of β_2 agonists. Hypokalaemia resulting from β_2-agonist therapy may be potentiated by xanthine derivatives, steroids or diuretics. Antidepressant drugs may potentiate cardiovascular effects.

ADVERSE EFFECTS AND ADVERSE REACTIONS These include tremor, anxiety, restlessness, dizziness, headaches, muscle cramps, palpitations, insomnia, tachycardia and an unusual taste in the mouth. Overdosage symptoms are those of excessive α- or β_1-adrenoceptor stimulation.

PRECAUTIONS Precautions are needed in patients with cardiovascular disease, diabetes or hyperthyroidism. Excessive use of bronchodilator aerosols, or lack of response, may indicate worsening hypoxaemia.

DOSAGE AND ADMINISTRATION The adult bronchodilator dose is 1–2 inhalations (100 mcg salbutamol, 500 mcg terbutaline), with the second inhalation at least 1 minute after the first, then again every 4–6 hours. Parenterally, a subcutaneous dose is administered in acute severe asthma.

BOX 32-1 MANAGING THEOPHYLLINE OVERDOSE

Treatment is supportive and symptomatic because there is no known specific antidote; overdose is potentially fatal.

To decrease drug absorption, administer an activated charcoal preparation orally or via a nasogastric tube. Institute gastric lavage early (within 1 hour of ingestion), or whole-bowel irrigation with a polyethylene glycol and electrolyte solution for very large overdoses of theophylline.

If the patient has seizures, establish an airway and administer oxygen. Diazepam or phenobarbitone IV may be administered to control the seizures.

Charcoal haemoperfusion may be necessary when the theophylline serum concentration is very high (greater than 40 mcg/mL in chronic overdose or if other risk factors are present, e.g. elderly patient, concurrent illnesses). Haemodialysis and peritoneal dialysis are less effective.

Monitor vital signs and provide supportive care as required to maintain circulation, respiration and fluid and electrolyte balance.

---

suppressant effects. Their exact mechanism in asthma is still poorly understood but involves:

- decreased activation of lymphoid cells and eosinophils
- decreased production and action of many cytokines, including interleukins involved in chemotaxis and bronchospasm
- decreased generation of vasodilator prostaglandins
- decreased histamine release from basophils
- decreased production of immunoglobulins IgE and IgG
- (long-term) decreased production of mast cells.

Overall, glucocorticoids reduce both the early and late (proliferative) stages of the inflammatory response. In asthma they have important clinical effects in reducing bronchial mucosal inflammation and bronchial hyperreactivity. They are administered both in treatment of acute severe attacks and prophylactically to reduce and prevent recurrent attacks; however, the airways wall remodelling and collagen deposition in some people with chronic asthma make them relatively resistant to the actions of glucocorticoids.

Daily administration of systemic (oral) corticosteroid therapy provides great therapeutic benefits, but the high incidence of adverse effects led to the use of the alternate-day schedule of treatment. Inhaled corticosteroids are more effective than alternate-day therapy with oral steroids. By chemically modifying the structural arrangement of the steroid molecule, compounds were developed to diminish systemic absorption from the respiratory tract. The products available now are **beclomethasone** (Drug Monograph 32-4), budesonide, fluticasone and ciclesonide. Chronic use of the steroid aerosols has resulted in a decrease in bronchial

---

Many remedies used to treat colds contain drugs with anticholinergic effects; many drugs (e.g. antihistamines, antidepressants) have atropinic adverse effects.

Prophylactic antiasthma drugs

These drugs are collectively known as **preventers**; they include the corticosteroids, mast-cell stabilisers (cromolyns) and newer drugs that prevent inflammatory responses.

Corticosteroids

Corticosteroids are used in chronic asthma to decrease airway obstruction. The adrenal cortex hormones are discussed in detail in Chapter 40; the actions useful in asthma are the glucocorticoid effects, i.e. anti-inflammatory and immuno-

DRUG MONOGRAPH 32-3 THEOPHYLLINE

Theophylline is the prototype of the xanthine derivative bronchodilators. It is most commonly prescribed as controlled-release tablets for treatment of severe asthma and COPD, and to avoid the need for an increase in the dosage of corticosteroids.

PHARMACOKINETICS The rate of absorption and therapeutic effects of theophylline products, especially slow-release products, can vary even if they have the same strength and active ingredient. The different dosage forms do not have proven bioequivalence and so should not be substituted.

Sustained-release (SR) tablets are formulated to optimise absorption: most provide a bioavailability of 100%, with peak levels 4–6 hours after dosage. Absorption is little altered by food. Protein binding is moderate (50%–70%) and theophylline distributes across the placenta (Pregnancy Category A) and into breast milk. Liver metabolism produces various uric acid and xanthine derivatives (some with low activity), which are excreted via the kidneys.

PLASMA LEVELS Theophylline has a narrow therapeutic window: plasma levels (trough concentration) for bronchodilator effects with theophylline are usually stated to be between 10 and 20 mg/L; however, therapeutic responses are variable and close supervision is necessary, with dosage adjustments according to the patient's therapeutic response or the presence of toxic effects. Plasma levels are also monitored if the drug regimen is altered or if there is prolonged fever.

DRUG INTERACTIONS The following effects may occur when xanthine products are given with the drugs listed below; many other drug interactions occur, so reference books should be consulted and therapy monitored closely.

ADVERSE REACTIONS These are related to the other main actions of xanthines (CNS and cardiac stimulation, and diuresis), and include nausea, headache, insomnia, increased anxiety, restlessness, gastric upset, vomiting, gastro-oesophageal reflux and increased urination. Tachycardia and convulsions may appear at high plasma levels (>30 mg/L).

Although the upper therapeutic level is 20 mg/L, theophylline toxicity may occur in some persons at 15 mg/L. Dosage adjustment with theophylline is necessary when concurrent factors affecting therapeutic effects are present (see Box 32-1).

PRECAUTIONS AND CONTRAINDICATIONS Use with caution in patients with fever, active gastritis, peptic ulcer disease or gastro-oesophageal reflux, arrhythmias, hypertension or heart failure. Avoid use in persons with theophylline or ethylenediamine hypersensitivity, heart failure, liver disease, hypothyroidism, sepsis, pulmonary oedema (acute), or convulsive disorders.

DOSAGE AND ADMINISTRATION The dosage of theophylline preparations must be tailored to the medical circumstances in each case. Monitoring is particularly recommended when dose levels exceed 1 g daily in adults or 24 mg/kg in children. The usual efficacy of a theophylline preparation depends on the attainment of a serum concentration of 10–20 mcg/mL ($\equiv$ mg/L; see previous comments on serum levels). Doses are increased gradually over several days while monitoring for adverse effects, e.g. 10 mg/kg/day for 3 days, then 13 mg/kg/day for 3 days, then 16 mg/kg/day for 3 days, at which stage plasma concentration should be measured. Sustained-release tablets are taken every 12 hours; steady state is achieved after about 4 days. SR preparations should never be chewed or crushed.

Drug	Possible effect and management
Phenytoin, and other enzyme inducers	Increased metabolism of xanthines. Decreased absorption of phenytoin with concurrent administration, leading to low plasma levels. Plasma levels of both drugs should be closely monitored, as dosage adjustments may be necessary
Sympathomimetic amines, β-adrenoceptor agonists	Synergistic effects with concurrent use; cardiac arrhythmias may result
Oral contraceptives; cimetidine, fluvoxamine, and quinolone antibiotics, including ciprofloxacin, and macrolides, including erythromycin	May decrease theophylline metabolism, resulting in elevated plasma levels of theophylline and possible toxicity. Monitor closely because dosage adjustments may be necessary
Smoking of tobacco or marijuana	May result in increased metabolism of xanthines, which may result in low plasma theophylline levels. Dosage increases of 50%–100% have been required in smokers
Nicotine replacements, e.g. gum	Smoking cessation may increase the therapeutic effects of the xanthines by decreasing metabolism; however, normalisation of xanthine levels may not occur for 3 months to 2 years after smoking cessation

---

DRUG MONOGRAPH 32-4
BECLOMETHASONE INHALED

INDICATIONS Inhaled corticosteroids are indicated for maintenance treatment and prophylaxis in persistent asthma.

PHARMACOKINETICS A considerable proportion (up to 80%) of an inhaled dose of beclomethasone is likely to be swallowed, then absorbed from the intestinal tract. Peak plasma concentrations are reached 3–5 hours after administration; the drug is subject to metabolism in the liver and excretion in faeces and urine.

ADVERSE DRUG REACTIONS Local adverse effects include dysphasia (changed voice), oropharyngeal candidiasis (oral thrush) and allergic reactions; systemic effects are rare.

DRUG INTERACTIONS None clinically significant; other antiasthma medications may be continued.

WARNINGS AND PRECAUTIONS Oral deposition of drug (and hence oral infections and systemic absorption) can be reduced by use of a spacer (see Figure 31-2) and by rinsing the mouth and throat after each dose. Correct inhaler technique is important. The drug is not useful for acute asthma attacks, as it is not a bronchodilator. If prescribed with an inhaled bronchodilator, the β_2 agonist or antimuscarinic should be inhaled (to open the airways) before the corticosteroid. Dosage should not be reduced or stopped unless advised.

CONTRAINDICATIONS Hypersensitivity to any ingredient.

DOSAGE AND ADMINISTRATION Dosage starts at levels likely to be effective, then is reduced to the minimum dose that controls symptoms and then is 'stepped down' by 25% every 3 months if possible. Dosage may be doubled if asthma worsens or respiratory tract infection occurs. Typical adult dosage is 50–400 mcg twice daily to a maximum of 800 mcg/day, but may be up to 2000 mcg daily in severe persistent asthma.

DRUG MONOGRAPH 32-5
ZAFIRLUKAST

INDICATIONS Leukotriene-receptor antagonists are indicated for the treatment and/or prophylaxis of chronic asthma; they may allow a reduction in dosage of inhaled corticosteroid.

PHARMACOKINETICS Administered orally, the drug is rapidly absorbed and highly bound to plasma proteins. Improvement in asthma symptoms should be noted within a few days. Zafirlukast is metabolised in the liver and excreted primarily in faeces.

DRUG INTERACTIONS Leukotriene-receptor antagonists may be given with other antiasthma medications. Concurrent administration of theophylline may result in a higher serum level of theophylline or a lower level of zafirlukast. Monitor serum levels closely. Zafirlukast inhibits some drug-metabolising enzymes and interacts with many drugs metabolised by the same enzyme systems.

ADVERSE EFFECTS AND ADVERSE REACTIONS The leukotriene-receptor antagonists appear to be well tolerated. Adverse effects include headache, nausea and abdominal upset or pain.

WARNINGS AND CONTRAINDICATIONS These drugs are not indicated for reversal of bronchospasm in acute asthma attacks. Use zafirlukast with caution in patients with alcoholism. Avoid use in persons with hypersensitivity to the drugs or in those with liver function impairment, and in pregnant or breastfeeding women.

DOSAGE AND ADMINISTRATION The dose for adults and children >12 years is 20 mg orally twice a day to a maximum of 40 mg twice daily.

---

theophylline cannot adequately control asthma. In emergencies, corticosteroids may be administered parenterally (e.g. IV hydrocortisone, dexamethasone). Daily doses above 10 mg oral prednisolone or 1–1.5 mg inhaled beclomethasone can cause systemic adverse effects, including adrenal suppression and growth suppression; altered deposition of muscle, fat, skin, hair and bone; ocular changes, infections, mineralocorticoid effects and psychological disturbances (see Chapter 40).

Appreciation of the great value of prophylactic use of inhaled corticosteroids in preventing the late-phase inflammatory response and decreasing bronchial hyperreactivity has recently revolutionised management of asthma. As a prototype drug, beclomethasone given by MDI is considered in detail (Drug Monograph 32-4). Budesonide is available via both MDI and nebuliser. The more recent fluticasone

hyperreactivity and symptoms. The maximum improvement in pulmonary function may take 1–4 weeks. Frequent use of inhaled corticosteroids, however, leads to a dose-related decrease in bone mineral density (BMD), with the increased risk of osteoporosis, so postmenopausal women taking inhaled steroids are advised to have their BMD monitored every 2 years.

Systemic corticosteroids are still used, e.g. short courses of prednisolone given orally when inhaled medications (corticosteroids, β_2 agonists, antimuscarinics) and oral

and ciclesonide may be less likely to cause systemic adverse effects.

COMBINATION THERAPY

A combined inhaler containing both salmeterol (a long-acting β_2-agonist symptom controller) and fluticasone (a corticosteroid preventer) became available in mid-2000 (Seretide). The combination is indicated for regular treatment of asthma when use of both drugs is appropriate, not for relief of acute symptoms. The pharmacokinetic parameters of each drug appear to be unaffected by coadministration, and the adverse reactions, precautions and interactions are as for each component drug. A similar new combination inhaler contains budesonide with eformoterol. The advantages are: convenience of using only one inhaler, cost advantage, better control of asthma, and regular use of a low-dose steroid.

Leukotriene-receptor antagonists

The first two drugs released in the newer category of **leukotriene-receptor antagonists** are montelukast and zafirlukast (Drug Monograph 32-5). These drugs block receptors for the leukotrienes (C_4, D_4 and E_4; Figure 32-3), which are components of slow-reacting substance of anaphylaxis (SRS-A), thought to be a mediator of inflammation in both early and late phases of asthma. These drugs can therefore reduce the inflammation, mucus secretion and bronchoconstriction associated with asthma. As this drug group is relatively new, clinical experience is not yet extensive; they are useful as 'add-on' therapy for patients inadequately controlled with inhaled corticosteroids.

5-lipoxygenase inhibitors

A new group of drugs under clinical trial act by inhibition of the enzyme 5-lipoxygenase, thus preventing synthesis of the leukotrienes from arachidonic acid. This mechanism is analogous to the inhibition of cyclo-oxygenase by non-steroidal anti-inflammatory drugs, preventing the synthesis of prostaglandins. Zileuton (the first of these drugs approved in the USA) thus interferes with the formation of leukotrienes that cause mucus plugs and constriction of bronchial airways. The late inflammatory response is also impaired; and similar drugs are being tested in prevention of cancer.

Mast-cell stabilisers (cromolyns)

Cromoglycate and nedocromil (Drug Monograph 32-6) are examples of **cromolyns** or **mast-cell stabilisers**,* anti-inflammatory agents that inhibit the release of histamine,

DRUG MONOGRAPH 32-6
CROMOGLYCATE AND NEDOCROMIL

INDICATIONS Cromoglycate and nedocromil are indicated for maintenance treatment in persistent asthma and for prevention of exercise-induced asthma. They can also prevent bronchospasm if given up to 30 minutes before exposure to allergens or exercise. In children, they are safer than inhaled corticosteroids. They are also indicated as prophylactic therapy against allergic rhinitis (by nasal spray) and allergic conjunctivitis (by eye-drops).

PHARMACOKINETICS The drugs have very low lipid solubility, and so are not absorbed orally. Administered by oral inhalation, only about 10% is absorbed in the lungs, and is excreted in the kidneys and bile. The onset of action is within 2–4 weeks.

ADVERSE REACTIONS These include cough, throat irritation, transient bronchospasm and GIT symptoms; adverse reactions are rare.

WARNINGS AND CONTRAINDICATIONS These drugs are not bronchodilators and should not be used in acute asthma. They are used prophylactically, and dosage should not be reduced unless advised. Avoid use in persons with hypersensitivity to the drug.

DOSAGE AND ADMINISTRATION The adult and child (≥ 5 years) oral inhalation dose of cromoglycate for prevention of asthma is 2–4 inhalations 4 times a day (8–80 mg/day). The dose for nedocromil is 2 inhalations 4 times a day (16 mg/day).

leukotrienes and other mediators of inflammation from mast cells, macrophages and other cells associated with asthma. The mechanism is not clear: they are said to stabilise mast cells but may also act by blocking chloride channels, suppressing activation of sensory nerves, desensitising neuronal reflexes and inhibiting release of cytokines. (Cromoglycate is also known as cromolyn sodium and as [di]sodium cromoglycate.) Inhaled before an attack, the overall effect of these drugs is to inhibit bronchoconstriction and reduce bronchial hyperreactivity. Neither drug has any bronchodilator effect, nor do they have any effect on any inflammatory mediators already released in the body.

Mast cell activation is also reduced by the new drug omalizumab, a recombinant human monoclonal antibody

---

*This group of drugs is sometimes referred to as inhaled non-steroidal anti-inflammatory drugs; however, this terminology is confusing, as it implies inhalation of aspirin-like NSAIDs. The collective terms 'cromolyns' and 'cromones' have also been coined.

that complexes with free IgE antigens to prevent their binding to mast cells. The drug has a slow onset and long duration of action after SC injection; it effectively reduces IgE concentrations and asthma symptoms in patients with allergic asthma, allowing reduction or cessation of steroid dosage.

New drugs for asthma

New drugs are constantly being developed and tested for use in asthma, particularly as more details of the actions of mediators of the inflammatory response are determined. Some currently in development include antagonists of cytokines (e.g. anti-interleukin-5 agents), antagonists of cell adhesion molecules, antagonists of platelet activating factor (disappointing thus far), neurokinin-receptor antagonists, and the antigout drug colchicine, which decreases the late-phase inflammatory response.

Overview of asthma management

Despite the availability of several groups of drugs for the treatment of asthma, many of which date back thousands of years, it is recognised that asthma therapy is frequently not optimal, and there is still an unacceptably high level of mortality and morbidity from asthma (see Clinical Interest Box 32-3). Possible reasons suggested for unsuccessful therapy include:

- overreliance on short-acting bronchodilator relievers
- underuse of inhaled corticosteroid preventers
- lack of objective measurements of severity of asthma
- inadequate monitoring of therapy and compliance.

In recent years, guidelines have been prepared and published by groups of specialist physicians (e.g. the Australian National Asthma Campaign, Therapeutic Guidelines: Respiratory Expert Group, the British Thoracic Society, and the Cochrane Airways Group) to encourage accurate and appropriate evidence-based treatment. The basis for the guidelines is stepwise management, with treatment stepped up as necessary to achieve good control of symptoms, and cautious stepping down after review of therapy. An example of the stepwise approach for management of adult asthma is shown in Figure 32-5.

Similar stepwise guidelines are available for childhood asthma, home management of acute asthma, and asthma in accident and emergency departments. Acute asthma is a life-threatening situation and may require systemic corticosteroids, adrenaline and aminophylline, oxygen, nebulised bronchodilators and close monitoring of lung function, blood gases and CNS function.

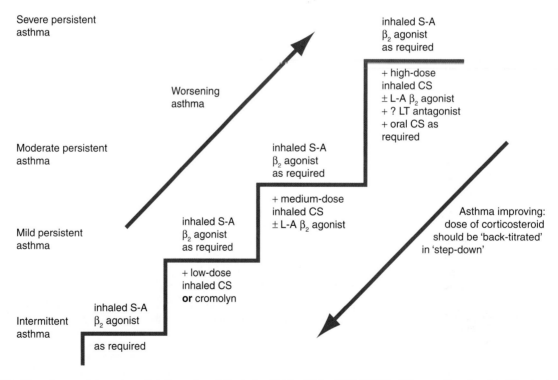

FIGURE 32-5 Stepwise maintenance of asthma in adults (after Table 19-1, AMH 2005). CS = corticosteroid; LT = leukotriene; L-A = long-acting; S-A = short-acting. Persistent: >3–4 attacks/week; moderate: asthma not controlled by low-dose inhaled CS + β_2 agonist.

Before treatment of chronic asthma begins, severity needs to be assessed and classified, and trigger factors identified and managed. Treatment is tailored to suit the patient and the severity. Inhaled corticosteroids are started at a dose sufficient to be effective, as monitored by peak-flow meter readings, then reduced to the minimum required to maintain control. Antibacterials are reserved for specific infections, antihistamines are rarely useful, and sedatives are contraindicated because of agitation from dyspnoea (Clinical Interest Box 32-6 includes a summary of drugs used in asthma).

Asthma action plans

Individualised written action plans are devised for each patient, including education and self-management aspects so that patients know how to recognise their own symptoms, start and step-up treatment, and promptly reach medical attention. Action plans may need to take into account factors such as closeness to hospital help, as rural patients may face added risk factors (isolation, lack of support networks, and seasonal high levels of environmental allergens).

A six-point action plan (proposed by several Australian and New Zealand groups through the National Asthma Campaign) advises carers to:
- assess the severity of the condition
- achieve best lung function (regularly monitor FEV_1)
- identify and avoid trigger factors
- optimise patients' medication programs (minimise the number of drugs, doses and adverse effects)
- develop an action plan
- educate the patient, and review lung function, compliance and inhaler technique regularly.

Special plans are developed for exercise-induced asthma, athletes, infants, the elderly, travellers, occupational asthma and for asthma in pregnancy (good asthma control is the priority, to maintain the health of the mother and fetus).

Patient information sheets help educate the patient and optimise therapy (see sample plan in Respiratory Expert Group 2005).

The Australian 'GP Asthma Initiative' promotes the 'Asthma 3+ Visit Plan' as the best-practice model for managing asthma. The plan involves at least three visits from a patient to a general practitioner (GP) over a short period (4 months) to improve the management of asthma. The visits incorporate diagnosis, assessment, and development and later reviews of a written asthma management plan. Brochures, proforma plans, guides and resources are made available to both GP and patient (see www.health.gov.au under keywords 'asthma 3+ visit plan').

DRUG TREATMENT OF CHRONIC OBSTRUCTIVE PULMONARY DISEASE (COPD)

COPD, also known as chronic obstructive airways disease (COAD) and as chronic airways limitation (CAL), is a disorder characterised by airflow obstruction that is not fully reversible. COPD is often associated with cough, emphysema, airway damage, excessive mucus and sputum production, and recurrent respiratory infections, so drugs used in respiratory tract infections are often indicated (see later).

COPD includes the three important disorders chronic bronchitis, emphysema, and chronic asthma with fixed airflow obstruction. Asthma (characterised by *reversible* airways narrowing) can coexist with COPD. COPD typically affects middle-aged and older people. Cigarette smoking is the major aetiological factor, and stopping smoking is the

---

CLINICAL INTEREST BOX 32-6 THERAPEUTIC TIPS FOR ASTHMA

- **Relievers:** Short-acting β_2-agonist drugs such as salbutamol and terbutaline provide the most rapid **relief** of acute asthma symptoms. These drugs have no anti-inflammatory effects but are very effective by inhalation in the treatment of acute bronchospasm. Subcutaneous injection is reserved for persons with a very severe dyspnoea that prevents them from responding to inhalation therapy.
- **Controllers:** Long-acting β_2-agonist drugs are administered by inhalation for symptom **control**.
- **Preventers:** Corticosteroid inhalation products such as beclomethasone are used as **preventive** therapy, to reduce inflammation and bronchial hyperreactivity; systemic adverse effects can occur.
- Theophylline is a bronchodilator used orally in severe

airways obstruction; pharmacokinetic variability means that patients require careful monitoring.
- Ipratropium may provide added bronchodilator effect in severe asthma. Leukotriene antagonists are being introduced to prevent inflammatory responses.
- Cromolyns (mast-cell stabilisers) decrease airway hyperreactivity; they have no bronchodilator effect and thus cannot be used for the treatment of acute asthma.
- Patients need to be taught about the proper techniques for use of an MDI and other inhaling devices as ordered. Spacer units are often suggested for young children and, at times, other patients also benefit from their use. Home use of peak-flow meters is also often recommended for early detection of airflow obstruction.

CLINICAL INTEREST BOX 32-7 SMOKING

Cigarette smoke is an aerosol, consisting of tarry particles suspended in a complex mixture of organic and inorganic gases, containing more than 4000 different known chemicals.

The gas phase (smoke) from burning cigarettes contains carbon monoxide, hydrogen cyanide, oxides of nitrogen, ammonia, volatile aldehydes, and vapours including benzene, acetone, acrolein and vinyl chloride.

The particulate phase of cigarette smoke contains nicotine (about 0.2–3.5 mg) plus many other potentially toxic chemicals including tar, metals, and carcinogenic hydrocarbons such as benzpyrene and nitrosamines.

The decreased respiratory efficiency of smokers is attributed to toxic effects of nicotine (causing broncho-constriction), carbon monoxide (reducing oxygen-carrying capacity of haemoglobin) and irritants (increasing mucus secretion and destroying cilia and alveolar sacs).

Many components of smoke are free radical species, some highly stable, including reactive oxygen and nitrogen species. These are responsible for much of the damage produced by smoking, including lipid peroxidation, lung damage and COPD.
(See also Chapter 22, section on tobacco and nicotine.)

only measure that slows progression of COPD. Inherited conditions such as deficiency of the α_1-antitrypsin enzyme predispose to alveolar collapse and exacerbate problems caused by smoking. Dyspnoea (difficult, laboured breathing) develops insidiously over many years and the FEV_1 is typically reduced to less than 70% of the forced vital capacity. Cardiac disease and disordered breathing during sleep are also common with COPD and need to be effectively treated.

Drug therapy of COPD

Drugs used in COPD and in acute exacerbations include:
• bronchodilators (by puffer with a spacer), especially long-acting drugs such as salmeterol and tiotropium
• oxygen therapy
• corticosteroids (short oral course if there is associated asthma)
• antibiotics (specific to the current pathogen)
• mucolytic agents
• annual influenza vaccination.

All these drug groups are considered in other sections. Respiratory rehabilitation, exercise programs and weight reduction are also effective and improve quality of life. Severe disease unresponsive to treatment may require lung transplantation.

However, the most important measure to improve COPD is smoking cessation. Smoking is described as 'the largest single preventable cause of death and disability

in Australia' (Respiratory Expert Group 2005). Smoking causes respiratory disease, particularly lung cancer, and increases the risks of cardiovascular, cerebrovascular and peripheral vascular diseases (see Clinical Interest Box 32-7). 'Quit Smoking' programs involve assessing dependency, education, support, monitoring of compliance, complementary therapies and pharmacological assistance with antidepressants and nicotine replacement therapy as patches, gum or inhaler. (The pharmacological effects of nicotine are discussed in Chapter 11, and the social use and abuse of nicotine in Chapter 22.)

DRUGS USED IN RESPIRATORY TRACT INFECTIONS

Drugs affecting cough
'Cough mixtures'

Cough is a protective reflex by which a sudden blast of compressed air from the bronchial tubes expels irritating, infective or obstructive material. The newly described 'cough receptors' are sensory nerves (part of the vagal afferents) with terminals in airway walls, which are activated by various stimuli including chemical irritants, inflammatory mediators, intraluminal material and mechanical stimulation to airway epithelium. Common causes of cough are pollutants including cigarette smoke, upper respiratory tract infections, asthma, COPD and gastro-oesophageal reflux.

While cough is a symptom common to most respiratory tract infections, it may also occur in more serious disorders such as bronchiectasis, asthma, lung cancer, gastro-oesophageal reflux or heart failure, also as an adverse effect of drug therapy (e.g. with ACE inhibitors) or of smoking. Such underlying disorders should be treated, rather than simply suppressing the cough with an antitussive (cough suppressant).

As well as a cough suppressant, 'cough mixtures' may include (with varying degrees of efficacy):
• expectorants and mucolytics (see earlier in this chapter)
• antihistamines
• antimuscarinics
• antipyretic analgesics
• sympathomimetic decongestants
• demulcent (soothing) liquids, flavouring and sweetening agents.

The combination of an antitussive (cough suppressant) and an expectorant (cough stimulant) in a cough mixture is illogical and should be avoided. If there is a component of bronchial hyperreactivity to the cough, an inhaled cromolyn

DRUG MONOGRAPH 32-7
CODEINE, DEXTROMETHORPHAN AND PHOLCODINE

INDICATIONS The opioid cough suppressants, such as codeine, are indicated for the symptomatic treatment of non-productive cough by their depressant actions on the medullary cough centre. They are generally formulated as oral liquids known as linctuses or 'cough mixtures'.

PHARMACOKINETICS After oral administration, the onset of action is rapid, with duration of action of 6–8 hours. Codeine is metabolised to morphine and norcodeine, and the metabolites are excreted by the kidneys.

DRUG INTERACTIONS Opioids interact with other CNS depressants, including antihistamines and alcohol, and concurrent use should be avoided.

ADVERSE REACTIONS These include drowsiness, respiratory depression, nausea and vomiting, and consti-pation. Adverse effects in the CNS, including dependence and withdrawal, are more likely with codeine. Excessive constipation tends to limit the use of codeine.

WARNINGS AND CONTRAINDICATIONS Patients should be warned of the risk of drowsiness and should not drive or operate machinery if affected. Avoid use in respiratory failure or asthma, in children under 2 years, or if the patient has a productive cough.

DOSAGE AND ADMINISTRATION The dosage of codeine for adults is 15–30 mg 4 times daily. (For com-parison, the analgesic dose of codeine in a Panadeine Forte tablet is 30 mg codeine phosphate.) Dosage should be reduced in renal or hepatic impairment and in the elderly.

CLINICAL INTEREST BOX 32-8
COMPLEMENTARY AND ALTERNATIVE THERAPIES IN RESPIRATORY DISORDERS

There are good pharmacological rationales for many of the traditional and complementary and alternative medi-cine (CAM) treatments for asthma: recommended herbal mixtures in chicken broth, garlic and horseradish contain several anti-allergy sulfur compounds and have a moisten-ing action on the airways; coffee and tea contain xanthine bronchodilators; saltpetre (potassium nitrate) is a smooth muscle relaxant; traditional Chinese medicine advocates the herb *Ephedra sinica* (ma huang), from which the broncho-dilator drug ephedrine was developed; and New Zealand green-lipped mussel has anti-inflammatory actions.

Many Australian native plants have long been used by indigenous people in symptomatic treatment of cough and respiratory tract congestion, either by inhalation or drinking a decoction (tea) containing aromatic or essential plant oils. The active ingredients are cineoles, which have mucolytic and decongestant properties. These are present in eucalypt species, especially the Tasmanian blue gum (*Eucalyptus globulus*), and in the liniment tree (*Melaleuca symphocarpa*), old man weed or common sneezeweed (*Centipeda cunninghamii*), lemon grasses (*Cymbopogon*) and river mint (*Mentha australis*). For treatment of breath-lessness and asthma, decoctions of the Queensland asthma plant (*Euphorbia hirta*) and the frangipani chain fruit (*Alyxia spicata*) have been used for their antispasmodic and antihistaminic-like properties.

Other CAM methods claimed to have benefit in asthma include:
- dietary methods: avoidance of allergenic foods, supplementation with fish oils, vitamin C, magnesium, selenium or zinc
- various Chinese, Japanese, Indian and Native American herbs, some of which may have steroidal components with anti-inflammatory activities
- homeopathic mixtures of botanical extracts at extremely low concentrations
- mind–body techniques, including meditation and biofeedback.

Echinacea extracts are the best-sellers in the herbal industry, particularly for treatment of coughs and colds, other upper respiratory tract infections and some inflammatory conditions. Clinical trials suggest that echinacea extracts are sometimes useful in reducing the duration and severity of symptoms, possibly by stimulating phagocyte activity in the non-specific immune system.

Volatile scented oils, discussed previously under Expectorants, are present in many cough and cold 'cures', and are sold in many alternative therapy outlets; they may also be present in proprietary elixirs. They may be inhaled in mists or sprays or vaporised over a candle. One popular OTC ointment, Vicks Vaporub, formulated to be applied topically to the chest or inhaled via steam, contains oils of menthol, camphor, thymol, eucalyptus, turpentine, nutmeg and cedarleaf.

Adapted from: Spencer & Jacobs 1999; Percival 2000; Braun & Cohen 2005.

---

or inhaled corticosteroid (e.g. beclomethasone) may be effective, as in asthma. There is little evidence of any efficacy greater than placebo for OTC cough preparations in children with acute cough.

Cough suppressants

Prescribing of **cough suppressants** is usually reserved for a non-productive (dry, hacking) cough that is inadequately controlled or unresponsive to OTC medications. Treatment of cough is secondary to treatment of the underlying disorder, i.e. the therapeutic objective is to decrease the intensity and frequency of the cough yet permit adequate elimination of tracheobronchial secretions and exudates. For example, cough secondary to gastro-oesophageal reflux may be reduced with histamine H_2-receptor antagonists and proton pump inhibitors.

OPIOID ANTITUSSIVE DRUGS

Opiates such as morphine potently suppress the cough reflex by direct depression of the medullary cough centre, a mechanism unrelated to their analgesic or respiratory depressant actions. Their clinical usefulness as antitussives, however, is limited by adverse effects. They also inhibit the ciliary activity of the respiratory mucous membrane, may cause bronchial constriction in patients with allergies or asthma, and cause drug dependence. Codeine, dextromethorphan and pholcodine (Drug Monograph 32-7) exhibit less pronounced antitussive effects than morphine but they also have fewer adverse effects. They are widely used and many products containing them are available over the counter. (See also Chapters 16 and 22.)

Treatment of colds and influenza
Upper respiratory tract infections

Most upper respiratory tract infections (URTIs) are caused by viruses, for which there are no safe, specific antiviral chemotherapeutic agents available. The recommended treatment is therefore usually symptomatic, as for the common cold.

Viral infections are notorious for lowering the body's immune defences and predisposing the patient to subsequent secondary bacterial infections, which may be dangerous in patients with other chronic conditions such as asthma, COPD or rheumatic heart disease. Such patients are often prescribed antibiotics appropriate for the specific infecting bacteria, following advice in the current *Antibiotic Guidelines* (Antibiotic Expert Group, 2003). For example, for *Streptococcus pyogenes* pharyngitis ('strep sore throat'), phenoxymethylpenicillin or roxithromycin are recommended and, for acute bacterial sinusitis, amoxycillin or doxycycline.

COMMON COLD (CORYZA)

The viruses most commonly responsible for the common cold are a group of RNA rhinoviruses, which are spread by contact and by droplets, often via the conjunctiva. The virus multiplies mainly in the cells lining the nostrils, and causes inflammation of the nose and throat, hence the common symptoms of redness and watery secretions of the nose, eyes and throat (see Table 32-1).

Development of vaccines against the common cold has been largely unsuccessful because of the many different and varying antigenic types of rhinoviruses. As there are no simple antiviral drugs effective against the cold virus, the Australian National Prescribing Service has mounted a campaign to discourage patients (and parents) from expecting to be prescribed antibiotics for colds; the punch-line is 'Antibiotics won't help a common cold; common sense will' (see www.gottacold.com). Treatment of the common cold is thus mainly symptomatic, with decongestants, antiseptics, expectorants,

---

> ### DRUG MONOGRAPH 32-8
> ### PSEUDOEPHEDRINE
>
> **Pseudoephedrine**, oxymetazoline and phenylephrine are sympathomimetic amines commonly administered as nasal sprays, cough mixtures, capsules or tablets and as eye-drops. Tolerance can occur rapidly to their α-receptor-mediated vasoconstrictor actions.
>
> **INDICATIONS** Decongestants are indicated for symptomatic relief of acute rhinitis caused by rhinoviruses and for treatment of red eyes.
>
> **PHARMACOKINETICS** Topically applied vasoconstrictors act rapidly, e.g. in the eyes or nose. If taken orally as tablets, pseudoephedrine is rapidly absorbed, and excreted largely unchanged, with a half-life dependent on urine pH (2–12 hours).
>
> **ADVERSE REACTIONS AND DRUG INTERACTIONS** Systemic sympathomimetic effects can occur, so pseudoephedrine should not be taken by patients with hypertension. Sympathomimetics should not be used by patients taking MAOIs, because of potentiation of effects.
>
> **WARNINGS AND CONTRAINDICATIONS** Patients should be advised that prolonged use of nasal vasoconstrictor sprays can cause rebound nasal congestion, and also that the drug may become less effective because of the development of tolerance— it is not simply that a cold is becoming worse. Sympathomimetics are contraindicated in hypertension and in concurrent use with MAOIs.
>
> **DOSAGE AND ADMINISTRATION** Pseudoephedrine is present in many 'cold cures'* and is commonly taken as tablets, e.g. Sudafed, containing a 60 mg dose. Nasal sprays are described in the later section on drugs affecting the nose.
>
> *This drug became infamous during the Sydney 2000 Olympic Games, when a gymnastics gold-medallist was disqualified for having taken pseudoephedrine, a stimulant, in a 'cold cure' medicine.

---

aspirin-like antipyretic analgesics and rest. Antihistamines, whisky or brandy and 'hot toddies' have no proven efficacy in colds, other than as sedatives or placebos. See Clinical Interest Box 32-8 for complementary and alternative therapies in respiratory disorders.

Vitamin C has long been recommended for the common cold, sometimes in massive doses (>1 g/day). Meta-analyses of trials of the effects of vitamin C overall indicate that vitamin C has no preventive effect in well-nourished persons,

TABLE 32-1 Colds, allergic rhinitis and influenza

AETIOLOGY, SIGNS AND SYMPTOMS	COMMON COLD	ALLERGIC RHINITIS	INFLUENZA
Causative factors	Usually viruses	Usually allergens	Usually viruses
Occurrence	Any time	Usually seasonal	Any time
Fever	Rare	Absent	Common: sudden onset
Aches and pains	Slight	Absent	May be severe
Sneezing	Usual	Common	Infrequent
Pruritus (itching)	Absent or rare	Common	Absent
Cough	Mild to moderate	Uncommon	Common
Headaches	Rare	Can occur	Prominent
Complications	Sinus congestion, earache	Uncommon	Bronchitis, pneumonia

DRUG MONOGRAPH 32-9 INFLUENZA VACCINE

Influenza vaccines are prepared from viral cultures that have been inactivated, purified and preserved.

INDICATIONS Administration of the current vaccine before winter induces antibodies against viral surface antigens and proteins, and provides protection against infection. Current Australian National Health and Medical Research Council recommendations are that the following groups be vaccinated annually:
- individuals over 65 years of age
- Aboriginal and Torres Strait Islander people over 50 years
- adults and children over 6 months with chronic debilitating diseases, including severe asthma and diabetes mellitus
- children with congenital heart disease or cystic fibrosis

- adults and children on immunosuppressant therapy
- residents of chronic care facilities.

ADVERSE REACTIONS Mild localised reactions, fever and malaise have been reported; very rarely, neurological reactions occur.

WARNINGS AND CONTRAINDICATIONS The vaccine is contraindicated during acute febrile illnesses, in persons with allergies to neomycin, polymyxin or gentamicin, and in those with allergies to egg proteins (as the virus vaccine is prepared in hen eggs).

DOSAGE AND ADMINISTRATION One or two doses are administered by deep SC injection.

but may slightly decrease the duration of colds and may lower the incidence of colds in people with low dietary vitamin C intake and those predisposed to respiratory tract infections.

DECONGESTANTS

Vasoconstriction in mucous membranes, leading to decongestion, may be achieved by the topical application of sympathomimetic amine **decongestants** such as **phenylephrine** (Drug Monograph 32-8), which stimulate α_1-adrenoceptors. This is the main clinical use of such drugs, which if administered systemically would cause generalised sympathetic effects, including hypertension and smooth muscle contraction (see Chapter 12). Decongestion may also be achieved by blocking muscarinic receptors, which mediate increased respiratory secretions, with atropinic drugs such as ipratropium.

INFLUENZA

Influenza is a common respiratory viral infection occurring during most winters, sporadically or in epidemics. Systemic symptoms of headache, myalgia, fever and chills occur 1–2 days before the respiratory symptoms (sore throat, cough, nasal obstruction). In an influenza epidemic, the incidence in crowded groups can reach as high as 70%, and mortality due to secondary bacterial infection is high among elderly and predisposed patients.

VACCINATION.   As with the rhinoviruses that cause the common cold, the influenza virus shows great antigenic variation, with frequent mutations. **Influenza vaccine** (Drug Monograph 32-9) for active immunisation must be prepared regularly against strains currently in circulation. To a certain extent, those of us living in the Southern Hemisphere are fortunate in that influenza strains cause flu epidemics in our southern winter 6 months after their appearance in the Northern Hemisphere, so vaccines can usually be prepared in time (see Clinical Interest Box 32-9). Vaccines are manufactured to conform with annual requirements of the Australian Influenza Vaccine Committee and the New Zealand Ministry of Health.

AMANTADINE. Amantadine is an antiviral drug that specifically inhibits the replication of the A2 (Asian) strain influenza virus. The dose is 100 mg orally twice daily for treatment in high-risk individuals and also prophylactically until 10 days after vaccination. There are many potential adverse drug reactions and precautions relating to the use of this drug, and dosage schedules are complicated, especially in the elderly and in renal failure.

Interestingly, amantadine is also used as an anti-parkinsonian agent, as it appears to have indirect dopamine-receptor agonist actions. Overdosage symptoms include neuromuscular disturbances and symptoms of acute psychosis.

NEURAMINIDASE INHIBITORS. Zanamivir and oseltamivir are new drugs for treating infections due to influenza viruses A and B (see Drug Monograph 32-10 and Clinical Interest Box 4-5).

Other respiratory tract infections
PNEUMONIA

Pneumonia is a condition of inflammation of the lower respiratory passages (bronchioles) and alveoli arising from infections, irritation or toxic material. The clinical features include fever and chills, shortness of breath and coughing of green or blood-stained sputum. It is most common at the extremes of life and is frequently the specified cause of death in frail elderly persons. Other significant risk factors include underlying cardiorespiratory disorders and immuno-deficiency states. A wide variety of pathogenic organisms may be involved. Community-acquired pneumonia is most commonly caused by *Streptococcus pneumoniae* and there is often occupational exposure, e.g. *Mycoplasma pneumoniae* in health-care institutions and *Legionella pneumophila* from air-conditioning systems. Pneumococcal vaccines are available, and are recommended for elderly people and those who are immunocompromised or at particular risk of contracting pneumococcal pneumonia.

Management is designed to preserve life and maintain lung function. It may entail resuscitative methods, drug therapy, postural drainage and physiotherapy, monitoring of blood gases and radiographic changes, and detection of associated lung diseases and complications.

Antimicrobial therapy depends on identifying the pathogenic organisms (usually bacteria), and careful selection of the appropriate antibiotics; for example, *Antibiotic Guidelines* recommends oral amoxycillin plus roxithromycin or doxycycline for mild community-acquired pneumonia, whereas severe pneumonia infections with *Legionella* species (Legionnaire's disease) require parenteral gentamicin plus erythromycin IV or ciprofloxacin IV.

The spectrum of potential pathogens causing hospital-acquired pneumonia differs from that in the community, and ill patients are often immunocompromised, so recommendations for antibiotic therapy vary. Organisms are emerging with significant levels of resistance to antibiotics, so current prescribing guidelines must be followed rigorously.

TUBERCULOSIS (TB)

Infection with *Mycobacterium tuberculosis* may be clinically manifest primarily in the lungs or in other organs, including lymph nodes, skin or bones. Pulmonary TB is the commonest form (around 75%); it is infectious and is a notifiable disease in Australia. It is estimated that one-third of the world's

---

DRUG MONOGRAPH 32-10   ZANAMIVIR (RELENZA)

Zanamivir is a new Australian-developed drug, introduced in 1999 (see Clinical Interest Box 4-5), which alleviates and reduces the duration of symptoms of influenza virus A and B infection. The mechanism of action of zanamivir is via selective inhibition of the viral surface enzyme neuraminidase; the effect is to inhibit replication and shedding of virus from respiratory epithelium. The drug is administered by oral inhalation of dry powder, twice daily for 5 days. It reduces the time to alleviation of symptoms by about 2.5 days. A similar drug, oseltamivir, can be taken orally.

INDICATIONS Zanamivir is indicated for treatment of influenza A and B viral infections in children 5 years and over and in adults. It can be used prophylactically (1 inhalation/day), but annual flu vaccination is recommended.

PHARMACOKINETICS After oral inhalation of the powder, the drug is distributed widely in the oropharynx and lung, with 10%–20% being absorbed systemically. It is excreted unchanged in the urine, with a half-life of 2.5–5 hours after oral inhalation.

ADVERSE REACTIONS AND DRUG INTERACTIONS Zanamivir appears to be well tolerated, with no more adverse drug reactions or drug interactions than placebo. Because of the short period over which zanamivir has been available for clinical use, clinical experience in children or the elderly is limited.

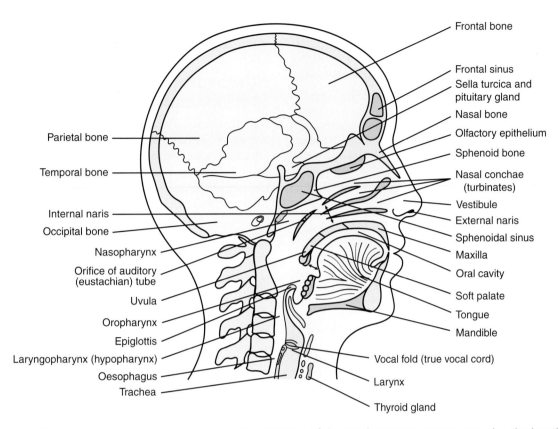

FIGURE 32-6 Sagittal section of head and neck showing the locations of the respiratory structures; note also the location of the pituitary gland, cradled in the sella turcica above the sphenoidal sinus. The sinuses are small cavities in the bones, that are open to the nasal cavity.

population is infected with TB; in Australia there are about 1100 new cases per year.

Because many strains of the causative organism have developed resistance to previously effective antibiotics, multi-drug regimens are necessary in all cases for several months. Pretreatment screening (visual acuity, renal function, liver function) is essential and compliance and treatment must be monitored. Standard short-course therapy consists of combination chemotherapy, with rifampicin, isoniazid and ethambutol. Regimens with daily, twice-weekly or thrice-weekly doses for 2–6 months have been devised, leading to cure in about 98% of cases.

CROUP

Croup is an acute syndrome of hoarse voice, barking cough and noisy breathing usually occurring at night. It is one of the more common respiratory tract infections of childhood. Most cases have a viral aetiology. Steroids, either systemic or inhaled, are effective in reducing symptoms of airway obstruction and respiratory distress and also reduce time spent in hospital.

DRUGS AFFECTING THE NOSE

While drugs administered by inhalation are commonly inhaled through the mouth, e.g. bronchodilators in treatment of asthma, they may also be administered by nasal inhalation for local effects (e.g. vasoconstrictors for decongestion), for systemic effects (e.g. inhaled general anaesthetic gases) and for effects on closely located tissues (e.g. desmopressin nasal spray for effects on the pituitary gland; see Figure 32-6 and Chapter 38).

Rhinitis and nasal obstruction

Obstruction to free air flow in the nose occurs very commonly as a feature of the common cold. It is due to rhinitis, or inflammation of the mucous membrane lining the nose. Overactivity of the mucus glands causes excessive mucus production and a watery discharge (rhinorrhoea, 'runny nose'). The condition may be due to viral infection, impaired nervous system control of blood vessels in the membrane (vasomotor rhinitis), hypersensitivity reactions (allergic rhinitis), hypertrophic or atrophic changes, drug adverse effects, or dietary factors.

Allergic rhinitis, or 'hay fever', is an atopic disorder (Type 1 hypersensitivity reaction) mediated by IgE antibodies. Sensitised mast cells and basophils release autacoids, including histamine, serotonin, prostaglandins and leukotrienes, which mediate the inflammatory and immune responses. The prevalence of allergic rhinitis is highest in children and young adults (20%). There is a strong association with asthma. Some inhaled allergens (e.g. grass or flower pollens and some moulds) cause seasonal symptoms, e.g. 'spring fever', whereas other allergens (e.g. house dust mites, animal fur and some foods) cause chronic or perennial rhinitis. Specific allergens can be identified by skin testing or in-vitro testing. Common symptoms include sneezing; nasal congestion and hypersecretion; itchy nose, palate and eyes; blocked ears; and irritated pharynx (see Table 32-1).

Management programs include attempts to identify and reduce exposure to specific allergens or environments, immunotherapy against antigens, and symptomatic drug treatment.

Nasal corticosteroids

The first-line treatment for rhinitis and nasal polyposis is now topical corticosteroids, administered intranasally by nasal spray or drops; several nasal formulations are available including beclomethasone, budesonide and mometasone. Nasal administration markedly reduces risk of systemic adverse effects, and reduces inflammation and mucus production.

They can be used as needed or regularly. The main adverse effects are local: nose bleeding, itching and sore throat.

H$_1$-receptor antagonists (antihistamines)

The other common drugs of choice in treating allergic rhinitis are the antihistamines (H$_1$-receptor antagonists). The many actions of histamine as an autacoid are discussed in Chapter 54 and the clinical uses of histamine-receptor antagonists in Chapters 34 and 55. H$_1$-antihistamines are indicated for the treatment of allergies and may also be useful for their antiemetic, sedative, antimuscarinic, local anaesthetic and antitussive effects.

In allergic rhinitis, the useful action of H$_1$-receptor antagonists is the blocking of histamine-induced vasodilation, decreasing capillary permeability, erythema and oedema. While released histamine normally contracts bronchial smooth muscle (bronchoconstriction), H$_1$-antihistamines are not useful bronchodilators and are not effective in asthma, as more powerful mediators (SRS-A, ACh, leukotrienes) are involved in allergic asthma.

The older H$_1$-antihistamines, such as promethazine and diphenhydramine, have powerful sedative effects,* which accounts for the common warning on packs of tablets 'Do not drive or operate machinery after taking this drug'. The newer, second-generation H$_1$-antihistamines, such as loratadine and fexofenadine, were developed to minimise this adverse effect. They are referred to as being 'less sedating', as they may still cross the blood–brain barrier and have slight sedative effects. The sedating antihistamines may be useful at night for hay-fever sufferers. The sedative effect common to older antihistamines is additive with other CNS depressants, including alcohol.

H$_1$-antihistamines are indicated for allergic rhinitis and are given orally (e.g. promethazine 10–25 mg 2–3 times daily) or intranasally (e.g. levocabastine nasal spray).

Other intranasal drugs for allergic rhinitis

Many drugs are formulated as nasal sprays or drops to be used topically in rhinitis; these have been considered earlier in this chapter and include:

- normal saline solutions, as nasal drops or spray (help relieve nasal congestion and sinusitis)
- nasal sympathomimetic decongestants (e.g. xylometazoline nasal spray or drops, 0.05% or 0.1% solutions), which decrease nasal blood flow and congestion by their vasoconstrictor actions via α-adrenoceptors

---

*This adverse effect may be appreciated by the parents of children given an antihistamine as an antiemetic to prevent travel sickness during long car journeys.

- nasal mast-cell stabilisers (e.g. cromoglycate nasal spray, 2% or 4% solutions); these must be used prophylactically to hinder release of inflammatory mediators
- nasal anticholinergics (e.g. ipratropium nasal spray, 21 or 42 mcg/dose), which dry up nasal secretions and reduce rhinorrhoea
- volatile oil decongestants, often administered as inhalation or chest rub: may include cineole, menthol, camphor, or oils of eucalyptus, peppermint, wintergreen (methyl salicylate), lavender or rosemary.

Sinusitis

Sinusitis, or inflammation of the mucous membranes lining the bone cavities (sinuses) of the face (see Figure 32-5), usually results from infection. Clinical features include feeling of fullness or pain in the forehead or cheeks, fever and nasal congestion. Bacterial infection causes purulent discharge. Specific antibiotics are prescribed if the infecting organism is bacterial: amoxycillin, doxycycline or cefaclor are usually suitable. Treatment with antipyretic analgesics (e.g. para-cetamol), saline irrigations and decongestants helps relieve symptoms.

PREGNANCY SAFETY	
ADEC Category	**Drug**
A	Aminophylline, budesonide, cromoglycate,* pholcodine, salbutamol, terbutaline, theophylline
B1	Cromoglycate,* ipratropium, ipratropium + salbutamol, montelukast, nedocromil, tiotropium, zafirlukast, zanamivir
B2	Acetylcysteine, influenza vaccine, pseudoephedrine
B3	Beclomethasone, eformoterol, fluticasone, fluticasone/salmeterol, ipratropium/ salbutamol
*Cromoglycate A or B1 depending on formulation.	

DRUGS AT A GLANCE 32: Drugs used in respiratory disorders

Therapeutic group	Pharmacological group	Key examples	Key pages
Respiratory gases		oxygen	524–7
		carbon dioxide	526–8
Respiratory stimulants	Analeptics		528
Mucoactive agents	Irritants	guaifenesin	529
	Mucolytics	acetylcysteine, dornase alfa	529, 30
Pulmonary surfactants	Surface-active agents	beractant, poractant alfa	530, 1
Antiasthma agents			531, 2
Relievers	Bronchodilators:		
	• short-acting β_2 agonists	salbutamol, terbutaline	534, 6
	• xanthines	theophylline	534–7
	• antimuscarinics	ipratropium, tiotropium	530, 5, 6
Controllers	Bronchodilators: long-acting β_2 agonists	salmeterol, eformoterol	534
Preventers	Corticosteroids (inhaled)	beclomethasone, budesonide	536, 8, 9, 48
	Leukotriene-receptor antagonists	zafirlukast, montelukast	538, 9
	Mast-cell stabilisers	sodium cromoglycate, nedocromil	539
Cough suppressants (antitussive agents)	Opioids	dextromethorphan, pholcodine	542–4
Decongestants	Sympathomimetics	pseudoephedrine	534, 5
Anti-influenza agents	Vaccine	influenza vaccine	545
	Neuraminidase inhibitors	zanamivir, oseltamivir	546

KEY POINTS

- Oxygen is a therapeutic gas that is essential to sustaining life and is used in many clinical situations, especially to treat hypoxia. Oxygen toxicity is a potential problem.

- Carbon dioxide gas is used for its effects on respiration, circulation and the CNS; in low concentrations it is a respiratory stimulant.

- Patients with abnormal or excessive respiratory tract secretions often need mucoactive drugs. These promote the removal of respiratory tract secretions by thinning hyperviscous secretions, thus enhancing the ciliary action of the respiratory tract. Mucolytics such as acetylcysteine may break down and reduce the viscosity of sputum. Expectorants aid in the removal of sputum.

- Pulmonary surfactant (natural or synthetic) can be administered intratracheally to infants with respiratory distress syndrome.

- Asthma is a major cause of morbidity and mortality in the community. Treating asthma involves educating the patient; regular monitoring of lung function, progress and compliance; avoiding trigger factors; and stepwise use of various antiasthma drugs.

- The main drug groups used in asthma are:
  - reliever (bronchodilator) medications (short-acting β_2 agonists, xanthines and antimuscarinic agents)
  - symptom controllers (long-acting β_2 agonists)
  - preventer medications (inhaled corticosteroids, leukotriene-receptor antagonists and mast-cell stabilisers).

- Cough suppressants such as the opioid antitussive drugs are used for non-productive coughs.

- Viral respiratory tract infections (cold, influenza, croup) are treated largely symptomatically.

- Bacterial RTIs (pneumonia, TB, and infections in COPD) are treated with antibiotics specific to the pathogenic organism.

- Drugs can be administered via the nose for local and/or systemic effects. Allergic rhinitis is treated with nasal corticosteroids, or oral or nasal antihistamines.

REVIEW EXERCISES

1 A patient with asthma has the following medications prescribed:
   - salbutamol (Ventolin CFC-free, 100 mcg/dose) 1–2 inhalations every 4 hours if necessary
   - fluticasone (Flixotide, 250 mcg/dose) two inhalations qid
   - salmeterol (Serevent, 25 mcg/dose) 2 inhalations twice daily.

   To obtain the maximum effects from the inhalers, what instructions would you give this patient on the sequence in which to use the drugs (first, second and third)? Describe additional therapeutic tips relevant to this drug regimen.

2 What are the indications, mechanism of action, pharmacokinetics and adverse reactions with the use of acetylcysteine?

3 Discuss the clinical use of expectorants, mucolytics and cough suppressants.

4 What are the mechanisms and signs and/or symptoms of oxygen toxicity?

5 Describe the actions of autacoid mediators of asthma, and explain the mechanisms of actions of the main groups of antiasthma drugs.

6 Outline the recommended stages in the stepwise management of asthma and the important components of an asthma management plan.

7 Discuss briefly the pharmacological treatment of common viral and bacterial respiratory tract infections.

8 Describe the pathology and pharmacological treatment of allergic rhinitis.

9 Discuss the administration of drugs via the nose, giving examples.

REFERENCES AND FURTHER READING

Abramson MJ, Walters J, Walters EH. Adverse effects of beta-agonists: are they clinically relevant? *American Journal of Respiratory Medicine* 2003; 2(4): 287–97.

Antibiotic Expert Group. *Therapeutic Guidelines Antibiotic, version 12.* Melbourne: Therapeutic Guidelines Limited, 2003.

Anonymous. Using β_2-stimulants in asthma. *Australian Prescriber* 1998; 21(1): 22–5.

Asthma Foundation of Victoria 2005. *All About Asthma*. www.asthma.org.au.

Australian Centre for Asthma Monitoring. *Health Care Expenditure and the Burden of Disease Due to Asthma in Australia*. Canberra: Australian Institute of Health and Welfare, 2005.

Australian Medicines Handbook 2006. Adelaide: AMH, 2006.

BOC Gases Group. *Medical Products Reference Manual*. Sydney: BOC Gases Aust., 1999.

Braun L, Cohen M. *Herbs and Natural Supplements: An Evidence-Based Guide*. Sydney: Elsevier Mosby; 2005.

Caswell A (ed.). *MIMS Annual June 2005*. Sydney: CMPMedica Australia, 2005.

Chapman S, Robinson G, Stradling J, West S. *Oxford Handbook of Respiratory Medicine*. Oxford: Oxford University Press, 2005.

Christiansen K. Pneumonia in the nineties. *Australian Prescriber* 1999; 22 (2): 37–9.

CSL. *Flu News*. 2nd edn. May 2000. Sydney: MediMedia Communications, 2000.

D'Souza WJ, et al. Asthma morbidity 6 years after an effective asthma self-management programme in a Maori community. *European Respiratory Journal* 2000; 15(3): 464–9.

Ducharme FM. Inhaled corticosteroids versus leukotriene antagonists as first-line therapy for asthma: a systematic review of current evidence. *Treatments in Respiratory Medicine* 2004; 3(6): 399–405.

Dunn CJ, Goa KL. Zanamivir: a review of its use in influenza. *Drugs* 1999; 58(4): 761–84.

Geelhoed GC. The management of croup. *Australian Prescriber* 1997; 20(4): 99–101.

Gibson PG. Management of chronic obstructive pulmonary disease (COPD). *Australian Prescriber* 2001; 24(6): 152–5.

Gibson PG. Outcomes of the Cochrane Airways Group International Conference. *Australian Prescriber* 2001; 24(4): 78–9.

Gillespie MB, Osguthorpe JD. Pharmacologic management of chronic rhinosinusitis, alone or with nasal polyposis. *Current Asthma and Allergy Reports* 2004; 4(6): 478–85.

Hall R. Influenza immunisation. *Australian Prescriber* 2002; 25(1): 5–7.

Halliwell B, Gutteridge JMC. *Free Radicals in Biology and Medicine*. 3rd edn. Oxford: Oxford University Press, 1999.

Hansel TT, Tennant RC, Tan AJ, Higgins LA, Neighbour H, Erin EM, Barnes PJ. Theophylline: mechanism of action and use in asthma and chronic obstructive pulmonary disease. *Drugs of Today* 2004; 40(1): 55–69.

Holt S, Pearce N. Asthma in New Zealand: myths and realities. *New Zealand Medical Journal* 2000; 113(1103): 39–41.

Howell M, Ford P. *The Ghost Disease and Twelve Other Stories of Detective Work in the Medical Field*. Harmondsworth: Penguin, 1986.

Jenkins C. An update on asthma management. *Internal Medicine Journal* 2003; 33(8): 365–71.

Murtagh J. *Cautionary Tales: Authentic Case Histories from Medical Practice*. Sydney: McGraw-Hill, 1992.

National Asthma Council. *Asthma Management Handbook 2002*. Melbourne: National Asthma Campaign, 2002.

New Zealand Ministry of Health. *Taking the Pulse: New Zealand 1996/97 Health Survey*. Wellington: Ministry of Health, 1999.

Page C, Lee LY. Summary: peripheral pharmacology of cough. *Pulmonary Pharmacology and Therapeutics*, 2002; 15(3): 217–9.

Percival SS. Use of echinacea in medicine. *Biochemical Pharmacology* 2000; 60(2): 155–8.

Poff CD, Balazy M. Drugs that target lipoxygenases and leukotrienes as emerging therapies for asthma and cancer. *Current Drug Targets* 2004; 3(1): 19–33.

Poole PJ, Black PN. Mucolytic agents for chronic bronchitis or chronic obstructive pulmonary disease. *Cochrane Database of Systematic Reviews* 2003; CD001287.

Redington AE, Morice AH (eds). *Acute and Chronic Cough*. Boca Raton: Taylor & Francis, 2005.

Respiratory Expert Group. *Therapeutic Guidelines Respiratory, version 3*. Melbourne: Therapeutic Guidelines Limited, 2005.

Schroeder K, Fahey T. Over-the-counter medications for acute cough in children and adults in ambulatory settings. *Cochrane Database of Systematic Reviews* 2004; CD001831.

Seale, JP. Anticholinergic bronchodilators. *Australian Prescriber* 2003; 26(2): 33–5.

Sears MR, Taylor DR, Print CG et al. Regular inhaled beta-agonist treatment in bronchial asthma. *Lancet* 1990; 336: 1391–6.

Spencer JW, Jacobs JJ. *Complementary/Alternative Medicine: An Evidence-Based Approach*. St Louis: Mosby, 1999.

Suresh GK, Soll RF. Overview of surfactant replacement trials. *Journal of Perinatology* 2005; 25 Suppl 2: S40–4.

Tattersfield AE. Use of β_2-agonists in asthma: much ado about nothing? Still cause for concern. *British Medical Journal* 1994; 309: 794–5.

van Asperen PP, Mellis CM, Sly PD. The role of corticosteroids in the management of childhood asthma. *Medical Journal of Australia* 2002; 176: 168–73.

Ward JA. Should antioxidant vitamins be routinely recommended for older people? *Drugs and Aging* 1998; 12(3): 169–75.

Watts RW. Asthma management in rural Australia. *Australian Journal of Rural Health* 1999; 7(4): 249–52.

Wormald PJ. Treating acute sinusitis. *Australian Prescriber* 2000; 23(2): 39–42.

Worsnop C. Combination inhalers for asthma. *Australian Prescriber* 2005; 28(2): 26–8.

Youngson RM. *Collins Dictionary: Medicine*. 2nd edn. Glasgow: HarperCollins, 1998.

ON-LINE RESOURCES

For specific New Zealand drugs, check Medsafe website: http://www.medsafe.govt.nz

Asthma 3+ visit plan, website: www.health.gov.au

National Asthma Council website: www.nationalasthma.org.au

National Prescribing Service campaign for optimising treatment of common cold: www.gottacold.com

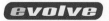   More weblinks at http://evolve.elsevier.com/AU/Bryant/pharmacology/

CHAPTER 33

Overview of the Gastrointestinal Tract

CHAPTER FOCUS

The gastrointestinal tract comprises the organs between the mouth and the anus, and includes the pharynx, oesophagus, stomach, and the small and large intestines. The primary functions of the gastrointestinal system—digestion and absorption—are aided by the motile and secretory properties of the tract and the associated accessory organs. This chapter provides an overview of the anatomy and physiology of the gastrointestinal tract, along with examples of disorders that affect each segment of the tract. An understanding of these factors provides the basis for the pharmacology of drugs that modulate gastrointestinal function.

OBJECTIVES

- To describe the functions of the various segments of the gastrointestinal tract.
- To describe the processes of mechanical and chemical digestion.
- To explain the process of gastric acid production and secretion.
- To describe the mechanical processes of vomiting and defecation.
- To describe the main functions of the liver and gallbladder.

KEY TERMS

chyme
constipation
defecation
deglutition
diarrhoea
digestion
dysphagia
gastrointestinal tract

gastrin
histamine (H_2) receptors
oesophagitis
parietal cells
pepsin
peristalsis
vomiting

KEY ABBREVIATIONS

CTZ	chemoreceptor trigger zone
ECL	enterochromaffin-like cells
GI	gastrointestinal
GIT	gastrointestinal tract

DISORDERS of the **gastrointestinal tract** (GI tract, GIT), such as indigestion, gastritis, peptic ulcers, diarrhoea and constipation, are very common problems reported by a large proportion of the population. The cause of many GI diseases remains unclear, and drug treatment is often focused on relieving symptoms rather than on control or cure. In this chapter, the anatomy and physiology of the GI tract are reviewed.

The digestive system has four main activities—**motility**, **secretion**, **digestion** and **absorption**—and is made up of the GI tract, also called the alimentary canal, and the accessory organs of digestion such as the teeth, tongue, biliary system (liver and gallbladder) and pancreas (Figure 33-1). The GI tract is an open-ended tube that extends from the mouth to the anus. Food consumed enters the tube and undergoes mechanical and chemical disruption (digestion) that breaks down large food particles into progressively smaller components. Mechanical digestion involves processes such as chewing and churning, while chemical digestion relies on secretion of digestive enzymes such as those in the mouth (salivary amylase), stomach (pepsin) and small intestine (pancreatic amylase). These processes aid absorption of nutrients, which may either be used as an energy source or stored, and the excretion of indigestible materials in the form of faeces. Movements by the smooth muscle fibres surrounding the GI tract mix the contents by segmental contractions and propel the material through the tract by peristalsis.

THE GASTROINTESTINAL TRACT

Neural innervation

The secretory and muscular activities of the GIT are regulated by both intrinsic and extrinsic neural mechanisms. The enteric nervous system, an interconnecting network of neurons, is located in smooth muscle and secretory cells of the GIT and relays information via the autonomic nervous system and via local reflexes. This intrinsic system is self-regulating and is capable of controlling exocrine gland secretions and muscular contractions independently of the central nervous system. Neurotransmitters in the enteric nervous system include acetylcholine, nitric oxide, 5-hydroxytryptamine (5-HT, serotonin) and substance P.

By contrast, the extrinsic innervation of the GIT is supplied by the divisions of the autonomic nervous system (see Chapter 10). These divisions coordinate activities among different regions of the GIT and also between this system and other parts of the body. The parasympathetic division sends nerve impulses via two branches of the vagus nerve and exerts mostly an excitatory action, which increases digestive secretions and muscular activity. The splanchnic nerves of the sympathetic division are primarily inhibitory nerves and depress digestive secretions and muscular activity. Under normal conditions, the two divisions of the autonomic nervous system and the enteric nervous system maintain a delicate balance of control over the functions of the GIT.

The mouth (buccal cavity)

The mouth, or buccal cavity, functions as the starting point of the digestive process. Ingested food is chewed and mixed with saliva that contains the enzymes amylase, which initiates the breakdown of disaccharide sugars and starches (polysaccharides), and lingual lipase, which initiates digestion of dietary triglycerides (fats).

Three pairs of salivary glands secrete saliva via ducts that empty into the mouth. The sublingual and submandibular salivary glands are located beneath the tongue; the largest pair is the parotid glands, which are found in front of and slightly below the ears. When food has been chewed and is reduced to a soft spongy mass in the mouth, it is swallowed. Swallowing (**deglutition**) is a complex process that begins as a voluntary movement but is continued as an involuntary muscular reflex as the bolus of food is propelled through the pharynx into the oesophagus.

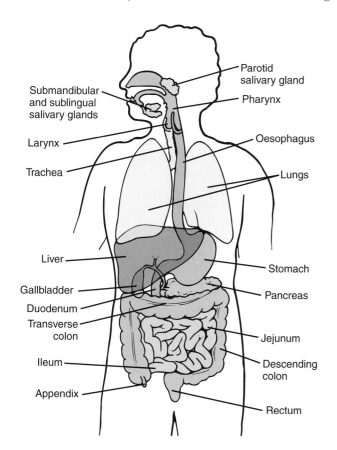

FIGURE 33-1 The gastrointestinal system.

Systemic diseases, nutritional deficiencies and mechanical trauma can cause irritation or inflammation of buccal structures. Dental disorders (e.g. caries and gingivitis) and bacterial, viral or fungal infections (e.g. candidiasis or herpes simplex) can affect the structures of the oral cavity, causing symptoms such as mouth blistering or other lesions, swelling, pain and inflammation. Mumps is an inflammation of the parotid glands by the mumps virus (myxovirus).

The pharynx

The pharynx (throat), a tube-like passageway connecting the mouth and the oesophagus, is important in swallowing. Food and fluid pass through the pharynx into the oesophagus. During this passage, the trachea is closed to prevent aspiration into the lungs and respiration is inhibited. The oral and pharyngeal phases of swallowing last less than one second.

Like the mouth, the pharynx can be affected by viral infections and become irritated and inflamed (e.g. due to sinusitis or the common cold). Neurological lesions and cerebrovascular accidents involving the medulla and the swallowing centre can result in difficulties in the pharyngeal phase of swallowing.

The oesophagus

The oesophagus is a collapsible muscular structure about 25 cm long that extends from the pharynx to the upper region (cardia) of the stomach. It passes through the diaphragm at the oesophageal hiatus into the abdominal cavity.

The oesophagus acts as a conduit for food and secretes mucus to aid lubrication but does not secrete digestive enzymes or absorb nutrients. The oesophagus continues the process of swallowing by involuntary muscular movements called **peristalsis**, which squeeze the food bolus towards the stomach. The lower oesophageal (cardiac) sphincter relaxes as a peristaltic wave approaches, allowing the bolus to pass into the stomach. The lower oesophageal sphincter then contracts to prevent reflux of the gastric contents into the oesophagus.

Oesophageal disorders are characterised by retrosternal pain (heartburn) and difficulty in swallowing (**dysphagia**). The sources of the pain are numerous; potential causes include diffuse oesophageal spasm, achalasia (failure of lower oesophageal sphincter to relax), pyloric or duodenal ulcers, postural changes (bending forward) and excessive alcohol ingestion. Heartburn commonly results from reflux **oesophagitis** (backflow of gastric contents into the oesophagus) (see Clinical Interest Box 33-1), or from hiatal hernia (protrusion of a part of the stomach through the diaphragm). Dysphagia can be a symptom, for example, of oesophageal obstruction, mechanical interference with or paralysis of the muscles of deglutition, carcinoma of the oesophagus, anxiety states or hysteria. Inflammation of the oesophagus can have many causes, e.g. reflux oesophagitis associated with hiatal hernia, irritant ingestion, infection, peptic ulceration or prolonged gastric intubation.

The stomach

The stomach is a J-shaped pouch-like structure lying below the diaphragm and has four divisions: the cardia, the fundus, the body and the pylorus. The pyloric sphincter controls communication between the stomach and the duodenum. The stomach wall is composed of the mucosa, which contains the gastric glands responsible for the secretion of pepsinogen, gastric lipase, hydrochloric acid and intrinsic factor, and the submucosa, which connects the mucosa to the underlying muscularis mucosae. The muscularis has three layers of smooth muscle: longitudinal, circular and oblique layers, which allow the stomach to churn and mix the contents. In general, vagal stimulation (parasympathetic) increases the force and frequency of contractions, while input from the sympathetic nervous system decreases both activities. When the stomach is empty, the mucosa forms large folds or rugae, which tend to flatten out when the stomach distends.

The stomach functions as a temporary storage site for food as it is being digested and is capable of holding 1500–2000 mL. When a bolus of food arrives, the proximal region of the stomach relaxes to accommodate the ingested meal. Gentle peristaltic movements pass over the stomach and the food is mixed with the gastric secretions to form a liquid called **chyme**. More vigorous mixing movements occur in the body of the stomach, and the velocity and force of contractions increase as the chyme is moved towards the pylorus. The contractions, which last 2–20 seconds and occur at a rate of 3–5 per minute, are responsible primarily for the mixing of the chyme with the digestive juices but they also assist the

---

**CLINICAL INTEREST BOX 33-1
GASTRO-OESOPHAGEAL REFLUX
DISEASE (GORD)**

GORD is extremely common and as many as 25% of the population experience symptoms on occasion. GORD differs from non-ulcer dyspepsia in that the predominant symptom is heartburn, or acid regurgitation. The results of a large international study of 5581 people, published in 1999, proved that the incidence of GORD-like symptoms strongly correlated with stressful life events and with psychiatric illness (Stanghellini 1999). Other risk factors for GORD include obesity, smoking, and consuming in excess of seven standard alcoholic drinks per week. Lifestyle modifications that may be beneficial include avoiding food known to cause symptoms, not eating at bedtime, limiting alcohol, stopping smoking, stress management, and intermittent use of an antacid when symptoms occur.
Source: Gastrointestinal Expert Group 2002.

propulsion of the chyme into the duodenum. As the peristaltic contraction approaches the pylorus, a small volume of the chyme is forced into the duodenum but the majority is forced back into the body of the stomach, where further mechanical and chemical digestion occurs. Only a limited amount of nutrient and drug absorption takes place in the stomach (see Chapter 6).

The time required for digestion in the stomach depends on the amount and type of food eaten. Normal gastric emptying time is 2–6 hours but certain drugs, physical activity of the individual and body position during digestion may affect this. Liquids empty more rapidly, whereas solids must be reduced in size to particles less than 2 mm^3 in volume before emptying occurs. Neural and hormonal reflexes control the balance between the gastric emptying rate and the processing capacity of the small intestine.

Gastric secretions

The stomach is a primary site of digestion of food, and the major stimulant to gastric acid secretion is protein. Gastric juice comprises four components, **pepsin**, hydrochloric acid, mucus and intrinsic factor. The secretion of hydrochloric acid by **parietal cells** kills bacteria in food, denatures protein and converts inactive pepsinogen into active pepsin, which aids further in protein degradation. Mucus and bicarbonate ions secreted by superficial mucosal cells form a gel-like layer that serves to protect the stomach from the acid environment and provides lubrication between the superficial cells and bulky undigested material. The parietal cells also secrete intrinsic factor, a protein essential for the binding of vitamin B$_{12}$ before its absorption in the ileum. The stimuli for gastric secretion and the cells involved are illustrated in Figure 33-2.

GASTRIC ACID SECRETION

The hormone **gastrin**, the neurotransmitter acetylcholine and the local hormone histamine directly stimulate acid secretion by parietal cells. In contrast, prostaglandins E$_2$ and I$_2$ inhibit acid secretion (see Chapter 34). The process of gastric acid production and secretion is illustrated in Figure 33-3. The exact mechanism is not clearly established but, in general, gastrin and acetylcholine (ACh) stimulate histamine release from enterochromaffin-like cells. Histamine then acts via **histamine (H2) receptors** on parietal cells to increase acid secretion. Additionally, gastrin, ACh and histamine stimulate their respective receptors on the parietal cells, which potentiates acid secretion.

Parietal cells secrete 1000–2000 mL hydrochloric acid per day, so maintenance of the gastric mucosal barrier is essential to prevent ulceration. Changes in mucosal blood flow, decreased secretion of protective mucus, bacterial infection and damage by agents such as alcohol and aspirin may all lead to weakening of the mucosal barrier and ulceration. Understanding the role of prostaglandins, the various hormones and neurotransmitters in regulating acid secretion provides the basis for the pharmacological management of peptic ulcer disease.

Disorders affecting the stomach

Acute gastritis is an inflammatory response of the stomach lining to ingestion of irritants, such as ethanol (alcohol) or non-steroidal anti-inflammatory agents (NSAIDs), including aspirin. Symptoms include epigastric discomfort, nausea, abdominal tenderness and GI haemorrhage. Treatment consists of lifestyle modifications and drugs such as antacids (see Chapter 34).

Chronic gastritis is a long-term inflammation of the stomach lining, generally with degeneration of the gastric mucosa, but its causes are not well established. It is more common in women, and the incidence increases with age, excessive smoking and ethanol use. Symptoms are non-specific but may include flatulence, epigastric fullness after meals, diarrhoea and bleeding. Treatment is the same as for acute gastritis. Iron deficiency anaemia and pernicious anaemia may result from chronic gastritis. Treatment of symptoms and elimination of possible causative or aggravating factors (e.g. aspirin use) comprise the usual therapeutic regimen.

Peptic ulcer disease is a broad term encompassing both gastric and duodenal ulcers. Although both types of ulcers produce a break in the gastric mucosa, the causes differ. With gastric ulcers, the ability of the gastric mucosa to protect and repair itself seems to be defective; in duodenal ulcers, hypersecretion of acid and pepsin is responsible for the erosion of the duodenal mucosa. Gastric colonisation with *Helicobacter pylori*, a common Gram-negative bacillus, has been identified as a major causative agent in individuals with peptic ulcer disease not caused by NSAIDs (see Clinical Interest Box 33-2).

CLINICAL INTEREST BOX 33-2
HELICOBACTER PYLORI

H. pylori is a Gram-negative bacterium that commonly infects around 30%–40% of Australian-born adults. There appears to be no difference between males and females in frequency of infection (Australian Gastroenterology Institute). It is a spiral (helical)-shaped organism that has evolved to inhabit the highly acidic environment of the stomach, particularly the pylorus. Once the bacterium adheres to the gastric epithelial cells, it breaks down endogenous urea, creating a protective cloud of ammonia and bicarbonate that enables it to protect itself against the effects of gastric acid. The ability of the bacterium to degrade urea and release carbon dioxide forms the basis of the *H. pylori* breath test, which is used to detect infestation and also to monitor the effectiveness of drug-mediated eradication. *H. pylori* has been established as a causal agent in the development of chronic gastritis, duodenal and gastric ulcers, and gastric cancer.

Treatment with various drug combinations results in healing and a low peptic ulcer recurrence rate (Bytzer & O'Morain 2005).

Duodenal ulcers are more common than gastric ulcers, accounting for nearly 80% of all peptic ulcers, and usually occur more frequently in younger persons. Overall, the reported incidence of peptic ulcers is much lower in females. In addition to various drug treatment regimens, diet and lifestyle modifications are equally important (see Chapter 34). Hereditary factors, use of some drugs (e.g. aspirin and cortico-

steroids), psychological factors, stress and diet have also been implicated in the development of peptic ulcer disease.

Vomiting

The induction of **vomiting** involves a complex coordinated response between two areas, the **chemoreceptor trigger zone (CTZ)**, located in the floor of the fourth ventricle of the brain, and the vomiting centre, or emetic centre, located in the medulla. The emetic centre receives inputs from:

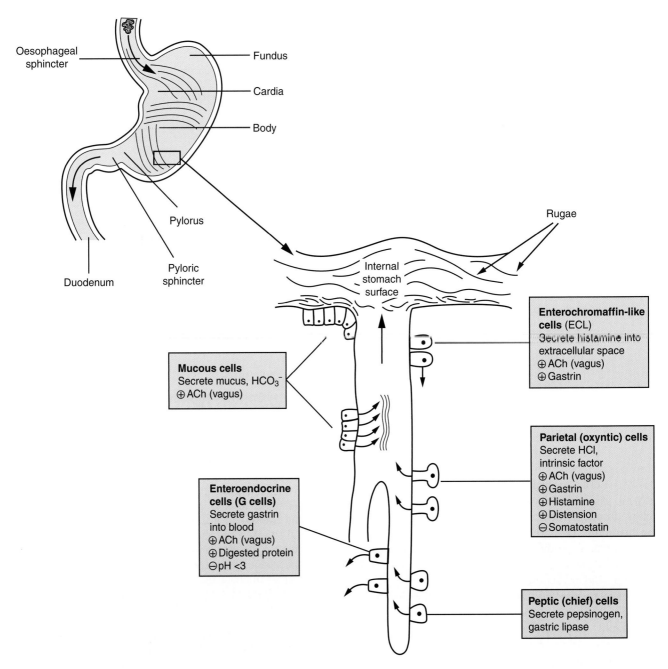

FIGURE 33-2 Schematic diagram of stomach, gastric gland and secretory cells. ACh = acetylcholine; HCl = hydrochloric acid; HCO_3^- = bicarbonate ions; ⊕ = stimulated by; ⊖ = inhibited by.

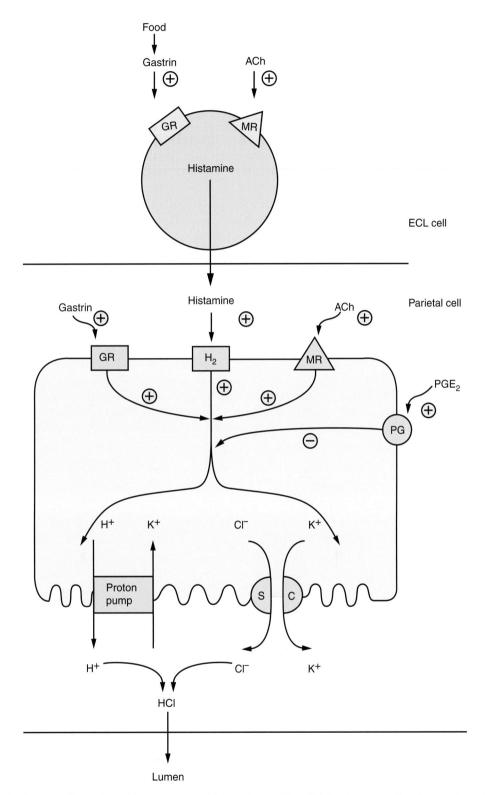

FIGURE 33-3 Schematic diagram of gastric acid secretion and interrelationship of histamine secretion from enterochromaffin-like cell (ECL) and the acid-secreting parietal cells. Pathways may be stimulated ⊕ or inhibited ⊖. ACh = acetylcholine; GR = gastrin receptor; H_2 = histamine (H_2) receptor; M = muscarinic receptor; PG = prostaglandin E_2 (PGE_2) receptor; proton pump = H^+–K^+-ATPase; SC = symport carrier. *Adapted from*: Rang HP, Dale MM, Ritter JM, Moore PK. *Pharmacology*. 5th edn. Edinburgh: Churchill Livingstone, 2003. By permission of the publisher.

- the CTZ
- the vestibular apparatus
- higher brain centres relaying sensory inputs such as pain, smell and sight
- organs such as the heart, testes and parts of the GI tract.

The CTZ (Figure 33-4) is an area of sensory nerve cells activated by blood-borne emetics such as chemical toxins and drugs, and by the neurotransmitter 5-HT, released from afferent nerve pathways from the stomach and small intestine. The CTZ itself is not able to induce vomiting but is stimulated by smells, strong emotion, severe pain, raised intracranial pressure, labyrinthine disturbances (motion sickness), endocrine disturbances, toxic reactions to drugs, GI disease, radiation treatments and chemotherapy. The CTZ then relays messages to the emetic centre through actions of the neurotransmitters acetylcholine, 5-HT, histamine and dopamine. Antagonism of transmission through these pathways forms the basis for the antiemetic effects of several drugs used clinically. Because the CTZ is close to the respiratory centre in the brain, it is difficult to completely control vomiting initiated from this site without affecting respiration. Discharge from both the sympathetic and parasympathetic nervous systems often leads to the accompanying symptoms of salivation, sweating, rapid breathing and cardiac arrhythmias.

Vomiting is characterised by forceful expulsion of the contents of the stomach (and sometimes that of the duodenum) through the mouth. This occurs as a result of impulses sent via efferent nerves from the emetic centre to the upper GI tract, diaphragm and abdominal muscles. Strong contraction of the abdominal muscles then forces the contents past the oesophageal sphincter and into the mouth. Relaxation of the abdominal muscles allows any material remaining in the oesophagus to empty back into the stomach. This cycle may be repeated many times. Although vomiting in many instances is a protective mechanism to rid the body of toxic substances, it may in severe cases lead to fluid and electrolyte disturbances.

The cerebral cortex is also involved in anticipatory nausea and vomiting, a conditioned response caused by a stimulus connected with a previous unpleasant experience. For example, unpleasant memories, such as receiving cancer chemotherapy that has resulted in vomiting, might make a person vomit at the sight of the hospital, the doctor or the nurse, even before treatment is started (Koda-Kimble & Young 1995).

The pancreas

Continued digestion and absorption of food in the small intestine relies on secretions from the accessory organs—the pancreas, liver and gallbladder. The pancreas (see Chapter 41) secretes about 1500 mL liquid daily, comprising water, sodium bicarbonate and enzymes such as pancreatic amylase, trypsin and chymotrypsin. The acidic duodenal chyme is neutralised by the aqueous component, which brings the pH within range

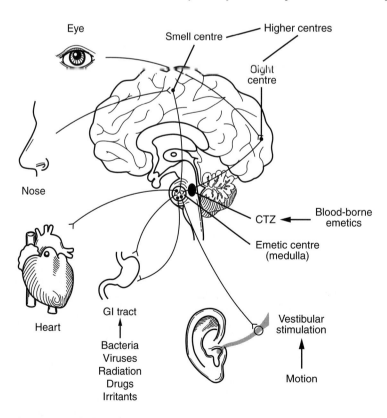

FIGURE 33-4 The chemoreceptor trigger zone (CTZ) and other sites activating the emetic centre.

for further digestion of nutrients by the pancreatic enzymes. Regulation of pancreatic secretion is complex; for example, to prevent erosion of the duodenal mucosa, the rate of delivery of acidic chyme into the duodenum is equalled by the rate of secretion of bicarbonate ions, which neutralise the chyme.

With the exception of diabetes mellitus (see Chapter 41), many pancreatic diseases have symptoms that are not readily diagnosed. Inflammation of the pancreas may be acute or chronic. Among the many causes are blockage of the pancreatic ducts, trauma to the pancreas, excessive alcohol consumption, drug use, and tumours, cysts or abscesses. Symptoms are non-specific but ultimately include severe pain. Carcinoma of the pancreas is as difficult to diagnose as other pancreatic disorders.

The liver

Immediately under the diaphragm and above the stomach is the largest gland in the body, the liver. It weighs around 1.5 kg and is metabolically an extremely important organ that performs over 100 different functions. The liver consists of two lobes that comprise multiple lobules of specialised cells called hepatocytes. The liver does not have capillaries; instead, the hepatocytes are arranged in an interconnecting network of canals through which blood flows. These canals are lined with endothelium and are called sinusoids. Blood from the hepatic artery and also the portal vein (which drains blood from the intestinal tract) flows into the sinusoids, where toxins and nutrients are extracted by the hepatocytes, and products manufactured in the hepatocytes are secreted into the blood. Sinusoidal blood drains into the central veins and passes to the hepatic vein.

The main functions of the liver are:
- carbohydrate metabolism
- lipid metabolism
- protein metabolism, synthesis and secretion
- drug and chemical metabolism
- excretion of bilirubin
- synthesis of bile salts
- storage of glycogen and the vitamins A, B_{12}, D, E and K
- storage of iron and copper.

Disorders affecting the liver include acute and chronic viral hepatitis, biliary and postnecrotic cirrhosis, primary hepatic carcinoma and chronic alcoholism.

The gallbladder

Hepatocytes secrete into the bile canaliculi 800–1000 mL bile per day, which flows into the gallbladder, a pear-shaped organ 7–10 cm long and 2.5–3.5 cm wide, lying on the undersurface of the liver. Bile, a yellowish-green liquid (pH 7.6–8.6), contains water, bile acids, bile salts, cholesterol, phospholipids and bile pigments such as bilirubin. The gallbladder stores and concentrates the bile and, after a meal,

CLINICAL INTEREST BOX 33-3 GALLSTONES

There are two types of gallstones: those that are composed principally of cholesterol (cholesterol stones), and a second type that are mainly a complex of unconjugated bilirubin and calcium (pigment stones). Normally, about 50% of the bile secreted during the course of a day is saturated with cholesterol. In people with cholesterol gallstones, the bile is supersaturated with cholesterol, which results in a crystal formation that leads to the development of gallstones. Pigment stones arise as a result of saturation of bile with unconjugated bilirubin that precipitates with calcium to form stones. Surgical removal of the gallbladder (cholecystectomy) is a common treatment for the condition.

contracts rhythmically, expelling bile into the duodenum. The bile salts aid in the emulsification and absorption of lipids in the small intestine.

Cholecystitis, i.e. inflammation of the gallbladder, is often associated with the presence of gallstones (cholelithiasis; see Clinical Interest Box 33-3). The stones lodge in the gallbladder neck or ducts, causing congestion and oedema as bile builds up. This may be an acute or a chronic condition. Malignant tumours of the gallbladder are infrequent.

The small intestine

The small intestine, comprising the duodenum, jejunum and ileum, begins at the pyloric sphincter, coils through the abdominal cavity and connects with the large intestine at the ileocaecal sphincter. The small intestine is actually about 6–7 m long but under normal conditions muscle tone keeps it to about 3 m in length. The contents of the small intestine are propelled forward by peristaltic waves, which are weak in comparison to those of the stomach. Chyme remains in the small intestine for 3–5 hours, during which time more than 90% of the nutrients and water are absorbed. Any undigested material passes to the large intestine. The small intestine is also the principal site of drug absorption (see Chapter 6).

Two disorders affecting the entire lower GI tract are diarrhoea and constipation. These are discussed in Chapter 34, along with the drugs used in their treatment. Other disorders affecting the small intestine include obstruction, malabsorption syndrome and blind loop syndrome. Symptomatic treatment is customary while the underlying causative factors are investigated.

The large intestine

The caecum, colon and rectum make up the large intestine, which is about 1.5 m long. The distal 2.5 cm of the rectum is known as the anal canal. The final stages of digestion in the large intestine occur through bacterial action, including fermentation of carbohydrate, with the release of carbon dioxide, hydrogen and methane gas. These bacteria also synthesise vitamin K, which is absorbed by simple diffusion in the colon. Around 400–800 mL water is also reabsorbed in the large intestine. Decomposition of bilirubin contributes to the brown colour of faeces. Secretion of mucus by the lining of the large intestine protects the bowel from the rough undigested faecal matter. Peristaltic movements push the faeces to the rectum, where they are expelled through the reflex action known as **defecation**.

Distension of the rectum by faeces stimulates stretch receptors. This sends sensory information to the central nervous system via the sacral segment of the spinal cord. Parasympathetic motor impulses to the colon, rectum and anus result in contraction of rectal muscles. This increases pressure in the rectum which, coupled with contraction of the diaphragm and abdominal muscles, relaxation of the internal sphincter and voluntary relaxation of the external sphincter, results in expulsion of faeces through the anus.

Diarrhoea is characterised by defecation of liquid faeces occurring as a result of decreased absorption by the small and large intestine, accumulation of non-reabsorbable solutes (osmotic diarrhoea) or excessive secretion in the small intestine and colon (secretory diarrhoea). In contrast, **constipation** results from either infrequent or difficult defecation of hard, dry faeces. Causes of constipation include disordered bowel habits, various disease states, lack of dietary fibre, inadequate fluid intake or certain drugs, such as codeine and morphine (see Chapter 16).

Other disorders affecting the large intestine include diver-

ticular disease, which has no specific therapy; inflammatory bowel disease (IBD), which is the collective term used to describe ulcerative colitis and Crohn's disease (see Clinical Interest Box 33-4); irritable bowel syndrome and carcinoma. Haemorrhoids (varicosities of the external or internal haemorrhoidal veins) are also common.

CLINICAL INTEREST BOX 33-4
CROHN'S DISEASE

Manifestations of Crohn's disease, described by Dr Burrill D. Crohn in 1932, occur as a result of a complex process that involves infiltration of the full thickness of the bowel wall with macrophages and lymphocytes. As the disease progresses, the lining of predominantly the terminal ileum and colon develop deep linear ulcers interspersed with normal tissue, which gives rise to the characteristic cobblestone appearance. Collagen deposition is common and this often leads to stricture formation.

Crohn's disease is a chronic recurring illness, but many people experience periods of remission when they are free of symptoms such as abdominal pain, diarrhoea, nausea and tiredness. Treatment of the disease involves the use of various drugs and in about 60% of cases surgery may be required to remove affected portions of the bowel. The cause of Crohn's disease is unknown but associations have been made with smoking, the increased intake of simple sugars, increased intestinal permeability, genetic factors and infection with *Mycobacterium paratuberculosis*. It is estimated by the Australian Crohn's and Colitis Association (ACCA) that around 43,000 Australians have IBD, of whom about 30,000 have Crohn's disease.

KEY POINTS

- The primary functions of the GI system are digestion and absorption. These processes are facilitated by the motile and secretory properties of the GI tract and associated organs.
- Digestion involves mechanical and chemical disruption. Mechanical digestion involves processes such as chewing and churning, while chemical digestion relies on the secretion of digestive enzymes.
- The secretory and muscular activities of the GI system are regulated by the autonomic and enteric nervous systems.
- Saliva is secreted by the sublingual, submandibular and parotid glands, and initiates the breakdown of sugars, starches and fats.
- Swallowing (deglutition) moves the food bolus to the stomach via the oesophagus.
- Mechanical and chemical digestion continues in the stomach. Various gastric glands secrete mucus, pepsinogen, gastric lipase, hydrochloric acid and intrinsic factor.
- Gastric acid secretion is regulated by neural (parasympathetic) and hormonal (gastrin, histamine) mechanisms.
- The small intestine comprises the duodenum, jejunum and ileum, and is the major site of nutrient and drug absorption.
- The caecum, colon and rectum make up the large intestine.
- The final stage of digestion in the large intestine occurs through bacterial action.
- Undigested faecal matter is expelled from the rectum through the reflex action of defecation.

- The accessory organs associated with the GI tract include the pancreas, the liver and the gallbladder.
- The liver is the second-largest organ of the body (after the skin) and performs over 100 different functions. These include carbohydrate, lipid and protein metabolism, and, importantly, drug and chemical metabolism.

REVIEW EXERCISES

1. List the functions of the buccal cavity, pharynx, oesophagus, stomach, liver, gallbladder, pancreas, and small and large intestines.
2. Describe the processes of mechanical and chemical digestion in the stomach.
3. Discuss the factors that regulate secretion of gastric juice.
4. How is gastric acid produced and what factors stimulate its release?

REFERENCES AND FURTHER READING

Bytzer P, O'Morain C. *Treatment of Helicobacter pylori. Helicobacter* 2005; 10 (Suppl. 1): 40–6.
Gastrointestinal Expert Group. *Therapeutic Guidelines: Gastrointestinal, version 3.* Melbourne: Therapeutic Guidelines, 2002.
Johnson LR. Part V: Gastrointestinal physiology. Chs 32–35 in: Johnson LR (ed.). *Essential Medical Physiology.* 2nd edn. Philadelphia: Lippincott-Raven, 1997.
Koda-Kimble MA, Young LY. Nausea and vomiting. In: Young LY, Koda-Kimble MA (eds). *Applied Therapeutics: The Clinical Use of Drugs.* 6th edn. Vancouver: Applied Therapeutics, 1995.
Lambert J. Testing for *Helicobacter pylori. Australian Prescriber* 1997; 20 (4): 96–7.
Podolsky DK. Inflammatory bowel disease. *New England Journal of Medicine* 1991; 325(13): 928–37.
Rang HP, Dale MM, Ritter JM, Moore PK. *Pharmacology.* 5th edn. Edinburgh: Churchill Livingstone, 2003 [ch. 24].
Selby WS. Current issues in Crohn's disease. *Medical Journal of Australia* 2003; 178(11): 532–3.
Stanghellini V. Relationship between upper GI symptoms and lifestyle, psychosocial factors and comorbidity in the general population: results from the Domestic/International Gastroenterology Surveillance Study (DIGEST). *Scandinavian Journal of Gastroenterology* 1999; 231 (Suppl.): 29–37.
Tortora GJ, Grabowski SR. *Principles of Anatomy and Physiology.* 9th edn. New York: Harper Collins, 2000 [ch. 24].

evolve   More weblinks at http://evolve.elsevier.com/AU/Bryant/pharmacology/

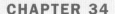

CHAPTER 34

Drugs Affecting the
Gastrointestinal Tract

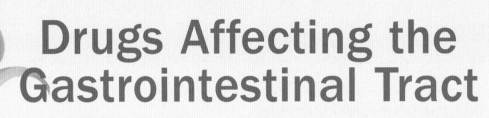

CHAPTER FOCUS

This chapter reviews the various topical and systemic medications that are used to treat illnesses or disorders affecting the upper and lower gastrointestinal (GI) tract. These include drugs that affect the mouth, stomach, vomiting reflex, GI tract and gallbladder. As many GI disorders—such as peptic ulcers, nausea, vomiting, constipation, diarrhoea, inflammatory bowel disease and irritable bowel syndrome—negatively affect a person's quality of life, the health-care professional needs to have knowledge of the drugs used in the treatment of GI tract disorders.

OBJECTIVES

- To describe the various drugs used to maintain oral hygiene.

- To review the use and adverse effects of antacids and antacid combinations.

- To discuss the modes of action of the various drugs used for nausea and vomiting.

- To discuss the mechanism of action of drugs used to treat peptic ulcer disease, and the role of *Helicobacter pylori* eradication drug regimens.

- To discuss the mechanism and sites of action of the various types of laxatives and antidiarrhoeal drugs.

- To review the use of drugs in the treatment of inflammatory bowel disease and irritable bowel syndrome.

KEY DRUGS

diphenoxylate
mesalazine
metoclopramide
misoprostol
nystatin
omeprazole
ondansetron
ranitidine
sucralfate

KEY TERMS

antacids
antidiarrhoeal
antiemetics
constipation
cytoprotective agents
inflammatory bowel disease
irritable bowel syndrome
laxatives
peptic ulcer disease

KEY ABBREVIATIONS

GORD	gastro-oesophageal reflux disease
IBD	inflammatory bowel disease
IBS	irritable bowel syndrome
NSAIDs	non-steroidal anti-inflammatory drugs
OTC	over-the-counter
PEG	polyethylene glycol

DRUGS THAT AFFECT THE MOUTH

MEDICATIONS generally have little effect on the mouth. Good oral hygiene, which includes brushing properly after meals and at bedtime, flossing and gum stimulation, has more influence on the tissues of the mouth than most drugs. Many mouth and throat preparations containing anti-inflammatory agents, anaesthetics and antiseptics are available for various disorders of the oral cavity, including chapped lips, sun and fever blisters, inflammatory lesions, ulcerative lesions secondary to trauma, gingival lesions, teething pain, toothache, irritation caused by orthodontic appliances or dentures, and oral cavity abrasions. Most topical agents that affect the mouth may be purchased over the counter (OTC).

Mouth-washes and gargles

Mouth-washes and gargles are dilute aromatic solutions that often contain a sweetener and an artificial colouring

agent. They may also contain an antiseptic (e.g. alcohol, cetylpyridinium chloride or chlorhexidine gluconate), an anaesthetic (e.g. benzocaine, lignocaine hydrochloride), an analgesic (e.g. benzydamine hydrochloride, choline salicylate) and an anticaries agent (sodium fluoride). Use of mouth-washes with high alcohol content may be problematic in some groups of the general population, e.g. children and people with cultural or religious objections to alcohol use (see Clinical Interest Box 34-1).

Products that inhibit plaque formation are available, and clinical trials have demonstrated some success with volatile oils, cetylpyridinium chloride and chlorhexidine. Commercial products that contain at least one of these active ingredients include Cepacol (cetylpyridinium chloride), Listerine (volatile oils) and Plaqacide (chlorhexidine gluconate). A detergent-type product to lessen plaque (Plax) is also available on the market. These products do not replace good oral hygiene but are recommended as an adjunct to proper brushing and flossing of the teeth (Flynn 1996).

Mouth-washes are often used for halitosis, or 'bad breath', or as gargles to treat colds or sore throats. They are generally not considered effective for such problems. Mouth-washes can improve mouth odour briefly but if such a problem persists, the underlying cause, such as poor dental hygiene or various gum diseases, needs to be identified and treated.

Sore throats are usually caused by infection, most often viral rather than bacterial. Symptomatic relief may be obtained using lozenges, sprays and gargles. Gargling might not reach the site of infection, which is often deep in the throat tissues. In addition to commercial preparations (e.g. Cepacaine, Betadine Sore Throat Gargle), sodium chloride solution (1/2 teaspoon of salt in an average-sized glass of warm water) has been commonly used as a gargle and mouth-wash.

CLINICAL INTEREST BOX 34-1 ALCOHOLIC MOUTH-WASH WARNING

PAEDIATRIC ALERT
The leading mouth-washes usually contain 7%–30% alcohol. As mouth-washes are in general not packaged in boxes with safety information inserts, parents of young children should be cautioned to store these products out of the reach of small children. The use of mouth-wash in young children is not recommended, as children often swallow the mouth-wash rather than expectorating it.

CLINICAL INTEREST BOX 34-2 FLUORIDATED WATER

Artificial fluoridation of water has been endorsed worldwide by more than 150 scientific and health organisations since the early observations that communities with naturally fluoridated water had lower incidences of dental caries. It has been estimated that two-thirds of the Australian population live in areas receiving fluoridated water. Exposure to fluoride is now even more widespread as exposure also occurs through ingestion of food grown in fluoridated areas, use of fluoridated toothpaste and ingestion of fluoride supplements. Fluoride toothpaste is sold widely in Australia and New Zealand.

In Australia, the natural fluoride concentration of water is <0.1 mg/L and all Australian capital cities except Brisbane have implemented water fluoridation. The nominal target level for fluoride in drinking water is 0.7–1.1 mg/L but water fluoridation is not widespread outside the metropolitan areas. In New Zealand, the fluoride content recommended

for drinking water by the Ministry of Health for oral health reasons is 0.7–1.0 mg/L with a maximum acceptable value of 1.5 mg/L.

Increased exposure to fluoride can cause enamel fluorosis, which can vary from whitish striations to pitting and staining of tooth enamel. Factors implicated in the increasing incidence of fluorosis in Australia include changes to tooth-brushing habits, use of fluoridated toothpaste, residence in fluoridated areas, prolonged use of infant formulae and ingestion of fluoride supplements. Use of fluoride supplements is not recommended for children under 3 years old. Compliance with Australian Drinking Water Guidelines ensures the quality of our water, including the level of fluoridation appropriate for conveying health benefits without any health risks (2004 Australian Drinking Water Guidelines; www.nhmrc.gov.au/publications/synopses/eh19syn.htm, accessed 29 August 2006).

Fluoridated mouth-washes

Several fluoride-containing preparations, including mouth-wash (Neutrafluor 900), toothpaste, tablets and solutions, are available for use as anticaries agents. The exact mechanism of action of fluoride in preventing caries is not fully understood; however, fluoride ions appear to exchange for hydroxyl or citrate (anion) ions and then settle in the anionic space in the surface of the enamel (Marcus 1995). This results in a harder outer layer of tooth enamel (a fluoridated hydroxyapatite) that is more resistant to demineralisation. Fluoridated mouthwashes have been used in communities with both limited fluoridated and unfluoridated water supplies, and their use has been associated with a significant decrease (17%–47%) in tooth decay (Flynn 1996).

Fluoridated mouth-washes are generally used once a day (rinsed for a minute and expectorated), preferably after brushing and flossing. Eating and drinking should be avoided for about 30 minutes after use.

Dentifrices

A dentifrice is a substance used to aid in cleaning teeth. Ordinary dentifrice contains one or more mild abrasives, a foaming agent and flavouring materials made into a powder or paste (toothpaste) to be used as an aid in the mechanical cleansing of accessible parts of the teeth. Fluoride dentifrices are effective anticaries agents.

Dentifrices are also available for the treatment of hypersensitive teeth. This usually occurs from exposed root areas at the cement–enamel junction, allowing access to nerve fibres in the pulp area of the tooth. Dentists often suggest desensitising dentifrices that contain potassium nitrate, such as Sensodyne toothpaste.

Drugs used to treat oral candidiasis

The term candidiasis ('thrush') is used commonly to refer to a superficial fungal infection; in the case of the mouth, rarely are fungi other than *Candida* involved. Local factors predisposing to an outbreak of visible oral fungal lesions include smoking, the wearing of dentures, decreased salivation and the use of inhaled corticosteroids. In some individuals, however, the precipitating factor may be associated with systemic antibiotic or corticosteroid use or cancer chemotherapeutic treatment regimens. Although there is a variety of antifungal agents, miconazole (oral gel) and nystatin (pastilles and oral suspension) are the most commonly used for oral candidiasis. In contrast, in severely immunocompromised patients, oral antifungal drugs such as fluconazole and ketoconazole are preferred. Only nystatin will be reviewed in this section (see Drug Monograph 34-1), as the azole antifungal agents are discussed in Chapter 52.

Saliva substitutes

Saliva substitutes such as Aquae are used for the relief of dry mouth caused by factors such as salivary gland dysfunction or occurring as a result of drug administration (e.g. anticholinergics). Available as solutions and as pump sprays, saliva substitutes contain electrolytes (potassium, magnesium, calcium and sodium chloride), potassium phosphate, saccharin, sorbitol solution and carboxymethylcellulose as the base.

Drugs used to treat mouth blistering

Acute viral diseases such as herpes simplex, herpes zoster and varicella are treated symptomatically with antipyretic analgesics such as paracetamol and aspirin. In worsening

---

DRUG MONOGRAPH 34-1   NYSTATIN

Nystatin is a product of *Streptomyces noursei* and was one of the first antibiotics to be discovered and used clinically.

MECHANISM OF ACTION It is thought to exert its effect by interacting with sterols in the cell wall and membrane, causing leakage of essential intracellular components such as ions, amino acids and sugars.

PHARMACOKINETICS Nystatin is not absorbed from mucous membranes of the mouth, (GI) tract and vagina or from the skin. Due to systemic toxicity, its use is limited to the treatment of mucocutaneous and intestinal candidiasis.

DRUG INTERACTIONS Nystatin is not metabolised and no drug interactions have been documented.

ADVERSE REACTIONS The most common adverse reactions of nausea, vomiting and diarrhoea occur more frequently with higher doses.

WARNINGS AND CONTRAINDICATIONS Nystatin is contraindicated in people with a previous history of hypersensitivity to the drug. As GI absorption is negligible, use in pregnancy is considered safe (ADEC category A).

DOSAGE AND ADMINISTRATION The dose ranges from 500,000 to 1,000,000 units 3–4 times daily and is taken as a suspension, tablet, capsule or lozenge. In general, the preparation should be held within the mouth for as long as possible to increase contact time with the mucosa.

cases and in recurrent herpetic infection, treatment with the antiviral drug aciclovir should be considered. Aciclovir acts to reduce viral shedding, time to crusting, duration of local pain, and severity of symptoms, and is available in oral and parenteral dosage forms. Aciclovir and other antiviral agents are covered in Chapter 52. In addition to viral infections, mouth lesions can be caused by local irritation, medications, radiation, dental manipulations or systemic disease. Instituting proper treatment involves initial identification of the causative factor.

DRUGS THAT AFFECT THE STOMACH

Conditions of the stomach requiring drug therapy include hyperacidity, ulcer disease, nausea, vomiting and hypermotility. Some of the drugs used for these conditions are not unique in their treatment of gastric dysfunction but are members of other major groups of drugs, such as anticholinergics, antihistamines and antidepressants.

Antacids

Antacids are chemical compounds that buffer or neutralise hydrochloric acid in the stomach and thereby raise the gastric pH. They have been used for centuries, often in the form of 'baking soda' (sodium bicarbonate), and are indicated for the relief of symptoms associated with **peptic ulcer disease**, gastritis, gastro-oesophageal reflux disease (GORD) and dyspepsia. The major ingredients in antacids include aluminium hydroxide, calcium carbonate, magnesium salts

and sodium bicarbonate, alone or in combination. Heartburn, indigestion and stomach upset are common and most antacids may be purchased as OTC preparations. These include Dexsal, Gastrogel, Gaviscon, Mylanta, Quick-Eze and Salvital.

Antacid combinations

Although there are many antacid preparations on the market, the magnesium–aluminium combinations (e.g. Mylanta, Gaviscon) are among the most common antacids selected by individuals and health-care professionals. Combination antacids have been formulated to reduce the risk of diarrhoea or constipation as an adverse effect. In some formulations, alginic acid or simethicone may also be included. Gaviscon contains alginic acid, which forms a viscous cohesive foam; this is thought to be beneficial in reflux oesophagitis by increasing adherence of mucus to the lower oesophageal mucosa. Simethicone, a defoaming agent, relieves flatulence by dispersing and preventing the formation of mucus-surrounded gas pockets in the GI tract.

Dosage and administration

The amount of antacid needed to neutralise hydrochloric acid depends on the individual, the condition being treated and the buffering capability of the preparation used. The acid-neutralising property of antacids varies and is defined as the quantity (milliequivalents [mEq]) of hydrochloric acid brought to a pH of 3.5 in 15 minutes (Table 34-1). The maximum dosages listed on antacid packages should be followed; however, many individuals exceed the recommendations, thus increasing the potential for producing many of the adverse reactions.

TABLE 34–1 Antacids: acid-neutralising capacity

ANTACID	PRIMARY INGREDIENTS	ACID-NEUTRALISING CAPACITY
Liquid preparations		**(mEq/5 mL)**
Dexsal Antacid Liquid	Calcium carbonate, simethicone	12.5
Gelusil	Aluminium hydroxide, magnesium hydroxide, simethicone	12
Mylanta Original	Aluminium hydroxide, magnesium hydroxide, simethicone	12.7
Mylanta Double Strength	Aluminium hydroxide, magnesium hydroxide, simethicone	25.4
Tablet preparations		**(mEq/tablet)**
Gelusil	Aluminium hydroxide, magnesium hydroxide, simethicone	11
Mylanta Original	Aluminium hydroxide, magnesium hydroxide, simethicone	11.5
Mylanta Double Strength	Aluminium hydroxide, magnesium hydroxide, simethicone	23
Andrews Tums	Calcium carbonate	10

Source: United States Pharmacopeial Convention 1998.

Antacids are considered either rapid-acting (e.g. sodium bicarbonate) or less rapid-acting (e.g. aluminium hydroxide). When administered in a fasting state, the antacid effect lasts 20–40 minutes. If administered 1 hour after meals, the effects may be extended for up to 3 hours. Liquid and powder dosage forms have been found to be more effective antacids than the tablet dosage form. Most tablets require chewing before swallowing to ensure complete dissolution of the antacid in the stomach. Absorption of antacids varies, and those that contain aluminium, calcium or magnesium are absorbed to a lesser extent than those containing sodium bicarbonate. Most of the unreacted insoluble antacids are excreted in the faeces.

In people with normal renal function, absorption of cations (e.g. Al^{3+}, Mg^{2+}, Ca^{2+}) causes little in the way of systemic problems; however, in the presence of renal insufficiency, absorption of, for example, Ca^{2+} may cause hypercalcaemia. As sodium bicarbonate is also absorbed in the intestine, prolonged use of this antacid should be avoided, particularly in people with heart failure or hypertension and those on sodium-restricted diets. Additionally, antacids should be avoided in the presence of coexisting conditions such as constipation (worsened by aluminium) or diarrhoea (aggravated by magnesium).

Antacids are generally considered safe for use in pregnancy if prolonged or high doses are avoided (ADEC category A). A concise list of adverse reactions is shown in Table 34-2.

Drug interactions

Antacid–drug interactions depend on the composition of the antacid used; in general, antacids have been reported most frequently to reduce or delay the absorption of many drugs. In some instances the reverse occurs and, in particular, antacids containing magnesium hydroxide can increase the absorption of some hypoglycaemic drugs, thus potentially placing the

DRUG INTERACTIONS 34-1 Antacids

Drug	Possible drug interactions
Captopril (angiotensin-converting enzyme inhibitor)	Decreased bioavailability. Separate the administration of these drugs by at least 2 hours
Quinolones	Aluminium- and magnesium-containing antacids can reduce absorption and effect of these drugs. Advise taking antacid at least 6 hours before or 2 hours after quinolone
Isoniazid	Aluminium hydroxide gel decreases the absorption of isoniazid. Separate the administration of these drugs by at least 2 hours
Ketoconazole	Increased gastric pH may decrease absorption of ketoconazole. Advise patients to take antacids at least 2 hours after ketoconazole
Tetracyclines (oral)	Antacids may combine with tetracyclines, decreasing their absorption in the GI tract. Advise patients to take antacids at least 3–4 hours before or after tetracycline

For a comprehensive list of interactions, see Maton & Burton 1999.

TABLE 34-2 Adverse reactions associated with antacids

CONSTITUENT OF ANTACID	ADVERSE REACTIONS*	CONTRAINDICATION/COEXISTING CONDITIONS
Aluminium hydroxide	Constipation, chalky taste, phosphate depletion, faecal impaction, intestinal obstruction, encephalopathy	Chronic renal failure because of increased risk of aluminium toxicity.
Calcium carbonate	Belching, flatulence, constipation, abdominal distension, hypercalcaemia, alkalosis, phosphate depletion, renal calculi, milk-alkali syndrome	Hypercalcaemia, hyperparathyroidism, renal impairment (increased risk of hypercalcaemia)
Sodium bicarbonate	Belching, abdominal distension, metabolic alkalosis (high doses), hyperventilation, hypokalaemia, hyperirritability, tetany, volume overload, pulmonary oedema	Metabolic or respiratory alkalosis, chloride depletion, hypoventilation, oedema associated with heart failure, renal failure or cirrhosis, renal impairment (increased risk of sodium retention)
Magnesium salts	Diarrhoea, chalky taste, belching, elevated plasma magnesium	Diarrhoea (may be aggravated), renal impairment (increased risk of raised plasma magnesium)

*Adverse reactions are listed in order of most common through to rare (AMH 2006).

person at risk of hypoglycaemia. Additionally, the urinary alkalinising (increased pH) effect of sodium bicarbonate can enhance the effect of amphetamines, quinidine, ephedrine and pseudoephedrine. Health-care professionals should be aware of the need for careful scheduling of antacids, as most medications need to be separated by at least 2 hours from an antacid. See the Drug Interactions table 34-1 for antacids.

DRUGS FOR NAUSEA AND VOMITING

There are numerous causes of nausea and vomiting, and treatment differs for acute situations such as pregnancy and gastroenteritis, chronic situations such as gastric or metabolic diseases, and psychogenic vomiting such as that occurring with bulimia. Control of vomiting is important and at times it can be very difficult, which can be distressing to the individual concerned.

Antiemetics

Vomiting is a complex process involving multiple nerve pathways and neurotransmitters (e.g. acetylcholine, histamine, dopamine, substance P and 5-hydroxytryptamine; see Chapter 33). **Antiemetics** act principally by blocking these neurotransmitters in the vomiting centre, the cerebral cortex, the chemoreceptor trigger zone (CTZ), or the vestibular apparatus. A variety of miscellaneous drugs are also used to control vomiting; these include corticosteroids (dexamethasone and methylprednisolone); benzodiazepines (lorazepam), which are used primarily for their sedative and anxiety-relieving actions; and the common spice ginger (*Zingiber officinale*).

The neurotransmitters and drugs used to control and prevent nausea and vomiting are summarised in Table 34-3.

Cancer chemotherapy-induced vomiting

Vomiting caused by cancer chemotherapy and radiotherapy can be severe enough that treatment can be delayed, and many individuals vehemently refuse further treatment. Often when cancer chemotherapeutic agents are used in combination, the emetogenic potentials of the agents are additive. Typically, vomiting starts within 4 hours of treatment, peaks towards 10 hours and subsides over the following 12–24 hours. Delayed vomiting can occur with high-dose cisplatin and can last 3–5 days. It is not surprising that anticipation of therapy and the sight and smell of the hospital can trigger nausea and vomiting in as many as 25% of individuals.

CLINICAL INTEREST BOX 34-3 MILK–ALKALI SYNDROME

The earliest record of a reaction to milk and alkali was described by Hippocrates more than 2000 years ago, but during the 1920s and 1930s, when 'Sippy' (antacid) powders were widely used for heartburn and indigestion, cases of milk–alkali syndrome were widespread. Reports continue to appear, and the characteristic features of the syndrome arising from prolonged and excessive intake of milk and antacids are irritability, distaste for milk, occasional nausea and vomiting, headache, mental confusion, anorexia, muscle ache, weakness and malaise. Impairment of renal function ensues, with elevated plasma calcium, phosphorus and bicarbonate. Calcium and phosphate precipitate in the kidney tubules, contributing to the renal damage. The syndrome has a reported mortality of around 5%.

TABLE 34-3 Drugs for controlling nausea and vomiting, and the associated neurotransmitters

NEUROTRANSMITTER AND RECEPTOR	DRUG CLASS	ANTIEMETIC AGENT
Dopamine acting via (D$_2$) receptors located in the stomach and CTZ	Dopamine antagonists	Domperidone, droperidol, haloperidol, metoclopramide, prochlorperazine
Acetylcholine receptors in the vestibular and vomiting centres. Overstimulation of the labyrinth (inner ear) results in the nausea and vomiting of motion sickness	Muscarinic receptor antagonists (anticholinergics)	Hyoscine
Histamine (H$_1$) receptors in vestibular and vomiting centres	H$_1$ receptor antagonists (antihistamines)	Dimenhydrinate, promethazine
5-hydroxytryptamine (5-HT$_3$) receptors in the GI tract, CTZ and vomiting centres	5-HT$_3$ receptor antagonists	Dolasetron, granisetron, ondansetron, tropisetron
Substance P acting via neurokinin-1 (NK$_1$) receptors located in CNS	NK$_1$ receptor antagonist	Aprepitant

Because antiemetics are usually more effective in preventing vomiting than they are in treating it, they should be administered (often in high doses) prophylactically before cytotoxic therapy. Chemotherapy-induced vomiting may also require several antiemetic agents with different sites of action for effectiveness, e.g. metoclopramide and lorazepam, metoclopramide and dexamethasone, or prochlorperazine and dexamethasone. In addition to drug therapy, behavioural and psychological support should be provided.

Dopamine antagonists

Drugs within this class include prochlorperazine and **metoclopramide** (see Drug Monograph 34-2). Prochlorperazine is a phenothiazine derivative with antiemetic effects, probably by an inhibitory action on the CTZ and vomiting centre. Phenothiazines are thought to act mainly as D_2-receptor antagonists but they also have antihistamine and antimuscarinic properties. Only their actions relevant to nausea and vomiting are discussed here; other information on phenothiazines and their use as antipsychotic drugs can be found in Chapter 19.

Prochlorperazine is indicated for the treatment of nausea and vomiting due to causes such as migraine and vertigo, as in Ménière's syndrome. Use is contraindicated where there is evidence of previous hypersensitivity to phenothiazines and in situations of CNS depression. Adverse reactions are common and include constipation, dry mouth, sleepiness, dizziness, blurred vision and extrapyramidal effects (parkinsonism in the elderly and dystonia in younger people). Less common reactions include skin rash, hypotension, peripheral oedema, agranulocytosis and cholestatic jaundice. Prochlorperazine (ADEC pregnancy category C) is considered safe for use during lactation. (For additional information, including phenothiazine warnings and contraindications, see Chapter 19.)

Muscarinic receptor antagonists (anticholinergics)

Hyoscine hydrobromide is a competitive antagonist of the actions of acetylcholine at muscarinic receptors and is used to prevent motion-induced (sea, air, car, train) nausea and vomiting by depressing conduction in the labyrinth of the

DRUG MONOGRAPH 34-2 METOCLOPRAMIDE

Metoclopramide is used for diabetic gastroparesis, gastro-oesophageal reflux, and parenterally for the prevention of nausea and vomiting secondary to emetogenic cancer chemotherapeutic agents, radiation and opioid medications. It is also used as an adjunct for GI radiological examinations because it hastens barium's transit through the upper GI tract by its stimulation of gastric emptying and acceleration of intestinal transit. Parenteral metoclopramide may be used to facilitate small-intestinal intubation.

MECHANISM OF ACTION Metoclopramide has both central and peripheral actions in preventing or relieving nausea and vomiting. Centrally it blocks dopamine (D_2) receptors in the CTZ (in high doses 5-HT_3 antagonism may be observed), while peripherally it accelerates gastric emptying, reduces reflux from the duodenum and stomach into the oesophagus, and enhances motility of the upper GI tract. These latter effects may be mediated through an action on muscarinic cholinergic systems within the GI tract.

PHARMACOKINETICS Metoclopramide is almost completely absorbed following oral dosing, and peak plasma concentrations occur 30–180 min after oral administration, 10–15 min after an IM dose and within 5–20 min of an IV dose. The half-life in plasma is 2.5–5 h. Metoclopramide is extensively metabolised by the liver (about 70%) and excreted in urine.

DRUG INTERACTIONS An additive CNS depressant effect is observed with a combination of metoclopramide and CNS depressant drugs. Avoid this combination or a potentially serious drug interaction could occur. Changes in absorption affect the plasma concentrations of cyclosporin and digoxin which should be monitored and dosage adjustments made if indicated. In surgical patients, metoclopramide can reduce inactivation of succinylcholine and hence prolong neuromuscular blockade.

ADVERSE REACTIONS These include diarrhoea, sleepiness, restlessness, dizziness, headache, extrapyramidal (parkinsonian) effects, hypotension, tachycardia and, rarely, agranulocytosis and tardive dyskinesia (see Chapter 19).

WARNINGS AND CONTRAINDICATIONS Metoclopramide is contraindicated where a previous reaction to dopamine antagonists has been reported, and in phaeochromocytoma because of a risk of a hypertensive crisis. The drug should be used with caution in Parkinson's disease and depression, as it can worsen the symptoms. Dosage reduction (25%–50%) should be considered in situations of severe renal impairment, and low doses used in children because of an increased risk of extrapyramidal adverse effects.

DOSAGE AND ADMINISTRATION To treat diabetic gastroparesis or gastro-oesophageal reflux in an adult, the oral dose of metoclopramide is 10 mg four times daily. The adult antiemetic dose (for chemotherapy-induced emesis) is 1–3 mg/kg by IV infusion over 15 min; 10–40 mg every 4 h by IV injection. Nausea and vomiting in children is treated with a dose of 0.15 mg/kg every 6–8 h as needed. The maximum dose is 0.5 mg/kg/day for all age groups.
Source: AMH 2006

inner ear. Overstimulation in this area is responsible for the nausea and vomiting of motion sickness common in ocean yacht races. Hyoscine is partially metabolised in the liver and excreted by the kidneys. The adverse effects of hyoscine are related to its anticholinergic effects; these include dry mouth, tachycardia, blurring of vision and, less commonly, constipation, mental confusion, fatigue and restlessness and irritability. Administration is recommended 30 minutes prior to travel. Travacalm contains dimenhydrinate, hyoscine hydrobromide and caffeine.

5-HT₃-receptor antagonists

Ondansetron, dolasetron, granisetron and tropisetron are selective 5-hydroxytryptamine (5-HT, serotonin) antagonists (see Drug Monograph 34-3). 5-HT receptors are located peripherally on the vagus nerve terminal and centrally in the CTZ. One theory is that cancer chemotherapeutic agents cause the release of stored 5-HT from the enterochromaffin cells of the GI tract (Veyrat-Follet et al 1997). The 5-HT stimulates 5-HT receptors located in the vagus nerve in the GI tract, which then stimulates 5-HT receptors in the CTZ, inducing vomiting. When ondansetron is administered before antineoplastic therapy, the 5-HT receptors in the brainstem and GI tract are blocked. As a result, 5-HT released in response to the administration of antineoplastic agents cannot bind with the 5-HT receptors and thus vomiting is prevented.

Aprepitant

Substance P, a neurotransmitter that acts on neurokinin-1 (NK_1) receptors, is widely distributed in the CNS. It is thought to be involved in pain transmission and emetic pathways. Aprepitant is a new oral NK_1 receptor antagonist that acts centrally to control, in particular, chemotherapy-induced vomiting. It is most effective when used in combination with a $5HT_3$ receptor antagonist and dexamethasone. Currently, its use in combination with other antiemetic drugs has not been fully investigated. As a consequence of its metabolism by CYP3A4, potential drug interactions are likely with agents such as ketoconazole (an inhibitor of CYP3A4) and dexamethasone (a substrate for CYP3A4). When aprepitant is used concomitantly with oral dexamethasone, the dose of dexamethasone is halved. At present there are no data for its use in severe hepatic impairment; in children; or in pregnancy (ADEC category B1) and lactation. Common adverse effects include diarrhoea, fatigue, headache, hiccoughs and, rarely, angio-oedema and urticaria.

Corticosteroids

Corticosteroids have been reported to be effective for chemotherapy-induced nausea and vomiting, either alone or when used in combination with other antiemetics. The mechanism of action is unknown, but it has been proposed that these drugs may inhibit prostaglandin synthesis and decrease 5-HT turnover in the CNS, which might be involved in cancer chemotherapy-induced vomiting. Research has indicated that certain prostaglandins (especially the E series) can induce nausea and vomiting.

Many studies with corticosteroids have involved the use of dexamethasone and methylprednisolone. Their effectiveness

as antiemetics was a serendipitous discovery—it was noticed patients receiving various chemotherapeutic regimens had less nausea and vomiting when corticosteroids were one of the agents administered. It has since been established that the addition of corticosteroids to an antiemetic regimen enhances overall the antiemetic effect and can diminish the severity of some of the adverse reactions, e.g. diarrhoea. A full discussion of the pharmacology of corticosteroids can be found in Chapter 40.

DRUGS USED TO TREAT PEPTIC ULCER DISEASE

Treatment regimens for peptic ulcer disease have varied enormously over the years and are still undergoing rapid change. Drugs used include antacids, anticholinergics, antidepressants, anxiolytics, H_2-receptor antagonists, proton pump inhibitors, and **cytoprotective agents** (substances that protect cells from damage) such as sucralfate and the prostaglandin analogue misoprostol. The following section is limited to those drugs not covered elsewhere in this book: proton pump inhibitors, H_2-receptor antagonists, prostaglandin analogues and cytoprotective agents. See the Geriatric Implications box for antiulcer therapies.

Helicobacter pylori treatment regimens

It is now well established that infection with *Helicobacter pylori* causes chronic active gastritis, is associated with the development of gastric and duodenal ulcers, and is implicated in the development of gastric carcinoma. Eradication of *H. pylori* is considered first-line treatment because it vastly improves the odds of non-recurrence of the ulcer. Early therapies involved use of a single drug such as an antibiotic, a proton pump inhibitor or bismuth, but monotherapy was found to be effective in less than 30% of people so combinations were developed. The first 'triple therapy', which included bismuth, metronidazole and tetracycline, was effective in eradicating *H. pylori* in about 90% of people, but adverse effects were common.

Undoubtedly the most successful therapy is three drugs administered twice a day for 1 week. However, there is still debate as to whether the duration of therapy for successful eradication (while limiting both drug resistance and adverse effects) should be increased to 10–14 days.

Current triple therapy regimens include:
- proton pump inhibitor (PPI), clarithromycin and amoxycillin (>90% eradication)
- PPI, clarithromycin and metronidazole (>80% eradication)
- PPI, amoxycillin and metronidazole (>80% eradication)

**GERIATRIC IMPLICATIONS
ANTIULCER THERAPIES**

Gastrointestinal symptoms are very common in elderly patients, and a thorough evaluation should be conducted before instituting drug therapy.

Acid secretion reaches its peak during sleep, between the hours of 10 pm and the early morning hours (Covington 1996). Therefore H_2-receptor antagonists prescribed as a daily dose are usually taken at bedtime.

Confusion and dizziness following administration of cimetidine are more commonly reported by the elderly than by younger adults. The acute confusional state usually resolves with discontinuation of the therapy.

For many antiulcer therapies, dosage adjustment may be necessary in elderly patients with impaired renal function.

When H_2-receptor antagonists are prescribed with antacids, schedule medications at least 2 hours apart, as absorption is reduced by concurrent administration.

- PPI, bismuth subcitrate, metronidazole and tetracycline (>70% eradication).

Within Australia, the most commonly prescribed twice-daily combination is omeprazole (20 mg), clarithromycin (500 mg) and amoxycillin (1000 mg) (Medicare Australia Health Statistics 2005). Combining the individual agents in a single packet helps simplify a complicated drug schedule, and omeprazole, clarithromycin and amoxycillin are available in Australia and New Zealand as a 'single script' combination pack (Klacid Hp7 and Nexium Hp7).

The success of *H. pylori* eradication hinges on adherence to therapy and susceptibility of the bacterium to the antibiotics. The 1-week regimens with lower instances of adverse reactions have a high adherence rate (>95%), whereas therapies over 10 days tend to have much higher discontinuation rates. Bacterial resistance is an ever-increasing problem, and resistance of *H. pylori* strains to clarithromycin hinders success in about 10% of the population in the United States, south-western Europe and Japan, and in about 20% of the Australian population (AMH 2006).

Proton pump inhibitors

Proton pump inhibitors suppress gastric acid secretion by inhibiting the hydrogen–potassium adenosine triphosphatase (ATPase) enzyme system at the secretory surface of the gastric parietal cells (see Figure 33-3). These drugs are weak bases that reach the parietal cells from the blood and diffuse into the secretory canaliculi of the parietal cells. There the drugs become trapped because of the addition of a hydrogen ion (protonation). When sufficient molecules of drug bind to the proton pump, they block the final step of acid production, inhibiting both basal and stimulated gastric acid secretion. The first of these drugs to be developed was **omeprazole** (see Drug Monograph 34-4), which binds irreversibly to the proton pump; others now developed and released in Australia include lansoprazole, pantoprazole, rabeprazole and esomeprazole.

H₂-receptor antagonists

Histamine, found in the mucosal cells of the GI tract, activates H₂ receptors to increase gastric acid secretion. The major components of gastric secretion include hydrochloric acid and intrinsic factor, produced by the parietal (acid-forming) cells; pepsinogen, synthesised by the chief cells; and mucus. The principal function of mucus is to protect the epithelial cells of the GI tract from attack by pepsin and irritation by the HCl secreted by the stomach. Pepsinogen, an enzyme, is the precursor of pepsin; HCl catalyses the cleavage of pepsinogen to active pepsin and provides a low-pH environment in which pepsin can initiate the digestion of proteins.

Gastric secretion is regulated by a neural mechanism, parasympathetic (vagus) fibres and the hormone gastrin. Activation of the vagus nerve causes secretion of vast quantities of pepsinogen and HCl. In contrast, the hormonal mechanism involves the actual presence of food, which distends the stomach and stimulates the antral mucosa to

---

DRUG MONOGRAPH 34-4 OMEPRAZOLE

Omeprazole, the prototype drug, is indicated for the treatment of peptic ulcer disease, severe erosive oesophagitis that occurs with gastro-oesophageal reflux, and long-term treatment of hypersecretory gastric conditions such as Zollinger–Ellison syndrome.

PHARMACOKINETICS After a single oral dose, omeprazole's onset of action as indicated by decreased gastric acid secretion is within 1 hour, its peak effect in 2 hours, and its duration of action is 3–5 days (time needed for return of secretory activity). It is almost completely metabolised in the liver by cytochromes P450 (CYP2C19 and CYP3A4), and the metabolites are excreted in urine (about 80%) and faeces (about 20%).

DRUG INTERACTIONS In view of its metabolism by cytochromes P450, interactions with other drugs should be expected. Concurrent administration of omeprazole with diazepam or phenytoin can lead to increased plasma concentrations, and dosage reduction might be necessary. Similarly, coadministration with warfarin can lead to increased anticoagulation, and monitoring of the INR should be considered (for a review of drug interactions see Andersson 1991).

ADVERSE REACTIONS Omeprazole is generally well tolerated. Minor adverse effects include abdominal pain, dizziness, headache, nausea, vomiting, diarrhoea, flatulence and skin rash. Rare adverse reactions include agranulocytosis, pancytopenia, thrombocytopenia and increased liver enzymes.

WARNINGS AND CONTRAINDICATIONS Avoid use in people with omeprazole hypersensitivity and during pregnancy (ADEC category B3). Care should be exercised in patients with impaired hepatic function because of risk of accumulation of the drug when high doses are used.

DOSAGE AND ADMINISTRATION The adult oral dose for gastro-oesophageal reflux is 20–40 mg daily for 4 weeks. For gastric hypersecretory conditions, the maintenance dose is 20–120 mg daily, adjusting as necessary. The capsule formulation should not be opened, crushed or chewed, as the drug will degrade in the acidic environment of the stomach.

TABLE 34-4 H$_2$-receptor antagonists pharmacokinetics (oral administration)					
Drug	Absorption	Time to peak plasma concentration	Half-life (h)	Duration of action (h)	% Metabolism excretion
Cimetidine	>90%	45–90 min	2	4–5 basal, 6–8 nocturnal	Liver (about 25%)/kidneys
Famotidine	40%–45%	1–3 hours	2.5–4	10–12 basal and nocturnal	Liver (5%)/kidneys
Nizatidine	>70%	0.5–3 hours	1–2	Up to 8 basal, up to 12 nocturnal	Liver (about 35%)/kidneys
Ranitidine	50%	1–3 hours	2–3	Up to 4 basal, up to 13 nocturnal	Liver (about 25%)/kidneys

DRUG INTERACTIONS 34-2
H$_2$-Receptor antagonists

Drug	Possible effect and management
Ketoconazole	Reduced effect. Choose another antifungal
Phenytoin/ carbamazepine	Risk of toxicity. Monitor plasma anticonvulsant concentration
Tricyclic antidepressants	Increased incidence of adverse reactions. Monitor patient
Theophylline	Risk of toxicity. Monitor plasma theophylline concentration
Warfarin	Increased anticoagulation. Monitor international normalised ratio (INR)

release gastrin. This hormone is then absorbed into the blood and carried to the parietal cells and chief cells that secrete HCl and pepsinogen, respectively. Histamine is believed to activate the gastric mucosa in much the same way as gastrin does. In addition, caffeine and alcohol are potent stimuli for gastrin release. When the pH of the gastric juice drops to 2, a negative feedback mechanism helps block production of gastric secretion from the parietal and chief cells. Inhibition of gastric gland secretion thus plays an essential role in protecting the stomach against excessively acidic secretions, which are responsible for causing peptic ulcerations.

Normally, the mucosal surface of the stomach and upper duodenum is protected from the irritation of gastric acid by a layer of mucus. If a circumscribed area of the mucosal surface is damaged and fails to repair rapidly, it can become eroded, forming an ulcer. Exposure of this inflamed region to gastric acid causes pain.

The H$_2$-receptor antagonists include cimetidine, **ranitidine**, famotidine and nizatidine. They competitively block histamine from stimulating the H$_2$ receptors located on the gastric parietal cells, thus reducing the volume of gastric acid secretion (from stimuli such as food, histamine, caffeine and insulin). These drugs are indicated for treatment of peptic ulcer disease, GORD and dyspepsia, and for stress ulcer prophylaxis. The pharmacokinetics of these agents are summarised in Table 34-4.

In general, these drugs are well tolerated. Common adverse reactions include diarrhoea, constipation, headache, dizziness, rash, and confusion in the elderly. Cimetidine can cause breast swelling, impotence and decreased libido. The less common and rare adverse effects include hypotension, hepatitis, agranulocytosis, thrombocytopenia and bradyarrhythmias.

Dosage varies, depending on the condition being treated (peptic ulcer disease, GORD, dyspepsia, stress ulcer prophylaxis). Consult the relevant drug information sources for dosing recommendations. If impaired renal function is a coexisting condition, dosage reduction may be necessary. Safety in pregnancy has not been established (ADEC category B1).

Drug interactions

Because cimetidine, unlike the other H$_2$-receptor antagonists, inhibits the metabolism of other drugs by the cytochrome P450 system, drug interactions have been noted with many drugs, including oral anticoagulants, phenytoin, theophylline, nifedipine, lignocaine and tricyclic antidepressants. See the Drug Interactions table 34-2 for H$_2$-receptor antagonists.

In addition, all the H$_2$-receptor antagonists reduce the bioavailability of drugs that require an acidic environment for absorption.

Cytoprotective agents

Protection of the gastric and duodenal mucosa is aided by secretion of bicarbonate ions into a mucus layer that protects the underlying epithelial cells against erosion from gastric acid. **Cytoprotective agents** enhance the protection afforded by the mucus layer by providing a physical barrier over the ulcerated surface. The two main agents are sucralfate and the prostaglandin analogue misoprostol.

Sucralfate

Sucralfate is composed of sulfated sucrose and aluminium hydroxide. In the presence of acid, it undergoes a chemical reaction that results in formation of a sticky, yellow–white gel that forms a protective, acid-resistant shield in the ulcer crater. This barrier hastens the healing of the ulcer by protecting the mucosa for up to 6 hours. The binding to the ulcer crater is thought to be the main therapeutic effect, but sucralfate also stimulates production of mucus and protective prostaglandins. It is administered orally with minimal systemic absorption (up to 5%) and is excreted primarily by the faecal route. This product is indicated for short-term (up to 8 weeks) peptic ulcer treatment and for the prevention of stress-induced ulcers.

See the Drug Interactions table 34-3 for sucralfate. The most common adverse reaction is constipation, which occurs in 1%–15% of patients. Infrequently, there are reports of nausea, vomiting, dry mouth, dizziness, back pain, rash and headache.

The adult dose for peptic ulcer disease is 1 g four times daily (1 hour before each meal and at bedtime; maximum 8 g daily) for 4–8 weeks, with a maintenance regimen of 1 g twice daily on an empty stomach. For prophylaxis of stress ulcers, 1 g every 4 hours.

Misoprostol

Misoprostol, a synthetic analogue of prostaglandin E_1, is indicated for the treatment of peptic ulcers and the prevention of gastric ulcers associated with the use of non-steroidal anti-inflammatory drugs (NSAIDs). Normally, prostaglandins of the E and I series (see Chapter 54) protect the stomach by decreasing gastric acid secretion and increasing gastric cytoprotective mucus and bicarbonate. The NSAIDs inhibit prostaglandin synthesis, which reduces the effectiveness of the protective mechanisms and can result in gastric ulcer formation. Misoprostol suppresses gastric acid secretion and thus helps to heal gastric ulcers.

Misoprostol is rapidly absorbed after oral administration and is metabolised by fatty acid oxidising systems to an active metabolite, misoprostol acid, which is further metabolised. Less than 1% of the dose is excreted as unchanged drug; renal elimination accounts for 75% and faecal elimination for about 15%. No significant drug interactions have been reported. Infrequent adverse reactions reported include constipation, gas, headache, nausea and vomiting. In about 30% of people, diarrhoea limits its usefulness.

As misoprostol can cause hypotension in patients with cerebrovascular and coronary artery disease, it should be used with caution in these groups. Importantly, as misoprostol can

DRUG INTERACTIONS 34-3 Sucralfate	
Drug	**Possible effect and management**
Antacids	Concurrent use can interfere with sucralfate binding, thus reducing its effect. Administer antacids at least 2 hours after sucralfate administration
Ciprofloxacin, norfloxacin, ofloxacin, tetracyclines	Decreased absorption and bioavailability of these antibiotics. Advise patients to take antibiotics 2–3 hours before sucralfate
Digoxin, theophylline, phenytoin	Decreased absorption and bioavailability. Avoid concurrent administration or advise patients to take these drugs at least 2 hours before sucralfate. Monitor plasma concentration of these drugs and adjust dose if necessary

induce premature labour and may be teratogenic in large doses, it should not be used in pregnant women or in those contemplating pregnancy (ADEC Category X).

For treatment of peptic ulcer disease, the adult dose is 0.8 mg daily in 2–4 divided doses for 4–8 weeks. For prevention of NSAID-induced ulcers, 0.4–0.8 mg daily (2–4 divided doses) is used for the duration of the NSAID treatment.

PANCREATIC ENZYME SUPPLEMENTS

The pancreas releases digestive enzymes and bicarbonate into the duodenum to help in the digestion of fats, carbohydrates and proteins. Bicarbonate neutralises acid and thus helps to protect the enzymes from both acid and pepsin. When acid chyme enters the duodenum, vagal stimulation regulates pancreatic secretion, and enzyme replacement therapy may be necessary for patients who have had the vagal fibres surgically severed or who have had surgical procedures that cause food to bypass the duodenum. In addition, replacement therapy is usually necessary in exocrine pancreatic enzyme deficiency states, chronic pancreatitis, cystic fibrosis, pancreatic tumours and pancreatic obstruction.

The supplements are all of porcine origin and contain principally lipase with protease and amylase. If possible, use enteric-coated products because the microsphere formulation resists gastric inactivation, so the enzymes reach the duodenum to hydrolyse fats into glycerol and fatty acids, proteins into peptides, and starch into dextrins and sugars.

The most common adverse reactions include nausea, vomiting and abdominal pain. Hyperuricaemia and intestinal obstruction occur rarely. Dosage should be adjusted as necessary to suit the individual, and is guided by the quality and quantity of stools. Use of these products should be avoided in people with hypersensitivity to pork proteins.

DRUGS THAT AFFECT THE BILIARY SYSTEM

Ursodeoxycholic acid is a minor constituent of human bile. Its administration results in a change in bile acid composition and an increase in bile acid output and bile flow. It is indicated for the treatment of chronic cholestatic liver disease and cholestasis related to cystic fibrosis. There are limited data on its use in children and pregnant women (ADEC category B3). Drugs such as cholestyramine, colestipol, charcoal and antacids can bind ursodeoxycholic acid, resulting in reduced absorption of the drugs. In contrast, ursodeoxycholic acid may increase the absorption of cyclosporin, leading to an increased cyclosporin plasma concentration. Diarrhoea is a common adverse reaction.

DRUGS THAT AFFECT THE LOWER GASTROINTESTINAL TRACT

Bowel function is often a major concern, particularly constipation in the elderly and diarrhoea in children and immunosuppressed patients. **Constipation** is defined as difficult faecal evacuation as a result of hardness and perhaps infrequent movements. Everyone has regular bowel movements that range from three per day to three per week. Changes to bowel habits should be investigated thoroughly and causative factors eliminated before instituting drug therapy.

Chronic constipation is sometimes simply caused by a lack of dietary fibre and reduced fluid intake. Often, however, the underlying cause is organic disease such as tumours; bowel obstruction; metabolic abnormalities, such as diabetes mellitus or hypercalcaemia; rectal disorders; diseases of the liver, gallbladder or muscles; neurological abnormalities, such as multiple sclerosis and Parkinson's disease; or pregnancy. Other factors that contribute to constipation include a failure to respond to defecation impulses, a sedentary lifestyle characterised by insufficient exercise, and impaired physical mobility. In addition, constipation is an adverse reaction of many commonly used drugs, and simply changing or stopping drug therapy may be all that is required to restore normal bowel habit. Drugs causing constipation include aluminium

antacids, anticholinergics, tricyclic antidepressants, opioids and the calcium channel blocker verapamil.

The elderly also appear to have a higher incidence of constipation, often because of multiple illnesses that require a variety of medications. The ageing process itself is associated with a decline in both physiological function and physical activity, and people who suffer from disorders of the GI tract frequently complain of constipation (see Geriatric Implications box). On the other hand, a person may complain of constipation when no organic disease or lesion can be found.

Laxatives

Laxatives are drugs given to enhance transit of food through the intestine. The duration of treatment with laxatives should be as short as possible, and the desirability of limiting reliance on laxatives should be discussed with the person. Box 34-1 and Figure 34-1 summarise the types of laxatives.

Bulk-forming laxatives

The laxatives constituting this group are natural plant gums such as psyllium (ispaghula) husk (see Drug Monograph 34-5), bran and *Sterculia* and semisynthetic cellulose derivatives such as methylcellulose. These agents are polysaccharide polymers that are not broken down by normal digestive processes.

BOX 34-1 SELECTED TYPES OF LAXATIVES

Bulk laxatives absorb water and increase the volume, bulk and moisture of non-absorbable intestinal contents, thereby distending the bowel and initiating reflex bowel activity.

Faecal softening agents act as dispersing wetting agents, facilitating mixture of water and fatty substances within the faecal mass, producing soft faeces.

Stimulant laxatives promote accumulation of water and increase peristalsis in the colon by irritating intramural sensory nerve plexi endings in the mucosa.

Osmotic laxatives are not absorbed and, because they exert an osmotic effect, they increase the volume of fluid in the lumen.

Saline laxatives retain and increase the water content of faeces by virtue of an osmotic effect and stimulate peristalsis.

DRUG MONOGRAPH 34-5 PSYLLIUM

Ispaghula consists of the dried ripe seeds of *Plantago ovata*, commercially known as Spanish or French psyllium seed. Psyllium hydrophilic mucilloid (Metamucil) is a powder that contains around 50% powdered husk (outer epidermis) of psyllium seeds and 50% dextrose or sucrose. The husk swells rapidly in water and this mixture is used to treat constipation because it promotes the formation of a soft, water-retaining, gelatinous residue in the lower bowel within 12–72 hours. In addition, it has a demulcent effect on inflamed mucosa. Large quantities can cause abdominal distension and there is a risk of intestinal obstruction. In general, the dosage is in the order of 4–7 g, administered 1–3 times daily with 250 mL liquid (refer to the product information for full details).

They stimulate peristalsis by increasing the bulk of the stool through absorption of water in the colon. This mechanism of laxative action is a normal stimulus and is one of the least harmful. These drugs do not interfere with absorption of food, but need to be administered with sufficient fluids to ensure an adequate effect.

The effect of these laxatives may not be apparent for 12–24 hours, and their full effect may not be achieved until the second or third day after administration. Some health-care practitioners maintain that bran and dried fruits (e.g. prunes, prune juice and figs) exert the same effect, and they prefer to suggest these foods rather than the bulk-forming laxatives. Although bulk-forming laxatives are indicated for constipation, they have also been found to improve stool consistency in diarrhoea and for colostomy and ileostomy patients. Adverse reactions are minimal, the most commonly reported being flatulence and bulky stools.

Faecal softening agents

The faecal softening agents include docusate, liquid paraffin and poloxamer. They are commonly used to treat acute constipation and to prevent straining, e.g. after bowel surgery.

Docusate acts like a detergent, permitting water and fatty substances to penetrate and to become well mixed with the faecal material. It may also inhibit water absorption from the bowel and stimulate water secretion into the GI tract. Softened stools are usually excreted in 1–3 days after oral administration and about 15 minutes after rectal administration. These agents may be used for patients with rectal impaction, haemorrhoids, postpartum constipation and painful conditions of the rectum and anus, and for people who should avoid straining during defecation (e.g. after rectal surgery). Docusate may be useful for immobile patients, especially children. Adverse reactions are infrequent, and oral formulations should be given with plenty of fluid.

Liquid paraffin, a mixture of liquid hydrocarbons obtained from petroleum, is not digested and absorption is minimal. Liquid paraffin penetrates and coats the faecal mass and prevents excessive absorption of water. Liquid paraffin is especially useful when it is desirable to keep faeces soft and when straining must be avoided, as after abdominal surgery, rectal operations, repair of hernias, eye surgery, aneurysm or myocardial infarction, or for prevention of haemorrhoidal tearing.

Liquid paraffin can impair the absorption of fat-soluble vitamins A, D, E and K. If liquid paraffin is taken with meals, gastric emptying time may be delayed. An objection to its use is that in large doses it tends to leak or seep from the rectum, which can cause anal pruritus and interfere with healing of post operative wounds in the region of the anus and perineum. This leakage is often an embarrassment to the patient. Although absorption of liquid paraffin is limited, after prolonged use it may cause a chronic inflammatory reaction in tissues where it is found.

Stimulant laxatives

The principal stimulant laxatives are bisacodyl, sodium picosulfate and preparations of senna. These agents promote accumulation of water and electrolytes in the lumen, and stimulate nerve endings to increase intestinal motility. The stimulant laxatives usually act in 6–12 hours. Their primary effect is on the small and large intestines, which explains their tendency to produce cramping. Stimulant laxatives are used in preparation for diagnostic and surgical bowel procedures. Adverse effects of stimulant laxatives include abdominal cramping and fluid and electrolyte imbalance.

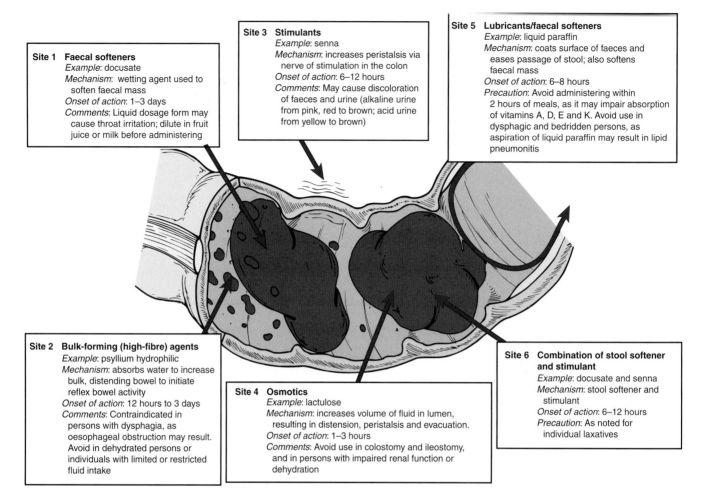

Site 1 Faecal softeners
Example: docusate
Mechanism: wetting agent used to soften faecal mass
Onset of action: 1–3 days
Comments: Liquid dosage form may cause throat irritation; dilute in fruit juice or milk before administering

Site 3 Stimulants
Example: senna
Mechanism: increases peristalsis via nerve of stimulation in the colon
Onset of action: 6–12 hours
Comments: May cause discoloration of faeces and urine (alkaline urine from pink, red to brown; acid urine from yellow to brown)

Site 5 Lubricants/faecal softeners
Example: liquid paraffin
Mechanism: coats surface of faeces and eases passage of stool; also softens faecal mass
Onset of action: 6–8 hours
Precaution: Avoid administering within 2 hours of meals, as it may impair absorption of vitamins A, D, E and K. Avoid use in dysphagic and bedridden persons, as aspiration of liquid paraffin may result in lipid pneumonitis

Site 2 Bulk-forming (high-fibre) agents
Example: psyllium hydrophilic
Mechanism: absorbs water to increase bulk, distending bowel to initiate reflex bowel activity
Onset of action: 12 hours to 3 days
Comments: Contraindicated in persons with dysphagia, as oesophageal obstruction may result. Avoid in dehydrated persons or individuals with limited or restricted fluid intake

Site 4 Osmotics
Example: lactulose
Mechanism: increases volume of fluid in lumen, resulting in distension, peristalsis and evacuation.
Onset of action: 1–3 hours
Comments: Avoid use in colostomy and ileostomy, and in persons with impaired renal function or dehydration

Site 6 Combination of stool softener and stimulant
Example: docusate and senna
Mechanism: stool softener and stimulant
Onset of action: 6–12 hours
Precaution: As noted for individual laxatives

FIGURE 34-1 Classification of laxatives according to site of action.

TABLE 34-5 Stimulant laxatives

NAME	ONSET OF ACTION (hours)	REMARKS
Bisacodyl	6–12 (oral)	To prevent premature dissolving of enteric coating and GI irritation, bisacodyl should not be taken with, or within 1 hour of ingestion of, milk or antacids
Sodium picosulfate	10–14	Often used in preparation for surgery
Senna	6–12	Crude senna may cause urine discoloration

With the exception of spinal patients, these agents are not recommended for regular use. Table 34-5 compares the stimulant laxatives in use today.

Bisacodyl is a relatively non-toxic laxative agent that stimulates peristalsis on contact with the mucosa of the colon. The enteric coating is formulated to dissolve in intestinal fluids and, when released, produces its stimulating effects on the colon. It should not be chewed, crushed or taken with milk or antacids because it can irritate the stomach, manifesting as severe abdominal cramps. If antacids are to be taken, they should be taken at least several hours apart from the bisacodyl. The tablets produce evacuation of the bowel in 6–12 hours, and suppositories and enemas act within 15–60 minutes. The suppositories may cause a burning sensation and proctitis.

Senna is obtained from the dried leaves of the *Cassia* plant. It produces a thorough bowel evacuation in 6–12 hours, and this may be accompanied by abdominal pain or gripping. It is found in proprietary remedies such as Laxettes, Sennetabs and Senokot.

DRUG MONOGRAPH 34-6 LACTULOSE

MECHANISM OF ACTION Lactulose is a semisynthetic disaccharide of galactose and fructose. In the GI tract, the normal colonic bacteria (*Lactobacillus* and *Bacteroides*, *Escherichia coli* and *Streptococcus faecalis*) metabolise lactulose to organic acids, primarily lactic, acetic and formic acids. These acids produce an osmotic effect, an increase in fluid accumulation, distension, peristalsis and bowel movement within 24–72 hours. Lactulose is indicated for constipation and is used to decrease blood ammonia levels in people with hepatic encephalopathy secondary to chronic liver disease. The latter effect is thought to result from the trapping by the lactulose of intestinal ammonia (as NH_4^+) and hence the excretion of excess ammonia in the faeces.

PHARMACOKINETICS Absorption is minimal (<1%) after oral administration; this exceedingly small dose is excreted via the kidneys.

DRUG INTERACTIONS The effectiveness of lactulose can be reduced if it is used concomitantly with an antibiotic that destroys the normal colonic bacteria. Conflicting reports exist regarding the concomitant use of neomycin and lactulose. Closer monitoring of patients should occur with concomitant oral antibiotic therapy.

ADVERSE REACTIONS These include flatulence, intestinal cramps, increased thirst and belching. Excessive doses might produce some diarrhoea and nausea (caused by the sweet taste).

CONTRAINDICATIONS Avoid use in people with intestinal obstruction or galactose or lactose intolerance.

DOSAGE AND ADMINISTRATION The adult dose is 15–30 mL daily to a maximum of 90 mL. If the sweet taste is a problem, suggest mixing with water, milk, fruit juice or a citrus-flavoured beverage.

CLINICAL INTEREST BOX 34-6 AUSTRALIAN MEDICINAL PLANTS

Australian Aborigines have long used plant-derived astringents such as mucilage or tannins for symptomatic treatment of GI tract disorders.

Astringents obtained from exudates, barks and roots of several plants, most commonly eucalypt and wattle species, can be used to treat diarrhoea and dysentery. Exudates, commonly known as *kinos*, provide a rich source of the astringent tannins. Kinotannic acid is thought to be the active ingredient. Exudates of the river red gum (*Eucalyptus camaldulensis*) are dissolved in water and drunk, as are those of the coastal she-oak (*Casuarina equisetifolia*) and sassafras (*Cinnamonium oliveri*). Queensland Aborigines use the inner roots, leaves and boiled fruits (named jelly boys) of the dysentery tree (*Grewia retusifolia*) for relief of gastric upsets. The fruits form a jelly-like substance, which is ingested. Similarly, the roots and stems of some species of orchid (*Cymbidium albuciflorum*) provide a rich source of mucilage or pseudostarch.

Stomach upsets of unspecified cause are treated with infusions of either the bark of black wattle (*Acacia mearnsii*) or the leaves of wild or native raspberry (*Rubus hillii*). Small balls of white clay, perhaps similar to kaolin, may be chewed, sometimes with pieces of termite mounds. The termite mound pieces might also provide nutritional benefit, as they are a rich source of iron, with levels as high as 2%.

Natural purgatives or laxatives include the mildly active ingredient mannitol, found in the sugary exudate of manna gum (*Eucalyptus viminalis*). The leaves and pods of the native senna (*Cassia pleurocarpa* or *Cassia australis*) also provide a laxative effect. Although the active constituents are not known, the leaves do contain triterpenes.

Osmotic and saline laxatives

The osmotic laxatives glycerol, lactulose (Drug Monograph 34-6) and sorbitol are not absorbed. By exerting an osmotic effect, they increase the volume of fluid in the lumen. This increased volume accelerates the transfer of the gut contents and leads to increased defecation. Glycerin suppositories are available in adult, child and infant sizes. These suppositories act as osmotic agents by absorbing water, but they also lubricate and increase stool bulk. Local irritation of the mucous membrane of the rectum may promote peristalsis, and evacuation occurs 5–30 minutes after insertion.

Saline laxatives are soluble salts (e.g. magnesium salts, sodium salts, polyethylene glycol [PEG] electrolyte solutions) that are only slightly absorbed from the alimentary canal. Because of their osmotic effect, they retain and increase the water content of faeces. The water in the intestinal lumen produces fluid accumulation and distension, leading to peristalsis and eventual evacuation of bowel contents. The result is a faecal mass of liquid or semiliquid stools. The laxative dose promotes laxation in 6–8 hours, whereas a cathartic dose works in less than 3 hours.

The intestinal membrane is not entirely impermeable to the passage of saline laxatives, and as much as 20% of the salt may be absorbed. Electrolyte disturbances have been reported with their long-term daily use, and sodium salts should be avoided in patients with congestive cardiac failure. Renal impairment can lead to the accumulation of magnesium and sodium ions, and hence significant electrolyte disturbances. A common formulation of magnesium sulphate is Epsom Salts.

Isosmotic solutions containing PEG and electrolytes are marketed as GI solutions specifically for bowel evacuation before surgery or GI diagnostic procedures. These powders (ColonLYTETLY, Movicol and Glycoprep-C) consist of a mixture of PEG (a non-absorbable osmotic substance) with sodium salts (sulfate, bicarbonate and chloride) and potassium chloride that is isosmotic with body fluids. The large volume of non-absorbable fluid, commonly 2–4 litres, leads to copious watery diarrhoea. Because it is isosmotic, dehydration does not occur. These products can cause failure of regular medication, e.g. the oral contraceptive pill. All the saline laxatives can cause nausea, vomiting, bloating and electrolyte disturbances, and are used with caution in people with intestinal obstruction or suspected perforation.

Antidiarrhoeal drugs

The term diarrhoea generally describes the increased passage of semiliquid or liquid stools. Causes are numerous. Diarrhoea may be acute, with a sudden onset in a previously healthy individual, lasting about 3 days to 1–2 weeks; this is usually self-limiting and resolves without sequelae. Chronic diarrhoea can last for 3–4 weeks or more, with recurring passage of liquid stools, and may be accompanied by fever, anorexia, nausea, vomiting, weight reduction and chronic weakness. In many instances, chronic diarrhoea in adults

BOX 34-2 CAUSES OF ACUTE AND CHRONIC DIARRHOEA

Causes of acute diarrhoea

Invasive organisms
Campylobacter fetus (jejuni)
Clostridium difficile
Escherichia coli (enteropathogenic)
Salmonella
Shigella dysenteriae
Staphylococcus
Non-invasive toxigenic organisms
Cholera (Vibrio cholerae) enterotoxin
Escherichia coli (enterotoxigenic) toxin
Toxin-mediated food poisoning
Bacillus cereus
Clostridium pertringens
Salmonella
Staphylococcus aureus
Viral
Adenoviruses
Coxsackievirus
Coronaviruses
Echoviruses

Norwalk agent
Rotavirus
Protozoa
Amoebic dysentery (Entamoeba histolytica), amoebiasis
Giardiasis (Giardia lamblia)
Nutritional
Allergy
Ingestion without discretion (spices, fats, roughage, seeds, preformed toxin)
Enteral nutrition
Other
Bile acids
Carcinoma
Diverticulitis
Fatty acids
Neurogenic
Psychogenic
Radiation therapy
Regional and ulcerative colitis
Stress

Causes of chronic diarrhoea

Addison's disease
Diabetic enteropathy or iatrogenic neuropathy
  Bacterial overgrowth
  Postsurgical
Inflammatory bowel disease
  Chronic ulcerative and granulomatous colitis
  Crohn's disease
Irritable bowel syndrome
Malabsorption syndrome
  Pancreatic adenoma—non-gastrin-secreting, such as syndrome of watery diarrhoea–hypokalaemia–achlorhydria (WDHA)
Pancreatic insufficiency
Thyroid—hyperthyroidism

Tumours
  Carcinoma of colon and rectum
  Intestinal
  Lymphoma
  Polyposis
  Villous adenoma
Other
  Blind loops, ileostomy, colostomy
  Carcinoid syndrome
  Enteritis
  Gardner's syndrome
  Gastrointestinal hormones
  Gluten enteropathy
  Zollinger–Ellison syndrome

signifies an underlying disease that necessitates definitive treatment directed to the organic cause. Persistent diarrhoea in any age group, but particularly in infants, can lead to significant fluid and electrolyte disturbances and circulatory collapse.

In some circumstances, specific anti-infective drug treatment is indicated but, in the main, the rationale for the use of **antidiarrhoeal** drugs relates to relief of symptoms and the prevention of fluid and electrolyte loss. These drugs should not be used in infants and children with acute diarrhoea, as their use may delay expulsion of organisms and does not reduce fluid and electrolyte loss (AMH 2006). Many OTC antidiarrhoeal drugs contain limited amounts of opioids (codeine, loperamide, **diphenoxylate**), aluminium hydroxide, attapulgite, kaolin, pectin and belladonna alkaloids (hyoscyamine, hyoscine and atropine).

In addition to the causes listed in Box 34-2, many drugs can cause diarrhoea; these include NSAIDs, antibiotics, cytotoxic agents, magnesium-containing antacids and laxatives.

Adsorbents

Adsorbents are said to act by coating the intestinal mucosa, adsorbing the bacteria or toxins causing the diarrhoea and passing them out with the stools. Definitive studies confirming their proposed mechanism of action and their usefulness in treating diarrhoea have not been conducted. Examples of OTC drugs in this class are activated aluminium hydroxide (Kaomagma), attapulgite (a highly adsorbent

DRUG MONOGRAPH 34-7 DIPHENOXYLATE*

MECHANISM OF ACTION Diphenoxylate is chemically related to pethidine and inhibits intestinal propulsive motility by acting directly on opioid (μ) receptors on intestinal smooth muscles. The addition of atropine has no therapeutic benefit but it is included in the formulation to discourage abuse.

PHARMACOKINETICS Peak plasma concentrations occur after 2 hours, and a half-life of 2.5 hours indicates rapid metabolism. Diphenoxylate undergoes hydrolysis and conjugation in the liver; the metabolites are excreted principally in bile and eliminated via the faeces. A small amount of unchanged drug is excreted via the urine.

ADVERSE REACTIONS Common adverse reactions include abdominal pain, nausea, vomiting and constipation. Rash, dizziness and paralytic ileus occur rarely. Accidental or deliberate overdosage can produce additional symptoms of flushing, hyperthermia, tachycardia, dry mouth, agitation, pinpoint pupils, lethargy, respiratory depression and coma.

DRUG INTERACTIONS The following effects can occur when diphenoxylate and atropine are given with the drugs listed.

Drug	Possible effect and management
Alcohol	Concurrent use can result in increased CNS-depressant effects of alcohol
Anticholinergics or other drugs with anticholinergic effects (e.g. tricyclic antidepressants)	An increase in anticholinergic effects may result. A dosage adjustment might be required
Monoamine oxidase inhibitors (MAO inhibitors)	Concurrent use with diphenoxylate can result in a hypertensive crisis. Avoid or a potentially serious drug interaction could occur

WARNINGS AND CONTRAINDICATIONS These include previous known hypersensitivity reaction to diphenoxylate/atropine and intestinal obstruction. Caution should be exercised where there is evidence of coexisting inflammatory bowel disease and severe hepatic impairment.

DOSAGE AND ADMINISTRATION For the treatment of acute diarrhoea in adults, the dosage is 5 mg 3 or 4 times daily, to a maximum of 20 mg daily.

*Diphenoxylate is available only in combination with atropine.

hydrated magnesium aluminium silicate, Diareze) and kaolin and pectin (Kaopectate).

Each of the formulations available has specific dosing information; in general, an initial higher dose is taken, followed by a further lower dose after each loose bowel movement until the diarrhoea has been controlled. Caution should be exercised if other medications are given concurrently with adsorbents, as they can bind to other drugs (e.g. antibiotics, anticoagulants, digoxin, salicylates, H$_2$-receptor antagonists and phenothiazines) and interfere with their absorption.

Opioid antidiarrhoeals

Loperamide and diphenoxylate are synthetic OTC opioids that activate opioid receptors in the gut wall, resulting in a reduction in secretions and inhibition of propulsive movements in the gut (see Drug Monograph 34-7). This slows the passage of intestinal contents and allows reabsorption of water and electrolytes, reducing stool frequency.

Both these agents are indicated for short-term treatment of diarrhoea and for reducing the frequency and fluidity of motions in people with an intestinal stoma. Adverse reactions are usually minimal, but combinations of diphenoxylate with atropine (Lomotil) can produce dizziness, dry mouth and blurred vision.

Inflammatory bowel disease

Inflammatory bowel disease (IBD) includes ulcerative colitis and Crohn's disease (see Clinical Interest Box 33-4). Genetic and environmental factors are thought to play a role in both of these conditions, and management includes not only drug therapy but also consideration of dietary and lifestyle factors. Excellent information can be obtained from the Australian Crohn's and Colitis Association (ACCA). Management is primarily aimed at inducing and maintaining remission of the disease state and preventing complications such as fistulae and abscesses. This in turn improves quality of life and ensures adequate nutrition. The latter is particularly important in children with irritable bowel syndrome, as adequate nutrition is essential to growth and sexual development.

Drug therapy for inflammatory bowel disease

Current therapy for both conditions includes corticosteroids (e.g. prednisolone), which are discussed in detail in Chapter 40; the 5-aminosalicylates, which include sulfasalazine, mesalazine and olsalazine; and the immunosuppressants, such as azathioprine, mercaptopurine, cyclosporin and methotrexate (discussed in Chapter 55). Newer agents such as immunoglobulins and interferons are also being investi-

---

CLINICAL INTEREST BOX 34-8 PEPPERMINT OIL

Peppermint (*Mentha x piperita*) belongs to the mint family (Labiatae). Peppermint oil is obtained by distillation from the fresh flowering tops and consists mainly of menthol (50%–60%), ketones (as menthone, 5%–30%) and 5%–10% esters.

Menthol is thought to act as the antispasmodic, relaxing intestinal muscle most probably through antagonism of calcium. Unlike peppermint tea, the oil can cause heartburn,

bradycardia, skin rash, allergic reactions, headache, muscle tremor and ataxia. Release of peppermint oil in the mouth can cause local irritation of the mouth and oesophagus, and capsules should not be broken or chewed. Mintec capsules contain 0.2 mL peppermint oil; the initial dosage is one capsule three times daily 30 minutes before food, increasing to 1–2 capsules three times daily (AMH 2006; Goh & Roufogalis 2001).

DRUG MONOGRAPH 34-8 MESALAZINE

MECHANISM OF ACTION The exact mechanism of action of mesalazine is unknown but it is thought to exert an anti-inflammatory effect by inhibiting the production of inflammatory mediators and reactive oxygen species.

PHARMACOKINETICS Disintegration of the enteric coating takes place about 5 hours after administration in the small bowel, and about 80% of the drug is available to exert its action on the intestinal mucosa. The majority of the drug is metabolised by acetylation, and 20%–40% of the dose is excreted in faeces and 30%–50% in urine. The plasma half-life is 0.5–1 hour.

ADVERSE REACTIONS These are more common with higher doses, and include headache, nausea, rash, abdominal discomfort and diarrhoea.

WARNINGS AND CONTRAINDICATIONS Mesalazine is contraindicated in people with known hypersensitivity to salicylates or sulfasalazine, and in the presence of impaired renal function.

DOSAGE A dose of 250–500 mg three times daily is recommended for acute exacerbations of ulcerative colitis and Crohn's disease, and 250 mg three times daily as a maintenance regimen.

gated for their use in IBD, and currently Crohn's disease is an indication for the use of infliximab, a new humanised antibody that targets tumour necrosis factor alpha.

AMINOSALICYLATES

Sulfasalazine consists of the sulfonamide antibiotic sulfapyridine, linked to the anti-inflammatory salicylate mesalazine. Sulfasalazine is poorly absorbed and in the colon it is split by bacteria into sulfapyridine and mesalazine, which is the active component effective in the treatment of IBD (see Drug Monograph 34-8). Olsalazine is two linked molecules of mesalazine and is split by bacteria in the intestine into two molecules of mesalazine.

Irritable bowel syndrome

The cause of **irritable bowel syndrome** (IBS) is unknown. The condition is considered 'the most common gastro-intestinal condition encountered by general practitioners' (Farthing 1998). IBS affects up to 20% of adults in the industrialised world.

Although IBS is often thought of as a predominantly female condition, symptoms are found equally in men and women. The female tag to the syndrome has probably arisen because women more frequently seek medical advice. Symptoms of IBS include long-term recurrent abdominal pain, change in bowel habits, anorexia, nausea, bloating and flatulence. The condition is often precipitated by stress and anxiety and may occur after severe intestinal infection.

Management of IBS varies enormously and no real consensus on treatment exists. Dietary manipulation (e.g. exclusion-type diets) and supplements (e.g. wheat bran,

fibre) are popular approaches, as is psychotherapy. The use of drug therapy is still debated and includes anti-spasmodic agents (e.g. hyoscine, hyoscamine), loperamide if diarrhoea predominates, and short-term use of laxatives if constipation predominates. It has been shown that IBS sufferers improved significantly when treated with Chinese herbal medicines. Among the many herbal medicines that have calming properties, peppermint oil has found its way into mainstream medicine (see Clinical Interest Box 34-8). Although conflicting studies have been published, the current balance of data tends to support a role for peppermint oil in the treatment of IBS.

PREGNANCY SAFETY

ADEC Category	Drug
A	Antacids, bisacodyl, docusate, liquid paraffin, metoclopramide, nystatin, senna, sulfasalazine
B1	Aprepitant, cimetidine, dolasetron, famotidine, granisetron, nizatidine, ondansetron, ranitidine, sucralfate
B3	Lansoprazole, loperamide, omeprazole, pantoprazole, tropisetron, ursodeoxycholic acid
C	Diphenoxylate, mesalazine, olsalazine, prochlorperazine
X	Misoprostol

DRUGS AT A GLANCE 34: Drugs affecting the gastrointestinal tract

Therapeutic group	Pharmacological group	Key examples	Key pages
Drugs for acid-related disorders	Antacids	aluminium hydroxide	565, 6
	Cytoprotective agents	sucralfate	573
	H₂-receptor antagonists	cimetidine	571, 2
		ranitidine	571, 2
	Proton pump inhibitors	esomeprazole	571
		lansoprazole	571
		omeprazole	571
Antiemetics	Dopamine antagonists	metoclopramide	568
		prochlorperazine	568
	5-HT₃ receptor antagonists	dolasetron	569
		ondansetron	569

DRUGS AT A GLANCE 34: Drugs affecting the gastrointestinal tract

Therapeutic group	Pharmacological group	Key examples	Key pages
Antidiarrhoeal drugs	Adsorbents	kaolin and pectin	579, 80
	Opioid antidiarrhoeals	diphenoxylate	579
		loperamide	580
	NK$_1$-receptor antagonist	aprepitant	570
Laxatives	Bulk-forming laxatives	psyllium	574, 5
	Stool softeners	docusate	575
		liquid paraffin	575
		poloxamer	575
	Stimulant laxatives	bisacodyl	575, 6
		senna	575, 6
		sodium picosulfate	575, 6
Drugs for inflammatory bowel disease	Aminosalicylates	mesalazine	580
		olsalazine	580
		sulfasalazine	581

KEY POINTS

- Drugs used for maintaining oral hygiene include mouth-washes, gargles, dentifrices, and topical antifungals and antiviral agents.
- Drugs affecting the stomach include antacids, antiemetics and agents used to treat peptic ulcers.
- Antiemetics, which include dopamine receptor antagonists, muscarinic receptor antagonists, 5-HT$_3$ receptor antagonists and NK$_1$ receptor antagonists, are given for the relief of nausea and vomiting, including that associated with cancer chemotherapy.
- The drugs used in the treatment of peptic ulcer include the proton pump inhibitors, H$_2$-receptor antagonists and cytoprotective agents.
- Use of *Helicobacter pylori* eradication regimens improves the odds of non-recurrence of peptic ulcers.
- Drugs affecting the lower GI tract include laxatives and antidiarrhoeal medications, and specific drugs used for the treatment of inflammatory bowel disease (e.g. mesalazine) and irritable bowel syndrome (e.g. peppermint oil).

REVIEW EXERCISES

1. Describe three significant antacid drug interactions of which health-care professionals should be aware.
2. Why does the treatment of peptic ulcer disease often include an *H. pylori* eradication regimen?
3. Why is it necessary in some circumstances to administer more than one antiemetic to prevent nausea and vomiting?
4. Describe the mechanism of action and effects of metoclopramide in nausea and vomiting. Explain why some patients might experience extrapyramidal reactions with this drug.
5. Why are proton pump inhibitors and H$_2$-receptor antagonists effective in peptic ulcer disease?
6. Discuss the mechanisms and sites of action of laxatives and antidiarrhoeal drugs.

REFERENCES AND FURTHER READING

Ahronheim JC. *Handbook of Prescribing Medications for Geriatric Patients.* Boston: Little Brown, 1992.

Andersson T. Drug interactions with omeprazole. *Clinical Pharmacokinetics* 1991; 21: 195–212.

Australian Medicines Handbook 2006. Adelaide: AMH, 2006.

Bensoussan A, Talley NJ, Hing M, Menzies R, Guo A, Ngu M. Treatment of irritable bowel syndrome with Chinese herbal medicine: a randomised controlled trial. *Journal of the American Medical Association* 1998; 280: 1585–9.

Brookes MJ, Green JRB. Maintenance of remission in Crohn's disease. Current and emerging therapeutic options. *Drugs* 2004; 64(10): 1069–89.

Caeiro JP, DuPont HL. Management of travellers' diarrhoea. *Drugs* 1998; 56: 73–81.

Carter MJ, Lobo AJ, Travis SPL. Guidelines for the management of inflammatory bowel disease in adults. *Gut* 2004; 53 (Suppl V): v1–v6.

Casburn-Jones AC, Farthing MJG. Management of infectious diarrhoea. *Gut* 2004; 53: 296–305.

Covington TR. *Handbook of nonprescription drugs.* 11th edn. Washington, DC: American Pharmaceutical Association, 1996.

Cribb AB, Cribb JW. *Wild Medicine in Australia.* Sydney: Collins, 1988.

Farthing MJG. New drugs in the management of the irritable bowel syndrome. *Drugs* 1998; 56: 11–21.

Flynn AA. Oral health products. In: Covington TR (ed.). *Handbook of Nonprescription Drugs.* 11th edn. Washington, DC: American Pharmaceutical Association, 1996.

Gastrointestinal Expert Group. *Therapeutic Guidelines: Gastrointestinal, version 3.* Melbourne: Therapeutic Guidelines Limited, 2002.

Gisbert JP, Pajares JM. *Helicobacter pylori* 'rescue' therapy after failure of two eradication treatments. *Helicobacter* 2005; 10: 363–72.

Goh PP, Roufogalis BD. Peppermint: a herb for calming irritable bowel? *Australian Pharmacy Trade* 2001; 8 February; 22–3.

Habib AS, Gan TJ. Evidence-based management of postoperative nausea and vomiting: a review. *Canadian Journal of Anesthetics* 2004; 51: 326–41.

Kovac AL. Benefits and risks of newer treatments for chemotherapy-induced and postoperative nausea and vomiting. *Drug Safety* 2003; 26(4): 227–59.

Lassak EV, McCarthy T. *Australian Medicinal Plants.* Sydney: New Holland Publishers, 2001.

Low T. *Bush medicine: A pharmacopoeia of natural remedies.* Sydney: Angus & Robertson, 1990.

Marcus R. Agents affecting calcification and bone turnover. In: Young LY, Koda-Kimble MA (eds). *Applied Therapeutics: The Clinical Use of Drugs.* 6th edn. Vancouver: Applied Therapeutics, 1995.

Maton PN, Burton ME. Antacids revisited: a review of their clinical pharmacology and recommended therapeutic use. *Drugs* 1999; 57: 855–70.

Mazzotta P, Magee LA. A risk–benefit assessment of pharmacological and nonpharmacological treatment for nausea and vomiting of pregnancy. *Drugs* 2000; 59: 781–800.

Neuvonen PJ, Kivisto KT. Enhancement of drug absorption by antacids: an unrecognised drug interaction. *Clinical Pharmacokinetics* 1994; 27: 120–8.

Olver IN. Aprepitant in antiemetic combinations to prevent chemotherapy-induced nausea and vomiting. *International Journal of Clinical Practice* 2004; 58P: 201–6.

Piper DW, de Carle DJ, Talley NJ et al. Gastrointestinal and hepatic diseases. In: Speight TM, Holford NHG (eds). *Avery's Drug Treatment.* 4th edn. Auckland: Adis International, 1997 [ch. 22].

Stieler JM, Reichardt P, Riess H, Oettle H. Treatment options for chemotherapy-induced nausea and vomiting: current and future. *American Journal of Cancer* 2003; 2: 15–26.

United States Pharmacopeial Convention. *USP DI: drug information for the health care professional.* 18th edn. Rockville: US Pharmacopeial Convention, 1998.

Veyrat-Follet C, Farinotti R, Palmer JL. Physiology of chemotherapy-induced emesis and antiemetic therapy. *Drugs* 1997; 53: 206–34.

Zola N, Gott B. *Koorie Plants, Koorie People: Traditional Aboriginal Food, Fibre and Healing Plants of Victoria.* Melbourne: Koorie Heritage Trust, Globe Press, 1992.

ON-LINE RESOURCES

Medicare Australia Health Statistics 2005: www.medicareaustralia.gov.au/stastics/dyn_plos/forms/pbs_tab1.shtml

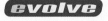 More weblinks at http://evolve.elsevier.com/AU/Bryant/pharmacology/

UNIT X
Drugs Affecting the Eye, Ear and Special Senses

CHAPTER 35

Drugs Affecting the Eye

CHAPTER FOCUS

Disorders that affect vision markedly impair a person's ability to function independently, and require early detection and treatment. Ophthalmic drugs have made a significant contribution to the treatment of eye disorders and the preservation of vision. Drugs are used to treat medical conditions such as glaucomas, infections, inflammations and muscular dysfunction, and to assist in ocular examination, diagnosis and surgery. Adverse reactions may be manifest in the eyes after ocular or systemic administration of drugs.

OBJECTIVES

- To describe clinical aspects of the anatomy and physiology of the eye.

- To describe the formulations used for ocular administration of drugs, the routes of administration, and how drugs are absorbed across the cornea.

- To contrast the autonomic innervation and muscles involved with miosis, mydriasis and cycloplegia, and drugs inducing these effects.

- To describe the mechanisms of action for the main drug groups used to treat glaucoma.

- To review the indications and mechanisms of action for ocular antimicrobial, anti-inflammatory, local anaesthetic and diagnostic agents, and drugs used in ophthalmic surgery procedures.

- To discuss the systemic adverse reactions induced by ophthalmic drugs, and ocular adverse reactions from systemic drugs.

KEY TERMS

accommodation
anticholinergic
aqueous humour
carbonic anhydrase
cataract
conjunctiva
contact lenses
cornea
cycloplegic
decongestant
eye-drops
eye ointments
glaucoma
intraocular pressure
local anaesthetics
miosis/miotic
mydriasis/mydriatic
nasolacrimal ducts
stains
sympathomimetic
trachoma

KEY DRUGS

aciclovir
atropine
botulinum toxin
brimonidine
chloramphenicol
dorzolamide
fluorescein
latanoprost
phenylephrine
pilocarpine
prednisolone
proxymetacaine
timolol
verteporfin

KEY ABBREVIATIONS

ACh	acetylcholine
ADR	adverse drug reaction
CA	carbonic anhydrase
CNS	central nervous system
IOP	intraocular pressure
LA	local anaesthetic
NSAID	non-steroidal anti-inflammatory drug
POAG	primary open-angle glaucoma

OVERVIEW OF THE EYE

THE EYE is the receptor organ for one of the most delicate and valuable senses—vision. The eyeball is protected in a deep depression of the skull called the orbit; it is moved in the orbit by six small extraocular muscles. The eyeball has three layers or coats (see Figure 35-1): the protective external layer (cornea and sclera), the middle layer (which contains the choroid, iris and ciliary body), and the light-sensitive retina.

The anterior covering of the eye is the **cornea**. The cornea is normally transparent, allowing light to enter the eye. The cornea is avascular (has no blood vessels) and receives its nutrition from the aqueous humour, and its oxygen supply by diffusion from the air and surrounding structures. The surface consists of a thin layer of epithelial cells, which are resistant to infection unless damaged. The cornea is also supplied with sensory fibres that elicit pain whenever the corneal epithelium is damaged. Seriously injured corneal tissue is replaced by scar tissue, which is usually not transparent and hence results in impaired vision. Increased **intraocular pressure (IOP)** also results in loss of transparency of the cornea.

The sclera, which is continuous with the cornea, is non-transparent; it is the white fibrous envelope of the eye (the 'white of the eye'). The **conjunctiva** is the mucous membrane lining the anterior part of the sclera and the inner surfaces of each eyelid.

The iris gives the eye its brown, blue, grey, green or hazel colour. It surrounds the pupil; the sphincter and dilator muscles in the iris alter pupil size. Pupil constriction normally occurs in bright light or when the eye is focusing on nearby objects. Pupil dilation normally occurs in dim light or when the eye is focusing on distant objects.

The lens, situated behind the iris, is a transparent mass of uniformly arranged fibres encased in a thin elastic capsule. Its protein concentration is higher than that of any other tissue of the body. The lens has suspensory ligaments called zonular fibres around its edge, which connect with the ciliary body. Their tension helps to change the shape of the lens to ensure that the image on the retina is in sharp focus and to adjust to variations in distance. **Accommodation** for near vision occurs readily in young people, but with age the lens becomes more rigid. The ability to focus on close objects is then lost and the near point (the closest point that can be seen clearly) recedes.

With age, the lens may also lose its transparency and become opaque; this is known as a **cataract**. Unless it can be treated or removed surgically, blindness can occur. If the opaque (cataract) portion is located peripherally in the lens, however, vision is not compromised.

Aqueous humour is formed by the ciliary body. It bathes and feeds the lens, iris and posterior surface of the cornea. After it is formed, it flows forward between the lens and the iris into the anterior chamber and drains out of the eye through drainage channels located near the junction of the cornea and sclera. A trabecular meshwork called the canal of Schlemm drains the aqueous humour into the venous system of the eye (see Figures 35-1 and 35-2).

Behind the lens is the vitreous humour, comprising about 80% of the eye volume. This is a gel-like viscous fluid–collagen matrix, which bathes the retina. The retina contains nerve endings and the rods and cones that function as visual sensory receptors. It is connected to the brain by the optic nerve, which leaves the orbit through a bony canal in the posterior wall. Trauma or inflammation may cause the retina to separate from the pigmented epithelium, leading to retinal detachment and loss of vision; this is an optical emergency.

Eyelashes, eyelids, blinking and tears all protect the eye. Each eye has about 200 eyelashes. A blink reflex occurs whenever a foreign body touches the eyelashes. The lids close quickly to prevent the foreign substance from entering the eye. Blinking, which is bilateral, occurs every few seconds during waking hours. It keeps the corneal surface free of mucus and spreads the lacrimal fluid evenly over the cornea. Tears are secreted by lacrimal glands at the rate of about 1–2 µL/min and contain lysozyme, a mucolytic enzyme with bactericidal action. Tears provide lubrication for lid movements and wash away noxious agents. By forming a thin film over the cornea, tears provide it with a good optical surface. Tear fluid is lost by evaporation and by draining into two small **nasolacrimal ducts** (the lacrimal canaliculi) at the inner corners of the upper and lower eyelids, and thence eventually into the throat and the systemic circulation. Through these ducts, drugs applied topically to the eye can reach the systemic circulation and cause systemic effects.

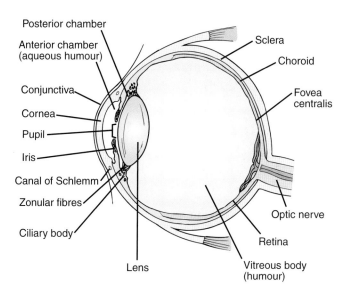

Posterior chamber
Anterior chamber (aqueous humour)
Conjunctiva
Cornea
Pupil
Iris
Canal of Schlemm
Zonular fibres
Ciliary body
Lens
Sclera
Choroid
Fovea centralis
Optic nerve
Retina
Vitreous body (humour)

FIGURE 35-1 Cross-sectional anatomy of the eye (lid not shown).

OCULAR ADMINISTRATION OF DRUGS

Drugs used to treat eye disorders can be divided into the following major groups: mydriatic and cycloplegic agents; drugs used to treat glaucoma; antimicrobial agents; anti-inflammatory and antiallergic agents; and ocular local anaesthetics (LAs). In addition, there are many miscellaneous agents used in the eye, such as preparations used during ophthalmic surgery, diagnostic agents to stain damaged tissue, and botulinum toxin, which is used to paralyse muscle. (Most of these drugs are used systemically in other conditions, so their pharmacology is covered in detail in other chapters.)

Drugs intended to treat eye conditions may be administered in three ways: systemically, by injection to the eye, or topically to the eye. Examples of systemic administration of drugs to act in the eye include oral or intravenous administration of acetazolamide to treat glaucoma, or of antibiotics in eye infections. In some acute serious conditions, drugs may be administered by direct injection to the eye, either by a periocular route (subconjunctival, or retrobulbar), e.g. antibiotics, corticosteroids or LAs; or by intravitreal route (into the vitreous humour), e.g. antibiotics for a severe infection. An LA may be required first to relieve the pain of the main injection.

Most commonly, drugs intended to act in the eye are administered topically to the eye, usually directly onto the conjunctival surface as eye-drops or ointment. Ocular administration requires some dexterity and may be difficult with children.

Some general points to note with respect to ocular administration of drugs are:

- most drugs used in the eye have marked effects elsewhere in the body when given systemically
- drugs can be applied topically to the conjunctival surfaces, may then be absorbed through the cornea and diffused through the aqueous humour
- drugs need to be both water-soluble, to dissolve in body fluids and the corneal stroma (framework tissue), and lipid-soluble, to pass cell membranes and the corneal epithelium
- non-polar, uncharged molecules penetrate the cornea most readily, leading to effective drug concentrations in the anterior segment (in front of the lens)
- absorption is likely to be enhanced if the cornea is damaged, and topical administration is not generally used in open eye injuries
- the drug (in eye-drops) is rapidly blinked or washed away; excess solution spills over or drains through the tear ducts to the nasal mucosa
- reflex tear production rapidly dilutes the drug within 1–2 minutes after application to the eye; thus it can be difficult to maintain a pharmacologically effective concentration of drug in the eye
- the vehicle and the formulation (i.e. solution in drops, ointment base, gel or plastic insert) can affect absorption of the drug.

Ocular formulations

There are many eye formulations available, including eye-drops, eye ointments, eye lotions and irrigating solutions, and inserts. The formulation of ocular preparations is a specialised branch of pharmaceutics, as the preparation must be sterile (see Clinical Interest Box 35-1), buffered to body pH and isotonic with body solutions so that it is non-irritant, and stable in solution. Consequently, ocular formulations may contain buffers, preservatives, pH adjusters, antioxidants, agents to increase viscosity (such as polyvinyl alcohol or hypromellose) and salts, all of which may affect tissues or cause allergies.

Eye-drops

Eye-drops are drugs formulated in aqueous or oily solutions, dispensed in a small dropper-bottle (usually 10–15 mL capacity) such that a small drop can be instilled into the conjunctival sac. Aqueous (watery) drops generally provide for quick absorption and effect, have a brief duration of action and produce little interference with eye examination. The effects may be variable because of spillage or blinking away of the drop, and systemic effects are possible after

---

CLINICAL INTEREST BOX 35-1
STERILITY OF OCULAR FORMULATIONS

Some of the eye tissues are relatively or completely avascular (notably the cornea and lens, hence their transparency), so they are at severe risk if infection or trauma occurs, as they have no immediate blood supply to provide immune defences. Thus it is important that all drugs administered to the eye, particularly during operations or when there is tissue damage, be provided in a sterile form and be maintained non-contaminated as far as possible. Most formulations of eye preparations contain preservatives to minimise bacterial growth; these preservatives can themselves impair healing or cause allergies.

The shelf-life of eye formulations is usually stated to be a maximum of 28 days after opening (in the home situation); in a clinic situation, 7 days is more appropriate. Every effort must be made to avoid contaminating the preparation by touching the tip of the dropper bottle or ointment tube onto any surface, including the conjunctival surface or the benchtop.

absorption, without the drug having passed through the liver first. Oily drops are less common, as they interfere more with vision, but provide longer retention time on the cornea, are more stable and are less likely to cause systemic toxicity.

The technique of administering eye-drops is important: the person should be instructed to wash the hands, shake the bottle gently, pull down the lower lid, instil one drop, then close the eyes gently and press on the inner corner of the eyelid for 3 minutes (this minimises systemic absorption of the drug). If another eye-drop preparation is also being used, wait at least 5 minutes before instilling the next drop.

There is little point in trying to add more than one drop to the eye, because the average volume of a drop from a dropper bottle is about 25–50 µL so it will overfill the conjunctival sac, which is estimated to have a capacity of 10 µL. The excess solution will simply overflow onto the cheek or drain or be blinked away.

To minimise the risk of contamination of formulations and consequent growth of microorganisms in solutions, eye-drops are also dispensed in single-dose containers (e.g. the Minim brand in Australia). These come as a tiny pack (0.5 mL) for one use only and are then discarded. The advantages are that the drop is always sterile, the solution need contain no preservative, there is a cost saving because there is less waste to be discarded, and there is no risk of cross-contamination between eyes or patients. Drugs available in single-dose eye-drop packs include sodium chloride, prednisolone, amethocaine, chloramphenicol, neomycin, atropine, pilocarpine and fluorescein with or without lignocaine.

NOTE ON DOSAGE OF EYE-DROPS

The strength of drug solutions in eye-drops is often expressed in percentage terms rather than as milligrams per millilitre or in molar units. Pilocarpine eye-drops, for example, are available in strengths ranging from 0.5% to 6%. In this context, '%' refers to % weight in volume (% w/v), i.e. grams weight of solid dissolved in 100 mL of solution. Thus 1% means 1 g/100 mL, which equates to 10 mg/mL. For some more modern drugs, the strength may be quoted in mg/mL, e.g. dorzolamide eye-drops are formulated as a 20 mg/mL solution.

Eye ointments and gels

Ointments are semisolid preparations intended for topical application to the skin or mucous membranes; the active drug is incorporated into an oily vehicle and is thinly spread on the surface to which it is applied. **Eye ointments** are supplied in small (e.g. 5 g) tubes and have short shelf-lives due to the risk

of contamination and infection: they should be discarded after 1 month (at home) or 1 week (in a practice or clinic).

The advantages of eye ointments over eye-drops are:
• they are more stable than aqueous solutions
• there is less absorption of drug into the lacrimal ducts
• there is a longer retention time of the drug on the conjunctival surface (important when prolonged contact time is required, e.g. with antiviral drugs)
• they are safer for home use with potent drugs
• due to the emollient (softening) effect of oily ointment bases, they are useful for protection and comfort at night.

The disadvantages of eye ointments are that they can be difficult to self-administer, they can cause blurred vision or interfere with ocular examination, and they cannot be used with contact lenses, as the greasy base forms an oily film over the lens. As with eye-drops, good hygiene is important to minimise contamination.

Gels are thick liquid or semisolid suspensions, usually aqueous (like a jelly) rather than oily; they are less likely to blur vision than are ointments, yet retain drug in contact with the corneal surface longer than do watery eye-drops. Timolol has been formulated in a gel eye-drop form, suitable for once-daily administration.

Other ocular formulations
EYE LOTIONS
Eye lotions or irrigating solutions are used to wash foreign materials from the eye. They should be sterile, at pH 6.6–9, and isotonic; in an emergency, 0.9% sodium chloride (normal saline) can be used. Some specific formulations are available, e.g. a solution of dihydrogen sodium versenate to be used if the eyes are splashed with lime (calcium oxide, a caustic powder). Buffered solutions of sodium hyaluronate and of salts are used during intraocular surgery.

OCULAR INSERTS
Various devices impregnated with drug can be applied to the conjunctival surface to encourage absorption of drug across the cornea. Such devices include lamellae (dissolvable discs), hydrophilic contact lenses and crescent-shaped polymer inserts that float below the pupil. They may be difficult to insert and remove, and may appear to become lost (temporarily) in the conjunctival sac. Absorbable gelatin implants are available for use in ocular surgery.

IONTOPHORESIS
Iontophoresis is a technique in which the drug solution is placed in an eyecup bearing an electrode; when held up against the eye the current 'drives' the drug in by altering its ionisation and enhancing absorption.

AUTONOMIC NERVOUS SYSTEM EFFECTS ON THE EYE

Autonomic innervation of ocular tissues

Because many drugs used in the eye act by effects on autonomic pathways and responses, it is important to review autonomic innervation of ocular tissues and the relevant neurotransmitters and receptors involved (see Unit III Peripheral Nervous System, Table 10-1 and Table 35-1).

The sphincter muscle, which encircles the pupil, is parasympathetically innervated; contraction, either alone or with relaxation of the dilator muscle, causes constriction of the pupil, or **miosis**. The dilator muscle, which runs radially from the pupil to the periphery of the iris, is sympathetically innervated; contraction of the dilator muscle or relaxation of the sphincter muscle causes dilation of the pupil, or **mydriasis**.

Accommodation (focusing for near vision) depends on two factors: (1) ciliary muscle contraction and (2) the ability of the lens to assume a more biconvex shape when tension on the ligaments is relaxed. The ciliary muscle is innervated by parasympathetic fibres; normal parasympathetic tone keeps the eye accommodated for near vision, with the pupil constricted in response to contraction of the sphincter muscle and the zonular fibres relaxed. In the unaccommodated eye (i.e. focused for distant vision), the ciliary muscle is relaxed, the zonular fibres are taut and the pupil dilates, resulting in sharp distant vision and blurred near vision.

Uses of autonomic drugs in ocular conditions

Drugs acting on the autonomic nervous system are frequently used in ocular conditions:

- to achieve mydriasis in eye examinations (with sympathomimetics or antimuscarinics)
- to achieve cycloplegia for diagnostic refraction, i.e. assessment of optical errors (with antimuscarinics)
- to achieve miosis, in treatment of glaucoma or to reverse the effects of a mydriatic (with parasympathomimetics)
- to achieve vasoconstriction, useful for a decongestant effect (with sympathomimetics)
- to decrease formation of aqueous humour in glaucoma (with sympathomimetics or β-blockers).

Mydriatic and cycloplegic agents
Mydriatics

Mydriatics are drugs that cause pupil dilation (mydriasis). They are primarily used to facilitate examination of the peripheral lens and retina in the diagnosis of ophthalmic disorders, and to prevent or break down posterior synechiae (adhesions) in iridocyclitis. Mydriasis can be achieved either by blocking acetylcholine (ACh) effects on muscarinic (ACh$_M$) receptors or by enhancing noradrenaline effects on α_1-adrenoceptors. The main clinical differences are that sympathomimetics are less likely to raise IOP and do not cause cycloplegia, so the pupillary light reflex is retained. Frequently, an antimuscarinic and an adrenergic agent are given together to cause faster and more complete mydriasis. The effects of these agents depend on the patient's age, race and colour of iris. Mydriatic agents evoke less of a response in people with heavily pigmented (dark) irises than in those with lighter-pigmented (blue) eyes, because the drug binds to melanin.

ANTICHOLINERGICS (ANTIMUSCARINICS, ATROPINIC AGENTS)

Anticholinergic agents reversibly block ACh$_M$ receptors on iris sphincter muscle and ciliary muscle, producing mydriasis (focusing for distant vision) and cycloplegia (paralysis of ciliary muscle). They are indicated to relieve ocular pain by relaxing inflamed intraocular muscles in inflammations such as uveitis and keratitis, and for relaxation of ciliary muscles

---

CLINICAL INTEREST BOX 35-2
OCULAR AUTONOMIC PATHOLOGIES

Autonomic effects in the eye are well demonstrated in two classic pathological conditions of the eye, Horner's syndrome and Adie's tonic pupil, and the tests used to diagnose them.

Horner's syndrome occurs in any oculo-sympathetic paralysis, i.e. interruption to sympathetic supply to the orbit; the lesion may be central, preganglionic or postganglionic. Common causes are trauma (especially in young people), tumours (in older people), infections, poliomyelitis, stroke and aneurysms. The signs are those of impaired autonomic innervation, including slow redilation of the pupil in dim light, miosis and ptosis (drooping of the eyelid). Diagnosis is by the cocaine test: slow or absent pupil dilation in response to cocaine (an indirect sympathomimetic agent). Management may be surgical, medical or neurological, depending on the aetiology.

Adie's tonic pupil syndrome is due to a unilateral lesion (often in the ciliary ganglion) with damage to postganglionic parasympathetic innervation to the constrictor pupillae and ciliary muscle. This leads to absent or slow responses to bright light or to near-vision effort. Diagnosis is by the pilocarpine test: the 'denervated' iris sphincter is hypersensitive to cholinergic agonists.

TABLE 35-1 Effects of autonomic stimulation on ocular tissues

OCULAR TISSUE	SYMPATHETIC	PARASYMPATHETIC
Smooth muscle of iris	Dilator pupillae (radial muscle) (α_1) causes mydriasis	Sphincter pupillae (circular muscle) (M_3) causes miosis and regulation of IOP
Ciliary muscle (adjusts curvature of lens)	Relaxation (β_2) causes focus for distant vision	Contraction causes accommodation for near vision and increases filtration angle, so drains aqueous humour; paralysis causes cycloplegia
Lacrimal gland		Secretion of tears
Blood vessels	Vasoconstriction (α_1) decreases formation of aqueous humour	
Muscle of upper lid	Contraction (α_1) widens eyes	

The main effects of stimulation of autonomic pathways to ocular tissues are shown; sympathetic effects are mediated by actions of noradrenaline on α- or β-adrenoceptors, and parasympathetic effects are mediated by acetylcholine actions on muscarinic (M) receptors.

for accurate measurement of refractive errors, which permits proper lens determination for eyeglasses.

Contraction of the iris sphincter can lead to an increase in IOP, hence glaucoma may be precipitated. Other adverse effects include increased glare (due to paralysed response to light), blurred vision and stinging (which may be relieved by prior administration of an LA eye-drop). Patients should be advised to wear dark glasses afterwards to reduce glare.

Systemic effects that may follow absorption via the nasolacrimal ducts include classical 'atropinic' effects: dryness of the mouth, tachycardia, decreased gastrointestinal tract functions and ataxia. Anticholinergic eye-drops should be used cautiously in patients with head injury or glaucoma, and in children.

Commonly used anticholinergic agents include **atropine**, tropicamide and cyclopentolate (see Table 35-2 for the pharmacokinetics and dosing of anticholinergic agents). Note that atropine eye-drops cause prolonged mydriasis and cycloplegia (for 7–14 days) and are too strong for routine use. Many other drugs have antimuscarinic effects and hence affect eyes. Examples of systemic drugs with atropinic effects include some antihistamines, phenothiazines, antiparkinson agents and antidepressants (see AMH 2005, Appendix A, Table A-3).

SYMPATHOMIMETICS (ADRENERGIC AGONISTS)

Topical **sympathomimetic** agents mimic (directly acting) or potentiate (indirectly acting) the α_1-receptor-mediated actions of noradrenaline on the dilator muscle of the iris. This results in mydriasis, vasoconstriction and decreased congestion of conjunctival blood vessels, an increase in outflow of aqueous humour and a decrease in aqueous humour formation, and relaxation of the ciliary muscle. Sympathomimetics do not affect accommodation or the pupillary light reflex.

Adrenergic drugs are used to produce mydriasis for ocular examination, to treat wide-angle glaucoma and glaucoma secondary to uveitis, and to relieve congestion and hyperaemia (red eyes). Adrenergic drugs are contraindicated in the treatment of narrow-angle glaucoma or abraded cornea because dilation of the pupil will further restrict ocular fluid outflow, which may cause an acute attack of glaucoma. As mydriatics, they are generally used as adjuncts with the anticholinergic mydriatics.

Serious systemic effects from these drugs are unusual, but can include brow ache, sweating, tremors and confusion; adverse effects are likely to be greater in children and in the elderly. Systemic absorption is a concern in patients with cardiovascular disease because tachycardia and elevated

TABLE 35-2 Anticholinergic agents: pharmacokinetics and dosing

DRUG	TIME TO MAXIMAL MYDRIASIS (min)	RECOVERY (days)	TIME TO MAXIMAL CYCLOPLEGIA	RECOVERY	USUAL ADULT DOSE
Atropine	30–40	7–10	3–6 hours	7–14 days	1%: 1 drop
Cyclopentolate	30–60	1	25–75 min	6–24 hours	0.5%, 1%: 1 drop
Homatropine	20–30	¼–4	30–60 min	½–2 days	2%, 5%: 1 drop
Tropicamide	20–40	6 hours	30–40 min	2–6 hours	0.5%, 1%: 1 drop

Based on data in AMH 2005 and Caswell 2005.

blood pressure can occur. Adverse drug interactions may occur with monoamine oxidase inhibitors and with α-adrenoceptor antagonists.

The primary adrenergic drugs used in ophthalmology include phenylephrine, dipivefrine (a prodrug metabolised to adrenaline), naphazoline and tetrahydrozoline (mild agents used as vasoconstrictors); and new α_2 agonists used in glaucoma, apraclonidine and brimonidine. Table 35-3 lists adrenergic ophthalmic drugs with their uses and usual adult dosages; note that the strengths of the solutions, and hence the dosages, vary widely depending on use (antiglaucoma, mydriatic or vasoconstrictor).

Cycloplegics

Cycloplegic agents are drugs that paralyse ciliary muscle, causing loss of accommodation. As explained earlier, cycloplegia is invariably accompanied by mydriasis, as it is induced by antimuscarinic agents, whereas mydriasis induced by adrenergic agonists is not accompanied by cycloplegia.

Cycloplegics are used:

• to prevent accommodation during refraction
• for pain relief in iridocyclitis
• to induce chemical occlusion for treatment of suppression amblyopia (failure of sharp visual images).

Cycloplegic agents are the antimuscarinics, i.e. **atropine**, homatropine, cyclopentolate and tropicamide; see again Table 35-2. Note that the same peripheral and central anticholinergic effects can occur; these agents are used only with great caution in children (particularly those with blue eyes, or people with disorders of the central nervous system [CNS]) due to the risk of central adverse effects.

Miotic agents

Miotics are drugs that constrict the pupil, i.e. cause miosis. Their clinical uses are to reverse mydriatic effects and to treat glaucoma (see later discussion). Because the main autonomic tone in the eye is parasympathetic, with constriction of pupils and accommodation for near vision, parasympathomimetic drugs act as miotics; however, they are likely to cause blurring of vision and spasm of accommodation. Drugs can enhance parasympathetic effects either by acting as agonists on ACh muscarinic receptors or by increasing the amount of ACh available to act.

Muscarinic agonists

Muscarinic agonists stimulate muscarinic receptors, including those in the circular muscle of the iris, causing contraction and thus pupil constriction. ACh itself can be used; however, it is subject to very rapid hydrolysis and inactivation by cholinesterase enzymes, so has a very brief action. It is occasionally used by injection into the anterior chamber for

TABLE 35-3 Adrenergic ophthalmic agents

DRUG	USES	USUAL ADULT DOSAGE
Naphazoline	V	0.01–0.1%: 1 drop every 3–4 hours as necessary
Phenylephrine	IOP, M	2.5%, 10%: 1 drop as necessary
	V	0.12%: 1 or 2 drops every 3–4 hours as necessary
Tetrahydrozoline	V	0.05%: 1 or 2 drops up to 4 times daily
Brimonidine	IOP	0.2%: 1 drop 2 times daily
Dipivefrine	IOP	0.1%: 1 drop 2 times daily
Apraclonidine	IOP	0.5%: 1 drop 3 times daily

IOP = reduction in intraocular pressure; M = mydriasis; V = vasoconstriction.

rapid miosis during surgery. Carbachol, a potent ACh 'lookalike' that is more stable to metabolism, is a quaternary amine (charged), so is poorly absorbed across the cornea and has fewer systemic or CNS effects. It is used for rapid miosis during surgery at a strength of 0.01% (injections) and in open-angle glaucoma.

Pilocarpine is a natural compound from various *Pilocarpus* species plants. Its vasodilator properties were described by Langley in 1875; it has been shown to mimic the effects of ACh in the parasympathetic nervous system. It is an uncharged molecule and so is well absorbed and likely to have CNS adverse effects. It has little effect on the ciliary muscle and thus does not markedly affect accommodation. It is an effective miotic, enhancing outflow of aqueous humour and decreasing IOP, hence its usefulness in glaucoma. To allow careful titration of doses, pilocarpine is available in a wide range of strengths (0.5%, 1%, 2%, 3%, 4%, 6%).

ANTICHOLINESTERASES

These drugs act by inhibiting the breakdown of ACh by cholinesterase enzymes, hence they allow a build-up of ACh at the neuroeffector junction and enhance its parasympathetic and neuromuscular actions. They have been used topically as miotics in the eye, where they also cause accommodation for near vision, increased lacrimation (tearing) and vasodilation. They were also used in treatment of glaucoma and squint. Until early 2002, the only anticholinesterase available in Australia for ocular use was the long-acting, 'irreversible' drug ecothiopate (formerly known as phospholine iodide); it has since been deleted.

Other anticholinesterases are used in treatment of myasthenia gravis (see Clinical Interest Box 21-4) and Alzheimer's disease. They have also been used as insecticides, as war gases and as 'trial' drugs (Clinical Interest Box 35-3).

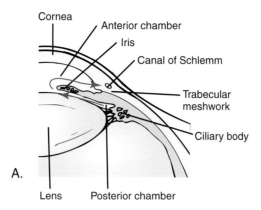

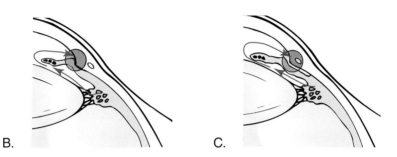

FIGURE 35-2 Main structures of the eye and enlargements of the canal of Schlemm, showing aqueous humour flow. **A.** Normal **B.** Closed-angle glaucoma. **C.** Open-angle glaucoma. *Note:* The 'angle' is the angle of the anterior chamber, effectively the angle between the iris and the cornea; it is the main region of drainage of the aqueous chamber.

Ocular decongestants

Drugs that are vasoconstrictors have useful '**decongestant**' effects in the eye (and nose: see Drug Monograph 32-8). These drugs are sympathomimetics, and their mechanism of action is as α-adrenoceptor agonists. By causing vasoconstriction, they reduce hyperaemia and fluid exudation, hence they reduce reddening and signs of inflammation. Vasoconstriction may also decrease the absorption of other drugs into the bloodstream.

Examples of drugs used as ocular decongestants are **phenylephrine**, naphazoline and tetrahydrozoline. Note that much lower doses are used for vasoconstrictor and

---

CLINICAL INTEREST BOX 35-3 TRIAL BY ANTICHOLINESTERASES

In primitive societies, a person accused of a crime or of witchcraft was often subjected to trial by ordeal, involving dunking in deep water or administration of a potentially poisonous plant extract; if the person survived he or she was presumed innocent. The trick with poisons was to swallow the dose rapidly in the hope that the powerful emetic effect of the poison would cause severe vomiting and thus remove the toxin. An innocent person might do this, whereas a guilty person might be more hesitant and hence absorb more of the toxin.

One of the plants used this way was *Physostigma venenosa*, which grew on the Calabar Coast of western Africa. Its fruit, known as Calabar bean, contains an active alkaloid named physostigmine (or eserine). British missionaries described its use as an ordeal drug in about 1840. The active ingredient of the Calabar beans, eserine, was studied in Edinburgh by botanists and pharmacologists who grew the plants from seeds supplied by missionaries.

After showing that the toxin caused death of animals by paralysis of heart and respiratory muscles, one valiant researcher (Robert Christison) tried an extract of seeds on himself. He described the effects as numbness, giddiness and, even after forced vomiting, feeble pulse and extreme pallor.

The major constituent of Calabar bean was purified and isolated in 1864, and named physostigmine. In 1875 it was used for the treatment of glaucoma, as it had been observed to reduce IOP and cause copious tears and a distinct contraction of the pupil. Its chemical structure was elucidated in 1925. Further pharmacological studies showed that physostigmine mimicked the actions of ACh, and eventually its mechanism was shown to be inhibition of breakdown of ACh by the acetylcholinesterase enzyme. Since then, longer-acting anticholinesterases have been developed, so physostigmine is now rarely used. *Source:* Mann 1992.

decongestant effects than are required for mydriasis (see Table 35-3). Decongestants are often formulated as eye-drops together with:

- an antihistamine (antazoline, pheniramine, levocabastine), to reduce itching and redness
- a corticosteroid, for anti-inflammatory effects
- an antibiotic, for antibacterial activity
- zinc sulphate, which assists healing.

ANTIGLAUCOMA AGENTS

Glaucomas

Glaucomas are a group of optic neuropathies involving damage to the optic nerve, changes in visual fields and abnormally elevated intraocular pressure (IOP) (>21 mmHg); this is sometimes referred to as 'ocular hypertension' (strictly speaking, hypertensive retinopathy). The raised IOP may result from excessive production of aqueous humour or diminished ocular fluid outflow, and is the third most common cause of blindness worldwide. Although it is primarily a disease of middle age, occurring in about 2% of all people aged 40 or over, it has also been diagnosed in younger adults and children. It is estimated that about a third of the population have a familial tendency to raised IOP and are predisposed to glaucoma.

Primary glaucoma includes closed-angle (acute congestive) glaucoma and open-angle (chronic simple, or wide-angle) glaucoma (Figure 35-2) Primary open-angle glaucoma (POAG) is the more common, occurring in about 90% of individuals with primary glaucoma, and in 2%–3% of the population aged over 70 years. It is a chronic, familial condition, with gradual insidious onset.

Acute closed-angle glaucoma is due to a physiological or anatomical predisposition to mechanical blockage of the trabecular network. This is a rare acute optical emergency, with severe pain and a rapid rise in IOP threatening vision. Emergency drug therapy with IV acetazolamide or mannitol, oral glycerol or topical pilocarpine is needed to control the acute attack, followed usually by surgery, such as iridectomy or laser surgery.

Secondary glaucoma may result from previous eye disease or cataract extraction, or may be secondary to inflammation (uveitis), trauma, tumour, adhesions (iritis) or drugs (corticosteroids, mydriatics, vasodilators, phenothiazines, antidepressants or antimuscarinics). Therapy for secondary glaucoma requires attention first to the primary cause and avoidance of precipitating factors if possible, then antiglaucoma drugs.

Treatment of glaucomas

The main medications used to treat glaucoma include β-adrenoceptor antagonists (β-blockers), prostaglandin agonists, carbonic anhydrase inhibitors, miotics (cholinergics) and sympathomimetics (see Tables 35-3 and 35-4); selection of a drug is determined largely by the requirements and individual response of the person. The efficacy of each drug may be checked in one eye first for 2–4 weeks, using the other eye as a 'control'; if the IOP in the treated eye decreases, the drug is applied to the other eye as well.

A suggested step-wise treatment approach to POAG is as follows:
1. start with mild topical agents: a prostaglandin agonist eye-drop
2. add a β-blocker
3. add a CA inhibitor or α agonist
4. add a miotic: pilocarpine drops (or carbachol)
5. consider surgery.

Some combination preparations are now available, such as eye-drops containing timolol plus dorzolamide, or timolol plus latanoprost. The target IOP is 30% below the original baseline reading. Patients with dark eyes may need higher doses, and it is important to teach patients to minimise systemic absorption of drugs by pressing on the nasolacrimal ducts for 2–3 minutes after administration of drops.

Ocular β-adrenoceptor antagonists

The β-blockers used in glaucoma include betaxolol, levobunolol and **timolol**, as 0.25% and 0.5% drops. The exact mechanism of action for these drugs is unknown; however, it is suggested that they block β-receptor-mediated stimulation of ciliary epithelium, leading to impaired aqueous humour formation. The advantages of β-blockers are their safety, their duration of action (meaning they need be given in only one or two doses per day) and their lack of effect on pupil size or accommodation.

Betaxolol, a cardioselective (β$_1$) blocking agent, is indicated for the treatment of POAG and ocular hypertension, and may be preferred for patients with airways disease, as it is less likely than non-cardioselective β-blockers to cause bronchoconstriction and asthma (see Chapter 12).

Adverse reactions are primarily local: burning, stinging or eye irritation. Rare effects include visual disturbances, pruritus or allergic reaction. Systemic absorption can lead to adverse effects including hypotension, asthma and depression; precautions need to be taken in patients with asthma or diabetes, and in the elderly and children. Table 35-4 lists β-blocking agents, times of action and dosing information.

TABLE 35-4 Antiglaucoma agents: pharmacokinetics and dosing

DRUG	ONSET OF ACTION (h)	PEAK EFFECT (h)	DURATION OF ACTION (h)	USUAL ADULT DOSAGE
α₂-adrenoceptor agonists				
Apraclonidine	N/A	N/A	N/A	0.5%: 1 drop 2–3 times daily
Brimonidine	rapid	2	8–12	0.2%: 1 drop 2 times daily
β-adrenoceptor antagonists				
Betaxolol	0.5	2	12–18	0.25%, 0.5%: 1 drop 2 times daily
Levobunolol	1	2–6	Up to 24	0.25%: 1 drop 2 times daily
Timolol	0.5	1–2	Up to 24	0.25%, 0.5%: 1 drop 2 times daily gel 0.1%: 1 drop daily
Carbonic anhydrase inhibitors				
Systemic				
Acetazolamide				
tablets	1–1.5	2–4	8–12	250 mg PO 1–4 times daily
IV injection	2 min	15 min	4–5	250–1000 mg/24 hours IV
Eye-drops				
Dorzolamide	N/A	N/A	8–12	2%: 1 drop 3 times daily
Brinzolamide	N/A	N/A	8–12	1%: 1 drop 2 times daily
Prostaglandin agonists				
Latanoprost	N/A	2	24–36	50 mcg/mL (0.005%): 1 drop in the evening
Bimatoprost	4	8–12	24–36	0.03%: 1 drop in the evening
Travoprost	2	>12	24–36	0.004%: 1 drop in the evening
Miotics (muscarinic agonists)				
Carbachol	0.25	4	4–12	1.5%, 3%: 2 drops 3 times daily
Pilocarpine	Up to 0.5	1–1.25	4–12	0.5%–6%: 1 drop up to 4 times daily

IV = intravenously; N/A = not available; PO = orally. See also Table 35-3.

Sympathomimetic agents (α-receptor agonists)

The **sympathomimetic** agents have been discussed earlier as mydriatics and decongestants, and are summarised in Table 35-3. When used in glaucoma, it appears that the α-receptor stimulation increases aqueous humour outflow via vasoconstriction and may also suppress aqueous humour formation. These agents are indicated for the treatment of POAG.

The older directly acting agents are dipivefrine, adrenaline and phenylephrine. Dipivefrine is a prodrug, a more lipophilic compound that penetrates well through the cornea into the anterior chamber of the eye, where it is converted to adrenaline by an enzyme. Newer sympathomimetic agents are the α₂-receptor selective agonists apraclonidine and brimonidine; these are related to the antihypertensive agent clonidine. Apraclonidine is indicated for short-term use only, for up to 3 months.

Adverse reactions are rarely troublesome; they include eye irritation, headache and mydriasis. Effects of systemic absorption are those of α-receptor stimulation: palpitations, hypertension, tremors and lightheadedness.

Carbonic anhydrase inhibitor agents

The enzyme **carbonic anhydrase** (CA) catalyses the interconversion of bicarbonate with carbon dioxide and water; its actions are necessary for the secretion of aqueous humour.

Drugs that inhibit this enzyme are used as mild diuretic agents, to treat epilepsy and raised intracranial pressure, and in glaucoma.

The most commonly used systemic CA inhibitor is acetazolamide. It is administered in glaucoma emergencies; given PO, IV or IM, it lowers IOP by decreasing the aqueous production to about half of its baseline measurement. Some new CA inhibitors are now available as topical eye-drops (see Table 35-4): **dorzolamide** and brinzolamide, which has a high affinity for the ocular enzyme and can be used twice daily. Currently they are recommended for short-term use only.

Important drug interactions can occur from systemically administered CA inhibitors, due to alkalinisation of the urine and hence decreased excretion of basic drugs such as amphetamines, ephedrine and quinidine.

Cholinergic agents (miotics)

Miotics contract the circular muscle of the iris, thus relieving obstruction to outflow of aqueous humour and reducing IOP in glaucoma. These drugs have been discussed earlier (Miotic agents). They are used much less commonly these days.

Adverse reactions to cholinergic agents such as carbachol and **pilocarpine** include visual blurring, eye irritation, myopia and headache. Miosis also makes it difficult to adjust quickly to changes in illumination; this may be serious in elderly people. Systemic effects include symptoms of parasympathetic stimulation, such as salivation, nausea, vomiting, diarrhoea, precipitation of asthmatic attacks and a fall in blood pressure.

Prostaglandin agonists (lipid-receptor agonists)

Latanoprost, bimatoprost and travoprost are the first synthetic prostaglandin $F_{2\alpha}$ agonists approved to treat POAG. They reduce IOP by increasing aqueous humour outflow; the precise mechanism of action is not yet well clarified (see Drug Monograph 35-1).

Adverse reactions include blurred vision, burning and stinging, itching, photophobia and conjunctival hyperaemia. The drugs may also permanently increase pigmentation (brown) of the iris. Their long duration of action enhances patient compliance.

Osmotic agents

Osmotic agents are non-absorbed chemicals that raise plasma osmotic pressure (OP); they are given intravenously or orally to reduce IOP. The rationale for their use in glaucoma is that these agents generally do not cross the blood–aqueous humour barrier into the anterior chamber of the eye. Consequently, the plasma OP exceeds intraocular OP, leading to dehydration

DRUG MONOGRAPH 35-1 LATANOPROST

Latanoprost is a prostaglandin $F_{2\alpha}$ analogue, which reduces intraocular pressure (IOP) by enhancing uveoscleral outflow of aqueous humour. It can reduce IOP by 27%–34%; no tolerance develops over at least 4 years.

INDICATIONS Latanoprost is indicated for patients with open-angle glaucoma, to reduce IOP and prevent the risk of optic nerve damage.

PHARMACOKINETICS Latanoprost is administered as eye-drops. Its onset of action is 3–4 hours, maximum effect occurs in 8–12 hours, and duration of action is >24 hours. It is a prodrug, an ester that is hydrolysed to the active form during passage through the cornea; it is distributed to the anterior segment of the eye, conjunctiva and eyelids. Following ocular administration, approximately 45% of the administered dose is absorbed systemically; it is metabolised in the liver to inactive metabolites, which are excreted in the urine. The elimination half-life is approximately 17 minutes.

DRUG INTERACTIONS Few data are available as yet on significant drug interactions. There are additive effects with timolol and other β-blockers, and the drug can be used effectively as adjunct therapy with most other antiglaucoma agents.

ADVERSE REACTIONS The most common adverse reactions are in the eye: stinging, blurred vision, conjunctivitis, red eye, itching and eye pain. An unusual side-effect is change in iris colour: people with hazel or yellow-brown eyes are particularly susceptible to darkening of the iris; this effect, if it occurs, usually starts within 8 months of commencing therapy. Latanoprost should be used with caution in patients with, or susceptible to, asthma or macular oedema.

WARNINGS AND CONTRAINDICATIONS Patients should be warned of the possible change in eye colour, especially if the drug is being applied only to one eye. It is contraindicated if there is known hypersensitivity to any ingredient; thus far there are few data on use in children or during pregnancy or lactation.

DOSAGE AND ADMINISTRATION One drop of latanoprost solution (50 mcg/mL) is administered to the eye daily, preferably in the evening; pressure should be applied to the tear duct to minimise systemic absorption. It is also available in a combination formulation with timolol (5 mg/mL) for use if either drug alone does not provide adequate reduction in IOP.

of the vitreous body and decreased formation and increased resorption of aqueous humour.

Examples are mannitol 20% solution IV, which is rapid and effective, and glycerol 50% solution for oral administration. They are used in emergency treatment of acute glaucoma, before surgery for cataract, and sometimes to reduce intracranial pressure.

Other drugs that reduce intraocular pressure

Other drugs that can decrease IOP include marijuana (Δ^9-tetrahydrocannabinol; see Chapter 22), tranquillisers, phenytoin and digoxin. These effects, however, are not sufficiently specific or safe for the drugs to be used in glaucoma.

ANTIMICROBIAL AGENTS

Because the eye (conjunctival surface) is open to the atmosphere and maintained in a moist condition, it is very prone to infection. Some parts of the eye are avascular, hence the body's natural defences cannot function there, and severe infections may damage the eye and impair vision. Thus eye infections require prompt treatment with antimicrobial agents; solutions (eye-drops) are preferred formulations, because ointment bases tend to interfere with healing.

Ocular infections

The common routes of transmission of infection to the eye include:

- congenital, during passage of the infant down the birth canal if infection is present (e.g. ophthalmia neonatorum, a gonococcal infection)
- direct contact (e.g. herpes simplex transmitted by fingers from 'cold sore' lesions)
- airborne: droplet transmission in aerosol (e.g. from coughing or sneezing)
- migration from other loci, especially from the nasopharynx
- trauma, especially penetrating eye injuries
- from infected contact lenses, instruments or contaminated ocular drug formulations (eye-drops, lotions, solutions or ointments).

Common ocular pathogens include bacteria (especially *Staphylococcus aureus*, streptococci and pneumococci), viruses (*Adenovirus*, herpes simplex virus), *Chlamydia* and protozoa (acanthamoeba). Diagnosis of infections may be difficult to differentiate from severe inflammation, as the signs and symptoms (pain, reddening, swelling, heat and loss of function) are similar. Conjunctivitis, for example, may be of infectious or inflammatory aetiology.

Common ocular infections

Some of the common ocular infections treated with antimicrobials are described briefly below.

Conjunctivitis is an acute inflammation of the conjunctiva resulting from bacterial or viral infection, or of allergic or irritative origin. Symptoms include redness and burning of the eye, lacrimation, itching and at times photophobia. Conjunctivitis is usually self-limiting. The eye should be protected from light. In severe cases, antibiotic eye-drops or ointment may be required.

Blepharitis (inflammation of the eyelids) may result from bacterial or viral infection, dandruff-type inflammation, or allergy; symptoms are crusting, irritation of the eye and red and oedematous lid margins. For seborrhoeic (dandruff-type) blepharitis, treatment is to wash lids gently with a mild soap (e.g. 'baby shampoo' or 'baby soap') or sodium bicarbonate solution. If the infection is staphylococcal, the lids are cleansed, then antibiotic eye ointment (tetracycline or chloramphenicol) is applied.

Hordeolum (stye) is an acute localised infection of the eyelash follicles and the glands of the anterior lid margin, resulting in the formation of a small abscess or cyst, usually effectively treated by drainage. An internal hordeolum may also require oral antistaphylococcal antibiotics, e.g. dicloxacillin.

Keratitis is corneal inflammation caused by bacterial or viral infection. Adenoviral keratoconjunctivitis is very contagious, but usually resolves simply. Herpes simplex keratitis, however, may cause corneal ulcers and scarring, and requires treatment with an ocular antiviral agent (aciclovir).

Infection with *Acanthamoeba* (a protozoon) occurs usually in wearers of soft contact lenses, from contaminated water and solutions. It causes redness, pain and photophobia, and can lead to corneal breakdown, scarring and loss of vision. Consequently, it requires early diagnosis and aggressive antimicrobial therapy, e.g. with an antiamoebic agent (propamidine) and an antibacterial (neomycin) and possibly an antifungal to prevent secondary infections.

Trachoma is an infection caused by the organism *Chlamydia trachomatis*, an intracellular microorganism, which in the eye produces keratoconjunctivitis. It can also infect the genital tract and cause sexually transmitted disease and sterility. Trachoma is a serious world health problem (estimated to affect 500 million people) and is the major cause of preventable blindness. There is a high incidence in hot dry areas with poor hygiene and crowded living conditions; it is a major public health problem in northern parts of Australia. It is common in children. Although it may appear mild, chronic infection can lead to visual loss in middle age; hence the importance of early detection, good public health education and effective compliance with therapy. Treatment is with one dose of oral azithromycin (1 g adult dose).

Toxoplasmosis is an infection with the unicellular organism *Toxoplasma gondii*; it is commonly contracted before birth or from domestic cats. If the eye is affected, posterior uveitis can lead to loss of sight. Immunocompromised patients are particularly at risk. Treatment is combination therapy with specific antimicrobials (such as clindamycin or pyrimethamine) plus corticosteroids to limit the damaging inflammatory response.

Antimicrobial chemotherapy of ocular infections

Selection of an antimicrobial for ocular infection is based on clinical experience, the nature and sensitivity of the organisms most commonly causing the condition, the disease itself, the sensitivity and response of the patient, and laboratory results. Prophylactic use of anti-infective agents in general is useless, wasteful and potentially dangerous due to the risk of resistance developing in microorganisms. Topical application of anti-infective agents can also interfere with the normal flora of the eye and encourage growth of other organisms.

Most antimicrobial agents do not easily penetrate the eye when applied. Some drugs, however, will penetrate the inflamed eye when the blood–aqueous humour barrier is impaired by injury or inflammation. Topically applied anti-infective agents can cause sensitivity reactions (stinging, itching and dermatitis) and an unpleasant taste following nasolacrimal drainage. Individuals sensitised to one drug may show cross-reactions to chemically related drugs (e.g. penicillins and cephalosporins).

The ideal properties of antimicrobials are that they should have the appropriate spectrum of antimicrobial activity; should have long-lasting, non-toxic actions; should not interfere with vision or healing; and should be available in sterile, single-dose containers. It is considered important that the antimicrobials used locally (whether in the eye or on the skin) be different from those used systemically. There is then less likelihood of inducing resistance in the organisms to the actions of the drug, or of possible sensitisation in the person to systemic antimicrobial drugs. In addition, drugs that are too toxic systemically can often be safely used locally. For local administration to the eye, these agents are administered topically or by ocular injection. In Australia, some topical antibiotics (ciprofloxacin, gentamicin and tobramycin) are preferentially reserved for ophthalmologists' use, either to reduce resistance or because the drugs are potentially toxic. (Antimicrobial drugs are considered in detail in Unit XIV, where their mechanisms of action and typical antimicrobial spectra of activity are discussed.)

Antibacterial agents used in ocular infections

Antibacterial antibiotics used in the eye include chloramphenicol, tetracycline, aminoglycosides (neomycin, gentamicin, framycetin and tobramycin), quinolones (ciprofloxacin and ofloxacin), and various miscellaneous agents (bacitracin, polymyxin B and gramicidin). Combination preparations may contain various combinations of these ingredients, such as 'triple antibiotic' ophthalmic ointment and drops (neomycin, polymyxin B and gramicidin ophthalmic ointment and drops).

Gramicidin is not used systemically because of its nephrotoxic effects. Topically, it is particularly useful in treating surface superficial infections caused by Gram-positive bacteria. The combination dosage form with neomycin and polymyxin B provides a bactericidal effect against many Gram-positive and Gram-negative organisms. It is indicated for the treatment of superficial ocular infections caused by susceptible organisms. A small amount (1 cm) of ointment is usually applied to the conjunctiva every 3–4 hours.

CHLORAMPHENICOL

A broad-spectrum bacteriostatic agent, chloramphenicol prevents peptide bond formation and protein synthesis in a wide variety of Gram-positive and Gram-negative organisms, and is a useful drug for ocular infections. Burning and stinging on administration have been reported. Irreversible aplastic anaemia has not been reported with topical chloramphenicol (as it has with oral administration).

AMINOGLYCOSIDES

Aminoglycosides (neomycin, gentamicin, framycetin and tobramycin) are used against a wide variety of Gram-negative organisms, including *Proteus* and *Klebsiella* organisms and *Escherichia coli*. They are applied as an ointment 2 or 3 times daily, or as 1 drop of solution every 4 hours.

Adverse reactions include ocular toxicity and hypersensitivity, including lid itching, swelling and conjunctival erythema. When topical aminoglycosides are used concurrently with systemic aminoglycosides, the total plasma concentration will be increased and should be monitored, as systemic toxicity (renal damage and ototoxicity) may occur from excessive use.

SULFONAMIDES

Sulfacetamide sodium is a sulfonamide, and as such blocks the synthesis of folic acid in susceptible bacterial organisms. The action of sulfonamides, however, is reduced by the presence of purulent exudate (pus), so lid exudate should be removed before the drug is instilled; sulfacetamide sodium is irritant, so its use is not recommended.

SYSTEMIC ANTIMICROBIALS

In severe eye infections, it may be necessary to administer antimicrobial agents systemically. Drugs are selected specifically for the organism cultured, e.g. cefotaxime or benzylpenicillin for gonococcal ophthalmia (in parents and newborn), or azithromycin for trachoma.

TOPICAL ANTIVIRALS

The only ophthalmic antiviral preparation available currently in Australia is **aciclovir** ointment, 30 mg/g, indicated for treatment of herpes simplex keratitis. For treatment of keratitis, a 1 cm ribbon of the aciclovir ointment is added to the lower conjunctival sac, five times daily. Aciclovir is well absorbed through the cornea, and effective concentrations appear in the aqueous humour. Adverse reactions include transient stinging, sensitivity reactions and occasionally reversible superficial corneal damage. Although antiviral agents are potentially teratogenic, aciclovir use during pregnancy is considered safe (Pregnancy Safety Category B3).

ANTISEPTICS

Many antiseptics that were used to treat infections of the eye before the advent of antibiotics are now obsolete. Inorganic mercuric salts such as yellow mercuric oxide have been used, but Golden Eye Ointment (1%) has recently been deleted.

Propamidine is an old drug with a new use. It was previously used in ointments and creams as a mild antiseptic and skin disinfectant, effective against skin flora including *S. aureus* and some streptococci and clostridia. Propamidine and its dibromo- derivative have been found to be very effective topically against *Acanthamoeba*, an infection transmitted via tap water to contact lens solutions and the eyes of wearers, with potentially sight-threatening consequences. Propamidine eye-drops (0.1%) and dibromopropamidine eye ointment (0.15%) are available for the treatment of *Acanthamoeba* keratitis and for mild acute conjunctivitis.

ANTI-INFLAMMATORY AND ANTIALLERGY AGENTS

Inflammation of the eye

Inflammation of the eyes, with reddening, tearing, itching and mild pain, is relatively common and may accompany infections, mechanical damage or allergies, or occur as an ocular adverse effect of systemic medications (see Table 35-6 for drugs that induce ocular effects). Inflammatory conditions include uveitis (intraocular inflammation), episcleritis and scleritis; these range in severity from common and mild to severe vision-threatening conditions. Treatment is with cold

> ### CLINICAL INTEREST BOX 35-4 THE FIRST COMMANDMENT OF EYE CARE
>
> An early classic textbook of ocular pharmacology, discussing 'The Ten Commandments of Eye Care', listed as the first commandment: 'Thou shalt not use cortisone'. The text went on to describe the many ocular inflammatory conditions in which steroid eye-drops and ointments give great relief, including allergic conjunctivitis and acute iritis.
>
> The point was well made, however, that steroids can result in corneal perforation in the presence of viral infection; can predispose to devastating bacterial and fungal infections, especially in the presence of a foreign body; and when used chronically, can induce blindness from cataract or glaucoma. It is now recommended that ocular steroids not be prescribed without the close supervision of an ophthalmologist to monitor the corneal epithelium and IOP.

compresses, decongestant drops, mydriatics, oral or ocular non-steroidal anti-inflammatory drugs (NSAIDs), and steroid drops if more severe.

A major potential risk involving inflammation of the eye is postoperative inflammation, which can occur, for example, after cataract surgery or after eye trauma, and lead to the formation of adhesions, which can threaten vision. To prevent adhesions, a decreasing course of topical corticosteroids is administered with antibiotic cover, e.g. steroid drops in the first week: 1 drop four times per day, reducing to 1 drop/day in the 4th week.

Ocular corticosteroids

Corticosteroids inhibit the inflammatory cascade and the functions of fibroblasts and keratocytes (see Chapter 40). Their anti-inflammatory and immunosuppressant effects are useful in many ocular conditions, including inflammations and allergies of the conjunctiva, cornea and anterior segment of the eye, such as contact dermatitis, allergic blepharitis and conjunctivitis, vernal conjunctivitis, keratitis, iritis and iridocyclitis, posterior uveitis, scleritis and optic neuritis. Corticosteroids are now also being trialled in posterior segment diseases such as age-related macular degeneration, diabetic retinopathy and macular oedema, because of their angiostatic actions in reducing growth of new blood vessels and their reduction in vascular permeability. They have major adverse effects (see Clinical Interest Box 35-4) and are contraindicated in ocular infections and glaucoma.

Many corticosteroids are available for ophthalmic use as topical solutions, suspensions or ointments. They include dexamethasone, fluorometholone, hydrocortisone and **prednisolone**, available in varying strengths and sometimes in combination with antibiotics (see Table 35-5).

TABLE 35-5
Potency of ocular corticosteroids

STEROID DROPS	POTENCY	RELATIVE TENDENCY TO RAISE INTRAOCULAR PRESSURE
Hydrocortisone	Low	++
Prednisolone sodium phosphate	Mid	+++
Fluorometholone	Mid–high	+++
Prednisolone acetate	High	++++
Dexamethasone	High	++++

Adverse reactions include burning, lacrimation, visual disturbances, eye pain, headaches, enlarged pupils, raised IOP and glaucoma, impaired healing and opportunistic infections. More rarely, corneal damage, refractive changes and cataracts can occur: these should be reported to the prescriber.

Non-steroidal anti-inflammatory agents

The NSAIDs are now available in formulations for ocular use (early drugs were too irritant to the cornea). Diclofenac (0.1%), flurbiprofen (0.03%), ketotifen (0.025%) or ketorolac drops (0.5%) are used in inflammatory conditions. They have the following indications:

- to inhibit intraoperative miosis (a debatable effect)
- to treat postoperative inflammation after a cataract extraction
- to treat conjunctivitis and seasonal allergic ophthalmic pruritus (itching associated with hay fever).

These agents, if absorbed, may produce systemic effects. Because they have the potential to cause increased bleeding, their use should be monitored closely in patients who are known to have bleeding tendencies. The most common adverse reaction reported is transient burning or stinging on application. Other minor symptoms of ocular irritation have also been reported, such as itching, redness and allergic reactions.

Ocular antiallergic agents

Allergic reactions of the eyelid and conjunctiva can lead to oedema, erythema, itching, crusting and contact dermatitis. Typical allergens are pollens, dust, bites and stings, food, cosmetics, jewellery, animals and chemicals. Drugs that are known to cause ocular allergies include some antibiotics, preservatives, topical antihistamines (a paradoxical effect) and timolol.

Treatment of ocular allergies is first to eliminate the allergen (if possible); then cooling, saline lotions and oral NSAIDs may bring relief. Topical treatment is with eye-drops:

- antihistamines (block H_1 receptors), e.g. levocabastine 0.05%, antazoline 0.5%, pheniramine 0.3%, olopatadine 0.1%
- NSAIDs, e.g. ketorolac 0.5%
- prophylactic mast-cell stabilisers, such as sodium cromoglycate 2%, lodoxamide 0.1%
- if allergy is severe, corticosteroids, e.g. prednisolone 1%.

Note that the combination of a decongestant with an antihistamine often leads to rebound conjunctivitis, with exacerbation of symptoms.

Vernal conjunctivitis ('hay fever')

Hay fever is often associated with extreme itching of the eyes, with blurring of vision and development of papillae (small projections of tissue from the conjunctiva). Prophylactic cromoglycate may be preventive; treatment is with antihistamines or prednisolone (tapering the dose off over 1–2 weeks).

MAST-CELL STABILISERS (CROMOLYNS)

Drugs such as sodium cromoglycate (cromolyn sodium) and lodoxamide inhibit degranulation of sensitised mast cells occurring after exposure to a specific antigen; this prevents the mediators of inflammation from producing their effects. The drugs are used for allergic eye disorders (vernal and allergic keratoconjunctivitis, papillary conjunctivitis and keratitis) that have symptoms of itching, tearing, redness and discharge.

Adverse reactions include stinging and burning sensation in the eyes. Concomitant use of corticosteroids may be necessary. For adults and children (over 4 years), 1 drop is instilled in each affected eye 4–6 times a day at regular intervals; the clinical effects may not be felt for some days.

OCULAR LOCAL ANAESTHETICS

Local anaesthetics (LAs) temporarily block nerve conduction by reducing membrane permeability to sodium. The first nerves blocked are small unmyelinated fibres, which carry the sensation of pain, hence these 'membrane-stabilising agents' are relatively selective at inhibiting transmission of pain impulses (see general discussion of LAs in Chapter 15). The order of loss of sensations is: pain, temperature, touch, then proprioception; muscle power may be lost last. A vasoconstrictor (adrenaline) is often added to the LA solution to localise the drug in the tissue into which it has been injected and prolong its actions. The indications for use of LAs are for minor surgery, and surgery in which the cooperation of the patient is required; thus they are particularly useful for ophthalmic surgery and to relieve pain associated with other ocular procedures and drug administrations.

LAs can be applied topically to the eye as drops; these will temporarily anaesthetise the conjunctival and corneal epithelium and provide short-term ocular anaesthesia. This is useful in foreign body removal, contact lens fitting, removal of sutures, some diagnostic procedures, painful irritations, in relieving stinging of other drops, and in tonometry (measurement of IOP) and gonioscopy (examination of the interior of the eye). LA solutions can also be injected subcutaneously or by retrobulbar technique, or around the pathway of specific nerves for nerve blocks, e.g. of the orbital or frontal nerve.

The ideal properties of an ocular LA are that it should have:
- quick onset of action (10–20 seconds)
- useful duration of action (10–20 minutes)
- no adverse effect on eye functions or healing
- no adverse interaction with other drugs likely to be used concurrently.

Ocular LAs usually increase the penetration of other drugs (eye-drops) applied around the same time, and commonly cause stinging and sometimes allergies. It has been recommended that a patient never be given LA drops to take home, as the person may overuse the drops without realising that the eye's normal protective reflexes (blinking, tear production) may be abolished, leading to risk of impaired healing and possibly ulceration.

The LAs available for ocular administration as eye-drops are amethocaine, oxybuprocaine and **proxymetacaine**. They have onset of action within 10–20 seconds, and duration of action about 20 minutes. One of the most commonly used is proxymetacaine (known as proparacaine in the USA); it has the advantages of remaining stable in solution, with rapid onset of action and short duration, while causing minimal adverse reactions, mydriasis or irritation. Adverse reactions from excessive use can include allergic contact dermatitis, pupillary dilation, cycloplegia, and damage to cornea and conjunctiva. It is more toxic if it enters the systemic circulation.

OTHER OPHTHALMIC PREPARATIONS

Diagnostic aids: stains

Stains are diagnostic agents that rapidly provide useful information due to their differential staining characteristics on cells and cell constituents. The ideal properties of an ocular stain are that:
- it is water-soluble and readily reversed or washed away
- it selectively stains certain cells while not staining skin, contact lenses, instruments or clothes
- it does not interfere with vision or have other pharmacological or adverse effects

- it is compatible with other drugs likely to be used concurrently.

The two stains used in the eye are fluorescein and rose bengal.

Fluorescein

Fluorescein is a non-toxic, orange-red, water-soluble dye that is used as a diagnostic aid; it fluoresces even when very dilute, and colours the tear film. Normal corneal epithelium is impermeable and hence is not stained; however, areas of abrasion or desquamation, which have a higher pH, show up intensely green. Thus when fluorescein is applied to the cornea, it permits detection of corneal epithelial defects caused by injury or infection.

Fluorescein is very commonly used for tonometry (measurement of IOP), to show corneal abrasions, in location of a foreign body, in detection of retinopathy, and to test whether the nasolacrimal drainage system is open.

Fluorescein solutions readily support growth of *Pseudomonas* colonies; however, the usual preservatives are incompatible with the dye. The dye is formulated in single-dose packages as eye-drops (1%, 2%) and as drug-impregnated paper strips (see Drug Monograph 35-2). Drops combining fluorescein with lignocaine are also available, to reduce the stinging caused by fluorescein.

Intravenous injection of a sterile solution of fluorescein is used in ophthalmic angiography to examine the fundus, vasculature of the iris and aqueous flow, and to determine time for blood circulation in the eye. Possible adverse reactions after IV injection include nausea, headache, abdominal distress, vomiting, hypotension, hypersensitivity reactions and anaphylaxis.

Rose bengal

Rose bengal is a reddish-brown fluorescein derivative (disodium tetrachlorotetraiodofluorescein). It is used as an ocular stain and has been used as a food dye. It stains dead cells in the cornea and conjunctiva, and is useful in diagnosis of dry eyes and infections, and in detection of minute foreign bodies. Rose bengal drops can cause severe stinging of the eyes.

Botulinum toxin

Botulinum toxin type A is a purified fraction of toxin from *Clostridium botulinum*, the organism that commonly causes food poisoning (botulism) from poorly cooked or preserved food. It is the most poisonous biological toxin known. The toxin blocks neuromuscular transmission by binding to membrane receptors on the nerve terminals and entering the cell, where peptidase enzymes in the toxin then cleave proteins involved in exocytosis and thus specifically inhibit

A blink is the shutting and opening of the eyelids, whereas a wink is a blink of one eye to convey a private message to another person. Thus blepharospasm, a dystonia characterised by involuntary sustained or spasmodic contractions of muscles leading to eyelid blinking or twitching, could be misconstrued and lead to embarrassing problems other than the clinical sequelae. The aetiology of blepharospasm is unknown; it is presumed to be due to irritation of the facial nerve by an artery or tumour.

Many treatments have been tried:
- complementary and alternative medicine methods: hypnosis, acupuncture, herbs, relaxation
- adjunctive drugs: benzodiazepines, levodopa, baclofen, haloperidol
- surgery to facial muscles.

Botulinum toxin has found a specific place in therapy of this disorder, with improvement in 70%–100% of patients in whom the toxin has been injected to paralyse the muscles undergoing spasm (pretarsal orbicularis oculi).

**DRUG MONOGRAPH 35-2
FLUORESCEIN STRIPS**

Fluorescein sodium is an orange-red dye, soluble in water and alcohol, which stains lesions of the cornea.

INDICATIONS It is used in diagnosis of eye damage, and in tonometry and fitting of contact lenses.

ADMINISTRATION AND PHARMACOKINETICS The fluorescein is impregnated into paper strips, which are provided dry and sterile. After the individually wrapped strip has been carefully opened, the coloured tip is moistened with 1–2 drops of sterile saline solution then touched to the conjunctiva. The patient blinks to distribute the fluorescein solution. There should be minimal systemic absorption of the drug, although there may be some staining of adjacent tissues (lids, tears, cheek).

There are no significant adverse reactions or drug interactions with normal clinical use. (With the lignocaine–fluorescein combination drops, there may be hypersensitivity reactions to the LA component, and precautions need to be taken to protect the anaesthetised eye.)

DOSAGE AND ADMINISTRATION Sufficient dye is applied to stain the required area; excess solution is wiped away or washed off with sterile saline solution.

ACh release (see Chapters 11 and 13, and Figure 13-2). It is used to treat muscle spasticity in many dystonic conditions, including blepharospasm (Clinical Interest Box 35-5) and strabismus, cerebral palsy, torticollis, hemifacial spasm, migraine and tension headaches, and in cosmetic surgery to tighten facial muscles (see Drug Monograph 35-3).

Verteporfin, a photosentiser

Many chemical compounds can act as photosensitisers, i.e. the molecules absorb energy from electromagnetic radiation or light, and form activated metabolites such as oxygen free radicals, which damage cell constituents. Examples of photosensitisers are the drug groups sulfonamides and phenothiazines, and the natural compounds porphyrins, which are products of haemoglobin biosynthesis and metabolism. This process can be exploited in photodynamic therapy, in which a photosensitiser plus light energy can be directed to ablate specific lesions.

Verteporfin is a porphyrin-type molecule that is being used as a photosensitiser in the treatment of macular degeneration, the condition in elderly people where the most sensitive part of the retina degenerates, new blood vessels are formed and central vision is lost. This has previously been treatable only by laser burns to seal the leaks into the retina. Verteporfin is a dark green-black chemical which is administered as an IV infusion over 10 minutes. At 15 min, non-thermal red light from a laser source is focused on the macular lesion (e.g. neovasculature) for about 80 seconds. Verteporfin is activated by the light to reactive oxygen free radicals, which cause local damage and vessel occlusion. It is indicated in treatment of age-related macular degeneration and choroidal neovascularisation due to other macular diseases. Adverse reactions include loss of visual acuity, field defects, haemorrhages, cataract, blepharitis and pain at the infusion site.

Contact lens products
Types of contact lenses

Contact lenses are classified as hard (including 'rigid gas-permeable' lenses) or soft.

Hard lenses are generally manufactured from polymethylmethacrylate, and rigid gas-permeable lenses (permeable to oxygen) are made from silicone resins. Hard (and rigid) lenses are less comfortable for wearers in the initial adaptation period, but have the advantages of being more durable, less adsorbent (hence drugs and other chemicals are less likely to bind) and better optically.

Soft contact lenses are made from materials such as hydrogels and silicone elastomers, and all contain more than 80% water, hence their softness. They have the advantages of being more comfortable, requiring a shorter adaptation period and allowing prolonged extended wear; more than 90% of new contact lens fits are with soft lenses. However, there are potential problems of chemicals (even systemically

DRUG MONOGRAPH 35-3
BOTULINUM TOXIN

The toxin is purified from a culture of the organism *Clostridium botulinum*, and is prepared as a dried complex of the high-molecular-weight toxin protein plus a haemagglutinin and albumin; it is reconstituted before use with sterile saline. When injected IM or SC, the toxin causes localised 'chemical denervation' and muscle paralysis, leading to muscle atrophy. The paralysis is slowly reversible over a period of months; the duration of action is 6 weeks to 6 months.

INDICATIONS In blepharospasm, botulinum toxin decreases excessive abnormal contractions of the muscle injected; care must be taken to avoid injecting the lower lid. In strabismus, the toxin causes atrophic lengthening of the injected muscle, and hence can be used to relieve squint.

PHARMACOKINETICS Studies in animals have shown that the toxin diffuses slowly from the injected muscle and is metabolised and excreted over a period of 1–2 days. It has a high affinity for cholinergic nerve terminals, and is transported in a retrograde manner back along the axons.

ADVERSE REACTIONS Adverse reactions include rashes, swelling, ptosis, pain and diplopia. Antibody production may lead to decreased effectiveness of the toxin. Muscle weakness is an expected effect. There have been rare fatalities associated with dysphagia or cardiovascular reactions. Overdosage can lead to difficulty in swallowing and muscle paralysis; long-term medical supervision is required.

DRUG INTERACTIONS Botulinum toxin can interact with any other drugs that interfere with neuromuscular transmission, including aminoglycoside antibiotics and skeletal muscle relaxants.

WARNINGS AND CONTRAINDICATIONS Anaphylactic reactions to the foreign protein can occur, and impaired ability to blink can lead to corneal exposure and damage. Long-term studies in children or pregnant or lactating women have not been carried out, so the drug is contraindicated in these people. It is contraindicated in patients with myasthenia gravis.

DOSAGE AND ADMINISTRATION As treatment with botulinum toxin is highly specialised, it is recommended that physicians be especially trained in the procedures. The dose is expressed in units of activity as measured by biological assay; in this case, a unit of activity is defined as the calculated median lethal intraperitoneal dose in mice. The dose may range up to 360 units over any 2-month period, depending on the muscle(s) being injected and the technique used.

CLINICAL INTEREST BOX 35-6
COMPLEMENTARY AND ALTERNATIVE THERAPIES IN OCULAR MEDICINE

Many alternative therapies have been tried in chronic ocular conditions, some with good pharmacological rationale.

In cataracts, antioxidants such as lipoic acid, vitamins E and C, and selenium are used as nutrients to increase glutathione concentrations within the lens. Other nutrients and herbs that may benefit cataract patients are vitamin A and carotenes, riboflavin, folic acid, melatonin and bilberry.

Diabetic cataracts are caused by raised concentrations of polyols in the lens, such as sorbitol formed from high concentrations of glucose by aldose reductase; natural aldose reductase inhibitors include flavonoids such as quercetin.

In glaucoma, vitamin C and glucosamines may improve glycosaminoglycan metabolism; high-dose vitamin C has an osmotic effect; *Ginkgo biloba* improves circulation; topical forskolin (from *Coleus forskohlii*) lowers IOP; IM *Salvia* injections improve vision; and various other nutrients and vitamins have been tried.
Sources: Head KA 2001; Braun & Cohen 2005.

administered drugs) binding to the lenses and staining them, and of microbial growth due to the high water content.

Both types of lenses can be used for bifocals or extended wear. If a person with contact lenses is prescribed eye-drops, it is recommended that the drops be instilled before the lenses are inserted in the morning and again after the lenses are removed in the evening. Oily drops or eye ointments should not be used because they may contaminate the lenses and obscure vision.

Many products (in fact, a bewildering array in most pharmacies) are available for care of contact lenses. These products must be selected carefully as they are not interchangeable between soft and hard lenses. As with all products intended for use in the eye, solutions should be sterile (initially), non-harmful to the lens or eye, simple to use and should have a reasonable shelf-life. Likely pathogens in solutions include *E. coli, S. aureus, Pseudomonas aeruginosa, Serratia, H. influenzae*, fungi, and acanthamoebae from tap water. Contact lens wearers are advised never to use saliva to clean their lenses; boiled water or sterile saline solution is preferred.

A typical routine is that after the lens is removed in the evening, it is cleansed by gentle rubbing with a few drops of cleaning solution, then rinsed and stored in a case in storage solution. Before insertion next morning it may be rinsed again. Wetting solutions and 'comfort drops' facilitate insertion and wearing; enzymatic solutions are used occasionally to remove deposits. Combination solutions for cleaning, wetting and storage are available and simplify lens care. Reaction-free one-bottle lens care systems have improved compliance and lens care.

Cleaning solutions

These loosen and remove debris from the lens, and may include detergents, surfactants or hydrogen peroxide. Typical bactericidal disinfectants are benzalkonium chloride or EDTA (ethylenediamine tetra-acetic acid).

Wetting solutions, 'comfort drops'

These promote spreading of water across the surface of the lens and hence facilitate its insertion. They include a surfactant (wetting agent) such as polyvinyl alcohol (PVA) or methylcellulose, plus a disinfectant.

Storage solutions

These solutions maintain the hydration of hydrophilic lenses in a bacteriostatic solution while not in the eyes, and help remove deposits; they contain disinfectants.

Enzymatic cleaners

These solutions are made up from tablets containing dried enzymes: non-specific lipases and/or proteolytic enzymes, which actively remove deposits of fat or protein that have built up on the lenses. The lenses are soaked in the enzymatic solution overnight; weekly use is recommended.

Artificial tear solutions and lubricants

Eyes can become excessively dry in conditions of hot winds, dry air-conditioning or heating, or due to inadequate tear production; the medical term for the condition is kerato-conjunctivitis sicca: dry eyes. It is common in older adults and contact lens users, and in dry areas. It can also occur as a drug adverse reaction. Lack of adequate tears causes a burning, scratchy sensation.

Lubricants or artificial tears are used to provide moisture and lubrication in diseases in which tear production is deficient, to lubricate artificial eyes and moisten contact lenses, to remove debris, and to protect the cornea during procedures on the eye. These agents may also be incorporated in ophthalmic preparations to prolong the contact time of topically applied drugs.

Such products may include a balanced salt solution (BSS; equivalent to 0.9% sodium chloride), buffers to adjust pH, preservatives to maintain sterility, and agents to increase viscosity and extend eye contact time, such as hypromellose (methylcellulose), propylene glycol, carbomers (polyacrylic acids), dextrans (polysaccharides), polyvinyl alcohol (PVA: a resin) and povidone (polyvinylpyrrolidone). Similar chemicals are also used in some contact lens solutions and blood volume expanders. These products are usually administered three or four times a day.

Ointment preparations are also used as ocular lubricants. They will help to protect the eye and lubricate the eye, e.g. during and after eye surgery. They are particularly valuable for patients who have an impaired blink reflex, and for night-time use.

Irrigating solutions

The sterile isotonic external irrigating solutions are used in tonometry, fluorescein procedures and removal of foreign material, and to cleanse and soothe the eyes of patients wearing hard contact lenses. These products do not require a prescription and are available as drops, irrigations and eye-washes.

Miscellaneous products used in ocular surgery

These products include:

- solutions of sodium hyaluronate or sodium chondroitin sulfate: these are transparent, non-antigenic, viscoelastic solutions in water at physiological pH, used as substitutes for aqueous or vitreous humour during ocular operations to protect exposed cell layers
- balanced salt solution (BSS), with or without glutathione: this solution maintains corneal integrity during surgery
- gelatin insert: an insert used to prevent formation of adhesions after surgery; it is absorbable over 1–6 months
- natural products used in treatment of cataract and glaucoma: see Clinical Interest Box 35-6.

SYSTEMIC DISEASES AND DRUGS AFFECTING THE EYE

Many systemic diseases can affect the eye; in general, the primary condition is treated first, then specific treatment for the ocular manifestations may not be required. Some of the major conditions commonly affecting the eye are described briefly below.

Cardiovascular diseases

Hypertension can cause damage to retinal arteries, with constriction, sclerosis, fibrosis and necrosis, leading to haemorrhages, papilloedema and loss of vision. Pharmacological treatment is with antihypertensive agents.

Atheroma in the internal carotid artery may embolise to the retinal circulation and cause transient or permanent blindness. Treatment with antihyperlipidaemic drugs can reduce the risk of atheroma and embolism.

Advanced congestive heart failure causes cerebral hypoxia and reduced blood supply to the eye. Pharmacological treatment is with drugs, including cardiac glycosides, which have important ocular adverse effects such as impaired vision and change in colour vision.

Endocrine disorders

Hyperthyroidism, especially Graves' disease, leads to major pathological changes in the eyes, and thyrotoxicosis may cause exophthalmos, orbital pain, photophobia, ocular muscle weakness and blurred vision. Treatment is by thyroid surgery or with antithyroid drugs such as carbimazole.

Ocular manifestations of diabetes mellitus include retinopathy, haemorrhages, detachment and oedema; morbidity is decreased by optimal control of diabetes, hypertension and hyperlipidaemia. Pharmacological treatment is with insulin (type 1 diabetes) or oral hypoglycaemic drugs (type 2). Photocoagulation of vessels or tissue relieves retinal oedema and haemorrhages.

Collagen diseases

Rheumatoid arthritis, systemic lupus erythematosus and Sjögren's syndrome may cause many ocular manifestations, e.g. dry eyes, scleritis, pain, uveitis, corneal opacity and retinopathy. Pharmacological treatment to the eye is with steroid drops and artificial tears; systemic steroids, NSAIDs and chloroquines are given as anti-inflammatory agents.

Ocular adverse drug reactions from steroids and chloroquine require monitoring.

Temporal arteritis, especially of the ophthalmic artery or central retinal artery, can cause sudden unilateral vision loss. Treatment is with steroidal anti-inflammatory agents.

Muscular diseases

Myasthenia gravis involves autoimmune reactions to ACh receptors at the neuromuscular junction; in more than 90% of cases, the ocular muscles are the first affected, with ptosis (the usual first sign) and diplopia. The specific diagnostic test is a positive improvement in ptosis in response to an IV dose of edrophonium (an anticholinesterase drug). Pharmacological treatment is with anticholinesterases (neostigmine, pyridostigmine), which raise the concentration of ACh to act at remaining functional ACh receptors.

OCULAR ADVERSE DRUG REACTIONS FROM SYSTEMIC DRUGS

With respect to the eye and adverse drug reactions (ADRs), there are several possible scenarios:
- drugs administered systemically to treat ocular conditions may have ADRs in the eye or elsewhere in the body
- drugs administered systemically to treat systemic conditions may have ADRs in the eye (Table 35-6)

CLINICAL INTEREST BOX 35-7 BEWARE OF THOSE EYE-DROPS!

The active ingredient in eye-drops can be absorbed systemically and may cause systemic ADRs, as evidenced by the following case study.

Violet was a 65-year-old former nurse with a history of mild hypertension, migraine and back pain; her medications were a thiazide diuretic daily and paracetamol as required. She presented with headaches resembling migraine, and as her blood pressure was elevated, a cardioselective β-blocker (metoprolol) was prescribed.

The headaches and hypertension were relieved, but Violet complained of severe nocturnal coughing. Examination revealed no abnormality, so a cough linctus was prescribed, but proved ineffective. Auscultation of her chest revealed wheezing, on which Violet commented that she had not suffered asthma since a child.

At this stage, it was apparent that the β-blocker had precipitated iatrogenic (drug-induced) asthma, so it was withdrawn and the hypertension treated with other drugs. The nocturnal cough persisted, responding to oral cortico-

steroids. A consultant specialist physician added more drugs and physiotherapy to the treatment regimen.

When Violet requested a referral to her ophthalmologist for review of her glaucoma, the missing piece of the jigsaw was found: unbeknown to her general practitioner, Violet was using timolol eye-drops prescribed by her eye specialist for glaucoma!

This case illustrates that:
- even topically applied β-blockers can precipitate asthma
- drugs can be absorbed from ocular formulations and produce systemic effects
- β-blocker eye-drops are contraindicated in glaucoma patients predisposed to asthma
- all drugs taken by a patient need to be queried and recorded
- better communication between health practitioners may avoid potentially dangerous drug reactions and interactions.

Adapted from: Murtagh 1992; used with permission.

- drugs administered topically to the eye may have ADRs in the eye.
- drugs administered topically to the eye may have ADRs elsewhere in the body after nasolacrimal absorption (Table 35-7).

Because of the potential for ADRs and drug interactions, patients being treated for ocular conditions should be asked about their drug therapy, including prescription drugs, over-the-counter drugs and complementary and alternative therapies. In particular, important parameters to consider are the drug's name, formulation, therapeutic index, dose, duration of therapy and the 'use-by' date of the formulation (usually 28 days after opening). Patient parameters include age, sex, eye health, eye colour, whether contact lenses are worn, tendency to allergies, and other medical conditions (see Clinical Interest Box 35-7).

The most common ocular ADRs are decreased tolerance to contact lenses, dry eyes, stinging or irritation from eye-drops, development of cataract, diplopia, retinopathy, raised IOP and impaired accommodation with or without mydriasis. Many of the important ADRs have been described in the context of particular groups of drugs and are summarised in Tables 35-6 and 35-7. In the next section, drugs causing particular ocular pathologies or impairment of vision are grouped together.

Drugs causing retinopathies
Ethanol

The ocular effects of alcohol, such as nystagmus (rapid jerky eye movements), are reversible. The closely related alcohol, methanol (as in methylated spirits), however, is highly toxic to the retina—as little as 10 g methanol can cause blindness. The toxicity is due to the metabolite formaldehyde (formalin), which inhibits cellular respiration and glycolysis in the retina, whereas the analogous metabolite of ethanol, acetaldehyde, is much less toxic.

Chloroquine and related antimalarial and anti-inflammatory agents

Chronic high doses of these drugs accumulate in the pigmentary epithelium of the retina, where they impair protein synthesis and vitamin A metabolism and can lead to irreversible damage. The maximum safe dose is considered to be about 250 mg per day for 1 year. All patients should be monitored for early detection of retinal changes.

Phenothiazine tranquillisers (antischizophrenic neuroleptic agents)

These drugs can bind to melanin and also cause lens deposits; high doses are retinotoxic.

TABLE 35-6 Ocular adverse effects induced by some systemic medications

DRUG	POSSIBLE OCULAR ADVERSE EFFECT INDUCED
Allopurinol	Retinal haemorrhage, exudative lesions
Anticholinergics	Dry eyes, mydriasis, glaucoma
Anticholinesterases	Cataracts
Antidepressants	Glaucoma
Aspirin	Allergic dermatitis, including keratitis and conjunctivitis
Barbiturates	Nystagmus
Busulfan	Cataracts
Cannabis, marijuana	Nystagmus, conjunctivitis, double vision, red eyes
Chloral hydrate	Eyelid oedema, conjunctivitis, miosis
Chloroquine	Lenticular and corneal opacity, retinopathy
Clomiphene citrate	Blurred vision, light flashes
Clonidine	Miosis
CNS depressants	Impaired vision, nystagmus, diplopia
Corticosteroids	Cataracts, raised IOP, papilloedema
Diazoxide	Oculogyric crisis
Digitalis glycosides	Scotomas, optic neuritis, changes in colour vision
Ethambutol	Optic neuritis
Ethanol	Nystagmus
Glyceryl trinitrate	Transient elevation in IOP
Guanethidine	Miosis, ptosis, blurred vision
Hydralazine	Lacrimation, blurred vision
Ibuprofen	Altered colour vision, blurred vision
Indomethacin	Mydriasis, retinopathy
Isoniazid	Optic neuritis
Lithium carbonate	Exophthalmos
Methanol	Retinopathy, blindness
Oestrogens	Vessel occlusion

TABLE 35-6 Ocular adverse effects induced by some systemic medications—cont'd

DRUG	POSSIBLE OCULAR ADVERSE EFFECT INDUCED
Opiates	Miosis, nystagmus
Oxygen	Retrolental hyperplasia, blindness (in infants)
Phenothiazines	Corneal and conjunctival deposits, cataracts, retinopathy, oculogyric crisis
Phenytoin	Nystagmus
Quinine	Blurring of vision, optic neuritis, blindness (reversible)
Thiazide diuretics	Acute transient myopia, yellow colouring of vision
Vincristine	Ptosis, paresis of extraocular muscles
Vitamin A overdose or toxicity	Papilloedema, increased IOP
Vitamin D toxicity	Calcium deposits in cornea

TABLE 35-7 Ophthalmic drugs: adverse systemic effects

OPHTHALMIC DRUG	REPORTED ADVERSE EFFECT
Antimicrobial agents	
Antibiotics	Secondary infections, drug resistance
Sulfacetamide	Stevens–Johnson syndrome, systemic lupus erythematosus
Anticholinergic drugs	
Atropine	Tachycardia, elevated temperature, fever, delirium
Cyclopentolate	Convulsions, hallucinations
Antiglaucoma medications	
β-blocking agents (timolol)	Bradycardia, syncope, low blood pressure, asthmatic attack, congestive heart failure, hallucinations, loss of appetite, headaches, nausea, weakness, depression
Parasympathomimetics (pilocarpine)	Nausea, stomach pain, increased sweating, salivation, tremors, bradycardia, lightheadedness
Adrenergic medications	
Phenylephrine (10%)	Hypertension, cerebral haemorrhage, arrhythmias, myocardial infarction

Oxygen in newborns, especially premature infants

Neonates with respiratory distress syndrome often need high levels of oxygen administered to prevent hypoxia; however, this can lead to permanent blindness (see Clinical Interest Box 32-2). Thus the levels of oxygen provided to these vulnerable infants must be restricted.

Other drugs

Other drugs that can cause retinal damage include digoxin, corticosteroids, chloramphenicol, cocaine and interferon.

Drugs causing development of cataracts

Many organic chemicals can induce development of **cataracts** (i.e. opacity in the crystalline lens), including:
- organophosphorus anticholinesterases (e.g. those used to treat myasthenia gravis or Alzheimer's disease): these can lead to the formation of vacuoles behind the lens
- corticosteroids: patients on chronic high doses of glucocorticoids, e.g. for rheumatoid arthritis or asthma or to prevent transplant rejection, have a high incidence of cataract; the mechanism of this adverse reaction is not well understood. Corticosteroids can also cause glaucoma and predispose to infections
- phenothiazines (tranquillisers): high doses can lead to pigment deposition and eventually to a polar cataract; it is suspected that the cause is a phenothiazine metabolite.

Other ocular adverse drug reactions
Photosensitivity

Photosensitivity is a hypersensitivity reaction in which UV light energy stimulates production of a hapten–protein complex between the drug and a natural protein, leading to damage to lysosomes and a photoallergy or phototoxicity, which may be manifest as severe sunburn or skin eruptions. (Photosensitivity can also be a symptom of porphyria.) The drugs most commonly implicated are the sulfonamides, tetracyclines, phenothiazines and thiazide diuretics. Note that mydriatics also increase the sensitivity of the eye to light.

Excessive tear formation

Lacrimators (better or more infamously known as 'tear gases') are chemicals that cause intense corneal and conjunctival irritation and pain, and hence induce reflex tear secretion and eyelid spasm. They are used as crowd controllers, 'harassing agents' and war gases, as the excessive tear production tends to inhibit people's interest in other activities. These agents also irritate other mucous membranes and induce coughing and nausea. If used in confined spaces, their toxicity can cause blindness and death. Many are highly reactive organic chemicals with cyano groups (carbon and nitrogen linked in a triple bond). Others include bromoacetone, acrolein (a compound produced from overheated cooking fats) and the organic sulfides present in onions and garlic.

PREGNANCY SAFETY

ADEC Category	Drug
A	Atropine, carmellose, chloramphenicol, hydrocortisone, prednisolone, sodium cromoglycate
B1	Azithromycin, brimonidine, cefotaxime, ketotifen, lodoxamide, olopatadine
B2	Acetylcholine, carbachol, cyclopentolate, dipivefrine, homatropine, phenylephrine, pilocarpine, proxymetacaine
B3	Acetazolamide, aciclovir, apraclonidine, bimatoprost, botulinum toxin, brinzolamide, ciprofloxacin, dexamethasone, dorzolamide, fluorometholone, latanoprost, levocabastine, ofloxacin, travoprost, tropicamide, verteporfin
C	Betaxolol, diclofenac, flurbiprofen, ketorolac, levobunolol, sulfacetamide, timolol
D	Bacitracin, framycetin, gentamicin, neomycin, polymyxin B, tetracycline, tobramycin
Unclassified	Amethocaine, antazoline, fluorescein, naphazoline, propamidine, rose bengal, sodium hyaluronate, tetrahydrozoline

Notes: (1) The drugs in the above list are the ocular formulations, wherever relevant. (2) The list of preparations exempt from Pregnancy Classification includes some ocular preparations, e.g. contact lens preparations, diagnostic agents (including stains), enzymes and herbal remedies.

DRUGS AT A GLANCE 35: Drugs for the treatment of eye conditions

Therapeutic group	Pharmacological group	Key examples	Key pages
Cycloplegic mydriatics	Anticholinergics (antimuscarinics)	atropine, tropicamide	588–90
Mydriatics	Sympathomimetics	phenylephrine (high-dose), dipivefrine	589, 90
Miotics	Muscarinic agonists	carbachol, pilocarpine	590, 1
Decongestants	Sympathomimetics	phenylephrine (low-dose), naphazoline	590–2
Antiglaucoma agents	α_2-adrenoceptor agonists	apraclonidine, brimonidine	592, 3
	β-adrenoceptor antagonists	betaxolol, timolol	592
	Carbonic anhydrase inhibitors • Systemic • Topical	acetazolamide dorzolamide, brinzolamide	593, 4
	Prostaglandin agonists	latanoprost, travoprost	593, 4
	Muscarinic agonists (miotics)	carbachol, pilocarpine	593, 4
	Osmotic agents (systemic)	mannitol, glycerol	594, 5

DRUGS AT A GLANCE 35: Drugs for the treatment of eye conditions—cont'd

Therapeutic group	Pharmacological group	Key examples	Key pages
Antimicrobial agents			
Antibacterials	Aminoglycosides	neomycin, framycetin	596
	Sulfonamides	sulfacetamide	596
Antitrachoma agents		azithromycin	595
Antivirals		aciclovir	597
Antiacanthamoeba agents		propamidine	595, 7
Anti-inflammatory agents	Corticosteroids	fluorometholone, prednisolone	597, 8
	Non-steroidal anti-inflammatory drugs (NSAIDs)	ketorolac	598
Antiallergy agents	Antihistamines	antazoline, olopatadine	598
	Mast-cell stabilisers (cromolyns)	sodium cromoglycate, lodoxamide	598
Local anaesthetics		amethocaine, oxybuprocaine, proxymetacaine }	598, 9
Miscellaneous	Stains	fluorescein, rose bengal	599
	Inhibitors of muscle contraction	botulinum toxin	599–601
	Photosensitisers	verteporfin	600
Artificial tears	Lubricants, viscosity enhancers	balanced salt solutions hypromellose, dextrans }	602
Surgery adjuncts	Aqueous/vitreous humour substitutes	hyaluronate, chondroitin sulfate	602
Contact lens products (used in storage packs)	Cleansers, wetting solutions, storage solutions, enzymes	various	600–2

All drugs in this table are administered topically unless otherwise indicated.

KEY POINTS

- Some knowledge of the anatomy and physiology of the eye is essential for understanding how drugs are administered to and act in the eye.
- Autonomic effects are important: sympathetic innervation leads to mydriasis, focus for distant vision and vasoconstriction, whereas parasympathetic effects include miosis, reduced IOP, accommodation for near vision and secretion of tears.
- Drugs are administered to the eye (as eye-drops, ointments or via inserts) for local effects in the eye after absorption across the cornea. Some systemic absorption can occur via the nasolacrimal ducts.
- Mydriatic agents dilate the pupil and are used to facilitate ocular examination. Drugs with mydriatic actions are anticholinergics, such as atropine (which also cause cycloplegia), and α-adrenergic agonists, such as phenylephrine; the latter drugs also have useful vasoconstrictor and decongestant effects in the eye.
- Miotic agents reduce pupil size and reduce IOP. Miosis is caused by muscarinic agonists (carbachol, pilocarpine) and anticholinesterases.

● Glaucomas are a group of conditions associated with raised IOP, which can threaten vision. Ocular administration of β-blockers, carbonic anhydrase inhibitors, α agonists, prostaglandin agonists or miotics is used to reduce IOP.

● Ocular infections can be caused by bacteria, viruses, protozoa or *Chlamydia*. Serious infections threaten vision and require treatment with antimicrobials specific to the pathogenic organism. Antimicrobials that are not commonly used systemically are preferred for topical use, including chloramphenicol, neomycin, aciclovir, propamidine and azithromycin.

● Minor ocular inflammations may be self-limiting; however, severe or chronic inflammations can cause scarring or retinal detachment and require treatment with anti-inflammatory agents, such as corticosteroids or NSAIDs.

● Allergic reactions in the eye are treated with antihistamines (e.g. levocabastine) or mast-cell stabilisers (sodium cromoglycate).

● Local anaesthetics are used in the eye for ophthalmic surgery, to facilitate examinations and procedures, and to treat pain. Proxymetacaine is particularly effective in the eye.

● The stains fluorescein and rose bengal are administered topically to show up areas of abrasion and cell damage.

● Botulinum toxin, a long-acting skeletal muscle paralysing agent, is used in blepharospasm and strabismus.

● Verteporfin is a new agent utilised in photodynamic therapy to occlude abnormal blood vessels in macular degeneration.

● Contact lenses (hard or rigid gas-permeable, or soft) require meticulous handling and regular care. Solutions for cleansing, soaking, wetting and enzymatic digestion of deposits are available.

● Other drugs used in the eye include artificial tear solutions, products used to facilitate eye surgery, and various complementary and alternative therapies (antioxidants, vitamins and herbal remedies).

● The eye can be affected in many systemic diseases, particularly cardiovascular, endocrine and musculoskeletal conditions. The primary disease needs to be treated first, to minimise ocular complications.

● Many adverse drug reactions occur in the eye, from both ocular and systemically administered drugs. Common adverse effects are ocular irritation, retinopathy, cataract, raised IOP and glaucoma, and photosensitivity. Agents that commonly cause ocular effects are methanol, chloroquine, corticosteroids, phenothiazines, sulfonamides, and oxygen in newborns. 'Tear gases' are used purposely to induce ocular irritation and pain.

REVIEW EXERCISES

1   Explain the theories on how timolol, pilocarpine, dipivefrine, latanoprost and dorzolamide lower IOP in glaucoma.

2   What are the indications for the use of anticholinergic and adrenergic agonist ophthalmic medications? Describe their mechanisms of action.

3   Describe the ocular adverse effects induced by chloroquine, corticosteroids, marijuana, digitalis glycosides, ethanol and ibuprofen.

4   Name the serious adverse systemic effects that may be induced by the following ophthalmic drugs: atropine, β-blocking agents and phenylephrine.

5   Discuss the ocular administration of local anaesthetics, anti-inflammatory agents and antiallergy drugs, describing the indications for their use and common adverse effects.

6   Discuss the use of antimicrobial agents in the treatment of common ocular infections.

7   Describe the types of solutions used in the care of contact lenses.

REFERENCES AND FURTHER READING

Antibiotic Expert Group. *Therapeutic Guidelines Antibiotic, version 12.* Melbourne: Therapeutic Guidelines Limited, 2003.
Australian Drug Evaluation Committee. *Prescribing Medicines in Pregnancy: An Australian Categorisation of Risk of Drug Use in Pregnancy.* 4th edn. Canberra: Therapeutic Goods Administration, 1999.
Australian Medicines Handbook 2005. Adelaide: AMH, 2005.
Bartlett JD, Jaanus SD. *Clinical Ocular Pharmacology.* 4th edn. Boston: Butterworth-Heinemann, 2001.
Braun L, Cohen M. *Herbs and Natural Supplements: An Evidence-Based Guide.* Sydney: Elsevier Mosby; 2005.
Caswell A (ed.). *MIMS Annual June 2005.* Sydney: CMPMedica Australia, 2005.
Ciulla TA, Walker JD, Fong DS, Criswell MH. Corticosteroids in posterior segment disease: an update on new delivery systems and new indications. *Current Opinion in Ophthalmology* 2004; 15(3): 211–20.
Distelhorst JS, Hughes GM. Open-angle glaucoma. *American Family Physician* 2003; 67(9): 1937–44.
Fraunfelder FT, Fraunfelder FW, Randall JA (eds). *Drug-Induced Ocular Side-Effects.* 5th edn. Boston: Butterworth-Heinemann, 2001.
Goldberg I. Drugs for glaucoma. *Australian Prescriber* 2002; 25(6): 142–6.

Guymer R. Drug treatment of macular degeneration. *Australian Prescriber* 2002; 25(5): 116–9.

Head KA. Natural therapies for ocular disorders, part two: cataracts and glaucoma. *Alternative Medicine Review* 2001; 6: 141–66.

Johnson EA. Clostridial toxins as therapeutic agents: benefits of nature's most toxic proteins. *Annual Review of Microbiology* 1999; 53: 551–75.

Mahant N, Clouston PD, Lorentz IT. The current use of botulinum toxin. *Journal of Clinical Neuroscience* 2000; 7: 389–94.

Mann J. *Murder, Magic and Medicine.* Oxford: Oxford University Press, 1992.

Murtagh J. *Cautionary Tales: Authentic Case Histories from Medical Practice.* Sydney: McGraw-Hill, 1992.

Ng P. Treatment of ocular toxoplasmosis. *Australian Prescriber* 2002; 25(4): 88–90.

Rakow PL. Current contact lens care systems. *Ophthalmology Clinics of North America* 2003; 16(3): 415–32.

Scott IU, Siatkowski MR. Thyroid eye disease. *Seminars in Ophthalmology* 1999; 14: 52–61.

Spencer JW, Jacobs JJ. *Complementary/Alternative Medicine: An Evidence-Based Approach.* St Louis: Mosby, 1999.

Tripathi RC, Parapuram SK, Tripathi BJ, Zhong Y, Chalam KV. Corticosteroids and glaucoma risk. *Drugs and Aging* 1999; 15: 439–50.

Youngson RM. *Collins Dictionary: Medicine.* 2nd edn. Glasgow: HarperCollins, 1998.

ON-LINE RESOURCES

For specific New Zealand drugs, check Medsafe website: http://www.medsafe.gvt.nz

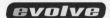   More weblinks at http://evolve.elsevier.com/AU/Bryant/pharmacology/

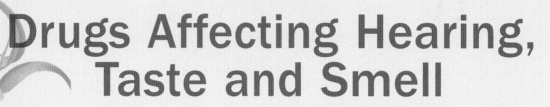

CHAPTER 36

Drugs Affecting Hearing, Taste and Smell

CHAPTER FOCUS

Knowledge of the anatomy and physiology of the
ear is necessary to understand the clinical use of
medications in treating ear disorders. People with ear
disorders may have ear pain, vertigo, deafness and
difficulty with communication. The pharmacological
agents used to treat ear disorders are limited (mainly
antimicrobial and anti-inflammatory agents); however,
many systemic agents can affect the ear adversely,
causing ototoxicity. The other special senses, taste
and smell, may also be impaired by drugs. This chapter
reviews these agents.

OBJECTIVES

● To describe briefly the anatomy of the ear (external,
   middle and inner ear) and the mechanisms of
   hearing and balance.

● To describe the most common ear disorders and
   their pharmacological management.

● To discuss the mechanisms of drug-induced
   ototoxicity, and the four main drug groups reported
   to cause ototoxicity.

● To review the chemical senses (taste and smell) and
   the drugs that can affect them adversely.

KEY TERMS

aminoglycoside antibiotics
auditory ossicles
cerumen
cochlea
eustachian (auditory) tube
external ear
gustation
inner ear
middle ear
olfaction
otic administration
otitis media
ototoxicity
tinnitus
vertigo

KEY DRUGS

acetic acid
chloramphenicol
framycetin
neomycin
triamcinolone

KEY ABBREVIATIONS

OM otitis media

ANATOMY AND PHYSIOLOGY OF THE EAR

THE ear consists of three sections: the **external ear**, **middle ear** and **inner ear** (Figure 36-1). The external ear has two divisions: the outer ear, or pinna, and the external auditory canal. The canal leads to the eardrum, or tympanic membrane, a thin transparent partition of tissue between the canal and the middle ear. The function of the external ear is to receive and transmit auditory sounds to the eardrum and to protect it from damage. The tympanic membrane in turn transmits sound to the bones of the middle ear and protects it from foreign substances.

The middle ear is an air-filled cavity in the temporal bone that contains three small bones called the **auditory ossicles**:* the malleus (hammer), incus (anvil) and stapes (stirrup). The tip of the malleus is attached to the surface of the tympanic membrane. Its head is attached to the incus, which in turn is attached to the stapes. The ossicles amplify (about tenfold) and transmit vibrations from sound waves to the inner ear. The middle ear is also directly connected to the nasopharynx by the **eustachian (auditory) tube**. The eustachian tube is usually collapsed except when the person swallows, chews, yawns, or moves the jaw. This tube joins the nasopharynx and the tympanic cavity, which allows for the equalisation of the air pressure in the inner ear with atmospheric pressure to prevent the tympanic membrane from rupturing. On airline flights, ear pain due to pressure changes is relieved by way of the eustachian tube by chewing, yawning or swallowing.

The inner ear, also referred to as the labyrinth because of its convoluted series of canals, has two main divisions. The bony labyrinth consists of the vestibule, **cochlea** and semicircular canals, and the membranous labyrinth consists of a series of sacs and tubes within the bony labyrinth. The cochlea, through which pass fibres of the cochlear division of the acoustic nerve, is the primary organ of hearing, while the vestibular apparatus is vital to maintaining equilibrium and balance. The inner ear transduces vibrations from sound waves, via movements of the hair cells in the cochlea, into electrical signals in the vestibulocochlear (acoustic) nerve. Action potentials generated are then transmitted along complex neuronal pathways to the acoustic areas in the temporal lobes of the cerebral cortex, where they are interpreted as sounds of varying pitch and loudness.

---

*These are in fact the smallest bones in the body, and the stapedius muscle, which damps the vibrations of the stapes and thus protects the ear against loud noises, is the smallest skeletal muscle. These are fully grown at birth, and the sense of hearing is already well developed.

COMMON EAR DISORDERS

The most common ear disorders include infections of the ear (bacterial or fungal), earwax accumulation, various other painful or inflammatory conditions, and deafness. Many ear disorders are minor and easily treated or are self-limiting. Persistent pain or ear problems should be professionally evaluated because some untreated disorders can lead to hearing loss.

External ear disorders

External ear disorders usually include trauma and subsequent infections, such as from lacerations or scratches to the skin of the ear canal, or from infected water entering the canal (see Clinical Interest Box 36-1). These are often minor and heal with time. If the injury results in bleeding and perhaps a haematoma, referral to a doctor may be necessary. Localised infections of the hair follicles may result in boils (furuncles associated with *Staphylococcus aureus*). Patients with recurring boils that do not respond to good hygiene and topical compresses may require surgical drainage and systemic antibiotics.

Dermatitis of the ear, itching, local redness, weeping and drainage must be evaluated individually, as the causes can vary, from inflammation induced by seborrhoea, psoriasis or contact dermatitis, to head trauma producing ear discharge. Self-medication should be discouraged when infection is suspected, in the presence of known injuries of the ear, or whenever effusion, pain and dizziness are present.

CLINICAL INTEREST BOX 36-1
SWIMMER'S EAR

Swimmer's ear is an infection of the ear canal (otitis externa) related to aquatic activities such as swimming, bathing or showering. It is often associated with overzealous use of cotton swabs or other implements to clean or dry the ear.

Bacteria may be introduced with water (especially if chlorination of pools is inadequate), and multiply in the warm moist environment of the ear canal. Debris can be generated, the canal lining invaded, and symptoms of otitis externa appear (pain, swelling, sensation of fullness in the ear, impaired hearing).

Prevention is assisted by excluding moisture from the canal, e.g. with ear plugs, and by desiccation and acidification of the canal with drying ear drops containing **acetic acid** or isopropyl alcohol.

Treatment is by gentle removal of debris with suction, drying with an astringent agent such as aluminium acetate, and may require topical antibiotics and anti-inflammatory agents.

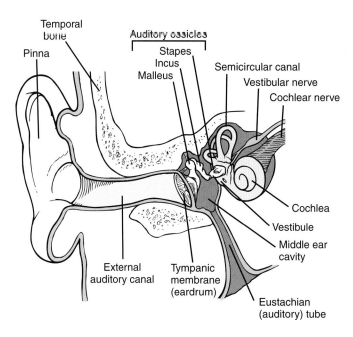

FIGURE 36-1 Anatomy of the ear.

Middle ear disorders

Middle ear disorders should not be treated with over-the-counter (OTC) medications because prescription-only treatment such as antibiotics may be required. The most commonly reported problem is middle ear inflammation, **otitis media**. This occurs most often in children with viral upper respiratory tract infections, and is one of the most common infections of childhood. Common bacterial pathogens are *Streptococcus pneumoniae* and *Haemophilus influenzae*. Pain, fever, malaise, pressure, a sensation of fullness in the ear and hearing loss are common symptoms. Such conditions should be treated promptly. Analgesia is required (e.g. ibuprofen or paracetamol), but systemic decongestants and antihistamines have no proven efficacy. Systemic antibiotics (amoxycillin, cefuroxime or cefaclor) may be required.

Persistent effusion of fluid in the middle ear (glue ear) with pain and hearing loss may resolve after some weeks or may require relief by drainage with a ventilating tube (grommet). Suppurative otitis media, in which the eardrum has become ruptured and purulent exudate (pus) appears in the external canal, may require surgical removal of the pus and treatment with topical combination ear-drops containing an anti-inflammatory agent (dexamethasone) and antibiotics (framycetin plus gramicidin).

Acute tympanic membrane perforation from foreign objects or from water sports (such as diving or water skiing) may result in pain at the time of injury that subsides, diminished hearing acuity, **tinnitus** (a ringing or buzzing sound in the ears), nausea, **vertigo**, and otitis media or mastoiditis. A physician's examination is vital when a perforated tympanic membrane is suspected.

Vertigo, the sensation that the environment or the body is rotating, can be so severe as to cause the sufferer to fall over. There are numerous causes, and the drug treatment varies accordingly: otological vertigo due to inner ear disorders is treated with anticholinergics, betahistine and benzodiazepines, whereas vertigo associated with migraine or strokes is treated with calcium channel antagonists, tricyclic antidepressants and β-blockers.

A new type of treatment for the vertigo and other balance disorders associated with Ménière's disease is that of transtympanic perfusion, i.e. administration through the eardrum, by means of a sustained delivery system, of the corticosteroid dexamethasone or the antibiotic gentamicin. The aminoglycoside antibiotics are known to cause hearing loss, and it is thought that the transtympanic administration of gentamicin has its effect by damaging hair cells and thus reducing vestibular function; the dose must be carefully judged so that hearing is not completely lost.

Inner ear disorders

Loss of hearing, especially unilateral hearing loss, may result from viral infection of the **inner ear**.

Untreated external and middle ear infections may also affect the hearing and balance functioning of the inner ear.

Other causes of ear disorders

Hearing deficits may be caused by genetic diseases or slowly progressive diseases such as otosclerosis or Ménière's disease (see Clinical Interest Box 36-2). Some drugs can cause ototoxicity as an adverse effect, which results in impaired hearing for the patient. These will be discussed later in this chapter.

DRUGS AFFECTING THE EAR

A wide variety of both single and combination products is used to treat impacted **cerumen** (wax), inflammation, bacterial or fungal infections, ear pain, and other minor or superficial problems associated primarily with the external ear canal. More serious problems, such as an earache secondary to an upper respiratory tract infection, ear discharge or drainage, persistent or recurrent otitis media, or ear pain caused by recent injury or head trauma, require prescribed drugs such as antimicrobial drops, corticosteroid anti-inflammatory agents and local anaesthetics, given by the otic or systemic routes.

Otic administration

Drugs are administered to the ear for local effects only and are not absorbed systemically (as they may be from the eye). Formulations for **otic administration** are ear-drops and ear ointments. Pharmaceutical aspects of these are basically similar to the requirements for eye-drops and eye ointments; however, there is not the same strict importance attached to sterility of preparations, as ear-drops and ointments cannot penetrate the middle or inner ear unless the eardrum is perforated, and the tissues of the ear are well vascularised. Some drops are formulated for either eye or ear use. **Acetic acid** is often used in ear-drops to return the ear canal to a mildly acidic environment after swimming or bathing. Ear-drops and sprays are often formulated with the active drug(s) dissolved in aqueous solvents such as isopropyl alcohol, saline solutions, glycerol, benzyl alcohol, polyethylene glycol or propylene glycol; or in oily solvents such as arachis (peanut) oil

Antimicrobial ear preparations

Antimicrobial ear preparations are used topically to treat infections of the external auditory canal surface (otitis externa). For serious middle or inner ear infections, systemic antibiotics are indicated. Antibiotics preferred for topical use are those that are not used systemically (because of systemic toxicity or adverse pharmacokinetics), such as chloramphenicol, framycetin, neomycin, gramicidin, ciprofloxacin and bacitracin. Nystatin is an effective antifungal agent. (These antimicrobial drugs are covered in detail in Unit XIV.)

Antibiotics

Chloramphenicol, a broad-spectrum bacteriostatic antibiotic, is used to treat external ear infections caused by *Staphylococcus aureus*, *Escherichia coli*, *Pseudomonas aeruginosa*, *Enterobacter aerogenes*, *Haemophilus influenzae* and other susceptible organisms. It is available as 5 mg/mL ear-drops. Potential

---

> ### CLINICAL INTEREST BOX 36-2
> ### MÉNIÈRE'S DISEASE
>
> Ménière's disease (named after the French physician Prosper Ménière, 1799–1862) is a progressive episodic inner ear disease caused by an increase in pressure and spontaneous bursts of activity within the labyrinth (the semicircular canals and the cochlea that make up the vestibular system). It involves recurrent attacks of vertigo, nausea, tinnitus and variable hearing loss.
>
> The motion sickness and dizziness are thought to be caused by a disparity in the proprioceptive information being received from the two sides of the head. This also occurs in motion sickness, for example when viewing outside stationary objects from within a moving vehicle, or when watching waves from a rolling ship. There are other causes of vertigo, both peripheral (rubella, mumps, acoustic neuroma, otitis media) and central (migraine, epilepsy, multiple sclerosis).
>
> Treatment in the acute phase is with 'labyrinthine sedation', using phenothiazine tranquillisers, benzodiazepines or an antihistamine, and a diuretic to reduce fluid load. Between attacks, restricted intake of salt, cigarettes, alcohol, and caffeine and other CNS stimulants may be prophylactic. A new treatment method is transtympanic administration of gentamicin, to reduce vestibular function.
>
> The distressing vertigo may also be helped by various manoeuvres in which the head is moved through different planes to attempt to remove fluid in the canals. Sometimes the only effective treatment is surgical: vestibular nerve section or removal of the balance mechanisms (labyrinthectomy) on the affected side; this also removes the sense of hearing from that side, causing deafness.

adverse effects include burning, redness, rash, swelling, or other signs of topical irritation that were not present before the start of therapy. The medication should be discontinued if this hypersensitivity reaction occurs. The usual dosage for adults and children is 4 drops inserted in the ear canal four times a day.

The aminoglycoside antibiotics (such as **framycetin** and **neomycin**) are also used in ear-drops but it must be noted that these drugs themselves are liable to cause ototoxicity. Framycetin is formulated as drops (5 mg/mL), ear ointment (5 mg/g) and also in combination preparations with other antibiotics and with corticosteroids.

Corticosteroid ear preparations

Corticosteroid anti-inflammatory agents used in the ear include **triamcinolone**, flumethasone, dexamethasone and hydrocortisone; corticosteroids combined with antimicrobials are also available (see Drug Monograph 36-1). The cortico-steroid is included for its anti-inflammatory, antipruritic and antiallergic effects, while the antibiotic treats external ear canal infections and mastoidectomy cavity infections. Note, however, that corticosteroids have immunosuppressant actions and hence predispose to infections. Corticosteroids applied intranasally have also been used in otitis media with effusion (glue ear), but without general success.

Other otic preparations

OTC otic preparations often contain acetic or boric acid, benzalkonium chloride, aluminium acetate (Burow's solution), isopropyl alcohol or propylene glycol (propylene glycol also enhances the acidity of acetic acid). Glycerin, mineral oil and olive oil are used as emollients to help relieve itching and burning in the ear.

Accumulations of **cerumen** (ear wax) can be softened and its removal encouraged ('ear toilet') with the topical application of oil-based or aqueous solutions. Ingredients include almond oil, olive oil, glycerin, chlorbutol, sodium bicarbonate and docusate sodium (a surfactant also used systemically as a laxative agent). Carbamide peroxide (urea hydrogen peroxide) is an antibacterial agent that releases oxygen to help remove wax.

Although most (OTC) otic preparations are considered safe and effective, patients should be advised to see a doctor if symptoms do not improve within several days of using these preparations or if an adverse reaction occurs.

Drug-induced ototoxicity
Manifestations and mechanisms of ototoxicity

Many medications reportedly cause **ototoxicity** in humans. The ototoxicity may affect the person's hearing (auditory or cochlear function), balance (vestibular function) or both. The most common symptom reported is **tinnitus**, 'ringing in the ears'. Ototoxicity is usually bilateral and may be reversible but can become irreversible if not recognised early enough to withdraw the offending medications.

Cochlear ototoxicity causes a progressive or continuing hearing loss. High-pitched tinnitus, or the loss of high tones, occurs first, then progresses to affect lower tones. Because of this slow progression, most patients are unaware it is occurring. Vestibular toxicity may start with a severe headache of 1–2 days' duration, followed by nausea, vomiting, dizziness, ataxia and difficulty with equilibrium. The person may feel as though the room is in motion (vertigo). Tinnitus is very difficult to treat; attempts have been made with retraining therapy, devices that mask the buzzing/ringing noises, and hearing aids. Drug therapy that has been tried includes local lignocaine, or systemic corticosteroids or benzodiazepines;

DRUG MONOGRAPH 36-1 ANTIBIOTIC–CORTICOSTEROID EAR-DROPS AND OINTMENTS

Combination ear-drops or ear ointments typically contain a corticosteroid (**triamcinolone** 0.1% or dexamethasone 0.05%) and two or three antibiotics (e.g. **framycetin** 0.5%, **neomycin** 0.25%, gramicidin 0.005%, bacitracin 400 IU/g and nystatin 100,000 U/g). Antimicrobial agents acting by different mechanisms (e.g. inhibiting protein synthesis, altering cell membrane permeability, antifungal actions) are usefully combined in 'triple antibiotic' formulations. The corticosteroid also has mild vasoconstrictor actions.

INDICATIONS These preparations are used as anti-inflammatory and antimicrobial agents to treat ear infections with sensitive organisms, such as otitis externa of bacterial or fungal origin, or chronic suppurative otitis media.

PHARMACOKINETICS The antibiotic components are not usually absorbed through intact skin. Corticosteroids and neomycin may be absorbed, particularly if the skin is inflamed, and can cause mild systemic effects. If absorbed, they are subject to normal elimination processes of metabolism and excretion (in urine and bile).

ADVERSE DRUG REACTIONS Prolonged use can lead to hypersensitivity reactions, skin irritations and contact dermatitis; corticosteroids can cause delayed healing and secondary infections, especially fungal infections.

DRUG INTERACTIONS As the drugs are not well absorbed through the skin, few interactions should occur.

WARNINGS AND CONTRAINDICATIONS Aminoglycosides are used with caution if the eardrum is perforated or ventilated (with a grommet), as inner ear damage and hearing loss can occur. Patients are advised to stop using the medication and contact their doctor if aural symptoms (tinnitus, hearing loss, unsteadiness or dizziness) appear.

There is a risk of fungal overgrowth if antibiotic–corticosteroid preparations are used for more than 7 days. Use in children should be limited to the minimal effective duration.

DOSAGE AND ADMINISTRATION Before otic administration, ear wax and debris should be gently removed. Dosage of ear-drops is usually 3 drops, 2–4 times daily. Cream or ointment is applied and the ear gently massaged 2–3 times daily.

Ginkgo biloba extracts have proven to be little better than placebo. The most recent pharmacological treatment is with transtympanic perfusion of corticosteroids or gentamicin, as for vertigo.

TABLE 36-1 Some drugs reported to cause ototoxicity

DRUG	COMMENTS
Analgesics	
Aspirin and other non-steroidal anti-inflammatory drugs (NSAIDs)	NSAIDs, especially in high doses, can cause tinnitus, vertigo and hearing loss. These adverse effects are generally reversible if drug use is reduced or discontinued, although some cases of irreversible hearing loss are documented.
Antibiotics	
Aminoglycosides	Incidence of ototoxicity is 1%–5% and may be irreversible; damage occurs to auditory and vestibular hair cells.
Clarithromycin	Hearing loss has been reported (usually reversible). It occurs more often in elderly women.
Erythromycin	Reversible hearing loss has been reported in people with liver and/or kidney impairment, in people 50 years of age and over, and in people who received high doses (>4 g/day). IV erythromycin has resulted in irreversible ototoxicity.
Vancomycin	Hearing loss has been reported, especially in people with kidney impairment or those receiving another ototoxic medication concurrently.
Antineoplastic agents	
Platinum compounds	Ototoxicity with tinnitus, hearing loss and possible deafness has been reported. This effect is especially severe in children under 12 years. The effect is cumulative, therefore audiometric testing is recommended.
Vinca alkaloids	Tinnitus and, less frequently, hearing loss and vertigo have been reported.
Loop diuretics	
Bumetanide, ethacrynic acid, frusemide	Reversible and irreversible hearing loss have been reported, usually with too-rapid IV injection, high diuretic dosages or concurrent use with other ototoxic medications, and in people with renal impairment; tinnitus and vertigo can also occur.

For full listing see Lee et al 2005.

Reactive oxygen and nitrogen species, including free radicals (see Chapter 32 under Oxygen), have been implicated in ototoxicity. Oxidative stress damages macromolecules such as DNA, proteins and lipids; oxidative damage to the sensory hair cells in the inner ear may be involved in the ototoxicity of aminoglycoside antibiotics, loop diuretics and cisplatin antineoplastic agents. Similar mechanisms of toxicity may explain how these same drug groups damage the cells of the proximal tubules in the kidneys. (Reduction of ototoxicity in animals by antioxidants and iron chelators supports this proposed mechanism.)

The patients most at risk of ototoxicity are the elderly, those with impaired renal function (due to impaired drug excretion processes, which is exacerbated by nephrotoxicity of the same drugs that cause ototoxicity), people working or living with high noise levels, and those taking ototoxic agents in high doses or for prolonged duration.

Drugs associated with ototoxicity

Although many drugs have been associated with toxic effects on the ears, most drug-induced ototoxicity is associated with the use of salicylate and other anti-inflammatory agents, aminoglycoside antibiotics, cisplatin antineoplastic agents and loop diuretics. Table 36-1 lists important drugs reported to induce ototoxicity.

AMINOGLYCOSIDE ANTIBIOTICS

The **aminoglycoside antibiotic** group includes the antibiotics amikicin, gentamicin, neomycin and tobramycin, commonly used for treatment of Gram-negative bacterial infections and mycobacterial diseases because of their high efficacy and low cost. Mechanisms proposed for the ototoxic actions are inhibition of mitochondrial protein synthesis, free-radical cell damage and activation of N-methyl-D-aspartate (NMDA) receptors. Susceptibility to ototoxicity is dose-related and

Chemicals from many different classes may taste sweet —even salts of beryllium and lead. However, the most important sweet-tasting compounds are sugars, synthetic sweet-tasting compounds such as aspartame and saccharin, and amino acids.

The sweetest known sugar is β-D-fructose but its sweetness decreases with increasing concentration, and at higher temperatures. In decreasing order of sweetness, other sugars rank as follows: sucrose, glucose, galactose = mannose = lactose, maltose, raffinose.

Amino acids (particularly the D-isomers, e.g. those of asparagine, histidine or tryptophan) often taste sweet whereas their L-forms may be bitter or tasteless.

Aspartame is about 180 times sweeter than sucrose (sugar); it contains phenylalanine, which is contraindicated in people with phenylketonuria. Aspartame has undeservedly been linked to various disorders, but the American Food and Drug Administration (FDA) considers aspartame 'one of the most thoroughly tested and studied food additives the agency has ever approved' (Henkel 1999).

Saccharin is about 300–400 times sweeter than sucrose but has a bitter aftertaste and has been shown to cause cancer in some laboratory animals. Cyclamates are 30–40 times sweeter than sucrose; these were banned by the FDA after being linked to increased risk of bladder cancer.

Newer sugar substitutes (artificial sweeteners) include acesulfame potassium, sucralose, and sugar alcohols such as xylitol and mannitol.

The leaves of the Indian plant *Gymnema sylvestre* contain steroidal compounds that specifically block sweet taste. After chewing the leaves of the plant, solutions of sugar, saccharin, cyclamates or D-amino acids are all tasteless. Various west African plants have the opposite effect: after chewing their berries or roots, a sweet taste is added to other foods such as lemons or sour bread; a glycoprotein is thought to be responsible.

The sensation of taste adapts rapidly: within about 90 seconds, the salty taste of a sodium chloride solution may be lost. People who load teaspoons of sugar into cups of tea or coffee presumably have raised thresholds to sweet taste, and may benefit from gradually reducing the sugar load until they become sensitive to much lower levels.
Adapted from: Bowman & Rand 1980; Henkel 1999; Weihrauch & Diehl 2004.

also sometimes idiosyncratic and genetically linked. Total aminoglycoside exposure of patients should be noted, and both ototoxicity and nephrotoxicity monitored in clinical usage. Once-daily administration may be useful in increasing efficacy and reducing toxicity. Prophylactic treatment with antioxidants has been trialled.

SALICYLATES AND OTHER ANTI-INFLAMMATORIES

Salicylates such as aspirin and methyl salicylate have long been known to cause auditory toxicity, especially after high doses (>4 g/day aspirin). Tinnitus, loss of acoustic sensitivity, and alterations of perceived sounds occur, particularly at high frequencies. The mechanisms of auditory changes and hearing loss are not well understood, but outer hair cells in the cochlea are known to be damaged. It is not known yet whether the very low antiplatelet doses of aspirin used in prevention of ischaemia (75 mg/day) will have a cumulative effect on hearing.

Drugs affecting taste and smell
Gustation—the sense of taste

Gustation (the sense of taste) is a chemical sense closely linked to smell but is much less sensitive. Substances that have strong tastes, including alcohols, sugars, salts and acids, may have no smell. Molecules dissolved in saliva in the mouth are sensed by gustatory receptors on taste buds (specialised epithelial cells) located mainly on the back of the tongue and also elsewhere in the mouth, throat and oesophagus. The chemical contacts a gustatory 'hair' passing through a pore on the surface of the cell, stimulating receptors on the membrane and inducing action potentials in the primary afferent sensory neurons that make contact with the receptor cells. The chemical information is transduced into cellular signals via stimulation of seven-transmembrane-helix receptors, coupled to G-proteins, second messengers, enzymes and ion channels. Subsequent neurons in the taste pathway run via the pons and medulla to the thalamus, thence to the taste centre in the parietal lobe of the cerebral cortex, where the taste is perceived. Trace metals, especially zinc and copper, are involved at the active site of taste receptors, and zinc deficiencies may cause loss or distortion of taste.

The **gustatory** receptors are sensitive only to four classes of taste: sour, sweet, bitter and salty (see Clinical Interest Box 36-3). The threshold for bitter tastes is the lowest: brucine is detectable at the level of about 0.4 parts per million. This sensitivity to bitter tastes may have developed as a protective function, as many potentially poisonous natural substances (including drugs such as quinine, strychnine, nicotine and cocaine) are very bitter.

Loss or decrease of taste sensation (ageusia, hypogeusia) may occur as a result of neuronal damage or as an adverse effect of drugs. In some conditions, the sense of taste is distorted (dysgeusia), giving unexpected tastes such as metallic, bitter, burned or rotten. While these conditions cannot readily be treated medically, zinc supplements have been shown in some trials to be effective.

TABLE 36-2 Drug effects on taste and smell

DRUG GROUP: EXAMPLE	SENSORY EFFECT		PROPOSED MECHANISM
	Taste	Smell	
Cardiovascular drugs			
ACE inhibitors: captopril	⇓, X	—	Zn chelation
Calcium channel blockers: nifedipine	⇓, X	X	Inhibit receptor events
Antiarrhythmics: procainamide	X	—	Inhibit receptor action potentials
β-blockers: propranolol	⇓, X	—	Antagonise adrenoceptors
Antimicrobials			
Penicillins: ampicillin	⇓	—	Inhibit receptor turnover
Quinolones: ofloxacin	X	X	Inhibit cytochrome P450
Antivirals: zidovudine	⇓, X	—	Inhibit receptor events
Drugs acting on the GI tract			
H_2-antagonists: cimetidine	⇓, X	⇓	Inhibit rceptor events
Anti-inflammatory agents			
NSAIDs: aspirin	⇓, X	—	Inhibit PGs; deplete Zn
Corticosteroids: prednisolone	⇓	⇓	Inhibit receptor membrane activity
Antirheumatics: penicillamine	⇓	—	Zn, Cu interactions
Endocrine drugs			
Antithyroid: carbimazole	⇓	⇓	Hypothyroidism, Zn interactions
Hypoglycaemics: insulin	⇓	—	Inhibit receptor events
Hypoglycaemics: sulfonylureas	X	—	Inhibit receptor events
Drugs affecting the CNS			
Antimigraine: triptans	X	X	Inhibit receptor events
Antidepressants: imipramine	⇓, X	—	Altered NA effects, dry mouth
Antidepressants: sertraline	⇓, X	—	Altered 5-HT effects
Anorectics: amphetamines	X	—	Altered NA effects
Antiparkinsonian drugs: levodopa	⇓, X	X	Enhanced DA activity
Autonomic drugs			
Nicotine	X	—	Binds to ACh receptor
α-agonists: phenylephrine		⇓	Inhibit receptor events
Antineoplastic drugs			
Antimetabolites: fluorouracil	X		Inhibit receptor turnover
Antimetabolites: methotrexate	⇓		Inhibit receptor turnover, stomatitis
Antibiotics: bleomycin	⇓		Inhibit receptor turnover, stomatitis

Sensory effects: ⇑ = increased sense; ⇓ = decreased sense; X = impaired sense; — = no effect or not known.
ACE = angiotensin-converting enzyme; ACh = acetylcholine; CNS = central nervous system; Cu = copper; DA = dopamine; GI = gastrointestinal; H_2 = histamine H_2-receptor; 5-HT = 5-hydroxytryptamine (serotonin); NA = noradrenaline; NSAID = non-steroidal anti-inflammatory drug; PG = prostaglandin; Zn = zinc.
Only drug groups in which the adverse effects are well documented for a group of drugs have been included. In most cases, the impaired sensation takes some days or weeks of chronic dosing to develop, and the impairment may persist for weeks or months. Doses at which the effects occur are very variable and many individual drugs have been omitted. (For details see Henkin 1994.)

Olfaction—the sense of smell

The receptors for **olfaction** (the sense of smell) are located in the olfactory epithelium at the top of the nasal cavity (see Figure 32-6). Specialised cilia projecting down from the dendrites of the olfactory receptor cells are stimulated by chemicals in the inhaled air, and initiate an action potential in the olfactory neurons. These synapse within the olfactory bulb and form the olfactory tract of the first cranial nerve, passing eventually to the lateral olfactory area of the temporal lobe of the cortex and to other regions of the limbic system and to the hypothalamus.

Humans have a much greater sensitivity to smell than to taste. Vanillin can be smelt in the air at a concentration about one millionth of the concentration of brucine that can just be tasted. Consequently, there is a great range of different types of smells,* and a wide variation (1000-fold) in the thresholds at which different people can sense smells.

Anosmia (lack of sense of smell) can occur as a genetic trait, and different specific anosmias exist; for example, some people cannot smell naphthalene, others menthol, thymol, iodine or vanillin. Hyposmia, a mild general defect in olfaction, is a common symptom of colds and rhinitis (see Chapter 32), due to inflammation and obstruction of the nasal passages. (Food often becoming tasteless during these conditions indicates that components of the flavour can no longer be smelled.) Hyperosmia occurs in cystic fibrosis, adrenal insufficiency and states of hysteria. In schizophrenia and

---

*Smells may be classified subjectively, e.g. as smelling like fruit, ether, mint, roses, citrus, vanilla, musk, onion, fish, sweat, faeces, urine, mould, jasmine, camphor. As Shakespeare put it so memorably: '   that which we call a rose By any other name would smell as sweet.'

(Romeo and Juliet, II, ii, 43)

PREGNANCY SAFETY	
ADEC Category	**Drug**
A	Dexamethasone, nystatin, triamcinolone
D	Framycetin, neomycin
Not classified	Acetic acid, benzocaine, carbamide peroxide, isopropyl alcohol, propylene glycol

Note: With combination preparations, the formulation takes the category of the least safe ingredient.

epilepsy, olfactory hallucinations may occur. As with disorders of taste, there are few specific medical treatments for these olfactory dysfunctions; zinc supplements may be useful.

Drugs affecting taste and smell

The sensations of taste and smell may be impaired in many situations, e.g. by ageing, radiation, dental treatment, poor oral hygiene, psychiatric disorders, tumours, trauma, epilepsy, migraine, hypothyroidism, infections, renal failure and deficiencies of vitamin B or zinc. A great variety of drugs have been noted to cause alterations in taste and smell as an adverse effect; these are summarised in Table 36-2. In most cases, the mechanism by which the chemical sense is altered is poorly understood; however, patients who notice that 'things are starting to smell different' may need reassurance that this is an acknowledged adverse effect of the drug, which is usually reversible after stopping treatment.

DRUGS AT A GLANCE 36: Drugs used to treat ear conditions

Therapeutic group	Pharmacological group	Key examples	Key pages
Drugs treating swimmer's ear	Acidifying/drying agents	acetic acid, isopropyl alcohol	611, 3
Antimicrobials	Antibacterials	chloramphenicol framycetin neomycin	613, 4
	Antifungals	nystatin	613
Anti-inflammatories	Corticosteroids	triamcinolone, dexamethasone	613, 4
Wax removal agents	Solvents	carbamide peroxide, docusate sodium	614

Note: This table excludes drugs causing adverse drug reactions to hearing, taste or smell; see Tables 36-1 and 36-2. For drugs used in treating rhinitis, see Chapter 32.

KEY POINTS

- Knowledge of the anatomy and physiology of the ear is necessary for understanding the pathology of conditions affecting the senses of hearing and balance.
- Conditions affecting the external ear are generally simply treated with ear-drops that dry out and mildly acidify the ear canal. Antibiotic ear-drops are used to treat severe infections.
- Infections and inflammation of the middle ear (otitis media) are treated with systemic analgesics and antibiotics. If the eardrum is ruptured, ear-drops containing antibiotics and anti-inflammatory agents are useful.
- Antiseptic aqueous or oily preparations are used topically to remove cerumen (ear wax).
- Systemic medications can cause ototoxicity by various mechanisms. The main drug groups causing ear damage are the salicylate anti-inflammatory agents, aminoglycoside antibiotics, cisplatin antineoplastic agents and loop diuretics.
- Other special senses are the chemical senses: taste and smell. Many drugs can cause impaired or altered taste and smell, which is usually reversible.

REVIEW EXERCISES

1 Describe the anatomy of the ear, explaining which parts of the ear are primarily involved in hearing and which function in equilibrium and balance.
2 Explain the function of the eustachian tube. What advice can you offer the airline traveller to reduce the problem caused by air pressure changes?
3 Discuss the use of topical antibiotic and anti-inflammatory agents in infections of the outer and middle ear.
4 Discuss the mechanisms by which drugs can cause toxic effects in the ear.
5 Give examples of drugs that commonly cause changes in hearing, taste or smell.

REFERENCES AND FURTHER READING

Antibiotic Expert Group. *Therapeutic Guidelines Antibiotic, version 12*. Melbourne: Therapeutic Guidelines Limited, 2003.
Australian Medicines Handbook 2006. Adelaide: AMH, 2006.
Bowman WC, Rand MJ. *Textbook of Pharmacology*. 2nd edn. Oxford: Blackwell, 1980 [chs 6, 30].
Caswell A (ed.). *MIMS Annual June 2005*. Sydney: CMPMedica Australia, 2005.
Cazals Y. Auditory sensori-neural alterations induced by salicylate. *Progress in Neurobiology* 2000; 62(6): 583–631.
Cohen-Kerem R, Kisilevsky V, Einarson TR, Kozer E, Koren G, Rutka JA. Intratympanic gentamicin for Ménière's disease: a meta-analysis. *Laryngoscope* 2004; 114(12): 2085–91.
Dodson KM, Sismanis A. Intratympanic perfusion for the treatment of tinnitus. *Otolaryngologic Clinics of North America* 2004; 37(5): 991–1000.
Doty RL, Bromley SM. Effects of drugs on olfaction and taste. *Otolaryngologic Clinics of North America* 2004; 37(6): 1229–54.
Evans P, Halliwell B. Free radicals and hearing: cause, consequence and criteria. *Annals of the New York Academy of Sciences* 1999; 884: 19–40.
Forge A, Schacht J. Aminoglycoside antibiotics. *Audiology & Neuro-Otology* 2000; 5(1): 3–22.
Gilbertson TA, Damak S, Margolskee RF. The molecular physiology of taste transduction. *Current Opinion in Neurobiology* 2000; 10(4): 519–27.
Hain TC, Uddin M. Pharmacological treatment of vertigo. *CNS Drugs* 2003; 17(2): 85–100.
Henkel J. Sugar substitutes: research on new and existing artificial sweeteners. *FDA Consumer* 1999; 33(6): 12ff.
Henkin RI. Drug-induced taste and smell disorders: incidence, mechanisms and management related primarily to treatment of sensory receptor dysfunction. *Drug Safety* 1994; 11(5): 318–77.
Humes HD. Insights into ototoxicity: analogies to nephrotoxicity. *Annals of the New York Academy of Sciences* 1999; 884: 15–18.
Lee CA, Mistry D, Uppal S, Coatesworth AP. Otologic side effects of drugs. *Journal of Laryngology and Otology* 2005; 119(4): 267–71.
Light JP, Silverstein H. Transtympanic perfusion: indications and limitations. *Current Opinion in Otolaryngology and Head and Neck Surgery* 2004; 12(5): 378–83.
Morris PS. Management of otitis media in a high risk population. *Australian Family Physician* 1998; 27(11): 1021–9.
Pichichero ME, Casey JR. Otitis media. *Expert Opinion on Pharmacotherapy* 2002; 3(8): 1073–90.
Smith PF. Are vestibular hair cells excited to death by aminoglycoside antibiotics? *Journal of Vestibular Research* 2000; 10(1): 1–5.
Weihrauch MR, Diehl V. Artificial sweeteners–do they bear a carcinogenic risk? *Annals of Oncology* 2004; 15(10): 1460–5.
Youngson RM. *Collins Dictionary: Medicine*. 2nd edn. Glasgow: HarperCollins, 1998.

ONLINE RESOURCES

New Zealand medicines and medical devices safety authority: www.medsafe.govt.nz

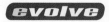 More weblinks at http://evolve.elsevier.com/AU/Bryant/pharmacology/

CHAPTER 37

Overview of the Endocrine System

CHAPTER FOCUS

The endocrine system comprises glands that produce hormones necessary for a variety of vital functions in the body. The endocrine glands secrete their hormones directly into the bloodstream, which carries the hormones to other organs or tissues that they affect, control or regulate. This chapter reviews the anatomy and physiology of the endocrine system.

OBJECTIVES

- To describe the general functions of hormones in the body and explain the common mechanisms of hormone action.

- To describe the various processes and levels of control of endocrine gland functions.

- To identify the major endocrine glands, name their hormones and explain their main functions in the body.

- To explain how hormone levels may be altered in pathological conditions and how hormones are commonly used in medicine.

KEY TERMS

binding protein
endocrine gland
hormone
hypothalamic factor
hypothalamic–pituitary–adrenal axis
international units
negative feedback
permissive effect
replacement therapy
steroid hormone
target gland
trophic hormone

KEY ABBREVIATIONS

ACTH	adrenocorticotrophic hormone (corticotrophin)
ADH	antidiuretic hormone (vasopressin)
FSH	follicle-stimulating hormone
GH	growth hormone (somatotropin)
IU	International Units
LH	luteinising hormone
TSH	thyroid-stimulating hormone (thyrotrophin)

HORMONES AND ENDOCRINE GLANDS

Hormones

HORMONES are active, natural chemical substances that are secreted into the bloodstream from the endocrine glands and initiate or regulate the activity of an organ or group of cells in another part of the body. They have specific, well-defined physiological effects on metabolism, growth, homeostasis and integration of bodily functions. The list of major hormones includes the **hypothalamic factors**, which stimulate or inhibit release of anterior pituitary hormones, the hormones from the anterior and posterior pituitary glands, the thyroid hormones, parathyroid hormone, pancreatic insulin and glucagon, several potent steroids from the adrenal cortex and the gonadal hormones of both sexes.

One of the major developments of the 20th century in the fields of biology and medicine was the recognition, isolation, purification and chemical and cellular investigation of most known hormones. Once their chemical structure was known, duplicating and mimicking hormones by chemical synthesis and/or genetic engineering techniques became possible.

Endocrine glands

Endocrine glands are groups of cells that produce and secrete hormones into the bloodstream; they are usually highly vascular, and the circulating blood collects and distributes the hormones to virtually all other cells in the body (see Figure 37-1). (Endocrine glands were originally known as 'ductless glands', to distinguish them from exocrine glands such as sweat glands, which secrete their products into ducts; see Clinical Interest Box 37-1.) Transport of hormone in blood is usually in a bound form and specific **binding proteins** exist, such as thyroxine-binding globulin. The process is closely analogous to that of protein binding of drugs; in each case, binding increases the transportability of the drug or hormone, decreases its movement across membranes in the kidney or across the blood–brain barrier, and acts as a reserve depot in the blood. Only the free, unbound hormone or drug is available to act at receptors or to cross membranes.

Chemical classes of hormones

The major types of hormones are the **steroid hormones**, amino acid-derived hormones, and polypeptides and simple proteins. Steroid hormones are secreted by the adrenal cortex and the sex glands (testes and ovaries). They are lipid-soluble cholesterol derivatives (see Figure 37-2); their physiological effects begin when the steroid enters the nucleus, with subsequent binding to the specific steroid receptor. Steroid hormones are usually secreted as they are synthesised, rather than being stored.

Thyroid hormones are iodinated derivatives of the amino acid tyrosine. The catecholamines secreted from the adrenal medulla, adrenaline and noradrenaline (sometimes considered hormones), are also tyrosine derivatives (see Figure 10-9).

Polypeptide hormones (<20 amino acid residues) include the posterior pituitary hormones, oxytocin and vasopressin, and some of the hypothalamic releasing factors. Protein hormones (>20 amino acids) include the classic hormones insulin, growth hormone and parathyroid hormone, and other releasing factors. Peptide and protein hormones are generally stored in cells in membrane-bound vesicles, and are released by exocytosis.

The main clinical significance of knowing the chemical class of a hormone is that it affects how the hormone is administered: peptide and protein hormones cannot be given orally, as they would be digested in the gastrointestinal tract, so they are administered by injection (parenterally) or sometimes as nasal sprays.

General functions of hormones

Hormones from the various endocrine glands work together to regulate vital processes, including:

- secretory and motor activities of the digestive tract

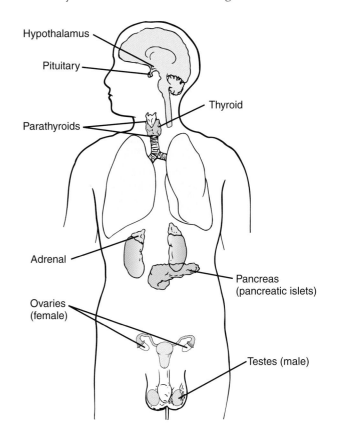

FIGURE 37-1 Locations of the major endocrine glands.

- energy production
- composition and volume of extracellular fluid
- adaptation, such as acclimatisation and immunity
- growth and development
- reproduction and lactation.

Interactions among hormones account for some of the very complicated effects seen in endocrine physiology; for example, the thyroid hormones have a **permissive effect** on the lipolytic action of adrenaline, increasing adrenaline actions. In other situations, two hormones can have opposing effects; thus glucagon can be considered to have anti-insulin actions.

Mechanisms of hormone actions

Research in endocrinology has advanced the concept of specific receptors within or on the surfaces of cells in target organs. This has led to knowledge of hormone specificity and the essential cellular mechanisms involved in the actions of the hormone–receptor complex. Only specific receptors recognise and bind a hormone to mediate its activity; the hormone has no effect on tissues that do not carry its specific receptors. The extent of effect of the hormone is determined by the concentration of the circulating active hormone.

Steroid hormones act intracellularly on specific steroid receptors in the cytosol or nucleus. Typically, the steroid enters the cell and activates the receptor, which up- or down-regulates gene expression, leading to altered transcription of DNA and hence protein synthesis; the newly synthesised proteins ultimately bring about the actions of the hormone.

Water-soluble hormones, such as peptides, proteins and catecholamines, cannot enter cells and instead act through receptors located in the cell membranes. The general mechanisms are similar to those for neurotransmitters and may involve second messenger systems such as adenylate cyclase and cyclic adenosine monophosphate, or cyclic guanine monophosphate, diacylglycerol or inositol triphosphate (see Chapter 5), which then activate protein kinases and phosphorylate other enzymes, leading to the physiological responses attributed to the hormone.

Control of hormone concentrations

To maintain the internal environment, physiological functions must be able to be increased or decreased; in the endocrine system there are multiple levels of control (see Figure 37-3). At the highest level, environmental, cognitive and emotional factors may influence hormone concentrations. The hypothalamus secretes several hypothalamic factors (or hormones) that either stimulate or inhibit release of hormones from the

> ## CLINICAL INTEREST BOX 37-1 DEATH FROM DUCTLESS GLANDS — OR WAS IT FROM DIGITALIS?
>
> The mystery opens in a gentlemen's club in post-World War I London. An elderly retired general is found to have died in his chair by the fire. His doctor declares the death to be from 'natural causes' after heart failure. The doctor explains that the general had been taking digitalis to 'relieve the feebleness of the heart's action', and had succumbed despite having taken a powerful dose not long before his death. Detective Lord Peter Wimsey, however, is not satisfied with the diagnosis...
>
> Soon after, Lord Peter is present at a literary cocktail party, at which the hostess explains to a guest that 'a new young man is going to read a paper on ductless glands [which] will be "news" in next to no time—ever so much more up-to-date than vitamins ... So very wonderful about glands, isn't it? ... those marvellous old sheep. Such a hope for us all. What young criminals really needed was a little bit of rabbit-gland or something ... all pineal or pituitary, and they come right again'.
>
> It seems that it is the general's doctor who is researching into endocrinology, and is planning to establish a new clinic 'to make everybody good by glands. It's the science of the future, it puts biology in quite a new light. We're on the verge of some really interesting discoveries . . . anything does for these women as long as it's new —especially if it's sexual'. A reporter notes that 'Glands are news, you know. He'll be one of these fashionable practitioners. Shrewd man—knows there's money in glands. If only he could start one of these clinics for rejuvenating people, he could be a millionaire'.
>
> Eventually, it transpires that the doctor had given his patient a lethal dose of digitalis in capsules, hoping thereby to gain sufficient wealth to establish his endocrine clinic. The morals of the story appear to be:
> - the long half-life of digoxin makes it a potentially toxic drug in elderly patients, especially those with poor renal function
> - fascination with endocrinology is no excuse for crime
> - even 80 years ago, clinical researchers had difficulty obtaining financial grants for funding research.
>
> *Source*: Dorothy L Sayers, *The Unpleasantness at the Bellona Club*, first published Victor Gollancz, London, 1921; New England Library, London, 1977.

anterior pituitary gland. The anterior pituitary hormones are referred to as **trophic hormones**, as they nourish or change the functions of the **target glands** where they act. (There is some confusion as to whether the term 'tropic' or 'trophic' is correct. 'Trophic' comes from the Greek root meaning nutrition or feeding, whereas 'tropic' comes from the root meaning to turn or change. In the context of endocrinology, the terms are sometimes used interchangeably. In this book, we have standardised on 'trophic' except where the approved name of the hormone used as a drug

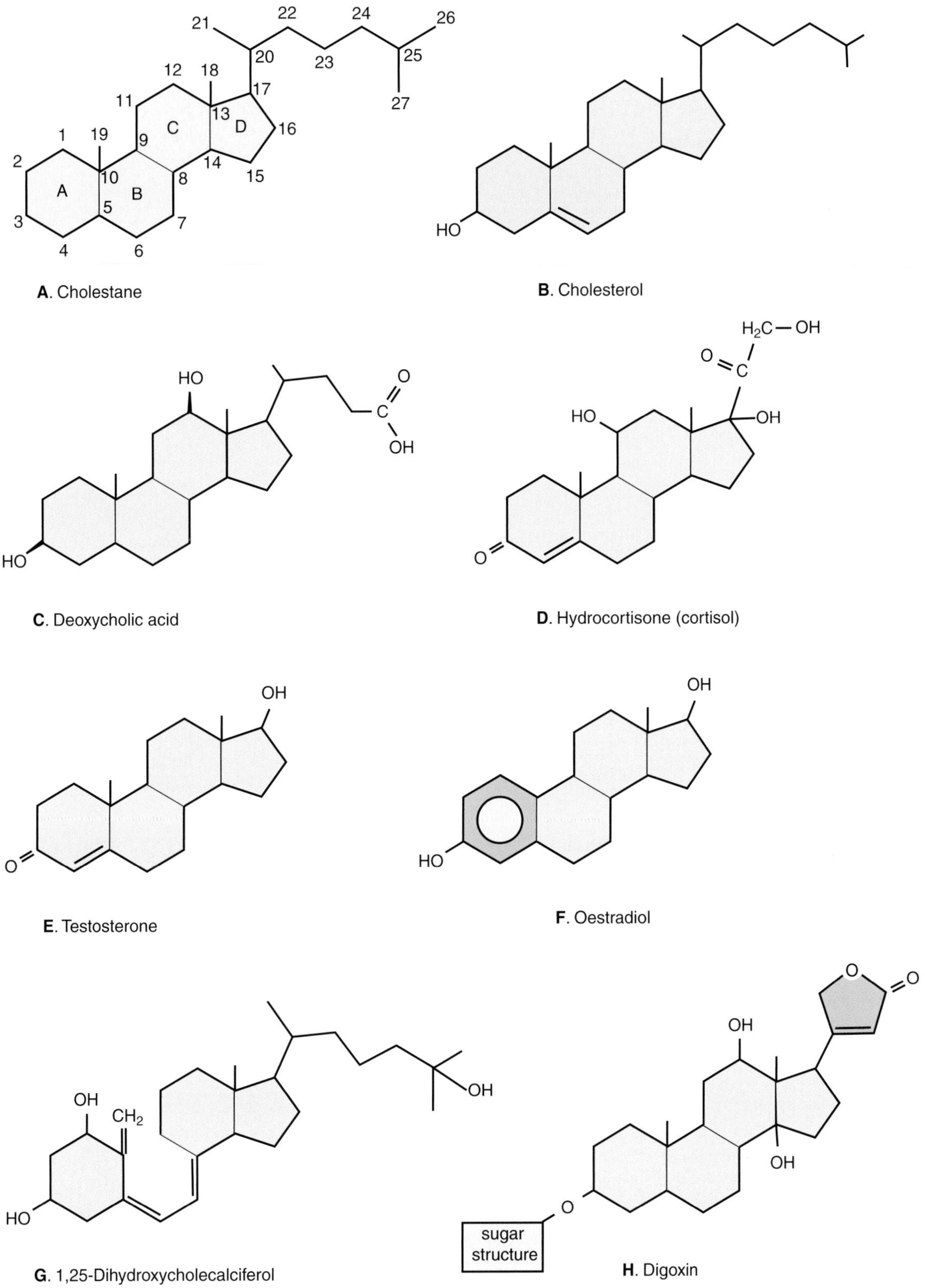

FIGURE 37-2 Chemical structures of some naturally occurring steroids. **A.** A typical steroid (cholestane), showing the conventional ring lettering and carbon atom numbering pattern. **B.** Cholesterol, a component of cell membranes and precursor to other steroids. **C.** Deoxycholic acid, a bile acid. **D.** Hydrocortisone, a glucocorticoid. **E.** Testosterone, a male sex hormone. **F.** Oestradiol, a female sex hormone. **G.** 1,25-dihydroxycholecalciferol, an active form of vitamin D. **H.** Digoxin, a cardiac glycoside.

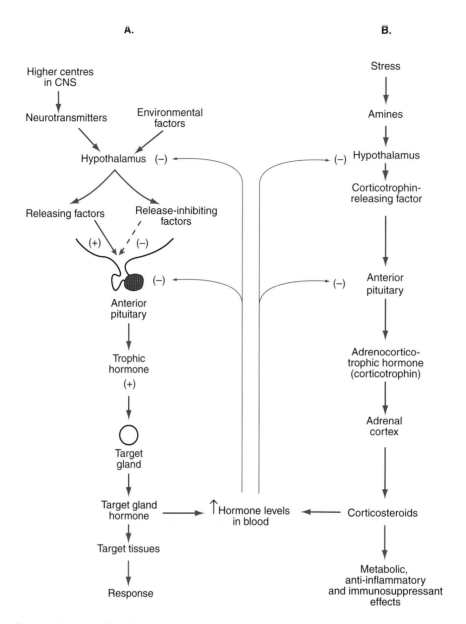

FIGURE 37-3 Levels of endocrine control. Various internal and external factors may inhibit or stimulate the hypothalamus to secrete inhibitory or releasing factors, which increase (+) or decrease (−) output of hormones from the anterior pituitary gland, and ultimately hormone release from target glands. Short and long negative feedback loops 'damp down' further release. **A.** Flowchart showing typical pattern of levels of controls. **B.** Example in the adrenal cortex.

is definitely otherwise, as in somatropin [recombinant or biosynthetic growth hormone] and follitropin [recombinant human follicle-stimulating hormone]. The natural hormones are somatotrophin, urofollitrophin, gonadotrophins etc.) The target glands may themselves release hormones that are transported via the blood to other tissues (e.g. the adrenal cortex responds to corticotrophin and produces various steroid hormones), or they may respond with generalised effects, such as bone and muscle growth in response to stimulation by growth hormone.

The hormones produced by the pituitary or the target glands may also act to inhibit the release of stimulating or trophic hormones earlier in the pathway. This self-regulating series of events is known as **negative feedback**, i.e. a hormone produces a physiological effect that, when strong enough, inhibits further secretion of that hormone, thereby inhibiting the physiological effect. Exogenous hormones given as drugs can also activate this negative feedback effect; thus corticosteroids administered chronically for asthma can switch off the **hypothalamic–pituitary–adrenal axis** (i.e. the linked functions of the hypothalamus, the anterior pituitary gland and the adrenal cortex) and leave the body less able to respond to stress or infections (see Clinical Interest Box 37-2).

Less commonly, there may be a positive feedback effect. An example is childbirth, when uterine contractions stimulate the posterior pituitary gland to release oxytocin, which stimulates increased uterine contractions; the cycle is ended by the birth of the baby. Hormone concentrations are also regulated by other hormones, by changes in plasma concentrations of ions and nutrients, and by nervous system effects. Secretion may thus be episodic, pulsatile, or follow a daily or monthly rhythm.

Hormones are not used up in exerting their physiological effects but must be inactivated or excreted if the internal environment is to remain stable. Inactivation occurs enzymatically in the liver, kidney, blood or target tissues. Excretion of hormone metabolites is primarily via the urine and, to a lesser extent, the bile. Most hormones are destroyed rapidly, having a half-life in blood of 10–30 minutes. Some, however, such as the catecholamines, have half-lives of seconds, whereas thyroid hormones have half-lives measured in days. Some hormones exert their physiological effects immediately, while others require minutes or hours before their effects occur. In addition, some effects end immediately when the hormone

---

CLINICAL INTEREST BOX 37-2 RESPONSES TO STRESS

The integrated responses of the body to stress are a good example of the complex relationships between the nervous systems and endocrine systems. Some of the processes involved in response to stress include:

- stimulation from the hypothalamus of sympathetic pathways to the adrenal medulla, causing release of adrenaline and noradrenaline, leading to:
- sympathetic fight or flight reactions, activating the cardiovascular system and energy supplies to skeletal muscle, and switching off digestive, reproductive and urinary functions
- secretion of hypothalamic factors that increase release from the anterior pituitary gland of the trophic hormones corticotrophin, growth hormone and thyrotrophin, hence:
- stimulation of the adrenal cortex to secrete glucocorticoids (altering metabolism, and decreasing inflammatory and immune responses)
- stimulation of the adrenal cortex to secrete mineralocorticoids (causing retention of sodium and water and raising blood pressure)
- alteration of metabolism in the liver, to use fats and glycogen for glucose and energy
- control of neuronal responses underlying behavioural adaptations to stress.

Thus overall the body is 'fired up' to overcome stress, meet emotional crises, perform strenuous tasks and resist blood loss. If excessively prolonged, however, the responses can lead to exhaustion, negative feedback effects and inability to respond to infection or immune challenge (see de Kloet et al 2005).

---

disappears from the circulation, while other responses persist for hours or days after hormone concentrations have returned to basal concentrations. The steroid hormones typically have slow actions because they induce synthesis of new proteins, and long half-lives because they are lipid-soluble and tend to be retained in the enterohepatic circulation. This wide range in times of onset and duration of hormonal activity contributes to the flexibility of the endocrine system.

Clinical aspects

Alterations in hormone secretion or hormone receptor responses may culminate in endocrine disease states. Hormone concentrations may be increased above normal (e.g. hyperpituitarism), often as a result of hormone-secreting tumours (adenomas), or may be decreased (e.g. hypothyroidism), due to gland atrophy or impairment of hormone synthesis. (The situation in which hormone concentrations are normal is given the prefix 'eu-', e.g. euthyroid.) Conditions involving hypersecretion of hormones may be treated by surgery or with antihormones. Hyposecretion can usually be treated simply by replacing the missing hormone with exogenous natural or synthetic hormone.

Certain cell-surface receptors can become antigenic and stimulate formation of antibodies that accelerate receptor destruction, block receptor function or mimic the action of the hormone. Among the receptor disorders are Graves' disease and insulin-resistant diabetes mellitus.

In medicine, hormones are generally used in three ways:

- for **replacement therapy**, exemplified by the use of physiological concentrations of insulin in diabetes or of adrenal steroids in Addison's disease
- for pharmacological effects beyond replacement, as in the use of larger-than-endogenous doses of adrenal steroids for their anti-inflammatory or immunosuppressant effects
- for endocrine diagnostic testing; for example, in the 'dexamethasone suppression test', a low dose of the corticosteroid dexamethasone (which normally suppresses pituitary ACTH release) is administered and plasma corticosteroid concentrations are subsequently measured to check the functionality of the hypothalamic–pituitary–adrenal axis.

Dosing: International Units or milligrams?

In the past, hormones produced for therapeutic use were extracted from animal (or human) cadaver tissues, then purified and tested biologically for pharmacological activity, so that the activity of the extracts was known. As it was not possible to be sure that the natural preparation was 100% pure, the activity of such an extract was compared in biological assays with international standard preparations, and the strength of the new preparation was quoted in terms of '**International Units**' (IU) of activity, rather than in milligrams of active extract. Thus insulin preparations, for example, were standardised to contain 100 IU hypoglycaemic activity per millilitre of solution.

Although many hormone preparations are now prepared purely synthetically or by recombinant DNA technology, and it is possible to ensure that they are 100% pure, such preparations may still have the doses quoted in IU rather than in absolute amounts.

Other hormones and endocrine tissues

By our definition, a multitude of endogenous active chemicals released into the bloodstream would be classified as hormones: the list has been suggested to range from ions such as sodium and calcium, through the neurotransmitters adrenaline and noradrenaline, to steroids such as vitamin D. Local hormones (paracrines, or autacoids) such as prostaglandins, histamine

and nitric oxide, which are secreted and released to act in the same or nearby cells and tissues, could also be included.

By the same token, many organs that are not usually considered as endocrine glands secrete into the bloodstream 'hormones' that act on distant tissues. Thus cells in the gastrointestinal tract secrete gastrin and cholecystokinin, helping regulate digestion; the pineal gland secretes melatonin, an autacoid similar to 5-hydroxytryptamine (5-HT, serotonin) and suspected of involvement in the body's biological clock and sleep–waking cycles (and used by some shift-workers and jet-setters to adjust daily rhythms); the thymus gland secretes thymic factors involved in T-cell functions and immunity; and the kidneys secrete erythropoietin, involved in red blood cell production (sometimes abused by athletes to enhance their endurance). During pregnancy, the placenta also has endocrine functions.

However, in this unit we concentrate on the 'classical' hormones and endocrine glands, as shown in Figures 37-1 and 37-4. The main functions of these hormones are summarised

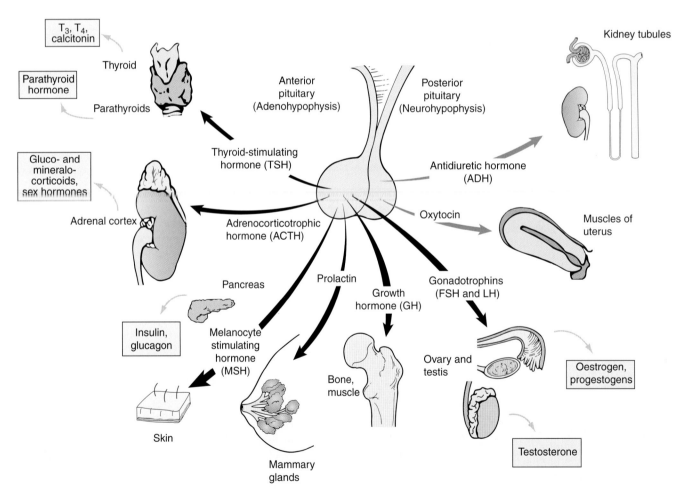

FIGURE 37-4 Pituitary hormones. Some of the major hormones of the adenohypophysis and neurohypophysis and their principal target organs; hormones produced by target glands are shown in boxes. Note that there are no pituitary trophic hormones for the pancreas or parathyroid gland, and that some target glands do not produce further hormones. FSH = follicle-stimulating hormone; LH = luteinising hormone; T_3 = tri-iodothyronine; T_4 = tetra-iodothyronine.

in this chapter to provide an overview of endocrine function. Details of control of the gland, individual hormone actions, and monographs on the hormones, their analogues and antagonists when used as drugs are discussed in subsequent chapters in this unit and in Unit XII.

THE MAJOR ENDOCRINE GLANDS
Pituitary gland

The pituitary gland is made up of two parts, quite distinct in embryological, anatomical and physiological terms.

Anterior pituitary hormones

Anterior pituitary function is regulated by hypothalamic releasing and release-inhibiting factors, and by negative feedback control from target gland hormones (Figure 37-3). The hormones of the anterior part of the pituitary gland exert important effects in regulating the secretion of other hormones; Figure 37-4 shows anterior pituitary hormones and their principal target organs. Note that four of the hormones (adrenocorticotrophic hormone, thyroid-stimulating hormone,

follicle-stimulating hormone and luteinising hormone) regulate the functions of other endocrine glands, whereas three (growth hormone, melanocyte-stimulating hormone and prolactin) act directly on target organs. The main functions of the hormones are listed in Table 37-1; common pathological conditions related to gland or hormone dysfunction are also indicated.

Posterior pituitary hormones

The neural-type tissue in the posterior pituitary gland secretes two hormones, closely related chemically: oxytocin (a hormone that stimulates the smooth muscle of the uterus to contract), and vasopressin (antidiuretic hormone, with antidiuretic and vasopressor actions).

Other endocrine gland hormones and functions

The other main endocrine glands (shown in Figure 37-1) are listed in Table 37-2, and their hormones and functions are summarised. These will be discussed in much greater detail, and their uses in endocrine medicine described, in subsequent chapters.

TABLE 37-1 The hormones secreted by the anterior pituitary gland, their functions and related pathological conditions

ANTERIOR PITUITARY HORMONE	FUNCTIONS	RELATED PATHOLOGIES
Thyroid-stimulating hormone (TSH, thyrotrophic hormone, thyrotrophin)	Stimulates the thyroid gland to produce thyroid hormones, hence regulates metabolic rate, growth and maturation; also affects central nervous system and cardiovascular functions; and calcium metabolism	Graves' disease, hyperthyroidism
Adrenocorticotrophic hormone (ACTH, corticotrophin)	Stimulates the cortex of the adrenal gland to produce glucocorticoids, mineralocorticoids and precursors to sex hormones, hence regulates metabolism and fluid balance	Cushing's disease, Addison's disease
Growth hormone (GH, somatotrophin)	Promotes growth in most tissues; regulates metabolism	Pituitary adenomas, acromegaly and gigantism, dwarfism
Follicle-stimulating hormone (FSH)	Stimulates the growth and maturation of the ovarian follicle, regulates menstruation or spermatogenesis	Dysmenorrhoea, infertility
Luteinising hormone (LH), also known as the interstitial cell-stimulating hormone (ICSH)	Regulates reproduction (ovulation, formation of the corpus luteum, or spermatogenesis; secretion of sex hormones)	Dysmenorrhoea, infertility
Prolactin	Proliferation and secretion of the mammary glands	Pituitary adenomas, galactorrhoea, gynaecomastia
Melanocyte-stimulating hormone (MSH)	Functions in humans are not defined; does darken skin	

TABLE 37-2 **The major endocrine glands (excluding the pituitary), their hormones and main functions**

GLAND	HORMONES	FUNCTIONS
Adrenal cortex	Glucocorticoids, mineralocorticoids and some sex hormones	Regulates carbohydrate and protein metabolism and fluid balance; also involved in inflammatory and immune responses
Corpus luteum, placenta	Progesterone	Menstrual cycle, pregnancy
Ovary, placenta	Oestradiol	Female sex organs and characteristics; menstrual cycle, pregnancy
Pancreas	Insulin; glucagon	Glucose uptake, fat synthesis; gluconeogenesis
Parathyroid	Parathyroid hormone	Calcium balance
Testes	Testosterone	Male sex organs, characteristics and behaviour
Thyroid	Thyroxine, tri-iodothyronine; calcitonin	Metabolism, growth, protein synthesis; calcium balance and bone resorption

KEY POINTS

● The endocrine system is involved with integrating and regulating body functions.

● The system is composed of specialised glands, which secrete into the bloodstream hormones that act on specific target cells to produce complex responses.

● Pathological conditions in this system usually involve the overproduction or underproduction of hormones, and are treated by surgery, antihormones or replacement hormone therapy.

REVIEW EXERCISES

1 Name six vital effects produced by hormones from different endocrine glands.

2 Maintenance of the internal environment is similar to the functioning of a thermostat. Explain with reference to the negative feedback mechanisms operating in the endocrine system.

3 Describe the major chemical classes of hormones and discuss the relevance of their chemical structure to their modes of action and routes of administration, giving examples.

4 Outline how the nervous system and endocrine system respond to stress.

REFERENCES AND FURTHER READING

Bolander FF. *Molecular Endocrinology*, 3rd edn. Amsterdam: Elsevier Academic, 2004.
Bowman WC, Rand MJ. *Textbook of Pharmacology*. 2nd edn. Oxford: Blackwell, 1980 [chs 1, 19, 20, 26].
de Kloet ER, Joels M, Holsboer F. Stress and the brain: from adaptation to disease. *Nature Reviews Neuroscience* 2005; 6(6): 463–75.
Endocrinology Expert Group. *Therapeutic Guidelines: Endocrinology, version 3*. Melbourne: Therapeutic Guidelines Limited, 2004.
Goodman HM. Part VI: Endocrine physiology. In: Johnson LR (ed.). *Essential Medical Physiology*. 2nd edn. Philadelphia: Lippincott-Raven, 1999 [chs 37, 42].
Kennaway D. Melatonin—what's all the fuss about? *Australian Prescriber* 1997; 20: 98.
Melmed S, Conn PM (eds). *Endocrinology: Basic and Clinical Principles*. Totowa NJ: Humana Press; 2005.
Tortora GJ, Grabowski SR. *Principles of Anatomy and Physiology*. 9th edn. New York: HarperCollins, 2000 [ch. 18].
Youngson RM. *Collins Dictionary: Medicine*. 2nd edn. Glasgow: HarperCollins, 1999.

evolve More weblinks at http://evolve.elsevier.com/AU/Bryant/pharmacology/

CHAPTER 38

Pharmacology of the Pituitary Gland and Hypothalamic– Pituitary Axis

CHAPTER FOCUS

This chapter describes the structure and function of the pituitary gland and how it is controlled by factors from the hypothalamus. Although the pituitary gland secretes many hormones, detailed discussion in this chapter is limited to two anterior pituitary hormones —growth hormone (and its release-inhibiting factor, somatostatin) and prolactin—and the posterior pituitary hormones vasopressin and oxytocin. Other hormones will be discussed in the appropriate chapters more directly involved with the endocrine glands affected.

OBJECTIVES

- To describe the structure and functions of the pituitary gland.

- To describe how the hypothalamus controls anterior pituitary function, and name the hypothalamic factors, their actions, characteristics and clinical uses.

- To name and discuss the main actions of the anterior and posterior pituitary hormones.

- To describe the mechanisms of action and clinical uses of growth hormone, somatostatin, prolactin, vasopressin and oxytocin.

- To describe briefly the clinical manifestations of disorders of the pituitary gland and explain how drugs are used in therapy of the disorders.

KEY DRUGS

desmopressin
growth hormone (and
   somatropin)
octreotide
oxytocin

KEY TERMS

adenohypophysis
adenoma
growth hormone (and somatropin)
growth hormone release-inhibiting factor
   (somatostatin)
hypersecretion
hyposecretion
hypothalamic factors
negative feedback
neurohypophysis
oxytocin
pituitary gland
prolactin
trophic hormone
vasopressin (antidiuretic hormone)

KEY ABBREVIATIONS

CRF   corticotrophin-releasing factor
GH   growth hormone
GHRIF growth hormone release-inhibiting factor
GnRH   gonadotrophin-releasing hormone
IGF-1 insulin-like growth factor 1
PRIF   prolactin release-inhibiting factor

THE PITUITARY GLAND

THE **pituitary gland** exerts important effects in regulating the function of other endocrine glands and hormones. The pituitary body is about the size of a pea and occupies a niche in the sella turcica of the sphenoid bone (see Figure 32-5, showing the anatomical relationship of the pituitary gland to the hypothalamus, the nose and the sphenoidal sinus).

It consists of an anterior lobe (**adenohypophysis**), a posterior lobe (**neurohypophysis**), and the smaller pars intermedia, composed of secreting cells, the function of which is not well understood. The two main lobes develop separately in the embryo and remain histologically and functionally distinct. The anterior lobe consists of ectodermal tissue derived from the roof of the buccal cavity, whereas the posterior lobe consists of neural tissue derived by downward projection from the floor of the third ventricle in the brain.

The variety of preparations available that affect or are secreted by the pituitary gland are generally used as replacement therapy for hormone deficiency or as drug therapy for specific disorders, to produce a therapeutic hormonal response, or as diagnostic aids to determine hypofunctional or hyperfunctional gland disorders.

Regulation of anterior pituitary function

The anterior pituitary and some of the target glands have a **negative feedback** relation, as shown in Figure 37-3. As the level of the target-gland hormone builds up in the bloodstream, it inhibits further secretion of the hypothalamic releasing factor and of the **trophic hormone** by the pituitary (the long negative feedback loops). The negative feedback concept alone, however, is not enough to account for changes in serum levels of target-gland hormones, especially those caused by changes in the external environment. Stress, for example, can induce release of corticotrophin (ACTH), and psychological factors can delay menstruation in women. The anterior pituitary hormone may also inhibit secretion of the specific hypothalamic factor that stimulates the anterior pituitary (the short negative feedback loop). The central nervous system is therefore believed to play a decisive role in regulating pituitary function to meet environmental demands.

Hypothalamic control of anterior pituitary functions

The central nervous system communicates with the anterior pituitary by secreting into the bloodstream (the hypothalamic–hypophyseal portal system) active proteins known as hypothalamic hormones, or factors. Several have been identified and at least two (and their analogues) are in clinical use (see Table 38-1). As in many new and active research areas, the complete picture has not yet emerged and the terminology is still variable and confusing.

The discovery of various hypothalamic factors is of great research and medical interest. These factors cause the release, or inhibition of release, of the various hormones from the anterior pituitary (see Figure 38-1). The process can be summarised as follows:
* central monoamine-containing neurons secrete neurotransmitters
* the neurotransmitters stimulate hypothalamic neuro-endocrine transducer cells
* these cells secrete releasing factors (or release-inhibiting factors) into the portal system
* these factors stimulate (or inhibit) anterior pituitary target cell secretion of trophic hormones
* the hormones circulate to target glands
* target glands are stimulated to respond and/or produce further hormones.

This has been described as a 'cascading amplifier' process, as at each stage the response (e.g. release of hormone or growth of tissues) is magnified many thousand-fold. Thus minute amounts of monoamine neurotransmitter may eventually lead to dramatic changes in behaviour or growth.

HYPOTHALAMIC FACTORS

A range of **hypothalamic factors** affecting anterior pituitary function has been identified, and many have been synthesised, including the following: growth hormone-releasing factor (GHRF), **growth hormone release-inhibiting factor** (GHRIF, **somatostatin**), thyrotrophin-releasing hormone (TRH), corticotrophin-releasing factor (CRF), gonadotrophin-releasing hormone (GnRH, gonadorelin) and prolactin release-inhibiting factor (PRIF, dopamine).

The hypothalamic factors are all peptides, ranging in size from a tripeptide (TRH) to large proteins. Their specificity

TABLE 38-1 Hypothalamic factors in medical use		
HYPOTHALAMIC FACTOR	**CHARACTERISTICS**	**CLINICAL USES**
GHRIF (somatostatin); also **octreotide** and lanreotide, analogues with longer half-lives	14-amino-acid peptide, inhibits release of GH; also inhibits release of TSH, insulin, glucagon and gastrointestinal hormones	Used in acromegaly and in therapy of various endocrine tumours
GnRH; also nafarelin and other analogues	10-amino-acid peptide, causes release of FSH and LH	Used in diagnosis, and in infertility, uterine disorders, prostate and breast cancers

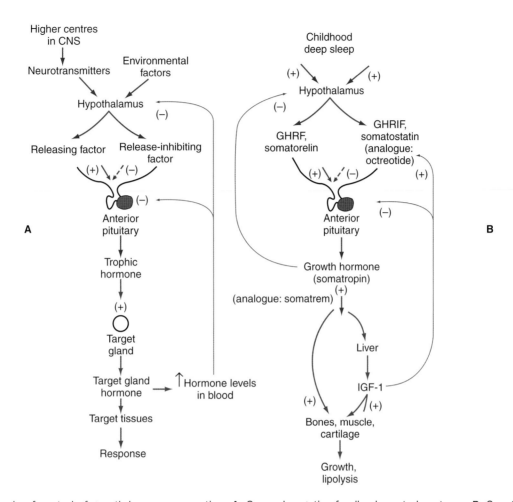

FIGURE 38-1 Levels of control of growth hormone secretion. **A.** General negative feedback control systems. **B.** Growth hormone controls. (+) indicates stimulation or increase, and (–) inhibition or decrease. GHRF = growth hormone-releasing factor; GHRIF = growth hormone release-inhibiting factor; IGF-1 = insulin-like growth factor 1.

of action is not absolute: for example, TRH can increase the release of prolactin as well as thyrotrophin, while GHRIF inhibits the release of GH, TSH, insulin, glucagon and various gastrointestinal tract hormones and autacoids. The medical uses of various hypothalamic factors are summarised in Table 38-1. Other releasing factors are sometimes used by specialist endocrinologists in diagnostic tests of pituitary or target gland functions.

Anterior pituitary hormones

The hormones produced by the anterior lobe of the pituitary gland are important physiologically and clinically; at least seven active extracts have been prepared in a pure state and their specific hormone actions identified. The hormones and their target organs are shown diagrammatically in Figure 37-4. The pharmacology of GH and prolactin will be discussed in detail in this section; TSH, ACTH and the gonadotrophins are considered in subsequent chapters.

Growth hormone

Growth hormone (and its recombinant form, somatropin) is the main growth factor influencing the development of the body. It promotes skeletal, visceral and general growth. Acromegaly, gigantism and dwarfism are associated with pathological conditions of this protein hormone. The anterior lobe of the pituitary gland in the average adult contains about 5–10 mg GH, the greatest amount of all pituitary hormones.

SECRETORY SYSTEM

The amount of GH secreted decreases during the lifespan: it is very high in the newborn and decreases progressively throughout childhood, puberty and adulthood. The levels of control of GH secretion are shown in Figure 38-1, and the sites of action of hormones and analogues used in pharmacological treatment of disorders of GH secretion are indicated. Normally, release of GH is pulsatile during the 24-hour cycle: levels can vary by factors of 10–100. Secretion is increased by GHRF and dopamine and during deep sleep in children, and decreased by GHRIF.

Growth hormone is unusual in that it is species-specific; thus, whereas beef or pork insulin can be used in human medicine, and ACTH from animals works in humans, animal GH does not. Hence GH for use in medicine originally had to be extracted from human cadavers. Some hypothalamic and pituitary factors to be used in medicine, including GHRIF, were also obtained from human cadaver material.

However, brain extracts were found to be able to transmit Creutzfeldt–Jakob disease, a slowly progressive fatal disease of the central nervous system. Use of human pituitary extracts resulted in the deaths of some patients many years after receiving these products.

Synthetic analogues, or human hormones prepared by recombinant DNA technology, are now available for use, including several formulations of somatropin (recombinant human GH [Drug Monograph 38-1]), and tetracosactrin (a synthetic analogue of ACTH), while octreotide, a synthetic analogue of somatostatin, is used to inhibit the release of growth hormone.

Other human tissues (i.e. not from the central nervous system) cannot transmit Creutzfeldt–Jakob disease, so human gonadotrophins can be safely prepared from the urine of pregnant or menopausal women, provided that precautions are taken against other transmissible agents such as HIV.

PHYSIOLOGICAL ACTIONS

Growth hormone's anabolic (growth-increasing) effects are indirect, being due to the effects of another mediator (somatomedin), now identified as insulin-like growth factor 1 (IGF-1). This is produced in the liver and is directly responsible for skeletal and soft tissue growth and increased protein synthesis in cartilage and bone. It is also involved in tissue hypertrophy and wound healing. A major pharmacological consequence of GH use is therefore an increase in growth, whereas a deficiency in growth hormone usually results in dwarfism (see Clinical Interest Box 38-2). Growth hormone is used to treat children deficient in GH (see Drug Monograph 38-1). When it is injected, children grow at a normal or faster-than-normal rate, and 'catch-up' growth brings them to the stature they would be expected to attain, as shown in Figure 38-2.

Growth hormone has many metabolic effects. It:
- decreases insulin sensitivity and may also affect glucose transport
- increases lipolysis
- promotes cellular growth through retention of phosphorus, sodium and potassium
- enhances protein synthesis through increased nitrogen retention.

Acromegaly, caused by excessive secretion of GH, can be treated with GHRIF (somatostatin) or its analogues (see Drug Monograph 38-2).

DRUG MONOGRAPH 38-1 SOMATROPIN, RECOMBINANT

Somatropin products are all synthesised by recombinant DNA technology and are identical in amino acid sequence to the human **growth hormone**. Somatropin is used to stimulate linear growth in patients who lack sufficient endogenous GH. The size of organs and size and number of muscle cells and red cell mass are also increased. An increase in cellular protein synthesis and lipid mobilisation resulting in a decrease in body fat stores has also been reported. A diabetogenic effect may follow insulin overproduction, due to insulin resistance.

INDICATIONS Somatropin is indicated for the treatment of growth failure in children caused by a pituitary growth hormone deficiency, or in Turner's syndrome or chronic renal insufficiency. It is sometimes abused by athletes seeking increased size and strength.

PHARMACOKINETICS As it is a protein, GH can only be administered parenterally. The maximum serum level occurs at about 5 hours and the elimination half-life of parenteral (SC) somatropin is about 4 hours.

DRUG INTERACTIONS When somatropin is given concurrently with glucocorticoids or ACTH, the growth-promoting effects of GH may be impaired. Doses of other replacement hormones require careful adjustment and monitoring.

ADVERSE REACTIONS Antibodies to GH have been reported but it is rare for a patient not to respond to therapy. An allergic-type reaction (rash and itching) and lipodystrophy have been reported at the site of injection. Hypothyroidism, arthralgia, 'growing pains' and intracranial hypertension can occur. Excessive doses may produce gigantism and acromegaly.

WARNINGS AND CONTRAINDICATIONS Use with caution in patients with hypothyroidism, diabetes or cancer. Avoid use in persons with GH hypersensitivity, intracranial tumour or closed epiphyses, and during pregnancy or lactation.

DOSAGE AND ADMINISTRATION The dosage of somatropin for children is individualised, 14–22 IU/m² weekly, divided into daily SC injections. The growth rate response is monitored after 3–6 months to determine whether dosage adjustment is necessary. Therapy is usually continued until epiphyseal closure occurs or there is no further response. One mg somatropin is equivalent to 3 IU.

CLINICAL INTEREST BOX 38-2 GIGANTISM, DWARFISM AND SHORT STATURE

GH-secreting pituitary **adenomas** cause the classical clinical syndromes of acromegaly and gigantism. Chronic GH **hypersecretion** causes excessive production of IGF-1, with overgrowth of bone and soft tissues and generalised systemic disorders.

If this occurs in adults (in whom the epiphyses of long bones have already fused), the manifestations include enlargement of the hands and feet and coarsening of facial features. Arthritis, hypertension, organomegaly (excessive growth of organs) and diabetes are common.

In childhood and adolescence, GH hypersecretion leads to gigantism, with striking acceleration of linear growth, plus the features of acromegaly. Despite being enormously tall, pituitary giants are not abnormally strong because of thyroid, cardiovascular, joint and vision problems. (Thus the Biblical giant Goliath would have been very susceptible to young David's slingshot.)

Treatment is with surgery, radiation therapy and octreotide, a somatostatin analogue.

Congenital GH deficiency leads to hypopituitary dwarfism, with early-onset growth failure and delayed onset of puberty. Treatment is with GH and appropriate gonadotrophins.

The use of GH to increase height in short children is controversial — the short height usually concerns the parents more than the child. In Australia, supplies of somatropin as a subsidised drug are restricted by the Growth Hormone Program of the Pharmaceutical Benefits Branch of the Department of Health & Ageing. Guidelines for GH prescription include that the child be in lower than the first centile for height, and lower than 25th centile for growth rate. Treatment is with GH injections SC 6–7 per week, with individualised dose, e.g. 0.1 IU/kg/day. GH is contraindicated after closure of the epiphyses.

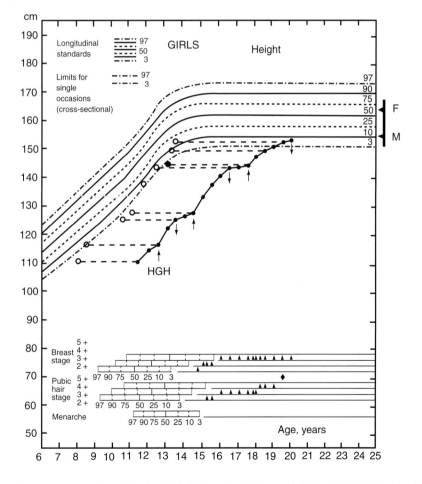

FIGURE 38-2 Effects of growth hormone treatment in GH deficiency, with catch-up following treatment with human growth hormone (HGH) given over three periods indicated by arrows for a girl with isolated growth-hormone deficiency. Open circles represent bone age. F and M are father's and mother's height centiles, and bar represents predicted height centile range for their children. Puberty ratings at each age are shown by arrowheads, lower section.
Source: Tanner 1989. Reproduced with permission from Castlemead Publications.

DRUG MONOGRAPH 38-2 OCTREOTIDE

Octreotide is a synthetic octapeptide analogue of GHRIF. It is a potent agent that also inhibits secretion of many gastrointestinal hormones, including insulin and glucagon. Lanreotide is an analogue with much longer-lasting activity.

INDICATIONS Octreotide is indicated for lowering blood levels of growth hormone and IGF-1 to normal in persons with acromegaly who are unable to have, or have not responded to, other therapies such as surgery or radiotherapy. It is also used to treat the symptoms associated with carcinoid tumours, such as flushing and severe diarrhoea.

PHARMACOKINETICS It is rapidly absorbed after SC injection, with an elimination half-life of about 1.5 hours; about 32% is excreted in the urine unchanged.

DRUG INTERACTIONS Due to its effects on fluid, electrolyte and glucose balance, octreotide can interact with many drugs. Concurrent use with the sulfonylurea antidiabetic agent glucagon, growth hormone or insulin may result in altered blood sugar levels and needs close monitoring.

ADVERSE REACTIONS These include local injection-site reactions and abdominal disorders.

WARNINGS AND CONTRAINDICATIONS Use with caution in patients with diabetes mellitus, gastro-intestinal tract tumours or severe kidney impairment, and in pregnancy. Thyroid function requires monitoring during long-term treatment. Avoid use in persons with octreotide hypersensitivity and gallbladder disease.

DOSAGE AND ADMINISTRATION Dosage depends on clinical use and on formulation administered, e.g. in acromegaly 50–100 mcg SC every 8–12 hours. Octretide is also available as a long-acting formulation, to be administered by deep IM injection once every 4 weeks.

Prolactin

A lactogenic factor (**prolactin** or mammotrophin) plays a part in the proliferation and secretion of the mammary glands of mammals. Prolactin is a protein hormone (198 amino acids in a single peptide chain), closely related chemically to GH and to the placental hormone human chorionic gonadotrophin (human placental lactogen). All three hormones appear to have evolved from a single ancestral gene. Females have about 1.5 times the male concentration of prolactin. The functions of the hormone in males and in non-lactating females are not clearly established.

SECRETORY SYSTEM

The main hypothalamic control over prolactin release is inhibitory, as the main hypothalamic factor is prolactin release-inhibiting factor (PRIF). There is good evidence that PRIF is in fact the neurotransmitter dopamine. Stimuli for release of prolactin include oestrogens, suckling, dopamine antagonists and TRH. Secretion is decreased by dopamine agonists such as bromocriptine and cabergoline.

PHYSIOLOGICAL ACTIONS (IN FEMALES)

Prolactin causes an increase in the amount of breast tissue during pregnancy (due to actions of oestrogens), and in milk production, and possibly 'nest-building behaviour'. Gonadotrophin release and ovulation are suppressed, which tends to have natural contraceptive effects, decreasing the likelihood of conception during breastfeeding.*

*While this is effective on a mass scale, such that the birth rate is generally low in countries in which women customarily breastfeed for extended periods, it is not sufficiently reliable as a contraceptive in individual women, as women can ovulate and become pregnant while breastfeeding.

Anterior pituitary disorders
Hyperpituitarism

Hypersecretion of anterior pituitary hormones is most commonly due to a pituitary **adenoma** (a hormone-secreting tumour). The clinical manifestations are both those of the 'space-occupying lesion' effects (raised intracranial pressure, compression of the brainstem and optic nerves) and those

CLINICAL INTEREST BOX 38-3 DOPAMINE AND LACTATION

Galactorrhoea (excessive production of milk other than after pregnancy) can occur in both men and women, and is due to hyperprolactinaemia. High prolactin levels are usually due to low levels of the hypothalamic inhibitory factor PRIF (dopamine). This can occur in hypothalamic lesions and tumours, and also after use of dopamine-blocking agents such as the phenothiazine antipsychotic drugs.

Treatment is with dopamine agonists, to stimulate hypothalamic dopamine receptors and hence decrease synthesis and release of prolactin in the anterior pituitary gland. Dopamine agonists used include apomorphine, levodopa and especially bromocriptine, cabergoline or pergolide. They are useful in pituitary adenomas and in preventing lactation (also in Parkinson's disease; see Chapter 21).

Because dopamine is a neurotransmitter in many pathways in both the central and peripheral nervous systems, there are many adverse reactions and adverse drug interactions whenever dopamine agonists or antagonists are used. Adverse effects occur particularly in the central nervous system, motor nervous system, cardiovascular system, endocrine glands and gastrointestinal tract.

of excess hormone levels (pituitary and/or target-gland hormones). Thus prolactin-secreting adenomas manifest as gynaecomastia, galactorrhoea and infertility; GH-secreting adenomas as gigantism or acromegaly; and ACTH-secreting adenomas as Cushing's syndrome.

First-line treatment is usually surgical removal of the tumour by a trans-sphenoidal approach. Prolactin-secreting tumours are effectively suppressed by the dopamine agonist bromocriptine, acting as a PRIF analogue.

Hypopituitarism

Deficiencies of pituitary hormones are most commonly due to non-hormone-secreting tumours; combination deficiencies are common. For diagnosis, levels of both pituitary hormones and target-gland hormones are measured to distinguish between primary pituitary **hyposecretion** and target-gland hypofunction or negative feedback effects. Treatment is usually lifelong and requires replacing all target-gland hormones; imbalance in adrenal cortex hormones is corrected first, as this can be life-threatening.

Posterior pituitary hormones

Two hormones obtained from the posterior lobe of the pituitary gland have been identified and chemically synthesised: **oxytocin** (a hormone that stimulates the smooth muscle of the uterus to contract), and **vasopressin (antidiuretic hormone)**. As described earlier, the posterior lobe of the pituitary gland, the neurohypophysis, consists almost entirely of glial cells and neurons, with their cell bodies in the paraventricular and supraoptic nuclei of the hypothalamus. The hormones are synthesised in the hypothalamus and stored in secretory granules that are transported down the axons to the nerve endings, from where they are released in response to neural stimuli.

Availability of these hormones in pure form has clarified their structures, actions and mechanisms of action, and has allowed better control of their therapeutic use. They are both nonapeptides (9-amino-acid residues), with very similar structures. Their effects are not specific; for example, a certain overlap of pharmacological actions exists even in the pure preparations: pure oxytocin has some antidiuretic activity and vice versa. The antidiuretic potency of vasopressin is much greater than its pressor (causing an increase in blood pressure) potency. The hormones are released together into the circulation but in varying proportions depending on the stimulus: thus during uterine contractions in the process of childbirth, and in response to suckling by the infant, mainly oxytocin is released, whereas in response to fluid loss, mainly ADH is released. (It is interesting to note that ethanol [alcohol] inhibits release of both ADH and oxytocin; hence its diuretic effect and also possible effects in slowing uterine contractions and milk letdown.

Nicotine, on the other hand, increases secretion of ADH, thus decreasing urine production—a useful drug interaction for drinkers who smoke, especially while listening to long after-dinner speeches.)

Vasopressin (antidiuretic hormone, ADH)

Vasopressin is released in response to raised plasma osmotic pressure. This may occur after haemorrhage, water deprivation or other factors that cause diuresis or decrease the circulating blood volume. Obtained from natural sources and originally named because of its effects in raising the blood pressure, vasopressin is not often used in medicine now that potent, more specific synthetic analogues have been developed. Derivatives such as felypressin (mainly vasoconstrictor) and desmopressin (mainly antidiuretic; Drug Monograph 38-3) have very little, if any, oxytocic activity.

MECHANISMS AND ACTIONS

Vasopressin has been shown to act by activation of vasopressin V_1 receptors (via inositol phosphate production) and V_2 receptors (via adenylate cyclase). It increases the permeability of renal distal tubule walls to water and hence leads to resorption of water, resulting in decreased urine volume with a higher osmolarity (i.e. antidiuresis). In 100-fold higher doses, vasoconstrictor effects occur, causing raised blood pressure and potentially angina. Vasopressin also has many non-renal actions, including smooth muscle contraction, platelet aggregation, raised factor VIII levels (hence its use in haemorrhage and haemophilia), and increased release of ACTH and hydrocortisone. It also has neuromodulator actions and may be involved in learning and memory.

CLINICAL ASPECTS

Vasopressin and its analogues are used as replacement therapy in pituitary diabetes insipidus (see Clinical Interest Box 38-4) and in bleeding conditions. They have been used for their antidiuretic effects in nocturnal enuresis (bed-wetting) and as vasoconstrictors in formulations of local anaesthetics. Because they are peptides, these hormones are rapidly metabolised by peptidases. They are best administered intranasally as a finely divided powder (a snuff) or as a nasal spray.

There are many drug interactions; for example, ADH sensitivity is increased by carbamazepine, while it is decreased by lithium and methoxyflurane.

OXYTOCIN

Oxytocin means 'rapid birth', a term derived from the hormone's ability to contract the pregnant uterus. When released during birth, it causes physiological-type contractions, i.e. regular and coordinated towards the cervix, with relaxation in between. The non-pregnant uterus is relatively

DRUG MONOGRAPH 38-3 DESMOPRESSIN

Vasopressin analogues include lypressin (lys-vasopressin, i.e. one of the original amino acids substituted with lysine) and felypressin (phe-lys-vasopressin), which are predominantly vasoconstrictors, and **desmopressin** (1-desamino-8-D-arg-vasopressin), a specific V_2-receptor agonist with potent ADH activity. Desmopressin has a longer duration of activity than the other agents, presumably because it is more resistant to usual metabolic inactivation.

INDICATIONS Desmopressin is used to treat pituitary diabetes insipidus. It is not effective for polyuria induced by renal impairment or for nephrogenic or drug-induced diabetes insipidus. Desmopressin is also used intranasally for primary nocturnal enuresis, while the parenteral dosage form is used to treat haemorrhage in patients with haemophilia A or von Willebrand's disease.

PHARMACOKINETICS About 10% of an intranasal dose becomes bioavailable, thus the nasal spray dose

is 10 times the parenteral dose. Desmopressin administered IM or SC has a half-life of 8–75 minutes; the duration of effect is 8–20 hours. The intranasal effect lasts 10–12 hours. The drug is excreted by the kidneys.

ADVERSE REACTIONS Headache, nausea, mild stomach cramps, pain and swelling at the injection site; rare: allergic reaction, water retention, intoxication and cardiac failure, hyponatraemia, convulsions. No significant drug interactions have been reported.

DOSAGE AND ADMINISTRATION The adult injection dosage is 1–4 mcg daily IM or SC when needed to treat central diabetes insipidus. The adult nasal spray dose is 10–40 mcg (1–2 sprays to one or both nostrils) when urination frequency increases or a significant thirst sensation occurs. Desmopressin is also available in oral tablet form, where because of its low oral bioavailability the dose is approximately 10 times that for the nasal spray.

CLINICAL INTEREST BOX 38-4 DIABETES INSIPIDUS

Diabetes insipidus is a rare disease characterised by lack of ADH, leading to polyuria and polydipsia, with a daily urine volume of 3–20 L (compared with the normal 1.5 L).

Diabetes insipidus of pituitary origin may be primary, due to a decreased number of neurons in the paraventricular nucleus or supraoptic nucleus of the hypothalamus (idiopathic or familial), or secondary, due to lesions (severe head injury, tumours, surgery) or drugs. In nephrogenic diabetes insipidus, ADH production is normal but kidney

tubules fail to respond appropriately.

Treatment is with ADH, vasopressin analogues or pituitary extract (IM, IV, as a snuff or nasal spray). Thiazide diuretics are effective (a paradoxical effect). Various other unrelated drugs, including carbamazepine, are also used.

Note that demeclocycline, a tetracycline antibiotic, is also an ADH antagonist and is used to produce diuresis in the syndrome of inappropriate secretion of ADH (SIADH).

insensitive to oxytocin but during pregnancy, uterine sensitivity to oxytocin gradually increases, with the uterus being most sensitive at term. Large amounts of oxytocin have been detected in the blood during the expulsive phase of delivery. A positive feedback mechanism may be operating: more forceful contractions of uterine muscle and greater stretching of the cervix and vagina result in more oxytocin release. Oxytocin acts directly on the myometrium, having a stronger effect on the fundus than on the cervix, and is used clinically to induce or enhance labour (see Drug Monograph 38-4).

Oxytocin also transiently impedes uterine blood flow and stimulates the mammary glands to increase milk excretion from the breast, although it does not increase the production of milk. Release of oxytocin during suckling by the infant helps reduce the uterus to pre-pregnancy size.

Because of its close similarity to ADH, oxytocin also has weak ADH-like actions but may have transient vasodilator (not vasoconstrictor) action. There is no distinct clinical syndrome related to oxytocin deficiency.

PREGNANCY SAFETY BOX

ADEC Category	Drug
A	Bromocriptine, oxytocin
B1	Cabergoline, somatropin (or B2)
B2	Desmopressin, vasopressin
B3	Quinagolide
C	Lanreotide, octreotide, pergolide
D	Tetracosactrin

Note: Hormones used chiefly in reproductive medicine are included in the relevant Pregnancy Safety boxes in Chapters 44–47.

DRUG MONOGRAPH 38-4 OXYTOCIN

INDICATIONS Oxytocin is administered IM or IV to induce, augment or manage labour when uterine muscle function is inadequate, to treat postpartum haemorrhage and to stimulate lactation. Uterine motility and fetal heart rate must be monitored. It is contraindicated if there is fetal distress or if vaginal delivery is contraindicated.

PHARMACOKINETICS This product is available parenterally and is usually given by IV infusion. Oxytocin is inactivated rapidly in the liver; it has a half-life of 1–6 minutes. After IV administration, its onset of action is immediate, although uterine contractions increase gradually over 15–60 minutes before they stabilise. Duration of action is until 1 hour after the infusion is stopped.

DRUG INTERACTIONS When used concurrently with sodium chloride or urea for intra-amniotic induction of labour or with other oxytocics, uterine rupture or severe cervical laceration may occur. Prostaglandins

and inhalational anaesthetics may enhance oxytocin's actions. Whenever such combinations are used, the patient and fetus should be closely monitored.

ADVERSE REACTIONS These include nausea, vomiting, hypotension, tachycardia and irregular heart rate with the parenteral drug. Prolonged therapy may result in water intoxication. Oxytocin may occasionally cause fetal bradycardia, dysrhythmias and neonatal jaundice. Careful monitored use of oxytocin has contributed significantly to the safety of childbirth; it has an Australian pregnancy safety classification of A.

DOSAGE AND ADMINISTRATION The dose to induce labour is 1–6 mU/min by IV infusion, increased at intervals of >30 min until a contraction pattern is established that simulates normal labour (up to a maximum of 48 mU/min). It is administered IM to manage the third stage of labour, sometimes in conjunction with ergometrine (see Chapter 46).

DRUGS AT A GLANCE 38: Drugs affecting the pituitary gland and the hypothalamic–pituitary axis

Therapeutic group	Pharmacological group	Key examples	Key pages
Hypothalamic factors	Growth hormone release-inhibiting factor (GHRIF)	somatostatin	630
	GHRIF analogues	octreotide } lanreotide	630, 4
	Gonadotrophin-releasing hormone (GnRH)	GnRH	630
	GnRH analogues	nafarelin	630
Pituitary hormones			
Anterior	Growth hormone (GH)	growth hormone somatropin	631–3 632
	Prolactin	prolactin	634, 5
Posterior	Oxytocics	oxytocin	635–7
	Vasopressin (antidiuretic hormone, ADH)	vasopressin } desmopressin	635, 6
Treatment of hyperprolactinaemia	Dopamine agonists	bromocriptine } cabergoline, pergolide	634, 5

KEY POINTS

- The pituitary gland consists of two main parts: the anterior lobe, which produces seven hormones, and the posterior lobe, producing two hormones.
- The pituitary hormones are secreted into the bloodstream and act on target glands or organs, which respond by secreting other hormones or regulating growth or metabolism.
- The functions of the anterior pituitary gland are controlled by hypothalamic factors, which may stimulate or inhibit release of anterior pituitary hormones, and by negative feedback loops from target-gland hormones.
- Various hypothalamic factors are used in medicine to diagnose endocrine disorders or treat dysfunction of the target glands.
- The pituitary hormones are usually used for replacement therapy in hormone deficiencies, such as drug therapy for a specific pituitary or target-gland disorder.
- Somatropin (growth hormone) is used for growth failure in children.
- Octreotide is similar to somatostatin, the growth-hormone-inhibiting agent, so it is used in acromegaly and in gastrointestinal tract tumours.
- Prolactin is hypersecreted in pituitary adenomas and as an adverse effect of antidopamine drugs. It can be suppressed by dopamine agonist drugs that mimic the prolactin-release-inhibiting factor.
- Vasopressin analogues such as desmopressin are used for central diabetes insipidus and to treat primary nocturnal enuresis or haemorrhage; felypressin is used as a vasoconstrictor.
- Oxytocin is administered to induce or manage uterine contractions during childbirth.

REVIEW EXERCISES

1 Name the hormones produced by the anterior and posterior lobes of the pituitary gland and describe their physiological effects.
2 Describe how the hypothalamus controls pituitary functions, name the hypothalamic factors and briefly describe their characteristics and uses.
3 Describe the mechanism of action underlying somatropin's anabolic effects. What metabolic effects does it have? What adverse reactions?
4 What effects does octreotide have in the body? What are its indications, pharmacokinetics and adverse reactions?
5 Compare the effects, indications and dosage and administration of vasopressin and oxytocin.
6 Describe the aetiologies, manifestations and treatment of hyperprolactinaemia.

REFERENCES AND FURTHER READING

Australian Medicines Handbook 2006. Adelaide: AMH, 2006.
Caswell A (ed.). *MIMS Annual June 2005.* Sydney: CMPMedica Australia, 2005
Endocrinology Expert Group. *Therapeutic Guidelines: Endocrinology, version 3.* Melbourne: Therapeutic Guidelines Limited, 2004.
Goodman HM. Part VI: Endocrine physiology. In: Johnson LR (ed.). *Essential Medical Physiology.* 2nd edn. Philadelphia: Lippincott-Raven, 1999 [chs 38, 44].
Greenspan FS, Strewler GJ. *Basic and Clinical Endocrinology.* 5th edn. Stamford: Appleton & Lange, 1997.
Rang HP, Dale MM, Ritter JM, Moore PK. *Pharmacology.* 5th edn. Edinburgh: Churchill Livingstone, 2003 [ch. 27].
Tanner JM. *Foetus into Man: Physical Growth from Conception to Maturity.* Ware: Castlemead, 1989.
Tortora GJ, Grabowski SR. *Principles of Anatomy and Physiology.* 9th edn. New York: HarperCollins, 2000 [ch. 18].
Youngson, RM. *Collins Dictionary: Medicine.* 2nd edn. Glasgow: HarperCollins, 1998.

ONLINE RESOURCES

New Zealand medicines and medical devices safety authority: www.medsafe.govt.nz

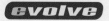 More weblinks at http://evolve.elsevier.com/AU/Bryant/pharmacology/

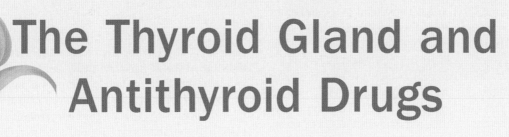

CHAPTER 39

The Thyroid Gland and Antithyroid Drugs

CHAPTER FOCUS

The thyroid hormones thyroxine and tri-iodothyronine increase oxygen consumption and basal metabolic rate; accelerate carbohydrate, lipid and protein metabolism; increase sensitivity to sympathetic stimulation and promote growth; and are required for normal development of the central nervous system. Disorders of thyroid function thus have major effects on virtually all aspects of bodily functions, including growth and development, energy levels, and nervous and reproductive systems. Replacement thyroid hormones or antithyroid drugs are useful in conditions of hypo- or hyperthyroidism, respectively, and health-care professionals need to be knowledgeable about these agents to ensure safe and effective management of their patients.

OBJECTIVES

- To describe the signs and symptoms associated with hypothyroidism and hyperthyroidism.

- To describe the synthesis, actions and clinical uses of thyroid hormones.

- To discuss the use of thyroid hormones in tests for assessment of thyroid function.

- To compare the effects and clinical uses of iodine (iodide ion), radioactive iodine, and thiourea (thionamide) drugs in treating hyperthyroidism.

KEY DRUGS

carbimazole
iodine
liothyronine
thyroxine
propylthiouracil
radioactive iodine

KEY TERMS

antithyroid agents
euthyroid
goitre
Graves' disease
hyperthyroidism
hypothyroidism
iodine
myxoedema
thyroglobulin
thyrotoxicosis

KEY ABBREVIATIONS

DIT	di-iodotyrosine
MIT	mono-iodotyrosine
T_3	tri-iodothyronine (liothyronine)
T_4	tetra-iodothyronine (thyroxine)
TRH	thyrotrophin-releasing hormone
TSH	thyroid-stimulating hormone (thyrotrophin)

THE THYROID GLAND

THE thyroid gland, one of the most richly vascularised tissues of the body, is located in the throat region, in front of the trachea (see Figure 37-1). It has two lateral lobes, linked by a narrow section; the small parathyroid glands (usually four) are located on the posterior surface of the thyroid lobes. The thyroid lobules contain follicles full of a viscid colloid secretion, enclosed by follicular cells, which produce thyroxine (tetra-iodothyronine, T_4) and tri-iodothyronine (T_3).

The gland also contains parafollicular cells, the source of calcitonin. Because of its role in calcium metabolism, calcitonin is discussed in the chapter on the parathyroid gland and calcium balance (Chapter 42). In this chapter, however, we generally use the term 'thyroid hormones' to refer only to T_4 and T_3 and not to calcitonin.

The history of discovery of thyroid gland functions and hormones is interesting. In 1883, it was found that cretinism and myxoedema might result from loss of thyroid function. (These conditions are described later in the section on hypothyroidism.) Very soon afterwards, experiments showed that extracts of thyroid glands could reverse the effects of thyroidectomy, i.e. that active substances found in the gland could be circulated and act elsewhere in the body and affect many aspects of homeostasis, growth and metabolism. In 1914, the main thyroid hormone, T_4, was purified and crystallised, allowing detailed studies of its actions and uses. It was not until 1952, however, that T_3 was discovered, and not until 1961 that calcitonin's actions were demonstrated. The roles and clinical uses of the hypothalamic factors, including thyrotrophin-releasing hormone (TRH), are still being studied and clarified.

Thyroid hormones
Synthesis, release and control

Thyroxine (T_4) and tri-iodothyronine (T_3) are amino acid hormones, being iodinated derivatives of tyrosine. They are usually stored in the thyroid gland and circulated in the bloodstream bound to proteins. The synthesis, storage, release, secretion and circulation of the hormones are complicated—during the process, the scene of action moves from the bloodstream into the follicle cell, thence into the follicle lumen, back into the cell, and finally into the blood again. A summary of the processes involved is given below, and the control mechanisms are shown diagrammatically in Figure 39-2. Because synthesis of the hormones requires **iodine**, the handling of iodine by the body is discussed first.

ROLE OF IODINE

Iodine is a non-metallic element in the halogen group, with an atomic mass of 127. The large amount of iodine in thyroid hormones, and the availability of radioactive iodine have led to detailed knowledge about thyroid physiology and its role in metabolism. Iodine is essential for thyroid hormone synthesis. Around 1 mg iodine is required by an adult each week; most of this is ingested in food, water and iodised table salt (see Clinical Interest Box 39-1). About two-thirds of this iodine is reduced in the gastrointestinal tract, enters the circulation as iodide and is excreted into the urine. The other third is taken up by the thyroid gland for hormone synthesis; thus the thyroid gland normally contains virtually all the iodide in the body. An iodide pump takes up iodide from the extracellular fluid, traps it and concentrates it to many times the level found in plasma. The ratio of iodide in the thyroid gland to that in the plasma (serum) is expressed as the T/S ratio;

CLINICAL INTEREST BOX 39-1
DISORDERS DUE TO IODINE DEFICIENCY

If iodide intake is low, thyroid hormones cannot be synthesised in sufficient quantities, and thyroid functions are impaired.

- This can occur in congenital hypothyroidism, due to maternal iodine deficiency or congenital defects in hormone synthesis; if untreated in the first few months of life, it leads to severe brain damage, neurological disorders and cretinism, which has been described since the Middle Ages. This is recognised by the World Health Organization (WHO) as the most common preventable cause of brain damage.
- Endemic goitre is usually due to low soil iodine levels (especially in inland hilly areas), leading to low levels of iodine in the food chain and decreased synthesis of thyroid hormones; compensatory high pituitary secretion of thyroid-stimulating hormone leads to enlarged thyroid gland (goitre).
- A double-blind, controlled trial carried out in New Guinea in 1966–1970 established the causal role of iodine deficiency in cretinism, and showed that cretinism can be prevented by injections of iodised oil prior to pregnancy; the Adelaide scientist Dr Basil Hetzel has been a world leader in this area of clinical nutrition.
- Unless children born with a thyroid deficiency are treated at once, permanent brain damage occurs; biochemical screening is routinely carried out.
- Prevention now is by addition of iodine to staple dietary components such as salt or bread, to provide about 200 mcg iodine daily. In 1996, WHO reported that 56% of the population of 83 developing countries now had adequate access to iodised salt, and by 1999 it was 68%.
- Iatrogenic goitre and hypothyroidism can occur after ingestion of toxic compounds (goitrins) in turnips or weeds, and after drugs, including p-aminosalicylic acid, lithium, remedies containing iodide (including amiodarone and cough mixtures containing potassium iodide as an expectorant), or antithyroid drugs.

Adapted from: Hetzel 2000; Delange & Lecomte 2000.

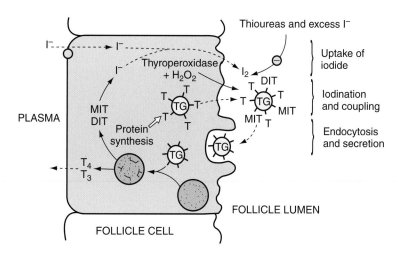

FIGURE 39-1 Synthesis of thyroid hormones. Iodide is taken up from the bloodstream into the thyroid cell, where it is bound to tyrosine residues (T), then coupled to form thyroid hormones, which are stored as thyroglobulin (TG) in the follicle lumen before release into the circulation (see text for details and abbreviations). *Adapted from*: Rang et al 2003, Figure 25-1; used with permission.

normally this ratio ranges from 20:1 to 39:1. (In hypoactivity of the gland the ratio may be 10:1; in hyperactivity it may be as great as 250:1.)

SYNTHESIS OF T_4 AND T_3

See Figure 39-1.

1. IODIDE TRAPPING. Iodide is removed from the blood by the iodide pump into the thyroid follicular cells. The uptake is blocked by antithyroid compounds such as thiocyanate and perchlorate, and by cardiac glycoside drugs.

2. SYNTHESIS OF THYROGLOBULIN. Meanwhile, also in the follicle cells, **thyroglobulin** is being synthesised. This is a large glycoprotein very rich in tyrosine (about 115 tyrosine residues per molecule of thyroglobulin), which is then released into the lumen of the follicle where it is the main component of the thick colloid gel.

3. OXIDATION OF IODIDE (I^-) TO IODINE (I_2). The iodide initially removed from the blood is usually as sodium or potassium iodide. In follicle cells, the enzyme peroxidase converts the iodides to iodine, which passes into the lumen.

4. IODINATION OF TYROSINE RESIDUES IN THYRO-GLOBULIN. Initially, one or two iodine atoms bind to tyrosine residues (yielding mono- or di-iodinated tyrosine, MIT or DIT); this process is known as 'organification' of iodine. The iodination process can be blocked by thiourea antithyroid drugs.

5. COUPLING OF MIT AND DIT. Two residues then couple, to form tri- or tetra-iodinated thyronine (T_3 or T_4). The thyroid hormones are thus incorporated into thyroglobulin molecules, mostly as T_4.

6. STORAGE OF THYROID HORMONES. The synthesised hormones (T_3 and T_4) in thyroglobulin are stored as colloid in the lumen of the follicle. About 30% of the thyroid mass is stored thyroglobulin, which contains enough thyroid hormone to meet normal requirements for 2–3 months without any further synthesis.

7. DIGESTION OF COLLOID IN FOLLICLE CELLS. Normally, thyroglobulin is not released into the circulation but undergoes proteolytic digestion back in the follicle cells, releasing the active thyroid hormones T_3 and T_4; iodine, MIT, DIT and peptide residues are reused.

8. SECRETION OF THYROID HORMONES. T_4 and T_3, being lipid-soluble amino acids, can diffuse from the thyroid cells via the membranes into the bloodstream.

9. CIRCULATION. T_4 is present as a large pool in the circulation. It is 99.95% protein-bound, to thyroxine-binding globulin and other proteins. This binding is decreased by salicylates, dicoumarol and other drugs. T_4 has a low turnover rate, with a half-life of about 6–7 days; as it circulates and enters cells, most T_4 is converted to T_3.

T_3 is present as a small pool, mainly stored intracellularly; it is more potent than T_4, less strongly protein-bound, and has a faster turnover rate, with a half-life of about 2 days.

CONTROL OF HORMONE SYNTHESIS AND RELEASE

Control of thyroid hormone levels is complicated, involving a complex negative feedback mechanism between the thyroid gland and the hypothalamic–pituitary axis, and depends on iodine levels and body temperature (see Figure 39-2).

Low levels of circulating thyroid hormones increase the release of thyroid-stimulating hormone (TSH) from the pituitary gland and appear to influence the secretion of TRH from the hypothalamus. Increased levels of TSH stimulate many aspects of thyroid gland function: TSH increases

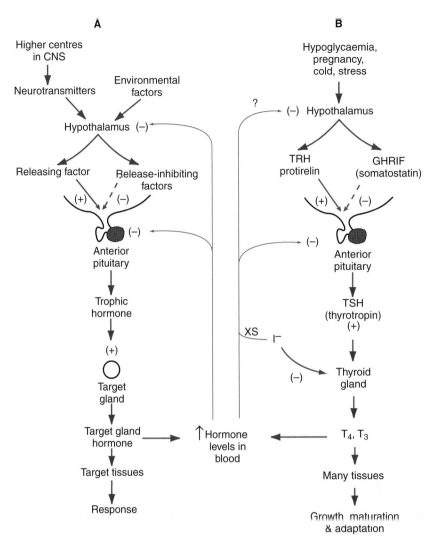

FIGURE 39-2 Secretion and control of thyroid hormones. **A.** General control mechanisms for hormone secretion. **B.** Control mechanisms for thyroid hormone secretion. Environmental factors influence secretion of the hypothalamic factors thyrotrophin-releasing hormone (TRH) and growth hormone release-inhibiting factor (GHRIF, somatostatin) to increase or decrease release from the anterior pituitary of thyrotrophin (TSH), which stimulates production in the thyroid glands of thyroxine (T_4) and tri-iodothyronine (T_3).

thyroid cell utilisation of glucose and oxygen, and increases blood flow to the thyroid gland. Iodide trapping by the gland, iodination and proteolysis of thyroglobulin are increased, which results in an increase in synthesis and release of hormones. Actions of TSH are triggered at the membrane of the thyroid cell, via activation of adenylate cyclase and then phosphorylation of enzymes. In the long term, an increase in TSH leads to both hypertrophy (greater size of cells) and hyperplasia (greater number of cells).

An increase in free, unbound thyroid hormone causes a decrease in the release of TRH and TSH. The negative feedback mechanism responds only slowly to changes in iodide levels: low levels make it difficult for sufficient hormones to be synthesised, while excessively high levels switch off production, via negative feedback and by acting directly at the organification step in hormone synthesis.

Mechanism of thyroid hormone actions

Tri-iodothyronine, the main active intracellular hormone, enters the nucleus of target cells and binds to specific receptors that act as transcription factors to activate or repress various genes. (There are at least three forms of the thyroid hormone receptor.) Production of mRNA is modified, and hence synthesis of specific proteins, e.g. Na^+–K^+-ATPase, is altered.

Physiological effects of thyroid hormones

The thyroid hormones T_4 and T_3 increase oxygen consumption and basal metabolic rate; accelerate carbohydrate, lipid and protein metabolism; promote normal gastrointestinal tract, cardiovascular, reproductive and temperature regulation functions; increase sensitivity to sympathetic stimulation; promote growth and development; and are required for normal development and functioning of the CNS. Four generalisations can be made about thyroid hormones:

- They have a diffuse effect and do not have one specific target organ; no special cells or tissues appear to be particularly affected by the thyroid hormones.
- Their long delay in onset of action and their prolonged action rule them out as minute-to-minute regulators of physiological function. Instead, their role is more likely to be that of establishing and maintaining long-term functions such as growth, maturation and adaptation.
- They are not necessary for survival in normal conditions, although reduced levels can affect quality of life.
- T_3 and T_4 appear to have the same physiological actions, although T_3 is more potent than T_4.

The growth-promoting actions of thyroid hormones are said to be 'permissive', i.e. a normal thyroxine level permits the cells of the body to function properly. Children who develop hypothyroidism after birth have increasingly slow bodily growth and delayed maturity.

TREATMENT OF HYPOTHYROIDISM
Hypothyroidism and goitre
Goitre

The synthesis of the thyroid hormones and their maintenance in the blood in adequate amounts depend largely on an adequate intake of iodine (see Clinical Interest Box 39-1). Prolonged iodine deficiency in the diet results in increased TRH and TSH, and hence enlargement of the thyroid gland, known as a simple **goitre**. The enlarged thyroid then removes residual traces of iodine from the blood. This type of goitre (simple or non-toxic) can be prevented by providing an adequate supply of iodine. Iodine is not abundant in most foods, except fish and seafood, and iodised salt is frequently the primary source of iodine in areas where seafood is expensive or not readily available.

Note that the presence of goitre is not diagnostic, as an enlarged thyroid may also be due to excessive stimulation of the gland in thyrotoxicosis.

Hypothyroidism

Patients with primary **hypothyroidism** have low T_3 and T_4 levels despite an elevated TSH level. Those with pituitary (secondary) hypothyroidism and hypothalamic (tertiary)

hypothyroidism have low levels of T_3, T_4 and TSH (see Clinical Interest Box 39-2).

INCIDENCE
Hypothyroidism is common, occurring in about 2% of the population, especially in middle-aged and elderly women; it is associated with autoimmune disorders, previous Graves' disease (and antithyroid therapy) and Down syndrome.

AETIOLOGIES
Aetiological factors include post-thyroidectomy, iodine deficiencies (simple non-toxic goitre), Hashimoto's disease (autoantibodies to thyroidal antigens), antithyroid drugs, and lithium and amiodarone.

DIAGNOSIS AND CLINICAL MANIFESTATIONS
The condition can easily be missed, as it has very variable and non-specific presentations and development is usually insidious; the TSH stimulation test is diagnostic. Clinical manifestations are seen in most systems of the body, and include bradycardia, infertility, muscle pain, cold intolerance, lethargy, husky voice, 'non-toxic goitre', hair loss, and neurological and psychiatric problems. There is decreased clearance of many drugs and increased sensitivity to digoxin.

Severe hypothyroidism in the adult is called **myxoedema**,

CLINICAL INTEREST BOX 39-2 DIAGNOSTIC TESTING FOR HYPOTHYROIDISM

TRH and TSH are used as diagnostic agents for assessing thyroid function. The TSH stimulation test is a very sensitive test used to diagnose and differentiate types of hypothyroidism. TRH is administered to measure the pituitary's response to TRH.

- In hypothalamic **hypothyroidism**, for example, the pituitary responds slowly to exogenous TRH and produces a slow but rising TSH.
- If the patient has hypothyroidism resulting from hypopituitarism, no response to TRH is expected.
- In patients with primary hypothyroidism (i.e. the dysfunction is in the thyroid gland), TSH basal levels are raised, and the pituitary is hyperreactive to TRH stimulation, but T_3 and T_4 levels remain low.

Thus the TSH stimulation test can differentiate a primary from a secondary hypothyroidism, and differentiate hypopituitary from hypothalamic hypothyroidism. See Figure 39-3 for an illustration of this thyroid feedback mechanism.

There are several other thyroid function tests, including the free T_4 index (FTI), T_3 resin uptake (T_3RU) test, and total or free (unbound) T_4 levels; the tests are used to determine the exact site of the dysfunction and hence to optimise therapy.

TABLE 39-1 Thyroid preparations: adult dosing schedules

DRUG	AVERAGE DAILY DOSE	ADULT DOSAGE SCHEDULES
Thyroxine	100–200 mcg (0.1–0.2 mg)	Orally: initially 25–50 mcg daily. Dose changes should be considered only every three to four weeks. Maintenance dose is lower in elderly people. Fine dose adjustments can be achieved with alternating doses of 50, 100 or 200 mcg.
Liothyronine	20–60 mcg (0.02–0.06 mg)	Orally: 20–60 mcg daily, in 2–3 divided doses. For myxoedema coma, treatment may be initiated with 60 mcg by stomach tube (under specialist supervision). For maintenance therapy of myxoedema, thyroxine is preferred.

Pregnancy safety for both thyroid products has been established as category A.

referring to the thickened skin caused by acid mucopolysaccharide accumulation. In the last stage of long-standing, inadequately treated, or untreated hypothyroidism, coma sets in accompanied by hypotension, hypoventilation, hypothermia, hyponatraemia and hypoglycaemia.

Hypothyroidism in the young child (formerly known as cretinism) is characterised by cessation of physical and mental development, which leads to dwarfism and mental retardation. Children with hypothyroidism usually have thick, coarse skin; a thick tongue; gaping mouth; protruding abdomen; thick, short legs; poorly developed hands and feet; and weak musculature. This condition may result from faulty development or atrophy of the thyroid gland during fetal life. Failure of development of the gland may be caused by lack of iodine in the mother (see Clinical Interest Box 39-1). In congenital hypothyroidism, thyroid hormone levels equal to or above those required for the adult must be established immediately after birth to prevent permanent mental and physical retardation.

GERIATRIC IMPLICATIONS THYROID HORMONES

Hypothyroidism, the second most common endocrine disease in the elderly, is often misdiagnosed. Only one-third of the geriatric patients exhibit the typical signs and symptoms of cold intolerance and weight gain. Most often, the symptoms are non-specific, such as failing to thrive, stumbling and falling episodes, and incontinence. If neurological involvement has occurred, a misdiagnosis of dementia, depression or a psychotic episode may be made.

Laboratory tests for plasma T_4 and TSH are used to confirm hypothyroidism.

T_4 is usually the drug of choice for thyroid replacement. Because the elderly are usually more sensitive to, and experience more adverse reactions (particularly cardiovascular effects) to, thyroid hormones than other age groups, it is recommended that thyroid replacement doses be individualised. In some people, the dose should be 25% lower than the usual adult dose, and slower dosage adjustments are required.

TREATMENT

People with hypothyroidism need to be informed of their lifelong need for replacement therapy. Therapy is simple: the thyroid hormones are safe, stable, cheap and available orally; dosage regimens can be adjusted in response to thyroid function test results. Treatment is with T_4, usually 100–200 mcg daily, with dosage adjusted upwards in pregnancy, and possibly decreased in the elderly and before surgery. In myxoedema coma, a medical emergency, treatment is with T_3, the more potent and rapidly acting hormone (see Table 39-1).

In children who develop hypothyroidism, the delay in growth and maturity can be reversed by administration of T_4. There is a rapid catch-up growth spurt, and eventually the expected adult height is attained (see Figure 39-3, and compare with Figure 38-2).

Thyroid hormone preparations

Individuals with hypothyroidism require thyroid replacement therapy. For many years, natural extract or desiccated thyroid tissue was used for replacement therapy, but the synthetic thyroid hormones available today are better standardised and more stable formulations, and so are generally prescribed. The preparations available in Australia are: **thyroxine** (levo-thyroxine, T_4; Drug Monograph 39-1) and **liothyronine** (tri-iodothyronine, T_3); the latter hormone is more potent and has a shorter half-life, so is preferred for emergency and short-term use. Table 39-1 illustrates average doses and the usual adult dosing schedules for thyroid products.

The goal of treatment of patients with hypothyroidism or myxoedema is to eliminate their symptoms and restore them to a normal physical and emotional state (i.e. render them **euthyroid**). Clinical response is more important than blood hormone level; however, laboratory assessments of T_3, T_4, plasma cholesterol and thyrotrophin levels are used as criteria for adequacy of therapy. Because of the long half-life and slow response time for T_4, plasma TSH concentrations are measured 2, 4 and 10 months after initiation of therapy, and annually thereafter for adults.

DRUG MONOGRAPH 39-1   THYROXINE SODIUM

Levo-thyroxine (**thyroxine**) is the thyroid T_4 hormone given exogenously as a drug; it has all the chemical and pharmacological properties of the natural hormone.

INDICATIONS Thyroid supplements are indicated for the treatment of hypothyroidism, treatment and prevention of goitre, replacement therapy after thyroid block in hyperthyroidism, and treatment of thyroiditis and thyroid carcinoma (high doses for suppressive effects).

PHARMACOKINETICS Thyroxine is adequately absorbed from the gastrointestinal tract (50%–75%) and is highly protein-bound in the circulation; there is some enterohepatic recycling. The plasma half-life is about 6–7 days in euthyroid people, so peak effect may not be reached for 3–4 weeks, and response to altered dosage is slow. The agent is metabolised in the same way as endogenous thyroid hormone — some in peripheral tissues and smaller amounts in the liver — and metabolites are excreted in bile and urine. Thyroxine can be dosed once daily and is given on an empty stomach, usually before breakfast.

DRUG INTERACTIONS The following effects can occur when thyroid hormone preparations are given with the drugs listed below:

Interacting drugs	Possible effect and management
Anticoagulants, oral (warfarin or phenindione)	Can enhance the therapeutic effects of the oral anticoagulant: a decrease in anticoagulant oral dosage may be required. Monitor coagulation time closely, using the international normalised ratio (INR)
Cholestyramine, colestipol, aluminium hydroxide, calcium carbonate, ferrous sulfate and sucralfate	Reduce the absorption of thyroxine from the gastrointestinal tract. A 4–5 hour interval is recommended between administration of these drugs and thyroxine

Interacting drugs	Possible effect and management
Sympathomimetics and tricyclic antidepressants	The effects of one or both medications may be increased; cardiovascular adverse reactions can result. Monitor closely, as dosage adjustments may be necessary
Digoxin	Levels and activity may be decreased by thyroid hormones; digoxin dose may need to be increased

ADVERSE REACTIONS Adverse effects generally correspond to symptoms of hyperthyroidism: tachycardia, elevated temperature, diarrhoea, hand tremors, increased irritability, weight loss and insomnia. A rare adverse reaction is an allergic skin rash. Adverse effects are dose-related and may occur more rapidly with T_3 than with T_4, mainly because the former has a faster onset of action.

The general signs of underdosage are those of hypothyroidism: coldness, dry skin, constipation, lethargy, headaches, drowsiness, tiredness, weight gain and muscle aching. During the early period of treatment, hair loss may occur in children.

WARNINGS AND CONTRAINDICATIONS Use with caution in patients with diabetes mellitus, adrenocortical or pituitary insufficiency, cardiac disease and malabsorption problems. Avoid use in people with hyperthyroidism, thyrotoxicosis or thyroid hypersensitivity.

DOSAGE AND ADMINISTRATION See Table 39-1 and the Geriatric Implications box. The stability of thyroxine tablets is limited; patients need to watch the 'use by' dates on their packs. The two Australian brands of thyroxine have equivalent bioavailability, but this cannot be assumed for overseas brands (see Roberts 2004).

TREATMENT OF HYPERTHYROIDISM

Hyperthyroidism (thyrotoxicosis)

Excessive formation of the thyroid hormones and their escape into the circulation result in a toxic state called **thyrotoxicosis**; this is not a distinct disease, but the clinical manifestations of tissue responses to excess thyroid hormone. This occurs in conditions including toxic multinodular goitre, toxic hot nodule, exophthalmic **goitre** (**Graves' disease**, see Clinical Interest Box 39-4), subacute thyroiditis, and as adverse reaction to some drugs (iatrogenic causes), including thyroid hormones, iodine load and amiodarone. (Amiodarone is an interesting drug: it is an antiarrhythmic agent with two atoms of iodine per drug molecule. It can cause either hypothyroidism, by blocking

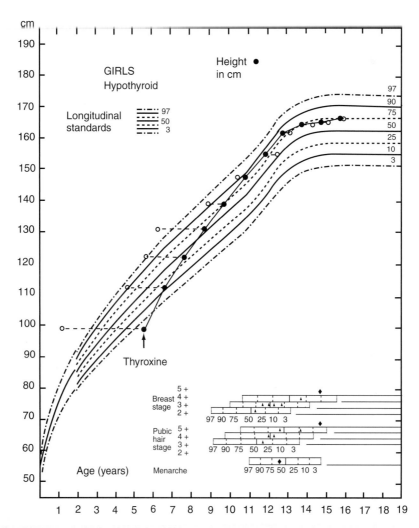

FIGURE 39-3 Effect of thyroxine on growth: response of 6-year-old hypothyroid girl treated with thyroxine. The short stature caused by hypothyroidism starting insidiously in childhood is readily reversed by regular exogenous administration of thyroxine, and the catch-up growth is usually marked and complete, as shown here. *Source*: Tanner 1990. Reproduced with permission from Castlemead.

release of T_3 and T_4, or hyperthyroidism by causing focal thyroiditis.)

Primary **hyperthyroidism** is characterised by elevated levels of T_3 and T_4 despite a decreased level of TSH. In pituitary (secondary) hyperthyroidism, levels of TSH, T_3 and T_4 all rise. Hyperthyroidism leads to symptoms the opposite of those seen in myxoedema (see Clinical Interest Box 39-3). The metabolic rate is increased, sometimes as much as 60% or more. The body temperature is frequently above normal, the pulse rate is fast, and the patient complains of feeling too warm. Other symptoms include restlessness, anxiety, emotional instability, muscle tremor and weakness, sweating and exophthalmos. The raised T_4 levels can cause cardiomegaly, tachycardia, congestive heart failure and hepatic damage. Drug clearances may be increased, so doses of other drugs might need to be increased. In thyroid storm, a sudden onset of exaggerated hyperthyroid symptoms occurs, especially those affecting the nervous and cardiovascular systems, because of elevated T_4 levels. Hyperthyroidism is a life-threatening condition, potentially leading to heart failure and coma.

Treatment

The aims of treatment are to decrease thyroid hormone overproduction and block peripheral effects of excess T_4. Before the advent of antithyroid drugs (carbimazole and propylthiouracil, the thioureas), treatment was limited to a subtotal resection of the hyperactive gland. Antithyroid drugs provide less rapid control of hyperthyroidism than do surgical measures. Typically, the stages of treatment are:
1. Rendering the patient euthyroid with an antithyroid drug.
2. Definitive treatment:
   • surgery (subtotal thyroidectomy), with high doses of iodine used pre-surgery to dampen down thyroid activity *or*

CLINICAL INTEREST BOX 39-3 HYPERTHYROIDISM AND HYPOTHYROIDISM: CLINICAL FEATURES

	Hyperthyroidism	Hypothyroidism
Eyes	Prominent	Eyelids oedematous; ptosis
Temperature	Intolerance to heat	Intolerance to cold
Weight	Appetite increases, weight loss	Appetite decreases, weight gain
Emotional	Increased nervousness, irritability, insomnia	Lethargic, depressed, increase in sleeping needs
Gastrointestinal	Diarrhoea	Constipation
Neuromuscular	Fast deep tendon reflexes; tremor	Slow or delayed deep tendon reflexes; myalgia
Extremities	Hot, moist skin; sweating	Cold, dry skin; myxoedema
Cardiovascular	Arrhythmias; heart failure	Bradycardia; ischaemic heart disease
Drug clearances	Increased	Decreased

- radioactive iodine therapy with ^{131}I (used primarily in treatment of middle-aged and elderly patients) *or*
- 'block and replace' therapy: continuing high dose of an antithyroid drug plus replacement therapy with thyroxine *or*
- high-dose antithyroid drug for 3–4 months, then adjustment to a maintenance dose

3. Maintenance of **euthyroid** state, monitoring and replacing as necessary.

Relapse is common, as is weight gain; hypothyroidism is treated as necessary with thyroxine. Treatment in pregnancy is difficult, as thioureas cross the placenta and can cause goitre and cretinism, and ^{131}I is contraindicated; careful monitoring is required.

β-adrenoceptor antagonists (e.g. propranolol) are frequently used as adjunctive therapy to provide relief of symptoms due to the peripheral effects of excess T_4, including tachycardia, tremor and sweating. Both cardioselective and non-selective β-blockers are effective; they should be used with caution in cardiovascular disease and are contraindicated in asthma.

Antithyroid agents

An **antithyroid** agent is a chemical that lowers the basal metabolic rate by interfering with the formation, release or action of thyroid hormones. Antithyroid drugs that interfere with the synthesis of the thyroid hormones are known as goitrogens; some occur naturally, e.g. in cabbages and turnips. A variety of compounds is included in the category of antithyroid drugs, but only iodine (iodide ion), radioactive iodine and thiourea (thionamide) derivatives are discussed here (Drug Monographs 39-2 and 39-3). Note that accurate diagnosis and optimal treatment of hyperthyroidism require careful monitoring with thyroid function tests.

CLINICAL INTEREST BOX 39-4 GRAVES' DISEASE

Graves' disease, 'exophthalmic goitre', is the commonest cause of hyperthyroidism in patients under 40 years old, affecting about 0.4% of the population; it is an autoimmune condition affecting women more often than men.

There are two main types of autoantibodies against thyroid antigens: thyroid-stimulating antibodies, which lead to the signs of hyperthyroidism, and thyroid-growth antibodies, which stimulate growth and hence lead to goitre. (In Hashimoto's thyroiditis, conversely, the autoantibodies are destructive and produce hypothyroidism.)

The first symptoms noticed may be fullness in the neck, difficulty in doing up the collar button and grittiness in the eyes; other signs and symptoms are as described in the text under 'Hyperthyroidism (thyrotoxicosis)'.

The classic sign, exophthalmos (i.e. protruding eyes), is due to fat deposition behind the eyeballs and oedema of the muscles controlling eye movements, leading to excessive fibrosis and eyelid retraction; corneal ulceration can occur.

As well as therapy of the thyroid dysfunction to render the patient euthyroid, immunosuppressants are required to minimise the autoimmune processes, and moisturising eye-drops are helpful.

Iodine and iodides

Iodine is the oldest of the antithyroid drugs. Although a small amount of iodine is necessary for normal thyroid function and to synthesise thyroid hormones, large amounts of iodine depress TRH and TSH release (see Figure 39-2). The response of the patient with thyrotoxicosis to high-dose iodine administration is inhibition of thyroid hormone synthesis and release from the hyperfunctioning thyroid gland. Thus large doses of iodides are generally used for 7–14 days before

CLINICAL INTEREST BOX 39-5
LUGOL'S SOLUTION

Lugol's solution, or Aqueous Iodine Solution BP, is a mixture of 5% iodine and 10% potassium iodide in water; the total iodine content is about 130 mg/mL. After oral administration, the iodine is converted to iodide in the gastrointestinal tract before systemic absorption.

Iodine solution is indicated to protect the thyroid gland from radiation before and after the administration of radioactive isotopes of iodine or in radiation emergencies, and in patients with hyperthyroidism, to suppress thyroid function and vascularity prior to thyroidectomy.

Adverse reactions include diarrhoea, nausea, vomiting, stomach pain, rash, swelling of the salivary gland and a metallic taste in the mouth.

It is used with caution in patients with tuberculosis, iodine or potassium iodide hypersensitivity, bronchitis, hyperkalaemia or kidney impairment, and in pregnancy.

The adult dose of Lugol's solution before thyroid surgery is 1 mL/day (in divided doses, administered in a full glass of water, fruit juice or milk), for 10–14 days to depress thyroid function.

Lugol's solution used to be a favourite 'extemporaneous product' for examiners at pharmacy colleges to include in practical dispensing examinations: the carelessness of students could be readily judged by the amount of purple staining of fingers and laboratory coats.

thyroid surgery to decrease the gland's size and vascularity, resulting in diminished blood loss and a less complicated surgical procedure (see Clinical Interest Box 39-5).

Radioactive iodine is preferred for people who are poor surgical risks, such as debilitated or elderly patients and those with advanced cardiac disease. It is also used for patients who have not responded adequately to drug therapy or who have had recurrent hyperthyroidism after surgery. The primary disadvantage of using surgery or radioactive iodine therapy, in addition to the risks involved with surgery and radiation, is the induction of hypothyroidism. It is now recognised that, in the long term, definitive therapy that produces hypothyroidism, followed by replacement with adequate thyroxine, is an easier regimen for maintaining euthyroidism than frequent changes of antithyroid drug doses.

Iodine is also used in medicine for its bactericidal, fungicidal and viricidal actions; solutions such as povidone–iodine are used as antiseptics, especially in podiatry to reduce fungal foot infections. Potassium iodide is present in many cough mixtures as an expectorant.

Radioactive iodine (^{131}I)

The ^{131}I radioactive isotope of iodine is chemically identical to iodine, so it has the same pharmacokinetic parameters. After oral administration, it is taken up actively by thyroid cells and accumulates in thyroid tissue, where the ionising beta radiation emitted selectively damages thyroid cells (see Drug Monograph 39-2).

Thiourea antithyroid drugs

The thioureas (also known as thionamide or thioureylene derivatives) **carbimazole** and **propylthiouracil** inhibit thyroid hormone synthesis by inhibiting the iodination of

DRUG MONOGRAPH 39-2
RADIOACTIVE IODINE

INDICATIONS Radioactive iodine (^{131}I) is indicated for the treatment of hyperthyroidism and thyroid carcinoma, and is also used in diagnostic thyroid function tests.

PHARMACOKINETICS Administered orally (usually as sodium iodide in a capsule), it has an onset of effect within 2–4 weeks; the peak therapeutic effect occurs between 2 and 4 months; and it is mainly excreted by the kidneys, 50% within 24 hours. It has a radionuclide half-life of about 8 days; principal types of radiation are beta and gamma rays.

ADVERSE REACTIONS These include sore throat, neck swelling or pain, temporary loss of taste, nausea, vomiting, gastritis and painful salivary glands. After treatment for hyperthyroidism, the patient may experience increased or unusual irritability or tiredness. There is a small increased risk of subsequent thyroid cancer. After treatment for thyroid carcinoma, the patient may experience fever, sore throat, chills (due to leucopenia) and increased bleeding episodes (thrombocytopenia).

If hypothyroidism occurs after treatment, symptoms should be monitored and thyroid function tests carried out for replacement therapy.

WARNINGS AND CONTRAINDICATIONS Use with caution in patients with diarrhoea, vomiting, kidney function impairment or severe thyrotoxic cardiac disease, especially the elderly. Avoid use in people with hypersensitivity to radiopharmaceutical preparations, and in pregnancy and breastfeeding.

Precautions for radioactivity safety must be observed; after high doses, patients' excretions are collected for safe disposal.

DOSAGE Dosage depends on the size and activity of the gland, and the indications for which it is being administered; dosage is in millicuries (mCi) or in the SI units megabecquerels (MBq, where 1 Bq = 2.7 × 10^{-11} Ci). For example, 5–15 mCi may be prescribed for hyperthyroidism, whereas 50–100 mCi is required for thyroid carcinoma.

DRUG MONOGRAPH 39-3 CARBIMAZOLE AND PROPYLTHIOURACIL

ACTIONS The thioureas act as antithyroid drugs by inhibiting synthesis of thyroid hormones; they concentrate in the thyroid gland and inhibit organic binding of I_2.

INDICATIONS These agents are indicated for the treatment of hyperthyroidism, either in a short course in thyroid storm or before surgery or radiotherapy, or in a long course as adjunct therapy for treatment of thyrotoxicosis.

PHARMACOKINETICS Thioureas are readily absorbed from the GIT. **Carbimazole** is a prodrug; it is rapidly converted in the body to the active metabolite, methimazole. The half-life of each thiourea drug is relatively short (2–6 hours); however, the effects may take some weeks to be maximal, as the body may already have large stores of preformed thyroid hormones. Thus the peak effect occurs in about 7 weeks with carbimazole and 17 weeks with **propylthiouracil**. They are metabolised in the liver and excreted by the kidneys; they cross the placenta and can cause fetal hypothyroidism and goitre, and are excreted in breast milk (Pregnancy Category C, and contraindicated during breastfeeding).

DRUG INTERACTIONS The following drug interactions can occur when carbimazole or propylthiouracil is administered with the drugs listed below:

Drug	Possible effect and management
Amiodarone, iodinated glycerol, lithium or potassium iodide	Increased or excess amounts of amiodarone, iodide or iodine can result in a decreased response to the antithyroid drugs. Iodine deficiency, however, may result in an increased response to the antithyroid medications. Monitor closely
Anticoagulants (warfarin or phenindione)	As thyroid status approaches normal, the response to anticoagulants may decrease or, if the thiourea produces a drug-induced hypoprothrombinaemia, the anticoagulant response may increase. Monitor closely because anticoagulant doses are adjusted based on INR test results

Drug	Possible effect and management
Digitalis glycosides	As thyroid status and basal metabolic rate approach normal, plasma levels of digoxin and digitoxin may increase. Monitor closely, as dosage adjustments might be necessary
Sodium iodide 131I	Thyroid uptake of 131I may be decreased by the antithyroid agents. Monitor closely

ADVERSE REACTIONS These include rash, pruritus, dizziness, loss of taste, nausea, vomiting, paraesthesias and stomach pain; fever, mouth ulcers and sore throat may be early indications of serious agranulocytosis. Overall, signs of thyrotoxicosis indicate inadequate dosing, and signs of hypothyroidism indicate possible overdosage (see Clinical Interest Box 39-3). Propylthiouracil is more likely to cause liver damage.

WARNINGS AND CONTRAINDICATIONS Use with caution in patients with a low leucocyte count; contraindicated during pregnancy.

Avoid use in people with a history of carbimazole or propylthiouracil hypersensitivity or liver impairment. Regular blood tests and liver and thyroid function tests are recommended.

DOSAGE AND ADMINISTRATION Dosage depends on usage: after initial 3–4 weeks of high-dose antithyroid therapy, either dosage is regularly adjusted to maintain euthyroid status, or high dosage is maintained and thyroxine added to restore thyroid function to normal ('block and replace' regimen).

The carbimazole oral adult dosage is initially 15–60 mg daily, reducing to a maintenance dose of 10–15 mg daily. In the 'block and replace regimen' the initial dose is continued with the addition of thyroxine 100–150 mcg as necessary. The propylthiouracil initial oral adult dosage is 200–400 mg daily in divided doses. The maintenance dose is 50–800 mg daily in divided doses.

In each case, treatment is continued with monitoring for about 2 years, as remissions do occur. Relapse, however, is frequent.

tyrosine residues in thyroglobulin. Propylthiouracil (but not carbimazole) also inhibits the conversion of T_4 to T_3 in peripheral tissues, which may make it more effective for treatment of thyroid crisis or storm. These drugs all contain a sulfur–carbon–nitrogen linkage; they are closely related chemically to the sulfonamide antibacterials and the sulfonylurea hypoglycaemic agents, both of which drug groups may also interfere with thyroid function.

CLINICAL INTEREST BOX 39-6 NATURAL ANTITHYROID COMPOUNDS: CABBAGES AND CELERY SEEDS

Many natural plants have **antithyroid** activity; this was discovered in 1928 when rabbits fed large amounts of cabbages and related plants (turnips, mustard plants) developed signs of hypothyroidism. The compound responsible was identified and named goitrin; it is chemically closely related to the thiourea antithyroid drugs. Goitrogenous compounds ingested in livestock feed by cows can find their way into the human food chain and thus cause increased incidence in endemic goitre.

More recently, there have been reports of patients previously stabilised on doses of T_4 becoming hypothyroid after taking celery seed preparations as natural remedies for arthritic conditions, gout, fluid retention and cystitis. It is possible that the celery seed extracts contain goitrins that interfere with synthesis of thyroid hormones, as do the thioureas.
Adapted from: Bowman & Rand 1980, ch. 19; Moses 2001.

PREGNANCY SAFETY

ADEC Category	Drug
A	Liothyronine, thyroxine
C	Carbimazole, propranolol, propylthiouracil

Note: Radioactive iodine is contraindicated in pregnancy or if there is a risk of pregnancy.

DRUGS AT A GLANCE 39: Drugs affecting the thyroid gland

Therapeutic group	Pharmacological group	Key examples	Key pages
Thyroid hormones	Tetra-iodothyronine (T_4)	thyroxine	644–6
	Tri-iodothyronine (T_3)	liothyronine	644
Micronutrient/trace element	Halogen element	iodine	640, 1, 7, 8
Antithyroid agents	Thioureas (= thionamides)	carbimazole, propylthiouracil	647–9
	Radioactive iodine	^{131}I	640
Symptomatic treatment of hyperthyroidism	β-blockers	propranolol	647

KEY POINTS

- The thyroid gland has important homeostatic and controlling effects in growth and development, metabolism and energy balance, and cardiovascular and nervous system functions.
- The main thyroid hormones are thyroxine (T_4) and liothyronine (tri-iodothyronine, T_3); calcitonin is also produced and is involved in calcium balance.
- Iodine is actively taken up from the circulation by the thyroid gland and incorporated in T_3 and T_4, which are stored in the thyroid follicles, bound in thyroglobulin.
- Hypothyroidism is manifest generally as slowed body activities; severe hypofunctioning in the adult leads to myxoedema, and in the infant to dwarfism and mental retardation.
- Replacement therapy with thyroid hormones is effective and safe.
- Hyperthyroidism (thyrotoxicosis) leads to speeding up of body functions, with potential damage particularly to the cardiovascular system and eyes.
- Hyperthyroidism is managed by means of a thiourea derivative that inhibits thyroid hormone synthesis, large doses of iodides to inhibit thyroid hormone release and reduce the size of the thyroid, radioactive iodine, or surgery.
- Regular testing of thyroid function is needed to monitor disease progression and therapy, and to optimise dosage regimens.

REVIEW EXERCISES

1 Describe the synthesis and physiological actions of the two main thyroid hormones.

2 Discuss the indications, pharmacokinetics, adverse effects and drug interactions of the thyroid hormones when used clinically.

3 Describe the pharmacological effects of iodine products and the thiourea derivatives on the thyroid gland.

4 Discuss the aetiologies, pathogenesis and treatment of hypo- and hyperthyroidism.

REFERENCES AND FURTHER READING

Anonymous. Managing subclinical hypothyroidism. *Australian Prescriber* 1999; 22: 132–4.

Australian Medicines Handbook 2006. Adelaide: AMH, 2006 [ch. 10].

Bowman WC, Rand MJ. *Textbook of Pharmacology*. 2nd edn. Oxford: Blackwell, 1980 [ch. 19].

Caswell A (ed.). *MIMS Annual June 2005*. Sydney: CMPMedica Australia, 2005.

Ceccarelli C, Bencivelli W, Vitti P, Grasso L, Pinchera A. Outcome of radioiodine-131 therapy in hyperfunctioning thyroid nodules: a 20 years' retrospective study. *Clinical Endocrinology* 2005; 62(3): 331–5.

Endocrinology Expert Group. *Therapeutic Guidelines: Endocrinology, version 3*. Melbourne: Therapeutic Guidelines Limited, 2004.

Delange F, Lecomte P. Iodine supplementation: benefits outweigh risks. *Drug Safety* 2000; 22: 89–95.

Gittoes NJ, Franklyn JA. Hyperthyroidism: current treatment guidelines. *Drugs* 1998; 55: 543–53.

Goodman HM. Part VI: Endocrine physiology. In: Johnson LR (ed.). *Essential Medical Physiology*. 2nd edn. Philadelphia: Lippincott-Raven, 1999 [ch. 39].

Greenspan FS, Strewler GJ. *Basic & Clinical Endocrinology*. 5th edn. Stamford: Appleton & Lange, 1997 [ch. 7].

Hetzel BS. Iodine and neuropsychological development. *Journal of Nutrition* 2000; 130 (2S Suppl): 493S–95S.

LaFranchi S. Congenital hypothyroidism: etiologies, diagnosis and management. *Thyroid* 1999; 9: 735–40.

Lazarus JH, Clarke S. Use of radioiodine in the management of hyperthyroidism in the UK: development of guidelines. *Thyroid* 1997; 7: 229–31.

Moses G. Thyroxine interacts with celery seed tablets? *Australian Prescriber* 2001; 24: 6–7.

Rang HP, Dale MM, Ritter JM, Moore PK. *Pharmacology*. 5th edn. Edinburgh: Churchill Livingstone, 2003 [ch. 28].

Roberts GW. Taking care of thyroxine. *Australian Prescriber* 2004; 27(3): 75–6.

Speight TM, Holford NHG (eds). *Avery's Drug Treatment*. 4th edn. Auckland: Adis International, 1997.

Sweetman SC (ed.). Martindale: The Complete Drug Reference (on-line resource). London: Pharmaceutical Press, 2005; accessed 31 January 2006.

Tanner JM. *Foetus into Man: Physical Growth from Conception to Maturity*. 2nd edn. Ware: Castlemead, 1990.

Tortora GJ, Grabowski SR. *Principles of Anatomy and Physiology*. 9th edn. New York: HarperCollins, 2000 [ch. 18].

Tuckwell KR. *MIMS Disease Index*. 2nd edn. Sydney: MIMS Australia, 1996.

Wallace K, Hofmann MT. Thyroid dysfunction: how to manage overt and subclinical disease in older patients. *Geriatrics* 1998; 53: 32–8.

Woeber KA. Update on the management of hyperthyroidism and hypothyroidism. *Archives of Internal Medicine* 2000; 160: 1067–71.

Wolf J. Perchlorate and the thyroid gland. *Pharmacological Reviews* 1998; 50: 89–105.

Youngson RM. *Collins Dictionary: Medicine*. 2nd edn. Glasgow: HarperCollins, 1998.

ONLINE RESOURCES

New Zealand medicines and medical devices safety authority: www.medsafe.govt.nz

evolve   More weblinks at http://evolve.elsevier.com/AU/Bryant/pharmacology/

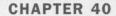

CHAPTER 40

Pharmacology of the Adrenal Cortex

CHAPTER FOCUS

This chapter describes the endocrine functions of the adrenal glands, including the synthesis, secretion and functions of the glucocorticoids and mineralocorticoids; and reviews the rhythms that influence glucocorticoid function. The medical approach to managing hyposecretion or hypersecretion states of the adrenal cortex is discussed. The glucocorticoids affect numerous normal and pathological processes in the body and are often used for their anti-inflammatory and immunosuppressant effects, so the health-care professional must have knowledge about the drugs that affect the adrenal cortex or mimic the actions of its hormones.

OBJECTIVES

- To describe the synthesis, release and actions of the main adrenal cortex hormones.
- To describe the major adverse effects of the glucocorticoids when used clinically.
- To discuss potentially serious drug interactions with corticosteroids.
- To discuss the routes of administration and clinical uses of glucocorticoids, and the recommended method for discontinuing corticosteroid treatment.
- To describe the clinical use of synthetic analogues of the mineralocorticoids.

KEY DRUGS

aminoglutethimide
fludrocortisone
hydrocortisone

KEY TERMS

Addison's disease
adrenal cortex
adrenal medulla
aldosterone
circadian rhythm
Conn's syndrome
corticosteroid
corticotrophin
cortisone
Cushing's syndrome
glucocorticoids
hydrocortisone
hypothalamic–pituitary–
   adrenal axis
mineralocorticoids

KEY ABBREVIATIONS

ACE	angiotensin-converting enzyme
ACTH	adrenocorticotrophic hormone (corticotrophin)
CBG	corticosteroid-binding globulin
CRF	corticotrophin-releasing factor
HPA	hypothalamic–pituitary–adrenal (axis)

GENERAL ASPECTS OF THE ADRENAL GLANDS

IT has probably been recognised for thousands of years that women suffering from chronic inflammatory conditions such as rheumatoid arthritis experience relief from their symptoms during pregnancy. The first suggestion that this effect might be due to a hormone was made in 1930. The so-called 'compound E' was shown in the 1940s to be the steroid hormone **cortisone**, produced in the adrenal glands from cholesterol; the levels of cortisone and its metabolites are indeed markedly elevated during pregnancy. The clinical benefits of the hormones were immediately recognised but they remained very rare and expensive until the 1950s, when chemical methods for the synthesis of the steroid structures were developed. Since then, hundreds of steroids have been synthesised and tested for specific anti-inflammatory and immunosuppressant effects, and for actions in various endocrine and reproductive glands.

The adrenal glands* are located just above the kidneys in the retroperitoneal space, in capsules of connective tissue (see Figure 37-1). Each adrenal gland consists of two separate endocrine organs: the inner medulla surrounded by the outer cortex. They differ in their embryological development, functions and control but share a common blood supply. The **adrenal medulla** can be considered best in relation to the sympathetic nervous system. The medulla is innervated by preganglionic sympathetic fibres and secretes the catecholamine hormones/neurotransmitters adrenaline and noradrenaline (see Unit III). In a situation of stress, both the adrenal medulla and adrenal cortex are 'fired up' to help the body respond and adapt, in different ways (see Clinical Interest Box 37-1 for the mechanisms involved). Normally, a reaction to serious stress causes a prompt and measurable increase in release of adrenaline, noradrenaline, hydrocortisone and aldosterone. These hormones operate together to maintain the cardiovascular tone essential to survival. In the absence of the adrenal cortex, survival of animals is possible only under rigidly controlled non-stressful conditions with available food and a high sodium intake.

The **adrenal cortex** synthesises three important classes of hormones based on the steroid structure—the **corticosteroids** (or adrenocorticoids):
• the glucocorticoids (e.g. cortisone), which have important metabolic, anti-inflammatory and immunosuppressant

effects; they are synthesised primarily in the zona fasciculata of the cortex and are under the control of adrenocorticotrophic hormone (ACTH, corticotrophin) from the pituitary gland
• the mineralocorticoids (primarily aldosterone), which help maintain blood volume, promote retention of sodium and water, and increase urinary excretion of potassium and hydrogen ions. They are synthesised specifically in the zona glomerulosa of the adrenal cortex, and are under the control of both ACTH and the renin–angiotensin system
• some androgens (primarily dehydroepiandrosterone) that are metabolic precursors to the sex hormones; they are synthesised in the zona fasciculata and the zona reticularis; androgens essentially enhance male characteristics.

This chapter discusses the glucocorticoids and mineralo-corti-coids. Androgens are discussed in Unit XII.

Synthesis of adrenal cortex hormones

Cholesterol, which the body uses for the biosynthesis of **corticosteroids**, is synthesised and stored in the adrenal cortex. The general pathways for synthesis of the adrenal cortex hormones are shown in Figure 40-1 (and the structures of typical steroids in Figure 37-2). Note that there is no large store of corticosteroids in the body, so the rate of synthesis from plasma cholesterol determines the rate of release. The rate-limiting step, the synthesis of pregnenolone from cholesterol, is regulated by ACTH. The synthetic pathways can be blocked if there are deficiencies of the enzymes required, and by enzyme inhibitors such as the drugs metyrapone (mainly of research and diagnostic interest) and aminoglutethimide (discussed later in this chapter).

Secretion of adrenal cortex hormones

Two rhythms appear to influence glucocorticoid release: circadian (diurnal, daily) rhythm and ultradian (less than daily) rhythm. A **circadian rhythm**, a pattern based on a 24-hour cycle with the repetition of certain physiological processes, is controlled by the dark–light and sleep–wakefulness cycles via the limbic system. Persons living a normal day–night cycle (sleeping in the dark at night) will have raised plasma hydrocortisone levels in the early morning hours that reach a peak after they are awake. These levels then slowly fall to very low levels in the evening and during the early phase of sleep. The importance of this rhythm is emphasised by the finding that corticosteroid therapy is more

---

*The adrenal glands have also been called the perinephric (meaning round about the kidneys) and the epinephric (over or beside the kidneys) glands, hence the American terms 'epinephrine' and 'norepinephrine' for the English terms 'adrenaline' and 'noradrenaline', the hormones from the adrenal medulla.

potent when given at midnight than when given at noon; daily doses are usually divided, with two-thirds given in the morning and one-third at night, to simulate the natural diurnal rhythm.

In humans, there are also 4–8 adrenal glucocorticoid bursts that occur over each 24 hours, which may follow bursts in the release of corticotrophin-releasing factor (CRF) and ACTH. These bursts are clustered close together and are very pronounced during the circadian rise in plasma glucocorticoid levels in the early hours of the morning. At other times, they may be so widely spaced that adrenal secretion is zero. Consequently, the adrenal cortex secretes glucocorticoids only about 25% of the time in unstressed individuals. Although the basal production rate averages 30 mg every 24 hours, under stressful conditions (trauma, major surgery or infection) there is a reserve capacity production of up to 300 mg daily. Increases in glucocorticoid production may be proportional to increases in the release of ACTH by the anterior pituitary gland.

The corticosteroids are transported in the plasma highly protein-bound to albumin and to corticosteroid-binding globulin (CBG). They are metabolised to hydroxy derivatives and then undergo conjugation and glucuronidation in the liver before excretion by the kidneys.

Control of adrenal cortex hormones

Corticosteroid synthesis depends on stimulation of the adrenal cortex by pituitary **corticotrophin** (ACTH), which is governed by CRF from the hypothalamus (see Figure 40-2 and Figure 37-3). Corticotrophin secretion fluctuates with a circadian rhythm, with high levels in the early morning and trough levels in the evening. The rhythms are disrupted by long transmeridian airline flights and take several days to be restored. This rhythm in turn determines the circadian rhythm in secretion of corticosteroids. Increased levels of corticosteroids, in the usual negative feedback fashion, inhibit the adrenal glucocorticoid system by inhibiting the release of CRF from the hypothalamus and hence inhibiting the release of ACTH from the anterior pituitary. This is referred to as suppression of the **hypothalamic–pituitary–adrenal** (HPA) **axis**.

Corticotrophin is a 39-amino-acid polypeptide. When administered clinically, it tends to be antigenic, hence a synthetic analogue tetracosactrin (24 amino acids) has been developed. It has similar actions to the natural hormone, i.e. it has trophic actions on adrenal cortex cells, increases the synthesis and release of corticosteroids (mainly glucocorticoids),

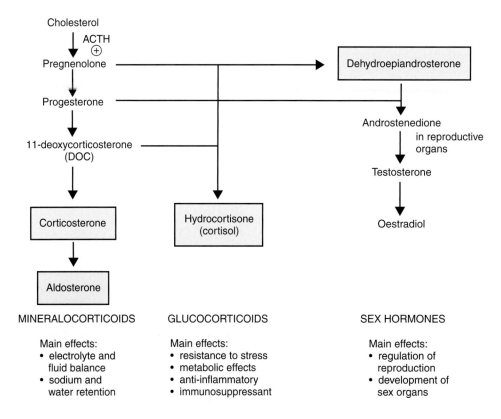

FIGURE 40-1 Biosynthesis of adrenal cortex hormones. Hormones shown in boxes are produced in the adrenal cortex in physiologically active amounts.

and regulates enzymes for steroidogenesis. It is administered parenterally in diagnostic tests of adrenal cortex function: administration should result in a rapid rise in cholesterol synthesis and release of hydrocortisone into the bloodstream.

GLUCOCORTICOIDS
Actions of glucocorticoids

Hydrocortisone (cortisol) is considered the key or prototype **glucocorticoid** hormone, and it and its synthetic analogues have similar effects in the body. These include general metabolic effects, anti-inflammatory and immunosuppressant actions, and negative feedback effects on the HPA axis. Some mineralocorticoid effects may also occur, as the specificity between the two types of steroids is not absolute.

Carbohydrate metabolism

Glucocorticoids decrease glucose uptake into cells and glucose utilisation, while increasing gluconeogenesis; thus they help to maintain the blood sugar level and liver and muscle glycogen content. This can produce hyperglycaemia and glycosuria, i.e. glucocorticoids are diabetogenic: they can aggravate diabetes, unmask latent diabetes and cause insulin resistance.

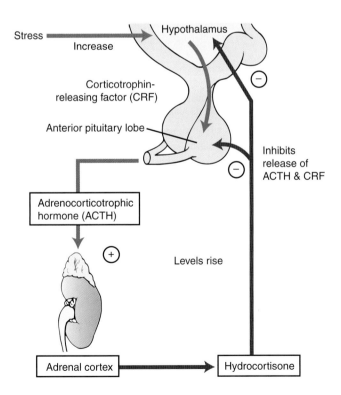

FIGURE 40-2 Glucocorticoid secretion. Refer to text for details and to Figure 37-3.

Protein metabolism

Glucocorticoids facilitate the breakdown of protein in muscle and extrahepatic tissues, which leads to increased plasma amino acid levels. Glucocorticoids increase the trapping of amino acids by the liver and stimulate the deamination of amino acids. Subsequent inhibition of protein synthesis can delay wound healing and cause muscle wasting and osteoporosis. In young people, these effects can inhibit growth.

Fat metabolism

Glucocorticoids promote mobilisation of fatty acids from adipose tissue, increasing their concentration in the plasma and their use for energy. Despite this effect, individuals taking glucocorticoids for long periods may accumulate fat stores ('moon face', 'buffalo hump') because of redistribution of fat. The effects of glucocorticoids on fat metabolism are complex and are thought to occur through metabolic actions of catechol-amines.

Maintenance of normal blood pressure

Glucocorticoids potentiate the vasoconstrictor action of noradrenaline, partly by inhibiting extraneuronal uptake of catecholamines. When glucocorticoids are absent, the vasoconstricting action of the catecholamines is diminished and blood pressure falls.

Stress effects

During stressful situations (e.g. injury and major surgery), corticosteroids are suddenly released and help maintain homeostasis. This sudden release is believed to be a protective mechanism for the individual: without steroid release (or administration), hypotension and shock may occur. Simultaneous release of adrenaline and noradrenaline from the adrenal medulla has a synergistic action with the corticosteroids.

Central nervous system

Corticosteroids affect mood and behaviour, and possibly cause neuronal or brain excitability. Some persons on exogenous corticosteroids report euphoria, insomnia, anxiety, depression and increased motor activity, or they may become psychotic.

Calcium balance

Glucocorticoids tend to decrease calcium absorption from the gut and increase its excretion via the kidneys, causing an overall negative calcium balance. In response, bone is resorbed by osteoclastic activity, raising blood calcium levels. Chronically, this can lead to osteoporosis.

Immunosuppressant actions

Glucocorticoids can cause atrophy of the thymus and decrease the number of lymphocytes, plasma cells and eosinophils in blood. By blocking the production and release of cytokines and other mediators, corticosteroids interfere with the integrated roles of T and B lymphocytes, macrophages and monocytes in immune and allergic responses.

Anti-inflammatory action

Glucocorticoids, especially hydrocortisone, in larger than physiological doses can stabilise lysosomal membranes and prevent movement of neutrophils and release of proteolytic enzymes during inflammation. They can also suppress virtually all the vascular and cellular events in the inflammatory response, both immediate events and late processes, including wound healing and repair. By stimulating the production of the mediator protein lipocortin, they inhibit phospholipase-A2, inhibiting the production from damaged cell membranes of many mediators, including prostaglandins, thromboxanes, prostacyclin and leukotrienes. Because phospholipase-A2 is involved much earlier in the pathways for synthesis of inflammatory mediators than is cyclo-oxygenase, the corticosteroids inhibit production of many more mediators than do the non-steroidal anti-inflammatory drugs (see Chapters 54 and 55).

Negative feedback effects on the hypothalamus and anterior pituitary

Decreasing secretion of CRF and ACTH suppresses the HPA axis, leading to decreased secretion of adrenal cortex glucocorticoids and, in the long term, atrophy of the adrenal cortex. This leaves the body unable to cope immediately with stress, infection or immune challenge.

Because the glucocorticoids have so many physiological actions, pathological conditions affecting the adrenal cortex in which there are deficiencies (**Addison's disease**) or excesses (**Cushing's syndrome**) of hormones have varied and potentially severe manifestations throughout the body (see Clinical Interest Box 40-1).

Mechanism of action

The general mechanism of action of the glucocorticoids is as for most steroids:
- entry into the target cell and the nucleus
- interactions with steroid-specific receptors in the cytoplasm and/or nucleus
- binding to DNA
- transcription or regulation of specific mRNAs
- induction or repression of particular genes
- increased or decreased synthesis of specific proteins
- generation or suppression of mediators.

**CLINICAL INTEREST BOX 40-1
ADDISON'S DISEASE AND CUSHING'S SYNDROME**

ADDISON'S DISEASE: DEFICIENCIES OF CORTICOSTEROIDS
- Aetiologies: autoimmune; tuberculosis (less common now); breast cancer; bilateral adrenalectomy; iatrogenic (resulting from HPA suppression).
- Manifestations: weakness, hypoglycaemia, depression, anorexia, excessive skin pigmentation, with or without aldosterone deficiency (hypotension, dehydration).
- Potentially a life-threatening crisis if there is trauma or severe infection.
- Treatment: glucocorticoid (life-saving), e.g. hydrocortisone 20 mg PO morning and 10 mg PO at night, with the dose increased 2× to cover illness or 5× to cover surgery.
- A mineralocorticoid (e.g. fludrocortisone) may be required.
- Other drugs are used with caution.

CUSHING'S SYNDROME: EXCESS OF CORTICOSTEROIDS
- Aetiologies: adrenal hypersecretion (e.g. pituitary or adrenal ACTH-secreting tumour); prolonged glucocorticoid administration.
- Manifestations: 'moon face', trunk obesity, 'buffalo hump', thin extremities, skin striae, hirsutism (due to excessive androgenic steroid production), osteoporosis, amenorrhoea, impotence, diabetes mellitus, stunted growth.
- Treatment: depends on aetiology, e.g. surgery for tumour, plus replacement corticosteroids afterwards.

In the case of the glucocorticoids, there is increased synthesis of various kinase enzymes and anti-inflammatory mediators, including lipocortin. At the same time, there is decreased synthesis of other enzymes, including cyclo-oxygenase-2 and collagenase, and hence suppression of pro-inflammatory mediators, including histamine, some cytokines, prostaglandins and leukotrienes.

Structure–activity relationships

Many thousands of steroid compounds have been synthesised and their pharmacological actions tested in attempts to enhance particular actions or pharmacokinetic properties. The synthesis of steroids with little or no mineralocorticoid activity was a great advance, as the most useful clinical effects are those of the glucocorticoids, i.e. anti-inflammatory and immunosuppressant actions. Mineralocorticoid effects such as hypokalaemia, hypertension and oedema are then adverse effects.

Hydrocortisone (cortisol) is taken as the 'gold standard' corticosteroid (see Drug Monograph 40-1), so relative affinities of other steroids at glucocorticoid receptors can be compared and relative potencies calculated; for example, three drugs of choice for glucocorticoid (anti-inflammatory) activity are prednisolone (4 times the potency of hydrocortisone), dexamethasone (30 times) and betamethasone (30 times)—all with minimal sodium-retaining activity. For mineralocorticoid activity, the drugs of choice are aldosterone (500 times the potency of hydrocortisone) and fludrocortisone (150 times), both having much lower anti-inflammatory activity. Table 40-1 lists the doses, relative potencies and some pharmacokinetic data for typical adrenocorticoids.

Pharmacokinetic aspects of glucocorticoids
Routes of administration

These very frequently used drugs have been administered by virtually every imaginable route and formulation, including PO, IM, IV, by inhalation, topically, locally and per rectum (enema and suppositories). Local administration to the site of action is preferred if possible, as this allows lower doses to be used, fewer systemic adverse effects are likely, and a more rapid and direct action occurs. Local routes include dermal, inhalational, intra-articular (into joints), into the eye or ear and intralesional. If glucocorticoids must be given orally, alternate-day therapy is preferred, as this minimises the risk of systemic adverse effects, especially suppression of

the HPA axis, growth suppression in children, raised blood sugar levels, protein catabolism, bone loss, infections and mineralocorticoid effects. A drug is selected from the short- or intermediate-acting corticosteroids and, when the patient's condition is stabilised on a particular dosage, the schedule is tapered down on one day and increased on the next until the patient is taking about 2–3 times the previous daily dose every alternate day.

Absorption

Glucocorticoids are well absorbed after oral, topical or local administration. Parenterally (IM) and topically, the soluble esters (phosphate and succinate) are rapidly absorbed, while the poorly soluble agents (acetate, acetonide, diacetate, hexacetonide and valerate) are slowly but completely absorbed and act as depots in the tissues for slow release of hormone. Rectally, about 20% of the drug is absorbed normally, but if the rectum is inflamed, absorption may increase by up to 50%.

Distribution

Steroids, being lipophilic, diffuse well into cells; they are transported around the body in the bloodstream bound to albumin and to corticosteroid-binding globulin (CBG).

TABLE 40-1 Relative potencies and pharmacokinetic properties of major adrenocorticoids

ADRENOCORTICOID	EQUIVALENT GLUCOCORTICOID DOSE (mg)*	RELATIVE GLUCOCORTICOID POTENCY†	RELATIVE MINERALOCORTICOID POTENCY ‡	PLASMA HALF-LIFE (h)	DURATION OF ACTION
Short-acting					
Cortisone	25	0.8	2	0.5	8–12 h
Hydrocortisone	20	1	2	1.5–2	8–12 h
Intermediate-acting					
Fludrocortisone	—	10	150	0.5–3	1–2 days
Methylprednisolone	4	5	0**	3–4	24–36 h
Prednisolone	5	4	1	3–4	24–36 h
Prednisone	5	3.5	1	1	24–36 h
Triamcinolone	4	5	0**	2–5	18–36 h
Long-acting					
Betamethasone	0.6	20–30	0**	3–6.5	2–3 days
Dexamethasone	0.5–0.75	25–50	0**	3–4	2–3 days

*Approximate dosages, applies to PO only.
†Refers to anti-inflammatory, immunosuppressant and metabolic effects.
‡Potassium excretion and sodium and water retention.
**Some hypokalaemia and/or sodium and water retention may occur, depending on dose and individual response.

Metabolism and excretion

The natural hormone cortisone must be hydroxylated to hydrocortisone before it is active; the same is true for the synthetic analogue prednisone, activated to prednisolone (thus cortisone and prednisone are prodrugs). As with most drugs, steroids are metabolised by sulfation and glucuronidation to inactive metabolites, which are eventually excreted in the urine. The fluorinated adrenocorticoids are more slowly metabolised than the other compounds.

Half-lives

The elimination half-lives of the drugs may be relatively short, as the administered drugs are rapidly metabolised (e.g. the half-life of hydrocortisone is about 90 min). The biological half-life and duration of action, however, may last for several hours or days, as the actions initiated by the hormone—enzyme activation and protein synthesis—continue in tissues long after the drug has activated the receptor and been eliminated (see Table 40-1).

Clinical uses

In low doses (physiological levels), glucocorticoids are used in replacement therapy, e.g. in Addison's disease, adrenal insufficiency or hypopituitarism. A typical daily adult dose of hydrocortisone is 10–30 mg, with two-thirds in the morning and one-third in the evening. Doses are increased (doubled or trebled) in times of stress, e.g. during intercurrent illness, before surgery and after trauma. In acute adrenal insufficiency, higher doses (100 mg every 4–8 hours) may be required IV.

Higher doses (pharmacological levels) such as 100 mg hydrocortisone are also used for the anti-inflammatory and immunosuppressant effects.

Indications

Corticosteroids have been tried in virtually every condition that may have an inflammatory or immune pathology, including:

- to prevent transplant rejection in patients with organ or tissue transplants
- in haematological malignancies such as lymphomas and leukaemia (to suppress white cells, induce lymphopenia and reduce the size of enlarged lymph nodes)
- in severe allergic reactions, including asthma, urticaria, anaphylactic shock and reactions to drugs and venoms
- in autoimmune disorders (systemic lupus erythematosus, rheumatoid arthritis)
- in chronic inflammatory conditions in the skin, gut, liver, eye etc.
- in neoplastic diseases, to decrease cerebral oedema, and for the euphoric effects.

They are also used as replacement therapy in patients with suppressed HPA axis (e.g. after several months of glucocorticoid therapy), before surgery or in times of stress.

Specialised uses
TOPICAL GLUCOCORTICOIDS

Dozens of topical steroid preparations are available, in many dosage forms (creams, gels, ointments, eye- and ear-drops, eye ointments, lotions, shampoos) and in many combinations, e.g. with antibacterials or keratolytics. Potencies of topically administered corticosteroids vary: fluorinated compounds are particularly potent, e.g. fluorometholone eye-drops.

Topical glucocorticosteroids are used for their anti-inflammatory and antimitotic actions, in inflammatory and pruritic eruptions, hyperplastic conditions and infiltrative disorders such as eczema, and psoriasis. There are many advantages of topical preparations, including broad applicability, rapid action, stable formulations, compatibility and ease of use, with no pain or odour and few systemic adverse effects.

The degree of absorption through the skin depends on the particular drug, its formulation, the site of application, the presence of any inflammation, and the use of occlusive dressings (this is discussed in greater detail in Chapter 56). Note that efforts to improve percutaneous absorption can lead to systemic adverse reactions, including 'cushingoid' effects, glaucoma and suppression of the HPA axis. Local adverse effects include vasoconstriction, skin striae, atrophy and infections.

INHALED GLUCOCORTICOIDS

The glucocorticoids are potent anti-inflammatory agents because of their actions in decreasing the degranulation of mast cells and in the synthesis of inflammatory mediators and new antibodies. They are also effective immunosuppressants, so they are extremely useful as preventers in asthma, in which corticosteroids are administered by inhalation to decrease bronchial hyperreactivity and minimise the pathophysiological changes (oedema, excess mucus) (see Chapter 32). Administration directly to the airways via a metered-dose inhaler or nebuliser decreases the incidence of systemic adverse reactions.

At least three inhaled corticosteroids are available: beclomethasone, budesonide and fluticasone. Note that corticosteroids do not bronchodilate, so they may be used after an inhaled bronchodilator, which increases penetration of the anti-inflammatory agent into the smaller airways.

INTRALESIONAL ADMINISTRATION

Glucocorticoids are used for musculoskeletal and joint pain (e.g. tennis elbow), usually by intralesional or intra-articular (joint) injection given by specialised practitioners. Long-acting corticosteroids are administered, but not more than 3–4 times per year or joint damage can occur.

DRUG MONOGRAPH 40-1   HYDROCORTISONE

Hydrocortisone is the prototype glucocorticoid, used clinically as replacement therapy for adrenocortical insufficiency and in many inflammatory and immune disorders (see above for Indications). It has some mineralocorticoid (salt-retaining) effects.

PHARMACOKINETICS After oral administration, hydrocortisone is readily absorbed and circulates bound to plasma proteins (>90%). It is metabolised in the liver and most body tissues by hydroxylation and glucuronidation, and metabolites are excreted in the urine. Peak plasma concentrations are reached in about 1 hour, the elimination half-life is about 1.5–2 hours, and the duration of action is 8–12 hours.

ADVERSE REACTIONS Adverse effects can occur in most systems and tissues (see above), including musculoskeletal, cardiovascular, gastrointestinal, dermatological, neurological, endocrine, immunological, haematological, ophthalmic and metabolic effects. Chronic administration leads to suppression of the hypothalamic–pituitary–adrenal axis.

WARNINGS Use with caution in patients with hypertension, colitis, diverticulitis, open-angle glaucoma, liver or kidney disease, oral herpes lesions, hyperlipidaemia, hypothyroidism, hypoalbuminaemia, psychotic tendencies, osteoporosis, systemic lupus erythematosus

or uncontrolled infections (and many other conditions). See the Pregnancy Safety box at the end of this chapter for pregnancy safety classifications of corticosteroids.

CONTRAINDICATIONS Avoid use in persons with corticosteroid hypersensitivity, HIV infection or AIDS, heart disease, heart failure, severe kidney disease, chickenpox, measles, peptic ulcer, oesophagitis, systemic fungal infection, diabetes mellitus, herpes simplex infection (eye), myasthenia gravis or tuberculosis. Corticosteroids transfer into breast milk, and may cause adverse effects in the infant.

DRUG INTERACTIONS (see also Table 40-2) Important interactions occur with hepatic-enzyme inducers, which shorten the half-life of hydrocortisone, and with oral contraceptives, which may prolong the half-life. Hydrocortisone (as with other mineralocorticoids) can increase potassium excretion, hence there are potential interactions with diuretics and digoxin (increased sensitivity).

DOSAGE AND ADMINISTRATION Dosage is individualised depending on the disease and the patient's response; a typical adult dosage is 20 mg PO in the morning and 10 mg at night. Dosage is increased to cover other illness or surgery; a mineralocorticoid may also be required.

RECTAL ADMINISTRATION

Prednisolone is formulated for rectal administration (as suppositories or a retention enema) for use in inflammatory bowel disease (ulcerative colitis, Crohn's disease) and other painful inflammatory conditions of the rectum and anus. Budesonide capsules are used for similar indications.

Adverse drug reactions and drug interactions of glucocorticoids

There are many adverse reactions from the use of glucocorticoids, especially after prolonged administration. Like the drugs' actions, they can be summarised as cushingoid effects mainly on metabolism; pituitary–adrenal suppression effects (adrenal atrophy, decreased growth, decreased response to stress or infection); and mineralocorticoid effects (hypertension, oedema). Suppression of the HPA axis also leads to hazards of sudden withdrawal of therapy, so doses should be reduced gradually.

Adverse reactions include euphoria, headache, insomnia, restlessness, anxiety, psychiatric changes, an increase in appetite (anorexia with triamcinolone), hyperpigmentation, increased hair growth, lowered resistance to infections, visual

disturbances (cataracts, glaucoma), increased urination or thirst, and decreased growth in children. Parenterally at an injection site, redness, swelling, rash, pain, tingling or numbness may occur.

Chronic use may result in abdominal pain, gastrointestinal bleeding, peptic ulcers, round face, acne, weight gain, muscle cramps, weakness, osteoporosis, irregular heart rate, nausea, vomiting, bone pain, increased bruising and difficulty in wound healing. Diabetes mellitus and hyperglycaemia can occur or be unmasked; masking of signs and symptoms of other pathological conditions can occur and confuse the diagnosis.

Potentially, adverse interactions can occur with many drugs. These are summarised in Table 40-2. Patients taking glucocorticoids chronically are advised to wear a 'Medic-Alert' bracelet and carry a steroid therapy card giving details of dosage and emergency instructions.

MINERALOCORTICOIDS

The other important steroid hormones secreted by the adrenal cortex are the **mineralocorticoids**, of which the main natural hormone is **aldosterone**. Its primary function is to regulate sodium and potassium balance in the blood. It is synthesised

TABLE 40-2 Potential drug interactions with glucocorticoids

The following effects may occur when a corticosteroid is given with the drugs listed below.

DRUG	POSSIBLE EFFECT AND MANAGEMENT
Aminoglutethimide	Suppresses adrenal function, therefore do not administer corticotrophin concurrently. When aminoglutethimide is given, glucocorticoid supplements are often prescribed. Aminoglutethimide can increase the metabolism of many drugs, reducing their half-lives significantly. Hydrocortisone is recommended because its metabolism does not appear to be affected by aminoglutethimide
Amphotericin B (parenteral)	May result in severe hypokalaemia. If given concurrently, monitor serum potassium levels closely. May also decrease the adrenal gland response to corticotrophin
Antacids	When given concurrently with oral prednisone or dexamethasone, a decrease in steroid absorption may result. Monitor closely, as steroid dosage adjustments may be necessary
Antidiabetic drugs (oral) or insulin	Glucocorticoids may elevate serum glucose levels (both during therapy and after, if the glucocorticoid is stopped); therefore a dosage adjustment of one or both drugs may be necessary
Antifungal agents (itraconazole, ketoconazole)	Reduce the metabolism and enhance the clinical effects of some glucocorticoids; chronic administration should be monitored and dosage of glucocorticoid may need to be reduced
Digitalis glycosides	May result in increased potential for toxicity (arrhythmias) associated with hypokalaemia
Diuretics	The sodium- and fluid-retaining effects of the adrenocorticoids may reduce the effectiveness of diuretic agents. Monitor closely for oedema and fluid retention. Potassium-depleting diuretics given with adrenocorticoids may result in severe hypokalaemia, whereas the effects of potassium-sparing diuretics may be decreased. Monitor serum potassium levels and patient response closely
Hepatic-enzyme-inducing agents	Barbiturates, carbamazepine, phenytoin and others may decrease the adrenocorticoid effect because of increased metabolism. Dosage increase may be necessary. Monitor serum hydrocortisone levels closely. A benzodiazepine is safer
Potassium supplements	These reduce the effect of either one or both medications on serum potassium levels. Monitor serum levels if given concurrently
Sodium-containing foods or medications	Concurrent use may result in oedema and hypertension. Monitor weight, intake and output and blood pressure closely
Vaccines, live virus and other immunisations	Generally, immunisations are not recommended for patients receiving pharmacological or immunosuppressant doses of glucocorticoids. Because corticosteroids inhibit antibody response, the immunisation effect will be reduced or ineffective and the patient may develop neurological complications or develop the viral disease

CLINICAL INTEREST BOX 40-2 ADRENAL INSUFFICIENCY AND CONN'S SYNDROME

In adrenal insufficiency, there is aldosterone deficit, sodium reabsorption is inhibited and potassium excretion decreases; hyperkalaemia and mild acidosis occur. With adrenalectomy, the loss of aldosterone leads to an overall reduction of sodium reabsorption and a powerful and uncontrolled loss of extracellular fluid. Plasma volume drops, and a state of hypovolaemic shock may ensue. This may cause death unless a mineralocorticoid, salt and water are administered.

On the other hand, in excessive doses aldosterone increases potassium excretion and, unless dietary intake compensates for the loss, hypokalaemia results.

Acidification of the urine then occurs, leading to metabolic alkalosis. **Conn's syndrome**, a condition of hyperaldosteronism occurring with a secretory adenoma, leads to similar problems, including hypertension and potassium depletion.

Treatment is with surgery, such as unilateral adrenalectomy, or with the competitive aldosterone antagonist spironolactone (also known as a potassium-sparing diuretic). Liquorice has significant indirect mineralocorticoid activity: persons 'addicted' to liquorice as a candy can suffer sodium retention and raised blood pressure.

in the adrenal zona glomerulosa, the outer edge of the adreno-cortical tissue below the adrenal capsule.

Aldosterone production is regulated primarily by the renin–angiotensin system and the concentration of circulating serum potassium (see Unit VI), rather than by stimulation of the adrenal cortex by ACTH. A drop in the circulating arterial volume or pressure stimulates receptors in the juxta-glomerular apparatus within the renal afferent arterioles (see Figure 28-2). As a result, renin (a proteolytic enzyme) is released and acts on angiotensinogen (an α_2-globulin synthesised by the liver) to form angiotensin I. When the angiotensin I passes through the pulmonary circulation, and also in the kidneys, two amino acids are cleaved from it by angiotensin-converting enzyme (ACE) to form angiotensin II,

an octapeptide. Angiotensin II stimulates the adrenal cortex zona glomerulosa to produce aldosterone. Aldosterone has two distinct actions: first, it is a potent vasoconstrictor; second, it promotes reabsorption of sodium (and, by the resulting osmotic pressure gradient, water) in the kidney at the distal convoluted tubule to preserve extracellular fluid volume. (Aldosterone acts on receptors in the kidneys, via altered DNA transcription, leading to increased activation of sodium channels, thus increased numbers of Na^+–K^+-ATPase molecules.) Hence renin release leads to two major actions that counteract the initiating decrease in blood pressure or volume—an important homeostatic mechanism.

In the normal patient, aldosterone secretion is stimulated by a decrease in circulating volume (e.g. loss of blood,

---

DRUG MONOGRAPH 40-2 FLUDROCORTISONE

Fludrocortisone has very potent mineralocorticoid activity, for which it is mainly used, with strong glucocorticoid effects as well. It acts primarily on the renal distal convoluted tubule to reabsorb sodium, enhance excretion of potassium and hydrogen, and raise blood pressure. It is indicated for the treatment of Addison's disease (adrenocortical insufficiency) and salt-losing adrenogenital syndrome, and is also used in orthostatic hypotension.

PHARMACOKINETICS Fludrocortisone has good oral absorption and a half-life of about 3.5 hours in the plasma, with a biological half-life of activity in the body of 18–36 hours and a duration of action of 24–48 hours. It is highly protein-bound, and metabolites produced in the liver and kidneys are excreted by the kidneys.

DRUG INTERACTIONS The following effects may occur when fludrocortisone is given with the drugs listed below:

Drug	Possible effect and management
Digitalis glycosides	Hypokalaemic effect may potentiate the risk for cardiac arrhythmias or digitalis toxicity. Monitor closely with electrocardiogram (ECG) and monitor serum potassium levels
Diuretics	Effectiveness of diuretics may be decreased with these medications. Concurrent use of potassium-depleting diuretics or hypokalaemic-inducing medications may produce severe hypokalaemia. Monitor serum potassium levels closely

Drug	Possible effect and management
Hepatic-enzyme inducers	Increased metabolism of mineralocorticoids may result in a decrease in their effectiveness
Sodium in food or medications	In renal tubular acidosis, concurrent use of sodium with fludrocortisone may result in hypertension, hypernatraemia and oedema. Monitor sodium intake closely and advise patients on safe consumption of foods and medications to avoid hypernatraemia

(See also adverse drug interactions with glucocorticoids [Table 40-2].)

ADVERSE REACTIONS These include severe or persistent headaches, hypertension, dizziness, oedema of the lower extremities, joint pain, hypokalaemia and increased weakness. Such adverse reactions should be reported immediately to the prescriber. At the low doses of mineralocorticoids usually used, serious glucocorticoid adverse effects are unlikely.

WARNINGS AND CONTRAINDICATIONS Use with caution in patients with peripheral oedema, acute glomerulonephritis, liver impairment, hypothyroidism, hyperthyroidism, chronic nephritis, infections or osteoporosis. Avoid use in persons with fludrocortisone hypersensitivity, heart disease, hypertension or kidney function impairment. During chronic administration, periodic monitoring of serum electrolytes, and dietary sodium restriction and potassium supplementation, are advisable.

DOSAGE AND ADMINISTRATION The adolescent and adult oral dosage is 100 mcg daily. The usual paediatric dosage is 50–100 mcg daily.

DRUG MONOGRAPH 40-3 AMINOGLUTETHIMIDE

Aminoglutethimide inhibits the enzymatic conversion of cholesterol to pregnenolone, thereby blocking the synthesis of all adrenal steroids, and may have other suppressive effects in the synthesis and metabolism of these steroids (see Figure 40-1). It acts by competitive binding to cytochrome P450. It also inhibits oestrogen production from androgens by blocking an aromatase enzyme in the peripheral tissues (particularly important in postmenopausal women), and may enhance oestrone metabolism; thus it is used to treat breast cancer.

INDICATIONS Aminoglutethimide is indicated for the treatment of Cushing's syndrome associated with adrenal carcinoma, ectopic ACTH-dependent tumours and adrenal gland hyperplasia, and in advanced breast cancer in postmenopausal women.

PHARMACOKINETICS Aminoglutethimide is rapidly absorbed orally and has a half-life of 13 hours, which is reduced to 7 hours after chronic therapy. The time to peak concentration is 1.5 hours, with adrenal function suppression occurring within 3–5 days of therapy. Aminoglutethimide is partly metabolised in the liver and excreted by the kidneys.

DRUG INTERACTIONS Aminoglutethimide increases its own metabolism and the metabolism of several

other drugs, including glucocorticoids, tamoxifen, oral anticoagulants and oral hypoglycaemic agents, thus reducing their effectiveness. If a glucocorticoid is necessary for a patient receiving aminoglutethimide, hydrocortisone is usually the drug of choice. Doses of other concomitant drugs may need to be adjusted.

ADVERSE REACTIONS These include ataxia, dizziness, sedation, anorexia, nausea, vomiting, a measles-like rash, and fever. Because adrenocortical function is suppressed, the patient may be at risk in stressful situations.

WARNINGS AND CONTRAINDICATIONS Therapy is usually initiated and dosage adjusted in the hospital setting. Use with caution in patients with liver or kidney function impairment or hypothyroidism. Avoid use in persons with aminoglutethimide or glutethimide hypersensitivity, chickenpox, herpes zoster and/or other infections.

DOSAGE AND ADMINISTRATION The adult oral dosage is 250 mg three or four times daily for about 14 days; the maintenance dosage is 250 mg every 6 hours maximum. Glucocorticoid and mineralocorticoid replacement may be required. A paediatric dosage has not been established.

---

excessive diuresis, low salt intake) and raised potassium levels. It restricts the loss of sodium and its accompanying anions, chloride and bicarbonate, and thereby helps to maintain extracellular fluid volume. It also maintains acid–base and potassium balance. However, aldosterone secretion is suppressed by an elevation of sodium levels in the blood, e.g. by excessive dietary salt intake.

PREGNANCY SAFETY

ADEC Category*	Drug
A	Betamethasone (topical), budesonide (topical), cortisone, dexamethasone, hydrocortisone (tablets), methylprednisolone, prednisone
B3	Budesonide (oral), fluorometholone (eye-drops), mometasone (topical)
C	Betamethasone (injection), fludrocortisone, hydrocortisone (injection), methylprednisolone (depot), prednisolone (eye/ear-drops), triamcinolone
D	Aminoglutethimide, tetracosactrin

*Note that the Pregnancy Category can depend on the type of formulation or route of administration.

Aldosterone is several thousand times more potent as a mineralocorticoid than is hydrocortisone. In adrenal cortex insufficiency, replacement of a glucocorticoid and sometimes a mineralocorticoid also is necessary. The clinical use of aldosterone has been limited because of its cost, short half-life and relative unavailability, and because it is best administered parenterally; hence synthetic analogues such as **fludrocortisone** are administered (see Drug Monograph 40-2). In high doses, aldosterone analogues have a negative feedback effect on the pituitary secretion of ACTH, and on adrenal cortex secretion of endogenous steroids (see Figure 37-3).

ADRENAL STEROID SYNTHESIS INHIBITORS

Aminoglutethimide and metyrapone are inhibitors of adrenal steroid synthesis, thus they inhibit or suppress adrenal cortex function (see Drug Monograph 40-3). The antifungal agent ketoconazole is also a powerful inhibitor of steroidogenesis (steroid synthesis), and of the cytochrome P450 3A4 system. While it is not used for this purpose, it is important to recognise that ketoconazole can potentially interact with hundreds of other drugs.

DRUGS AT A GLANCE 40: Drugs acting on the adrenal cortex

Therapeutic group	Pharmacological group	Key examples	Key pages
Adrenocorticosteroids	Glucocorticoids	hydrocortisone dexamethasone beclomethasone	655–9 657 658
	Mineralocorticoids	aldosterone fludrocortisone	659–62 657, 61
Inhibitors of adrenocorticosteroid synthesis	Inhibitors of cholesterol hydroxylation	aminoglutethimide	662

Note: See also Table 40-2 for significant drug interactions.

KEY POINTS

- The corticosteroids (glucocorticoids and mineralocorticoids) are steroidal hormones that are synthesised in and released from the adrenal cortex.
- Release of corticosteroids is controlled by the hypothalamus and pituitary gland, and is subject to circadian rhythms.
- The many important pharmacological actions of the glucocorticoids (metabolic, anti-inflammatory and immunosuppressant) have led to their extensive use in medicine.
- The mineralocorticoids act in the kidneys to reabsorb sodium and water, and enhance the excretion of potassium and hydrogen.
- The actions of these agents are vitally important in helping the body to maintain homeostasis, particularly in times of stress.
- Long-term administration of the glucocorticoids can cause many adverse reactions, including Cushing's syndrome and suppression of the HPA axis.
- Mineralocorticoid agents are used in replacement therapy in adrenocortical insufficiency and in hypotension; aldosterone antagonists are used as diuretics.
- The adrenal steroid synthesis inhibitor aminoglutethimide is used for the treatment of Cushing's disease and for breast cancer.

REVIEW EXERCISES

1 Name the three types of steroid hormones produced by the adrenal cortex and review the primary functions of the glucocorticoids and mineralocorticoids.
2 Discuss the control of adrenal cortex steroid synthesis and release, and the relationship of circadian rhythms to plasma hydrocortisone levels.
3 Describe the mechanisms of the anti-inflammatory and immunosuppressant effects of the glucocorticoids.
4 What effects does stress have on the adrenal gland generally?
5 When hydrocortisone is prescribed, what is the suggested dosing schedule? Name three additional points to be discussed with the patient concerning the clinical use of an oral corticosteroid.
6 Outline the pathways of synthesis of the adrenal steroids.
7 Explain the advantages of local administration of glucocorticoids and describe four specialised uses.
8 Discuss the clinical use of fludrocortisone as a typical mineralocorticoid.

REFERENCES AND FURTHER READING

Australian Medicines Handbook 2006. Adelaide: AMH, 2006.
Bowman WC, Rand MJ. *Textbook of Pharmacology.* 2nd edn. Oxford: Blackwell, 1980 [ch. 19].
Caswell A (ed.). *MIMS Annual June 2005.* Sydney: CMPMedica Australia, 2005.

Endocrinology Expert Group. *Therapeutic Guidelines: Endocrinology, version 3*. Melbourne: Therapeutic Guidelines Limited, 2004.

Goodman HM. Part VI: Endocrine physiology. In: Johnson LR (ed.). *Essential Medical Physiology*. 2nd edn. Philadelphia: Lippincott-Raven, 1999 [ch. 40].

Greenspan FS, Strewler GJ. *Basic & Clinical Endocrinology*. 5th edn. Stamford: Appleton & Lange, 1997 [ch. 16].

Mann J. *Murder, Magic and Medicine*. Oxford: Oxford University Press, 1992.

Morand E. Corticosteroids in the treatment of rheumatologic diseases. *Current Opinion in Rheumatology* 1997; 9(3): 200–5.

Pelaia G, Vatrella A, Cuda G, Maselli R, Marsico SA. Molecular mechanisms of corticosteroid actions in chronic inflammatory airway diseases. *Life Sciences* 2003; 72(14): 1549–61.

Rang HP, Dale MM, Ritter JM, Moore PK. *Pharmacology*. 5th edn. Edinburgh: Churchill Livingstone, 2003 [ch. 27].

Rogerson FM, Brennan FE, Fuller PJ. Mineralocorticoid receptor binding, structure and function. *Molecular and Cellular Endocrinology* 2004; 217(1–2): 203–12.

Speight TM, Holford NHG (eds). *Avery's Drug Treatment*. 4th edn. Auckland: Adis International, 1997.

Stanbury RM, Graham EM. Systemic corticosteroid therapy: side effects and their management. *British Journal of Ophthalmology* 1998; 82(6): 704–8.

Tortora GJ, Grabowski SR. *Principles of Anatomy and Physiology*. 9th edn. New York: HarperCollins, 2000 [ch. 18].

Youngson RM. *Collins Dictionary: Medicine*. 2nd edn. Glasgow: HarperCollins, 1998.

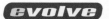 More weblinks at http://evolve.elsevier.com/AU/Bryant/pharmacology/

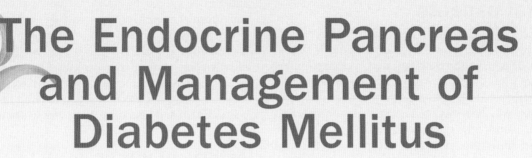

CHAPTER 41

The Endocrine Pancreas and Management of Diabetes Mellitus

CHAPTER FOCUS

The pancreas is a gland with both exocrine and endocrine functions; its major hormones are insulin and glucagon. Their main physiological effects are the regulation of nutrient storage and blood sugar levels. Inadequate production of insulin causes diabetes mellitus, a common disorder of carbohydrate metabolism that affects about 2% of the population and has serious long-term complications due to vascular disease, impaired circulation and damage to kidneys, eyes and feet. Pharmacological treatment of diabetes depends on the type: patients with type 1 diabetes are dependent on exogenous parenteral administration of insulin, whereas patients with type 2 may be treated with improved diet or maintained on oral hypoglycaemic agents, sometimes with additional insulin. Health-care professionals should be well informed on the pathophysiology, overall management and pharmacological treatment of diabetes mellitus.

OBJECTIVES

- To discuss the endocrine functions of the pancreas and the physiological roles of its hormones, insulin and glucagon.

- To review the normal regulation of blood glucose levels.

- To discuss the contrasting features of type 1 (insulin-dependent) and type 2 (non-insulin-dependent) diabetes mellitus and their general management.

- To describe the different sources and formulations of insulin and their clinical uses.

- To discuss the mechanisms of action and clinical use of the various oral hypoglycaemic agents.

- To explain the aetiology of hypoglycaemia and describe the hyperglycaemic medications, including their indications, mechanisms of action and adverse reactions.

KEY DRUGS

acarbose
glibenclamide
glucagon
insulin
metformin
repaglinide
rosiglitazone

KEY TERMS

blood glucose level
diabetes mellitus
glucagon
hyperglycaemia
hypoglycaemia
insulin
islets of Langerhans
ketoacidosis
lipodystrophy
oral hypoglycaemic agents
sulfonylureas
type 1 diabetes
type 2 diabetes

KEY ABBREVIATIONS

BGL   blood glucose level
BMI   body mass index
DCCT   Diabetes Control and Complications Trial
DKA   diabetic ketoacidosis
IDDM   insulin-dependent diabetes mellitus
IU   International Units
NIDDM   non-insulin-dependent diabetes mellitus
OHA   oral hypoglycaemic agent
SMBG   self-monitored blood glucose
UKPDS   United Kingdom Prospective Diabetes Study

THE ENDOCRINE PANCREAS

General aspects

THE pancreas is a gland that lies transversely across the abdomen, in close contact with the duodenum. It secretes into the duodenum, via the pancreatic duct, a clear, colourless fluid (about 1200–1500 mL/day) containing mainly water, sodium bicarbonate, salts and digestive enzymes that digest proteins, fats, carbohydrates and nucleic acids—these are the exocrine functions of the gland (see Unit IX).

Scattered among the clusters of exocrine cells are small pockets of endocrine tissue known as the pancreatic islets, or **islets of Langerhans**, making up about 2% of the weight of the pancreas. These cells have endocrine functions: they produce hormones that are secreted into the bloodstream and are involved in nutrient balance, particularly blood glucose levels, and gastrointestinal (GI) functions. Different cell types produce specific hormones: insulin is produced by beta cells, glucagon by alpha, or A, cells, and somatostatin (GHRIF) by delta, or D, cells. (Somatostatin is considered in Chapter 38; it has significant effects in inhibiting not only the release of growth hormone but also of insulin and glucagon.)

Insulin

Insulin can be considered as the body's main fuel storage hormone; it is secreted by the pancreatic beta cells in response to raised levels of glucose in the blood. Insulin's overall functions are to ensure that the tissues have sufficient chemical substrates for energy, storage, anabolism and repair.

Insulin is a protein hormone consisting of two polypeptide chains joined by disulfide bridges; the chains contain 51 amino acids, the exact sequence of which is known. It is synthesised in the beta cells from a larger protein known as proinsulin, which acts as the storage form of the hormone.

Release and circulation of insulin

Insulin is released via capillaries into the portal circulation to the liver. There is a low basal level of release, in pulses every 15–30 minutes, with increased release in response to stimuli. Release occurs via depolarisation of cell membranes and calcium influx. The most important physiological stimulus is raised blood glucose level: within 30–60 seconds, there is increased release of insulin, with a rapid initial rise due to release of stored insulin, then a slower delayed phase over 60–90 minutes when both stored and newly synthesised insulin are released to deal with the raised sugar level in the blood. Other stimuli include glucagon, nutrients (amino acids, fatty acids), GI tract hormones, vagal and β-adrenoceptor stimulation, and the antidiabetic sulfonylurea drugs.

Insulin release is inhibited by somatostatin and by adrenaline (via α_2 receptors). Deficiencies of release occur in pancreatic disorders (diabetes mellitus, pancreatitis) and other endocrine disorders (Cushing's disease, acromegaly), and can be caused by drugs, including alloxan (of mainly experimental interest) and the thiazide diuretics.

Insulin is circulated bound to β-globulin; being a protein, it is rapidly digested in the gut if given orally, with a half-life of only a few minutes (this explains why the hormone must be administered parenterally to treat diabetes). It has much longer biological duration of action (2–4 hours), however, as it is taken up and bound by the tissues where it acts.

Actions of insulin

Overall, insulin facilitates removal of glucose from the blood into cells and promotes storage of metabolic fuels. The mechanism by which insulin stimulates glucose uptake into muscle and fat cells is primarily by recruiting glucose transporters from intracellular storage pools to the cell membrane, where they facilitate the active uptake of glucose into the cell.

A great variety of biochemical reactions and processes are mediated by insulin: in summary, it affects uptake,

---

CLINICAL INTEREST BOX 41-1
UNITS OF INSULIN ACTIVITY

All early preparations of **insulin** were purified extracts of animal pancreas (beef or pig), and the content could not be guaranteed to be 100% pure insulin. Hence the only way to quantify the insulin level in the extract was by means of a bioassay, i.e. an experiment in which the activity of the extract in lowering blood sugar levels of an experimental animal (such as a rabbit) was compared with that of a known standard preparation of insulin.

A standard 'unit of insulin activity' had to be defined and used, rather than an absolute unit such as milligrams. The International Unit (IU) of insulin activity was, for example, at one stage defined as 'the hypoglycaemic activity present in 0.04167 mg of the 4th International Standard Preparation' (of ox and pig pancreas extract). Calculation will show that this highly purified extract contained about 24 IU/mg.

Using these units, it can be calculated that the human pancreas normally contains about 200 IU insulin and that about 50 IU of insulin are secreted each day. This maintains the fasting glucose concentration of about 6 mmol/L (0.8–1.2 mg/mL).

Insulin can now be prepared synthetically or by genetic engineering techniques so that we know it is 100% pure, hence amounts and doses could be expressed in milligram terms. The IU of activity is, however, so well known and accepted that it remains with us. Thus all insulin preparations in Australia are standardised to contain 100 IU/mL. This facilitates dosing and minimises errors.

utilisation and storage of carbohydrates, fats and protein in liver, adipose and muscle cells, so that nutrients are stored as glycogen, triglycerides and fatty acids, and proteins. It thus controls intermediary metabolism, promotes the anabolic state (building up) and has long-term effects on cell proliferation and growth regulation.

The mechanism of action is via binding to cell surface receptors and activation of a tyrosine kinase enzyme. This initiates cascades of phosphorylation reactions leading to many kinase and phosphatase activities, as well as DNA transcription and cell replication.

The actions of insulin are physiologically antagonised by the catabolic hormones, i.e. adrenocorticotrophic hormone (ACTH) and the glucocorticoids, adrenaline, growth hormone (GH) and thyroxine. Hence low insulin levels (and diabetes) can occur secondary to other endocrine disorders, including acromegaly and Cushing's disease.

Glucagon

Glucagon, another pancreatic hormone, is a product of the alpha cells of the islets of Langerhans. It is a 29-amino-acid polypeptide, and was discovered in 1923 as a contaminant of insulin preparations. It can be considered a fuel-mobilising hormone, in contrast with the fuel-storage functions of insulin; it has been called an 'anti-insulin'. Glucagon acts primarily by mobilising hepatic glycogen and converting it to glucose, which produces an elevation in the concentration of glucose in the blood.

Secretion of glucagon is stimulated by low blood sugar levels (**hypoglycaemia**) and high-protein meals, and by exercise and stress, including infections. Secretion is inhibited by insulin and **hyperglycaemia**. (In diabetes, the lack of insulin leads to increased release of glucagon, which contributes to the markedly raised blood sugar levels and eventually to the state of ketosis.)

Glucagon also increases release of GH and ACTH, and (paradoxically) of insulin. It is used clinically to treat insulin-induced hypoglycaemia (see the section on Hyperglycaemic agents at the end of this chapter).

Control of blood glucose

Both the primary hormones released by the pancreas have major roles in control of **blood glucose levels**. Carbohydrate metabolism is controlled by a finely balanced interaction of several endocrine factors, in the adrenal, anterior pituitary and thyroid glands; these processes are summarised in Figure 41-1.

When plasma blood glucose declines, released glucagon facilitates the catabolism of stored glycogen in the liver, resulting in glycogenolysis, or the conversion of glycogen to glucose. Increased gluconeogenesis (new synthesis of glucose from precursors such as pyruvate, glycerol, lactic acid and amino acids) occurs, also increasing blood glucose. The release of glucagon stimulates insulin secretion, which then inhibits further release of glucagon. This feedback mechanism keeps the plasma glucose level around the optimum.

When blood glucose increases, glycogenesis (the conversion of excess glucose to glycogen for storage in skeletal muscle and the liver) occurs, gluconeogenesis is slowed and glucose uptake into cells is facilitated, thus lowering blood glucose levels.

DIABETES MELLITUS

The most important disease involving the endocrine pancreas is **diabetes mellitus**, which is characterised by polyuria associated with a chronic disorder of carbohydrate and lipid metabolism, and an inappropriate rise in glucose level in the blood, due to a relative or absolute lack of insulin.

CLINICAL INTEREST BOX 41-2 HISTORY OF DIABETES MELLITUS

The condition has been known for thousands of years; Egyptian references describe flesh melting into urine, unquenchable thirst and inevitable early death.

1788: the involvement of the pancreas was described.

1889: Minkowski and von Mering demonstrated that a pancreatectomised dog produced large volumes of urine with a high sugar content.

1900: diabetic patients were shown to have pancreatic lesions in the islets of Langerhans.

1904: the concept of hormones secreted from a gland into the bloodstream developed.

1921: Banting and Best extracted insulin from islet tissue and successfully treated pancreatectomised dogs; this was such a major breakthrough in the treatment of diabetes that the Toronto scientists received the 1923

Nobel Prize for Medicine for their work.

1923: insulin was first available clinically.

1936 onwards: as people with diabetes could be treated and hence live longer, the long-term complications were noted—renal and vascular problems and retinopathy.

1945–1955: the amino acid sequence and structure of insulin were determined by Sanger.

1954: the first oral hypoglycaemic agent became available.

1982: recombinant human insulin was produced by genetic engineering techniques.

Currently, the primary cause of type 1 diabetes is still not definite—viral infection leading to autoimmune destruction of the pancreatic islet cells is postulated.

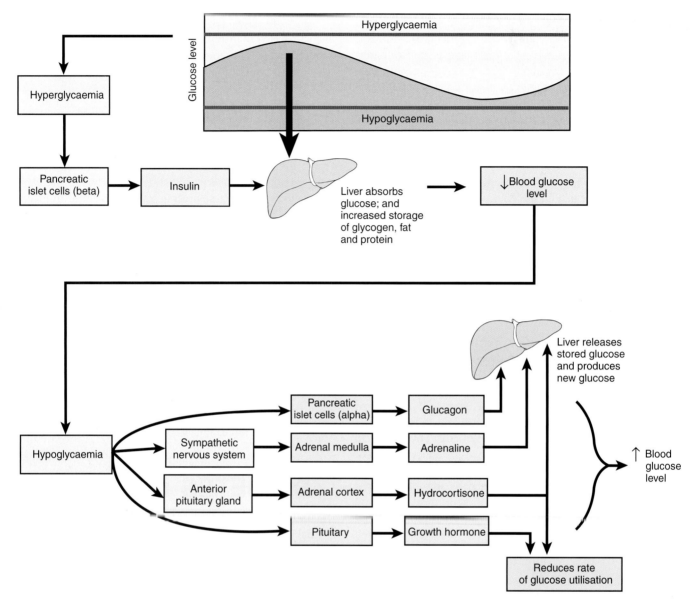

FIGURE 41-1 Control of **blood glucose levels**. Raised blood glucose levels cause the pancreas to release insulin, which causes the liver to absorb excess blood glucose and leads to storage of glycogen, fat and protein. When blood glucose levels are low, the alpha cells in the islets of Langerhans secrete glucagon, which stimulates liver glycogenolysis and gluconeogenesis. The sympathetic nervous system signals the adrenal medulla to secrete adrenaline, while the anterior pituitary gland signals the adrenal cortex to release hydrocortisone. Both substances enhance gluconeogenesis, while adrenaline also increases glycogenolysis, and hydrocortisone slows down the rate of glucose utilisation and raises the plasma level of amino acids available for glucose production. The pituitary secretes growth hormone, which decreases cellular glucose utilisation and promotes glycogenolysis.

The term 'diabetes mellitus' refers to the 'copious urine, sweet or honey-tasting', distinguishing it in earlier times from diabetes insipidus, in which the copious urine was dilute and tasteless. There are many causes and forms of diabetes mellitus, but all lead to hyperglycaemia and a wide range of metabolic and cardiovascular problems (see Clinical Interest Box 41-2 for a brief outline of the history of diabetes).

Epidemiology

The prevalence of diabetes mellitus in the adult Australian population is around 5%, thus it is estimated that nearly a million Australians have the condition; however, there may be as many people again in whom the disorder has not been diagnosed. Diabetes is the sixth leading cause of death in Australia (Australian Bureau of Statistics 2003). In 1999,

CLINICAL INTEREST BOX 41-3
DIABETES IN THE AUSTRALIAN ABORIGINAL AND TORRES STRAIT ISLANDER POPULATION

Aboriginal and Torres Strait Islander Australians have a much higher prevalence of type 2 diabetes and coronary heart disease than do Australians of European descent. Diabetes occurs at a younger age and lower body mass index (BMI, an index of obesity).

A recent follow-up study in two remote Australian Aboriginal communities showed that over a period of 8 years, the population diabetes incidence rate was 20.3 cases per 1000 person–years. Risk of developing diabetes was closely associated with BMI, with the BMI-associated diabetes incidence among the highest in the world. The risk of diabetes in the lowest BMI category was 2–5 times greater than in corresponding non-Aboriginal people.

Renal disease and infections (lungs, skin and urinary tract) are the most common complications.

It has been suggested that whereas the high level of insulin resistance among Aboriginal and Torres Strait Islander Australians would have protected them on a traditional low-fat/high-fibre diet, this insulin resistance is unsuited to a Westernised high-carbohydrate diet.

Poor access to nutritious affordable food and quality health services, and inadequate understanding of the role of diet and obesity in diabetes are barriers to optimal diabetes management in isolated communities.

Hyperglycaemia in type 2 diabetes is best controlled with weight loss, adequate diet and exercise, reduced alcohol consumption and use of oral hypoglycaemic agents. Establishment of local registers of people with diabetes, and regular assessment and screening are recommended.

Based on: Daniel et al 1999; National Prescribing Service 2001.

CLINICAL INTEREST BOX 41-4
DIABETES IN NEW ZEALAND

Diabetes mellitus is a major and increasing health problem in New Zealand. According to the New Zealand Health Survey 2002/3, 4.3% of adults have been diagnosed with diabetes. The Ministry of Health estimates that as many as 50% of New Zealanders with diabetes remain undiagnosed. Although the ethnic make-up of New Zealand is predominantly European/Pakeha, the Polynesian population, consisting mainly of indigenous Maori and more recent immigrants from other Pacific Islands, is increasing rapidly. Maori and Pacific Island people were more than twice as likely to have been diagnosed with diabetes than European/Pakeha people. The prevalence of obesity in these Polynesians is also high. These factors plus an ageing population are increasing the incidence and prevalence of type 2 diabetes in New Zealand. For reasons unknown the incidence of type 1 diabetes is also rising. Studies of diabetes in inner urban communities in Auckland have shown high prevalence among Maori, Pacific Islander and some Asian ethnic groups there. Diagnosed diabetes occurred up to four times more frequently where people were living in more deprived areas and with lower incomes.

Diabetic nephropathy is the most common cause of end-stage renal failure in New Zealand. Polynesian people with diabetes, particularly Maori, have a very high rate of diabetic nephropathy and develop renal failure at a more rapid rate than European/Pakeha patients.

The propensity for Maori patients with type 2 diabetes to develop renal failure may relate to a genetic susceptibility to nephropathy, the younger age at which they develop diabetes, and socio-economic or cultural factors leading to less adequate medical care. A study carried out in South Auckland among people with diabetes who had poor blood glucose control, including a high proportion of Maori and Pacific Island people, showed that presenting medi-cations in blister pack forms led to significant improve-ments in glycaemic control and systolic blood pressure measurements.

Metformin, the biguanide oral hypoglycaemic agent used in type 2 diabetes, remains a major cause of drug-associated mortality in New Zealand. Of 12 cases of lactic acidosis associated with metformin reported to the New Zealand Centre for Adverse Reactions Monitoring, eight had a fatal outcome, mostly in patients with pre-disposing factors such as renal insufficiency, chronic hepatic disease and conditions associated with hypoxia, including surgery, sepsis, increasing age, dehydration and alcoholism.

Sources: Simmons et al, 1999; *Taking the Pulse: New Zealand 1996/97 & 2002/3 Health Survey*. Ministry of Health 1999 & 2005.

Diabetes Australia launched a major community awareness campaign to focus on detection of type 2 diabetes among the estimated one-third of a million Australians who have diabetes but do not realise it. Uncontrolled diabetes is a devastating disease that is a major cause of blindness, end-stage renal disease, neuropathies, accelerated atherosclerosis and lower limb amputations. Diabetes affects males and females equally; the prevalence of diabetes increases with age, and the incidence of type 2 diabetes is increasing in older people (7.2% of people over 25 years old), in the Aboriginal and Torres Strait Islander population (see Clinical Interest Box 41-3) and in the Polynesian population in New Zealand (Clinical Interest Box 41-4). The cost to the Australian community of treating diabetes in 2000/01 was estimated to be about $784 million. In developing countries, the mortality rate is unacceptably high, often due to inadequate, expensive and irregular supplies of insulin.

TABLE 41-1 Features of type 1 and type 2 diabetes

FEATURE	TYPE 1	TYPE 2
Synonyms	IDDM, juvenile-onset	NIDDM, maturity-onset
Age of onset	Usually <20 years	Usually >35 years
Onset of symptoms	Sudden (symptomatic)	Gradual (usually asymptomatic)
Body weight	Usually non-obese	Obese (80%)
Family history	Usually negative	Often positive
Incidence (% all diabetes)	15%	85%
Insulin levels	Low, then absent	May be low, normal or high (insulin resistance)
Insulin-dependent	Yes	Usually not (may progress to be)
Insulin resistance	No	Yes
Insulin receptors	Normal	Usually low or defective
Complications	Frequent	Frequent
Ketoacidosis	Prone to	Rare
Dietary modifications	Mandatory	Mandatory

Pathology

The two general classifications for diabetes mellitus are **type 1 diabetes** (formerly known as insulin-dependent diabetes mellitus, IDDM, or juvenile-onset) and **type 2 diabetes** (non-insulin-dependent diabetes mellitus, NIDDM, mature-onset). The features of the two types are summarised in Table 41-1.

The complex disorder of carbohydrate, fat and protein metabolism is primarily a result of a complete lack of insulin (type 1), or a relative lack of insulin or defects of the insulin receptors (type 2). In either type of diabetes, because of the lack of effective insulin, glucose cannot be readily taken up into cells and glycogen fails to store in the liver, although the conversion of glycogen back to glucose and the formation of glucose from other substances (gluconeogenesis) are not necessarily impaired. As a result, the blood glucose level rises rapidly. When it exceeds a critical level (the renal threshold), the excess is secreted by the kidney (glycosuria). Symptoms include increased appetite (polyphagia), thirst (polydipsia), weight loss, increased urine output (polyuria), weakness (fatigue) and itching (e.g. pruritus vulvae).

Diagnosis is by the signs and symptoms described above and by measurement of high **blood glucose levels** (casual ≥11.1 mmol/L, fasting ≥7.0 mmol/L). Glucose tolerance testing is a more stringent criterion, in which a standard dose (75 g) of glucose is administered after overnight fasting, and the level of glucose is measured in a venous blood sample 2 hours later (≥11.1 mmol/L indicates diabetes).

Type 1 diabetes

This type of diabetes usually occurs before the age of 20 and was previously called juvenile-onset diabetes; it accounts for about 15% of all diabetes. It is thought that a viral infection (possibly unnoticed) sets up an autoimmune response by antibodies against islet cells, causing pathological changes and fibrosis in the tissue, which leads to a critical lack of insulin and abrupt onset of symptoms. There is some evidence of an inherited predisposition to **type 1 diabetes**.

The derangement of carbohydrate metabolism results in an abnormally high breakdown of proteins and fats. The ketone bodies (acetoacetic acid, acetone and β-hydroxybutyric acid) that result from oxidation of fatty acids accumulate faster than they can be oxidised, resulting in ketosis and acidosis; they can often be smelt (sweet and fruity) on the breath of people with diabetes. Diabetic **ketoacidosis** (DKA) occurs most commonly in type 1 diabetes and is a medical emergency requiring specialist care. Treatment includes rehydration, insulin replacement, potassium replacement and sometimes bicarbonate to reverse acidosis. Patients are also prone to muscle cramps, faintness, cardiac arrhythmias and infections. Exogenous insulin therapy is required, lifelong, for survival.

Type 2 diabetes

Type 2 diabetes was previously known as maturity-onset diabetes because the onset is usually after age 35. About 85% of the diabetic population has type 2 diabetes. Generally, people with this type of diabetes have some functioning islet cells, so they are not fully dependent on insulin for survival. There is impaired insulin secretion (especially the early phase after glucose load) and/or insulin resistance because of receptor and postreceptor defects.

Type 2 diabetic patients are typically middle-aged to elderly, overweight or obese; other risk factors include positive family history and physical inactivity. The condition comes on gradually, with glucose intolerance often associated with hypertension and hyperlipidaemia. Although older at the time of diagnosis, patients with type 2 diabetes are still at risk of long-term complications and of hyperosmolar coma, but DKA is rare.

Course and complications

The course of untreated diabetes mellitus is progressive. The symptoms of diabetic coma and acidosis are directly or indirectly the result of the accumulation of acetone, β-hydroxybutyric acid and acetone. Respiration becomes rapid and deep, the breath has an odour of acetone, the blood glucose level is elevated, the patient becomes dehydrated, and stupor and coma develop unless treatment is prompt.

The long-term complications of diabetes mellitus can lead to an increase in morbidity and mortality, despite treatment with insulin (type 1) or oral hypoglycaemic agents (type 2). Most of the complications have been shown to be due to thickening of the basement membrane of small blood vessels (microangiopathy), leading to ischaemia, neuropathies, nephropathy and diabetic retinopathy, which can include vitreal haemorrhage, retinal detachment and blindness. Macrovascular disease (atherosclerosis and thrombosis of larger vessels) may result in coronary artery disease, strokes, gangrene leading to amputations, and cardiomyopathy leading to heart failure. There is increased risk of infections (due to poor circulation and high blood glucose levels) and impaired wound healing.

MANAGEMENT OF DIABETES MELLITUS
General management plans

The general rationale for treatment is to replace insulin to physiological levels; to obtain metabolic control with insulin, oral hypoglycaemic drugs, or exercise and dietary regimens; and to avoid or delay acute symptoms and long-term complications.

Large-scale trials were carried out from the 1970s to the 1990s to assess the importance of control of blood glucose levels in delaying development of complications of diabetes. The Diabetes Control and Complications Trial (DCCT) in type 1 diabetes proved conclusively that tight control of blood glucose reduces the microvascular risks of retinopathy, nephropathy and neuropathy (Keen 1994). The United Kingdom Prospective Diabetes Study (UKPDS) in type 2 diabetes revealed that intensive therapy with oral hypoglycaemic agents and insulin, and good blood pressure control, reduce the risk of cardiovascular complications (UKPDS Group 1998). Overall, these trials showed that tight control of blood sugar levels in diabetes markedly decreases the progression to severe complications, so the aim of therapy for diabetes is to avoid frequent large swings in blood sugar levels.

Diabetes Australia has published targets for treatment, including specified maximum levels for blood glucose, cholesterol, blood pressure, body mass index (BMI), protein excretion and alcohol intake. Patients are strongly advised to give up cigarette smoking, as the combined effects of cigarettes and diabetes on the vascular system are potentially disastrous.

The treatment plan for diabetes mellitus usually involves a multidisciplinary team, including an endocrinologist, specialist nurse, podiatrist, diabetes educator and dietitian, with referrals to specialists (e.g. for ophthalmic care) and specialised care during pregnancy, concurrent illness, surgery, travel and other stressful times. Lifestyle aspects such as diet, exercise, education and monitoring of signs and symptoms need to be addressed, and patients taught to self-administer insulin or an oral hypoglycaemic agent as necessary to help control blood glucose levels.

Standard pharmacological treatment plans are, for type 1: daily insulin, with doses determined by monitored blood glucose levels (BGLs); and for type 2: dietary and weight control and/or oral hypoglycaemic agent (OHA) and insulin as necessary. Recent advances in diabetic therapy include:
* the synthesis of human insulin by bacteria genetically altered by recombinant DNA technology
* islet cell or pancreas transplantation
* external or implanted continuous insulin infusion pumps
* new oral hypoglycaemic agents.

Type 2 diabetes occurs often in association with hypertension and hyperlipidaemia; both can compound the risks of coronary heart disease and cerebrovascular disease. For all diabetes patients, vascular risk factors need to be assessed, lifestyle measures implemented and treatment with antihypertensives and lipid-lowering drugs optimised.

Glucose monitoring

To maintain euglycaemia (defined as normal level of glucose in the blood: 3.5–8 mmol/L), blood sugar levels are regularly determined by blood glucose monitoring (SMBG: self-monitored blood glucose), which has been simplified by the availability of both visual test strips and strips used in blood glucose meters or instruments. Such devices allow patients to monitor their diabetes and make the necessary adjustments with medication, diet and exercise, as instructed by their physician or health-care provider. The visual glucose

CLINICAL INTEREST BOX 41-5
SYMPTOMS OF HYPOGLYCAEMIA AND HYPERGLYCAEMIA

People administering insulin, and family and friends of patients with diabetes, should be aware of the signs and symptoms of hypoglycaemia and hyperglycaemia, and know what action to take if they occur.

Hypoglycaemia: Increased anxiety, blurred vision, chilly sensation, cold sweating, pallor, confusion, difficulty in concentrating, drowsiness, headache, nausea, increased pulse rate, shakiness, increased weakness, increased appetite.

Hyperglycaemia: Drowsiness; red, dry skin; fruity breath odour; anorexia; abdominal pain; nausea and vomiting; dry mouth; increased urination; rapid, deep breathing; unusual thirst; rapid weight loss.

TABLE 41-2 Drugs reported to cause hyperglycaemia or hypoglycaemia

HYPERGLYCAEMIA	HYPOGLYCAEMIA
Atypical antipsychotics (some)	Anabolic steroids
Corticosteroids	Beta-blockers (non-selective)
Glucagon	Disopyramide
Growth hormone	Ethanol (alcohol)
Progestogens (oral contraceptives)	Guanethidine
Quinolone antibiotics (floxacins)	Insulin
Sympathomimetics (adrenaline, salbutamol)	Octreotide
Thiazide diuretics	Oral hypoglycaemics Quinolone antibiotics (floxacins)
Thyroid hormones	Salicylates (aspirin; high doses)

Source: AMH 2006.

testing strips are less expensive than the testing instruments; however, the meter readings from the latter are much more precise (if properly calibrated). Thus people with visual problems or those who need a more accurate blood glucose reading will benefit from using a blood glucose meter. Urine tests are simpler and less invasive but less reliable, and are now used mainly for detection of ketone bodies in the urine.

Patients need to become aware of impending hypoglycaemia, which can occur rapidly from excess insulin or OHA dosage, unexpectedly high levels of exercise, inadequate food intake or other factors that impair blood glucose control. Common early symptoms of a 'hypo' are faintness, sweating and tremor; if untreated with an oral rapidly absorbed glucose source, this can lead to coma and death (see Clinical Interest Box 41-5). Hyperglycaemia, on the other hand, can lead to diabetic ketoacidosis and hyperosmolar coma; treatment is with rehydration and insulin.

Other drugs, both prescribed and over-the-counter, and social drugs, can all affect blood glucose levels and hence alter diabetic control. Table 41-2 and Clinical Interest Box 41-6 describe some of these effects.

Chronic hypoglycaemia is particularly dangerous for young people with diabetes, as the developing brain is dependent on glucose as an energy source; management of children with diabetes thus errs on the side of hyperglycaemia. Parents and carers of young people with diabetes need to be aware of the sugar content of medicines as well as that of foods; many medicines formulated for children have a high sugar content to encourage compliance (as Mary Poppins sang so engagingly, 'A spoonful of sugar helps the medicine go down'). Syrup, elixir and suspension formulations frequently have 50%–70% w/v (g/100 mL) sucrose, and may contain other caloric sweetening agents such as sorbitol or honey. The carbohydrate content of these mixtures may have to be considered in the diet, particularly if the medicines are for another chronic condition requiring long-term therapy, such as epilepsy or asthma. The sugars can also have deleterious effects on teeth

if taken chronically. Not all sweetening agents are sugars (see Clinical Interest Box 36-3), and other sweeteners may be more appropriate for people with diabetes or those on a strict diet. Lists are sometimes published of the sugar content of medicines, or of sugar-free formulations; however, such lists go rapidly out of date; see Clinical Interest Box 41-7 for some 'sugar-free' liquid formulations.

Insulins

By the time of diagnosis of type 1 diabetes, there is usually no functioning islet tissue remaining in the pancreas, and patients are thus totally dependent on an exogenous source of insulin as life-saving, lifelong therapy (hence the term 'insulin-dependent diabetes mellitus'). OHAs cannot be used in these patients, as the oral agents all depend for their actions on there being some remaining islet tissue that secretes some insulin.

Insulin formulations
SOURCES

Insulin preparations available in Australia now are either bovine insulin (derived from beef pancreas) or human insulin (synthesised in the laboratory by chemical alteration of pork insulin or by recombinant DNA technology). Beef insulin differs from human insulin by three amino acids, whereas the

CLINICAL INTEREST BOX 41-6
EFFECTS OF COMMONLY ABUSED DRUGS ON DIABETES MANAGEMENT

Many drugs can raise or lower blood glucose levels, but rarely are the commonly abused drugs reviewed in relation to diabetes. Because substance abuse by a person with diabetes can be very problematic, the most commonly abused drugs are reviewed here.

ALCOHOL

Alcohol promotes hypoglycaemia and blocks the formation, storage and release of glycogen. It can also interact with many other drugs, including oral hypoglycaemic agents such as chlorpropamide. In alcoholics who have decreased their food intake, alcohol can cause a serious drop in blood glucose levels, leading to a need for acute intervention.

CENTRAL NERVOUS SYSTEM (CNS) STIMULANTS

Amphetamines, sympathomimetics, anorexics, cocaine, psychedelic drugs and others can result in hyperglycaemia and an increase in liver glycogen breakdown. Large amounts of caffeine in products such as coffee, tea and cola drinks can also raise blood glucose levels.

MARIJUANA

Marijuana may increase appetite and food consumption. Heavy use may produce glucose intolerance leading to hyperglycaemia.

CIGARETTES

Nicotine in cigarettes is a potent vasoconstrictor. It can decrease the absorption of subcutaneous insulin, raise blood glucose levels and decrease response to insulin. Heavy smokers may need insulin requirements increased by 15%–30%. Smoking is also a risk factor for the development of ischaemic disorders, including diabetic nephropathy and peripheral vascular diseases.

OTHER EFFECTS OF CNS-ACTING DRUGS

CNS-acting drugs (e.g. stimulants, depressants, sedative-hypnotics, opiates, marijuana and alcohol) can impair judgement and alter perceptions (time and place) and thus interfere with the individual's control of the diabetic state.

CLINICAL INTEREST BOX 41-7
'SUGAR-FREE' ORAL MIXTURES

The sugar and calorigenic contents of medications are changed often by the manufacturers, so the best advice is to check the list of contents every time a medication is purchased. Patients with diabetes should be advised always to read bottle labels or check with their pharmacists before buying medications. The following is a listing of some medications that are currently sugar-free (active ingredients are given in brackets).

ANTIMICROBIALS

Amoxil Syrup SF (amoxycillin)
Bactrim Oral Suspension (trimethoprim/sulfamethoxazole)
Cilamox SF Syrup (amoxycillin)
Fungilin Lozenges (amphotericin)
Septrin SF Suspension (trimethoprim/sulfamethoxazole)

CNS-ACTIVE AGENTS

Dymadon Suspensions (paracetamol)
Epilim SF Liquid (sodium valproate)

COUGH AND COLD PREPARATIONS

Nucosef Liquid (dextromethorphan)

OTHERS

Bricanyl Elixir (terbutaline)
Ventolin Syrup SF (salbutamol)
Adapted from: Caswell 2005.

Although these formulations are claimed to be 'sugar-free', they may contain significant amounts of sorbitol, which has calorific value and can disturb diabetic control. SF = sugar-free.

---

pork insulin differs from human insulin by a single amino acid. The human (or recombinant) insulin is identical to the insulin produced by the human pancreas.

Many diabetic patients are effectively treated with beef insulin if they have not developed insulin resistance, insulin allergies or lipodystrophy (a breakdown of subcutaneous fat occurring after repeated injections) at the insulin injection sites. There is a higher degree of immunogenicity reported with beef insulin than with human insulin. Subcutaneously administered human insulin may be absorbed faster and have a shorter duration of action than the animal insulins. It is standard practice now to prescribe human insulin whenever possible, because of the decreased allergenic effects and decreased resistance reported with human insulin. Patients switched from an animal to human insulin should be closely monitored initially because a dosage adjustment may be

necessary. When human insulin was introduced, there was some suggestion that patients found it harder to predict when a 'hypo' (i.e. a hypoglycaemic state) was coming on; however, this has not been proven to be a problem clinically.

New, fast-acting synthetic insulin analogues, insulin lispro and insulin aspart, have been developed. In these insulins the sequence of two amino acids in human insulin is reversed. The primary advantage of the new insulins is that they have a more rapid onset of action than regular insulin; therefore they are administered as a 'bolus' immediately before a meal. They also have an earlier peak effect and shorter duration of action, so people with type 1 diabetes will usually require concurrent use of an intermediate- or long-acting insulin product as well.

Recently, two new insulin analogues have been approved for use as 'basal' insulins, as their long, flat absorption profiles give them a long-acting effect more reproducible than those of the older long-acting formulations (insulin zinc suspension [IZS] and NPH). Insulin glargine has a slightly different amino acid sequence, which makes it soluble in the acidic solution in the vial, but after injection, microcrystals form in the tissues, from which insulin is slowly released. This form of insulin must not be mixed with other insulins. Insulin detemir is a form in which a fatty acid compound is attached to the insulin molecule; after administration, the complex binds to albumin in the plasma and tissues, and insulin is slowly released.

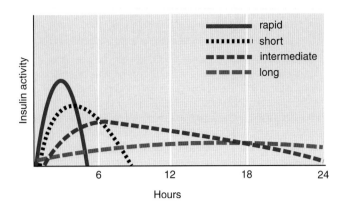

FIGURE 41-2 Insulin pharmacokinetics (see also Table 41-3). Curves indicate approximate times of onset, peak and duration of hypoglycaemic activity of the main types of insulin formulations.

INSULIN FORMULATIONS

Insulins, whether bovine or human, have been formulated in many different ways to alter the pharmacokinetic properties of the mixture; the formulations are described as ultra-short-acting, short-acting, intermediate-acting or long-acting (all contain 100 IU/mL). The wide range of formulations available allows careful titration of dosage to maximise blood sugar level control and minimise fluctuations.

The chemical nature of the protein is not changed (except in the 'bolus' and 'basal' analogues), only the rate at which it acts and is inactivated. Table 41-3 lists some types of insulin formulations, their approved names and pharmacokinetic characteristics; the formulations are also compared graphically in Figure 41-2. (Note that the time-course of action may vary among individuals or at different times in the same individual, and is dependent on the site of injection, blood supply, body temperature, physical activity etc.) Premixed formulations are also available, i.e. 20/80, 30/70 and 50/50 mixes of short- and intermediate-acting types, giving a wide range of possible insulins.

Insulin stocks not in use are normally stored in the refrigerator, but the vial or cartridge currently in use is stable at room temperature. Freezing the solution denatures and inactivates the protein. Note that whereas the older-type insulin formulations were all chemically compatible and could be mixed together, some newer forms cannot, especially insulin glargine.

TABLE 41-3 Characteristics of insulin preparations after subcutaneous administration

INSULINS	ONSET (hours)	PEAK EFFECT (hours)	DURATION OF ACTION (hours)
Ultra-short-acting			
Insulin lispro and insulin aspart	0.25	1–3	3–5
Short-acting			
Insulin injection (regular, neutral, soluble insulin)*	0.5	2–5	6–8
Intermediate-acting			
Isophane insulin suspension (NPH Insulin)	1–2.5	4–10	16–20
Insulin zinc suspension (Lente Insulin)	1–3	6–12	16–24
Long-acting			
Insulin zinc suspension crystalline (Ultralente Insulin)	2–6	10–20	24–36
Insulin glargine (basal insulin analogue)	3	5–15	24
Insulin detemir (basal insulin analogue)	3	3–14	24
Combinations			
Neutral human insulin (20%) and isophane insulin (80%) (Mixtard 20/80)	0.5–1	2–8	24
Neutral human insulin (30%) and isophane insulin (70%) (Humulin 30/70)	0.5–1	2–12	24
Neutral human insulin (50%) and isophane insulin (50%) (Mixtard 50/50)	0.5–1	4–8	24

*These soluble insulins may be administered IV. Intravenously, the onset of action is within 10–30 minutes, peak effect within 15–30 minutes, and duration of action 30–60 minutes.
Sources: AMH 2006; Caswell 2005; product information from Novo Nordisk.

Insulin administration

Insulin is usually administered 'ac, SC', i.e. before meals (15–30 minutes before), subcutaneously. Injection sites are altered, rotating around the abdomen and thighs, to minimise local effects from the injections. In an emergency (diabetic ketoacidosis), short-acting insulins can be administered IV by infusion, or IM.

Insulins are supplied in vials, all in the strength 100 IU/mL. Some formulations are also available prepacked in cartridge 'pens', which facilitate injection and improve convenience and compliance with therapy. Vials or cartridges of insoluble preparations (i.e. all except regular insulin) should be rotated between the hands and inverted gently before a dose is withdrawn, to resuspend the protein; the container should not be shaken vigorously because this could denature the protein.

Portable insulin pumps have improved the metabolic state of some type 1 patients who did not have adequate diabetic control after intensive dietary restrictions and multiple daily injections of insulin. The insulin pump is battery-operated and connected to a small computer that is programmed to release small amounts of insulin per hour. It does not analyse the blood glucose level; however, it is programmed based on the individual's daily insulin needs, diet and physical exercise. The patient can also push a button that releases a bolus dose to cover each meal consumed. Pumps are expensive, subject to mechanical failure, and require careful maintenance.

Clinical trials of oral, nasal and inhaled insulin formulations are continuing; an effective non-injected form would be a wonderful improvement for people with diabetes.

Insulin dosage

There is no standard dose of insulin for the diabetic person; requirements depend on many factors, including lifestyle, weight, diet, exercise levels, stress, illness and pregnancy. (During pregnancy, insulin is the drug of choice to control diabetes; insulin requirements may drop for 24–72 hours after delivery and slowly return to pre-pregnancy levels in about 6 weeks.) Each patient's needs must be determined individually to avoid hypoglycaemia and hyperglycaemia. A typical daily dose might be in the order of 0.7 IU/kg per day, split into 2–4 injections and possibly 2 or 3 different types of insulin.

Insulin dosages should not be considered to be a fixed regimen; the dosage may need adjustment as a result of

---

DRUG MONOGRAPH 41-1 HUMAN INSULIN

Human **insulin** has all the properties and actions of the natural hormone.

INDICATIONS Insulin is indicated for the treatment of type 1 diabetes, and for treatment of type 2 diabetes during emergencies, in stress situations, during pregnancy or as an adjunct to treatment with oral hypoglycaemic agents.

PHARMACOKINETICS The wide variety of insulins available (including combination mixtures) allows sufficient blood glucose control to meet the diabetic patient's individual need and lifestyle. The onset, time to peak and duration of action depend on the particular type and proportions of insulin used. Insulin injected SC will be gradually leached from the injection site into the bloodstream, and will circulate to tissues where it acts, especially in the liver, muscles and fat. Insulin is metabolised and inactivated rapidly in most tissues of the body; the disulfide bonds are cleaved, then the peptide chains are broken down into amino acids.

ADVERSE REACTIONS Rare with human insulin; allergic reactions and **lipodystrophy** can occur. Overdose is indicated by symptoms of hypoglycaemia: faintness, sweating and tremor.

DRUG INTERACTIONS Many prescribed drugs can interact with insulin and impair diabetes control, in particular corticosteroids, β-blockers, thiazide diuretics and phenytoin (see Table 41-2); dosage adjustments of insulin may be necessary. β-blockers (including eye preparations) can mask the symptoms of hypoglycaemia, such as increased pulse rate and lowered blood pressure, and may prolong hypoglycaemia by blocking gluconeogenesis. Cardioselective β-blockers in low dosages, such as metoprolol and atenolol, cause fewer problems than do non-selective blockers.

Many other medications, or the sugar content in them, can also cause hyperglycaemia or hypoglycaemia or interfere with diabetes management, so the patient's medication regimen should always be closely monitored (see Clinical Interest Boxes 41-5 and 41-6).

WARNINGS AND CONTRAINDICATIONS Insulin should be used with caution in patients with liver or kidney disease, high fever, severe infection, hyperthyroidism, inadequately controlled adrenal or pituitary disorders, diarrhoea, intestinal obstruction or vomiting, and in patients who have had recent surgery or trauma. Insulin is contraindicated in patients with hypoglycaemia or with hypersensitivity to human insulin solutions. Changes in type, brand or species of insulin should be made cautiously.

DOSAGE AND ADMINISTRATION Dosage is dependent on the patient's weight, diet and lifestyle, and on the type of insulin and regimen used; dosage is individualised by monitoring blood glucose.

physical growth (child growing into adulthood), illness, the development of anti-insulin antibodies, concomitant administration of certain medications, changes in lifestyle, missing a meal or doing unexpected exercise. Specific instructions may be required regarding insulin administration for the preoperative patient because of the alteration in the patient's dietary patterns and metabolic requirements as the result of the surgical procedure. Treatment programs need to be reviewed regularly and adjusted as necessary, with the prescriber, other health-care professionals and patient working closely together to manage hypoglycaemia and hyperglycaemia and, if possible, avoid long-term complications.

DOSAGE REGIMENS

As described earlier, the DCCT and UKPDS trials showed the importance of tight control of blood glucose levels, and hence techniques ('insulin algorithms') were developed to help determine the exact amount of insulin required at any

time. Patients are taught to carry out self-monitoring of blood glucose (SMBG), and to adjust their insulin doses if the SMBG values are too high or low.

'BASAL–BOLUS' REGIMEN. A dose of short-acting insulin is given before each meal, plus some intermediate- or long-acting insulin at bedtime. This regimen is demanding, but it mimics well the body's natural rhythms of insulin release, i.e. a low basal level, with peaks in response to carbohydrate loads from meals.

'SPLIT–MIXED' REGIMEN. The total daily dose in units is estimated, and this is split between 1/3 short-acting, 2/3 intermediate- or long-acting insulins, with 2/3 of the total mixture given before breakfast and the other 1/3 before dinner.

New therapies

Inhalation is a potentially viable route for administration of insulin, as it is for some other protein hormones (e.g.

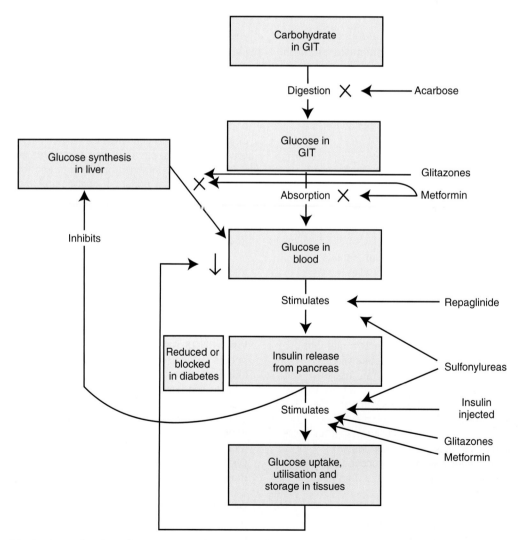

FIGURE 41-3 Mechanism of action of oral hypoglycaemic agents (and injected insulin). X = indicates process is reduced by drug; GIT = gastrointestinal tract.

vasopressin, given as a snuff). This method is being tested and it has been shown that insulin is absorbed into the systemic circulation if delivered to the alveoli via an aerosol formulation. Further studies of safety and efficacy are ongoing.

Transplantation of pancreatic islet tissue from cadaver donors has been investigated extensively for some years; there are problems, however, with supply and with rejection episodes. An alternative is to use stem cells with the ability to differentiate into islet cells; such cells have been shown to be effective in animal models of diabetes, and may become useful in human medicine.

Oral hypoglycaemic agents
Management of type 2 diabetes

Weight reduction with diet control and increased exercise are important in therapy and may be all that is required to prevent progression from the condition of impaired glucose tolerance to overt type 2 diabetes. If symptoms persist after weight reduction, patients may also require OHAs and, when necessary, insulin; the target is a blood glucose reading below 10 mmol/L. The UKPDS trial showed that patients with type 2 diabetes benefited from tight control of both blood glucose and blood pressure, and from attention to other cardio-vascular risk factors, including hyperlipidaemia, sedentary lifestyle and smoking. Metformin is recommended as first-line therapy unless contraindicated (as in renal, hepatic or cardiac impairment, and in the very elderly). A sulfonylurea is alternative or additional therapy, and insulin is added or sub-stituted if OHAs do not adequately control hyperglycaemia. It is now recognised that the introduction of insulin in type 2 diabetes should not be a last resort but may be implemented early in management, especially in young people, to minimise development of long-term complications. A regimen of daytime oral drug(s) with bedtime intermediate-acting insulin is recommended as simple, acceptable and resulting in rapid improvement in glycaemic control.

Cardiovascular risk factors, obesity and insulin resistance are so prevalent with type 2 diabetes that this combination has been called 'diabesity' or the 'metabolic syndrome'. A high proportion of such patients will not only be on metformin, with or without insulin, but also are likely to be taking antihypertensive agents (especially an ACE inhibitor), aspirin (for its antiplatelet effects) and a statin (to treat hypercholesterolaemia). As the beneficial effects of all these medications are additive, it has been suggested that a 'type 2 tablet' could be produced containing metformin, aspirin, a statin and an ACE inhibitor. However, such a multi-drug formulation would suffer the disadvantage common to all combinations: that the dose of an individual agent cannot be adjusted relative to the others. Equally, lifestyle changes suitable for preventing type 2 diabetes, such as healthy eating, regular exercise, healthy body weight, limited alcohol intake and ceasing cigarette smoking, will bring about major improvements in control of most cardiovascular diseases—a 'type 2 lifestyle plan'.

Oral hypoglycaemic agents

The **oral hypoglycaemic agents** (OHAs) are useful only in type 2 diabetes, as they generally depend for their action on some residual insulin secretion from the pancreas. The OHAs act by various mechanisms, summarised in Figure 41-3; they may stimulate further insulin release, lower insulin resistance, sensitise cells to the actions of insulin, reduce glucose load or alter absorption of carbohydrates.

Until the 1990s, there were only two main groups of OHAs: the sulfonylureas and the biguanides. Recently, new types of agents, including acarbose, glitazones and repagli-nide, have been trialled and used clinically; however, the definitive place of the new agents in the management of type 2 diabetes has not yet been clearly established. One agent, troglitazone, looked useful but had only a brief clinical life: it was approved in Australia in 1998 for restricted use in type 2 diabetes, was closely monitored due to concern about adverse hepatic effects, and withdrawn in 2000. Although OHAs are sometimes called 'oral insulins', this description is incorrect, as chemically they are completely different from insulin, and they differ from insulin in mode of action (see Table 41-4 for a summary of the OHAs, their pharmacokinetic parameters and usual adult doses).

The choice of drug depends on several factors, including the patient's pancreatic, renal and liver functions, and response to trialled drugs. It is estimated that 50% of type 2 diabetics will require insulin within 10 years of diagnosis; typically, the patient is stabilised on an OHA, and an intermediate- or long-acting insulin is administered at night.

Sulfonylureas

The **sulfonylureas** were developed as a spin-off from the sulfonamide antibacterial agents: it was noticed that some patients taking sulfonamides had lowered blood sugar levels. The sulfonylureas enhance the release of insulin from the beta cells in the pancreas, and increase the cellular sensitivity to insulin in body tissues; hence they decrease glycogenolysis and gluconeogenesis and reduce blood glucose concentration in people with a functioning pancreas.

The first-generation sulfonylureas included chlorpro-pamide and tolbutamide, both of which have now been withdrawn. The second-generation agents include **gliben-clamide** (see Drug Monograph 41-2), glipizide and gliclazide, and are more potent than the earlier drugs. All are taken with meals, to minimise risk of hypoglycaemia. Choice is made on the basis of pharmacokinetic parameters, as those with long half-lives are more risky in elderly patients, those that are excreted as active drug or metabolites are more risky in

TABLE 41-4 Oral hypoglycaemic agents: pharmacokinetics and usual adult doses

DRUG	PEAK IN PLASMA (hours)	DURATION OF ACTION	HALF-LIFE (hours)	PROTEIN BINDING	USUAL ADULT MAINTENANCE DOSE*	COMMENTS
Sulfonylureas						
Gliclazide	4–6	Medium	12	94%	40–320 mg/day	(H) (R)
Glipizide	1–3	Short	2–4	95%	5–40 mg before meals in divided doses	(H) (R)
Glibenclamide	2–6	Medium–long	2–10	99%	2.5–20 mg/day	(H) (R) (A)
Other OHAs						
Alpha-glucosidase inhibitor						
Acarbose	N/A	N/A	N/A	Not absorbed	50–100 mg tid with meals	Most effective if given with high-fibre diet
Biguanide						
Metformin	2–3	Medium	3	Not bound	500–1000 mg bid or tid	Risk of lactic acidosis. Take with food to reduce nausea and vomiting. (R) Not metabolised
Other						
Repaglinide	1	Short	1	>98%	0.5–4 mg before each meal	Take within 15 min of meal. Excreted via bile. (H)
Rosiglitazone	1	(6–8 weeks)	3–4	>99%	4–8 mg/day	Liver function should be monitored. (A) (pioglitazone)
Pioglitazone	2–4		5–23	>99%	15–30 mg/day	

Adapted from: Salerno 1999, *MIMS Annual* 2005; AMH 2006.
*May be given as divided doses. A = active metabolites; H = hepatic impairment leads to increased risk of hypoglycaemia; N/A = not available or not applicable; R = renal impairment leads to increased risk of hypoglycaemia.

patients with renal disease, and those that are eliminated mainly by hepatic inactivation are more risky in people with liver disease. Common adverse effects include hypoglycaemia, weight gain, GIT disturbances and rashes. Interactions are common with drugs that are metabolised by similar pathways, including sulfonamides, non-steroidal anti-inflammatory drugs, coumarins, alcohol and monoamine oxidase inhibitors, and with drugs that compete for protein-binding sites.

Biguanides: metformin

A non-sulfonylurea OHA for the treatment of type 2 diabetes is **metformin**, classified as a biguanide. The first drug released in this chemical category was phenformin, but it was withdrawn from the market due to its association with lactic acidosis. Metformin has been associated only rarely with this complication; however, the drug is contraindicated in patients who are at risk, i.e. those with liver or kidney disease, the elderly, and those taking alcohol or drugs that raise metformin levels.

Metformin decreases glucose production in the liver and increases glucose utilisation in peripheral tissues; it may also decrease absorption of glucose. It does not affect the pancreatic beta cells; therefore it does not increase insulin release and is unlikely to cause hypoglycaemia. It is preferred to sulfonylureas in overweight patients as it is less likely to cause weight gain and improves the plasma lipid profile. It has a short half-life and is excreted unchanged in the urine. Metformin is now available in combination tablet formulations with glibenclamide

Drug interactions occur with alcohol, β-adrenoceptor-blocking agents and drugs that compete for renal transport mechanisms (including cimetidine, calcium channel blockers, digoxin, morphine, procainamide, quinidine, quinine, ranitidine, triamterene, trimethoprim and vancomycin). Blood glucose levels should be monitored, as drug dosage adjustment may be necessary.

Adverse reactions include GI upsets and, rarely, anaemia, hypoglycaemia and lactic acidosis. Metformin is used with caution in patients with GIT problems and conditions

DRUG MONOGRAPH 41-2
GLIBENCLAMIDE

Glibenclamide is a sulfonylurea oral hypoglycaemic agent. It increases pancreatic insulin secretion and possibly lowers insulin resistance; hence it increases storage of carbohydrates, fats and proteins, and decreases blood glucose.

INDICATIONS Glibenclamide is indicated for the treatment of uncomplicated type 2 diabetes in patients whose diabetes cannot be controlled by diet alone.

PHARMACOKINETICS Glibenclamide is inactivated in the liver and has a variable elimination half-life (2–10 hours) (see Table 41-4).

ADVERSE REACTIONS The most serious adverse effects are hypoglycaemia and weight gain; GI effects (nausea, vomiting, abdominal distress) and rashes are also common.

WARNINGS AND CONTRAINDICATIONS Use with caution in patients with concurrent illness, and in elderly patients and those with hepatic or renal impairment.

Avoid use in people with hypersensitivity to antidiabetic drugs, sulfonamides or thiazide-type diuretics, with any conditions that may cause hyperglycaemia (e.g. high fevers and severe infection), or severe liver function impairment. Avoid use in patients in diabetic coma (or with ketoacidosis), in those undergoing surgery, and in pregnancy or lactation (insulin administration is substituted).

DRUG INTERACTIONS See text under Sulfonylureas, and Table 41-2 and Clinical Interest Box 41-6.

DOSAGE AND ADMINISTRATION Average dosage is 2.5–20 mg/day before breakfast, but for doses over 10 mg daily the remainder is taken before the evening meal. Dosage is individualised on the basis of blood glucose determinations. Australian Pregnancy Safety classification is C: it is recommended that pregnant women requiring hypoglycaemic therapy use insulin.

CLINICAL INTEREST BOX 41-8
COMPLEMENTARY AND ALTERNATIVE THERAPIES IN DIABETES MELLITUS

Patients with type I diabetes are dependent on insulin and must continue taking adequate doses. Various CAM therapies, however, are effective in helping to lower blood glucose levels or to improve glucose tolerance, allowing reduced doses of insulin or oral hypoglycaemic agents, or improving quality of life. Effective techniques include:
- dietary modifications: Pritikin diet (vegetarian, low-fat), low-calorie diet (calories as protein), Oslo diet (high in fish, low in fat), dietary supplements (magnesium, chromium, zinc, vitamin C)
- mind–body therapies: lifestyle changes, yoga, biofeedback, exercise and qi gong
- herbal remedies: *Artemisia herba-alba* (wormwood), *Gymnema sylvestre*, *Trigonella* (fenugreek), *Momordica charantia* (bitter melon), evening primrose oil (from *Oenothera biennis*) and *Scutellaria laterifolia* (skullcap).

Acupuncture has generally been shown to be ineffective in the treatment of diabetes.

Patients should also be warned about taking products when they do not know the active ingredients. Several brands of Chinese 'herbal remedies' sold as antidiabetes treatments have been found to be adulterated with synthetic prescription hypoglycaemic agents such as glibenclamide and phenformin. Taking these remedies as adjuncts to prescribed drugs could lead to a dangerous drop in blood glucose levels.
Adapted from: Spencer & Jacobs 1999.

be discussed briefly; their pharmacokinetic characteristics and mechanisms of action are summarised in Table 41-2 and Figure 41-3, respectively. Complementary and alternative medicine methods relevant to the treatment of diabetes are discussed in Clinical Interest Box 41-8.

α-GLUCOSIDASE INHIBITOR: ACARBOSE

Acarbose is an oral α-glucosidase inhibitor that delays digestion and absorption of carbohydrates in the small intestine; therefore after a meal a smaller increase in blood glucose is noted. Thus any insulin produced by the pancreas in type 2 diabetes has a smaller glucose load to handle. It is indicated as an adjunct to diet for the treatment of type 2 diabetes; it may be given alone or in combination with a sulfonylurea to lower blood glucose. It does not increase insulin secretion or cause lactic acidosis or weight gain.

PHARMACOKINETICS. Acarbose absorption is intentionally minimal (around 2%) as its actions are in the gut; later, metabolites (35%) may be absorbed from the GIT (for half-life, peak effect and duration of action, see Table 41-2). Drug interactions occur particularly with drugs that affect absorption in the intestine, such as digestive enzymes and cholestyramine. The most frequent adverse reactions are

affecting blood sugar levels. Use is avoided in people with metformin hypersensitivity, severe liver or kidney disease, lactic acidosis, cardiac disorders, severe burns, dehydration or severe infections, in people in diabetic coma or with keto-acidosis, and in those who have recently had major surgery or trauma.

Other oral hypoglycaemic agents

The miscellaneous OHAs include an α-glucosidase inhibitor (acarbose), repaglinide and the 'glitazones'. These drugs will

DRUG MONOGRAPH 41-3 GLUCAGON

Glucagon is a natural 29-amino acid polypeptide hormone secreted by pancreatic alpha cells in response to hypoglycaemia. It is released to maintain plasma levels of glucose by stimulating hepatic glycogenolysis and gluconeogenesis (the conversion of glycerol and amino acids to glucose) and by inhibition of glycogen synthesis. Glucagon's effects are accelerated by stimulation of the synthesis of cyclic 3´,5´-adenosine monophosphate (cyclic AMP). Hepatic and adipose tissue lipolysis is enhanced, producing free fatty acids and glycerol, which stimulate ketogenesis and gluconeogenesis. Glucagon does not mobilise muscle glycogen. It stimulates release of catecholamines and hence inhibits tone and motility in GIT smooth muscle, and may have other sympathomimetic effects.

INDICATIONS Glucagon is indicated for the treatment of severe hypoglycaemia in people with diabetes, and to terminate insulin coma. It is useful in hypoglycaemia only if liver glycogen is available; thus it is ineffective for chronic hypoglycaemia, starvation and adrenal

insufficiency. It is also used as an adjunct for GI radiography, as it produces relaxation and decreases peristalsis, improving the outcome of the examination.

PHARMACOKINETICS As glucagon is a protein, it must be parenterally administered (IM, IV or SC). It has a half-life of 5–10 minutes and an onset of action (hyperglycaemic) according to route of administration: IV, 5–20 minutes; IM, 15 minutes; and SC, 30–45 minutes. Its duration of action is 1.5 hours. It is bound in the liver, kidneys and other organs, and is metabolised in the blood and organs.

CLINICAL ASPECTS No significant drug interactions are reported. Adverse effects are mild, and may include nausea or vomiting and an allergic reaction. It is contraindicated in people with glucagon hypersensitivity, phaeochromocytoma or a history of insulinoma. The adolescent and adult dose for hypoglycaemia is 0.5–1 mg IM, IV or SC, repeated in 20 minutes when necessary.

disturbed gut functions. If hypoglycaemia occurs, it should be treated with glucose rather than sucrose, as the absorption of sucrose will be impaired by the drug. As the drug is relatively new, use in pregnancy, lactation and renal impairment is not advised.

REPAGLINIDE

Repaglinide is a novel non-sulfonylurea hypoglycaemic agent, introduced in Australia in 2000. It stimulates the beta cells of the pancreas to produce insulin and improves insulin secretion in response to raised glucose levels, acting by a mechanism similar to that of the sulfonylureas (affecting the ATP-sensitive K+ channels) but at a different binding site. It is short-acting and is given with meals; it can cause hypoglycaemia and other GIT disturbances. Dosage may need to be decreased in liver impairment. Safety in pregnancy and lactation has not yet been established. New related agents are mitiglinide and nateglinide.

GLITAZONES (= THIAZOLIDINEDIONES)

Two new agents for use in treatment of type 2 diabetes are **rosiglitazone** and pioglitazone. These drugs enhance the sensitivity of peripheral tissues and the liver to insulin and thus reduce insulin resistance, which is common in type 2 diabetes. Reductions in blood glucose levels occur soon after starting treatment, but the full effect on insulin sensitivity is not seen for several weeks. The drugs can be used in combination with metformin and sulfonylureas, and are recommended in type 2 diabetes uncontrolled by diet alone. Adverse effects include anaemia, oedema and weight gain. An

earlier drug in this class (troglitazone) was withdrawn due to hepatic toxicity, so patients taking the newer glitazones are monitored carefully in case this adverse effect occurs.

NEW APPROACHES TO TREATMENT OF DIABETES

New types of small molecules are being tested as novel OHAs; potential biological targets include:
* enzymes that act as insulin sensitisers
* inhibitors of gluconeogenesis
* inhibitors of lipolysis or of fat oxidation
* control of energy expenditure (β_3-adrenoceptor agonists)
* alternative routes of glucose disposal in cells
* treatment of diabetic complications.

Immunosuppressant drugs are also being trialled, to delay the onset of diabetes.

Oral drugs that effectively and safely control hyperglycaemia will revolutionise treatment of diabetes and obviate the discomfort and adverse effects of regular injections of insulin.

HYPERGLYCAEMIC AGENTS

Hypoglycaemia can occur in starvation, when meals are missed or diet is inadequate. It is also a common consequence of many diabetes treatments, as use of hypoglycaemic agents inevitably (almost by definition) leads to swings in blood glucose levels around the normal values. The risks and benefits of hypo- and hyperglycaemia must be balanced. The DCCT and UKPDS trials have proved that maintaining euglycaemia is important in minimising diabetic complications, so patients need education with respect to treatment of hypoglycaemia without getting into vicious cycles of swinging blood glucose levels. The symptoms (see Clinical Interest Box 41-5) are similar to those due to sympathetic nervous system overactivity or impaired CNS activity.

In mild to moderate hypoglycaemia, a readily available sugar source should be taken, such as jelly beans, honey or a sweet drink. This must be followed by a complex carbohydrate, which is more slowly absorbed, such as bread or dried fruit. In severe hypoglycaemia, in which the patient is unconscious or cannot take oral glucose, **glucagon** 1 mg (adult) or 0.5 mg (children <5 years) is administered SC or IM (see Drug Monograph 41-3). It is recommended that all patients at risk of developing hypoglycaemia carry a glucagon injection with them, and their families or carers should know how to administer it. In the hospital or clinic situation, glucose 50% or 10% solution is administered IV. Unconscious patients with hypoglycaemia should wake within 4–6 minutes of these therapies.

PREGNANCY SAFETY	
ADEC Category	**Drug**
B2	Glucagon, insulin lispro
B3	Acarbose, insulin aspart, insulin detemir, insulin glargine, pioglitazone, rosiglitazone
C	Glibenclamide, gliclazide, glimepiride, glipizide, metformin, repaglinide

Glucose

Glucose is a monosaccharide that is absorbed from the intestine and then either used or stored by the body. It is indicated to treat or manage hypoglycaemia and is administered orally or parenterally. It is also present in many oral and parenteral electrolyte solutions, peritoneal dialysis solutions, formulations for rehydration, food supplements and blood glucose monitoring kits. In adults, about 10–20 g is administered orally and repeated in 10 minutes if necessary.

The only adverse effects have been some reports of nausea. No significant drug interactions are reported.

DRUGS AT A GLANCE 41: Drug treatment of diabetes mellitus; hyperglycaemic agents

Therapeutic group	Pharmacological group	Key examples	Key pages
Insulins	Ultra-short-acting	insulin lispro insulin aspart	673, 4
	Short-acting	neutral insulin	672–6
	Intermediate-acting	isophane insulin; insulin zinc suspension	674
	Long-acting	insulin zinc suspension crystalline-ultralente; insulin glargine; insulin detemir	674 673, 4
	Biphasic insulins	mixtures with various ratios of neutral/isophane insulins	674
Oral hypoglycaemic agents (OHAs)	Sulfonylureas	glibenclamide glipizide	677–9
	Biguanides	metformin	678, 9
	α-glucosidase inhibitors	acarbose	678–80
	Glitazones (= thiazolidinediones)	rosiglitazone pioglitazone	680
	Non-sulfonylureas	repaglinide	680
Hyperglycaemic agents	Pancreatic hormones	glucagon	667, 80–1

Note: See also Table 41-3, Figure 41-2 (insulins), and Table 41-4 (oral hypoglycaemic agents).

KEY POINTS

● The primary hormones of the pancreas are insulin and glucagon; both are involved in regulation of blood glucose levels and storage of nutrients as fuels.

● Normally, when blood glucose levels fall, glucagon release is increased, which facilitates the breakdown of glycogen stored in the liver to raise and restore blood glucose levels. In addition, the release of glucagon stimulates insulin secretion, inhibits the release of glucagon and maintains the homeostasis of carbohydrate metabolism.

● Insulin facilitates the uptake of glucose into cells and promotes the storage of glycogen, lipids and protein.

● Diabetes mellitus is a disorder of carbohydrate metabolism that results from a relative or absolute insulin deficiency or insulin resistance. Diabetes mellitus is classified as type 1 (insulin-dependent diabetes mellitus, or juvenile-onset diabetes) and type 2 (non-insulin-dependent diabetes mellitus, or maturity-onset diabetes). Long-term complications can be severe and are minimised by tight control of blood glucose levels.

● People with type 1 diabetes require lifelong insulin replacement; diet and lifestyle factors must also be controlled, and a multidisciplinary clinical team is usually involved.

● Various formulations of human or beef insulins are available, with differing pharmacokinetic characteristics; dosage regimen is determined by results of self-monitored blood glucose estimations.

● Type 2 diabetes is managed by dietary treatment, weight reduction and, if necessary, oral hypoglycaemic agents. People with type 2 diabetes may require insulin at some stage.

● Oral hypoglycaemic agents (including sulfonylureas) that act by different mechanisms are available; the choice of agent is made depending on the patient's weight and liver and kidney functions.

● Glucagon and glucose are hyperglycaemic agents available for the treatment of hypoglycaemia.

REVIEW EXERCISES

1 Explain the roles of insulin and glucagon in the regulation of blood glucose levels.

2 Describe the pathogenesis and the major complications of uncontrolled diabetes mellitus.

3 Why is human insulin preferred over animal-based insulins? In switching a patient to human insulin, what precautions need to be taken?

4 Describe the different classes of insulin formulations and the regimens by which they are administered.

5 List several important drugs that may cause hyperglycaemia or hypoglycaemia.

6 What are the symptoms of hypoglycaemia and hyperglycaemia? How is each treated?

7 Describe how a choice is made between sulfonylurea agents in treatment of type 2 diabetes.

8 What are the mechanisms of action of the different groups of oral hypoglycaemic agents?

REFERENCES AND FURTHER READING

Alexander WD. Human insulin: lessons from the UK? *Medical Journal of Australia* 1993; 159: 75–6.
Australian Bureau of Statistics. Causes of Death Australia 2002. ABS Cat. No. 3303.00 Canberra: ABS, 2003.
Australian Institute of Health and Welfare. Costs of Diabetes in Australia, 2000-1. *Australian Institute of Health and Welfare Bulletin* 2005; 26: 1–17.
Australian Medicines Handbook 2006. Adelaide: AMH, 2006.
Bowman WC, Rand MJ. *Textbook of Pharmacology*. 2nd edn. Oxford: Blackwell, 1980 [ch. 19].
Caswell A (ed.). *MIMS Annual June 2005*. Sydney: CMPMedica Australia, 2005.
Daniel M, Rowley KG, McDermott R, Mylvaganam A, O'Dea K. Diabetes incidence in an Australian aboriginal population: an 8-year follow-up study. *Diabetes Care* 1999; 22: 1993–8.
Dunning T. Insulin delivery devices. *Australian Prescriber* 2002; 25(6): 136–8.
Endocrinology Expert Group. *Therapeutic Guidelines: Endocrinology, version 3*. Melbourne: Therapeutic Guidelines Limited, 2004.
Gan SK. Hyperlipidaemia in diabetes. *Australian Prescriber* 1999; 22: 67–9.
Goodman HM. Part VI: Endocrine physiology. In: Johnson LR (ed.). *Essential Medical Physiology*. 2nd edn. Philadelphia: Lippincott-Raven, 1999 [chs 37, 42].
Greenfield JR, Chisholm DJ. Thiazolidinediones: mechanisms of action. *Australian Prescriber* 2004; 27(3): 67–70.
Greenspan FS, Strewler GJ. *Basic & Clinical Endocrinology*. 5th edn. Stamford: Appleton & Lange, 1997.
Holmwood C, Philips P. Insulin and type 2 diabetes: last resort or rational management? *Australian Family Physician* 1999; 28: 429–35.

Jung CY, Lee W. Glucose transporters and insulin action: some insights into diabetes management. *Archives of Pharmacal Research* 1999; 22: 329–34.

Keen H. The Diabetes Control and Complications Trial (DCCT). *Health Trends* 1994; 26: 41–3.

Klonoff DC. Inhaled insulin. *Diabetes Technology and Therapeutics* 1999; 1: 307–13.

MacIsaac RJ, Jerums G. Clinical indications for thiazolidinediones. *Australian Prescriber* 2004; 27(3): 70–4.

McDermott RA, Schmidt BA, Sinha A, Mills P. Improving diabetes care in the primary healthcare setting: a randomised cluster trial in remote Indigenous communities. *Medical Journal of Australia* 2001; 174: 497–502.

Ministry of Health. *Taking the Pulse: New Zealand 1996/97 Health Survey*. Auckland: Ministry of Health, 1999.

Mooradian AD, Chehade J. Implications of the UK Prospective Diabetes Study: questions answered and issues remaining. *Drugs and Aging* 2000; 16: 159–64.

National Prescribing Service. *NPS Newsletters 15 & 17*: Managing type 2 diabetes. Sydney: NPS, 2001.

National Prescribing Service. *NPS Newsletter 39*: Reducing risk in type 2 diabetes. Sydney: NPS, 2005.

Pekarsky B, Ewald B. Can we afford intensive management of diabetes? *Australian Prescriber* 2002; 25(5): 102–3.

Phillips P. Insulins in 2002. *Australian Prescriber* 2002; 25(2): 29–31.

Phillips P, Braddon J. The type 2 tablet: evidence based medication for type 2 diabetes. *Australian Family Physician* 2003; 32(6): 431–6.

Plumridge RJ. *The Sugar Content of Liquid Pharmaceuticals in Australia*. Melbourne: SmithKline Beecham, 1992.

Proietto J. The management of type 2 diabetes. *Australian Prescriber* 1997; 20: 65–7.

Rang HP, Dale MM, Ritter JM, Moore PK. *Pharmacology*. 5th edn. Edinburgh: Churchill Livingstone, 2003 [chs 5, 50].

Shaw JE, Chisholm DJ. Epidemiology and prevention of type 2 diabetes and the metabolic syndrome. *Medical Journal of Australia* 2003; 179(7): 379–83.

Simmons D, Harry T, Gatland B. Prevalence of known diabetes in different ethnic groups in inner urban South Auckland. *New Zealand Medical Journal* 1999; 112: 316–19.

Simpson RW, Shaw JE, Zimmet PZ. The prevention of type 2 diabetes: lifestyle change or pharmacotherapy? *Diabetes Research and Clinical Practice* 2003; 59(3): 165–80.

Soria B, Skoudy A, Martin F. From stem cells to beta cells: new strategies in cell therapy of diabetes mellitus. *Diabetologia* 2001; 44: 407–15.

Speight TM, Holford NHG (eds). *Avery's Drug Treatment*. 4th edn. Auckland: Adis International, 1997.

Spencer JW, Jacobs JJ. *Complementary/Alternative Medicine: An Evidence-Based Approach*. St Louis: Mosby, 1999.

Tortora GJ, Grabowski SR. *Principles of Anatomy and Physiology*. 9th edn. New York: HarperCollins, 2000 [ch. 18].

Turner RC. The UK Prospective Diabetes Study: a review. *Diabetes Care* 1998; 21 Suppl 3: C35–38.

UK Prospective Diabetes Study Group. Intensive blood glucose control with sulphonylureas or insulin compared with conventional treatment and risk of complications in patients with type 2 diabetes (UKPDS 33). *Lancet* 1998; 352: 837–53.

Vajo Z, Duckworth WC. Genetically engineered insulin analogs: diabetes in the new millennium. *Pharmacology Reviews* 2000; 52: 1–9.

Wagman AS, Nuss JM. Current therapies and emerging targets for the treatment of diabetes. *Current Pharmaceutical Design* 2001; 7: 417–50.

Weeks JC, Dutt A, Robinson PG. Promoting sugar-free medicines: evaluation of a multi-faceted intervention. *Community Dental Health* 2003; 20(4): 246–50.

Wong J. Starting insulin treatment in type 2 diabetes. *Australian Prescriber* 2004; 27(4): 93–6.

Youngson RM. *Collins Dictionary: Medicine*. 2nd edn. Glasgow: HarperCollins, 1998.

ONLINE RESOURCES

Australian Institute of Health and Welfare: www.aihw.gov.au/diabetes/index.cfm
Diabetes Australia: www.diabetesaustralia.com.au
New Zealand medicines and medical devices safety authority: www.medsafe.govt.nz

evolve   More weblinks at http://evolve.elsevier.com/AU/Bryant/pharmacology/

CHAPTER 42

The Parathyroid Glands and Calcium Balance

CHAPTER FOCUS

The parathyroid glands have a major role in control of the body's calcium balance via the actions of parathyroid hormone and interactions with calcitonin and vitamin D. Impaired calcium balance or bone mineral homeostasis can lead to severe bone pathologies. Various hormones, vitamin D and bisphosphonate drugs are used to treat bone pathologies. Health-care professionals need to be knowledgeable about these conditions and preparations to ensure safe and effective management of their patients.

OBJECTIVES

- To describe the signs and symptoms associated with hypoparathyroidism, hyperparathyroidism, hypocalcaemia and hypercalcaemia, and the management of these conditions.

- To describe the homeostatic mechanisms that maintain calcium and bone minerals at appropriate levels in the body.

- To describe the pathogenesis of common bone disorders and discuss the current approved drug prophylaxis and treatment of these disorders.

KEY DRUGS

alendronate
bisphosphonates
calcitriol
salcatonin
strontium ranelate
teriparatide
vitamin D

KEY TERMS

bone remodelling
calcitonin
calcium
hypercalcaemia
hyperparathyroidism
hypocalcaemia
hypoparathyroidism
mobilisation
osteomalacia
osteoporosis
Paget's disease
parathyroid hormone
rickets
vitamin D

KEY ABBREVIATIONS

HRT   hormone replacement therapy
PTH   parathyroid hormone
RDI   recommended daily intake
SERM selective (o)estrogen receptor modulator

THE PARATHYROID GLANDS

LYING behind the thyroid gland are bean-shaped glands known as the parathyroid glands. Humans usually have two pairs—one pair on the dorsal surface of each lobe of the thyroid gland—but the number can range from two to six. They are small and easily damaged during throat surgery. The adult glands consist of encapsulated masses of cells, between which are abundant adipocytes and vascular channels. Removal of the parathyroid glands (as frequently happened in surgery on the thyroid gland before the significance of the parathyroid glands was recognised) results in severe hypocalcaemia, leading to tetany and death.

The primary function of the parathyroids is to secrete **parathyroid hormone** (PTH), which maintains adequate levels of calcium in the blood and extracellular fluid. The cells of the parathyroid gland have specialised calcium sensors (G-protein-coupled receptors) in their membranes. When calcium levels in the extracellular fluid are low, the para-thyroids are stimulated to synthesise and secrete PTH, which acts to conserve calcium. When plasma calcium levels are high, binding of calcium to the receptor activates G-proteins, leading to activation of phospholipase C enzymes and eventually to inhibition of further PTH secretion.

Note that the parathyroid glands are not subject to higher control from the pituitary gland or hypothalamus (see Figure 37-4) but respond directly to, and help control, blood cal-cium levels (analogous to the pancreas responding to and controlling blood glucose).

Parathyroid hormone

PTH is a polypeptide of 84 amino acids. The active compo-nent has a half-life of 2–4 minutes; smaller peptide fragments produced in the liver and kidneys have longer half-lives. PTH has multiple effects, ultimately culminating in raised plasma calcium levels (see Figure 42-1). It also reduces phosphate concentration, permitting more calcium to be mobilised. The main effects are:

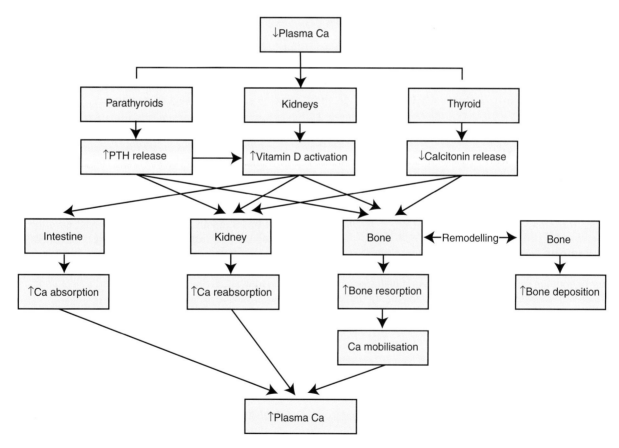

FIGURE 42-1 Calcium balance. Flowchart summarising the main factors regulating plasma calcium levels. Low calcium levels trigger increased release of PTH and vitamin D, and inhibit release of calcitonin, leading to conservation of calcium from the intestine, kidneys and bone, hence raising plasma calcium. Other factors involved (not shown) include phosphate levels, growth hormone, glucocorticoids, oestrogens, prolactin, and bone morphogenic proteins. Ca = calcium; PTH = parathyroid hormone. *Adapted from*: Grills 2002.

- in the kidneys, PTH increases the reabsorption of calcium in the distal convoluted tubule; conversely, reabsorption of phosphate and bicarbonate is inhibited
- in the intestine, calcium absorption is increased; this is an indirect effect, via increased activation of vitamin D in the kidneys
- in bone, PTH stimulates bone resorption by osteoclasts, thus **mobilising** calcium from bone.

By these integrated effects, PTH acts to increase inflow of calcium into extracellular fluid and protect against hypocalcaemia. Thus it is evident that the 'bottom line' in calcium balance is the level of calcium in the blood, as this provides the source for all calcium functions in the body; in this context, bone merely acts as a depot of calcium to be mobilised.

The mechanism of PTH action in the bone or kidney is incompletely understood; cAMP or calcium may mediate the cellular effects of PTH. Patients with hyperparathyroidism may be resistant to PTH action on kidney and bone. The decreased number of these receptors, not their altered affinity, produces a reduction in PTH-stimulated adenylate cyclase activity.

The new drug teriparatide, which consists of the active fragment (amino acids 1–34) of PTH, has recently become available for treatment of osteoporosis; see Drug Monograph 42-1.

Hypoparathyroidism

Hypoparathyroidism may be surgical (after surgery on the throat), autoimmune, familial or idiopathic. The signs and symptoms of hypoparathyroidism are those of hypocalcaemia (decreased serum calcium levels) and tetany; serum phosphate levels are raised (due to loss of PTH's phosphaturic effect). The symptoms include muscle spasms, convulsions, gradual paralysis with dyspnoea, and death from exhaustion. Before death, gastrointestinal haemorrhages and haematemesis often occur and at death the intestinal mucosa is congested.

The symptoms of tetany are relieved by administration of calcium salts (see Clinical Interest Box 42-1); PTH itself has too short a half-life to be useful clinically. Usually, vitamin D levels are low, so large doses of vitamin D also help to restore the normal calcium level in the blood and relieve tetany. The patient is hospitalised because frequent assessment of blood calcium and phosphate levels is essential.

Hyperparathyroidism

Primary **hyperparathyroidism** is the most common parathyroid disorder; it is hyperactivity of the parathyroid glands, with excessive secretion of parathyroid hormone. Generally, it is caused by a parathyroid adenoma or by spontaneous hyperplasia. PTH elevations produce increased resorption of calcium from the skeletal system and increased absorption of calcium by the kidneys and the gastrointestinal system. Elevated plasma levels of calcium with high urine phosphate levels can lead to renal stones, bone pain with skeletal lesions and, possibly, pathological fractures.

DRUG MONOGRAPH 42-1 TERIPARATIDE

A new drug to treat osteoporosis is **teriparatide**, a recombinant form of the active fragment of human PTH. It is referred to as a 'bone formation agent', as it activates osteoblasts via binding to specific PTH cell surface receptors.

INDICATIONS Teriparatide is indicated for treatment of osteoporosis in men and postmenopausal women, when other agents are unsuitable and there is a high risk of fractures. Calcium and vitamin D supplements are administered concurrently. Teriparatide has been shown to reduce the risk of new bone fractures and increase bone mineral density in the spine.

PHARMACOKINETICS Teriparatide is administered by SC injection; it has a high bioavailability and rapid absorption and elimination, with a half-life of approximately 1 hour. Metabolism is believed to occur in the liver and kidney.

DRUG INTERACTIONS As this is a very new drug, the range of drug interactions has not yet been identified.

ADVERSE REACTIONS In animal studies, high doses of teriparatide caused a higher incidence of osteosarcomas. The relevance of this finding to humans has not been determined; however, currently the lifetime maximum duration of teriparatide treatment has been set at 18 months, and all patients must have the possible risks explained and must give informed consent before treatment. Hypercalcaemia may be exacerbated. Other adverse reactions include nausea, headache, dizziness, leg cramps, arthralgia and hyperuricaemia.

WARNINGS AND CONTRAINDICATIONS
Teriparatide is contraindicated in hyperparathyroidism, hypercalcaemia and Paget's disease of bone. It is not recommended for use in pregnancy, lactation or in children.

DOSAGE AND ADMINISTRATION Teriparatide is formulated as an injection and provided in a preloaded disposable delivery device ('pen'), which can be used for up to 28 days and should be stored refrigerated. The usual daily dose is 20 mcg SC once daily.

Adapted from: AMH 2006; Caswell 2005.

Because tumours may cause this syndrome, surgery is usually the first-line treatment. In patients with mild hypercalcaemia or mild hyperparathyroidism, a thorough examination by a physician determines whether or not surgery is indicated. High serum levels of calcium may require immediate treatment (see below under Hypercalcaemia).

Secondary hyperparathyroidism occurs commonly in renal osteodystrophy associated with chronic renal insufficiency, and often requires parathyroidectomy. Prophylactic low doses of vitamin D and calcium may prevent the parathyroid cell hyperplasia that occurs to compensate for low plasma calcium levels resulting from inadequate renal activation of vitamin D.

A new treatment for hyperparathyroidism is cinacalcet, termed a 'calcimimetic agent', as it modulates the calcium-sensing receptors, increasing the receptors' sensitivity to calcium and thus reducing PTH secretion. Calcium and phosphorus levels are also reduced. Cinacalcet is indicated in some cases of primary hyperparathyroidism, in patients with chronic kidney disease on dialysis with secondary hyperparathyroidism, and in hyperparathyroidism secondary to hypocalcaemia. The low bioavailablity of the drug from tablets is increased by taking with food; once-daily dosing is effective.

CALCIUM BALANCE AND MINERAL HOMEOSTASIS

Calcium

Calcium serves an important central position in cellular physiology and metabolic regulation; although 99% of body calcium is in bone, the remaining 1% of body calcium has major roles in:

- stabilising excitable cell membranes
- release of neurotransmitters and formation of secretions
- second-messenger functions inside cells
- muscle contractility
- exocytosis of hormones and other regulators
- blood coagulation and platelet aggregation.

The level of extracellular and intracellular calcium is tightly controlled. Calcium homeostasis has to maintain exact levels of calcium, despite varying amounts of absorption in the diet and excretion via the kidneys and faeces. It must provide for calcium in bones and teeth, and maintain a gradient across cell membranes such that the level of calcium inside cells is only 1/10,000 of that outside. The hormones regulating calcium balance are PTH (see above), calcitonin and vitamin D (see Figure 42-1).

The recommended daily intake (RDI) of calcium is 0.3–2 g/day; requirements are higher in pregnancy and in postmenopausal women (to prevent osteoporosis—see later discussion). The main sources of calcium in the diet are dairy produce, soybeans, spinach, yeast products and nuts. Many milk products now have 'high calcium' to encourage adequate intake; for example, while normal whole milk contains about 120 mg calcium per 100 mL (and 3.4 g fat), low-fat milk contains about 138 mg calcium and 0.1 g fat per 100 mL, and high-calcium milk contains 175 mg calcium and 0.1–1.3 g fat per 100 mL. (Clinical Interest Box 42-1 lists some calcium salts present in calcium supplement tablets or capsules.)

Hypocalcaemia

The main cause of low calcium levels is hypoparathyroidism, as explained above. Kidney problems can cause renal osteodystrophy because of low vitamin D levels. **Hypocalcaemia** leads to hyperexcitability of nerves, manifest as paraesthesias ('pins and needles'), spasms (including arrhythmias, dysphonia and dysphagia), tetany and fits.

Treatment in the acute situation is with calcium. Moderate hypocalcaemia can be controlled with the vitamin D analogue calcitriol. Calcium is also used to prevent and treat osteoporosis. It is given orally and also IV, but not IM or SC, as solutions are irritant. Calcium can interact adversely with other drugs, including digoxin (causing arrhythmias), bisphosphonates (decreasing their absorption), calcium channel blockers (a physiological antagonism), and tetracyclines (causing yellow discoloration of teeth and bones). Table 42-1 lists drugs used to treat hypocalcaemia.

Hypercalcaemia

The most common cause of **hypercalcaemia** is hyperparathyroidism, due to an adenoma of the parathyroid gland causing excessive secretion of PTH. Excess vitamin D also causes excess calcium to be retained and, in various malignancies, osteolytic bone metastases and hypercalcaemia occur. Excess calcium may also be consumed as calcium salts in other medications, including antacids. The manifestations are weakness, arrhythmias, nausea and vomiting, constipation and ectopic calcification, e.g. as kidney stones. Treatment is by rehydration and with calcitonin or bisphosphonate drugs. Table 42-2 describes typical recommendations for treatment of hypercalcaemia.

Calcitonin

Calcitonin, the third major hormone product of the thyroid gland, was discovered in 1961. It is a polypeptide secreted by thyroid C cells when there is a high calcium concentration in the blood, especially when this is due to conditions of increased bone resorption. Calcitonin inhibits bone resorption and calcium reabsorption in the kidney, hence lowering

CLINICAL INTEREST BOX 42-1 CALCIUM SUPPLEMENTS

With the general recognition of the importance of **calcium** in bone structure and in prevention of osteoporosis in our ageing population, calcium has become 'trendy' and calcium supplements abound. Formulations available in supermarkets and health food shops, marketed as multivitamin or mineral preparations, may contain very little calcium (range: about 1.8 mg/tablet to 200 mg/tablet); average amount appears to be about 40–80 mg. Tablets marketed as mineral supplements may contain much higher levels, e.g. 300–600 mg, even up to 1 g calcium/tablet. Note that as some of the salts contain only a small proportion of calcium (e.g. calcium gluconate: 9% calcium), it is important to check the dose on bottle labels as mg calcium rather than mg calcium salt.

The activity of calcium depends on calcium ion (elemental) content. The approximate calcium contents of typical calcium supplements are listed as milligrams Ca per gram salt, milliequivalents Ca per gram salt, or percentage of calcium in the salt. The average number of tablets providing 1.5 g calcium (RDI for postmenopausal women) is also calculated.

Preparation	Calcium (mg/g)	Calcium (meq/g)	% Calcium	Calcium/salt in tablet (mg)	Tablets needed to provide 1500 mg calcium
Calcium carbonate	400	20.0	40	80/200	19
				140/350	11
				500/1250	3
				600/1500	3
Calcium citrate	211	10.5	21.1	164/780	9
				250/1190	6
Calcium gluconate	90	4.5	9	45/500	33
				1.8/20	>830
Calcium lactate	130	6.5	13	42/325	36
Calcium phosphate				115/500	13
Dibasic (CaHPO$_4$)	230	11.5	23	140/600	11
Tribasic (Ca$_3$(PO$_4$)$_2$)	380	19	38	16/40	>90
				220/570	7
				1000/2500	1.6
Calcium amino acid chelate	?	?	20	100/500	15

CLINICAL INTEREST BOX 42-2
GETTING ENOUGH CALCIUM

Good **calcium** intake, especially in adolescence and pregnancy, is important for building and maintaining strong bones and preventing osteoporosis. The main dietary sources of calcium for the New Zealand population are milk, cheese and other dairy products (53% of all calcium). The 1997 New Zealand National Nutrition Survey, carried out by staff of the University of Otago, conducted home interviews with 4636 New Zealand adults, including 704 Maori, with the following findings related to calcium and dairy food intake:
- a high proportion of young Maori and Maori women of all ages had inadequate intakes of calcium
- fewer Maori women (29%) consumed yoghurt at least once per week, compared with Pakeha women (49%)
- fewer Maori consumed cheese at least once per week, compared with Pakeha women
- only 15% of Maori chose trim or low-fat milk most often (the majority, 83%, preferred the standard milk with lower calcium content)
- both Maori and Pakeha reported similar consumption of ice cream, milk puddings, custard and other dairy foods.

Adapted from: Russell et al 1999.

plasma calcium levels. Calcitonin can thus be considered as a natural antagonist of the actions of PTH and vitamin D (see Figure 42-1). It has also been reported to have analgesic activity, possibly mediated by endorphins.

TABLE 42-1 Treatment of hypocalcaemia

DRUG	USUAL ADULT DOSE
Calcium gluconate	IV: 10–20 mL of 10% solution given slowly over 5–10 minutes (magnesium may also be required); then oral calcium 1.5–4 g/day in three divided doses
Vitamin D analogues	
Cholecalciferol (vitamin D$_3$)	Available only in low dose (100–400 IU, 2.5–10 mcg) in multivitamin or mineral preparations
Calcitriol	Oral: 0.25 mcg daily, increased every 2–4 weeks if necessary IV: 0.5 mcg three times a week, increased every 2–4 weeks if necessary
Ergocalciferol (vitamin D$_2$)	Oral: individualised dosing; prophylaxis dose is 5–10 mcg daily; the only formulation available is a 25 mcg (1000 IU) capsule

TABLE 42-2 Treatment of hypercalcaemia

Increase calcium excretion

Saline rehydration and diuresis	Infuse normal saline (100–200 mL/h) to increase calcium excretion. Monitor fluid intake, output and electrolytes. Watch closely for evidence of fluid overload.

Inhibit bone resorption

Salcatonin	Slow IV infusion/injection: 4–8 IU/kg every 6–12 hours. Tolerance can develop in 24–72 hours, so corticosteroids may be prescribed concurrently.
Pamidronate	Slow IV infusion: normally 60 mg/hour; has the advantage of being effective in a single dose.

Adapted from: AMH 2006; Tuckwell 1996.

CLINICAL INTEREST BOX 42-3 VITAMIN D

'Vitamin D' refers to a group of molecules derived from cholesterol. These sterols can be metabolised in the body to the active compound (1,25-dihydroxycholecalciferol), hence they are not, strictly speaking, vitamins. Many sterol sources and tissues are involved in the production of vitamin D:

- in the skin, cholesterol-derived provitamin D is converted to vitamin D$_3$ (cholecalciferol) by the action of UV rays in sunlight
- in the diet, a plant ergosterol derivative is present in some foods and added to fortified dairy products
- in the gut, ergocalciferol (vitamin D$_2$) is absorbed from the diet into the bloodstream
- in the liver, vitamin D is hydroxylated to 25-hydroxy-vitamin D (calcifidiol)
- in body fat, 25-hydroxyvitamin D is stored as the depot form
- in the kidneys, vitamin D is converted to its most active form, **calcitriol** (1,25-dihydroxycholecalciferol).

The significance of understanding this complicated pathway is that in various pathological conditions (e.g. malabsorption, liver disease, kidney failure) and in countries where people are not exposed to sufficient sunlight (due to long winters or highly protective clothing), sufficient active vitamin D cannot be produced, so calcium balance is impaired and hypocalcaemia can result. This leads to the conditions **rickets** (in children) and **osteomalacia** (in adults), marked by defects in bone mineralisation, with bone weakness, bending and distortion. It is prevented or treated with a vitamin D compound (ergocalciferol or calcitriol); this is effective in relieving hypocalcaemia but cannot correct already deformed bones.

Nutritional rickets, thought to have been cured in the early part of the 20th century when vitamin D and its role in bone strength were discovered, has made an unexpected return in recent years throughout the world. Even in sunny Australia, there are increasing numbers of case reports, thought to be due to low dietary intake of vitamin D and decreased sunshine exposure, particularly in children and women who wear long protective clothing, and in the elderly who are house-bound or in residential care (see Abrams 2002; Wark 2003).

Sources of calcitonin used in the past have included active extracts of porcine, human and salmon thyroid tissue. The salmon hormone is particularly potent, has a slightly longer half-life and has been given the approved name **salcatonin** (Drug Monograph 42-2). Porcine and human products have been discontinued in Australia.

Vitamin D

'Vitamin D' is really a family of steroid-type hormones derived from the diet and metabolised and activated in the body (see Clinical Interest Box 42-3 and Figure 37-2G). It is involved in calcium, phosphate and magnesium metabolism in bone and the gastrointestinal tract. Its actions are to raise the plasma calcium level by increasing calcium absorption (in the intestine), by reabsorption (in the kidney distal tubule), and mobilisation (from bone)—actions similar to those of PTH. Vitamin D's mechanism of action is similar to that of the steroid hormones: it enters the nucleus and sets in train a series of reactions leading to gene transcription and synthesis of calcium-binding proteins and bone matrix proteins. Vitamin D also has a permissive role in PTH actions. Requirements are increased during growth, pregnancy and lactation (Drug Monograph 42-3).

BONE MINERAL HOMEOSTASIS AND PHOSPHATE LEVELS

Bone has three major functions:
- providing rigid support for the body and cavities
- acting as levers and sites of attachment for muscles in locomotion
- providing a reservoir of ions, especially calcium, phosphate, magnesium and sodium.

Bone is constantly renewing itself in the process of **remodelling**, as old bone is resorbed by osteoclast cells and new bone deposited by osteoblasts. Until the age of about 20–25 years, bone mass increases and stabilises as the bone growth achieved during childhood and adolescence is consolidated; thereafter, during adulthood, bone is lost slowly. Elderly people are likely to suffer from osteoporosis (softened bones), leaving them at higher risk of fractures.

The process of bone remodelling is integrated by many endocrine and other factors, including those already discussed, such as vitamin D, PTH, calcitonin and plasma calcium levels (see Figure 42-1). Many other factors are still being identified and studied, including 'bone morphogenic proteins' (e.g. osteocalcin and osteonectin) and various growth factors and neuropeptides. The daily turnover of calcium in and out of bone is estimated to be at least 500 mg, i.e. about half of the average daily dietary requirements for calcium. Increased bone resorption (stimulated by PTH and vitamin D) leads to **mobilisation** of calcium from bone, i.e. calcium is released into the extracellular fluid and made available for physiological actions.

Phosphate balance

Bone resorption also mobilises phosphate from the calcium phosphate present in bone, mainly as hydroxyapatite. Phosphate is involved in many biochemical pathways, e.g. energy balance and phosphorylation of enzymes; as a component of nucleic acids, phospholipids and proteins; and in buffering systems in body fluids. Although the specific mechanisms regulating phosphate levels are not well identified, overall, vitamin D and PTH tend to increase calcium reabsorption from the kidney tubules while increasing phosphate excretion, thus conserving calcium but removing phosphate. Phosphate is present in many foods, so phosphate supplements are rarely needed.

BONE PATHOLOGIES
Rickets and osteomalacia

These conditions have been described above as deficiencies of vitamin D (Clinical Interest Box 42-3). They are characterised by demineralised bones, which are weak and soft; treatment is with vitamin D.

DRUG MONOGRAPH 42-2 SALCATONIN (SALMON CALCITONIN)

Calcitonin is the calcium-lowering hormone. The salmon extract **salcatonin** has the same physiological actions as the human hormone; it is now produced synthetically.

INDICATIONS Salcatonin is indicated for the treatment of Paget's bone disease and hypercalcaemia.

PHARMACOKINETICS Because it is a peptide, calcitonin cannot be administered orally; it is usually given SC, but also IM and IV. The elimination half-life is 60–90 minutes but the biological half-life is considerably longer. The peak effect in hypercalcaemia occurs in 2 hours and the duration of action is 6–8 hours. Tachyphylaxis develops over several days. Excretion of metabolites is via the kidneys.

Onset of the therapeutic effect in Paget's disease may range from 6 to 24 months of regular treatment, although some improvement (measured by a decrease in serum alkaline phosphatase levels) may occur within the first few months.

ADVERSE REACTIONS AND DRUG INTERACTIONS No significant drug interactions have been reported. Adverse effects include flushing or a tingling sensation of the face and hands, increased urinary frequency, nausea, vomiting, and pain or swelling at the injection site. Allergic reactions and antibody development can occur.

CONTRAINDICATIONS Avoid use in people with a history of protein allergy or calcitonin hypersensitivity. Few data are available on use in children, pregnancy or lactation.

DOSAGE AND ADMINISTRATION The usual salcatonin adult dosage for Paget's disease is 5 IU/kg daily, increasing to 10 IU/kg daily; treatment for months or years is required. To reduce the occurrence of nausea or flushing, bedtime administration is suggested; if necessary, a reduction in dosage may be initiated.

DRUG MONOGRAPH 42-3 CALCITRIOL

There are several forms of **vitamin D** available. Vitamins D_2 and D_3 require activation in the liver and kidney, and have a slow onset (4–8 weeks) and long duration of action (8–16 weeks). They are useful for preventing vitamin D deficiencies in people with adequate kidney function. **Calcitriol** is the preactivated form of the vitamin.

INDICATIONS Calcitriol is indicated in vitamin D deficiencies, hypocalcaemia, hypoparathyroidism, renal osteodystrophy, chronic renal dialysis (which may remove calcium or vitamin D) and postmenopausal and corticosteroid-induced osteoporosis.

PHARMACOKINETICS Calcitriol is well absorbed from the intestine, requiring bile salts for absorption. It enters the enterohepatic circulation and metabolites (some active) are excreted in the faeces and urine; some are stored in fat. The elimination half-life is about 3–6 hours but the effects of a single dose last for several days. It is transported across the placenta (ADEC Pregnancy Safety Category B3) and into breast milk, hence it is contraindicated during pregnancy and lactation.

ADVERSE DRUG REACTIONS AND INTERACTIONS
The main adverse effects are those of hypercalcaemia, i.e. gastrointestinal disturbances, polyuria and ectopic calcification (see above). Significant interactions occur with digoxin (arrhythmias), cholestyramine (impaired absorption) and thiazide diuretics (hypercalcaemia).

DOSAGE AND ADMINISTRATION Calcitriol is usually administered orally. It is highly potent, the average dosage being 0.25 mcg twice daily. Concurrent multi-vitamin preparations and calcium supplements should be avoided because of the risk of hypercalcaemia.

Paget's disease of bone (osteitis deformans)

Paget's disease is a focal disorder of bone remodelling, with greatly increased rates of bone turnover and disorganised remodelling, leading to soft, poorly mineralised bone; hypercalcaemia; bone pain; limb deformities; fractures; deafness* and neurological problems. The aetiology is unknown but a viral cause is suspected. It is estimated to affect 3%–4% of middle-aged to elderly Australians but only a small proportion (5%) of these may require treatment.

Treatment is with calcitonin analgesics and bisphosphonates (see below). A cytotoxic antibiotic, plicamycin (mithramycin), which inhibits osteoclastic activity, was formerly used in Paget's disease and hypercalcaemia but has been withdrawn because of excessive toxicity. Serum and urine markers of bone turnover are monitored and surgery may be necessary to free entrapped nerves or in cases of spinal cord compression.

Osteoporosis

Osteoporosis refers to increased bone fragility and consequent risk of fracture due to reduced bone density—the lower the bone density, the greater the risk of low-trauma bone fracture, especially fractures of the vertebrae, hip or forearm. Osteoporosis is an important health problem: as described earlier, bone strength is lost progressively during the adult

---

* This is thought to have been the cause of the total deafness of famous composer Ludwig van Beethoven (1770–1827); on autopsy, he was shown to have a dense skull vault and shrivelled auditory nerves due to compression by proliferated bones. He also suffered from severe depression, and liver, kidney and pancreatic disease (Wolf 1994).

years, so osteoporosis has an increasing prevalence in our community as the proportion of the population aged 65 and over increases. (It is estimated that by the year 2050, people aged over 65 will comprise 22% of the Australian population; the incidence of vertebral wedge fractures in women over 70 years is 20%–25%). Fractures contribute significantly to morbidity, mortality and growing health-care costs.

There are many risk factors for osteoporosis in women: late menarche (first menstrual period), episodic amenorrhoea and early menopause. These all indicate the protective effect oestrogens normally have on bones. Low calcium intake, excessive phosphate, no or excessive exercise, tobacco, caffeine and excessive alcohol are also contributing factors. Drugs such as long-term glucocorticoids or thyroid hormones, antacids, anticonvulsants, antidepressants and sedatives are all implicated. Malabsorption syndromes, hyperparathyroidism and other endocrine disorders can also impair calcium balance.

Management involves assessing risk factors and contributing conditions, measures to reduce the risk of falls, measuring bone density by densitometry techniques, and attention to diet, vitamin D and calcium intake (recommended 1–1.5 g/day in postmenopausal women). The imperative to treat increases with increasing age, declining bone mineral density, history of previous fragility fracture and the presence of multiple risk factors for osteoporosis.

The primary aim of treatment for osteoporosis is to reduce the risk of fragility fractures. First-line therapies for osteoporosis are those with the best evidence in reducing fragility fractures, namely the potent bisphosphonates (alendronate and risedronate), raloxifene, strontium ranelate and teriparatide. Some of the available therapies for osteoporosis include:

- calcium 1.5 g/day to maintain bone minerals. Calcium should be adjunctive therapy for all people with osteoporosis, unless contraindicated (e.g. hypercalcaemia)

DRUG MONOGRAPH 42-4   ALENDRONATE, A BISPHOSPHONATE

Alendronate has the actions of the bisphosphonates: it impedes bone resorption and reduces bone turnover.

INDICATIONS Alendronate is indicated in Paget's disease, for the prevention and treatment of postmenopausal osteoporosis, and for preventing and treating corticosteroid-induced osteoporosis. Other drugs in the group may also be indicated for hypercalcaemia associated with cancer, heterotopic ossification and osteolytic metastases (bone metastases).

PHARMACOKINETICS Alendronate has most unusual pharmacokinetic characteristics: it has virtually zero bioavailability, zero plasma levels and no metabolism, and a (terminal) half-life of more than 10 years! This is because the drug is taken up 50% into the bones, where it forms a stable depot for several weeks; the remaining 50% of an oral dose is excreted in the urine unchanged.

DRUG INTERACTIONS Oral medications, including antacids and mineral supplements, and food or beverages may interfere with the absorption of alendronate. Administration of the medications should

be separated by at least 2 hours. Alendronate increases the risk of gastric ulceration with NSAIDs, so the combination should be avoided.

ADVERSE REACTIONS These include gas production, acid regurgitation, oesophageal ulcer, gastritis, dysphagia, constipation, diarrhoea, muscle pain and headaches.

WARNINGS AND CONTRAINDICATIONS Use all bisphosphonates with caution in patients with gastrointestinal diseases and kidney impairment, or if the patient is reportedly hypersensitive to them.

DOSAGE AND ADMINISTRATION Because of the risk of oesophagitis, it is recommended that bisphosphonates be taken with a full glass of liquid and that the patient remain upright for at least the next 30 minutes, to facilitate delivery of the dose to the stomach.

The usual adult dosage of alendronate for Paget's disease is 40 mg daily (at least 30 minutes before breakfast) for 6 months; for osteoporosis, the dosage is 5–10 mg once daily.

- potent bisphosphonates (alendronate and risedronate) to decrease bone resorption and fracture risk
- raloxifene, a selective oestrogen receptor modulator (SERM),* decreases bone resorption. It is used for the treatment and prevention of postmenopausal osteoporosis
- parathyroid hormone or teriparatide stimulates bone formation. It is used for the treatment of severe osteoporosis when the risk of fracture is extremely high, or if other effective therapies are unsuitable
- strontium ranelate stimulates bone formation and inhibits bone resorption to reduce fracture risk in postmenopausal women
- hormone replacement therapy (HRT), especially oestrogens, to oppose PTH actions on bone resorption and calcium mobilisation. Presently, only short-term therapy is recommended and HT is not recommended as sole therapy for fracture prevention
- calcitonin, to inhibit bone resorption (hence less calcium is mobilised so calcium may be lowered)
- vitamin D preparations, to increase plasma calcium if osteomalacia is present or if there is evidence of vitamin D deficiency (but bone resorption may be increased). Supplemental calcium is not usually recommended with therapies that increase plasma calcium.

*We are using the English spelling for oestrogen rather than the American (estrogen); however, the accepted abbreviation for the selective oestrogen receptor modulator group of drugs is SERM.

EFFECTS OF DRUGS ON BONE

Oestrogens

During their reproductive years, women have low risk of osteoporosis. This is attributed to the protective effects of oestrogens, which may oppose the actions of PTH on bone (PTH increases resorption and mobilises calcium).

The SERM raloxifene has partial agonist and partial antagonist oestrogenic properties. It has positive effects on bone and lipid metabolism and antagonistic effects on the uterus and breast, minimising the risk of oestrogen-dependent cancers. Consequently, raloxifene prevents bone resorption without stimulating breast or uterine tissue. Recent evidence is emerging that raloxifene is as effective as tamoxifen, another SERM, at preventing oestrogen-receptor positive breast cancer in women at increased risk of breast cancer (Vogel et al 2006). This group of drugs is considered in the chapter on the female reproductive system (Chapter 44).

Corticosteroids

Corticosteroids are known to increase the risk of osteoporosis, which is an adverse effect of long–term glucocorticoid use; osteoporosis-related fractures occur in 30%–50% of patients receiving long-term glucocorticoids. Several mechanisms have been proposed: glucocorticoids impair transcription of the collagenase gene and block induction of the osteocalcin (calcium-binding) gene by vitamin D, reduce intestinal calcium absorption, increase urinary excretion of calcium and inhibit osteoblasts.

Bisphosphonates

The bisphosphonates have been designed to decrease bone turnover. They are enzyme-resistant analogues of pyrophosphate (i.e. the basic structure P–O–P), which is a natural inhibitor of bone mineralisation. The bisphosphonates have the general structure P–C–P, with two phosphonate groups linked by carbon rather than oxygen, making them more resistant to enzymatic inactivation.

It appears that the drugs are incorporated into bone, where they form a depot for some months, and act to inhibit normal and abnormal resorption, primarily by decreasing the activity of osteoclasts. The early drugs in the group, especially etidronate, in high doses reduced bone formation, making them less useful in treating disorders of bone. Later drugs (alendronate [Drug Monograph 42-4], clodronate, pamidronate and risedronate) inhibit bone resorption without inhibiting bone formation, so they are useful for decreasing abnormal bone growth in Paget's disease. Clodronate, pamidronate and zoledronic acid are especially indicated for treatment of hypercalcaemia of malignancy (a condition caused by PTH-like protein secreted by various tumours, including renal and breast carcinomas).

Strontium and strontium ranelate

Strontium, an element with chemical properties very similar to those of calcium, has long been known to have 'bone-seeking' roles: at moderate supplementation levels strontium

PREGNANCY SAFETY	
ADEC Category	**Drug**
B2	Salcatonin, tiludronate
B3	Alendronate, calcitriol, cinacalcet, clodronate, etidronate, pamidronate, risedronate, strontium ranelate, teriparatide, zoledronic acid
X	Raloxifene
Not classified	Calcium salts (e.g. calcium gluconate), cholecalciferol, ergocalciferol, phosphate supplements, vitamin D

Note: The bisphosphonates, being strongly alkaline, are usually present as their sodium or disodium salts; for simplicity, the drugs are referred to by just the basic form, '-dronate'.

promotes calcium uptake into bone, whereas at higher dietary levels strontium has rachitogenic (causing rickets) actions. A derivative, strontium ranelate, was approved in Australia in July 2005 for use in treatment of osteoporosis. The ranelate radical is an unusual five-membered ring with sulphur and cyanide substituents, and four carboxyl 'arms' which act as carriers of calcium or strontium; thus the molecule has a unique mode of action, decreasing bone resorption and increasing bone formation.

After oral administration, the molecule dissociates and strontium is taken into bone; it is slowly released and eventually excreted (half-life: 60 hours) by the gut and kidney. Clinically, strontium ranelate has been shown to be effective, in postmenopausal women with a history of bone fractures, in reducing incidence of new fractures and increasing bone mineral density. Adverse reactions include headache, nausea, diarrhoea, increased risk of venous thromboembolism, and neurological problems.

DRUGS AT A GLANCE 42: Drugs affecting the parathyroid gland			
Therapeutic group	**Pharmacological group**	**Key examples**	**Key pages**
Drugs treating hypocalcaemia	Calcium salts	calcium carbonate, calcium gluconate	687, 8
	Vitamin D analogues	calcitriol ⎫ ergocalciferol ⎭	689–91
Drugs treating hypercalcaemia	Calcitonin analogues	salcatonin	687, 90
Drugs treating osteoporosis	Bisphosphonates	alendronate, pamidronate	692, 3
	Parathyroid hormone analogues	teriparatide	685, 6
	Calcium uptake promoters	strontium ranelate	693
Drugs treating hyperparathyroidism	Calcimimetic agents	cinacalcet	687
	Phosphate supplements	phosphates	690

KEY POINTS

- The parathyroid glands synthesise and secrete parathyroid hormone (PTH), a peptide hormone that maintains appropriate calcium levels in the extracellular fluid.

- In hypoparathyroidism, severe hypocalcaemia and tetany can occur; the use of vitamin D and calcium supplements will usually restore the calcium and phosphorus levels to normal.

- In hyperparathyroidism, the primary approach is usually surgery; hypercalcaemia also responds to rehydration, calcitonin and bisphosphonate drugs.

- Calcium has important roles in the body both in physiological processes and in bone structure; calcium balance is tightly controlled by PTH, calcitonin and vitamin D.

- Bone undergoes continual remodelling; bone resorption leads to mobilisation of both calcium and phosphate from bone components.

- Impaired bone formation and remodelling leads to the pathological states of Paget's disease, osteoporosis, rickets and osteomalacia; dietary deficiencies and administered drugs can also lead to bone diseases.

- Calcium, PTH, calcitonin, vitamin D, oestrogens and the bisphosphonate group of drugs (which decrease bone turnover) are used to treat bone diseases.

- Generally, these therapies provide hormone replacement or hormone inhibition, so close patient monitoring is necessary to avoid over- or undertreatment of the pathological state and to maintain appropriate calcium balance.

REVIEW EXERCISES

1   Describe the condition and treatment for hypoparathyroidism and for primary hyperparathyroidism.

2   Summarise the mechanisms in the body that regulate blood calcium levels.

3   Describe the actions, indications, drug interactions, major adverse effects and adverse reactions, and dosage and administration for salcatonin, calcitriol and the bisphosphonates.

4   Discuss the actions of drugs that cause adverse effects in the bones.

5   Describe the aetiology, epidemiology and management of osteoporosis.

REFERENCES AND FURTHER READING

Abrams SA. Nutritional rickets: an old disease returns. *Nutrition Reviews* 2002; 60(4): 111–5.

Australian Medicines Handbook 2006. Adelaide: AMH, 2006.

Barman Balfour JA, Scott LJ. Cinacalcet hydrochloride. *Drugs* 2005; 65(2): 271–81.

Beckerman P, Silver J. Vitamin D and the parathyroid. *American Journal of the Medical Sciences* 1999; 317(6): 363–9.

Brown EM, Pollak M, Hebert SC. The extracellular calcium-sensing receptor: its role in health and disease. *Annual Review of Medicine* 1998; 49: 15–29.

Caswell A (ed.). *MIMS Annual June 2005.* Sydney: CMPMedica Australia, 2005.

Ebeling PR. Bisphosphonates—clinical applications in osteoporosis. *Australian Prescriber* 2000; 23(6): 133–6.

Endocrinology Expert Group. *Therapeutic Guidelines: Endocrinology, version 3.* Melbourne: Therapeutic Guidelines Limited, 2004.

Gaudio A, Morabito N. Pharmacological management of severe postmenopausal osteoporosis. *Drugs and Aging* 2005; 22(5): 405–17.

Greenspan FS, Strewler GJ. *Basic & Clinical Endocrinology.* 5th edn. Stamford: Appleton & Lange, 1997 [ch. 8].

Grills B. Osseous structure and function: study guide. Melbourne: La Trobe University, 2002 [unpublished].

Hory B, Drueke TB. The parathyroid–bone axis in uremia: new insights into old questions. *Current Opinion in Nephrology and Hypertension* 1997; 6(1): 40–8.

Jones G, Strugnell SA, DeLuca HF. Current understanding of the molecular actions of vitamin D. *Physiological Reviews* 1998; 78(4): 1193–231.

Kleerekoper M (ed.). *Drug Therapy for Osteoporosis.* London: Taylor & Francis, 2005.

Marie PJ. Strontium ranelate: a novel mode of action optimizing bone formation and resorption. *Osteoporosis International* 2005; 16 Suppl 1: S7–10.

Martin TJ. Bisphosphonates—mechanisms of action. *Australian Prescriber* 2000; 23(6): 130–2.

Nguyen TV, Center JR, Eisman JA. Osteoporosis: underrated, underdiagnosed and undertreated. *Medical Journal of Australia* 2004; 180 (5 Suppl): S18–22.

Pors Nielsen S. The biological role of strontium. *Bone* 2004; 35(3): 583–8.

Russell D, Parnell W, Wilson N et al. *NZ Food: NZ People. Key results of the 1997 National Nutrition Survey.* Wellington: New Zealand Minstry of Health, 1999.

Sambrook P, O'Neill S, Diamond T et al. Postmenopausal osteoporosis treatment guidelines. *Australian Family Physician* 2000; 29(8) 751–8.

Sambrook PN. Steroid-induced osteoporosis. *Annals of the Academy of Medicine, Singapore* 2002; 31(1): 48–53.

Seeman E, Eisman JA. Treatment of osteoporosis: why, whom, when and how to treat. *Medical Journal of Australia* 2004; 180(6): 298–303.

Speight TM, Holford NHG (eds). *Avery's Drug Treatment*. 4th edn. Auckland: Adis International, 1997.

Tuckwell K (ed.). *MIMS Disease Index*. 2nd edn. Sydney: MediMedia Australia, 1996.

Vogel VG, Constantino JP, Wickerham DL et al. Effects of tamoxifen vs raloxifene on the risk of developing invasive breast cancer and other disease outcomes: the NSABP Study of Tamoxifen and Raloxifene (STAR) P-2 trial. *Journal of the American Medical Association* 2006; 295: 2727–41.

Wark JD. Calcium supplementation: the bare bones. *Australian Prescriber* 2003; 26(6): 126–7.

Willhite L. Osteoporosis in women: prevention and treatment. *Journal of the American Pharmaceutical Association* 1998; 38(5): 614–24.

Wolf PL. If clinical chemistry had existed then … . *Clinical Chemistry* 1994; 40(2): 328–35.

ON-LINE RESOURCES

New Zealand medicines and medical devices safety authority: www.medsafe.govt.nz

evolve   More weblinks at http://evolve.elsevier.com/AU/Bryant/pharmacology/

UNIT XII
Drugs Affecting the Reproductive Systems

Overview of the Female and Male Reproductive Systems

CHAPTER FOCUS

This chapter reviews the anatomy and physiology of the female and male reproductive systems and their control by higher centres, as groundwork for the next four chapters, which discuss the drugs affecting the reproductive systems. Because privacy and cultural sensitivities often influence perceptions of reproductive disorders, care for patients with dysfunctions of the reproductive system is particularly challenging for the health-care professional. Thus, knowledge of reproductive anatomy and physiology and of the drugs that affect them is required for sensitive and appropriate health care, teaching and counselling.

OBJECTIVES

- To review the hypothalamic factors and anterior pituitary gland hormones that influence the female and male reproductive systems.

- To identify the primary male and female sex hormones and discuss their physiological functions.

- To describe hormonal influences on the uterus during the various stages of the menstrual cycle.

- To trace the transport of sperm in the male body from production to ejaculation.

- To describe the physiological responses in the human male and female during sexual intercourse.

KEY DRUGS

human chorionic gonadotrophin (hCG)

KEY TERMS

androgens
fertilisation
follicle-stimulating hormone (FSH)
gametes
gonadotrophins
gonadotrophin-releasing hormone (GnRH)
gonads
luteinising hormone (LH)
menstrual cycle
menstruation
oestrogens
ovulation
progestogens
sexual reproduction
sexual response
testosterone

KEY ABBREVIATIONS

FSH	follicle-stimulating hormone
GnRH	gonadotrophin-releasing hormone
hCG	human chorionic gonadotrophin
HRT	hormone replacement therapy
ICSH	interstitial cell-stimulating hormone
LH	luteinising hormone
OC	oral contraceptive

ENDOCRINE GLANDS

SEXUAL reproduction is the process by which organisms produce offspring to perpetuate the species by means of male and female germ cells **(gametes)**. **Fertilisation** of the female gamete (egg, or ovum) by the male gamete (sperm cell, or spermatozoon) results in a cell containing one set of chromosomes (numbered 1–23) from each parent, making 23 pairs, or a total of 46 chromosomes. In human beings, the reproductive process is highly complex, involving reproductive organs, ducts and supporting structures specialised for producing gametes, facilitating fertilisation and sustaining the growth of the embryo and fetus. The reproductive system of the human female consists of the ovaries, oviducts (fallopian tubes), uterus and vagina (Figure 43-1). The major organs of the male reproductive system consist of the testes, seminal vesicles, prostate gland, bulbourethral glands and penis (Figure 43-2).

The human sex chromosomes (chromosome 23) determine the sex of the embryo (an 'X' chromosome from each parent resulting in a female [XX], or an X from the mother and a 'Y' chromosome from the father resulting in a male [XY]), and later also the development of the **gonads**, the primary sex organs (testes in males, ovaries in females), which produce the gametes, secrete sex hormones and form endocrine secretions. The main functions of the sex hormones are to:

- regulate the development of the accessory sex organs (including seminal vesicles, prostate gland, breasts, uterus and vagina) and secondary sexual characteristics (differences in skeletal and muscle size, body fat deposition, distribution of hair, pitch of voice, development of breasts)
- control ovulation and the menstrual cycle or maintain pregnancy
- stimulate spermatogenesis and regulate growth and anabolism.

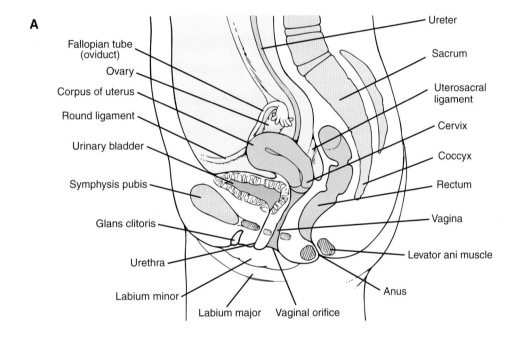

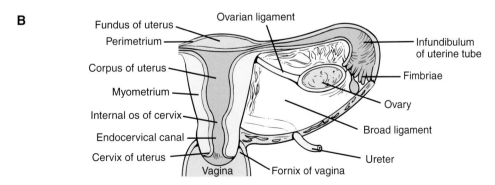

FIGURE 43-1 The female reproductive system. **A.** Sagittal section of pelvic area. **B.** Anterior section of the uterus, adnexa and upper vagina. *Modified from:* Salerno 1999.

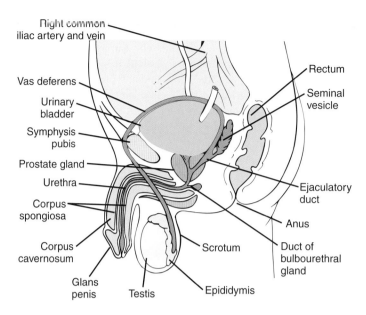

FIGURE 43-2 The male reproductive system, sagittal section. *Modified from*: Salerno 1999.

The main (gonadal) hormones concerned with reproduction in males are **androgens** (testosterone, dihydrotestosterone) and, in females, **oestrogens** (oestradiol, oestrone, oestriol) and **progestogens** (progesterone, hydroxyprogesterone). (Details of the actions of these hormones and their use as drugs will be covered in subsequent chapters; this chapter gives an overview of their functions and control systems.)

As with most other endocrine glands, there are several levels of control. The hypothalamus secretes a releasing factor (**gonadotrophin-releasing hormone [GnRH, gonadorelin]**), which stimulates the anterior pituitary gland to release **gonadotrophic hormones** (follicle-stimulating hormone [FSH] and luteinising hormone [LH]). These circulate in the bloodstream and act on target endocrine organs—the gonads (see Chapter 37, and Figures 37-1, 37-3 and 37-4, and Tables 37-1 and 37-2). Other hormones involved in reproduction include prolactin and oxytocin, from the anterior and posterior pituitary gland, respectively; the gonadal hormones; inhibin (which decreases secretion of FSH and LH); and hormones secreted during pregnancy by the placenta (chorionic gonadotrophin, and placental lactogen).

Later in life, gonadal function decreases. Women undergo menopause, or cessation of menses. Men have a decrease in sex hormone production, which may lead to physiological and psychological changes sometimes called the male climacteric.*

There has long been a dream of a 'fountain of youth' that would prevent the complex physical, mental and hormonal changes of ageing; many hormones, drugs and natural remedies have been tried. Hormone replacement therapy has been trialled in both women and men, with some positive results but also some adverse effects. Currently the best evidence is for prevention of hip fractures in predisposed older women by administration of vitamin D supplements and oestrogen (Horani & Morley 2004).

HYPOTHALAMIC AND PITUITARY CONTROL OF REPRODUCTIVE FUNCTIONS

Hypothalamic releasing factors

Gonadotrophin-releasing hormone (GnRH)

Formerly called FSH-releasing hormone or LH-releasing hormone, **GnRH** is a 10-amino-acid peptide secreted from the hypothalamus. GnRH has a similar role in the control of sex hormone release (Figures 43-3 and 43-4) to that of corticotrophin-releasing factor (CRF) in the control of adrenal cortex steroids. The actions of GnRH depend on how it is administered: at low (physiological) doses, and given in a pulsatile intermittent dose schedule, it stimulates pituitary synthesis and release of the pituitary gonadotrophins FSH and LH. By contrast, continuous administration in higher doses results in desensitisation and ultimately in decreased pituitary

---

*The term 'male menopause' is inappropriate, as 'menopause' literally means cessation of menstruation.

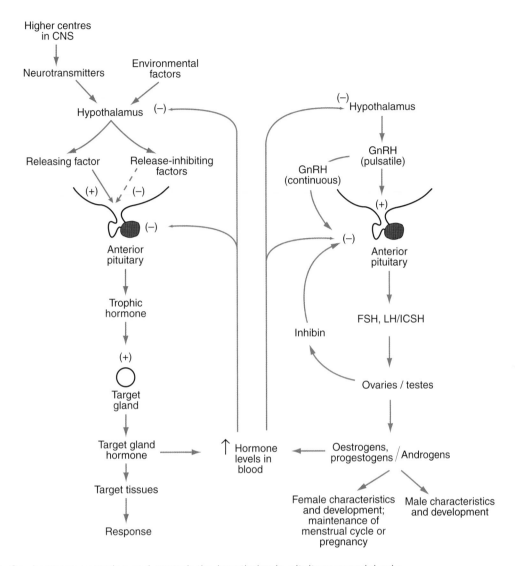

FIGURE 43-3 Sex hormone secretion and control: the hypothalamic–pituitary–gonadal axis.

production of LH and FSH; hence, there is suppression of production of sex hormones in the target glands (ovaries, testes), which can be used to inhibit growth of steroid-dependent tumours.

Gonadorelin was a synthetic form of GnRH identical to the natural hormone. It was used to induce ovulation and as an adjunct to other tests to diagnose hypogonadism in both males and females. There are also various synthetic GnRH analogues, with slightly different amino acid sequences, which are more potent and have longer durations of action. These are used at higher doses to suppress the pituitary (see Table 43-1).

GnRH inhibitors

Danazol is a compound that inhibits release of GnRH and is used to suppress the pituitary–ovarian axis, suppress menstruation and inhibit ovulation. It has complicated actions: it also alters sex hormone metabolism, interacts with sex hormone receptors and has weak androgenic and anabolic effects. It is mainly used in endometriosis, menorrhagia and fibrocystic breast disease. Common androgenic adverse effects include acne, hirsutism, vaginal dryness and hair loss. Danazol is contraindicated in pregnancy and lactation, cardiovascular disease and liver or kidney impairment. Another GnRH inhibitor, gestrinone, is also used in endometriosis, as it has no oestrogenic activity (although it does have some partial agonist actions at both progestogen and androgen receptors).

Two gonadotrophin-releasing hormone antagonists have recently been released for use by specialist physicians in assisted reproduction programs: cetrorelix and ganirelix. These drugs compete with GnRH for binding sites in the pituitary gland and prevent the surge in gonadotrophins that causes ovulation, so they can allow programmed timing of ovulation and harvesting of follicles.

TABLE 43-1 Characteristics of GnRH analogues

	GnRH ANALOGUE
Example	Goserelin, leuprorelin, nafarelin
Administration	Continuous, e.g. SC or IM depot, or nasal spray
Rationale	To suppress pituitary gonadotrophin release
Indications	Treatment of prostate or breast cancers, endometriosis, uterine fibroids, and before controlled ovarian stimulation
Half-life (roughly)	3–4 hours
Adverse reactions	Impaired fertility, decreased bone density; males: impotence, gynaecomastia; females: hot flushes, headache, pain, menstrual problems, hypercalcaemia
Precautions	Pregnancy, lactation

Pituitary gonadotrophic hormones

The pituitary **gonadotrophins**, FSH and LH, are glycoprotein hormones responsible for the development and maintenance of sexual gland functions. They can be purified and used clinically in male or female infertility and hypogonadism, and in combination with hCG for stimulation of multiple oocyte development in ovulatory patients who are using other technologies to conceive, such as gamete intrafallopian transfer (GIFT) or in-vitro fertilisation (IVF).

Prescribing of these hormones is usually restricted to specialists, such as endocrinologists and physicians involved in assisted reproduction clinics, as close monitoring of hormone levels and responses is essential.

Follicle-stimulating hormone stimulates the development of the Graafian ovarian follicles up to the point of ovulation in the female, which in turn brings on the characteristic changes of oestrus (menstruation in women); in the male, FSH stimulates the development of the seminiferous tubules and promotes spermatogenesis.

Luteinising hormone, also known in the male as interstitial-cell-stimulating hormone (ICSH), acts in the female to promote the maturation of the follicle, the formation of the corpus luteum and the secretion of oestrogen. In the male, ICSH stimulates spermatogenesis, the growth of interstitial cells in the testes and the formation of the androgenic hormones.

Other natural gonadotrophins include **human chorionic gonadotrophin (hCG)**, secreted by the chorion (the outer membrane enveloping the fetus); this hormone is measurable in the urine of pregnant women within a few days of fertilisation and is the antigen detected in pregnancy tests. hCG has mainly LH-type actions and is used to induce ovulation and to treat hypogonadism (see Drug Monograph 43-1). New recombinant forms of chorionic gonadotrophin are choriogonadotropin alfa and lutropin alfa; these are used

for their LH activities.

Other gonadotrophins prepared by recombinant DNA technology are follitropin alfa and beta. They are used for their FSH-type actions.

THE FEMALE REPRODUCTIVE SYSTEM

The anatomy of the organs, ducts and glands that constitute the female reproductive system is shown in Figure 43-1.

Hormonal control of the female reproductive system

The hypothalamic factor GnRH, which regulates anterior pituitary release of gonadotropic hormones, has been discussed in the previous section, as have the general actions of the gonadotrophins. Inhibin, a protein hormone secreted by the growing follicle and corpus luteum, inhibits secretion of FSH and LH by an action on the anterior pituitary. Figure 43-4 shows in more detail the specific effects of FSH and LH on the ovaries and their secretion of oestrogen and progesterone.

After about the age of 10 years, hormonal changes start to occur in both sexes; during puberty, there is increased output of GnRH, with pulsatile release occurring throughout the day, causing gradual development of secondary sexual characteristics. The pituitary gland is stimulated to produce increased levels of FSH and LH, and the ratio of LH:FSH secretion stimulates the ovaries to produce oestrogen and progesterone, leading to a surge of LH that causes ovulation. The oestrogenic steroids stimulate maturation of the female reproductive organs, development of secondary sexual characteristics and

DRUG MONOGRAPH 43-1 HUMAN CHORIONIC GONADOTROPHIN (hCG)

The action of **human chorionic gonadotrophin** is nearly equivalent to that of the pituitary's LH, with few or no follicle-stimulating effects. This drug is administered to make up for a deficiency in LH.

INDICATIONS hCG is indicated for:
- treating prepubertal cryptorchidism and hypogonadotrophic hypogonadism: stimulating androgen production in the testes may enhance descent of the testes and development of the secondary male sex characteristics
- treating male and female infertility: in females, it is combined with other drugs, such as GnRH analogues; men may receive it alone or in combination
- stimulating ovulation in infertility and assisted reproduction techniques.

PHARMACOKINETICS Administered IM, the drug has a half-life of 12–36 hours; in the female, ovulation usually occurs within 32–36 hours of administration. It is excreted by the kidneys within 24 hours. It has no significant drug interactions.

ADVERSE REACTIONS These include mood changes, aggression, headache, tiredness, oedema, precocious puberty, gynaecomastia, ovarian hyperstimulation and arterial thromboembolism; multiple pregnancies can occur.

WARNINGS AND CONTRAINDICATIONS Use with caution in breastfeeding women and in people with epilepsy, migraine headaches, asthma or heart or kidney disease. Avoid use in people with chorionic gonadotrophin hypersensitivity, precocious puberty and prostate cancer, and in pregnant women.

DOSAGE AND ADMINISTRATION The adult dosage for male hypogonadotrophic hypogonadism is 500–1000 units IM 2–3 times a week for several weeks to months or in some cases indefinitely. For boys with prepubertal cryptorchidism, the dose is also 500–1000 units IM 2 times a week. For induction of ovulation, a dose of 5000–10,000 units IM is administered, usually after suppression of endogenous LH levels by GnRH.

accelerated growth, followed by closure of the epiphyses of the long bones.

The first menstrual period (menarche) is closely correlated with a skeletal age of 13 years, but may occur some years earlier or later (range 9–15 years). The actual 'clock' that switches on reproductive development and function is unknown. It has been suggested that the clock is a timer of maturation, and that the prolonged period of childhood in humans allows a long period of learning before the onset of reproductive life. The clock depends on stimulus from the nervous system and can be affected by stress and emotion. After puberty, the female hormones are involved with regulation of the menstrual cycle or of pregnancy until about the age of 50, when levels of oestrogens decrease and menstruation ceases (the menopause).

The menstrual cycle

Figure 43-5 illustrates the effects of the pituitary gonadotrophic hormones and the ovarian hormones, and uterine changes occurring during the **menstrual cycle**. The physiology of the cycle will not be discussed in great detail—only insofar as it forms the basis for the pharmacology of the female reproductive system, and for clinical use of exogenous hormones, as described in subsequent chapters.

The endometrium, the inner layer of the uterus, contains glands, blood vessels and lymphatics in connective tissue. It undergoes cyclical changes (destruction and regeneration) during a woman's childbearing years, governed by changes

in levels of oestrogens and progestogens from the ovary, regulated by gonadotrophins. The menstrual cycle is marked by periods (about 5 days) of 'bleeding', when the uterine lining is shed. The menstrual fluid includes about 30–40 mL blood, plus mucus and cells from the degenerating endothelium. The stages of a 'typical' 28-day cycle are as follows:
- Days 1–5: **menstruation**. The onset of menses is (arbitrarily) labelled as day 1 of the menstrual cycle, and day 5 usually signifies the end of menstruation. During this time, FSH is stimulating follicular growth in the ovary and also stimulating the ovary to produce oestrogen, which is low at the beginning of the cycle
- Days 4–14 (roughly): the proliferative stage. As oestrogen levels rise, FSH levels fall. The rising oestrogen levels are preparing the uterus for a fertilised ovum; during this stage there is resumed growth of the selected follicle, growth of the glandular surface of the endometrium, and production, by the endocervical glands, of a more plentiful viscous mucus that contains nutrients that can be used by sperm. As the FSH level is falling, the LH level is rising. There is a sharp rise in oestradiol level just before ovulation, which stimulates the pituitary gland to produce the preovulatory surge in LH production (by positive feedback), and, later, the midcycle FSH surge
- About day 14: **ovulation** occurs when the mature follicle ruptures and releases its ovum
- Days 13–16: the fertile period; the ovum travels through the oviduct to the uterus. If fertilised, it implants in the uterine wall and continues to divide and grow

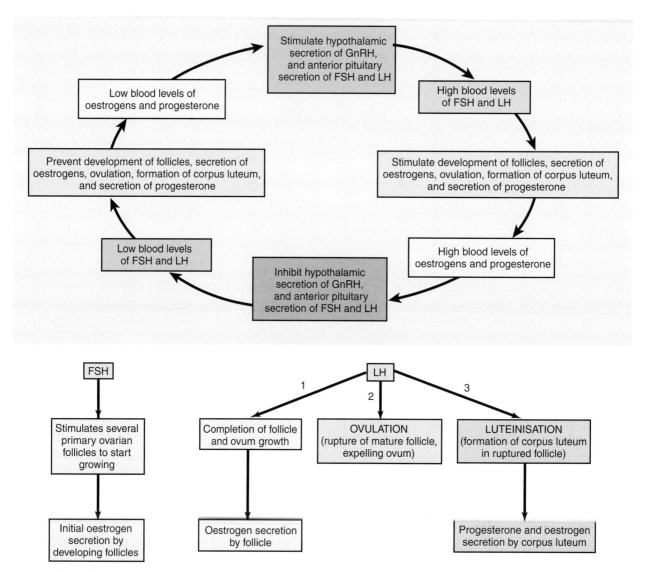

FIGURE 43-4 Hypothalamic and pituitary regulation of female sex hormones, and gonadotrophin effects on the ovaries. *Modified from*: Salerno 1999.

- Days 15–25: the secretory phase. LH causes luteinisation —changing of the ruptured follicle capsule into the corpus luteum, which releases oestrogen and progesterone. Both ovarian hormones increase secretion by the glands of the endometrium (to nourish a fertilised ovum). Progesterone, the 'progestational' or propregnancy hormone, maintains the endometrium to facilitate implantation and suppresses further ovulation to prevent subsequent pregnancy. Inhibin from the follicle and corpus luteum inhibits secretion of FSH and LH

- Days 25–28: if fertilisation (pregnancy) occurs, the corpus luteum continues to produce progesterone and maintains the endometrium and pregnancy, and secretion of hCG begins. Levels of oestrogens and progestogens continue to rise and all the other changes of pregnancy begin to occur or:

- Days 25–28: the premenstrual period. If fertilisation does not occur then, in the absence of hCG to 'rescue' the corpus luteum, the luteal cells become less responsive to LH, the levels of oestrogen and progesterone fall, the endometrium degenerates and is sloughed off, resulting in menstruation

- Day 28/Day 1: the next menstrual period.

Most women experience month-to-month variations in length of their menstrual cycles,* therefore ovulation is not

---

*Interestingly, the cyclical nature of the menstrual periods is regulated by the ovaries and by the time required for development of the follicle and the functional lifespan of the corpus luteum, rather than by any cyclical release of hypothalamic or pituitary hormones.

always predictable. The previous description of the menstrual cycle is based on a 28-day cycle, but ovulation varies and occurs on different days in cycles of different lengths (25–31 days). (Physiologically, this is the primary reason for the unreliability of the 'rhythm' or 'safe period' method of contraception, which depends on predicting the day of

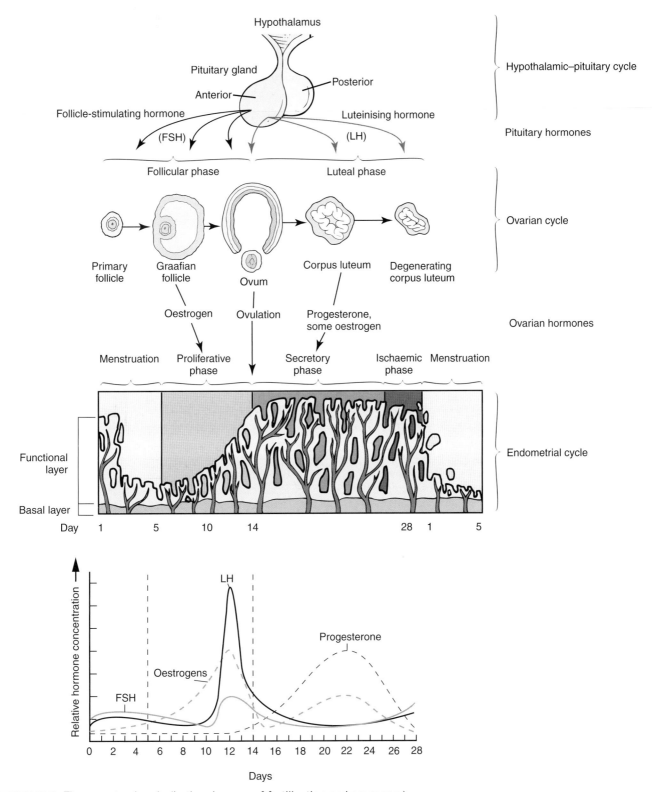

FIGURE 43-5 The menstrual cycle (in the absence of fertilisation and pregnancy).

ovulation, based on previous menstrual cycles. Ovulation most predictably occurs 14 days before the next menstrual period, which requires a very regular cycle to be reliable.)

The cyclical nature of secretion of oestrogens and progesterone is critical to normal female reproductive functions, and needs to be mimicked if the hormones are given exogenously, e.g. in the oral contraceptive (OC) pill or postmenopausal hormone replacement therapy (HRT) formulations. (Disorders of menstruation, and their treatments,

are described in Clinical Interest Box 43-1; the debate about whether menstruation should be optional is summarised in Clinical Interest Box 43-2.)

The female sexual response

In animals, sexual behaviour and the **sexual response** (mating) is more likely during oestrus (the recurring period of sexual receptivity in female mammals), which coincides with

---

CLINICAL INTEREST BOX 43-1   DISORDERS OF MENSTRUATION

- Amenorrhoea: absence of menstruation, which is physiological before menarche, during pregnancy and lactation, and after menopause; pathological causes include stess and endocrine tumours.
- Menorrhagia: excessive menstrual bleeding; menstruation may be regulated and excessive swings in hormone levels minimised by use of OC pill preparations.
- Dysmenorrhoea: painful menstruation occurs in about 40% of young women and is painfully incapacitating in about 3%. The pain and spasms of uterine muscles are thought to be due to prostaglandins (e.g. $PGF_{2\alpha}$) released from the degenerating endometrium. Treatment is with a non-steroidal anti-inflammatory agent, especially naproxen, which also has

analgesic actions and decreases the contractions, symptoms and blood loss. OC preparations are also useful.
- Premenstrual syndrome (PMS): breast tenderness, backache, depression or anxiety, headache, nausea, and oedema in the 2–3 days before the onset of menstruation, possibly due to the predominance of progestogens over oestrogens. Diuretics, dietary modifications and an OC preparation are effective.
- Metrorrhagia: bleeding from the uterus other than during a normal menstrual period; although strictly speaking not a disorder of menstruation, it is significant as a warning sign for cancer of the uterine cervix or endometrium.

CLINICAL INTEREST BOX 43-2   SHOULD MENSTRUATION BE OPTIONAL?

Modern women menstruate during their reproductive lives probably 2–3 times more overall than did women in earlier centuries, when women reached menarche later, had earlier first births, had more pregnancies, breastfed for long periods, and had shorter life expectancies. Yet menstruation can be easily and safely suppressed by the OC pill (by continuing to take active tablets every day of the month). Why are women not informed of this possibility, and encouraged to try it?

Reasons to suppress menstruation:
- menstruation is painful, messy, sometimes embarrassing to young women, expensive to deal with and potentially debilitating
- menstrual disorders are the leading cause of gynaecological morbidity
- time lost through menstrual disorders is costly to industry (estimated at about 8% of the total annual wage bill)
- suppressing menstruation decreases the problems related to anaemia, premenstrual syndrome, endometriosis and some reproductive cancers
- menstrual problems can be suppressed with OC tablets just as easily as menopausal problems can be suppressed with HRT

- women who have trialled suppression of menstruation (e.g. during their honeymoons, or as athletes) enjoy not having menstrual periods
- to view painful debilitating menstruation as normal and necessary inflicts regular pain on half the population
- to expect women to put up with painful periods and PMS may be allowing discrimination against them because of time periods of suboptimal performance.

Reasons to continue menstruation:
- menstruation is natural, the 'holy grail of womanhood'
- menstruation is a useful indicator of lack of pregnancy, and of proper female physiological functioning
- to view menstruation as medically controllable implies it is a pathological condition, whereas for some women it is merely a nuisance.

Menstrual control with OC preparations could substantially improve the health and quality of life of many women. Women should at least know that this safe, simple, inexpensive option is available to them if they prefer not to menstruate every month.
Adapted from: Thomas & Ellertson 2000.

peak levels of LH and ovulation, implying maximal likelihood of conception.

Sexual behaviours in animals may be inhibited by a rise in brain 5-hydroxytryptamine (5-HT, serotonin) levels, and by centrally acting muscarinic agonist drugs. These findings have implications for influencing human sexual behaviours with drugs such as selective serotonin reuptake inhibitors and anticholinergic agents. Catecholamine neurotransmitters are also involved, both in neuroendocrine integration (dopamine acting as the prolactin-release-inhibiting factor) and in vascular control; however, in humans, the basic endocrine and neuronal effects are usually overridden by psychological, social, cognitive and emotional influences. For both men and women, psychological stimulation and local sexual stimulation are necessary for a satisfactory sexual experience. Sexual desire is also affected by increasing levels of oestrogen secretion, especially during the preovulatory period; there is evidence of increased frequency of intercourse during the middle third of the menstrual cycle.

During the phase of sexual excitement, physical and psychological stimulation cause similar responses in both sexes and can enhance sexual sensations. In the female, the clitoris is very sensitive and its stimulation can initiate a sexual sensation. Erectile tissue is located in the vaginal opening and clitoral areas. These tissues are under parasympathetic nerve control; in early arousal, the parasympathetic nerves dilate the arteries located in the erectile tissues, leading to venous compression and engorgement of the erectile tissue, the labia, the breasts and the nipples, and tightening of the vagina. The parasympathetic nerves also stimulate the Bartholin's glands, situated near the labia minora, which results in increased mucus secretion inside the vagina. This secretion, in addition to mucus from the vaginal epithelium, serves as a lubricant during sexual intercourse.

The female climax, or orgasm, is reached when the local sexual stimulation reaches the maximum sensation or intensity. There may be 3–15 rhythmic contractions of the vagina, uterus and perineal muscles, caused by bursts of sympathetic nerve impulses. This is considered analogous to emission and ejaculation in the male, and may help to promote passage of sperm and seminal fluid and fertilisation of the ovum. It has been theorised that orgasm and reflex release of oxytocin from the posterior pituitary gland produce rhythmical uterine contractions and fallopian tube motility, and may result in cervical canal dilation for up to 30 minutes; however, conception can occur without orgasm.

The intense sexual sensations and sympathetic discharge that develop during orgasm also result in an increase in muscle tension throughout the body. There is tachycardia, a rise in blood pressure and increased respiration rate and depth. After the sexual activity, this tension subsides into relaxation or feelings of satisfaction, sometimes referred to as resolution. The genital tissues, cardiovascular and respiratory systems and muscle tone return to the unaroused state.

THE MALE REPRODUCTIVE SYSTEM

The effects of FSH and LH (or ICSH) in the male were described in the section on pituitary gonadotrophic hormones. Briefly, FSH from the anterior pituitary gland stimulates the seminiferous tubules to increase production of spermatozoa, while LH/ICSH stimulates the interstitial cells to increase secretion of testosterone. In some cells (e.g. in the seminal vesicles and prostate gland), testosterone is converted to a more potent metabolite, dihydrotestosterone. A high level of testosterone will inhibit the pituitary's release of FSH and ICSH (see Figure 43-3).

Testosterone, an androgen, performs numerous functions in the male. It aids in developing and maintaining the male secondary sex characteristics and male accessory sex organs, such as the prostate, seminal vesicles and bulbourethral glands. Testosterone promotes adult male sexual behaviour and spermatogenesis, as well as regulating metabolism and protein anabolism, resulting in the growth of bone and skeletal muscles and eventual closure of the epiphyses of long bones. Anabolic androgenic hormones including testosterone are abused in sport to increase muscle bulk but have major adverse effects (see Chapter 57).

Transport of sperm in the male

The male pelvic organs and the anatomy of the male reproductive system are shown in Figure 43-2. Sperm produced in the testes mature during a period of 1–3 weeks in the epididymis. The sperm, in seminal fluid, then travel through the epididymis (ducts that lie around the top of the testes), where motility is increased, to the vas deferens. The vas deferens, a ductal extension of the epididymis, extends over the bladder surface posteriorly to the ampulla to form the ejaculatory duct. (Thus a vasectomy, or severing of the vas deferens, will make a man sterile primarily because it interrupts the passage of sperm to the ejaculatory duct and urethra. Sperm are still produced, but they degenerate and are resorbed by phagocytes. Because the blood vessels are not cut, gonadotrophins continue to stimulate testosterone production, so libido and sexual performance are not impaired.) Sperm can be stored in the vas deferens for several months without loss of viability, depending on sexual activity. The vas deferens then passes within the spermatic cord, through the prostate to the urethra, from which semen (sperm and seminal vesicle secretions) is ejaculated during sexual response.

The male sexual response

Penile erection is a parasympathetic response that occurs during the phase of sexual excitement or arousal. It consists of dilation of the arteries and arterioles in the penis, which compresses the veins in this area; thus, more blood enters the penis than leaves, the cavernous tissue of the penis becomes engorged with blood and erection occurs. The stimulus that initiated erection will also help to move the sperm and secretions (semen) from the genital ducts to the prostatic urethra. Orgasm, the climax of the sexual act, moves the semen through the ejaculatory ducts. Emission and ejaculation of the sperm in semen is a reflex response, requiring sympathetic stimulation and powerful contractions of muscles that enable the transfer of sperm from male to female during coitus (intercourse). Cardiovascular, respiratory and muscular responses are similar to those already described for the female sexual response.

KEY POINTS

- Disorders of the reproductive systems cause physical and emotional distress. To assist patients with complex health issues in this area, health-care professionals require sound knowledge of the anatomy and physiology of these systems and sensitive understanding of their dysfunction.
- The primary organs associated with reproduction are the ovaries (female) and testes (male); these endocrine glands produce the sex hormones—oestrogens and progestogens, and androgens, respectively.
- The sex hormones regulate the development of sexual characteristics, and sexual behaviour and functions.
- The production of the sex hormones is under the control of gonadotrophins released from the anterior pituitary gland when stimulated by gonadotrophin-releasing hormone (GnRH) from the hypothalamus.
- GnRH can be used clinically to stimulate or suppress the release of pituitary gonadotrophins, depending on whether it is given in low pulsatile doses or high continuous doses.
- The pituitary gonadotrophic hormones FSH and LH regulate the development and maintenance of sex gland functions.
- Gonadotrophins are administered clinically to treat hypogonadism and infertility.
- Female reproductive functions are regulated by the menstrual cycle, in which cyclical changes in ovarian and pituitary hormone levels lead to monthly periods of regeneration and destruction of the uterine lining (if fertilisation and pregnancy do not occur).
- Disorders of menstruation can be treated by regulating hormone levels with oral contraceptive pill preparations.
- Reproductive functions in the male are also regulated by pituitary gonadotrophins and androgens from the testes.
- Sexual response in both sexes is under hormonal, neuronal, social and psychological controls. The sexual response involves mainly parasympathetic stimulation of erectile tissue, leading to engorgement, and sympathetic stimulation leading to muscular and cardiovascular responses.

REVIEW EXERCISES

1 Name the hypothalamic factor and pituitary gonadotrophins involved in regulating sex hormone activities and describe their actions.
2 Describe the feedback mechanisms controlling follicle-stimulating hormone (FSH) and luteinising hormone (LH/ICSH) and explain their effects on the primary sex organs.
3 Discuss the clinical use of GnRH and its analogues, and of gonadotrophins.
4 Describe the levels of hormones and changes in the uterus during the phases of the menstrual cycle.
5 Discuss the autonomic nervous system effects involved in the male and female sexual responses. Suggest why the autonomic-ganglion-blocking agents never gained great favour as antihypertensive agents.

REFERENCES AND FURTHER READING

Australian Medicines Handbook 2006. Adelaide: AMH, 2006.
Bowman WC, Rand MJ. *Textbook of Pharmacology.* 2nd edn. Oxford: Blackwell, 1980 [ch. 20].
Caswell A (ed.). *MIMS Annual June 2005.* Sydney: CMPMedica Australia, 2005.
Endocrine Expert Group. *Therapeutic Guidelines: Endocrinology, Version 3.* Melbourne: Therapeutic Guidelines Limited, 2004.

Goodman HM. Part VI: Endocrine physiology. Chs 45 & 46 in: Johnson LR (ed.). *Essential Medical Physiology*. 2nd edn. Philadelphia: Lippincott-Raven, 1999.

Greenspan FS, Strewler GJ. *Basic & Clinical Endocrinology*. 5th edn. Stamford: Appleton & Lange, 1997 [chs 12, 13, 15].

Horani MH, Morley JE. Hormonal fountains of youth. *Clinics in Geriatric Medicine* 2004; 20(2): 275–92.

Salerno E. *Pharmacology for Health Professionals*. St Louis: Mosby, 1999 [chs 38, 39, 43].

Tanner JM. *Foetus into Man: Physical Growth from Conception to Maturity*. Ware: Castlemead, 1989.

Thomas SL, Ellertson C. Nuisance or natural and healthy: should monthly menstruation be optional for women? *Lancet* 2000; 355 (March 11): 922–4.

Tortora GJ, Grabowski SR. *Principles of Anatomy and Physiology*. 9th edn. New York: HarperCollins, 2000 [ch. 28].

Youngson RM. *Collins Dictionary: Medicine*. 2nd edn. Glasgow: HarperCollins, 1998.

evolve More weblinks at http://evolve.elsevier.com/AU/Bryant/pharmacology/

CHAPTER 44

Drugs Affecting the Female Reproductive System

CHAPTER FOCUS

Drugs that affect the female reproductive system therapeutically are analogues or antagonists of the ovarian hormones oestrogen and progesterone. They are administered to mimic or suppress the biological effects of endogenous hormones, to supplement inadequate production (e.g. in the menopause), to correct hormonal imbalance (e.g. dysfunctional bleeding), to reverse abnormal processes (endometriosis, anovulation and infertility), and for contraception. Whatever the indication, the health-care professional needs to be knowledgeable about these drugs to support the patient's need for intervention and instruction.

OBJECTIVES

- To discuss the functions of the primary female sex hormones.
- To discuss the clinical uses, adverse reactions and drug interactions of oestrogens and progestogens.
- To list drugs affecting the female reproductive system and describe their clinical use.
- To compare and contrast continuous, monophasic, biphasic, triphasic and depot hormonal contraceptives.
- To discuss the use of HRT in the menopause.
- To describe drug therapy of common conditions affecting the female reproductive system.

KEY DRUGS

medroxyprogesterone acetate
oestradiol valerate
progesterone
raloxifene

KEY TERMS

emergency contraception
endometriosis
hirsutism
hormone replacement therapy
menopause
minipill
oestrogen receptors
oestrogens
oral contraceptives/contraception
osteoporosis
phyto-oestrogens
progestogens
selective oestrogen receptor
  modulators

KEY ABBREVIATIONS

DES	diethylstiboestrol
DVT	deep venous thrombosis
EE	ethinyloestradiol
ER	(o)estrogen receptors
FSH	follicle-stimulating hormone
HDL	high-density lipoproteins
HRT	hormone replacement therapy
IUD	intrauterine device
LDL	low-density lipoproteins
LH	luteinising hormone
MPA	medroxyprogesterone acetate
OC	oral contraception/contraceptive
PMS	premenstrual syndrome
SERM	selective (o)estrogen-receptor modulator

FEMALE SEX HORMONES

THE ovaries, in addition to producing ova, synthesise and secrete hormones that control female secondary sex characteristics, the reproductive cycle and the growth and development of the accessory reproductive organs in the female. Two main types of hormones are secreted by the ovary: the oestrogenic, or follicular, hormones (oestrogens)* produced by the cells of the developing Graafian follicle; and the progestational, or luteal, hormones (progestogens) derived from the corpus luteum that is formed in the ovary from the ruptured follicle. The periodic cycling of the female sex hormones depends on interactions between hypothalamic gonadotrophin-releasing hormone (GnRH), the pituitary gonadotrophins (follicle-stimulating hormone [FSH] and luteinising hormone [LH]) and the ovarian hormones oestrogen and progesterone (see Figures 43-3, 43-4 and 43-5). This results in a menstrual cycle that normally continues throughout reproductive life, except during pregnancy, from menarche until menopause.

Oestrogens

Although **oestrogens** are primarily secreted by the ovarian follicles, some may also be synthesised from androgens secreted by the adrenal glands, and by the corpus luteum, placenta (up to 100 times the pre-pregnancy levels), liver and testes. The structures of representative steroids are shown in Figure 37-2 and the biosynthetic pathways of adrenal cortex steroids from cholesterol are shown diagrammatically in Figure 40-1. It can be seen that the 'A' ring of oestrogens is an aromatic ring, unlike that of most other steroid hormones. There are three main endogenous (occurring naturally in women) oestrogens: oestradiol, oestrone and oestriol; oestradiol is metabolised in the body to oestrone and oestriol.

The physiological actions of oestrogens are:
- assisting in the follicle development
- stimulating the midcycle LH surge
- stimulating the growth of the myometrium and endometrium
- stimulating mucus production in the cervix

- involvement in 'metabolic' actions: retention of salt and fluid, mild anabolic actions, decreased risk of atheroma (increased high-density lipoprotein–cholesterol [HDLc], decreased low-density lipoprotein–cholesterol LDLc), increased coagulability of blood and decreased rate of bone resorption
- inhibiting secretion of FSH and LH from the pituitary gland (elevated oestrogen serum levels), which results in inhibition of ovulation and lactation, and the development of a proliferative endometrium.

The mechanism of the actions is through activation of **oestrogen receptors** (ERs) in oestrogen-responsive target tissues, especially in the uterus, vagina and breast. As with other steroid hormones, oestrogens enter the nucleus and bind to specific receptors (in this case, ERs). After recruitment of coactivators of the receptor, there is interaction with DNA and activation of gene transcription, leading to altered synthesis of proteins.

Oestrogen receptors have been classified into alpha- and beta-subtypes (ERα, ERβ); however, identification of these types in various tissues, and characterisation of them as acting via different transduction mechanisms or causing specific effects, is not yet clear.

Oestrogens used as drugs are available from natural sources (e.g. the urine of pregnant mares) in conjugated dosage forms known as conjugated equine oestrogens, and include oestradiol, oestriol and oestrone. These natural oestrogens are rapidly metabolised in the liver, so esterified or semisynthetic derivatives (e.g. **oestradiol valerate**, ethinyloestradiol (EE), mestranol) have been prepared, which are active orally because they are less rapidly metabolised. The natural oestrogens tend to be used in hormone replacement therapy (HRT) formulations (see Drug Monograph 44-1), which require only

---

*The term 'oestrus' is derived from the Greek word meaning the sexual heat period of animals. The English spelling of related words (oestrogen, oestradiol) retains the initial oe-diphthong, whereas the American spelling drops the 'o-' to become estrogen, estradiol etc. This can lead to confusion when consulting a dictionary or index, or when abbreviating compound words to an acronym, e.g. the accepted abbreviation for selective oestrogen receptor modulator is SERM, not SORM, and for oestrogen receptor is ER, not OR.

CLINICAL INTEREST BOX 44-1
CLINICAL USES OF OESTROGENS

Clinically, **oestrogens** are used very often. A large number of the world's female population take them daily for many years, either in oral contraceptive pill preparations or as hormone replacement therapy in the menopause. Other indications include:
- disorders of menstruation, e.g. endometrial hyperplasia, dysfunctional uterine bleeding, amenorrhoea
- replacement therapy (cyclical administration) in oestrogen deficiency, atrophic vaginitis or female hypogonadism
- in prostatic cancer, some breast cancers (metastatic breast carcinomas in postmenopausal women with tumour oestrogen-negative receptors), and selected male breast carcinomas
- as an emergency postcoital contraceptive
- in hirsutism (excessive androgen-dependent hair growth).

low doses, whereas the synthetic hormones, especially EE, are used in oral contraceptive (OC) preparations.

Oestrogens are administered by many routes: as tablets, implants, injections, patches, creams, nasal inhalations or pessaries. Being lipid-soluble, they are well absorbed orally and pass readily through membranes. They are circulated in the bloodstream bound to albumin and globulin. There is some enterohepatic recycling (as is usual with steroids). They are metabolised rapidly in the liver, with a high first-pass effect; metabolites are excreted in the urine and bile as conjugates. Conjugated oestrogens, a mixture of oestrogenic substances (especially oestrone and equilin), are available in oral, parenteral and vaginal cream dosage forms.

Dosages of oestrogens must be individualised according to diagnosis, clinical use, route of administration and therapeutic response, e.g. for treatment of breast cancer or vasomotor symptoms associated with menopause. Typical ethinyloestradiol daily doses may be 20–50 mcg in the OC pill and 1–3 mg in breast cancer treatment.

Oestrogenic adverse reactions are dose-dependent and include nausea and vomiting, dizziness, fluid retention, irregular menstrual bleeding and breast tenderness. In high doses (such as were present in early formulations of the OC pill), there was increased incidence of thromboembolic disorders such as deep vein thrombosis (DVT) and stroke. Because of this risk, the OC pill is not recommended for women over 35 years who smoke. In previous decades (1950s to 1980s), diethylstilboestrol was prescribed to pregnant women in an attempt to decrease the risk of spontaneous miscarriage in women for whom this was a problem. It was shown to cause increased incidence of cancer of the vagina or cervix in their daughters 15–20 years after their birth (i.e. the fetus was affected by DES in utero), so it has been withdrawn from use.

Selective oestrogen receptor modulators—raloxifene

Knowledge about the oestrogen receptor and mechanisms by which drugs may activate or repress oestrogen-dependent gene transcription is helping in the development and clinical use of new anti-oestrogens and **selective oestrogen receptor modulators (SERMs)**. The aim is to find tissue-specific modulators that lower the risk of oestrogen-dependent cancers (breast and endometrial) yet have positive effects on bone, the cardiovascular system, liver function, CNS function and menopausal symptoms.

The SERM class of drugs, of which **raloxifene** is the first clinically used example, have agonist actions at some oestrogen receptors (particularly in bone) and on lipid metabolism, and antagonistic actions on other oestrogen receptors (in breast and uterus). Hence SERMs are potentially useful in the long term for menopausal symptoms, to protect against osteoporosis and cardiovascular disease, while not

increasing the risk of breast or uterine cancers. In clinical use raloxifene has been shown to increase bone mineral density, reduce bone resorption and improve the blood lipid profile, with no stimulation of the endometrium or breast tissue; however, the hot flushes associated with menopause may be exacerbated, so it should be used in postmenopausal women. It is contraindicated in pregnancy (Category X).

Tamoxifen, long used as an anti-oestrogen in breast cancer (see below), is now recognised as a SERM. These SERMs have potential uses in many oestrogen-dependent gynaecological conditions. New SERMs include lasofoxifene and basedoxifene

Anti-oestrogens

Tamoxifen is an oestrogen antagonist (anti-oestrogen): it binds to oestrogen receptors but does not stimulate transcription and so has few oestrogenic actions. It is used in postmenopausal oestrogen-dependent breast cancers (see Drug Monograph 49-3).*

Clomiphene acts by rather different mechanisms: it inhibits oestrogen binding in the hypothalamus and pituitary gland, reducing the negative feedback effects of circulating oestrogens so that more GnRH is produced, which has the effect of increasing the release of gonadotrophins, especially LH. The raised oestrogen levels from the stimulated ovaries induce ovulation. The drug is therefore useful to treat female infertility. However, there are major risks: multiple pregnancies, ovarian enlargement, and oestrogenic adverse effects.

Progesterone and progestogens

Progesterone produced by the ovaries is the main naturally occurring **progestogen**, along with hydroxyprogesterone. LH secreted from the anterior pituitary stimulates the synthesis and secretion of progesterone from the corpus luteum, mainly during the latter half of the menstrual cycle. Progesterone is also formed during pregnancy (in the placenta, from steroid precursors), when it functions to promote breast development, maintain pregnancy and prevent further ovulation.

The normal physiological actions of progesterone are to:
- stimulate the secretory phase of the menstrual cycle
- maintain the endometrium to prepare for the implantation and nourishment of the embryo (i.e. 'progestational' effects that sustain pregnancy)
- cause relaxation of the uterine smooth muscles
- decrease levels of LH and of oestrogen receptors.

---

*If used in premenopausal women, it would be swamped by the large amounts of circulating oestrogens.

DRUG MONOGRAPH 44-1 OESTRADIOL VALERATE

Oestradiol valerate is an ester derivative of the natural hormone and has the pharmacological actions of oestrogens on the ovary and uterus. It is used in HRT to treat oestrogen deficiency symptoms after ovariectomy or menopause.

PHARMACOKINETICS Oestradiol valerate is a prodrug, a precursor of oestradiol-17β. It is rapidly and completely absorbed and is quickly metabolised in the liver to oestradiol, then to various metabolites, of which oestriol and oestrone have oestrogenic activity.

Oestradiol is highly protein-bound and has a half-life of about 24 hours. Metabolites are excreted in the liver and bile. Bioavailability is about 3%.

DRUG INTERACTIONS See table below for effects that may occur when oestradiol valerate is given with the drugs listed.

SIDE-EFFECTS AND ADVERSE REACTIONS These include typical oestrogenic effects: breast pain and enlargement, changes in menstrual bleeding, headaches, nausea, vomiting, a change in female libido (and decrease in male sex drive), oedema of the lower extremities and chloasma (darkened patches of skin on the face). There is an increased risk of thromboembolism.

WARNINGS AND CONTRAINDICATIONS Oestrogens should be used with caution in smokers and in patients with endometriosis, diabetes, migraine and epilepsy. Avoid use in pregnancy (see Pregnancy Safety box at the end of this chapter) and lactation, and in women with oestrogen hypersensitivity, thromboembolic disorders, breast cancer, severe liver disease, hypercalcaemia or severe cardiovascular disease. Oestrogens reduce lactation and are excreted in breast milk, so administration of oestrogens to nursing mothers is not recommended.

Drug	Possible effect and management
Enzyme inducers (barbiturates, antiepileptics)	May accelerate metabolism of oestrogens and reduce their activity

Drug	Possible effect and management
Antibiotics (e.g. ampicillin)	May reduce potency of oestradiol because of metabolism by altered gut flora
Some anti-convulsants, anticoagulants	Antagonism of effects may occur; doses may need to be increased
Tobacco (smoking)	Tobacco smoking increases the risk of serious cardiac adverse reactions, such as cerebrovascular accident, transient ischaemic attacks, thrombophlebitis, and pulmonary embolism. The risk is higher in women over 35 who smoke. Avoid or a potentially serious drug interaction may occur

DOSAGE AND ADMINISTRATION The lowest effective dose of oestrogens should be administered for the shortest time period to reduce the possibility of overstimulation of oestrogen-sensitive tissues. A cyclical dosing schedule of 3 weeks of oestrogen administration and 1 week off, or the addition of a progestogen for the last 10–13 days of the cycle, will most closely approximate the natural hormonal menstrual cycle. The progestogen must be added to a schedule of HRT in postmenopausal women with an intact uterus to avoid the possibility of endometrial hyperplasia or carcinoma. (The schedule is different for oophorectomised women or patients with cancer who are receiving hormonal therapy.) When continuous therapy is required, the prescriber should re-evaluate the patient at least annually.

Transdermal oestradiol is also used for women with oestrogen deficiency, particularly as HRT in menopause. Applied topically to intact skin, either 50 mcg (0.05 mg) or 100 mcg (0.1 mg) is released daily from the transdermal patch. It should be replaced twice weekly and is usually worn continuously. Sensitivity reactions at the application site often occur.

Progesterone is also thermogenic, i.e. it raises the core body temperature.[†] Progestogens are commonly used clinically in hormonal contraception (both combined with an oestrogen, and in progestogen-only formulations), in endo-

metriosis (to suppress the ovaries), and in HRT (in women with an intact uterus, to oppose oestrogen's actions).

Progesterone itself is inactive orally, as it is very rapidly metabolised in the liver; it can be administered IM or per vagina to avoid this first-pass effect. When used to treat amenorrhoea caused by hormonal imbalance, the dosage is 5–10 mg IM daily for 6–10 days. Bleeding will usually occur within 2–3 days of the last injection; normal menstrual cycles may then follow. Progesterone is also formulated as a

---

[†]This is the basis for attempting to time the day of ovulation in the 'rhythm' method of contraception, by monitoring the woman's body temperature: a rise of about 0.5°C occurs after ovulation, due to the rising levels of progesterone.

gel or pessary for per vaginal (PV) administration in assisted reproduction technologies.

Orally active derivatives, collectively called progestogens, have now been developed and have similar pharmacological effects in the body to those of the natural hormones. The advantages with these synthetic progestogens are the availability of an effective oral or sublingual dosage form, and a longer duration of action.

Progestogens commonly used include:

- **medroxyprogesterone**: active orally and IM (see Drug Monograph 44-2)
- testosterone derivatives, e.g. norethisterone, which is active orally. These have some androgenic and oestrogenic action and so may cause androgenic adverse effects (e.g. acne, hirsutism)
- cyproterone, another testosterone derivative, with significant antiandrogenic actions, used mainly as an OC and in HRT in women suffering masculinisation effects
- megestrol, a synthetic progestogen used for its anti-tumour activity in breast cancer and endometrial cancer
- other progestogens used commonly in combined OC formulations: levonorgestrel, desogestrel, drospirenone and gestodene.

Antiprogestogens

Mifepristone (RU486) is a partial agonist that binds strongly to progesterone receptors and prevents the activity of endogenous progestogens. It also has antiglucocorticoid activity and sensitises the uterus to prostaglandins. It has been used as an emergency contraceptive and in combination with a prostaglandin (gemeprost) for early termination of pregnancy.

ORAL CONTRACEPTIVES

The most effective form of reversible birth control currently available is oral hormonal contraception, i.e. oral administration of an oestrogen–progestogen combination in cyclical regimens. Since the 1960s, millions of women have used **oral contraceptives** (OCs) for decades during their reproductive lives. Through this experience, an enormous amount of information has been collected about the specific drugs, their effectiveness and the relationship of risk factors and contraindications to adverse reactions, drug interactions and morbidity and mortality. (Other types of contraception [non-drug, and non-oral] are discussed in Chapter 47.)

History

The rationale for the use of oestrogens and progestogens as reversible contraceptive agents was based on the fact that ovulation does not occur during pregnancy, when levels of oestrogens and progestogens are high. Advances in steroid chemistry during the 1930s allowed chemical synthesis of steroid hormones, but they were in short supply and very expensive. Research into methods of chemically modifying plant hormones to mass-produce compounds with oestrogenic or progestogenic activity led to the development of some orally active preparations. By the late 1940s, even the oestrogens that were difficult to synthesise were becoming available for clinical trials. Combinations of mestranol and norethynodrel as OCs were tested in large-scale clinical trials in the 1950s in Puerto Rica and Haiti, and were proven to provide successful reversible contraception with acceptable levels of adverse reactions.

The first OC preparation marketed was in the USA in 1960; it was a combination containing mestranol 150 mcg and ethynodiol diacetate 10 mg. It was realised at the time that this heralded not only a pharmacological revolution but also sexual and social revolutions. For the first time in history, women now had a reliable and safe method of controlling their own fertility, which provided them with opportunities to separate career choices from family planning and to compete more equally with men in the workforce.

Early preparations contained what are now recognised as unnecessarily large amounts of oestrogenic component (e.g. EE 100–150 mcg per tablet) plus 1–4 mg norethisterone. EE is a highly potent oestrogen with about 1000 times the potency of natural oestrogens. Current formulations include only 20–50 mcg EE plus 0.5–1 mg norethisterone or equivalent.

Actions of components

The aim of most OC formulations is to mimic closely the sequence and relative levels of oestrogen and progestogen in the menstrual cycle (see Figure 43-5). Thus oestrogen levels are low early in the cycle, high in midcycle, and medium late in the cycle; progestogen levels are very low or absent until after the midcycle surge of gonadotrophins, then rise in the latter half of the cycle. In the typical 21/7 combined OC regimen, withdrawal of the active hormones after 21 days (when placebo tablets or no tablets are substituted for active tablets) precipitates the withdrawal bleed, i.e. the next menstrual cycle. (Note that menstruation can be effectively suppressed by continuous taking of the active tablets [see Clinical Interest Box 44-2].)

Much research has gone into identifying the actions of the hormones that together bring about contraceptive effects. Current views are that the oestrogen component causes decreased FSH release and thus impaired selection of a dominant ovarian follicle and impaired follicle development, with consequent decreased likelihood of ovulation and decreased chance of implantation. The actions of the progestogen component are to modify the secretory activity of the uterine cervix, decrease LH release, impair ovulation and

DRUG MONOGRAPH 44-2 MEDROXYPROGESTERONE ACETATE

Medroxyprogesterone acetate (MPA) is a typical synthetic progestogen.

INDICATIONS Progesterone and progestogens are indicated for oral contraception (alone or combined with an oestrogen); in long-term contraception (as an IM depot preparation); in postmenopausal HRT; and in the treatment of female hormonal imbalance in amenorrhoea, dysmenorrhoea, endometriosis and specific carcinomas (breast, endometrial, renal cell; specialist oncologist use only).

PHARMACOKINETICS MPA is rapidly absorbed after oral administration and has an apparent half-life of about 30 hours. It is metabolised in the liver, with metabolites excreted by the kidneys.

DRUG INTERACTIONS The following effects may occur when MPA is given with the drugs listed below:

Drug	Possible effect and management
Aminoglutethimide	Concurrent use with oral or parenteral MPA has resulted in a fall in serum levels of MPA. Patients should be monitored closely; alternative contraception may be necessary
Liver-enzyme-inducing drugs such as carbamazepine, phenobarbitone, phenytoin and rifamycins	Concurrent use may decrease the effectiveness of some progestogens, resulting in contraceptive failure. Monitor patients closely; alternative contraception may be necessary

ADVERSE REACTIONS These include menstrual irregularities (amenorrhoea, breakthrough bleeding), breast pain, weight gain, stomach pain and cramps, swelling of face and lower extremities, headache, mood alterations including depression, nausea, hyperglycaemia, chloasma and galactorrhoea. Progestogens that are synthetic testosterone derivatives may cause androgenic and adrenocorticoid effects (virilisation, acne, libido changes, fluid imbalance).

WARNINGS AND CONTRAINDICATIONS Use with caution in patients with asthma, cardiac insufficiency, epilepsy, hypertension, migraine, kidney or liver function impairment, central nervous system disorders, diabetes mellitus, hyperlipidaemia, thrombophlebitis and uterine, genital or urinary tract bleeding (undiagnosed).

Avoid use in persons with progestogen hypersensitivity, breast or genital tract cancer (contraceptive use), severe liver disorders or thromboembolic disease, and in pregnancy.

DOSAGE AND ADMINISTRATION Low physiological dosages are used for progestational effects in replacement therapy, and high dosages to suppress ovulation and menstruation and inhibit gonadotrophin production. Because dosage and method of administration for progestogens can vary according to indications and current standards of practice, current package inserts or reference texts need to be consulted for the most recent recommendations. The following are examples of selected dosing regimens:
- in combined HRT formulations: 2.5–10 mg/day, depending on the type of cycle
- for endometriosis: 10 mg three times daily for 90 days
- for amenorrhoea or abnormal bleeding: 2.5–10 mg/day for 10 days in the second half of the cycle
- for inoperable endometrial or renal cell carcinoma: 200–400 mg/day
- for breast carcinoma: 500 mg/day.

CLINICAL INTEREST BOX 44-2 PHASED OC HORMONES

In order to optimise the relative levels of oestrogenic and progestogenic components of their combined OC pill preparations, and most closely mimic the body's natural hormone levels, two drug companies manufacture formulations containing the following daily doses (in one month's calendar pack):

Cycle day	Number of tablets	Ethinyloestradiol dose (mcg)	Levonorgestrel dose (mcg)
6–11	6	30	50
12–16	5	40	75
17–26	10	30	125
27, 28; 1–5	7 (inactive)	0	0

Withdrawal bleeding usually occurs 2–3 days after starting the inactive tablets. Thus this regimen mimics the natural surge in oestrogen levels midcycle, and the progesterone surge in late cycle.

impair tubal motility, decreasing likelihood of fertilisation.

Taken together over a few cycles, the combined OC pill* effectively inhibits secretion of hypothalamic GnRH, pituitary FSH and LH, and endogenous ovarian steroids. This causes production of a thickened cervical mucus that impairs sperm transport; decreases endometrial proliferation, secretions and menstrual flow; and reduces likelihood of ovulation and implantation. Overall, pregnancy does not occur.

Clinical use of oral contraceptives

Oral contraceptives are indicated for use in menstrual disorders and premenstrual syndrome as well as for contraception. In addition, they can be used (as described below) for emergency contraception (the 'morning-after pill'). For detailed information on the pharmacokinetics, adverse effects, drug interactions and contraindications of the component drugs, see the drug monographs for typical oestrogens (oestradiol valerate) and progestogens (medroxyprogesterone acetate) in earlier sections.

Before prescribing OC therapy, the prescriber should perform a thorough history and physical examination, including breast examination and a complete drug history. Teaching and monitoring of patients are also necessary. In particular, a woman needs to know:

• when to start taking a pack of tablets (day 1 of the cycle, i.e. the first day of menstrual bleeding)
• what to do if one or more active tablets are missed or if she suffers from vomiting or diarrhoea (if more than 12 hours late or a tablet may not have been absorbed, other contraception should be practised for 7 days)
• the greater risks of adverse effects if she is a smoker
• what adverse effects to watch out for and report (severe chest pain or headache, vision changes, leg pain or swelling)
• how to change formulations if prescribed (skip the inert tablets for the first cycle and keep taking the active tablets)
• that the pill does not protect against sexually transmitted diseases
• that it is very important to take the 'minipill' and other low-dose formulations at the same time each day.

---

*Early OC formulations were indeed pills—small spherical or ovoid masses containing pharmacologically active ingredients, prepared by rolling techniques. For many decades now, the drugs have been formulated as tablets (compressed powders, punched out as cylinders); however, the term 'pill' has stayed with us in the OC context.

Types of contraceptive formulations

Although the use of exogenous oestrogenic substances alone will inhibit ovulation, undesirable bleeding frequently occurs during the latter phase of the cycle. If oestrogen levels are increased to prevent this, severe nausea, breast tenderness and thromboembolic adverse reactions may occur. This is why progestogens are combined with oestrogens in OCs. Most formulations (99%) in Australia contain ethinyloestradiol; the only other oestrogen used is mestranol.

Because naturally occurring progesterone is inactivated or extremely weak in its effect when taken orally, and must be given by injection to be effective, synthetic progestogens with stronger actions were developed. Several are used in OC preparations: norethisterone, levonorgestrel, cyproterone (with antiandrogen activity), gestodene or drospirenone. Norethisterone is sometimes recommended for women having excess adverse reactions from oestrogen, such as greater weight gain and amenorrhoea; and cyproterone for women with oily skin, acne, hirsutism or breakthrough bleeding; see Clinical Interest Box 44-3.

Many different types of OC formulations are available, with different combinations and sequences of semisynthetic hormones selected to optimise activity and minimise adverse effects. See the 'Guide to Contraceptives' in early pages of MIMS bimonthly issues for current information.

Combination formulations

Combined products contain an oestrogen and progestogen, usually 3 weeks of active tablets (in one, two or three phases) and one week of placebo or no tablets. Phasic dosing was used in the belief that it might interfere less with a woman's normal metabolism but this has not been substantiated clinically. The low-dosage progestogen-only type (minipill) was developed for women unable to take oestrogens, e.g. during lactation. Table 44-1 lists the compositions, doses and brand names of some typical OCs used in these methods; however, formulations change often, so current reference texts should be consulted. Table 44-2 lists recommendations for prescription or selection of an OC formulation.

Combination oestrogen and progestogen contraceptives are divided into the following three types:

MONOPHASIC OCs

Monophasic OCs contain a fixed ratio of oestrogen and progestogen and are taken for 21 days of the normal menstrual cycle. These are generally found to be less confusing than the phasic types, provide good protection against mood swings and can be used to extend the cycle, e.g. to put off the next menstrual period until after sporting competitions or examinations.

TABLE 44-1 Selected hormonal contraceptives

BRAND NAME	OESTROGEN (mcg)	PROGESTOGEN (mg)
Monophasic		
Microgynon 20 ED (28†), Loette	Ethinyloestradiol 20	Levonorgestrel 0.1
Brenda-35 ED	Ethinyloestradiol 35	Cyproterone acetate 2.0
Norinyl-1 (28)	Mestranol 50	Norethisterone 1.0
Minulet	Ethinyloestradiol 30	Gestodene 0.075
Triphasic		
Triphasil, Logynon ED, Trifeme, Triquilar ED		
Phase 1 (6 tablets)	Ethinyloestradiol 30	Levonorgestrel 0.05
Phase 2 (5 tablets)	Ethinyloestradiol 40	Levonorgestrel 0.075
Phase 3 (10 tablets)	Ethinyloestradiol 30	Levonorgestrel 0.125
Progestogen-only (oral)		
Locilan 28, Micronor, Noriday 28	None	Norethisterone 0.35
Microlut, Microval	None	Levonorgestrel 0.03
Progestogen-only (depot)		
Depro-Provera	None	Medroxyprogesterone acetate 150 mg IM every 3 months
Implanon implant	None	Etonogestrel 68 mg subdermal every 3 years
Mirena intrauterine device	None	Levonorgestrel 52 mg; replaced every 5 years

Source: Caswell 2005.
†28s and ED (extended-dosage) formulations have seven placebo tablets.

TRIPHASIC OCs

Triphasic OCs most closely simulate the normal oestrogen and progesterone levels during the menstrual cycle. The dose of oestrogen is kept at a low level during the 21-day dosing period, or may increase in the middle of the cycle, while the progestogen is progressively phased up (increased twice) to mimic the natural release of hormones (see Clinical Interest Box 44-2). Because the lowest dosages of hormones possible are used in this type of formulation, the incidence and severity of adverse reactions reported are lower than with the monophasic or biphasic formulations; however, controlled trials show little difference in cycle control compared with monophasic types.

The minipill

Low-dosage progestogen-only OCs (the **minipill**) do not contain an oestrogen (see Table 44-1). They are generally prescribed for 28 days of the menstrual cycle, are usually slightly less effective than the combination products, and

have a higher incidence of breakthrough bleeding. Advantages are that they generally do not cause the more serious adverse reactions associated with oestrogen therapy, and that they can be taken by women who are breastfeeding, as there is no oestrogen component that might inhibit lactation. It is also indicated for women with a history of thromboembolic disorders or those who smoke. Because the dose is low, the timing of taking the tablet each day is critical; it is recommended that if the tablet is delayed by more than 3 hours, an additional method of contraception should be used for the next 48 hours.

Emergency contraception (the 'morning-after pill')

Emergency contraception is indicated for use within 72 hours of unprotected intercourse or in possible failure of contraceptive method in women not wanting to conceive. It is prescribed to reduce the frequency of unwanted pregnancies and abortions, especially in very young women. One 750 mcg

TABLE 44-2 Recommendations for selecting an oral contraceptive

CONDITIONS	CONTRACEPTIVE MANAGEMENT
Age	
Sexually active women (teenagers to age 35)	Low oestrogen (30–35 mcg)/low progestogen. Discourage smoking
Heavy smokers,[†] women >35 y and non-smokers >40 y	Increased risk of serious cardiovascular adverse reactions. Use alternative methods of contraception
Concurrent conditions	
Cancer (breast, uterus, cervix, liver)	Oral contraceptives contraindicated
Cerebrovascular disease, coronary artery disease or thromboembolic disorders	Oral contraceptives contraindicated
Liver impairment; smokers age >35; history of CVA, uncontrolled hypertension and migraine	Progestogen-only minipill
Breastfeeding women	Progestogen-only minipill
Epilepsy (or taking other enzyme-inducing drugs)	Higher doses of OC may be required: depot medroxyprogesterone recommended
Diabetes, hypertension, depression, jaundice, hyperlipidaemias, surgery	Existing condition may be exacerbated—monitor closely; possible additional risk of thrombosis
Management of adverse reactions	
Acne, oily skin, hirsutism, sebaceous cysts, weight gain	Trial OC with low progestogen dose, or use cyproterone as the progestogen component
Breakthrough bleeding	Early to midcycle bleeding or bleeding that never completely stops after menses is usually due to oestrogen deficiency, while late breakthrough bleeding is due to progestogen deficiency. Prescribers often continue with the same OC for 3–4 months because intermenstrual bleeding usually decreases with continued use; if bleeding continues, oestrogen and/or progestogen dosage may be adjusted to minimise effects; other possible causes of bleeding should be checked
Withdrawal bleeding absent	First, rule out pregnancy; if no pregnancy, then an OC with a low progestogen dose or higher oestrogen may be prescribed

Source: AMH 2006
†>15 cigarettes/day. CVA = cerebrovascular accident (stroke).

levonorgestrel tablet is followed 12 hours later by one more.

The main contraindication to these regimens is known pregnancy. This preparation is available in Australia without prescription, as the benefits far outweigh the risks; the method prevents 86% of expected pregnancies. (An alternative non-drug method of emergency contraception is insertion of a copper-impregnated intrauterine device [IUD], effective up to 5 days after unprotected intercourse.)

Progestogen depot preparations

Depot injections of progestogen (e.g. MPA 150 mg given IM every 3 months) have the lowest failure rate of all reversible contraceptive methods. Progestogen depots inhibit gonado-trophin secretion, thus preventing follicular maturation and ovulation, resulting in contraception. This method is suitable for women who do not want to take a daily tablet or who cannot take oestrogens. There may be a period of infertility for some months after completing the course. Adverse reactions include vaginal bleeding, irregular periods and weight gain.

A subdermal depot implant containing a progestogen was approved for use in Australia at the end of 1999.* It consists of a polymer rod (4 cm long, 2 mm diameter) impregnated with 68 mg etonogestrel. It is implanted using aseptic procedures under the skin of the inner aspect of the upper arm, and is left in place for 3 years, during which there is a gradually reducing rate of release of active drug (from 60–70 to 25–30 mcg/day). The contraceptive effect is due mainly to inhibition of ovulation. It is then removed and a new rod is inserted if continuing contraception is desired. Fertility will return after removal of the implants, with rapid return to normal menstrual periods.

A plastic IUD impregnated with 52 mg levonorgestrel, a slow-release progestogen, is also available. It is useful for long-term contraception (5 years), to treat menorrhagia and to provide the progestogen content of continuous combined HRT.

Risk–benefit analysis

Because OC preparations are taken by millions of women for most of their reproductive lives, it is crucial that long-term safety studies be carried out and risks and benefits identified. The risks need to be compared with those of pregnancy and childbirth, particularly in countries where obstetric care is inadequate, and with the risks of abortion in the case of unwanted pregnancy. Major long-term studies over millions of woman–years have demonstrated that the newer low-dose OCs have:

- a lower risk for adverse cardiovascular effects than earlier, higher-dose oestrogen formulations
- a higher risk for thromboembolic disease and myocardial infarction, especially in smokers and women aged over 35 years who take the pill (see Weisberg 2002)
- a lower rate of ectopic pregnancies
- a lower risk of ovarian cysts, ovarian cancer and endometrial cancer
- fewer bacterial sexually transmitted diseases
- protection against endometriosis and fibroids
- less acne and hirsutism
- a higher risk of cervical or liver cancer, or gallbladder disease
- reduced menstrual bleeding and hence reduced incidence of iron-deficiency anaemia; reduced pain.

Absolute contraindications for the use of OC are: thromboembolic disease, coronary artery disease, stroke, active liver disease, oestrogen-dependent cancers, focal migraine, porphyrias and pregnancy. OC is relatively contraindicated in hypertension, diabetes, previous cholestasis, undiagnosed vaginal bleeding, elective surgery within 4 weeks, sickle cell disease and severe depression, and in women over 35 years with risks for coronary artery disease.

Common adverse reactions and drug interactions are described under Oestrogens and Progestogens; see Table 44-2 on recommendations for selection of OC preparations.

---

*A similar contraceptive implant, but containing GnRH, is in use in some of Australia's koala population in areas where koalas are breeding excessively. The rod is inserted in the flap of skin behind the neck of adult females, and continuous release of GnRH effectively inhibits release of pituitary gonadotrophins, decreasing fertility for many months.

MENOPAUSE AND HORMONE REPLACEMENT THERAPY

Menopause

Menopause is loosely defined as the end of the reproductive period of a woman's life; it is a process rather than an event. As with puberty, there is no exact chronological age of initiation, rather a transitional period during which changes occur relatively quickly. The timing varies with ethnicity, geographical regions, socioeconomic status, extremes of body weight, smoking status, amount of heavy exercise, and a woman's menstrual, gynaecological and surgical history. The basis for the menopausal transition is the depletion of oocytes from the ovaries, and ovulation and menstruation cease.

The term 'climacteric' is used to refer to the signs, symptoms and consequences of the perimenopause, i.e. the period around the menopause. The stages are:
- the menopausal transition:
  — early: menstrual cycles of variable length
  — late: at least two skipped cycles: at least 60 days of amenorrhoea
- the final menstrual period
- menopause: considered definite after 12 months of amenorrhoea after the final menstrual period
- postmenopause:
  — early: the 5 years after the final menstrual period
  — late: subsequent years.

The menopausal transition occurs over a wide age range— from 42 to 58 years of age. The average age of the last menstrual period, around 51, has not changed significantly in recorded history (except that it is earlier in women who smoke), despite the increasingly younger onset of menarche and improved living conditions. Until about 1900, the median survival age for women was about 45 years, hence a large proportion of women never reached menopause. The average lifespan of women in developed countries is now over 80, so most women can expect to spend over one-third of their lives in menopause.

The changes occurring during menopause are considered to be due to the depletion of the stock of ova and follicles (estimated to be 0.2–2 million at birth) by decades of ovulation and atresia. Gonadotrophins are still released but the ovaries are less responsive, so there is a relatively sudden decrease in secretion of oestrogens and hence decreased ovulation and menstruation, decreased progesterone production, atrophy of genital organs and breasts, and reduced protein anabolism. Diagnosis is confirmed by low blood levels of oestrogens and progestogens despite high levels of FSH (due to reduced

CLINICAL INTEREST BOX 44-3
'THE PILL'

More than 40 years of worldwide clinical experience have shown the OC to be safe and effective. Provided that risk factors (smoking, hypertension, thromboembolic disease or obesity) are minimised, combined OCs are safe for most women for most of their reproductive lives.

Possible disadvantages are:
- weight gain (anabolic effects)
- breast tenderness and skin changes (oestrogenic effects)
- general symptoms (nausea, depression)
- short-term amenorrhoea after cessation
- increased risk of thrombosis or hypertension
- impaired glucose tolerance
- possible association with breast cancer, cervical cancer, liver cancer and rheumatoid arthritis.

Beneficial effects include:
- avoidance of unwanted pregnancy and pregnancy related morbidity and mortality
- less risk of atheroma and thyroid disease
- less risk of menstrual problems, anaemia, premenstrual tension, benign cysts, pelvic inflammatory disease and ovarian cancer.

On balance, the life-threatening risks associated with using modern low-dose OC formulations are statistically lower than those of having a baby or driving a car.

CLINICAL INTEREST BOX 44-4
HRT—WHY? WHY NOT? HOW? AND HOW LONG?

WHY?

Compared with women not using HRT, those taking oestrogen HRT after the menopause have been shown to have:
- significant relief from menopausal symptoms such as flushes, fatigue and vaginal dryness
- improved bone density and reduced risk of osteoporotic fractures
- reduced incidence of colorectal cancer.

HRT is also effective for the treatment of vaginal atrophy and associated sexual problems.

WHY NOT?

Possible disadvantages of HRT include:
- breast tenderness, nausea and fluid retention
- after long-term treatment, there are slightly increased risks of incidence of stroke, breast cancer and venous thromboembolism, and of endometrial or breast cancer, which is reduced by the progestogen added for women with an intact uterus
- likely cyclical uterine bleeding (especially in the first few years after the menopause) if cyclical progestogen is taken.

Relative contraindications include liver disease, thrombo-embolism and hypertension.

HOW?

Many HRT formulations are available:
- oral: calendar packs of oestrogen or oestrogen–progestogen (continuous)
- calendar packs of oestrogen-only for 11–14 days then oestrogen–progestogen for 10–14 days
- transdermal patches of oestrogen only for 4 weeks, or 2 weeks then oestrogen–progestogen for 2 weeks
- subcutaneous implants of oestrogen
- vaginal oestrogen creams or pessaries.

HOW LONG?

There is considerable debate about how long women can continue taking HRT:
- the risk–benefit ratio changes with time and patients should be reviewed annually
- longer-term therapy may be appropriate for the prevention and treatment of osteoporosis when first-line therapies are unsuitable or contraindicated
- the lowest effective dose should be prescribed.

Adapted from: MacLennan 2000 and 2003; RANZCOG 2004.

negative feedback from ovarian oestrogens and inhibin), LH and GnRH. There is still some production of oestrone and of androstendione, and libido and sexual performance are not necessarily decreased.

Many women suffer some unpleasant symptoms during the early years of menopause: hot flushes (during which there is a sudden rise in temperature and excessive sweating, thought to coincide with bursts of release of GnRH), nausea, insomnia, vaginitis, palpitations, increased risk of ischaemic heart disease, fatigue, depression, breast tenderness and **osteoporosis** (overall bone calcium content decreases by 1%–2% per year). The increased incidence of osteoporosis can decrease both quality and length of life but can be effectively reduced with replacement oestrogen therapy, with or without cyclical progesterone, or with other bone-protecting drugs (see discussion of osteoporosis in Chapter 42).

Hormone replacement therapy

Postmenopausal **hormone replacement therapy** involves daily low doses of a natural oestrogen (e.g. oestradiol), possibly for many years. It has become recognised that in women with an intact uterus, i.e. those who have not undergone surgical hysterectomy, it is important that a dose of a progestogen also be given 10–12 days per month to prevent endometrial hyperplasia and the risk of endometrial cancer;

this is known as 'opposed' therapy. The adverse reactions, drug interactions and contraindications are generally as for the constituent oestrogen and progestogen, but the oestrogen dose is considerably lower than in OC preparations, so fewer adverse reactions are expected.

Early studies on the effects of long-term HRT showed a reduced risk of heart disease in women using it; however, a recent very large trial of the risks and benefits of combined oestrogen plus progestogen in healthy postmenopausal women (Writing Group for the Women's Health Initiative Investigators 2002), which studied over 160,000 women with intact uteri, showed the following results:

- slightly increased hazard ratios (risks) for coronary heart disease, breast cancer, stroke and pulmonary embolism
- reduced risk of colorectal cancer, endometrial cancer and hip fractures
- overall, no significant effect on total mortality or total incidence of cancers, with reduced risk (0.76 ratio) of fractures and higher risk (1.22) of cardiovascular disease.

The consensus at present appears to be that HRT is useful in the short term to relieve menopausal symptoms and to prevent osteoporosis, but its safety in the long term is less definite and may depend on the woman's family history of, and predisposition to, cardiovascular disease, osteoporosis and specific cancers (breast, endometrial, colorectal). The need for continued use should be reviewed annually (MacLennan 2003).

Administration and formulations

The natural oestrogens are preferred because of their lower potency and fewer adverse reactions. Oral oestrogen preparations include conjugated equine oestrogens, oestriol and oestradiol valerate (see Drug Monograph 44-1). A low dose is taken daily, e.g. oestradiol valerate 1–2 mg orally. The oral progestogen used most commonly in HRT is MPA (see Drug Monograph 44-2); most of the progestogens used in the OC pill formulations are also used, at similar dosage levels, e.g. norethisterone 0.5–1 mg 12 days/month.

Transdermal oestrogen may be preferred, as it bypasses the liver, avoids first-pass metabolism and is considered more physiological in terms of the oestradiol:oestrone ratio. It is more expensive than tablets, however, and many women (10%–20%) suffer unpleasant skin reactions (redness, irritation, itchiness). A combination patch formulation has been released, with four patches containing oestradiol 4 mg, and four patches with norethisterone acetate 30 mg and oestradiol 10 mg. The recommended regimen is one of the first type of patch every 3–4 days for 2 weeks, then one of the second type every 3–4 days for 2 weeks. (This mimics the natural menstrual cycle, with low oestrogens in the first 2 weeks, then higher oestrogen and progestogen in the next 2 weeks.) This schedule is indicated for women intolerant of oral oestrogens or who prefer not to take daily tablets.

As there are many types and formulations of HRT available, subject to frequent changes, it is recommended that a current reference such as *Australian Medicines Handbook* be consulted for specific details and comparisons.

Other oestrogens: SERMs and phyto-oestrogens

Selective oestrogen receptor modulators (SERMs [see earlier notes under Oestrogens]), also known as tissue-specific oestrogens, are currently being tested for their effects in menopause. It is hoped that because of their selectivity on oestrogen receptors in bone and on metabolic processes, they will have an advantageous spectrum of pharmacological activities. Clinical trials have shown that they effectively decrease bone resorption and improve the blood lipid picture, while not stimulating breast or endometrial tissue growth.

Phyto-oestrogens (plant compounds with oestrogenic activity) are also of great interest, especially as they are advertised as being more 'natural' than white tablets in calendar packs (see Clinical Interest Box 44-5). They are isoflavones, coumestans and lignans occurring in plants and seeds, especially in clovers and soya beans.* Pharmacologically, they are best classified as SERMs, as they have varying agonistic and antagonistic activities in oestrogen-responsive tissues, and also have oestrogen enzyme-modulating and antioxidant activities. They could potentially be useful in control of menopausal symptoms but clinical trials so far have shown little if any benefit over placebo. In Australian indigenous medicine, berries of the 'kangaroo apple', *Solanum aviculare*, have been used for contraception. Active extracts contain steroids, alkaloids and solasadine, and have been used in the synthesis of oral contraceptives and cortisone.

Tibolone

Tibolone is an interesting drug found useful in treating menopausal symptoms, especially in protecting against bone resorption and in elevating mood and libido. It is neither an oestrogen nor a SERM but is classified as a 'gonadomimetic', with oestrogenic, anti-oestrogenic, progestogenic and androgenic effects.

Tibolone has a steroid structure that is rapidly metabolised, after oral administration, to active metabolites that have oestrogenic effects in the vagina, bone and thermoregulatory centre, and progestogenic and androgenic actions in the breast and bloodstream. It appears not to stimulate the endometrium, so it is potentially a good alternative to

---

*Japanese women have a low rate of breast cancer, attributed to high intakes of phyto-oestrogens in soybean paste soup. Genistein, from an Australian subterranean clover, has been held responsible for low fertility and high abortion rates in sheep grazing on these pastures. Phyto-oestrogen compounds are chemically related to both oestrogens and the coumarin anticoagulants.

HRT in women with an intact uterus. Overall, tibolone is useful in treating menopausal symptoms of hot flushes and vaginal dryness, and in preventing reduced bone mineral density. Adverse reactions are mild and rare, and include headache, dizziness, excess hair growth and acne. Results from studies of long-term administration of tibolone are still being accumulated.

TREATMENT OF GYNAECOLOGICAL DISORDERS

Hirsutism

Many gynaecological disorders can be treated with combinations of the sex hormones, to either stimulate or inhibit normal endocrine functions. The main drug groups—oestrogens, progestogens, hormone inhibitors, hypothalamic factors and pituitary hormones—have already been considered in detail.

Hirsutism, or excessive hair growth in women, can be distressing and require treatment. It may be an inherited trait or an adverse reaction to certain drugs, including phenytoin, minoxidil or steroids such as the progestogens based on the testosterone structure. Hirsutism can also be due to a relative androgen excess at the hair follicles, especially on the lower face and midline of the trunk. The androgens may come from hyperactive ovaries (e.g. polycystic ovaries), from the adrenal cortex or from other virilising endocrine disorders.

Possible treatments include suppression of ovarian functions, e.g. with OC preparations; suppression of the adrenal cortex, e.g. with dexamethasone; or administration of anti-androgens such as cyproterone or spironolactone.

Dysfunctional uterine bleeding

Dysfunctional uterine bleeding (DUB) occurs in about 5% of menstruating women and may be related to ovulation or to anovulatory cycles. It is relatively common around puberty and menopause, and in association with platelet dysfunction, cervical cancer, endocrine disorders or in women with low body-fat mass or who do excessive exercise. The primary causes should be sought and anaemia monitored. Pharmacological treatment of DUB associated with ovulation may include antianaemic drugs (iron, folic acid), non-steroidal anti-inflammatory drugs (e.g. naproxen) to relieve symptoms, tranexamic acid (an antifibrinolytic agent), the OC pill or depot progestogen. Less frequently, danazol or GnRH agonists are used. Treatment of anovulatory DUB

> ### CLINICAL INTEREST BOX 44-5
> ### COMPLEMENTARY AND ALTERNATIVE THERAPIES IN WOMEN'S CONDITIONS
>
> In menopausal symptoms, including hot flushes, various results have been obtained in clinical studies of complementary and alternative medicine methods:
> - dietary and herbal phyto-oestrogens are effective because of the oestrogenic components: natural oestrogens include ginseng, isoflavones, lignins and coumestans found in plants such as chick peas, grains, soybeans and clovers, and *Cimicifuga racemosa* (black cohosh)
> - techniques with variable results (not always proven effective) include acupuncture, respiratory modifications, relaxation and exercise
> - vitamin E therapy has been shown to be ineffective.
>
> In nausea and vomiting of pregnancy, acupressure, ginger and vitamin B_6 have been shown to be effective. The herb dong quai (*Angelica sinensis*) has long been used in traditional Chinese medicine for treating menstrual disorders, among other conditions. It has a volatile oil constituent that relaxes the uterus, and a non-volatile constituent that produces strong uterine contractions. Overall, the effects depend on the functional state of the uterus.
>
> In breast cancer, some relief of symptoms (nausea, pain, depression) has been obtained with acupuncture, mind–body therapies, and mistletoe and other herbs that may enhance immune functions.
>
> In premenstrual syndrome, symptoms of breast tenderness and neuropsychological symptoms such as anxiety and depression have been shown in some studies to be reduced with use of black cohosh, chaste tree berries, evening primrose oil or *Gingko biloba*; however, the evidence is not strong.
> *Adapted from*: Spencer & Jacobs 1999; Braun & Cohen 2005.

---

depends on the cause but usually involves balancing progestogen and oestrogen levels with OC or HRT preparations. Surgical treatments include dilatation and curettage of the uterus, laser endometrial ablation and, as a last resort, hysterectomy.

Dysmenorrhoea and premenstrual syndrome are treated similarly with NSAIDs, OCs and sometimes also vitamin B_6, or a selective serotonin reuptake inhibitor such as fluoxetine.

Endometriosis

Endometriosis is the location of endometrial tissue at unusual (ectopic) locations, e.g. within the oviducts, ovaries, myometrium or pelvis. It is relatively common, occurring in about 10% of women during their lifetime. As all endometrial tissue is subject to stimulation by gonadotrophic and ovarian hormones, ectopic tissue will also undergo cyclical changes during the menstrual period and produce menstrual fluid that cannot escape the abdominal cavity or other location. This can lead to ovarian cysts, pain and chronic inflammation, scar formation, infertility, dysmenorrhoea and painful intercourse.

First-line treatment is surgical, to remove ectopic endometrial tissue. Pharmacological treatments include progestogens, OC preparations, danazol (to inhibit GnRH and block LH surge) or GnRH analogues (continuous dose for gonadal suppression), with NSAIDs to reduce inflammation and pain.

PREGNANCY SAFETY

ADEC Category	Drug
B1	Oestradiol valerate;* oestriol
B3	Clomiphene, tamoxifen, many combined OC preparations†
D	Conjugated oestrogens, cyproterone, danazol, dydrogesterone, gestrinone, norethisterone, progesterone, tibolone
D	*Many HRT combinations (e.g. MPA–oestradiol valerate) and OC combinations (e.g. oestradiol valerate–norethisterone); high-dose levonorgestrel
X	Raloxifene

*Note that while some individual hormones (e.g. oestradiol valerate) may be in the higher (i.e. safer) categories, the OC or HRT combined products may be in a lower category.
†While OCs are contraindicated in pregnancy, there is no increased risk of birth defects if pregnancy occurs and OCs are taken during the early stages.

DRUGS AT A GLANCE 44: Drugs affecting the female reproductive system

Therapeutic group	Pharmacological group	Key examples	Key pages
Female sex hormones Oestrogenic compounds	Oestrogens	oestrogen oestradiol valerate ethinyloestradiol (EE)	709–11 709, 11 709
	Selective oestrogen receptor modulators (SERMs)	raloxifene	710, 19
Anti-oestrogens	Anti-oestrogens	tamoxifen; clomiphene	710
Female sex hormones Progestogenic compounds	Progestogens	progesterone medroxyprogesterone acetate (MPA)	710–12 712, 13
Antiprogestogens	Progesterone antagonists	mifepristone	712
Oral contraceptives	Combined oral contraceptives (COCs)	various combinations of EE or mestranol with levonorgestrel or norethisterone	712–6
	Progesterone-only (oral)	norethisterone; levonorgestrel	715–7
Depot contraceptives	Progesterone-only (depot)	MPA; levonorgestrel	716, 7
Hormone replacement therapy (HRT)	Natural oestrogens Progestogens Gonadomimetics	oestradiol valerate MPA; norethisterone tibolone	718, 9 719 719, 20

Note: See also Table 44-1 for a range of hormonal oral contraceptives, and CIB 44-3.

KEY POINTS

- Oestrogens and progesterone are the natural ovarian hormones and are very commonly used in medicine.
- Oestrogens stimulate and maintain the regular menstrual cycle, have metabolic actions and inhibit the release of pituitary gonadotrophins.
- Oestrogens are used in oral contraceptive preparations; in hormone replacement therapy after menopause; for disorders of menstruation, treating breast (and prostatic) carcinomas; hirsutism; and for preventing osteoporosis in postmenopausal women.
- Anti-oestrogens and selective oestrogen receptor modulators are used in breast cancers, infertility and menopausal problems.
- Progesterone stimulates the secretory phase of the menstrual cycle and facilitates and maintains pregnancy.
- Synthetic progestogens are orally active and are indicated for hormonal replacement therapy, treating endometriosis and specific carcinomas, and for preventing pregnancy.
- Oral contraception with combinations of an oestrogen and a progestogen is the most effective reversible form of birth control currently available.
- Types of oral contraceptive formulations include combined continuous and phased preparations, progestogen-only tablets and implants and emergency contraception regimens.
- Risk–benefit analysis shows that for most women, use of oral contraception is safe, effective, reversible and inexpensive, and protects against many gynaecological problems. Adverse reactions are generally mild with low- or no-oestrogen formulations.
- Because oral contraceptives are primarily for self-administration, the emphasis for the health-care professional is on patient education for accurate and safe administration and for early recognition of adverse reactions, particularly thromboembolism.
- Cessation of menstruation at the menopause may be associated with symptoms of low oestrogen levels, and brings increased risk of cardiovascular disease and osteoporosis.
- Hormone replacement therapy, i.e. regular use of low-dose natural oestrogen with cyclical progesterone, suppresses menopausal symptoms and protects against some cancers and bone disease. HRT may be administered orally or transdermally.
- Long-term use of HRT may cause a slightly increased risk of some conditions (e.g. stroke, breast cancer, venous thromboembolism), and reduced risk of others (osteoporotic fractures, colorectal cancer, dementia and diabetes).
- Other gynaecological disorders (hirsutism, dysfunctional bleeding and endometriosis) are treated with agonists or antagonists of oestrogens and progestogens.
- Because all these drugs may affect sexual functioning, the health-care professional must be sensitive to the patient's needs and alert to cues that reflect problems, such as a disturbance of sexual functioning and self-concept.

REVIEW EXERCISES

1 Name the three endogenous oestrogens and discuss the typical approach for dosage and administration of oestrogen products.
2 Describe the physiological actions of progesterone, then name four progestogens and discuss their primary indications and clinical uses.
3 Discuss why an oestrogen is combined with a progestogen in oral contraceptives. Describe the main types of combination oestrogen and progestogen contraceptives.
4 Discuss the indications, advantages, disadvantages and precautions with use of combined oestrogen–progestogen HRT during menopause.
5 Discuss the use of hormones and hormone antagonists in treating hirsutism, dysfunctional bleeding and endometriosis.

REFERENCES AND FURTHER READING

Australian Medicines Handbook 2006. Adelaide: AMH, 2006.

Bath PM, Gray LJ. Association between hormone replacement therapy and stroke: a meta-analysis. *British Medical Journal* 2005; 330(7487): 342–4.

Bluming AZ. Hormone replacement therapy: the debate should continue. *Geriatrics* 2004; 59(11): 30–1, 35–7.

Bowman WC, Rand MJ. *Textbook of Pharmacology*. 2nd edn. Oxford: Blackwell, 1980 [ch. 20].

Braun L, Cohen M. *Herbs and Natural Supplements: An Evidence-Based Guide*. Sydney: Elsevier Mosby, 2005.

Caswell A (ed.). *MIMS Annual June 2005*. Sydney: CMPMedica Australia, 2005.

Drew A. Dong quai. *Current Therapeutics* 2000; June 2000: 97–8.

Ellertson C, Trussell J, Stewart FH, Winikoff B. Should emergency contraceptive pills be available without prescription? *Journal of the American Medical Women's Association* 1998; 53 (5 Suppl. 2): 226–32.

Endocrinology Expert Group. *Therapeutic Guidelines: Endocrinology, version 3*. Melbourne: Therapeutic Guidelines Limited, 2004.

Evans A, Vollenhoven B, Healy D. Modern antioestrogens and the coming revolution in women's health care. *Australian & New Zealand Journal of Obstetrics & Gynaecology* 1999; 39(3): 334–40.

Finn M, Bowyer L, Carr S et al (eds). *Women's health: a core curriculum*. Sydney: Elsevier Mosby, 2005.

Fraser IS. Forty years of combined oral contraception: the evolution of a revolution. *Medical Journal of Australia* 2000; 173: 541–4.

Goodman HM. Part VI: Endocrine physiology. Ch. 46 in: Johnson LR (ed.). *Essential Medical Physiology*. 2nd edn. Philadelphia: Lippincott-Raven, 1999.

Greenspan FS, Strewler GJ. *Basic & Clinical Endocrinology*. 5th edn. Stamford: Appleton & Lange, 1997 [ch. 13].

Haynes B, Dowsett M. Clinical pharmacology of selective estrogen receptor modulators. *Drugs & Aging* 1999 ;14(5): 323–36.

MacLennan AH. Long-term hormone replacement therapy. *Australian Prescriber* 2000; 23(5): 90–2.

MacLennan AH. Hormone replacement therapy: where to now? *Australian Prescriber* 2003; 26(1): 8–10.

MacLennan AH, Wilson DH, Taylor AW. Hormone replacement therapy use over a decade in an Australian population. *Climacteric* 2002; 5(4): 351–6.

McDonnell DP. The molecular determinants of estrogen receptor pharmacology. *Maturitas* 2004; 48 Suppl. 1: S7–12.

Neeskens P. The evidence–relevance gap: the example of hormone replacement therapy. *Australian Prescriber* 2002; 25(3): 60–2.

Nilsson S, Koehler KF. Oestrogen receptors and selective oestrogen receptor modulators: molecular and cellular pharmacology. *Basic and Clinical Pharmacology and Toxicology* 2005; 96(1): 15–25.

Rang HP, Dale MM, Ritter JM, Moore PK. *Pharmacology*. 5th edn. Edinburgh: Churchill Livingstone, 2003 [chs 5, 50].

Riddoch G. The combined oral contraceptive pill: a practical review of current options. *Australian Family Physician* 2000; 29(11): 1039–44.

Soules MR, Sherman S, Parrott E et al. Executive summary: stages of reproductive aging workshop. *Fertility & Sterility* 2001; 76(5): 874–8.

Spencer JW, Jacobs JJ. *Complementary/Alternative Medicine: An Evidence-Based Approach*. St Louis: Mosby, 1999.

Stevenson JC. Hormone replacement therapy: review, update and remaining questions after the Women's Health Initiative Study. *Current Osteoporosis Reports* 2004; 2(1): 12–6.

Tortora GJ, Grabowski SR. *Principles of Anatomy and Physiology*. 9th edn. New York: HarperCollins, 2000 [ch. 28].

Tuckwell K (ed.). *MIMS Disease Index*. 2nd edn. Sydney: MediMedia Australia, 1996.

Vollenhoven B. *Contraception*. Melbourne: Monash University, 2000 [unpublished review].

Weisberg E. Progestogen-only methods of contraception. *Australian Prescriber* 1999; 22(1): 6–8.

Weisberg E. Contraception, hormone therapy and thrombosis. *Australian Prescriber* 2002; 25(3): 57–9.

Wilson JD, Foster DW, Kronenberg HM, Larsen PR. *Williams Textbook of Endocrinology*. 9th edn. Philadelphia: Saunders, 1998 [Sect. 5].

Writing Group for the Women's Health Initiative Investigators. Risks and benefits of estrogen plus progestin in healthy postmenopausal women: principal results from the Women's Health Initiative Randomized Controlled Trial. *Journal of American Medical Association* 2002; 288(3): 321–33.

Youngson RM. *Collins Dictionary: Medicine*. 2nd edn. Glasgow: HarperCollins, 1998.

ON-LINE RESOURCES

New Zealand medicines and medical devices safety authority: www.medsafe.govt.nz

RANZCOG. Advice to medical practitioners regarding the use of postmenopausal hormone therapy. Consensus statement, August 2004. Available: www.jeanhailes.org.au/issues/hrt_benefits_con.htm, accessed 4 September 2006.

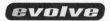 More weblinks at http://evolve.elsevier.com/AU/Bryant/pharmacology/

CHAPTER 45

Drugs in Pregnancy, Childbirth and Lactation

CHAPTER FOCUS

In this chapter, the physiology of pregnancy is reviewed
briefly and the use of drugs in pregnancy discussed,
including risks of fetal effects and teratogenesis.
Drugs affecting uterine smooth muscle activity
include those that induce labour (oxytocics) or inhibit
premature labour (tocolytics). These, and analgesics
and anaesthetics, are the typical medications used
during labour and delivery in women. Lactation can be
affected by drug therapy, as can the infant if drugs pass
across into breast milk; guidelines for use of drugs by
lactating mothers are described.

OBJECTIVES

- To describe the hormonal changes during pregnancy
  and the physiological changes that may impinge on
  drug pharmacokinetics.

- To discuss drug use during pregnancy and the risks
  associated with it.

- To describe drugs that affect the uterus and how
  they are commonly used during labour.

- To discuss maternal drug use during the perinatal
  period and describe drug effects on the neonate and
  on lactation.

KEY DRUGS

dinoprostone
ergometrine
nifedipine
oxytocin
salbutamol

KEY TERMS

ergot alkaloids
lactation
oxytocics
perinatal period
pregnancy
prostaglandins
teratogenesis
thalidomide
tocolytics

KEY ABBREVIATION

PG prostaglandin

DRUGS IN PREGNANCY
Hormone levels in pregnancy

IF implantation of a fertilised ovum occurs during the second stage of a woman's cycle, i.e. if she becomes pregnant, the chorionic gonadotrophin (see Drug Monograph 43-1) secreted 'rescues' the corpus luteum, which continues to secrete progesterone (the pro-pregnancy hormone), so menstruation does not occur and all the changes of **pregnancy** commence. By the second and third month, the placenta is maturing and acts as an autonomous endocrine gland, secreting large amounts of progesterone, oestrogens, chorionic gonadotrophin and human chorionic somatomammotrophin (also called human placental lactogen). Other hormones, including growth hormone, adrenocorticotrophic hormone and thyroid-stimulating hormone, can also be secreted by the placenta. Various hormone actions are important in pregnancy, and are summarised below.

Progesterone levels from the corpus luteum and placenta continue to rise sharply throughout pregnancy, to about 10 times the amount in late menstrual cycle. Progesterone relaxes the myometrium, ensures the cervix remains closed, assists oestrogens in development of breast tissue, and has an immunosuppressant effect, ensuring that the maternal immune system does not reject the (immunologically 'foreign') fetus.

Oestrogens (oestradiol, oestriol and oestrone) are secreted in increasing amounts, to about 10 times pre-pregnancy levels. Oestrogens stimulate breast development, encourage a 20-fold increase in weight of the uterus (excluding the conceptus), and cause skin changes. There is a further sharp rise in oestriol levels in the last few weeks of pregnancy, which enhances haemostatic mechanisms and may mediate dilation of the birth canal early in labour.

Human chorionic gonadotrophin levels are very high for the first 2–3 months, then decrease rapidly. This hormone has effects similar to those of luteinising hormone (the chorion is the outermost of the two membranes that enclose the embryo; the inner membrane is the amnion).

Human chorionic somatomammotrophin levels rise steadily throughout pregnancy. This hormone is related to growth hormone and hence has somatotrophic-type actions: it helps prepare the mammary glands for lactation, enhances maternal growth, and alters protein, fat and glucose metabolism so that more glucose and amino acids are available for the fetus (a consequence is exacerbation or precipitation of diabetes mellitus in the mother).

Prolactin levels from the anterior pituitary rise steadily throughout pregnancy and prepare the breasts for lactation.

Relaxin, a peptide hormone produced by the corpus luteum and later the placenta, increases the flexibility of the pelvic bones and joints during pregnancy and helps dilate the uterine cervix during labour and delivery.

Corticotrophin-releasing factor is secreted by the placenta, especially late in pregnancy, and may help control the timing of childbirth. It also increases the secretion of adrenal cortex hormones, which help maturation of the fetal lungs and production of surfactant (see Chapter 32).

Hormone levels can be readily measured during pregnancy (e.g. in maternal urine), which allows for close monitoring of how the pregnancy is progressing, and treatment if required.

Common conditions in pregnancy

Maternal adaptations to pregnancy include anatomical changes due to the expanding fetus putting pressure on the mother's internal organs, and weight gain due to the fetus, placenta, amniotic fluid and enlarged uterus. There are also physiological adaptations, which may affect how the mother responds to drugs or how her body handles drugs. In the cardiovascular system, for example, cardiac output, stroke volume, heart rate and blood volume all increase by 15%–30%. Similarly, pulmonary function increases to meet the demands of the fetus for oxygen, and pressure on the urinary bladder increases frequency of urination. Decreased gastrointestinal tract motility and increased risk of nausea and vomiting may delay absorption of nutrients and drugs.

Common conditions occurring in pregnancy include nausea, heartburn and 'morning sickness'. These can be severe enough to threaten the health of the mother and fetus, so antiemetic drugs may be required. Anaemias are common because of the increased demand for iron and blood cell functions, so iron and folic acid are frequently prescribed. Urinary tract infections are also more common. Other chronic conditions that the mother suffered before the pregnancy, such as diabetes, epilepsy, asthma, hypertension, peptic ulcer, migraine, depression, thyroid disorder or urinary tract infection, will need careful monitoring and treatment to optimise the mother's (and fetus's) health.

Miscarriage, or spontaneous abortion, before 20 weeks may be a natural rejection of an abnormal embryo or fetus. Threatened abortion later in pregnancy can sometimes be successfully delayed by tocolytic drugs. Therapeutic abortion, sometimes carried out if there is a threat to the life or health of the mother, is assisted by oxytocic drugs (see later sections).

Pre-eclampsia (toxaemia of pregnancy) is a potentially dangerous combination of hypertension, proteinuria and oedema, thought to be due to renal ischaemia. It can occur at any time in the second half of pregnancy, and complicates 2%–8% of pregnancies. Treatment is with magnesium sulphate by IV infusion or slow IM injection, to control convulsions. Large doses (several grams of magnesium sulphate over a period of hours) are given and can lead to magnesium toxicity, manifest by loss of reflexes and respiratory and cardiovascular collapse. Pre-eclampsia is a warning sign for the dangerous complication eclampsia, a condition carrying a high maternal and fetal mortality. The only safe treatment of eclampsia, which can cause convulsions, coma and death, is delivery of the baby.

Australian categorisation of drug risks in pregnancy

Other complications of pregnancy or conditions occurring during pregnancy may also dictate the use of medications, such as those to treat diabetes and systemic infections. The pharmacology of these drugs and their use are discussed in the appropriate sections of this textbook. Because most drugs taken by a pregnant woman can cross the placenta (see Chapter 8) and affect the fetus, it is important to know the relative risks of known harmful effects of medicines on the developing fetus, and balance these against the need of the pregnant woman for drug therapy. The Australian Drug Evaluation Committee has categorised drugs on the basis of their potential for harmful effects during pregnancy (see Table 8-1).

New drugs are not tested in pregnant women during clinical trials, so it is difficult to establish safety. Consequently, reference texts usually advise that 'use in pregnancy is not recommended' or give similar warnings. This makes it difficult for doctors (and their patients) wanting to use new drugs in pregnant women. Epidemiological studies and post-marketing studies of drug use in wide populations may establish the safety of drugs in pregnant women.

On the other hand, many pregnancies are unplanned or not verified for some months, which implies that pregnant women may be unwittingly exposed to many drugs during the early months. Fear of fetal damage, or misinformation, may lead such women to seek termination of pregnancy unnecessarily.

The general rules on drug use in pregnancy are:
- avoid all drugs in pregnancy if possible, especially in the first 12 weeks
- pregnant women should be counselled to avoid exposure to all unnecessary drugs and chemicals
- the risk to the fetus must be balanced against the health of mother (and fetus); for example, the dangers to mother and fetus of uncontrolled epilepsy far outweigh the risks of abnormalities caused by antiepileptic drugs
- if a drug is essential to the wellbeing of the mother or fetus, the lowest effective dose should be used for the shortest possible duration
- drugs shown to be safe for use in nausea and vomiting of morning sickness include metoclopramide, doxylamine and diphenhydramine.

Many drugs are **teratogenic** (i.e. can cause congenital malformations) at clinical dose levels in animals, including antineoplastics, sex hormones (androgens, stilboestrol), phenytoin, chloroquine, lithium, cannabis, aspirin and glucocorticoids. Results from animal studies, however, cannot always be extrapolated to humans. Of the drugs that have been shown to be teratogenic in humans, only a few are still in clinical use, for their efficacy in otherwise serious disorders. Such drugs include the antineoplastic agents methotrexate and cyclophosphamide; antiepileptics carbamazepine, valproic acid and phenytoin; endocrine agents including antithyroid drugs, danazol and oral hypoglycaemic agents; and ACE inhibitors, lithium, retinoids, tetracycline, **thalidomide** and warfarin. These drugs are listed in categories D or X in Pregnancy Safety Classifications, and their use during pregnancy is usually contraindicated unless the potential benefits are considered to outweigh markedly the teratogenic risks. Other precautions can also be instituted: e.g. the drug isotretinoin and its analogues (used to treat severe acne and psoriasis) are teratogenic at normal dose levels and have long half-lives; in women of childbearing age, they must be used only after a (negative) pregnancy test and provided the woman is using effective contraceptive measures.

Despite careful testing and warning, problems still occur, both from use of contraindicated drugs and from non-use of safe drugs. The combination of doxylamine, dicyclomine and pyridoxine, for example, taken for nausea and vomiting of pregnancy, was withdrawn in the 1980s following a scare about possible teratogenic effects. These were later disproved, but in the meantime the rate of hospitalisation of pregnant women in the USA for severe nausea and vomiting was doubled, putting the health of the women and their infants at risk. At the other extreme, the retinoid compounds, useful for treatment of severe acne unresponsive to milder drugs (see Drug Monograph 56-2), are known teratogens, causing CNS, cardiovascular and craniofacial defects. They are labelled appropriately and only very carefully prescribed; however, there have been cases of defects caused by women taking them without realising they were pregnant, or ignoring warning labels.

DRUGS AFFECTING THE UTERUS

The uterus is a highly muscular organ that exhibits a range of characteristic properties and activities. The smooth muscle fibres extend longitudinally, circularly and obliquely in the organ. The uterus has a rich blood supply; however, blood flow is diminished when the uterine muscle contracts. The myometrium undergoes rhythmical contraction; the contractions originate in muscle, with the myometrial cells in the fundus (the inner surface of the dome of the uterus) acting as pacemakers. During the menstrual cycle, contractions are weak on days 6–14, then become gradually larger and more prolonged, until during menstruation (days 1–5) the contractions are strong and coordinated and can lead to cramping pain. Drugs that act on the uterus include oxytocics, which increase uterine contractility, and tocolytics, which decrease it (from the Greek stem *tokos*: birth).

Control of uterine activity is via excitatory and inhibitory sympathetic fibres: noradrenaline (acting at α_2 receptors) causes stimulation of muscle contraction, and adrenaline (at β_2-adrenoceptors) causes inhibition, i.e. relaxation of uterine muscle, hence the use of salbutamol (a β_2-receptor stimulant) as a tocolytic. Adrenoceptor antagonists appear to have no effect on uterine muscle activity.

Profound changes occur in the uterus during pregnancy: it increases in weight from about 50 g to around 1000 g, its capacity increases 10-fold in length and new muscle fibres may be formed. The rhythmical contractions of the myometrium are depressed during pregnancy by the high concentrations of progesterone and oestrogens. These changes may be accompanied by changes in response to drugs.

Parturition (childbirth)

During the last few weeks of pregnancy, painless uterine contractions become increasingly frequent and the lower uterine segment and cervix become softer and thinner. The key event stimulating labour in women is still not determined; it appears to involve complex interactions of several placental, fetal and maternal hormones. Suggested factors causing initiation of labour include:

- a rise in the oestrogen:progesterone ratio (which increases the number of oxytocin receptors)
- increased sensitivity of the uterus to oxytocin
- prostaglandins produced from the amnion and chorion
- decreased levels of nitric oxide (a uterine smooth muscle relaxant)
- catecholamines, especially α_2-receptor agonists
- sudden changes in intrauterine pressure.

After labour has been initiated, regular uterine contractions moving downwards from the fundus of the uterus help expel the fetus. The process of birth usually takes several hours, with the stages of dilation of the cervix (6–12 hours) and expulsion (delivery of the baby, 10 minutes to several hours) taking much longer than the third stage, delivery of the placenta (10–30 minutes). The birth process is stressful on both mother and baby. The fetal adrenal medulla responds by secreting high amounts of catecholamines, and the adrenal cortex by secreting corticosteroids, all of which help prepare the infant for independent existence, clear the lungs, provide surfactant for breathing, mobilise nutrients and promote increased blood flow to the brain and heart.

Because many drugs are available for use during labour and delivery, it is important to consider the benefit versus risk to the fetus. The pharmacokinetics of drugs may be altered during labour and delivery: e.g. during labour, gastric emptying is delayed and vomiting may result, which would alter drug absorption. Vomiting may also be exacerbated by the use of opioid analgesics. Because oral drug absorption is unpredictable at this time, parenteral routes should be used. Drug metabolism and excretion may be altered and prolonged during labour and, although clinical data are currently sparse, the potential for inducing adverse or undesirable effects is always a concern. If a drug such as an opioid analgesic or sedative is potentially harmful to the fetus, then the smallest possible dose for the mother should be used.

Oxytocics

Agents that stimulate contraction of the smooth muscle of the uterus, resulting in contractions and labour, are **oxytocics**. The most commonly used oxytocics are synthetic oxytocin, alkaloids of the plant fungus ergot, and prostaglandins of the E and F series. Many other drugs may have some effect on the contractility of uterine smooth muscle, but their effects are too non-specific to be clinically useful. Oxytocics are used to induce labour, to reduce postpartum haemorrhage and to terminate pregnancy.

Oxytocin

Oxytocin is one of two hormones secreted by the posterior pituitary; the other hormone is vasopressin, or antidiuretic hormone (see Chapters 37 and 38). Oxytocin means 'rapid birth', a term derived from its ability to contract the pregnant uterus. It also facilitates milk ejection during lactation. The non-pregnant uterus is relatively insensitive to oxytocin, but uterine sensitivity to oxytocin gradually increases during pregnancy, with the uterus being most sensitive at term. Oxytocin secretion may precede and possibly trigger delivery of the fetus. Large amounts of oxytocin have been detected in the blood during the expulsive phase of delivery. A positive feedback mechanism may be operant: more forceful contractions of uterine muscle and greater stretching of the cervix and vagina result in more oxytocin release. Oxytocin acts directly on the myometrium, having a stronger effect on the fundus than on the cervix, thus helping propel the fetus down the birth canal. Oxytocin also transiently impedes uterine blood flow and stimulates the mammary gland to increase milk excretion from the breast, although it does not increase the production of milk.

The clinical use of oxytocin is described in Drug Monograph 38-4.

Ergot alkaloids

The **ergot alkaloids** are naturally occurring compounds that have varied effects in the body through their actions on several types of receptors (see Clinical Interest Box 45-1). **Ergometrine** produces prolonged, strong contractions of the uterus, especially postpartum, and has vasoconstrictor actions, so is useful in treatment of postpartum haemorrhage (see Drug Monograph 45-1).

Prostaglandins

Prostaglandins are produced in the endometrium and myometrium; $PGF_{2\alpha}$ is a vasoconstrictor, while PGE_2 and prostacyclin are vasodilators. Both PGEs and PGFs contract uterine smooth muscle and are implicated in disorders of menstruation. The uterus becomes increasingly sensitive to PGs during pregnancy, so the prostaglandins can be used to produce abortion.

In obstetrics, prostaglandins are used to soften and dilate the cervix ('uterine priming') and to stimulate uterine contractions, as follows:

- gemeprost, a PGE_1 analogue, as an abortifacient in second trimester, given by pessary
- dinoprostone, a PGE_2 analogue, for induction or augmentation of labour at term, given by vaginal gel or pessary
- dinoprost, a $PGF_{2\alpha}$ analogue, for intractable postpartum haemorrhage, or termination of first- or second-trimester pregnancy, by intravaginal or intrauterine administration.

The prostaglandin analogues are used only where emergency gynaecological care is available. They are also used to prevent dyspepsia and peptic ulceration induced by non-steroidal anti-inflammatory agents, and in the treatment of erectile dysfunction in men.

Premature labour inhibitors (tocolytics)

Preterm labour, or labour that occurs before the 37th week of pregnancy, is a major problem in obstetrics. It occurs in 10%–15% of all pregnancies. Premature birth increases the possibility of neonatal morbidity and mortality. Drugs that relax the uterus, and hence delay labour or inhibit threatened abortion, are described as **tocolytics**. If considered medically desirable to prevent premature labour, they are administered to prolong the time of the fetus in utero, to allow time for maturation of the fetus or administration of corticosteroids to the mother to facilitate fetal production of lung surfactant, and/or to allow transport of the mother to a special centre for delivery of a significantly preterm infant. The main drugs used as tocolytics are the β_2-adrenoceptor agonist salbutamol, the calcium channel blocker nifedipine, and the oxytocin antagonist atosiban (not available in Australia). Other drugs that may relax uterine smooth muscle include progestogens, general anaesthetics, alcohol, magnesium sulfate, direct vasodilators and non-steroidal anti-inflammatory drugs (NSAIDs) (by their actions inhibiting prostaglandin synthesis).

The preferred drug for delaying labour is now **nifedipine**; this is a new use for this calcium channel blocker, which is usually indicated in the treatment of hypertension and angina. In threatened preterm labour, standard 20 mg tablets can be given every 3–8 hours until contractions cease or labour becomes too well established to stop.

The clinical use of **salbutamol** as a bronchodilator in asthma has already been described (Drug Monograph 32-2). When used as a tocolytic, salbutamol is usually administered by IV infusion or IM injection, for management of uncomplicated preterm labour (24–34 weeks' gestation). Tocolytics are not

---

DRUG MONOGRAPH 45-1 ERGOMETRINE

Ergometrine increases the force and frequency of uterine contractions by direct stimulation of the smooth muscle of the uterine wall. The increased contractions and muscle tone and the vasoconstriction of bleeding vessels at the placental site arrest haemorrhage. It is indicated to prevent and treat postpartum haemorrhage. Because the cervix of the uterus is contracted as well as the fundus, the fetus can become compressed and distressed, thus ergometrine is contraindicated during the first two stages of labour or to induce labour.

PHARMACOKINETICS Ergometrine has unpredictable bioavailability, so is given parenterally. It is formulated for IM administration (or, in emergency, IV). It has a rapid onset of action, within 1–3 minutes. The duration of uterine contraction after IM injection is about 3 hours. The drug is metabolised in the liver and excreted mainly in the faeces.

DRUG INTERACTIONS Ergometrine has significant interactions with many drugs that also affect receptors for noradrenaline or 5-HT. The effects of other vasoconstrictors are enhanced, whereas those of anti-anginal agents are antagonised. Drugs that reduce the metabolism of ergometrine (e.g. erythromycin, clarithromycin and some antivirals) may cause ergotism and ischaemia.

ADVERSE REACTIONS These include nausea, vomiting, hypertension, headache, and rarely infarction, pulmonary oedema and gangrene. A dose-related effect is abdominal cramping.

WARNINGS AND CONTRAINDICATIONS Use with caution in patients with hypocalcaemia. Avoid use in women with ergometrine or other ergot alkaloid hypersensitivity, cardiac or vascular disease, eclampsia or pre-eclampsia, sepsis, or liver or kidney function impairment. Contraindicated in pregnancy, during the first two stages of labour or to induce labour.

DOSAGE AND ADMINISTRATION Parenterally, 0.5 mg is administered IM or IV; the IV route is usually recommended only in emergencies or in patients with excessive uterine bleeding.

Ergometrine (0.5 mg/mL) is also formulated in combination with oxytocin (5 IU/mL) for active management of the third stage of labour.

CLINICAL INTEREST BOX 45-1   ERGOT, ST ANTHONY, DALE AND LSD

Ergot is a fungus (*Claviceps purpurea*) that grows on the grain rye. Poisoning (ergotism) occurs from eating bread made from ergot-infected rye.

Symptoms of ergotism are mainly related to ergot's vasoconstrictor actions: dry cold skin, ischaemic pain in muscles, gangrene of the extremities, dizziness, and CNS depression or convulsions; powerful contractions of the uterus can cause abortion.

In Europe in the middle ages, victims of ergotism travelled to St Anthony's Shrine near Vienne, in France, to pray for cure. The intense pain from ischaemic limbs was thus referred to as 'St Anthony's fire', as St Anthony was considered to have special powers to protect against fire, infections and epilepsy. Often the pilgrims were healed, possibly because they had removed themselves from the area where the grains were infected with ergot. The infamous 'bewitchings' that occurred in Salem, Massachusetts, in December 1691 are also thought to have been due to ergotism, as the previous summer had been hot and wet, conducive to good growth of fungi on grain.

An early British pharmacologist, H.H. Dale, studied the activity of ergot extracts in the early 1900s. Dale showed that ergot extracts contain, in addition to active amines such as histamine, acetylcholine and tyramine, alkaloids that antagonise some actions of adrenaline.

The ergot alkaloids (i.e. nitrogen-containing active principles of ergot) are derivatives of lysergic acid amide. They have varied (and confusing) effects on many receptors and tissues.

Ergotamine and dihydroergotamine have partial agonist and antagonist actions on both α-adrenoceptors and 5-hydroxytryptamine (5-HT, serotonin) receptors, and have been used in treating migraine.

Ergotoxine (a mixture of alkaloids) has mainly oxytocic activity, and is used in obstetrics. Dihydroergotoxine on the other hand relaxes uterine muscle and is a vasodilator, so has been used to treat vascular insufficiency.

Ergometrine (known as ergonovine in the USA) is the most powerful oxytocic of the group and may be used by injection to prevent or treat postpartum haemorrhage.

The ergot alkaloids also act as emetics by stimulating the chemoreceptor trigger zone.

Other ergot derivatives include methysergide (a powerful 5-HT antagonist used prophylactically in migraine), bromocriptine (a dopamine agonist used to inhibit prolactin secretion) and lysergic acid diethylamide, the psychedelic hallucinogen better known as LSD. (See Chapter 22 and Figure 22-4.)

---

used in conditions in which prolongation of pregnancy is hazardous for the fetus or mother. Most tocolytics are effective in stopping labour for 2–3 days; however, many studies have shown that they do not themselves improve perinatal outcomes or decrease the rate of preterm delivery. Responses of both fetus and mother (heart rate, glycaemia) must be carefully monitored.

DRUGS IN THE PERINATAL PERIOD

Drugs given to the mother in the **perinatal period** (i.e. the period around childbirth, defined as from week 28 of pregnancy to the end of the first week of the infant's life) may affect the fetus or infant, due to drug passage across the placenta or into breast milk. Infants are born with immature hepatic and renal functions, so drugs given to them are cleared more slowly than in older people and may reach toxic concentrations. Another problem is that the immature blood–brain barrier of a premature or very young infant may allow passage into the CNS of drugs (and normal metabolites including bilirubin), which may have central effects or adverse effects. (These pharmacokinetic aspects are discussed in Chapter 8; the pharmacodynamic and clinical aspects are covered in chapters on the drug groups.)

Drugs commonly used in the perinatal period include:
- analgesics used for pain relief in childbirth: opioids such as pethidine (IM, IV) are strong analgesics, but can depress respiration in the infant (treated with the narcotic antagonist naloxone) and cause constipation in the mother
- anaesthetics used for pain relief in childbirth: the most common is nitrous oxide ('gas') 50% in oxygen, self-administered by the mother; this has little depressant effect on the infant
- epidural local anaesthetics such as lignocaine and bupivacaine, administered via the lumbar or caudal epidural space (an opioid and a local anaesthetic can be coadministered epidurally for the most effective obstetric analgesia); these can be used for caesarean section as well as vaginal delivery
- a benzodiazepine such as temazepam, for antianxiety or sedation during early labour.

Other drugs used by the mother may have the predictable effects in the neonate, e.g. β-blockers depress the infant's cardiovascular system, oral hypoglycaemic agents cause hypoglycaemia, and antithyroid drugs can cause goitre. 'Social drugs' can also affect the infant; for example, babies born to women who smoke are smaller and have an increased incidence of jaundice, and babies born to women dependent on narcotic analgesics such as heroin suffer a withdrawal syndrome after birth, which can be alleviated by administration of an opioid. Alcohol consumption during pregnancy can cause severe abnormalities; see Clinical Interest Box 8-1.

LACTATION

Lactation, i.e. secretion and ejection of milk from the mammary glands (breasts), is initiated and maintained by the anterior pituitary hormone prolactin (see Chapter 38). During the late months of pregnancy, high levels of progesterone and oestrogens inhibit the actions of prolactin, so lactation commences when levels of progesterone and oestradiol drop rapidly after birth. Suckling at the breast by the infant increases secretion of prolactin by neural reflexes, which act via the hypothalamus and pituitary gland, and triggers the milk letdown reflex, with oxytocin as a mediator.

Prolactin release is inhibited by the hypothalamic prolactin release-inhibitory factor (PRIF, dopamine), hence dopamine agonist drugs may decrease lactation, while dopamine antagonists such as the phenothiazine psychotropic agents may cause gynaecomastia and galactorrhoea (see Clinical Interest Box 38-3).

Lactation promoters

Prolactin, as its name implies, is the natural lactation promoter, and suckling or mechanical stimulation of the nipple are the best stimulators of prolactin secretion. The dopamine antagonist metoclopramide, normally prescribed as an antiemetic or to stimulate motility of the upper GI tract, has been used (10 mg doses three times daily) to stimulate lactation.

Lactation inhibitors

Oestrogens in combination contraceptive pill formulations are known to inhibit lactation, hence the use of progestogen-only minipill formulations for contraception in breastfeeding women. In the past, oestrogens such as chlorotrianisene (a prodrug with long-acting oestrogen effects) have been used to treat postpartum breast engorgement. This use of oestrogens has declined over the years, mainly because the incidence of painful engorgement is considered low, and studies have indicated that analgesics and other conservative measures such as breast binding and ice packs are effective. The prescriber must also weigh the benefit of using oestrogens for this purpose against the risks, particularly of inducing thromboembolism or uterine bleeding.

It may be necessary, for clearly defined medical reasons, to inhibit lactation, e.g. if the mother must take essential drugs that would be harmful to the infant when ingested in breast milk. The dopamine agonists bromocriptine and cabergoline inhibit the release of prolactin from the anterior pituitary gland, resulting in suppression of lactation.

Drugs and breastfeeding

Drugs can enter breast milk and be absorbed by the infant in sufficient amounts to cause pharmacological or toxic effects. In particular, very lipid-soluble drugs will partition into the lipid component of milk and so may cause problems, e.g. CNS depressants may sedate the baby and depress suckling (see Chapter 8). Alternatively, drugs given to the mother may depress lactation. It is essential for the welfare of the infant, however, that the mother's health be maintained, so drug therapy may need to be instituted or continued.

For these reasons, it is often necessary to know how a drug affects lactation and whether it is safe for a breastfeeding mother and child. Guidelines have been drawn up, based on clinical experience in breastfeeding mothers (see *Drugs and Breastfeeding*, from the Royal Women's Hospital, Melbourne), and including advice on specific drugs. In general, it is suggested that:

- the benefits of breastfeeding to both infant and mother are important
- optimising the mother's health is in the best interests of the infant
- older drugs that appear to be safe should be prescribed in preference to new drugs with which there is little clinical experience
- because many oral drugs reach maximum plasma concentrations within about 2–3 hours, and babies tend to feed at 4–6-hour intervals, taking a drug immediately after a feed will minimise the traces of drug in breast milk
- only essential drugs should be taken by breastfeeding women; if possible, surgery could be delayed
- breastfeeding mothers requiring surgery generally can continue to feed, provided adequate hydration is maintained and the first quantity of milk after surgery is discarded
- a drug should be selected within a group so that the drug least likely to transfer into milk is prescribed
- local administration will minimise dosage and plasma concentrations of drug, hence minimise transfer into milk
- give the mother a drug dose before the infant's longest sleep period
- withhold feeding (or give expressed milk) if a one-off drug is needed, e.g. diagnostic agent
- for some drugs, the milk to plasma ratio has been determined; if this is high, e.g. with antidepressants, some β-blockers and some NSAIDs, the drug may not be recommended, or recommended only with caution and monitoring of the infant (see Box 8-2).

PREGNANCY SAFETY	
ADEC Category	Drug
A	Oxytocin, salbutamol
B3	Gemeprost
C	Dinoprost, dinoprostone, ergot alkaloids, nifedipine
X	Misoprostol

DRUGS AT A GLANCE 45: Drugs in pregnancy, childbirth and lactation

Therapeutic group	Pharmacological group	Key examples	Key pages
Drugs stimulating uterine contractions	Oxytocics • Hormonal • Ergot alkaloids • Prostaglandin analogues	oxytocin ergometrine dinoprostone	727 727–9 728
Drugs inhibiting uterine contractions	Tocolytics • β-adrenoceptor agonists • Calcium channel blockers	salbutamol nifedipine	728, 9 728, 9
Lactation promoters	Hormones Dopamine receptor antagonists	prolactin metoclopramide	730 730
Lactation inhibitors	Dopamine receptor agonists	bromocriptine cabergoline }	730
Drugs contraindicated in pregnancy	Teratogenic agents • Antineoplastics • Antiepileptics • Androgens • Angiotensin-converting enzyme inhibitors • Retinoids • Tetracyclines • Oral anticoagulants	 methotrexate cyclophosphamide phenytoin carbamazepine testosterone captopril tretinoin tetracycline warfarin	 726

KEY POINTS

- During pregnancy, hormones secreted by the mother, fetus and placenta interact and maintain pregnancy.
- Changes occurring in the mother can affect the pharmacokinetics of drugs administered to her.
- Drugs taken by the mother pass across into the fetal circulation and may cause pharmacological effects, including teratogenesis; great care must be taken with drug use during pregnancy.
- Drugs affecting uterine smooth muscle activity include those that induce labour (oxytocics), such as oxytocin. Ergometrine induces strong sustained uterine contraction that is useful in controlling postpartum haemorrhage, and is only ever given after delivery. Tocolytics inhibit premature labour and include nifedipine and salbutamol.
- These, and analgesics and anaesthetics, are the typical medications used during the perinatal period; they can transfer across the placenta and into breast milk, and may affect the fetus or neonate.
- Lactation can be affected by drug therapy of the mother, as can the infant if drugs are excreted in breast milk; guidelines for use of drugs by lactating mothers are described, including careful drug use and timing of doses to minimise drug concentrations in milk.

REVIEW EXERCISES

1 Discuss the risks for the mother and the fetus of drugs taken during pregnancy.
2 Define the term 'teratogenesis' and list drugs known to be teratogenic.

3 Describe the effects of oxytocin on the non-pregnant and pregnant uterus.

4 Describe briefly the pharmacological and clinical uses of the ergot alkaloids.

5 Discuss the mechanisms of action, indications and clinical use of salbutamol and nifedipine in obstetrics.

6 Why has the use of lactation inhibitors declined over the years?

7 Describe how drugs can pass into breast milk, and outline guidelines for use of drugs by lactating women.

REFERENCES AND FURTHER READING

Australian Drug Evaluation Committee. *Prescribing Medicines in Pregnancy: An Australian Categorisation of Risk of Drug Use in Pregnancy.* 4th edn. Canberra: Therapeutic Goods Administration, 1999.

Australian Medicines Handbook 2006. Adelaide: AMH, 2006.

Bowman WC, Rand MJ. *Textbook of Pharmacology.* 2nd edn. Oxford: Blackwell, 1980 [ch. 20].

Caswell A (ed.). *MIMS Annual June 2005.* Sydney: CMPMedica Australia, 2005.

Chandraharan E, Arulkumaran S. Acute tocolysis. *Current Opinion in Obstetrics and Gynecology* 2005; 17(2): 151–6.

Endocrine Expert Group. *Therapeutic Guidelines Endocrinology, version 3.* Melbourne: Therapeutic Guidelines, 2004.

Gardiner SJ. Drugs in pregnancy. *New Ethicals Journal* 2002; 5(6):61–3.

Goodman HM. Part VI: Endocrine physiology. In: Johnson LR (ed.). *Essential Medical Physiology.* 2nd edn. Philadelphia: Lippincott-Raven, 1999 [ch. 47].

Greenspan FS, Strewler GJ. *Basic & Clinical Endocrinology.* 5th edn. Stamford: Appleton & Lange, 1997 [ch. 16].

Ilett KF, Kristensen JH. Drug use and breastfeeding. *Expert Opinion on Drug Safety* 2005; 4(4):745–68.

Katz VL, Farmer RM. Controversies in tocolytic therapy. *Clinical Obstetrics and Gynaecology* 1999; 42: 802–19.

King J, Flenady V, Cole S, Thornton S. Cyclo-oxygenase (COX) inhibitors for treating pre-term labour. *Cochrane Database of Systematic Reviews* 2005; (2): CD001992.

Lu JF, Nightingale CH. Magnesium sulfate in eclampsia and pre-eclampsia: pharmacokinetic principles. *Clinical Pharmacokinetics* 2000; 38: 305–14.

Mann J. *Murder, Magic and Medicine.* Oxford: Oxford University Press, 1992.

Royal Women's Hospital, Melbourne. *Drugs and Breastfeeding 2004.* Melbourne: Royal Women's Hospital, 2004.

Tortora GJ, Grabowski SR. *Principles of Anatomy and Physiology.* 9th edn. New York: HarperCollins, 2000 [ch. 29].

Wade A (ed.). *Martindale: The Extra Pharmacopoeia.* 27th edn. London: Pharmaceutical Press, 1977.

Winkler M, Rath W. A risk–benefit assessment of oxytocics in obstetric practice. *Drug Safety* 1999; 20: 323–45.

Youngson RM. *Collins Dictionary: Medicine.* 2nd edn. Glasgow: HarperCollins, 1998.

ON-LINE RESOURCES

Medications in Mother's Milk, by T. Hale: www.iBreastfeeding.com

New Zealand medicines and medical devices safety authority: www.medsafe.govt.nz

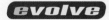 More weblinks at http://evolve.elsevier.com/AU/Bryant/pharmacology/

CHAPTER 46

Drugs Affecting the Male Reproductive System

CHAPTER FOCUS

Androgens, primarily testosterone, are male sex hormones used for replacement therapy in androgen deficiency and for treatment of advanced stages of breast cancer. Benign prostatic hyperplasia is a very common disorder that occurs in older men. The use of α_1-adrenoceptor antagonists and finasteride for treating this condition is discussed. Antiandrogens such as flutamide are indicated for treatment of prostatic cancer.

OBJECTIVES

- To compare the pharmacokinetics of oral and parenteral forms of testosterone and its ester derivatives.
- To describe the physiological actions and clinical uses of testosterone.
- To discuss the adverse reactions of androgen therapy and anabolic steroids in males and females.
- To discuss the relative effects and benefits of surgical and medical treatments for benign prostatic hyperplasia.
- To describe the various drugs that have antiandrogen effects, and the use of these in prostatic cancer.

KEY DRUGS

finasteride
flutamide
prazosin
testosterone

KEY TERMS

alpha-blockers
anabolic agents
androgens
antiandrogens
benign prostatic hyperplasia
hypogonadism
5α-reductase inhibitors
testosterone

KEY ABBREVIATIONS

BPH — benign prostatic hyperplasia (or hypertrophy)
DHT — dihydrotestosterone
GnRH — gonadotrophin-releasing hormone

THE MALE REPRODUCTIVE SYSTEM

THE hypothalamic and pituitary control of the testes are discussed in Chapter 38, and the anatomy and physiology of the male reproductive system have been reviewed in Chapter 43 (see Figures 43-2 and 43-3). To summarise:

- the main pituitary hormones involved in the male reproductive system are follicle-stimulating hormone (FSH), causing gametogenesis, and interstitial-cell-stimulating hormone (ICSH, luteinising hormone [LH]), stimulating production of androgens
- ICSH is downregulated by hypothalamic gonadotrophin-releasing hormone (GnRH) when given continuously; this effect is useful as 'chemical castration' in treating prostate cancer
- production of androgens occurs in the testis, stimulated by ICSH and decreased by oestrogens; production is not cyclical
- androgens are also produced in the adrenal cortex, stimulated by ACTH.

Androgens

Androgens, primarily **testosterone**, are the male sex hormones necessary for the normal development and maintenance of male sex characteristics. The actions of androgens are mediated in cells in androgen-sensitive tissues after conversion of testosterone by the 5α-reductase enzyme to the more active metabolite dihydrotestosterone (DHT). DHT binds to high-affinity androgen receptors and then activates nuclear receptors, which stimulate androgen-dependent RNA and protein synthesis. Androgenic effects include promotion of sexual maturation and growth, development of male secondary sexual characteristics, maturation of spermatozoa, anabolic effects and male sexual behaviour.

Testosterone, the naturally occurring androgenic hormone produced primarily by the testes, has a high first-pass effect when given orally as a drug, being rapidly metabolised in the liver to androstenedione, then excreted via the urine, with a half-life of only 5–20 minutes. Consequently, it is formulated as ester compounds to prolong the drug's duration of action. In the body tissues, the esters are rapidly hydrolysed to the active drug form. For example, testosterone undecanoate, formulated for oral administration in capsules, produces hormonal effects for 2–3 days. Testosterone enanthate as an oily solution for depot IM injection is much longer-acting, usually administered once every 2–4 weeks (see Drug Monograph 46-1). Testosterone pellets are available for subcutaneous implantation. This form will also provide an extended duration of action; depending on the number of

pellets used, effects may extend from 2 to 6 months before replacement pellets are necessary. Other synthetic androgens effective orally in tablet form include mesterolone, nandrolone and oxandrolone. Transdermal testosterone systems are available for application to the skin as gel or patches. Because androgens are used for replacement therapy in conditions of androgen deficiency that are usually chronic, lifelong therapy may be required, hence the importance of long-acting derivatives and depot preparations.

Androgen replacement therapy

Testosterone, its derivatives and synthetic agents are commonly used as replacement therapy for males who lack the hormone (see Drug Monograph 46-1). In males with **hypogonadism** or eunuchoidism (a deficiency of male hormone) or delayed puberty, the androgens produce marked changes in growth of the male sex organs, body contour, voice, and other secondary sex characteristics.

Androgen deficiency is relatively common (1 in 200 men) and may be due to disorders of the hypothalamus, pituitary

---

**CLINICAL INTEREST BOX 46-1
AKHENATON: A PHARAOH WITH FRÖHLICH'S SYNDROME?**

The Egyptian Pharaoh ruling in about 1369–1352 BC was Akhenaton, a powerful ruler and social reformer who overthrew the priestly caste and their gods. True-to-life statues at Karnak of the god-king in his later life show him with elongated and deformed skull, protruding lower jaw and stomach, narrow shoulders and arms, fat buttocks and thighs and prominent breasts (feminine physical characteristics), and no external male genitalia.

There has been much debate about Akhenaton, including suggestions that 'he' was a female masquerading as a male, that he had been castrated or that he suffered from rickets, pathological obesity, or a pituitary tumour or infection.

The overgrowth of skull bones suggests an early excess of growth hormone from the pituitary gland, while the obesity and feminisation suggest a lack of male hormones. Overall, it is most likely that he suffered from a hypothalamic or pituitary disorder, maybe an infestation of tapeworm in the pituitary gland or a pituitary tumour. Fröhlich's syndrome, or dystrophia adiposogenitalis, could account for the hypopituitarism and hypogonadism. However, Akhenaton was married to the famously beautiful Queen Nefertiti, who bore him six daughters, so hypogonadism and sterility are unlikely unless the tumour struck him after he had fathered several children. Until a mummy is found and identified with absolute certainty as Akhenaton's, medical experts and archaeologists will continue to dispute the cause of his unusual representations in statues.
Based on: Leavesley 1984, chapter on 'Akhenaton'.

DRUG MONOGRAPH 46-1 TESTOSTERONE ENANTHATE DEPOT INJECTION

Testosterone enanthate has long-acting and intense androgenic actions.

INDICATIONS Testosterones are indicated for:
- treatment of androgen deficiency, such as testicular failure caused by cryptorchidism (failure of one or both testes to descend into the scrotum), orchitis (inflammation of the testes), orchidectomy (surgical removal of one or both testes), or pituitary–hypothalamic insufficiency
- treatment of delayed male puberty when not induced by a pathological condition.

PHARMACOKINETICS The duration of action depends on the dose and the ester formulation administered. The longest duration of action for testosterone preparations is with the enanthate ester: after IM injection, the effects last for 2–4 weeks. Testosterone is metabolised in the liver, and metabolites are excreted by the kidneys.

DRUG INTERACTIONS Significant drug interactions have been reported when testosterone was given concurrently with oral anticoagulants (coumarin or indanedione), leading to enhanced anticoagulant effects, or with antidiabetic agents (enhanced hypoglycaemic effects).

ADVERSE REACTIONS Severe adverse effects occur particularly after inappropriate use in women, children and athletes. In females, the most frequent adverse reactions are an increase in oily skin or acne, deepening of the voice, increased hair growth and/or alopecia, enlarged clitoris and irregular menses. The deep voice or hoarseness may not be reversed, even when the medication is stopped. The adverse reactions reported in males are urinary urgency, breast swelling or tenderness (gynaecomastia), frequent or continuous erections, testicular atrophy and impaired spermatogenesis. In children, there is impaired growth due to early closure of the epiphyses of the long bones. Other general adverse reactions include hair loss and balding, decreased gonadotrophin release and consequent impaired fertility, salt and fluid retention, hepatotoxicity and aggressive behaviour (see the Pregnancy Safety box at the end of this chapter for pregnancy safety categories).

DOSAGE AND ADMINISTRATION Various testosterone esters are formulated for depot IM injection, as capsules (PO), implants, or transdermal gel or patches. The choice of dosage and length of therapy depend on the diagnosis, the patient's age and sex, and the intensity of the adverse reactions. For male hypogonadism, the usual IM dosage is initially 250 mg every 2–3 weeks, then, for maintenance, 250 mg every 3–6 weeks. The paediatric dosage for delayed puberty in males is 50–100 mg monthly for about 4–6 months.

or testis, or to androgen-receptor defects (see Clinical Interest Box 46-1). Partial androgen deficiency may also occur in ageing men. This has been termed the male climacteric, or andropause, but there is no clearcut event analogous to the sudden drop in oestrogen production at the menopause. While androgen replacement therapy may slow down deterioration in bone and muscle function, there is as yet no general recommendation for androgen replacement in ageing men.

Androgens are also used in breast cancer in women and (in conjunction with an oestrogen) to treat severe osteoporosis in women.

Anabolic steroids

Anabolism refers to the metabolic processes in which small molecules are combined to form larger molecules and complex tissues, e.g. proteins from amino acids, or polysaccharides from simple sugars. This definition is extended to imply generalised increased building up of tissues and, in the context of pharmacology, to drugs that increase the bulk of the body, particularly muscle mass.

Androgens are potent **anabolic agents**; they stimulate the formation and maintenance of muscular and skeletal protein. Steroids used particularly for their anabolic effects include nandrolone, oxandrolone and stanozolol.* They bring about retention of nitrogen (essential to the formation of protein in the body) and enhance storage of inorganic phosphorus, sulfate, sodium and potassium. Adverse reactions are those of excessive androgenic actions. Weight gain may be caused by fluid retention, an adverse effect of androgen therapy. Other potential adverse reactions include testicular atrophy, sterility, gynaecomastia, increased risk of coronary heart disease, liver disease, mood swings and aggressiveness ('steroid rage'), and induction of psychotic disorders. Women run the additional risks of virilisation, including irreversible voice changes. In the past, anabolic steroids have been used for improving appetite, wellbeing and libido in people with 'wasting diseases', including osteoporosis, anaemia, adverse effects of

---

*One of the few drugs with a name ending in '-olol' that is not a β-blocker; it is a veterinary steroid often abused by weightlifters and banned in sport. Note that other groups of drugs may have anabolic activity, notably the β₂-adrenoceptor agonists such as salbutamol and salmeterol, which increase lean body mass (muscle) and decrease fat by metabolic actions. These drugs are banned in sport as anabolics but permitted for use in inhaler form for bronchodilation by people with notified asthma. The β₂ agonists are sympathomimetic amines in structure, so by definition are not anabolic steroids.

corticosteroid therapy, and terminal cancers. Given the lack of proof of efficacy and the availability of safer drugs with more specific actions, they are no longer recommended for such indications.

Athletes have used androgens to increase weight, musculature and muscle strength, especially for endurance events requiring stamina. The potential risk of developing major serious adverse reactions from androgens far outweighs the advantages to be gained in athletic events. Several elite athletes (accused of using steroids) competing in international events, including long-distance cycling, have suffered death from cardiovascular collapse. Many major sporting events disqualify athletes whose use of such products is proved; some were removed from the Sydney 2000 Olympic Games. (Additional information on the abuse of drugs can be found in Chapters 22 and 57.)

BENIGN PROSTATIC HYPERPLASIA

Testicular androgens are believed to have a permissive role in the development of benign adenomas of the prostate, i.e. **benign prostatic hyperplasia** (BPH), the hyperplasia of the glandular and connective tissue in the portions of the prostate that surround the urethra (see Figure 43-2 and Figure 27-2). This is considered a normal age-related change that begins around age 40 in men. By age 70, about 75% of men will develop BPH symptoms severe enough to require professional intervention. BPH does not lead on to prostate cancer, but both types of hypertrophy are stimulated by androgens.

BPH obstructs the bladder neck and compresses the urethra, which results in urinary retention, increasing the risk of bacteriuria. If untreated, it may affect the ureters and kidneys and result in hydroureter, hydronephrosis and renal failure. The symptoms of BPH include hesitancy (difficulty starting the urinary stream); a decrease in the diameter and force of the stream; inability to terminate urination abruptly, resulting in postvoid dribbling; and a sensation of incomplete bladder emptying, resulting in frequency and nocturia. Mild BPH does not require immediate treatment and benefits from watchful waiting. Surgical treatment reduces the size of the prostate gland and is recommended for severe BPH, but many men are reluctant to submit to surgery in this area.

Because the pathophysiology of BPH may also include increased smooth muscle tone in the bladder outlet and the prostate, mediated by α_1-adrenergic receptors, pharmacological treatment of BPH with α_1-**adrenoceptor blockers** has been tried. The antihypertensive drugs **prazosin** (Drug Monograph 12-2), terazosin, tamsulosin and analogues are used for their smooth muscle relaxant actions in BPH and can improve urine flow rate; if effective, long-term therapy is required. Common adverse effects are those typical of

vasodilators, i.e. headaches, dizziness and hypotension.

The natural herbal remedy from *Serenoa repens* (saw palmetto extract) has been demonstrated in clinical trials to be effective in increasing urine flow in BPH and may owe some of its efficacy to inhibition of α_1-adrenoceptors and of 5α-reductase enzyme activity. Another herbal remedy is extract of bark of the African tree *Pygeum africanum*. The extract contains three active ingredients that reduce inflammation and enlargement of the prostate gland.

Finasteride, a **5α-reductase inhibitor**, is a drug available for the treatment of BPH (Drug Monograph 46-2). This drug acts by a very different mechanism: it is a specific inhibitor of the 5α-reductase enzyme, which in the prostate metabolises the conversion of testosterone to dihydrotestosterone (DHT), a more potent androgen responsible for prostate gland growth (see Figures 37-2 and 40-1). Finasteride is highly effective at reducing the levels of DHT in the bloodstream and in the prostate, and so markedly reduces the hypertrophy of the gland and reduces urinary outflow resistance. It does not reduce the synthesis of testosterone and so does not have

---

DRUG MONOGRAPH 46-2   FINASTERIDE

INDICATIONS Finasteride is indicated for mild to moderate symptoms of BPH with clinically demonstrated prostatomegaly, when surgical treatment is contraindicated or refused. It is also used to treat androgenic alopecia (hair loss) in men.

PHARMACOKINETICS Finasteride is well absorbed after oral administration, with maximum plasma concentrations being reached in about 2 hours; about 90% is bound to plasma proteins. Finasteride is inactivated in the liver, and metabolites are excreted in the urine, with an elimination half-life of about 6 hours. No dosage adjustments are required for elderly patients.

DRUG INTERACTIONS No significant drug interactions have been reported.

ADVERSE REACTIONS These include decreased libido, impotence, a decreased amount of ejaculate, gynaecomastia and allergic reactions.

WARNINGS AND CONTRAINDICATIONS Avoid use in patients with liver disease, obstructive uropathy or finasteride hypersensitivity. Finasteride is not indicated for use in women or children.

Finasteride will reduce serum levels of prostate-specific antigen (PSA); hence it may interfere with diagnosis of prostate cancer.

DOSAGE AND ADMINISTRATION The drug is administered orally, 5 mg daily. Clinically useful effects may take 6–12 months to develop.

antiandrogenic actions. It appears to be most effective in men with large prostates and may take up to 1 year for clinical improvement to be demonstrated.

Antiandrogens

Antiandrogen activity may be exhibited by many types of drugs: agents that block receptor sites for androgens, decrease release of gonadotrophins, physiologically antagonise androgenic effects or inhibit enzymes for androgen synthesis. Cyproterone, for example, has weak antiandrogen activity and also has progestogen activity (hence its use in some oral contraceptives and hormone replacement therapy products); continuous administration of GnRH decreases gonadotrophin release; and oestrogens and progesterone suppress gonadotrophin secretion. Danazol has weak androgenic activity but mainly suppresses the pituitary–ovarian axis and is used in female reproductive disorders such as endometriosis.

Antiandrogen agents have the following uses—low doses: acne, hirsutism in women; medium doses: hypersexuality in men; high doses: prostatic cancer. They have also been tested as male contraceptives. They are teratogenic, as they can cause feminisation of a male fetus.

Flutamide and analogues (nilutamide, bicalutamide) are more specific as orally active antiandrogens, which act by inhibiting androgen uptake or binding to receptors. They are used in advanced prostatic cancer, in combination with orchidectomy (removal of the testes) or as a GnRH analogue. They can cause hepatic impairment, so liver function must be monitored. There is as yet no consensus on the issue of the optimal treatment for prostate cancer: surgery, radiation, and chemical castration with GnRH analogues or antiandrogens appear to be about equally effective. All carry the risks of impotence, decreased libido, osteoporosis and gynaecomastia.

PREGNANCY SAFETY	
ADEC Category	**Drug**
B2	Prazosin, terazosin
B3	Cyproterone (B3 or D)
D	Androgens, including testosterone and ester derivatives, bicalutamide, oxandrolone
X	Finasteride, mesterolone

Note that flutamide and other 5α-reductases are indicated for use only in men, so no studies have been done in pregnant or lactating women; thus no classification is available.

DRUGS AT A GLANCE 46: Drugs affecting the male reproductive system

Therapeutic group	Pharmacological group	Key examples	Key pages
Male sex hormones	Androgens	testosterone enanthate nandrolone	734, 5
	Anabolic steroids	nandrolone oxandrolone	734–6
Drugs treating benign prostatic hyperplasia (BPH)	α₁-adrenoceptor antagonists 5α-reductase inhibitors Antiandrogens	prazosin finasteride flutamide	736, 7 737

KEY POINTS

- Testosterone is the male sex hormone (androgen) necessary for the normal development and maintenance of male sex characteristics.
- Testosterone is indicated for hormonal replacement therapy in males with androgen deficiency and for the treatment of advanced breast carcinoma. Because of its high first-pass effect, testosterone is usually administered as one of its ester derivatives in depot formulations or for transdermal administration.
- Androgens are anabolic steroids and are sometimes abused by athletes in endurance sports.
- The adverse reactions to androgens, such as cardiovascular disease, gynaecomastia in males, and virilism in females, may be troubling to some individuals and even fatal. The monitoring and support of health-care professionals is important for such patients.
- Benign prostatic hyperplasia is a common condition in older men; it can be treated by surgery or by drugs from the terazosin or finasteride groups.
- Antiandrogens such as cyproterone or flutamide are used in conjunction with other therapies in prostatic cancer.

REVIEW EXERCISES

1 Discuss the similarities and differences between different formulations of testosterone and its ester derivatives.

2 What are the effects, mechanism of action, clinical uses and adverse effects of testosterone?

3 Describe the pathophysiology and treatment of benign prostatic hyperplasia.

4 Discuss the problems associated with the abuse of anabolic steroids by athletes.

5 Describe several different mechanisms whereby drugs may have antiandrogenic actions.

REFERENCES AND FURTHER READING

Australian Medicines Handbook 2006. Adelaide: AMH, 2006.

Australian Sports Drugs Drug Agency. *Anti-Doping Information Handbook 2005*. Canberra: Australian Sports Drugs Drug Agency, 2005.

Caswell A (ed.). *MIMS Annual June 2005*. Sydney: CMPMedica Australia, 2005.

Drew A. An alternative stream: *Serenoa repens* for benign prostatic hypertrophy? *Australian Prescriber* 2000; 23(4): 79.

Endocrinology Expert Group. *Therapeutic Guidelines Endocrinology, version 3*. Melbourne: Therapeutic Guidelines Limited, 2004.

Fletcher PJ (ed.). New drugs: tamsulosin. *Australian Prescriber* 2000; 23(3): 65–6.

Goepel M, Hecker U, Krege S et al. Saw palmetto extracts potently and noncompetitively inhibit human alpha1-adrenoceptors in vitro. *Prostate* 1999; 38(3): 208–15.

Greenspan FS, Strewler GJ. *Basic & Clinical Endocrinology*. 5th edn. Stamford: Appleton & Lange, 1997 [chs 12, 22, 25].

Klein EA, Thompson IM. Update on chemoprevention of prostate cancer. *Current Opinion in Urology* 2004; 14(3): 143–9.

Leavesley JH. *Medical By-Ways: Famous Diseases and Diseases of the Famous*. [Chapter 'Akhenaton']. Sydney: Australian Broadcasting Corporation/William Collins, 1984.

Tuckwell K (ed.). *MIMS Disease Index*. 2nd edn. Sydney: MediMedia Australia, 1996.

Youngson RM. *Collins Dictionary: Medicine*. 2nd edn. Glasgow: HarperCollins, 1998.

ON-LINE RESOURCES

Australian Sports Anti-Doping Authority: www.asada.gov.au

New Zealand medicines and medical devices safety authority: www.medsafe.govt.nz

evolve More weblinks at http://evolve.elsevier.com/AU/Bryant/pharmacology/

CHAPTER 47

Drugs Affecting Fertility or Sexual Functioning

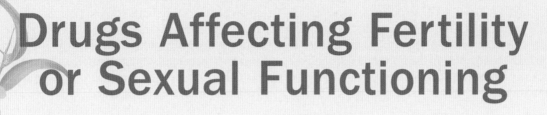

CHAPTER FOCUS

In this chapter, two important aspects of reproductive endocrinology are considered more specifically: fertility and sexual functioning. Reproductive and sexual behaviour and function are integral parts of an individual's identity. Many drugs can influence both sexuality and sexual function. Whenever possible, the health-care professional should be aware of all medications (legal and illegal, prescribed and over-the-counter) that patients are taking, so that useful information on the drugs' actions, interactions and adverse effects on these systems can be provided, and their effects on treatment taken into account.

OBJECTIVES

● To describe the common causes of infertility in men and women, and the drugs used to treat infertility.

● To describe the various methods of contraception, for men and women, with drugs, devices and 'natural' methods, indicating their relative rates of use and failure.

● To review the nervous control of sexual functions and describe the effects of common drugs that enhance or impair sexual functioning.

KEY DRUGS

clomiphene citrate
sildenafil

KEY TERMS

contraception
erectile dysfunction
impotence
infertility
intrauterine devices
libido
ovulatory stimulants

KEY ABBREVIATIONS

ANS	autonomic nervous system
ED	erectile dysfunction
FSH	follicle-stimulating hormone
GnRH	gonadotrophin-releasing hormone
5-HT	5-hydroxytryptamine
hCG	human chorionic gonadotrophin
IUD	intrauterine device
IVF	in-vitro fertilisation
LH	luteinising hormone
LSD	lysergic acid diethylamide
OC	oral contraceptive
PDE	phosphodiesterase
PGE	prostaglandin E
STD	sexually transmissible disease

DRUGS THAT AFFECT FERTILITY

FERTILITY in humans requires effective, coordinated and appropriately timed functioning of several processes: production of viable gametes, deposition and motility of sufficient spermatozoa, fertilisation of a mature oocyte, then its implantation and development in the primed uterine mucosa, and maintenance of pregnancy. Defects in any step can lead to infertility in a couple.

Infertility

Infertility is defined as the absence of conception after more than 1 year of regular sexual intercourse without contraception. It affects 10%–15% of all cohabiting couples, and the causes are estimated to be attributed to male factors in about 40% of cases, female factors in about 40% of cases and couple factors in 20% of cases. Infertility can cause great emotional distress to a couple hoping to conceive. Effective treatment requires careful assessment of possible causes in both partners and, if possible, identification of the specific cause. In men, common problems are abnormalities of sperm production, duct obstruction, hypothalamic or pituitary dysfunction, disorders of ejaculation or exposure to radiation. In women, cycles may be anovulatory due to hyperprolactinaemia, hypothalamic or pituitary dysfunction or ovarian dysfunction; or, if ovulation is normal, conception may be impossible due to tubal damage, endometriosis, or uterine or vaginal abnormalities. Diagnosis of the cause of infertility in a particular couple, and its treatment, are highly specialised areas of medicine, usually provided in clinics attached to teaching hospitals. Only general aspects can be considered here.

Treatment of female infertility

Some conditions causing female infertility are treatable with hormone replacement or stimulation, and have been discussed previously. Pulsatile administration of gonadotrophin-releasing hormone (GnRH), for example, will stimulate pituitary production of gonadotrophins, or the gonadotrophins themselves (follicle-stimulating hormone [FSH] and luteinising hormone [LH]) can be administered to stimulate normal functioning of the ovaries. In some cases, the treatment of choice may be microsurgery or assisted conception techniques, such as in-vitro fertilisation (IVF) or gamete intrafollicular transfer. The technical aspects of such procedures are beyond the scope of this text.

Ovulatory stimulants

Anovulation, the absence of ovulation, is physiological in women who are pregnant, breastfeeding or postmenopausal.

It becomes a suspected pathological condition in women with abnormal bleeding or infertility. The incidence of anovulation is unknown and cannot readily be ascertained, but diagnostic tests may determine its presence.

Clomiphene (Drug Monograph 47-1) and urofollitrophin are **ovulatory stimulants** used to treat anovulatory infertility in women. These treatments carry the risks of excessive stimulation leading to multiple pregnancies or potentially fatal ovarian hyperstimulation syndrome, and therefore are carried out only in specialist centres of reproductive medicine. Pregnancy must first be excluded.

Controlled ovarian stimulation is carried out to harvest multiple eggs for IVF procedures. This involves sequential use of first a GnRH antagonist (cetrorelix or ganirelix) to prevent premature ovulation in preparation for controlled ovarian stimulation, then the gonadotrophins FSH (e.g. follitropin) to recruit and mature follicles, then LH (as human chorionic gonadotrophin [hCG], see Drug Monograph 43-1; or lutropin alfa) to induce ovulation and luteinisation. Other drugs sometimes used as adjunct therapies in female infertility include progesterone (for its usual actions to aid implantation of the embryo and maintain pregnancy), dexamethasone or oral contraceptives, and an insulin-sensitising agent such as metformin. In women with anovulation due to hyperprolactinaemia, the dopamine agonist bromocriptine is used to suppress prolactin release from the pituitary gland (see Chapter 38).

Treatment of male infertility

Many cases of male infertility are due to anatomical abnormalities or problems with sexual functioning or technique, or to inadequate numbers or quality of sperm. Endocrine causes such as hyper- or hyposecretion of thyroid or adrenal glands usually respond to appropriate hormone therapy. **Erectile dysfunction (ED)** may also require treatment, and drugs that impair sexual functioning need to be avoided (see discussions later in this chapter). Aspiration of sperm and direct injection in vitro into the oocyte's cytoplasm, using the technique of intracytoplasmic sperm injection, is an effective IVF treatment for extreme oligospermia.

In gonadotrophin-deficient men, gonadotrophin therapy can induce spermatogenesis and hence increase fertility. Human chorionic gonadotrophin (which has mainly ICSH [interstitial cell-stimulating hormone] activity) is given 2–3 times weekly for several months, then, if necessary, FSH is added for several months. Semen analysis is used to assess sperm numbers, and pregnancy is often achieved despite low sperm count (oligospermia).

Contraception

For many couples, an ongoing problem is not conception but **contraception**, i.e. prevention of pregnancy after sexual

DRUG MONOGRAPH 47-1 CLOMIPHENE CITRATE

Clomiphene is a non-steroidal anti-oestrogen with some partial oestrogenic effects. Although its exact mechanism of action is unknown, it has been postulated that its competition with oestrogen for receptor sites in the hypothalamus inhibits the action of the stronger oestrogens and thus interferes with the normal negative feedback effect, allowing increased release of the pituitary gonadotrophins FSH and LH (see Figure 43-3). The result is ovarian stimulation, maturation of the ovarian follicle and development of the corpus luteum. A single course of therapy (5 days) usually results in a single ovulation. If the first course is unsuccessful, i.e. sexual intercourse does not result in conception, further courses are tried or the dose is doubled to increase the likelihood of ovulation.

INDICATIONS Clomiphene is indicated to treat female anovulatory infertility.

PHARMACOKINETICS It is well absorbed orally and recirculated in the enterohepatic system, which may account for its prolonged duration of action in the body. It has a plasma half-life of 5–7 days, with ovulation usually occurring 6–12 days after a course of treatment. Clomiphene is metabolised in the liver and excreted in the faeces and bile.

DRUG INTERACTIONS It has no known significant drug interactions.

ADVERSE REACTIONS These include hot flushes, abdominal pain or gas, visual disturbances, ovarian enlargement or cyst formation, abnormal uterine bleeding and hyperstimulation syndrome. There is an increased incidence of multiple pregnancies.

CONTRAINDICATIONS Avoid use in women with clomiphene hypersensitivity, liver function impairment, ovarian cyst or enlargement that is not associated with polycystic ovary syndrome, abnormal vaginal bleeding (undiagnosed) or fibroid tumours in the uterus.

DOSAGE AND ADMINISTRATION The dose for female infertility is 50–100 mg orally daily for 5 days, starting on the fifth day of the menstrual period if bleeding occurs, or at any time in women who have no recent uterine bleeding. This cycle is repeated until conception occurs, for a maximum of six cycles.

Assuming there is no other reason for infertility in the couple, about 70% of women will ovulate and 30% conceive after clomiphene therapy. If this treatment is unsuccessful, then the more complicated gonadotrophin therapy is tried, with sequential use of an exogenous FSH analogue (e.g. follitropin) then LH (e.g. hCG).

intercourse. The average rate of pregnancy following a year of regular unprotected intercourse is about 85%. It was estimated in 2000 that worldwide each day there were about 100 million acts of sexual intercourse, leading to about 910,000 conceptions (of which 25% were unwanted) and about 150,000 abortions. These days, 50% of couples use some contraceptive technique, yet the rates of abortion and unplanned pregnancies remain high.

An ideal contraceptive technique should be safe, 100% effective, immediately functional, not interfering with sex life, easy to use and rapidly reversible. Although no technique totally fulfils these criteria, many methods have remarkably low failure rates when used correctly by a couple with high motivation. Table 47-1 lists the failure rates of several methods, showing the range of pregnancy rates.

Data on contraceptive method usage from different countries are not readily comparable. However, Table 47-2 shows estimates of usage of various methods for worldwide data and for Australian couples (Vollenhoven, 2006).

Contraceptive methods in women

See Figure 47-1.

ORAL CONTRACEPTIVE PILL

The various formulations of the oral contraceptive pill (OC pill) have been described in detail in Chapter 44 and

are summarised in Tables 44-1 and 44-2. Combination and sequential formulations contain an oestrogen and a progestogen in various doses for a typical 28-day cycle, and mimic the normal physiological pattern of hormone secretion in the menstrual cycle (see Drug Monographs 44-1 and 44-2). The progestogen-only 'minipill' is commonly used by lactating women. There are also progestogen-only depot preparations (IM injection or solid rod implants); there can be loss of bone density due to lack of protective oestrogens. The 'morning-after pill' consists of high doses of oestrogen plus progestogen, or an even higher dose of progestogen only, as emergency contraception.

DIAPHRAGM/SPERMICIDAL AGENTS

An occlusive vaginal diaphragm may be used in conjunction with a spermicidal gel as a non-hormonal, physical method of contraception. The gel is applied to the surface of the diaphragm in contact with the cervix and around the rim before placement. The diaphragm should remain in situ for 6–8 hours after sexual intercouse. A fresh application of spermicidal gel should be made (using an intravaginal applicator) for subsequent sexual activity during this time frame. Neither diaphragms nor spermicides protect against sexually transmissible diseases. Spermicidal gel contains surfactants. Adverse effects may include mild irritation or dermatitis.

INTRAUTERINE DEVICES

Intrauterine devices (IUDs) impregnated with copper or progestogen are used for long-term (5–8 years) reversible contraception (see Drug Monograph 47-2). They alter the intrauterine environment to decrease sperm motility and viability, inhibit nidation (attachment of the embryo in the endometrium) and inhibit or decrease ovulation and follicular development. They can cause dysmenorrhoea, pelvic inflammatory disease or uterine perforation, and the IUD can be expelled from the uterus; they do not protect against sexually transmissible diseases (STDs) (see Drug Monograph 47-2).

OTHER METHODS

Other methods tested or under trial in women include continuous administration of GnRH drugs that inhibit luteinising hormone-releasing hormone; luteolytic agents, including prostaglandin $F_{2\alpha}$; vaccines against hCG, GnRH or sperm antigens; vaginal rings that release a progestogen and an oestrogen; and an intradermal implant releasing a progestogen (etonogestrel).

The non-oral hormonal methods (depot injections, transdermal patches, vaginal rings and depot IM rods) have many advantages over oral formulations:
- they avoid problems with impaired oral absorption (e.g. from vomiting)
- they avoid hepatic first-pass metabolism, so lower oestrogen doses are effective
- controlled-release formulations readily achieve steady plasma concentrations
- no daily action (or memory) required
- improved compliance
- scant or no menstrual bleeding or pain.

The main reasons given by women for discontinuation of these methods are the irregularity of bleeding and unpredictable return of ovulation.

New pharmacological methods currently under investigation include contraceptive vaccines, selective progesterone receptor modulators, and suppression of oocyte maturation.

Contraceptive methods in men

Male contraceptive methods involving drugs include androgens, antiandrogens, FSH inhibitors, progestogens or GnRH analogues to inhibit gonadotrophin secretion, the so-called 'male pill' (see Clinical Interest Box 47-1) and chlorinated sugar compounds. Immunological methods include vaccines against various hormones and against components of the reproductive tract or of spermatozoa.

In traditional Chinese medicine, gossypol, a natural anti-fertility agent in cottonseed oil, has been found to be effective. This is a naphtholphenol derivative (see Figure 1-1F for structure) that decreases the number and motility of sperm and impairs spermatogenesis after 2 months of daily oral administration. Adverse effects include fatigue and decreased libido, and the effects are not always reversible.

Non-drug contraception

Non-drug methods (except for condoms) generally have much lower success rates in preventing pregnancies. Barrier methods or occlusive devices have the advantage of offering some protection against STDs and cervical cancer; condoms are especially effective for this purpose. They are safe and inexpensive, and have been widely used throughout history.

'Diaphragms' inserted in the vagina prevent access of sperm to the cervical canal. They are most effective when used

TABLE 47-1 Failure rates for contraceptive methods

CONTRACEPTIVE METHOD	CONTRACEPTIVE FAILURE RATE* (= % women with pregnancy during 1 year of use)
No method	85
OC pill: combination	0.2–3
OC pill: progestogen-only	0.5–4
IUD + levonorgestrel	0.2
IUD + copper	0.1–1
Combined hormone vaginal ring	1–2
Depot IM progesterone	0.1–0.3
Implant etonogestrel	0.07
Sterilisation (male)	0.1–0.15
Sterilisation (female)	0.2–0.4
Spermicides	6–26
Diaphragm + spermicide	6–18
Periodic abstinence ('rhythm method')	9–20
Withdrawal ('coitus interruptus')	4–18
Male condom	3–14
Cap or diaphragm	10–20
Female condom	5–20

*Ranges are lowest expected (best) rate to typical rate in normal use. IUD = intrauterine device; OC = oral contraceptive. *Sources*: Speroff & Darney 1992; AMH 2006.

CLINICAL INTEREST BOX 47-1 THE 'MALE PILL'

Testosterone has a negative feedback effect on gonadotrophin production and hence decreases spermatogenesis and causes oligospermia; however, high doses of weekly testosterone enanthate IM in men are required to prevent pregnancy, and libido may also be decreased. Combinations of IM testosterone with a low daily oral dose of a progestogen or cyproterone (an antiandrogen) are effective contraceptive regimens. Preliminary trials have shown a high success rate for (reversible) contraception in some ethnic groups. Another approach has been to search for selective androgen receptor modulators that maintain desired anabolic effects (and male sex characteristics), while reducing specific androgenic actions such as high gonadotrophin and testosterone levels and spermatogenesis.

The methods are unlikely to gain universal appeal, partly because many men prefer not to take drugs that they feel may interfere with their virility, or prefer to leave contraception to the female partner, and because studies have shown that many women do not trust men to take contraceptive medication regularly, and prefer to rely on their own pill-popping to prevent pregnancy.

The male pill may gain acceptance as a niche method, e.g. for couples in a stable relationship who are highly motivated to space pregnancies, and when the female partner cannot use the female methods of contraception.

DRUG MONOGRAPH 47-2 INTRAUTERINE DEVICE WITH COPPER

The contraceptive intrauterine device (IUD) with copper consists of a Y-shaped flanged polyethylene device with copper wire wound around the stem; there are threads attached to facilitate checking of position. The device is supplied in an insertion tube, all sterile. The copper is radio-opaque, which allows its detection by imaging techniques.

Studies of the mechanism of action of the device have shown that it induces an inflammatory reaction to the foreign body in the uterus, with increases in leucocyte counts. The copper also hinders transport of sperm and ova. Overall, the viability and union of the sperm and ova are impaired, thus reducing the likelihood of conception after intercourse.

INDICATIONS The IUD with copper is indicated for contraception, in both nulliparous and multiparous women (i.e. those who have never been pregnant and those who have). It may be used during breastfeeding.

PHARMACOKINETICS After the device is inserted into the uterus, it slowly releases copper over the period (up to 5 years) that it is left in place. Any absorption into the systemic circulation is too low to raise the levels of copper in the plasma, as the average daily release is estimated to be less than 1% of the average daily copper intake via the diet.

ADVERSE REACTIONS Adverse effects occurring during insertion or removal include syncope (fainting) and slowed heart rate. In the first few weeks after insertion, bleeding and cramps can occur. In the long term, there may be urticarial skin reactions to copper, embedding of part of the IUD in the uterus wall or cervix, penetration of the abdominal cavity, expulsion of the device, heavier menstrual bleeding and hence anaemia, and higher risk of pelvic inflammatory disease and thus reduction in future fertility.

WARNINGS AND CONTRAINDICATIONS Use with caution in women with valvular heart disease. If pregnancy occurs despite the use of IUDs, there is higher risk of abortion, sepsis, or ectopic pregnancy and its associated dangers.

Avoid use in women with copper hypersensitivity, during pregnancy, and in women with current or previous disorders of the uterus or of menstruation, pelvic or genital inflammation or infection, or sexually transmitted diseases.

DRUG INTERACTIONS There are no clinically significant drug interactions.

DOSAGE AND ADMINISTRATION The copper wire in the device is 29 cm long (when unwound), and 0.4 mm in diameter; it provides a copper surface area of 375 mm^2.

The IUD must be inserted using strict aseptic procedures and following manufacturer's instructions closely. Its correct position should be checked soon after insertion, thence every 6 months. If there are no problems, it can be left in place for up to 5–8 years, then removed and another IUD inserted if contraception is still desired.

---

with a spermicidal cream, inserted before intercourse and left in place for at least 6 hours afterwards. Complications include irritation or pain, and allergic reactions.

Condoms—thin rubber sheaths stretched over the erect penis before intercourse—prevent sperm from entering the vagina and effectively protect against STDs. When used properly and regularly, they are 97% effective as contraceptives, especially when used with spermicides.

The female condom consists of a thin rubber pouch that is inserted in the vaginal canal. It also protects against STDs.

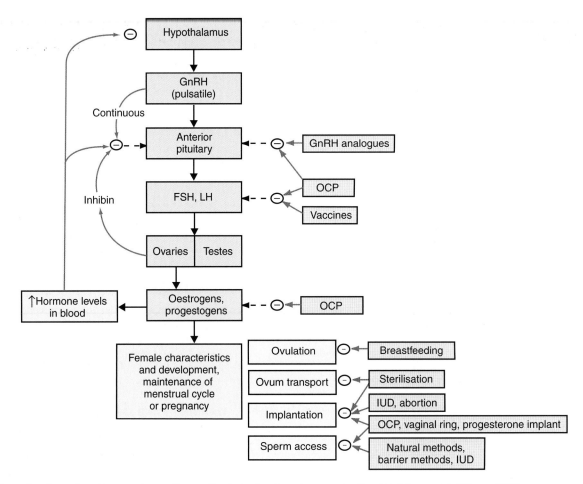

FIGURE 47-1 Sites of action of various contraceptive methods in the female reproductive tract (compare Figure 43-3). ⊖ = effect decreased or inhibited; GnRH = gonadotrophin-releasing hormone; IUD = intrauterine device; OCP = oral contraceptive pill

TABLE 47-2 Who uses what contraceptive method?		
CONTRACEPTIVE METHOD	**WORLDWIDE USAGE (2000)***	**AUSTRALIAN USAGE (2001)†**
Combined OC	9%	26.8%
Barrier method	5.3%	23.4%
Sterilisation (male/female)	20%	20%
Withdrawal/natural	6.9%	9.9%
Depot MPA	?	1.9%
IUD	10.6%	1.2%
Infertility	?	10.4%
Other or none	47%	32.8%

*Worldwide data for couples of reproductive age.
†Australian data for women aged 18–49 years.
OCP = oral contraceptive pill; MPA = medroxyprogesterone acetate; IUD = intrauterine device.
Data from: Assoc. Prof. Beverley Vollenhoven, Department of Obstetrics & Gynaecology, Monash University, Melbourne 2006; adapted with kind permission.

CLINICAL INTEREST BOX 47-2 'RHYTHM METHODS' FOR NATURAL FAMILY PLANNING

Natural family-planning methods are commonly used by people who for various reasons prefer not to use devices or drugs to prevent conception. They rely on attempts to predict the day of ovulation, and avoidance of intercourse for several days before and after ovulation (as the ovum is viable for about 2 days and sperm for up to 7 days after intercourse).

The method works only if the woman has regular periods and can predict the time of ovulation (usually 14 days before the next period).

The methods require abstinence from sex for at least half the cycle (days 8–20 in a 28-day cycle); e.g. safe days in an average 28-day cycle might be from day 21 of one cycle through the menstrual period to day 7 of the next cycle.

Accuracy in predicting the day of ovulation can be improved by measuring the small rise in basal body temperature that occurs in response to the rise in progesterone midcycle, or by identifying changes in mucus secretions, abdominal pain, breast tenderness, or cervix or mood changes before, during and after ovulation.

The unreliability of such methods has contributed to the high birth rates or high abortion rates in societies in which these methods are relied on.

The 'natural' methods of family planning or contraception include periodic abstinence from sexual activity (see Clinical Interest Box 47-2), withdrawal of the penis before ejaculation ('coitus interruptus'), and reliance on prolactin's antiovulation effects during breastfeeding.

Sterilisation, while not (usually) reversible, is virtually 100% effective as a contraceptive method and is the most widely used form of contraception in the world. The most common techniques in women involve ligation or clipping of the fallopian tubes, and in men, vasectomy, i.e. surgical interruption of the vas deferens to prevent transport of sperm. Severe complications are rare.

Other physical methods used in men rely on the fact that sperm are inactivated by higher temperatures than those in the scrotum. The thermal effects of hot water, microwaves, ultrasound and infrared heat have been trialled to cause azoospermia (absence of viable sperm).

DRUGS THAT AFFECT SEXUAL FUNCTIONING

Sexuality and sexual behaviour have physiological, psychological and social ramifications that reflect a higher level of complexity than this discussion of drugs affecting sexuality could encompass. Many contributing factors are involved, such as self-esteem, general health, partner availability, appropriate environment, religious beliefs, society's standards and lifestyle factors. Because drugs can affect sexual activities or sexual identity, health-care professionals should be aware of patients' needs and problems in this area.

Various drugs can produce one or more adverse effects on sexual function, such as:
• lower levels of testosterone, which is normally present in both sexes and enhances libido, or sexual drive
• higher or lower levels of oestrogen

• clinical depression, which may limit interest in or response to sexual stimuli
• autonomic nervous system blockade, which may interfere with lubrication, erection or ejaculation.

(Chapter 43 provides more detailed descriptions of the structure and function of the reproductive systems.)

Many physiological functions significant to sexual pleasure are controlled by higher centres in the central nervous system (CNS) and by the autonomic nervous system (see also Unit IV). The male and female sexual organs are composed of homologous tissues—although the shapes of the organs differ, they correspond, part for part, in structure, position and embryological origin. The embryo is characteristically female initially and does not differentiate until fetal androgens begin to masculinise tissues (7th to 12th weeks of pregnancy). Thus it is not surprising that the mature organs function in analogous ways and can be influenced by hormones of both sexes. Female hormones generally increase sexual functions in women and decrease them in men, and male hormones do the opposite. Central involvement in sexual functioning includes both behavioural and endocrine effects, with stimuli integrated via nuclei in the thalamus and hypothalamus. Many drugs that affect dopaminergic transmission have effects on hypothalamic–pituitary pathways, and any drugs with CNS-depressant effects may depress sexual interest or functions.

In the male, parasympathetic stimulation controls penile erection. This response results from vasodilation and congestion of the vascular sinuses in the penile corpora, caused by parasympathetic nerve action mediated by release of nitric oxide, which relaxes smooth muscle and hence dilates arterioles. (Priapism, a state of persistent painful erection without sexual excitation, is due to failure of drainage of blood from the penis; it requires urgent treatment, as blood clotting can cause permanent damage.) Drugs that interfere with parasympathetic neurotransmission, such as atropinic anticholinergic drugs, can cause erectile dysfunction. Because many drugs have atropinic effects, this is a common problem.

Sympathetic (adrenergic) impulses in the male produce emission and ejaculation by causing contraction of the vas deferens and seminal vesicles and of prostatic smooth muscle, along with effects on the bulbocavernosus and ischiocavernosus muscles. Ejaculation is a spinal reflex, with sympathetic stimulation causing rapid muscular contractions and expulsion of semen, and simultaneous cardiovascular stimulation that increases heart rate and blood pressure and constricts arterioles, which leads to waning of the erection. Impotence, or impotency, is the inability of a man to achieve or maintain a penile erection to allow normal vaginal sexual intercourse. Drugs that block adrenergic impulses can impair ejaculatory function through sympathetic blockade. In addition, ganglionic blocking agents, which may block both sympathetic and parasympathetic nerve transmission, can cause complete impotence and impaired sexual functioning. Androgens are required for normal seminal fluid content and volume, and play important roles in libido and erections, and responsiveness to erotic stimuli.

In the female, parasympathetic (cholinergic) impulses cause arterial dilation and venoconstriction, which produce clitoral erection and vasocongestion of the vulva, transudation (oozing of a fluid through pores) of lubricating secretions from the vaginal walls, and swelling of the introitus (vaginal opening). Continued sexual stimulation may then produce orgasm, with sudden skeletal muscle contractions, increases in heart rate and blood pressure, and intense pleasurable sensations. Oestrogens and progestogens are involved in sexual behaviour and responsiveness, and androgens are involved in enhancing libido in women as well as in men. Anticholinergic actions of drugs may depress the parasympathetic responses and hence decrease sexual functioning.

Drugs that may enhance sexual functioning

Substances that will increase **libido** (sexual potency or drive) have been sought throughout history. Inscriptions in the ruins of ancient cultures have described the preparation of 'erotic potions', and an endless number of 'aphrodisiacs' have been described since then. In contemporary society, many drugs and chemicals that modify mood and behaviour are claimed to have aphrodisiac properties.

In reality, very few drugs specifically enhance libido or sexual performance, and chemicals taken for this purpose without medical advice, and especially in combination with other drugs, pose the danger of adverse reactions, drug interactions or overdose. Many pharmacologically active agents, however, temporarily modify both physiological responsiveness and subjective perception to enhance the enjoyment, if not the fulfilment, of the sex act. Some of these agents are considered in this section; most are of psycho- or ethnopharmacological interest only and are not available clinically.

Yohimbine

One of the few compounds with proven activity is yohimbine, an alkaloid derived from the west African tree *Coryanthe yohimbe* and related chemically to the ergot alkaloids. Yohimbine produces a competitive α-adrenergic block, leading to vasodilation, enhanced erection and increased ejaculatory reflexes. There is no convincing evidence that it acts as a sexual stimulant, and it has no medical use as it has low efficacy.

Opioids and psychoactive agents

The use of drugs such as morphine, heroin, cocaine, marijuana, lysergic acid diethylamide (LSD) and amphetamines as aphrodisiacs has become widespread in contemporary society (see Chapter 22). These agents can, in certain circumstances, enhance the enjoyment of the sexual experience for some people. More commonly, however, sexual function decreases. Responsiveness varies because these agents have no particular properties that specifically increase sexual potency—rather they tend to affect the user according to expectations. Thus the user's state of mind, the amount consumed and the surrounding environment contribute considerably to the effect achieved. Like alcohol, these drugs act on the CNS to weaken inhibitions, which are often the cause of problems involving sexual behaviour. Taken in excess or too often, however, these drugs have the opposite effect and inhibit sexual drive and function. Because of these variations, researchers are sceptical of their clinical value.

Opioids such as morphine, pethidine and heroin are general CNS depressants and cause disorientation and mental confusion. They are said to have an 'orgasmic effect', but habitual users have low libido and impaired potency.

Marijuana (cannabis), an extract of the *Cannabis sativa* plant, is considered by many to be a sexual stimulant. Its effects, however, like those of alcohol, result indirectly from relaxation and release of inhibitions surrounding sexual activity. The active ingredient in marijuana is tetrahydrocannabinol. The pharmacological effects resulting from smoking marijuana depend on the expectations and personality of the user, the dose and the prevailing circumstances. Usually, the effects of marijuana are time distortion and enhanced suggestibility, producing the illusion that sexual climax is somewhat prolonged. Thus the expectation that marijuana is an aphrodisiac may enhance enjoyment of the sex act. Studies of marijuana for a specific effect on sexual behaviour, however, have shown that it has no such enhancing effect. On the contrary, there is evidence that marijuana smokers have a higher incidence of decreased libido, impaired potency and fertility than non-users do, possibly because of its oestrogenic-type effects and a decrease in release of the gonadotrophins FSH and LH. In addition, chronic intensive use of marijuana depresses plasma testosterone levels and produces gynaecomastia in some male users, and decreases prolactin levels and ovulation in women. Chromosomal breaks have also been reported, with the risk of congenital abnormalities.

LSD is another drug that, although considered an aphrodisiac by some, has potentially untoward effects on sexual function and behaviour. As with marijuana, any alteration of sexual performance produced by LSD is principally subjective. This drug acts almost entirely on the CNS, acting as an agonist at 5-hydroxytryptamine (5-HT, serotonin) receptors and causing facilitated sensory input, altered sensations and improved mood. The repeated use of LSD may produce serious psychological problems, which could overall adversely affect sexual interest or activity. Teratogenic effects have also been reported.

Amphetamines ('speed') have also been used to stimulate sexual function. These drugs release catecholamines from neuronal stores and inhibit their reuptake. They also have a powerful central stimulant action at dopamine and 5-HT receptors, and peripheral α- and β-sympathomimetic effects. The main effects are wakefulness and alertness, mood elevation, increased motor and speech activity, often elation and euphoria, and decreased fatigue. The effects of amphetamines on sexual performance, however, are inconsistent and may be attributed to overcoming feelings of shyness or inadequacy, or to delaying sleep.

Nicotine is a CNS stimulant and has complex peripheral effects due to its actions at nicotinic acetylcholine receptors in autonomic ganglia and skeletal muscle. Overall, it tends to increase heart rate and vasoconstriction, inhibit spinal reflexes and increase release of ADH and oxytocin. No clear-cut effect on sexual functions is evident.

Organic nitrates

Vasodilators such as the organic nitrates (glyceryl trinitrate, isosorbide mononitrate) might be expected to be useful in dilating blood vessels in the penis and improving erections; however, such drugs have powerful adverse effects, causing headaches, hypotension and fainting, which would be counter-productive. Amyl nitrite, a drug used in the past to treat angina pectoris, is alleged to enhance sexual activity in humans and has been reported to intensify the orgasmic experience for men if inhaled at the moment of orgasm. No effect of amyl nitrite on libido has been reported, but loss of erection or delayed ejaculation may result. Women generally experience negative effects on orgasm when taking this drug.

Other drugs that may stimulate sexual behaviour

Hormones involved in the reproductive systems have effects in sexual functions; thus oestrogens and androgens increase sexual activity in people of the appropriate sex. Oxytocin appears to have roles in mating and parenting behaviours in humans as well as in animals studied.

Levodopa, useful in treating parkinsonism by enhancing dopamine transmission in the CNS, is reported to increase libido and has caused priapism. Elderly men have been observed to have a sexual rejuvenation, and studies with younger men complaining of decreased erectile ability have shown that levodopa increases libido and incidence of penile erections. Overall, however, these effects are short-lived and do not reflect continued satisfactory sexual function and potency. Thus levodopa is not a true aphrodisiac, but the increased sexual activity experienced by parkinsonian patients treated with levodopa may reflect improved well-being and partial recovery of normal sexual functions impaired by Parkinson's disease.

Vitamin E compounds (the tocopherols) act as antioxidants and have metabolic roles, and have been postulated to be involved in sexual functions because deficiencies of the vitamin impair reproductive ability. Much has been said about the positive effects of vitamin E on sexual performance and ability in human beings, but beneficial effects are not proven. Because sexual performance is often influenced by mental attitude, a person who believes vitamin E improves sexual prowess may actually find improvement.

Cantharidin ('Spanish fly')

Cantharidin, a legendary and notorious reputed sexual stimulant, is a powerful irritant, vesicant (blistering agent) and potent corrosive systemic poison. It is a powder made from dried beetles (*Lytta vesicatoria*, formerly called *Cantharidin vesicatoria*, the blistering beetle, or Spanish fly) found in southern Europe. Cantharidin can produce severe illness characterised by vomiting, diarrhoea, abdominal pain, corrosion of mucous membranes and shock. When taken internally, it causes irritation and inflammation of the genitourinary tract and dilation of the blood vessels of the penis and clitoris, sometimes producing prolonged erections (priapism) or engorgement, usually without increased sexual desire. Deaths have been reported from the abuse of cantharidin as an aphrodisiac. The most infamous user of cantharidin was the French nobleman the Marquis de Sade (after whom sadism was named). He was convicted in 1772 of several counts of poisoning prostitutes and guests at his banquets with sweets dipped in cantharadin, administered as an aphrodisiac to inflame their sexual desires and encourage their participation in orgies of sexual perversions. Many of his victims died of corrosive poisoning and shock. It is currently recognised that cantharidin is not an effective sexual stimulant.

DRUG MONOGRAPH 47-3 SILDENAFIL

Sildenafil (Viagra) is a selective inhibitor of cGMP-specific PDE5 (phosphodiesterase type 5). After oral administration, it is active particularly in the penis, where it potentiates the vasodilator actions of nitrates released during sexual excitement.

INDICATIONS Sildenafil is indicated for erectile dysfunction in men, except for those taking nitrates or for whom sexual intercourse is inadvisable.

PHARMACOKINETICS Sildenafil is rapidly absorbed after PO administration and peak blood concentrations are reached after about 60 minutes; bioavailability is around 40%. Absorption is delayed by a high-fat meal. The drug and its major metabolite (also active as a PDE5 inhibitor) are highly protein-bound and widely distributed in tissues. Metabolites are mainly excreted in faeces, with a terminal half-life of 3–5 hours. Clearance is reduced in patients with severe liver or kidney disease.

DRUG INTERACTIONS Do not use with nitrate preparations, as the hypotensive vasodilator effects are synergistic. The PDE5 inhibitors are metabolised mainly by CYP3A4, so there may be interactions with all other drugs that inhibit or induce these enzymes, including many anticonvulsants, corticosteroids, hypoglycaemic agents, antibiotics, antivirals, antifungals, warfarin and grapefruit juice; reference lists should be consulted for specific interactions and doses varied accordingly. Other vasodilators may cause additive effects leading to hypotension.

ADVERSE REACTIONS These include typical vasodilator effects such as headache, facial flushing, nasal congestion, dizziness and cardiovascular events (e.g. angina pectoris, tachycardia and hypotension). Gastric distress, diarrhoea, allergic reaction and priapism can occur, and at higher doses the drug may cause some visual changes, including a blue–green colour tinge in the field of vision, light sensitivity and blurred vision.

WARNINGS AND CONTRAINDICATIONS Use with caution in patients with cardiovascular diseases, bleeding disorders, retinal disorders, Peyronie's disease (an anatomical abnormality of the penis) or conditions that predispose to priapism, such as multiple myeloma, leukaemia and sickle cell anemia. Avoid use in men with sildenafil hypersensitivity or concurrent use of organic nitrates.

DOSAGE AND ADMINISTRATION The usual adult dose is 50–100 mg, taken about 1 hour before sexual activity to a maximum of 100 mg in any day.

Treatment of erectile dysfunction (impotence)

Erectile dysfunction (ED), or **impotence**, is the condition in which a man is consistently unable to attain or maintain an erection long enough for sexual intercourse, or is unable to ejaculate. It is estimated that 25% of men over 55 years of age are impotent, as are most men over 50 after 20 years of tobacco smoking. Very few, however, present for treatment, because of embarrassment or denial. There are many possible causes of impotence:

- medical (diabetes mellitus, arterial disease, hypertension, uraemia, abnormalities of the reproductive system, infections such as syphilis)
- psychogenic (stress, fear of pregnancy or STD, religious or social inhibitions, emotional immaturity)
- neurogenic (autonomic dysfunction)
- hypogonadal (endocrine deficiencies)
- iatrogenic (see below under Drugs that decrease sexual functioning)
- lifestyle factors (smoking, excess alcohol)
- idiopathic (no obvious cause).

Attention to psychological factors and treatment of any underlying disorder are important in all cases.

The final common pathway leading to impotence is a lack of the vasodilator mediator nitric oxide (NO), which relaxes the smooth muscle of the penile arteries and allows congestion. Sildenafil (which rapidly became renowned worldwide by its trade name Viagra) specifically improves erectile function and treats impotence (see Drug Monograph 47-3). Released in 1998, sildenafil was the first oral medication approved for efficacy in treating impotence; later drugs in this group are tadalafil and vardenafil. The mechanism of action is secondary to sexual stimulation, which increases the release of NO. This activates the enzyme guanylate cyclase, thus increasing the levels of cyclic guanosine monophosphate (cGMP), a smooth muscle relaxant. Sildenafil enhances the NO effects by inhibiting phosphodiesterase type 5 (PDE5), an enzyme (found primarily in the penis) that degrades cGMP. The increased levels of cGMP in the corpus cavernosum enhance the smooth muscle relaxation and inflow of blood, and maintain erection. Sildenafil has no effect in the absence of sexual stimulation.

Since sildenafil's release and public acceptance (Clinical Interest Box 47-3), postmarketing surveillance has disclosed various adverse reactions, and several reports of fatality have been associated with its use; however, other current medications or disease states may have been involved in these deaths. There is now a warning that sildenafil should not be taken with concomitant administration of an organic nitrate (also vasodilators). This contraindication is based on the combination causing severe hypotension and possibly a decrease in coronary perfusion, which may result in myocardial ischaemia and infarction. Health-care professionals should be aware that a man without a history of angina who takes sildenafil for sexual impotence and develops his first angina attack should not receive any nitrate products in the emergency room. This includes glyceryl trinitrate tablets, patches or ointments, and other nitrates or nitrites. Men need advice as to treatment of priapism if it occurs: if the erection lasts more than 2 hours, pseudoephedrine (2 × 60 mg tablets) is useful as a vasoconstrictor; more than 4 hours becomes a medical emergency.

Other drugs used to treat erectile dysfunction

Other drugs used to treat ED are testosterone derivatives, prostaglandins and papaverine. All must be given parenterally, hence the major advantage of oral sildenafil. Alprostadil, a synthetic form of prostaglandin E_1 (PGE_1), is given by penile injection (into the corpora cavernosa) or transurethral application; it dilates the cavernosal arteries and thus assists erectile function. Testosterone implants or IM depot injections are tried if the ED is due to androgen deficiency (see Drug Monograph 46-1). Papaverine, a smooth muscle relaxant, is given by intracavernosal injection; it relaxes all vascular components of the penile erectile system.

Bromocriptine is effective in patients in whom the cause of ED is hyperprolactinaemia. The local anaesthetic lignocaine is available in a spray formulation as a local surface penile desensitiser in situations of premature ejaculation.

Drugs that decrease sexual functioning

As described earlier, effective sexual activity depends on adequate CNS, autonomic nervous system (ANS) and endocrine system functions, as well as behavioural, social and lifestyle aspects. Not surprisingly, many drugs can impair sexual functioning, libido or sexual gratification. In particular, drugs that depress the CNS and ANS, and hormone antagonists, are likely to have adverse effects on sexual functions; these are summarised below. (The pharmacology of the drugs is described fully in relevant chapters.)

Antihypertensives

Early antihypertensive drugs, especially ganglion blockers and adrenergic neuron-blocking agents, had such severe deleterious effects on sexual functions and potency in men that compliance with the therapy was often very poor. More modern, more specific drugs cause fewer problems in this area.

GANGLION-BLOCKING AGENTS

These drugs occupy nicotinic acetylcholine receptor sites at all autonomic ganglia, and block the actions of released acetylcholine. They thus block all sympathetic and parasympathetic responses and effectively 'wipe out' the entire ANS. Because of their widespread actions and severe adverse effects, including hypotension, inhibition of gut functions, urinary retention and impairment of both erectile capability and ejaculatory function, they are no longer used. Examples were hexamethonium and mecamylamine.

ADRENERGIC NEURON-BLOCKING AGENTS

Adrenergic neuron-blocking agents act by decreasing release of adrenergic transmitter (noradrenaline) and depleting transmitter stores. They thus impair sympathetic nervous system functions, causing vasodilation and hypotension, and ejaculatory disturbances and impotence. Reserpine, a drug affecting central transmitter stores of catecholamines and 5-HT, was formerly used as an antihypertensive drug and in psychiatry, but is no longer used because of its many adverse effects.

OTHER ANTIHYPERTENSIVE AGENTS

Centrally acting α₂-agonists used as antihypertensives, such as methyldopa and clonidine, have been associated with frequent reports of impotence and sexual dysfunction, and decreased libido and gynaecomastia. The α-blocker phenoxybenzamine, an effective hypotensive drug, decreases ejaculation. (This drug has been referred to as the male contraceptive: interestingly, it has been used successfully in men with premature ejaculation problems.) Beta-blockers such as propranolol and metoprolol have also been reported to cause impotence and sexual dysfunction, as have calcium channel blockers (nifedipine, verapamil) and angiotensin-converting enzyme inhibitors (captopril).

Antianxiety and psychotropic drugs

A wide variety of centrally acting agents affect sexual interest and capability both directly and indirectly. The phenothiazines and other neuroleptics, antidepressants, benzodiazepines and barbiturates are often associated with sexual dysfunction.

The phenothiazine tranquillisers, such as chlorpromazine, prochlorperazine, thioridazine and fluphenazine, are commonly prescribed antischizophrenic agents that are thought to act by inhibiting dopaminergic transmission in the CNS. They very frequently have endocrine-type adverse effects mediated through their stimulation of prolactin release, causing gynaecomastia (in men) or galactorrhoea (in women), and through their decreased release of pituitary gonadotrophins and thus of sex hormones, causing priapism and ejaculatory disorders or impaired menstruation and ovulation. The phenothiazines are very 'dirty' drugs, affecting many transmitter systems (see Tables 19-1 and 19-2), and can also block α receptors (causing hypotension and ejaculatory disorders) and cholinergic receptors (causing ED). They have general CNS-depressant effects, including sedation, which may partly account for decreased sexual interest in people undergoing phenothiazine therapy. There have been some reports of enhanced libido, particularly in women. Because of the many serious adverse reactions, patient compliance with phenothiazine therapy is often low.

Other non-phenothiazine neuroleptic (antischizophrenic) agents may cause similar adverse effects, because all appear to act by inhibiting dopamine transmission. Such drugs include the thioxanthenes (flupenthixol and analogues), haloperidol and droperidol, and pimozide. The 'atypical' neuroleptics, clozapine and olanzapine, appear to be less problematic than all other neuroleptics in these respects.

Antidepressant drugs generally elevate mood and thus may increase sexuality, as depression is often associated with diminished sexual interest, drive and activity (see Chapter 19). Unfortunately, however, antidepressants can influence sexual behaviour adversely by causing impotence, menstrual disorders, ejaculatory disturbances or gynaeco-mastia. All groups of antidepressants have been implicated: tricyclic antidepressants such as imipramine and amitriptyline (possibly related to their peripheral anticholinergic effects); monoamine oxidase (MAO) inhibitors such as phenelzine and moclobemide; and even the more specific selective serotonin reuptake inhibitors (SSRIs) such as fluoxetine (Prozac).

Benzodiazepine compounds (diazepam, alprazolam etc) are commonly prescribed antianxiety medications that are also useful as skeletal muscle relaxants. The sedative and relaxing effects of these drugs may account for the reported decreased interest in sexual activity, anorgasmia in men and women, and ejaculation failure. Alternatively, the judicious use of benzodiazepines has been considered of value in the treatment of sexual impotence and other problems involving sexual performance where excessive anxiety was a factor in decreased sexual performance. Buspirone, a non-benzodiazepine antianxiety agent, has also been associated with reports of increased or decreased libido and (rarely) with impotence or delayed ejaculation.

Barbiturates such as phenobarbitone and thiopentone are sedative–hypnotic drugs that have general depressant effects on all nervous tissues. They are used variously as antiepileptics, sedatives or induction anaesthetics. These drugs, in prescribed dosage, produce relaxation, hypnosis and sleep, with depression of various body functions, including sexual performance and ability.

Ethyl alcohol

Ethanol is, for its effects on human sexual function and behaviour, a drug of individual and unique notoriety (see Chapter 22, and Drug Monograph 22-3). Revered for centuries as a sexual stimulant and cure of all ills, alcohol is in fact a CNS depressant, but in moderate amounts may enhance sexual activity by relieving anxieties and loosening the inhibitions that often shroud sexual behaviour. In the often-quoted words of Shakespeare (the porter at the gate, in *Macbeth*, Act II, Scene III, in response to Macduff's question 'What three things does drink especially provoke?'):

Lechery, sir, it provokes and it unprovokes:
it provokes the desire, but it takes away the
performance: therefore, much drink may be said
to be an equivocator with lechery: it makes him,
and it mars him…

Or, as William Osler put it (quoted by Bowman & Rand 1980): "Alcohol does not make people do things better, it makes them less ashamed of doing them badly".

Beyond a certain limit, however, neither desire nor potency will overcome the depressed physical capability that alcohol causes. The CNS is more affected by alcohol than is any other system of the body. Electrophysiological studies show that alcohol first depresses the part of the brain responsible for integrating the various activities of the nervous system, causing impaired sensorimotor performance. The first mental processes affected are related to sobriety and self-restraint, producing a less inhibited and less restrained approach to sexual behaviour and other activities normally inhibited by previous training or experience. With continued consumption of alcohol, cerebral functions become depressed, reflexes become slowed, blood vessels are dilated and the capacity for sexual function is diminished. In addition, alcohol produces a potent diuretic effect, which can also interfere with sexual function.

Typically, the male alcoholic after years of chronic alcoholism experiences delayed ejaculation and impotence after drinking. Vascular changes, peripheral neuropathy and lower testosterone levels because of liver damage are thought to cause the impotence. Body image changes such as testicular atrophy, 'beer gut' and gynaecomastia compound the problems.

Diuretics

The thiazide diuretic hydrochlorothiazide may induce sexual dysfunction through its hypotensive and vasodilator actions. Spironolactone, an aldosterone antagonist, has both diuretic and endocrine effects, and has been associated with impotence, gynaecomastia and a decrease in libido.

Antihistamines

The classical antihistamines act as competitive inhibitors of histamine at H_1-receptor sites; these drugs include diphenhydramine, promethazine and chlorpheniramine. They are commonly taken as antiemetics and mild sedatives, and for the control of allergy symptoms and travel sickness. Most antihistamines cause anticholinergic effects such as dry mouth, urinary retention and constipation. Continuous use of these drugs may interfere with sexual activity.

The histamine H_2-receptor antagonists such as cimetidine and ranitidine, used to treat peptic ulcers, have been reported to cause gynaecomastia and impotence in men in high doses; ranitidine is probably the safer drug in this respect.

Hormones and derivatives

Sex hormones act on the endocrine system, CNS and other body organs to influence reproductive functions and sexual and aggressive behaviours, as well as mood and emotional outlook. Thus variations in female hormones may produce the anxiety, irritability and depression associated with premenstrual syndrome, whereas male hormones are associated with aggression and increased sexual interest (libido). Sexual drive may be influenced by sex hormone treatment.

The anabolic steroids are derived from or related to the male sex hormone testosterone. They have been misused by athletes and other people to promote muscle growth and endurance. As adverse effects, these drugs in women cause virilisation, hirsutism, libido changes and clitoral enlargement; in men, testicular atrophy, impotence, chronic priapism and oligospermia (see Chapters 46 and 57 and Drug Monograph 46-1).

Sex hormones, as well as being used in endocrine and reproductive medicine, are sometimes used in oncology to suppress the growth of hormone-dependent tumours. Thus androgen-dependent prostate tumours may be treated with antiandrogens, oestrogens or GnRH analogues. Breast tumours dependent on oestrogens may (depending on the tumour stage and patient factors) be treated with antioestrogens, androgens, progestogens or GnRH analogues. In each case, adverse reactions related to the normal actions of the hormone are possible and may impair sexual functioning. Antiandrogens (e.g. cyproterone) are also used to reduce sexual drive in overaggressive men.

Other drugs

Ketoconazole, an antifungal agent, may cause transient decreases in testosterone levels, with oligospermia and decreased libido in men. Various other medications have been reported rarely to cause sexual dysfunction; these effects would be listed in reference texts of adverse drug reactions or interactions.

Premature ejaculation, the occurrence of a male orgasm too early in sexual intercourse, is a condition that impairs sexual functioning in many relationships. A topical spray or cream formulation of the local anaesthetic lignocaine is available; it is used to desensitise the surface of the penis and prolong time to ejaculation.

Many of the drugs described earlier as reputedly having aphrodisiac or sexual stimulating actions (including opioids, marijuana, LSD, nitrates and cantharidin) have been shown to be more likely to cause sexual dysfunction, and so should probably be included in this rather than the previous section.

PREGNANCY SAFETY	
ADEC Category	**Drug**
A	Bromocriptine, human chorionic gonadotrophin
B1	Sildenafil, tadalafil
B2	Follitropin beta
B3	Choriogonadotropin alfa, clomiphene, lutropin alfa, papaverine, vardenafil
D	Follitropin alfa

Note: Alprostadil, used only in men and contraindicated in women, does not have a Pregnancy Safety category.

DRUGS AT A GLANCE 47: Fertility and sexual functioning

Therapeutic group	Pharmacological group	Key examples	Key pages
Ovulatory stimulants	Anti-oestrogens (partial agonist)	clomiphene	740, 1
	Gonadotrophins · Follicle-stimulating hormone · Luteinising hormone	follitropin chorionic gonadotrophin, human (hCG) }	} 740
	Dopamine agonist	bromocriptine	
Spermatogenesis stimulant	Interstitial cell-stimulating hormone (ICSH) activity	hCG	740
Contraceptives	Combined oral contraceptives (see Chapter 44)		741, 4
	Intrauterine devices (IUD)	IUD with copper	742, 3
Drugs treating erectile dysfunction (impotence)	Phosphodiesterase-5 inhibitors	sildenalfil, vardenafil, tadalafil }	748, 9
	Androgens	testosterone }	
	Prostaglandin agonists	alprostadil }	749
	Smooth muscle relaxants	papaverine ⌟	

KEY POINTS

- Infertility is a common problem in the community and has many possible causes. There are many types of treatments, including pharmacological and IVF methods.
- Anovulatory infertility in women may be treated with ovulatory stimulants, such as clomiphene, or with gonadotrophins.
- Male infertility is also treated with gonadotrophins (if the cause is hypogonadal).
- Contraception is practised by about 50% of couples to limit their fertility or plan their family. Drug and non-drug methods are available for the female or male partner, with varying usage rates, failure rates and degrees of reversibility. 'Barrier' methods are most effective at preventing STDs.
- Many medications, both legal and illegal, can affect sexuality and sexual behaviour.
- Although many drugs have been postulated or tried as sexual stimulants (aphrodisiacs), very few are actually active and none prescribed for this purpose. Psychoactive agents, including social drugs and hallucinogens, tend merely to suppress inhibitions or alter sensations.
- Erectile dysfunction (ED; impotence) in men is a common and distressing disorder; the most effective drug treatments are the oral PDE5 inhibitors such as sildenafil, which potentiates the natural vasodilation caused by nitric oxide. Other drugs used to treat ED include injected alprostadil or papaverine.
- Many groups of drugs are likely to impair sexual functioning; common drugs with this effect are antihypertensives, diuretics, antihistamines, antipsychotics, antidepressants, hormones and CNS depressants, including alcohol.
- Health-care professionals need to be aware of their patients' needs and sensitivities in the areas of fertility control and sexual functioning, and, when necessary, provide the appropriate medical intervention or information.

REVIEW EXERCISES

1   Describe the common causes of female or male infertility and the use of ovulatory stimulants or gonadotrophins in therapy.

2   List the main types of drug and non-drug contraception methods and discuss the advantages and disadvantages of each method.

3   List drugs that have been reputed to act as aphrodisiacs and discuss their pharmacological effects on sexual functions.

4 Discuss the main groups of drugs that have adverse effects on sexual functioning, explaining their mechanisms of action.

5 Describe the effects of ethanol on sexual function and behaviour.

6 Describe the clinical use of sildenafil in treatment of erectile dysfunction and explain its advantages over previous types of therapy.

REFERENCES AND FURTHER READING

Australian Medicines Handbook 2006. Adelaide: AMH, 2006.

Beck JI, Boothroyd C, Proctor M, Farquhar C, Hughes E. Oral anti-oestrogens and medical adjuncts for subfertility associated with anovulation. *Cochrane Database of Systematic Reviews* 2005; (1): CDs002249.

Bowman WC, Rand MJ. *Textbook of Pharmacology*. 2nd edn. Oxford: Blackwell, 1980 [chs 20, 42].

Caswell A (ed.). *MIMS Annual June 2005*. Sydney: CMPMedica Australia, 2005.

Chen J, Hwang DJ, Bohl CE, Miller DD, Dalton JT. A selective androgen receptor modulator for hormonal male contraception. *Journal of Pharmacology and Experimental Therapeutics* 2005; 312(2): 546–53.

Crosignani PG, Bianchedi D, Riccaboni A, Vegetti W. Management of anovulatory infertility. *Human Reproduction* 1999; 14 Suppl. 1: 108–19.

Dinsmore WW. Available and future treatments for erectile dysfunction. *Clinical Cornerstone* 2005; 7(1): 37–45.

Endocrinology Expert Group. *Therapeutic Guidelines Endocrinology, version 3*. Melbourne: Therapeutic Guidelines Limited, 2004.

Greenspan FS, Strewler GJ. *Basic and Clinical Endocrinology*. 5th edn. Stamford: Appleton & Lange, 1997 [chs 12, 13].

Guillebaud J. *Contraception: your questions answered*. 4th edn. Edinburgh: Churchill Livingstone, 2004.

Razvi K, Chew S, Yong EL, Kumar J, Ng SC. The clinical management of male infertility. *Singapore Medical Journal* 1999; 40: 291–7.

Richardson D, Green J, Ritcheson A, Goldmeier D, Harris JR. A review of controlled trials in the pharmacological treatment of premature ejaculation. *International Journal of STD and AIDS* 2005; 16(10): 651–8.

Speroff L, Darney P. *A Clinical Guide for Contraception*. Baltimore: Williams & Wilkins, 1992.

Tortora GJ, Grabowski SR. *Principles of Anatomy and Physiology*. 9th edn. New York: HarperCollins, 2000 [ch. 28].

Vollenhoven B. *Contraception*. Unpublished review. Melbourne: Monash University, 2005.

Weisberg E. Progestogen-only methods of contraception. *Australian Prescriber* 1999; 22: 6–8.

Wilson JD, Foster DW, Kronenberg HM, Larsen PR. *Williams Textbook of Endocrinology*. 9th edn. Philadelphia: Saunders, 1998 [chs 18, 19].

Youngson RM. *Collins Dictionary: Medicine*. 2nd edn. Glasgow: HarperCollins, 1998.

ON-LINE RESOURCES

New Zealand medicines and medical devices safety authority: www.medsafe.govt.nz

evolve   More weblinks at http://evolve.elsevier.com/AU/Bryant/pharmacology/

CHAPTER 48

Overview of Neoplasia and Cancer Chemotherapy

CHAPTER FOCUS

Although progress in antineoplastic chemotherapy has helped many people diagnosed with cancer, cancers are a leading cause of death in Australia. The antineoplastic agents have a low therapeutic index: that is, they possess both useful therapeutic effects and significant adverse reactions. A thorough knowledge of clinical aspects of antineoplastic chemotherapy is important for the health-care professional. In this chapter, an overview is given of tumour cell biology, and of the principles and clinical aspects of oncology, as background to understanding the types of drugs used in treating cancers. Drug groups are dealt with in more detail in Chapter 49, and sample drug monographs are given there.

OBJECTIVES

● To describe the stages involved in cell cycling and its regulation, the pathways for macromolecular synthesis, and the processes of carcinogenesis and growth of cancers.

● To identify phases in the cell cycle at which checkpoints occur and antineoplastic agents act.

● To describe the main modalities used in treating cancers, and to discuss important principles of antineoplastic chemotherapy.

● To explain the mechanisms of action of the main groups of cytotoxic drugs and hormones used in cancer treatment, and to identify potential targets for new drugs.

● To discuss the importance of combination chemotherapy and safe handling of cytotoxics, and to outline typical treatment regimens in cancer chemotherapy.

● To describe the commonest adverse effects of antineoplastic chemotherapy, and to explain why they occur.

● To discuss age-related considerations for treatment of cancer in children, people of reproductive age and the elderly.

KEY DRUGS

alkylating agents
antimetabolites
antineoplastics
cytotoxic agents
mitotic inhibitors

KEY TERMS

antineoplastic agents
apoptosis
cancer
carcinogen
cell cycle
cell-kill fraction
checkpoints
chemotherapy
combination chemotherapy
cytotoxic agents
macromolecular synthesis
metastasis
mutagen
neoplasia
oncogenes
purines, pyrimidines
safe handling
signal transduction

KEY ABBREVIATIONS

DNA	deoxyribonucleic acid
G_1, G_2	gap or growth phase 1, 2
GF	growth factor
M	mitosis phase
MOPP	mustine, Oncovin (vincristine), procarbazine, prednisone
RNA	ribonucleic acid
S	synthesis phase

NEOPLASIA (the process of growth of tumours) refers to a group of conditions that are characterised by uncontrolled proliferation and spread of abnormal forms of the body's cells. The tissue growth is uncoordinated and persists after the end of the stimulus provoking the growth (unlike hypertrophy of cardiac muscle or growth of the endometrium during the menstrual cycle). Other characteristics of tumours are that their presence is not useful; there may be dedifferentiation of cells, leading to loss of specialised functions; and the characteristics of the abnormal cells are inherited indefinitely by successive cells. Benign tumours may cause problems by their excessive growth and may kill by putting pressure on critical adjacent organs.

Malignant tumours (**cancers**) are more dangerous to the body because, in addition to the above properties, they are generally more rapidly growing and have the ability to spread by invading adjacent tissues and seeding secondary tumours to distant organs (**metastasis**). Malignant cells may have abnormal or unstable numbers of chromosomes and/or mutated genes (a varied genotype), and their properties may vary over time (varied phenotype).

It has been estimated that about 40% of people will develop cancer during their lifetime. Many people fear cancer because of the likelihood of pain and adverse treatment effects, and because it is difficult to accept that a small lump or mole that has the potential for rapid growth may lead to serious illness or death. Therefore education and early treatment are imperative to improve success rates in treatment of cancer, which is second only to cardiovascular disease as a cause of death in most developed countries.

Statistically, the chances of developing cancer and dying from cancer are greater now than ever before. As diseases that were formerly fatal earlier in life (such as childhood infections, complications of childbirth, diabetes and hypertension) have become treatable, the population is ageing and so a higher proportion will succumb to progressive conditions that occur later in life, such as cancers (see Clinical Interest Box 48-1).

This chapter discusses the principles of antineoplastic chemotherapy and the use of chemotherapeutic drugs in the treatment of cancer. To understand better the mechanisms and sites of action of cancer chemotherapeutic agents, it is important first to have a basic understanding of tumour cell biology and the development of cancers.

TUMOUR CELL BIOLOGY
Cell kinetics
The cell cycle

Appropriate control of cell growth is essential for steady-state tissue and physiological functioning, for replacement of cells as required, and in response to stimulation and increased demands for function. The **cell cycle** of division

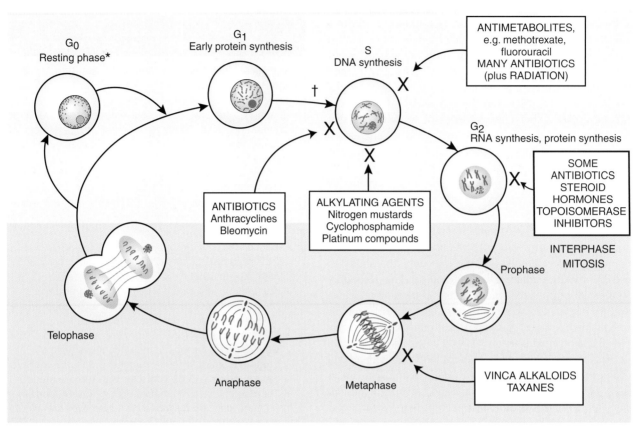

FIGURE 48-1 Phases of a cell cycle. Drugs (in boxes) are identified, showing the main site at which they exert their effects. *Adapted from*: Beare & Myers 1998. * = commitment to cell division: leads to cell enlargement, DNA replication and mitosis; † = first checkpoint if damaged DNA cannot be repaired, cell undergoes apoptosis: G_0 = resting phase, cells not cycling; G_1 = first gap, between previous nuclear division and beginning of DNA synthesis (duration highly variable); G_2 = second gap, between DNA replication and nuclear division (about 3 hours); M = mitosis (about 1 hour); S = period of DNA synthesis (8–20 hours).

and proliferation is essentially the same for normal and cancer cells (Figure 48-1). In the presynthesis 'gap' or growth phase (G_1), synthesis of RNA and protein occurs in preparation for the next (synthesis) phase. Also during this phase, the decision for cell replication or cell differentiation is determined. The cell progresses to the synthesis phase (S), during which its genetic material (DNA) doubles in preparation for cell division (see macromolecular synthesis, below). During the second gap phase (G_2), the postsynthesis or premitotic phase, DNA synthesis ceases but RNA and protein synthesis continues, to prepare the cell for mitosis (M), spindle formation and cell division. During the M phase, cells divide into two completely new 'daughter' cells that may continue to cycle, or may leave the cell cycle to develop into differentiated cells that perform a specialised function (such as neurons or hepatocytes [these cells no longer undergo cell division]) or become either temporarily or permanently non-proliferative (G_0 phase). Cells in the G_0 or resting phase, a type of 'neutral gear', may remain in this phase (as do fibroblasts until required for healing), may be recruited later to re-enter the cell cycle, or may mature and die. The average time for a

mammalian cell cycle is about 12–20 hours, depending on the time spent in the S phase.

REGULATION OF THE CELL CYCLE

Regulatory factors determine the progression of cells through the cell cycle by activation of receptors on the cell membrane followed by **signal transduction** (see Figure 48-2), by which growth stimulatory signals are passed on to the nucleus in cascades of biochemical reactions, where they trigger activation or repression of various genes required for DNA replication, cell division and proliferation. Factors that stimulate the replication and division of cells include growth factors, various types of GTP-binding proteins (such as Ras, Raf, Erk), and a family of intracellular proteins called cyclins.

Growth factors (GFs) involved in these signal transduction pathways include epidermal GF, fibroblast GF, transforming GF, insulin-like GF and many more, each with its related receptor. Cyclins may be activated after phosphorylation by a protein kinase known as p34 (of molecular weight 34,000 daltons, hence its name). Cyclins control mitosis via effects

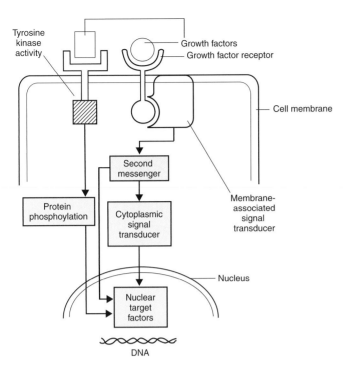

FIGURE 48-2 Diagram representing simplified mechanisms of growth factors in activation of target factors in the cell nucleus. On the left-hand side, a growth factor is shown binding to a membrane-associated receptor, leading to activation of a tyrosine kinase (a phosphorylating enzyme), which phosphorylates and thus activates a protein that enters the nucleus, where it targets factors involved in cell replication. On the right-hand side, binding of the growth factor activates a signal-transducing protein, which may bind with G-proteins and/or stimulate second messengers, eventually leading to effects inside the nucleus. *Reproduced from*: Souhami & Tobias 2005, with permission.

on cyclin-dependent kinases, which control the enzymes involved in the cell cycle. Genetic aberrations and mutations that result in continuous activation of cell-cycle progression are found in many human tumours.

Checkpoints are stages in the cell cycle at which cells may be 'checked', to ensure completion of phase-specific steps in the biochemical pathways before passage into the next phase of the cycle. Thus it is hypothesised that after checking at the G_1/S transition, S phase, G_2/M transition or at mitosis, the replication of mutated DNA can be blocked and the mitotic division of mutated chromosomes inhibited, leading to elimination of mutated cells. Human tumours often contain mutations in genes involved in these checking processes, explaining the uncontrolled proliferation of altered cells. The commonest mutation leading to loss of G_1 checkpoint function is genetic alteration of the gene coding for the p53 protein, which is a major regulator of the G_1 checkpoint in response to cellular stress.

The cyclins can be inhibited by negative regulatory factors, including proteins synthesised by two particular tumour

suppressor genes (the p53 gene and the retinoblastoma gene). These inhibitory factors usually halt the cell cycle at checkpoints and allow for repair of damaged DNA. The retinoblastoma family of proteins are thought to act as an 'emergency brake' to prevent cell-cycle progression when activated. Mutations that impair this signalling pathway and thus allow unscheduled progression of cells from the G_1 to the S phase have been shown to occur in nearly every type of adult cancer.

The p53 protein and its associated gene has been referred to as 'the guardian of the genome' (Cavalli et al 2004). p53 is a phosphoprotein in the nucleus that regulates the cell cycle; it has a molecular weight of 53 kD (kilodaltons). The p53 gene is often mutated in sporadic cancers of many types, leading to loss of normal 'braking mechanisms' and hence to uncontrolled growth.

Macromolecular synthesis (synthesis of proteins and nucleic acids)

For cells to proliferate, the genetic material deoxyribonucleic acid (DNA) must be replicated once every cell cycle. DNA, a large double-stranded helical molecule, is composed of four kinds of serially repeating nucleotide bases: **pyrimidines** (cytosine and thymine) and **purines** (adenine and guanine); see Figure 48-3. Particular nucleotide sequences make up the genes, the biological units of inheritance occupying precise positions on a chromosome. When genes are expressed, DNA is 'transcribed' into messenger ribonucleic acid copies, which are transported out of the nucleus into the cytoplasm and there act as templates to direct the amino acid sequence in the synthesis of enzymes and structural and other kinds of proteins from amino acids. The enzymes determine the structure, biochemical activity, growth rate and functions of the cell. Many anticancer agents act at different stages in the pathways of **macromolecular synthesis**; these are described briefly later (under types of antineoplastic agents), and in more detail in Chapter 49.

DUPLICATION OF DNA AND CHROMOSOMES

DNA REPLICATION AND TOPOISOMERASES. Packaging of DNA into the chromosomes visible in the nucleus during mitosis involves 'supercoiling' of the DNA fragments, i.e. regions where the double-stranded DNA helix is twisted on itself. This requires the actions of enzymes known as topoisomerases (one type of which was previously called gyrase), which have the ability to control the number and amount of twist in the supercoils, by cutting one or both strands, twisting them about each other and resealing the ends. These actions are essential to the complete replication of DNA and controlled growth of cells. Agents that selectively inhibit these enzymes have become useful anticancer drugs.

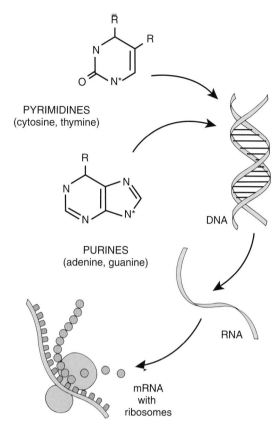

FIGURE 48-3 Synthesis of macromolecules (nucleic acids and proteins). In the general structures shown for the purine and pyrimidine bases, R stands for an oxygen (=O) or amine (–NH₂) group. In the polymers of DNA or RNA, each base is linked via the N* nitrogen atom to a sugar molecule (deoxyribose or ribose), and the sugar molecules are linked via phosphate groups to form long chains. In DNA, two complementary strands are twisted into the famous double-helix shape.

DUPLICATION OF CHROMOSOMES AND IMMORTALISATION OF CANCER CELLS. Normal cells appear to be able to undergo only a limited number of divisions. This is thought to be because the telomeres (the sections of DNA forming the ends of chromosomes) can be replicated only a limited number of times because a small fragment of 'junk' DNA is shaved off each time. An enzyme called telomerase (telomere terminal transferase), however, can reform the telomeres, thus preventing the shortening of the chromosome. This enzyme is present in about 90% of human cancers (and in immortal cell lines) but not in fully differentiated normal cells, so it is thought that the presence of the enzyme may confer immortality to cancer cells. Inhibition of telomerase activity is thus another possible mode of action of anticancer agents.

Apoptosis

If DNA repair fails during a cell-cycle checkpoint, an altered cell normally undergoes programmed cell death or **apoptosis**,

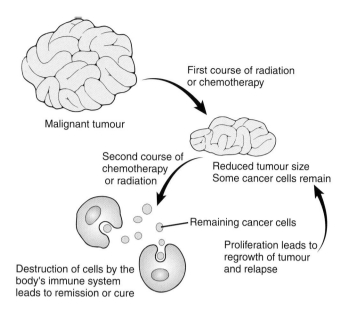

FIGURE 48-4 Response of cancer cells to therapy. *Adapted from*: Beare & Myers 1998.

a useful process that eliminates damaged, redundant or abnormal cells via a series of genetically programmed biochemical reactions. Apoptosis involves rounding up of the cell, shrinkage, then fragmentation and digestion. This process occurs constantly, for example, in the shedding of intestinal mucosal cells or skin cells, and in the expiry of red blood cells, and is also an important defence against malignant cells. Apoptosis involves a cascade of reactions involving endopeptidases that cleave proteins and enzymes, including deoxyribonucleases. It is thought that apoptosis is the 'fallback' position, automatically triggered at cell-cycle checkpoints unless inhibited by the many trophic factors, hormones, and growth factors necessary for cell cycling and survival.

The p53 gene can also mediate apoptosis via complicated pathways involving signalling proteins, growth factors, 'death receptors', specialised enzymes called caspases, and all their related genes (including PIGs: p53-inducible genes). The precise mechanisms and details of these pathways are still being elucidated. This fascinating area of molecular biology will be crucial in the design of new anticancer drugs, but details are beyond the scope of this textbook.

Cell-kill fraction

Studies in animals with leukaemias and lymphomas have shown that chemotherapeutic drugs given in adequate doses to the host will kill a constant proportion of the cancer cells; this is known as the **cell-kill fraction**. A drug or drug combination capable of killing 99.9% of the cells would leave 0.1% surviving and thus would only reduce a 10^{10} cell burden to 10^7 cancer cells. Each course of chemotherapy or radiation therapy may reduce cancer cells to levels that can eventually be controlled by the patient's immune system (Figure 48-4 and Table 48-1). This reduction may produce a remission but, if further therapies are not instituted or the immune system response is inadequate, the remaining cells may multiply and grow into another detectable tumour, i.e. cause recurrence and relapse. The aim of each cycle of cancer therapy is therefore to achieve total cancer cell kill if possible.

TABLE 48–1 cancer cell growth

NUMBER OF CELLS PRESENT		CLINICAL SIGNIFICANCE
10^0	1	Subclinical disease (undetectable by physical examination)
10^1	10	
10^2	100	
10^3	1000	
10^4	10,000	
10^5	100,000	
10^6	1,000,000	
10^7	10,000,000	
10^8	100,000,000	
10^9	1,000,000,000	~1 g: clinical symptoms appear
10^{10}	10,000,000,000	Regional spread
10^{11}	100,000,000,000	
10^{12}	1,000,000,000,000	Metastases
10^{13}	10,000,000,000,000	Lethal

Notes: In the very early stages, immune mechanisms may be effective at removing altered cells. The rate of cell proliferation slows as tumour size increases; i.e. tumour growth is non-exponential, or Gompertzian.

Carcinogenesis and cancer growth
Development of cancer cells

As described above, normal cells grow and divide in an orderly fashion, with the body's homeostatic mechanisms controlling the entire cell growth process, the process of cell adhesion inhibiting the movement of the newly formed cells, and apoptosis removing expendable cells.

Carcinogenesis (the development of cancers, also known as oncogenesis) is known to be a multicausal, multi-step process. Cancer cells may arise from a hereditary or genetic predisposition or from contact with certain environmental conditions. Many **carcinogens** (agents that cause the development of or increase the incidence of cancer) have been identified, e.g. the Epstein–Barr virus in Burkitt's lymphoma, cigarette smoking in many cancers, and asbestos in mesothelioma. Genetic inheritance also plays a role in some cancers (e.g. breast or colon cancer). The retinoblastoma gene is involved in many cancers; it is thought that if a person inherits a defective copy of the gene from one parent and the other copy of the gene is then damaged or altered, then there is loss of the 'brake' effect, the oncogenic potential of other proteins cannot be suppressed, and tumours result. Physical effects such as ionising radiation may cause mutations, and wherever there are higher rates of mitosis, e.g. during the monthly cycle of growth and regression of cells in breast and endometrial tissue, or during repeated physical injury, there is higher risk of mutations and potentially an increased frequency of cancer.

Many carcinogenic chemicals have been identified, including tars and other polycyclic hydrocarbons, phorbol esters, nitrosamines and aflatoxins. These may act synergistically, with some chemicals acting as initiators of tumours and others as promoters. Chemicals such as benzopyrene and aflatoxin from fungi, and UV radiation, act as mutagens and carcinogens by activating p53 signalling, also causing cross-links and mutations in the p53 gene and thus impairing checkpoint functions. Cells with defective checkpoint functions may, however, be more sensitive to anticancer agents; thus checkpoints may become a new target for anticancer drug. **Mutagens**, agents that induce a genetic mutation or increase the mutation rate, may increase the risk of development of cancers, as shown in Clinical Interest Box 48-2.

Much research effort has gone into studying any relationship between diet and cancer, particularly the Western

CLINICAL INTEREST BOX 48-2 PROCESSES IN THE TYPICAL DEVELOPMENT OF CANCERS

1. Exposure of a cell to a mutagen, or inheritance of a mutated gene, leads to:
2. alteration of the cell's DNA, which:
3. changes a proto-oncogene into an oncogene, or inactivates tumour suppressor genes, so that:
4. the transformed cell (clone) is no longer subject to cell-cycle control and thus:
5. has growth advantages over non-transformed cells and proliferates, which:
6. activates other proto-oncogenes and:
7. produces more growth factors and tumour-specific proteins, leading to:
8. uncontrolled cancer growth, such that cells become invasive and metastatic.

diet, which is generally high in animal fats. In the early 21st century it has been accepted that there is very little evidence for any relationship between diet and cancer, except for proven carcinogens such as aflatoxins, nitrosamines and salted fish, and associations with alcohol and obesity in increasing the risk of many cancers. By comparison, tobacco is known to contribute to 33% of all cancer deaths, and infection with microorganisms to 15%. A recent review of cancer epidemiology (Peto 2001) concluded that "Avoidance of overweight and prevention or treatment of oncogenic infections are the most important aims for non-smokers; but it is absurd for smokers in the West to worry about anything except stopping smoking".

ONCOGENES

Oncogenes are altered genes that are able to transform normal cells to malignant cells. They may initially occur as part of an oncogenic virus or may derive from an altered cellular counterpart of a viral oncogene (a proto-oncogene). They are named with a 3-letter italic designation, e.g. *src*, *ras* or *jun*; the related proto-oncogene is designated with an initial c-, thus c-*ras* or c-*jun*.

Oncogenes are probably all derived from growth-controlling genes, as oncogene proteins are known to interact with four types of growth-controlling systems in cells:
1. growth factors (e.g. epidermal growth factor, EGF)
2. growth factor receptors (e.g. the *neu* oncogene causes the EGF receptor to remain continuously activated)
3. intracellular transducers (e.g. *ras* proteins are involved in intracellular transduction mechanisms with cyclic AMP and inositol pathways in the cytoplasm; mutations may delete GTP-ase activity so Gs proteins (stimulatory G-proteins) are continuously activated)
4. nuclear transcription factors (proteins that allow new genes to be expressed, or modify expression of current genes; examples are fos, jun and myc).

To anchor proteins to the plasma membrane, the proteins may have a covalently bound lipid group. This is known as prenylation of the protein, and the lipid group may be a geranyl or farnesyl molecule. For example, the *ras* proteins have a farnesyl group attached (farnesyl is a 15-carbon unit normally involved in the synthesis of steroids and carotenoids). This 'farnesylation' is an essential lipidation step that allows the oncogene proteins to transform normal cells into tumour cells. The enzyme involved, farnesyl transferase, is a potential target for anticancer agents.

CHROMOSOMAL ABNORMALITIES

Chromosomal abnormalities are very common in tumours. Tumour cells may have an abnormal number of chromosomes (aneuploid); may contain translocations of parts of genes, which modify or activate proto-oncogenes; or may have localised duplications or deletions of DNA fragments.

GROWTH OF CANCERS

Neoplastic cells may lack the cellular differentiation of the tissues in which they originate and therefore may be unable to function like the normal cells around them. Cancer growth is enhanced by an increased rate of cell proliferation that lacks the body's normal system of control on cellular growth patterns. Because of the genetic differences, cancer cells lack the cell–cell or cell–basement membrane adhesive properties of normal cells, which may lead to metastasis, or spread of the cancer.

The growth of a cancer is usually rapid and exponential in the early stages but, as the tumour enlarges, the centre may outgrow its blood and nutrient supply and become necrotic. The growth rate then decreases or reaches a plateau phase for the tumour; this is referred to as Gompertzian growth kinetics. To continue to grow, the tumour must develop new blood vessels (angiogenesis) and requires the actions of specialised enzymes (metalloproteinases), which allow space for new cells and blood vessels. Inhibition of angiogenesis is another target for new anticancer drugs.

A tumour cell burden of 10^9 cells is usually the smallest (quantitative size) that is physically detectable (palpable). At this point, the individual has about 1 billion cancer cells, which is equivalent to a tumour about the size of a small grape and weighing around 1 g. This is the point at which clinical symptoms usually first appear (see Table 48-1). If untreated, the malignant tumour will continue to grow in size until it is fatal. An overall scheme for the development of cancers is shown in Clinical Interest Box 48-2.

Tumours are not homogeneous, even tumours of the same cell type in the same organ. They may vary in cell-cycling time, the proportion of cells cycling, their vascularity, susceptibility or resistance to the actions of particular drugs, and their size and extent of spread. Tumours are commonly 'staged' by the 'TNM' method to indicate the size of the primary tumour and extent of spread to lymph nodes and distant metastases. In some cases, the growth of the tumour can be monitored by measuring levels of a (relatively) specific marker, such as prostate specific antigen (PSA) for prostate cancers, or monoclonal immunoglobulins for multiple myeloma.

TREATMENT OF CANCER
Treatment modalities

The three main treatment modalities in cancer are surgery, irradiation and drugs (and, in slowly growing cancers, watchful waiting). If it is possible to remove all of a cancer surgically, this is obviously the first choice and may be curative. When this is not possible (e.g. with a large inoperable tumour in a vital organ, a tumour that is difficult to access or non-solid tumours such as leukaemias or lymphomas), then irradiation and/or drugs are used. Immunotherapy is also sometimes used to enhance the immune response against neoplastic cells. Adjuvant therapy may include drug treatment of adverse effects and related conditions such as depression or anxiety, and complementary and alternative therapies such as massage, behavioural therapy and counselling.

Radiation therapy uses X-rays, targeted to minimise damage to non-cancer cells, or radiopharmaceuticals, which are drugs or chemicals containing radioisotopes emitting gamma rays that damage cells. Radiation therapy has been shown to be important in reducing the risk of metastases (e.g. of leukaemias to the head and neck areas).

Radiopharmaceuticals include:

- iodine-131 (^{131}I) used in thyroid cancer (see Drug Monograph 39-2)
- phosphorus-32 (^{32}P), which is concentrated in the bones, where it is toxic to bone marrow cells and hence used to reduce excess production of red cells in polycythaemia vera
- strontium-89, a gamma-ray emitter, used to reduce metastatic bone lesions secondary to prostate cancer
- samarium-153, which emits beta and gamma rays and concentrates in areas of high bone turnover, providing relief of bone pain in patients with osteoblastic metastases.

Other radiopharmaceuticals, used in radiographic diagnostic procedures rather than treatment of cancers, are those containing the isotopes technetium-99, gallium-67 and thallium-201.

Drug therapy of cancer may include the use of antineoplastic agents, hormones, immunostimulating agents and specific drugs to treat adverse effects of anticancer drugs.

Principles of chemotherapy

Chemotherapy is defined as the clinical use of drugs that, in low concentrations, inhibit the growth of microbial or neoplastic cells. Chemotherapy usually relies on finding and exploiting a difference in the biochemical pathways between the host cell or normal cell, and the microbial cell or neoplastic cell; this is referred to as selective toxicity. In the context of treatment of cancers, to obtain optimal therapeutic effects with an antineoplastic agent or with combination cancer chemotherapies, several principles should be considered.

Cancer chemotherapy is most effective against small tumours because they usually have an efficient blood supply and therefore drug delivery to the cancer site is increased. Also, small tumours generally have a higher percentage of proliferating cells so that a higher cell-kill fraction is possible.

Removing large localised tumours by surgery reduces the tumour cell burden and thus contributes to the success of the adjuvant chemotherapy. The major use of adjuvant chemotherapy is to help eradicate the micrometastases (the migration of cancer cells via the bloodstream or lymphatic system to grow in organs, bone or tissues far from the primary site) of cancer after surgery or irradiation.

In general, combinations of cancer chemotherapeutic agents have a higher cancer cell-kill fraction than treatment with a single drug agent, and specific drug toxicities may be reduced. The toxicity of anticancer drugs needs to be anticipated and, if possible, organs need to be protected and treatment for adverse effects administered.

Types of antineoplastic agents
Cytotoxic agents

The formation of macromolecules (the nucleic acids DNA and RNA and, ultimately, proteins) requires pyrimidines and purines (nitrogen-containing 'bases') as the building-block materials for nucleic acids (see Figure 48-3). **Antineoplastic** agents known as **cytotoxic agents** (drugs that are toxic to cells, specifically those used to kill cancer cells) act by inhibiting the synthesis of macromolecules. Some drugs have more than one specific site of action.

Antimetabolites have structures similar to those of necessary building blocks for the formation of DNA, e.g. similar to folic acid or to a purine or pyrimidine base. This 'false building block' is accepted by the cell as the necessary ingredient for cell growth but, because it is an impostor, it interferes with the normal production of DNA.

Alkylating agents are drugs that substitute an alkyl chemical group for a hydrogen atom in DNA. This results in a cross-linking between strands of DNA, preventing cell division. Alkylator-like drugs are chemically different agents that are believed to have an action similar to those of the alkylating agents.

Antitumour antibiotic agents interfere with DNA functioning by blocking the transcription of DNA to RNA. In addition, they may delay or inhibit mitosis.

Mitotic inhibitors, such as vinblastine and vincristine, are plant alkaloids that block cell division in metaphase.

CELL CYCLE SPECIFICITY

The cytotoxic agents have different sites of action on the dividing cell cycle (see Figure 48-1), but they all inhibit cell replication and are thus antiproliferative. Agents that are most effective in one specific phase are referred to as cell-cycle-phase-specific agents. Antimetabolites, for example, are most active impairing DNA synthesis in the S-phase of the cell cycle, so these drugs are considered S-phase cell-cycle-specific agents. The podophyllotoxins, which inhibit topoisomerase II activity, are S- and G_2-phase-specific; the topoisomerase I inhibitors, the -tecans, are S-phase-specific. The vinca alkaloids generally act against mitosis and so are M-phase-specific.

Some antineoplastic agents that act on cycling cells, but not on a specific phase, are called cell-cycle-specific agents; examples are most alkylating agents and some antibiotics, which inhibit at many sites such as DNA, RNA and protein synthesis.

Antineoplastic agents that are active against both proliferating and resting cells are called cell-cycle-non-specific agents. The platinum compounds, some alkylating agents (the nitrosoureas), the anthracycline antibiotics and agents that enhance apoptosis are examples of this group (see Table 49-1).

Antineoplastic classifications are an important consideration in selecting the appropriate drug or drugs for a specific cancerous state. Methotrexate, for example, an agent active predominantly in the S-phase of the cell cycle, is not very effective in treating large tumour masses, which generally have slowly dividing cancer cells. Some clinicians consider it important to select and combine chemotherapeutic agents that act at different phases, in order to have synergistic effects and to reduce the development of drug resistance.

Hormone anticancer agents

The growth of some tumours is dependent on the stimulation of neoplastic cells by particular hormones. Breast cancer is stimulated by oestrogens, prostate cancer by androgens, and thyroid cancer by thyroid-stimulating hormone. These cancers may be effectively suppressed by antihormones (hormones having opposite effects to those stimulating the tumour), by drugs that suppress synthesis or secretion of the hormone, or by surgical removal or irradiation of the gland producing the hormone.

Other antineoplastic agents

Some miscellaneous antineoplastics do not conveniently fit into only one classification of mechanism of action, e.g. the enzyme crisantaspase, the hydroxyureas, DNA-intercalating agents and interferons.

Relatively new agents, and those currently under investigation and development, include chemicals and processes that target specific sites in the cell cycle and in tumour cell functions (described earlier), such as:
- inhibitors of specific enzymes (farnesyltransferase, thymidylate synthetase, ribonucleotide reductase, protein tyrosine kinases, cyclin-dependent kinases, matrix metalloproteinases, telomerase, histone deacetylase, proteasomes)
- inhibitors of biosynthesis of polyamines involved in differentiation
- neutralisation of growth factors or their receptors
- inhibitors of synthesis of growth factors or of their receptors

---

CLINICAL INTEREST BOX 48-3
A TREATMENT REGIMEN FOR LUNG CANCER

A typical regimen of chemotherapy for early stage lung cancer is:
- carboplatin AUC 5, by IV infusion over 1 hour, day 1
- plus gemcitabine 1 g/m² by IV infusion over 30 mins, days 1 and 8, repeated every 21 days.

As alternatives to gemcitabine, either vinorelbine (25 mg/m² IV days 1 and 8) or paclitaxel (175 mg/m² IV infusion, day 1) may be substituted, and the combination repeated every 3–4 weeks.

For patients with more advanced lung cancer, or otherwise not able to tolerate the above regimens, carboplatin is not administered; either gemcitabine or vinorelbine alone is used, with slightly different doses and regimens.

Management should be individualised for each case after consultation with a specialist radiation oncologist. Patients should be informed of the risks of treatment-induced adverse reactions.

Note that potent anticancer drugs are usually dosed in units of *mg drug/m² body surface area* (see explanation in Chapter 8). Carboplatin is most unusual in that its dosage (mg) is calculated by reference to the target area under the curve (AUC), based on individual patient pharmacokinetics, taking into account the patient's renal glomerular filtration rate and creatinine clearance (see AMH 2006 for details).
Personal communication: Dr Michael Michael, Division of Haematology and Medical Oncology, Peter MacCallum Cancer Centre, Melbourne 2005; see also Vinorelbine Italian Study Group 1999

- proteins to restore retinoblastoma gene-suppressor functions
- drug enhancement of apoptosis and activation of caspase enzymes
- anti-sense oligonucleotides to impair actions of specific gene protein products
- improved delivery of cytotoxic agents specifically to cancer cells
- monoclonal antibodies against growth factors, to potentiate effects of cytotoxics
- cytokines, such as interleukins or tumour necrosis factor, for synergistic actions with cytotoxic agents
- enhancers of the host's immune responses against cancer cells, e.g. interferons
- vaccines, e.g. against cervical cancer in women
- agents that inhibit angiogenesis (i.e. suppress development of new blood vessels that provide nutrients to the tumour)
- gene therapy, whereby genes can be introduced to reverse neoplastic changes or reverse acquired resistance to antineoplastic agents

- enhancement of known effects, e.g. whereby non-steroidal anti-inflammatory drugs that selectively inhibit cyclo-oxygenase-2 (COX-2 inhibitors) reduce the occurrence of colorectal cancers, or retinoids have antiproliferative and prodifferentiation actions in many cancers
- complementary and alternative therapies, e.g. nutritional, vitamin and herbal remedies (see Clinical Interest Box 49-3).

Clinical aspects
Cure and remission

In the context of cancer, the term 'cure' is used rather differently from the way it is understood in acute conditions that can be totally eradicated. Cancer cure may be defined as the disappearance of any evidence of tumour for several years, with a high probability of a normal lifespan. This definition, referring as it does to a statistical probability, implies the difficulty of complete certainty of removing every malignant cell and recognises the possibility of recurrence of cancer cell proliferation.

Patients are said to go into remission if the tumour and signs and symptoms of its presence are no longer detectable, whereas if the patient relapses, the tumour and/or its signs and symptoms are again detectable. Hence there may be remission after a course of chemotherapy, then a relapse some months or years later, and further remission after another course of therapy (see again Figure 48-4).

Tumours with a high growth fraction are most responsive to chemotherapy, as most of their cells are undergoing active cycling and can therefore be targeted by drugs that impair macromolecular synthesis or cell division. Examples are choriocarcinoma, a malignant tumour of fetal origin that is usually sensitive to methotrexate or dactinomycin, and Burkitt's lymphoma, usually sensitive to cyclophosphamide. Other tumours, including large solid tumours of internal organs such as lung, kidney and colon, may be more difficult to treat, although antineoplastic drugs may prolong and improve the quality of life.

Treatment regimens

Treatment regimens are often complicated, with patients being administered 2–4 cytotoxic agents on various days for 2 weeks, followed by a drug-free period (to allow white cells to recover), then another course of therapy, possibly with surgery and/or radiation therapy (see Clinical Interest Box 48-3). Drugs may also be given to treat adverse effects, and fluids administered to rehydrate the patient and 'flush out' the kidneys, where cytotoxic agents may concentrate.

As cancer treatment is a highly specialised and rapidly advancing area of medicine, patients are usually treated in a specialised oncology (cancer) unit or clinic, attached to a major hospital. Patients are often enrolled in clinical trials,

---

CLINICAL INTEREST BOX 48-4
WHAT PATIENTS WANT TO KNOW

The information patients want or need to have about any prescribed drug can be summed up in three questions. In the context of antineoplastic agents, the following sample answers help provide information and counselling.

1. What is it for?
   - Anticancer drugs are aimed at slowing or stopping the growth and spread of tumours.
   - Some anticancer drugs can cure the disease, others may control or slow symptoms, or help you feel better.
   - Antihormones are drugs used to slow the growth of tumours of the reproductive system, e.g. prostate or breast.
   - Some additional medicines may be given to control side-effects of anticancer drugs, e.g. antiemetics to prevent vomiting.

2. What will it do to me?
   - The drugs will slow down or stop the growth of the tumour, and help relieve the symptoms you're feeling.
   - Some side-effects may occur, such as allergies and rashes, infections, vomiting, sore mouth or throat, bleeding, hair loss, or temporary or permanent sterility.
   - Discuss these issues with your doctor, as there are medicines, procedures and people to help deal with them.

3. How do I take it?
   - Usually these drugs are injected while you are in the hospital or clinic; some are taken by mouth.
   - Often there are complicated 'courses' of treatment, with several drugs taken over weeks or months.
   - If you take them at home, it is important that the drugs be taken exactly as prescribed by your doctor.
   - Avoid going out into the sun without sunscreen and protective clothing.
   - Avoid use of aspirin or similar drugs, or over-the-counter or complementary medicines, unless your doctor has approved them.
   - You may be asked to come into the clinic for regular blood tests to check how your condition is progressing.
   - (if relevant) Use effective contraception and/or avoid breastfeeding while taking these drugs.

---

as new drugs are continually being developed, and can only be trialled in patients with the specific condition. Multicentre trials are usually coordinated from one large cancer institute but with investigators, physicians and patients in many centres around the world. This increases the number of patients enrolling in trials and, it is hoped, shortens the time taken for results (safety and efficacy of the new treatment) to become apparent. For some cancers (hepatoma, renal cell carcinoma) there are no definitive optimal therapies, and patients are given adjuvant therapy and enrolled in clinical trials of new agents as appropriate.

Treatment should always be individualised to the patient, with careful monitoring of efficacy and toxicity of therapies administered. The aims of the treatment (curative or palliative) need to be discussed with the patient (see Clinical Interest Box 48-4), and adjuvant therapies added as required (e.g. analgesics, laxatives, antimicrobials, antianxiety agents and sedatives).

COMBINATION CHEMOTHERAPY

In the late 1960s, **combination chemotherapy**, the use of two or more anticancer drugs at the same time, was initiated for treating acute lymphoblastic leukaemia and Hodgkin's disease. When the complete response rates for single agents were compared with those for combination drugs, it was evident that drugs can have synergistic therapeutic effects, with less development of resistance and lower toxicities. Oncologists therefore often use combination therapy in antineoplastic treatment. Table 48-2 lists some commonly prescribed drug combinations.

The response rates for the treatment of advanced Hodgkin's disease with mustine, Oncovin (vincristine), procarbazine and prednisone (MOPP) are a classic illustration:

Drug	Complete response rates
M (mustine)	20%
O (Oncovin [vincristine])	<10%
P (procarbazine)	<10%
P (prednisone)	<5%
MOPP combination	80%

The following principles are used to select the drugs for combination chemotherapy:

- each drug when used alone should be active against the specific cancer
- each drug should have a different mechanism of action
- the regimen should contain cell-cycle-phase-specific and cell-cycle-non-specific agents
- each drug should have a different organ toxicity or, if the toxic effect is similar, it should occur at different times after drug administration.

When these principles are applied to MOPP drug therapy, the concept of combination chemotherapy can be understood. First, the list illustrates the effectiveness of each drug against Hodgkin's disease. Second, the sites of major activity for each antineoplastic agent are believed to be different, and both cell-cycle-specific and cell-cycle-non-specific agents are included.

Mustine is an alkylating agent that can interfere with the replication, transcription and translation of DNA. Vincristine inhibits mitosis by interfering with the mitotic spindle. Procarbazine inhibits the synthesis of DNA, RNA and protein and also interferes with mitosis; its antineoplastic action is believed to occur during the S-phase (it is also a weak monoamine oxidase inhibitor and central nervous system depressant). Prednisone has lympholytic properties and so is useful in white-cell tumours, and may produce an antifibrotic effect that would be useful in treating cancer metastases surrounded by fibrous materials. It also improves appetite and general feelings of wellbeing.

The fourth principle, that of different organ toxicity or toxicities that occur at different times, has also been substantiated for the MOPP combination. The dose-limiting toxicity of bone marrow suppression is a property of both mustine and procarbazine, but the nadir, or the lowest depression point for this effect, occurs about 10 days after drug administration for mustine and 21 days after for procarbazine. The additive myelosuppressant effects from this combination are thus essentially avoided. Also, vincristine does not have bone marrow-suppressing effects but does exhibit a dose-limiting neurotoxicity. Prednisone does not demonstrate bone marrow suppression or neurotoxicity.

Adverse drug reactions

Most of the currently available antineoplastic agents appear

TABLE 48–2: Examples of combination chemotherapeutic regimens

CANCER	ACRONYM	DRUGS
Breast*	CMF(P)	Cyclophosphamide–methotrexate–fluorouracil (+/– prednisolone)
	CFPT	Cyclophosphamide–5-fluorouracil–prednisone–tamoxifen
Colon	FL	5-fluorouracil–Leucovorin (folinic acid)
Lung	CAV	Cyclophosphamide–adriamycin (doxorubicin)–vincristine
	CE	Cyclophosphamide–etoposide
Stomach	ELF	Etoposide–Leucovorin–5-fluorouracil

*Note: Chemotherapy of breast cancer is complicated, and choice of drug(s) depends on whether the woman is pre- or postmenopausal, whether or not there is lymph node involvement, what histological cell type is involved, whether the tumour tests positive or negative for oestrogen receptors and progesterone receptors, whether the woman has undergone mastectomy or lumpectomy, and whether there are any cardiovascular risk factors.

to act on similar metabolic pathways in both normal and malignant cells. This lack of tumour-cell specificity is a major limitation of cancer drugs. Because the target of most cytotoxic drugs is cell proliferation, it follows that normal tissues in the body are also vulnerable when their cells are proliferating. The most rapidly dividing cells in the body, which are in the bone marrow, hair follicles and gastrointestinal tract, are therefore generally most adversely affected by anticancer drugs.

Drug toxicities or adverse reactions may be divided into adverse reactions common to antineoplastic agents generally, and dose-limiting effects specific to particular drugs. A dose-limiting effect is a response to a drug that indicates that the maximum tolerable dose has been reached and that the drug dose should be decreased or discontinued.

The commonest adverse effects are alopecia (hair loss), gastrointestinal distress (nausea, vomiting, anorexia, diarrhoea), and mucositis and stomatitis (inflammation of the mucous membranes of the gastrointestinal tract and mouth). The nausea and vomiting can be so severe as to become dangerous and discourage the patient from continuing with chemotherapy (see Table 48-3); potent antiemetic drugs may be required for relief. Other general adverse effects include fever, extravasation (dispersal of IV solution out of vessels into the tissues, with subsequent necrosis reactions), delayed healing, and hyperuricaemia (from breakdown products of damaged cells; see under tumour lysis syndrome, below).

Bone marrow suppression (myelosuppression) is the major dose-limiting adverse reaction most often encountered in cancer chemotherapy: suppression of white cells (leucopenia) or of platelets (thrombocytopenia) can lead to serious and even life-threatening infections and haemorrhage, respectively. For this reason, cytotoxic agents are usually dosed to the limit of tolerance, with subsequent drug-free periods to allow recovery of white cell functions.

Long-term toxicities that need to be considered and monitored follow from cytotoxic agents impairing various stages in cell division and proliferation; they may thus cause infertility or may possibly be mutagenic, carcinogenic or teratogenic. Patients need to be warned of these potential dangers, as do health professionals handling the drugs or patients' excreta, as the agents may be absorbed through the skin (see Clinical Interest Box 48-5).

Specific dose-limiting effects are adverse reactions that should indicate to the prescriber that the maximum tolerated dose has been delivered and that the drug needs to be discontinued or reduced. Fortunately, this occurs only with certain drugs. Drugs that can produce hepatotoxicity include methotrexate, mercaptopurine, lomustine and carmustine (CCNU, BCNU), dacarbazine (DTIC) (see Table 48-3 for definitions) and doxorubicin (adriamycin).

Renal problems can occur from the high levels of these toxic agents that can accumulate in the kidney and renal tubules during drug excretion. Because dehydration increases the risks, adequate fluid intake is important when these

agents are administered. Haemorrhagic cystitis is associated with cyclophosphamide, and renal tubular necrosis with methotrexate, cisplatin and related drugs.

Cardiac toxicity is reported with both doxorubicin and daunorubicin. Cardiotoxicity increases in patients who receive more than 550 mg/m² body surface (total accumulated dosage given throughout therapy). Toxicity is also greater in elderly patients and in children under 2 years. As this effect is cumulative if either drug is given, the amount of one drug already received by the person must be considered when planning therapy with the other drug.

Neurological toxicity may range from tingling of the hands and feet and loss of deep tendon reflexes to ataxia, footdrop, confusion and personality changes. Drugs reported to produce neurological effects include vincristine and the other vinca alkaloids and methotrexate. Ototoxicity and peripheral neuropathy have been reported with cisplatin and related compounds.

Tumour lysis syndrome refers to the massive release of breakdown products from tumour cells killed by chemotherapeutic agents; it occurs most commonly in leukaemias and lymphomas. In particular, urate may

---

CLINICAL INTEREST BOX 48-5
SAFE HANDLING OF CYTOTOXIC AGENTS

Cytotoxic agents are inherently toxic and, if lipid-soluble, may be readily absorbed through the skin of people handling the drugs or coming into contact with the excreta and vomitus of patients who have been administered such agents. Consequently, **safe handling** guidelines have been developed to protect pharmacists, doctors and nurses and also patients' families and carers. Suggested precautions include:

• Drugs are prepared and dispensed in a cytotoxic drug safety cabinet, a dedicated laminar flow cabinet with the air filtered before being vented to the atmosphere.
• Staff handling the drugs use protective clothing and equipment, including masks and gloves; techniques must be developed to avoid inhaling droplets or powders or spilling solutions.
• Excess drug, and waste secretions and contaminated equipment, are disposed of by high-temperature incineration.
• The health of staff is monitored by means of blood tests and tests for liver and kidney functions.
• Labelling of equipment and solutions, and containment and transport of drugs after dispensing, must be carefully controlled.
• After administration of the cytotoxic agents, the patient's body fluids are treated as if mutagenic.
• Guidelines must be followed for dealing with spillages and care of contaminated staff and facilities.

Adapted from: the Peter MacCallum Cancer Institute 1999.

accumulate and precipitate in the renal distal tubules; to prevent this occurring, the urine may be alkalinised and/or hydration increased and allopurinol administered prophylactically. Hyperkalaemia, hyperphosphataemia and hypocalcaemia also occur.

Treatment of adverse drug reactions

Most adverse effects are treated symptomatically, e.g. infections with appropriate antimicrobial agents, mouth ulcers with mouth washes and zinc solutions, and fever with antipyretic analgesics. Many patients find the loss of hair most distressing; this can be helped with sensitive encouragement and use of hairpieces, wigs and scarves; usually the hair regrows after cessation of cytotoxic chemotherapy. More specific treatments of adverse drug reactions are discussed in Chapter 49.

TABLE 48-3 Emetic potentials of selected chemotherapeutic agents

High emetic potential	Cisplatin, cyclophosphamide (IV), dacarbazine (DTIC), dactinomycin, nitrogen mustards, nitrosoureas (BCNU, CCNU), streptozotocin
Intermediate emetic potential	Carboplatin, cyclophosphamide (oral), daunorubicin, doxorubicin, etoposide, gemcitabine, ifosfamide, irinotecan, methotrexate (>250 mg/m²), mitomycin, teniposide, topotecan
Low emetic potential	Busulfan, chlorambucil, fluorouracil, 6-mercaptopurine, methotrexate (<250 mg/m²), bleomycin, taxanes, vinblastine, vincristine

Adapted from: Peter MacCallum Cancer Institute Melbourne 2000; AMH 2006.
BCNU = 1,3-bis-(2-chloroethyl)-1-nitrosurea;
CCNU = N-(2-chloroethyl)-N'-cyclohexyl-N-nitrosurea;
DTIC = dimethyltriazenyl imidazole carboxamide.
Note that emetic potential may depend on doses administered.

Development of drug resistance

Just as microorganisms can develop resistance to antimicrobial drugs (see Figure 50-1 and related text) and pass the genes for drug resistance to other organisms, leading, for example, to the spread of multi-resistant strains of *Staphylococcus aureus*, so neoplastic cells can develop resistance to anticancer drugs and pass this acquired characteristic on to daughter cells. The cancer then becomes resistant to specific drugs. Some of the mechanisms by which cells develop resistance are:

- defective activation of a drug, e.g. cyclophosphamide and methotrexate are prodrugs, normally activated in cells to the active anticancer form

- enhanced inactivation of a drug, e.g. highly reactive compounds may be 'scavenged' by cell-protective mechanisms
- decreased accumulation of a drug, either by decreased uptake into cells or increased removal of drug from cells
- altered DNA repair, e.g. repair mechanisms may be enhanced such that DNA damaged by cytotoxic agents is partly repaired
- increased synthesis of precursor molecules, e.g. of purine or pyrimidine bases to circumvent the incorporation of antimetabolites into DNA
- altered or decreased level of target molecule, e.g. an enzyme form less sensitive to a drug, or an alternative bio-chemical pathway less dependent on an inhibited enzyme
- gene amplification, e.g. increased production of an enzyme targeted by a drug.

As with antimicrobial drug therapy, minimising anticancer drug usage will help to minimize development of drug resistance. Methods include use of the most specific drugs available to target the particular neoplastic cell, use of chemotherapeutic agents in rotation or cyclic patterns, and use of combinations of drugs acting at different stages of the cell cycle.

Age-related considerations
CANCER IN CHILDREN

Cancer in children is relatively uncommon, with fewer than 1% of new cancers occurring in children under 15 years (in Victoria, Australia).* The commonest cancers occurring in children under 15 in Victoria are leukaemias and lymphomas, then brain and central nervous system cancers. Carcinomas (malignant tumours of epithelial tissues such as breast, gastrointestinal tract, lung and skin), which are common in adults, are rare in children, while sarcomas (malignant tumours of connective tissues such as bone and muscle) are more common in children than adults. Because tumours in children grow rapidly, childhood cancer is generally more responsive to chemotherapy than is cancer in an adult. Children also tend to tolerate the acute adverse effects of chemotherapy better than adults. Of all children with cancer, 50% become long-term survivors or are actually cured.

CANCER IN THOSE OF REPRODUCTIVE AGE

Antineoplastic agents may have deleterious effects on reproduction, at different stages of life; factors to be considered carefully are as follows:

*For comparison: In Victoria in 2004, there were 180 postnatal deaths in children aged 0–14 years; the commonest causes of death were birth-related causes (41%), then unintentional injury (i.e. accidents, 16%), and malignancies (16%). Of the latter, approximately one-third were leukaemias/lymphomas and one-third CNS malignancies. (Consultative Council on Obstetric and Paediatric Mortality and Morbidity 2005).

- Children treated with cytotoxic agents, especially alkylating agents, may show infertility in later years.
- Alkylating agents administered to adults may cause lowered sperm count in men, and infertility due to ovarian failure in women.
- Other cyctotoxics, anti-oestrogens or radiation to the pelvis may also cause female infertility.
- Most cytotoxic agents are mutagenic and potentially teratogenic, and should not be taken during pregnancy; effective contraception should be practised if either partner is being administered antineoplastic agents.
- Most drugs can be secreted into breast milk, and antineoplastic agents are likely to be toxic to a baby; breastfeeding should be avoided unless indicated safe by the oncologist.

CANCER IN THE ELDERLY

Cancer in the elderly is a serious disease and its incidence increases sharply with age, with about 69% of new cancers occurring in people aged 60 and over. The elderly have more concurrent illnesses and less efficient homeostatic mechanisms than younger cancer victims, which may decrease their ability to withstand the effects of cancer or of antineoplastic therapies. Other factors to be considered when managing regimens for elderly persons are the possibility of impaired liver or kidney functions, concurrent administration of many other drugs (polypharmacy), reduced independence and income, and loss of friends and family support.

Often, compromises in treatment are made because of a person's advanced age; however, data suggest that a dosage reduction of chemotherapy based on age alone is not always appropriate and that the efficacy of chemotherapy is not age-dependent. A treatment approach should be based on the individual cancer and the physiological parameters noted in the elderly person. Because new drugs are usually not tested in elderly persons, more clinical trials are needed to examine the relation between cancer chemotherapy responsiveness and the person's age.

KEY POINTS

- Tumours are a common cause of morbidity and mortality in the community. Cells in malignant tumours are usually rapidly dividing, dedifferentiated, and have the ability to invade and metastasise.
- Research in tumour cell biology is elucidating the detailed biochemical pathways involved in cell cycling, regulation of cycling, checkpoints, stimulators and inhibitors of cell growth, tumour-suppressor genes, synthesis of macromolecules, duplication of genetic material, and apoptosis.
- In the development of cancers, normal cells may be transformed to neoplastic cells by viruses, carcinogenic chemicals, genetic influences, radiation, or oncogenes and their products. Small tumours and those undergoing rapid cycling are most responsive to treatment.
- The main modalities for cancer treatment are surgery, radiation and chemotherapy. In many cases, cure or remission is possible; however, cancers may relapse.
- Chemicals targeting specific enzymes, proteins, receptors, genes and cytokines in these pathways may prove useful as new anticancer drugs.
- The cytotoxic agents used in chemotherapy generally have antiproliferative effects by impairing macromolecular synthesis (antimetabolites, alkylating agents, antitumour antibiotics) or by disrupting mitosis (vinca alkaloids, taxanes).
- Tumours that depend on hormones for growth may be treated with antihormones or by suppressing secretion of the trophic hormone.
- Chemotherapeutic regimens usually combine cytotoxic agents acting by different mechanisms at different phases of the cell cycle, with different specific adverse effects; this minimises toxicity and the development of drug resistance.
- Typical 'chemo' regimens involve several courses of therapy, with drug-free weeks to allow bone marrow recovery.
- Adverse drug reactions common to cytotoxic agents include damage to other rapidly dividing cells (bone marrow, hair, skin, gastrointestinal mucosa), severe nausea and vomiting, kidney tubule damage and hyperuricaemia. Treatment of these adverse effects involves use of specific drugs and hydration with IV fluids.
- Long-term adverse effects include the risks of mutagenic, carcinogenic and teratogenic actions (hence the importance of safe handling of cytotoxic agents) and the development of drug resistance.

REVIEW EXERCISES

1 Explain the concept of cell cycling, its importance in tumour cell biology and the actions of antineoplastic agents.
2 Describe the pattern of growth of cancers. About how many cancer cells are present before clinical symptoms first appear?

3 Describe three considerations used to select drugs for combination antineoplastic chemotherapy. Discuss the MOPP treatment for advanced Hodgkin's disease and how it meets the principles for combination chemotherapy.

4 Discuss the adverse effects common to cytotoxic agents.

5 Set up a class 'consultation' in which you counsel a patient who has just been told s/he will need cancer chemotherapy.

REFERENCES AND FURTHER READING

Anonymous. A glossary of medical genetics. *Australian Prescriber* 1998; 21(3): 69–71.

Australian Institute of Health and Welfare (AIHW) & Australasian Association of Cancer Registries (ACCR). Cancer in Australia 2001. AIHW cat. No. CAN 23. Canberra: AIHW (Cancer Series No. 28), 2004. Available: www.aihw.gov.au/publications/index.cfm/title/10083, accessed 13 September 2006.

Australian Medicines Handbook 2006. AMH, 2006.

Beare PG, Myers JL. *Adult Health Nursing.* 3rd edn. St Louis: Mosby, 1998.

Bowman WC, Rand MJ. *Textbook of Pharmacology.* 2nd edn. Oxford: Blackwell, 1980 [ch. 3].

Buolamwini JK. Novel anticancer drug discovery. *Chemical Biology* 1999; 3(4): 500–9.

Caswell A (ed.). *MIMS Annual June 2005.* Sydney: CMPMedica Australia, 2005.

Cavalli F, Hansen HH, Kaye SB (eds). *Textbook of Medical Oncology.* 3rd edn. London: Taylor & Francis, 2004.

Consultative Council on Obstetric and Paediatric Mortality and Morbidity. *Annual Report for the Year 2004.* Melbourne: Victorian Department of Human Services, 2005.

Evan GI, Vousden KH. Proliferation, cell cycle and apoptosis in cancer. *Nature* 2001; 411: 342–8.

Favoni RE, de Cupis A. The role of polypeptide growth factors in human carcinomas: new targets for a novel pharmacological approach. *Pharmacological Reviews* 2000; 52(2): 179–206.

Flatt PM, Pietenpol JA. Mechanisms of cell-cycle checkpoints: at the crossroads of carcinogenesis and drug discovery. *Drug Metabolism Reviews* 2000; 32(3&4): 283–305.

Gibbs JB. Mechanism-based target identification and drug discovery in cancer research. *Science* 2000; 287: 1969–73.

Kelland LR. Telomerase inhibitors: targeting the vulnerable end of cancer? *Anti-Cancer Drugs* 2000; 11(7): 503–13.

Le Fanu J. *The Rise and Fall of Modern Medicine.* London: Little, Brown, 1999.

Lichtman SM, Skirvin JA. Pharmacology of antineoplastic agents in older cancer patients. *Oncology (Huntington)* 2000; 14(12): 1743–55.

Lodish H, Berk A, Zipursky SL, Matsudaira P et al. *Molecular Cell Biology.* 4th edn. New York: Freeman, 2000.

Olver I. Chemotherapy for elderly patients with advanced cancer: is it worth it? *Australian Prescriber* 2000; 23(4): 80–2.

Palliative Care Expert Group. *Therapeutic Guidelines: Palliative Care, version 2.* Melbourne: Therapeutic Guidelines, 2005.

Pawlik TM, Keyomarsi K. Role of cell cycle in mediating sensitivity to radiotherapy. *International Journal of Radiation Oncology, Biology, Physics* (2004); 59(4): 928–42.

Peter MacCallum Cancer Institute. *Guidelines for the Safe Handling of Cytotoxic Agents.* 5th edn. Melbourne: Peter MacCallum Cancer Institute, 1999.

Peter MacCallum Cancer Institute, 2000. *Standard Treatment Guidelines, January 2000.* Melbourne: Medical Oncology Unit.

Peto J. Cancer epidemiology in the last century and the next decade. *Nature* 2001; 411: 390–5.

Rang HP, Dale MM, Ritter JM, Moore PK. *Pharmacology.* 5th edn. Edinburgh: Churchill Livingstone, 2003 [chs 5, 50].

Rowinsky EK. The pursuit of optimal outcomes in cancer therapy in a new age of rationally designed target-based anticancer agents. *Drugs* 2000: 60(Suppl1): 1–14.

Senderowicz AM. Targeting cell cycle and apoptosis for the treatment of human malignancies. *Current Opinion in Cell Biology* 2004; 16(6): 670–8.

Seymour L. Novel anti-cancer agents in development: exciting prospects and new challenges. *Cancer Treatment Reviews* 1999; 25(5): 301–12.

Souhami R, Tobias J. *Cancer and its Management,* 5th edn. Malden, MA: Blackwell, 2005.

Smith AD (ed.). *Oxford Dictionary of Biochemistry and Molecular Biology.* Revised edn. Oxford: Oxford University Press, 1997.

Staples M, Marks R, Giles G. Trends in the incidence of non-melanocytic skin cancer (NMSC) treated in Australia 1985–1995: are primary prevention programs starting to have an effect? *International Journal of Cancer* 1998; 78: 144–8.

Stern M, Herrmann R. Overview of monoclonal antibodies in cancer therapy: present and promise. *Critical Reviews in Oncology/Hematology* 2005; 54(1): 11–29.

Stewart ZA, Westfall MD, Pietenpol JA . Cell-cycle dysregulation and anticancer therapy. *Trends in Pharmacological Sciences* 2003; 24(3): 139–45.

Tuckwell K (ed.). *MIMS Disease Index.* 2nd edn. Sydney: MediMedia Australia, 1996.

Vinorelbine Italian Study Group. Effects of vinorelbine on quality of life and survival of elderly patients with advanced non-small-cell lung cancer. *Journal of the National Cancer Institute* 1999; 91(1): 66–72.

Youngson RM. *Collins Dictionary: Medicine.* 2nd edn. Glasgow: HarperCollins, 1998.

Zalatnai A. Potential role of cell cycle synchronizing agents in combination treatment modalities of malignant tumours. *In Vivo* 2005; 19(1): 85–91.

Zock PL. Dietary fats and cancer. *Current Opinion in Lipidology* 2001; 12(1): 5–10.

evolve More weblinks at http://evolve.elsevier.com/AU/Bryant/pharmacology/

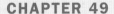

CHAPTER 49

Antineoplastic Agents

CHAPTER FOCUS

Cancer is a leading cause of death in developed countries. Solid tumours are generally treated with surgery and/or radiation, while disseminated cancers and some localised cancers are treated with antineoplastic agents, often as adjunctive therapy after surgery and irradiation. Antineoplastic drugs (in particular the cytotoxic agents) have many significant adverse effects, and many new antineoplastic agents are released annually, so health-care professionals should be well informed on the pharmacology, toxicity and clinical use of these drugs.

As oncology is a highly specialised area of medicine, antineoplastic drugs are usually administered only in specialist cancer hospitals or oncology units of major hospitals. Many new antineoplastic agents are available only under special access schemes or on a clinical trial basis. Consequently, we deal with the anticancer drugs in rather less detail than for other areas of pharmacology where the drugs are more widely available or used. To keep this area of pharmacology in perspective, it should be remembered that overall cancer survival, following all kinds of treatment, is approximately 63%. While many leukaemias

and childhood cancers have high cure rates, the contribution of chemotherapy to adult survival from cancer is considerably less than that of surgery or radiation.

OBJECTIVES

- To describe the mechanisms of action and clinical uses of the cytotoxic agents (alkylating agents, antimetabolites, antibiotic antitumour agents and mitotic inhibitors) and other miscellaneous antineoplastic agents.

- To discuss the use of hormones, antihormones and inhibitors of hormone synthesis and release in the treatment of cancer.

- To review the common adverse effects and dose-limiting adverse reactions of antineoplastic agents, and describe how they are treated.

- To describe the use of supportive adjunctive therapy, including palliative care, immunostimulatory agents, and drugs used to protect bone, kidneys and blood cells during cancer therapy.

KEY DRUGS

calcium folinate
cisplatin
colaspase
cyclophosphamide
doxorubicin
fluorouracil
flutamide
goserelin
mercaptopurine
methotrexate
tamoxifen
vincristine

KEY TERMS

alkylating agents
antibiotic antitumour agents
antimetabolites
antioestrogens
breakthrough pain
cytotoxic agent
immunostimulatory agents
mitotic inhibitors
palliative care

KEY ABBREVIATIONS

BCG	Bacille Calmette–Guérin, or the *Mycobacterium bovis* bacillus
ER	(o)estrogen receptor
FU	(5-)fluorouracil
G-CSF	granulocyte colony-stimulating factor
GnRH	gonadotrophin-releasing hormone
MTX	methotrexate

ANTINEOPLASTIC agents, i.e. drugs that are used to treat neoplasia, include cytotoxic drugs, hormones and antihormones, and various other agents that impair tumour growth by miscellaneous mechanisms. The general mechanisms by which these drugs affect neoplastic cells, particularly their actions in the cell cycle and on macromolecular synthesis, are discussed in Chapter 48; in this chapter, the drug groups and their clinical uses are described in more detail and drugs used as supportive or adjunctive therapies are also considered. This is a rapidly changing area of pharmacology, with new drugs and treatment regimens being introduced continually; individual drug information and treatment protocols from specialist oncology units should be consulted for the latest information on indications, doses, administration techniques, combination regimens, adverse drug reactions, precautions and contraindications.

CYTOTOXIC AGENTS

Cytotoxic agents do not directly kill tumour cells: they act by interfering with cell proliferation or replication. The cytotoxic agents are divided into various classes based on their probable major mechanisms of action (see Table 49-1 for classifications, indications and major adverse effects); many drugs act by more than one mechanism, and for some drugs the precise mechanisms have not yet been clarified.

Alkylating agents

Alkylating agents are often used for anticancer chemotherapy and were the first class of drugs applied clinically in the modern era of antineoplastic drug therapy (see Clinical Interest Box 49-1).

Mechanisms and groups

These drugs contain alkyl groups (e.g. methyl, ethyl) and form highly reactive chemical structures that react rapidly with an electron donor group, such as a nitrogen atom in a guanine base of DNA, forming strong bonds as the alkyl group is 'donated' (see Figure 49-1). Because the alkylating agents usually are bifunctional, i.e. have two active 'arms', they can link across or along the strands of DNA chains, effectively tying the double helix together—like a zipper that has become stuck by having thread caught in it and cannot be unzipped. This interferes with the unwinding of the DNA strands in the processes of transcription to RNA and replication of DNA. Thus the cell cycle (Figure 48-1) is blocked mainly at the S phase, before the G_2 phase, and cell proliferation is slowed or stopped. Some alkylating agents are considered cell-cycle-specific, others are cell-cycle-non-specific.

Various types of alkylating agents are available, such as the nitrogen mustards (including chlorambucil,

cyclophosphamide [Drug Monograph 49-1 and Figure 49-1], melphalan and ifosfamide) and nitrosoureas (carmustine, fotemustine and lomustine). Nitrosoureas are highly lipophilic alkylating agents that readily cross the blood–brain barrier and are thus useful for treating primary brain tumours. Other alkylating agents include busulfan, dacarbazine (and its orally active analogue temozolomide) and thiotepa.

CLINICAL INTEREST BOX 49-1 HISTORY OF ANTINEOPLASTIC CHEMOTHERAPY

While natural products have been used for thousands of years in medicine, the era of scientific anticancer chemotherapy can perhaps be dated to 1865, when a patient with leukaemia was administered potassium arsenite solution, with some positive results.

A group of chemical warfare agents developed as blistering agents and used during World War I included the sulphur mustards, such as 'mustard gas', known as Kampfstoff. Related compounds, the nitrogen mustards, were also synthesised and studied during later military campaigns, and antidotes were developed, but neither side dared to use them during WWII because of their toxicity.

After WWII, a clinical trial was published by Goodman, Gilman and colleagues with results of the effective use of nitrogen mustards in cancer chemotherapy against lymphomas. Patients were treated cautiously with these agents, and with considerable success. These are powerful **alkylating agents** and resulted in 'spin-offs' of effective anticancer drugs such as lomustine and **cyclophosphamide**.

The next lines of research were into agents that impair the co-factor functions of folic acid, used in the formation of new blood cells; the analogue aminopterin was shown in the 1940s to cause striking remissions in childhood leukaemia. This led to the development of **methotrexate**, still an important anticancer drug (see Drug Monograph 49-2).

Another approach was to study the pathways whereby nucleic acids are synthesised. This led to the purine and pyrimidine analogues, such as **6-mercaptopurine** and **5-fluorouracil**, thought to act by being incorporated into false nucleotides or by inhibiting enzymes in the pathways.

Along the way, some natural compounds from plants and fungi have been found with useful anticancer actions (see Clinical Interest Box 49-2). More recent research is targeting growth factors and their receptors; oncogenes and their product proteins; regulatory processes in cell biology, including signal transduction, apoptosis, cell cycle checkpoints and tumour-suppressor genes; and pharmaceutical and pharmacokinetic techniques to deliver agents directly to tumour cells or activate them there.

TABLE 49-1 Cytotoxic drugs

DRUG	PRIMARY INDICATIONS	MAJOR TOXICITIES*
Alkylating agents *Nitrogen mustards*		
Chlorambucil	CLL, Hodgkin's and non-Hodgkin's lymphomas	Bone marrow suppression
Cyclophosphamide	(See Drug Monograph 49-1)	Bone marrow suppression, haemorrhagic cystitis
Ifosfamide	Testicular tumours, sarcomas, lymphomas	Bone marrow suppression, nausea, vomiting, encephalopathy
Melphalan	Multiple myeloma, malignant melanoma	Bone marrow suppression, allergic reactions
Fotemustine	Melanoma	Bone marrow suppression, reversible neurotoxicity
Nitrosoureas		
Carmustine	Primary brain tumours, multiple myeloma	Bone marrow suppression, lung fibrosis, nephrotoxicity
Lomustine	Glioma, Hodgkin's lymphoma	Bone marrow suppression, anorexia, nausea, vomiting
Other		
Busulfan	CML	Bone marrow suppression, hyperpigmentation, gynaecomastia
Dacarbazine, procarbazine	Melanoma, sarcomas, glioma, lymphomas	Bone marrow suppression, GIT disorders
Oxaliplatin	Colorectal	Neurotoxicity, vomiting, diarrhoea, anaemia
Temozolamide	Gliomas, melanoma	Bone marrow suppression, neurological disorders
Thiotepa	Bladder cancers, lymphomas, malignant effusions	Bone marrow suppression
Antimetabolites		
Capecitabine	Breast, colorectal	GIT, skin disorders
Cladribine	Leukaemias	Bone marrow suppression, fever
Cytarabine	AML, ALL, lymphomas	Bone marrow suppression, anorexia, oral and GI ulceration
Fluorouracil	Solid tumours, GIT, breast, pancreas	Diarrhoea, stomatitis, bone marrow suppression
Fludarabine	CLL	Bone marrow suppression, fever, chills, nausea, vomiting, infection
Gemcitabine	Pancreas, lung, bladder	Bone marrow suppression, oedema
Mercaptopurine	ALL, AML, CML	Bone marrow suppression, cholestasis
Methotrexate	(See Drug Monograph 49-2)	Bone marrow suppression, diarrhoea, stomatitis, liver and lung toxicity
Permetrexed	Some lung cancers	Bone marrow suppression, skin rashes
Raltitrexed	Colorectal	Fever, GIT disorders, flu-like symptoms
Thioguanine	AML, CML	Bone marrow suppression

TABLE 49-1 Cytotoxic drugs—cont'd

DRUG	PRIMARY INDICATIONS	MAJOR TOXICITIES*
Antibiotics		
Bleomycin	Squamous cell carcinoma, lymphomas, testicular cancer	Chills, fever, pneumonitis, mucositis, lung fibrosis, skin reactions
Dactinomycin	Wilms' tumour, Ewing's sarcoma, choriocarcinoma, rhabdomyosarcoma	Bone marrow suppression
Daunorubicin	HIV–Kaposi's sarcoma, leukaemias	Bone marrow suppression, cardiomyopathy, severe mucositis, hair loss
Doxorubicin	Sarcomas, breast, endometrium, carcinoid	(as for daunorubicin)
Epirubicin	Breast, sarcomas	Bone marrow suppression, GIT, skin disorders
Idarubicin	AML, ALL, breast cancer	Severe bone marrow suppression, infection, alopecia, nausea, vomiting, mucositis
Mitomycin	Disseminated adenocarcinoma of pancreas or stomach; palliation	Bone marrow suppression
Mitozantrone	Breast, lymphoma, leukaemias	Cardiotoxicity, severe myelosuppression
Mitotic inhibitors		
Docetaxel, paclitaxel	Ovary, breast, lung	Bone marrow suppression, cardiovascular, GIT, neurological disorders
Vinblastine	Bladder, testis, Kaposi's sarcoma, lymphomas	Gastrointestinal bleeding, respiratory and CNS disorders
Vincristine	Wide range of solid and haematological malignancies	Mild to severe paraesthesias, jaw pain, ataxia, muscle wasting, constipation
Vinorelbine	Non small cell lung cancer, breast	Bone marrow suppression, nausea, vomiting, asthenia
Topoisomerase I inhibitors		
Irinotecan	Colorectal	Bone marrow suppression, diarrhoea, respiratory disorders
Topotecan	Ovary, lung	(As for irinotecan)
Topoisomerase II inhibitors		
Etoposide	Refractory testicular tumours, small-cell lung cancer, leukaemias, lymphomas	Bone marrow suppression, alopecia, GIT disorders
Teniposide	ALL, lymphomas, glioma, bladder	Bone marrow suppression, mucositis, alopecia
Other cytotoxic agents		
Carboplatin	Head and neck carcinomas, lung, nasopharynx	Bone marrow suppression, nausea, vomiting, neurotoxicity, neuropathies, ototoxicity
Cisplatin	Head and neck, cervix, lung, bladder, germ cells	Nephrotoxicity, severe nausea and vomiting, bone marrow suppression, electrolyte disturbances

ALL = acute lymphoblastic leukaemia; AML = acute myelogenous leukaemia; CLL = chronic lymphocytic leukaemia;
CML = chronic myelocytic leukaemia; GIT = gastrointestinal tract.
*Note that most cytotoxic agents can cause nausea and vomiting, gastrointestinal tract and reproductive disturbances, and alopecia.

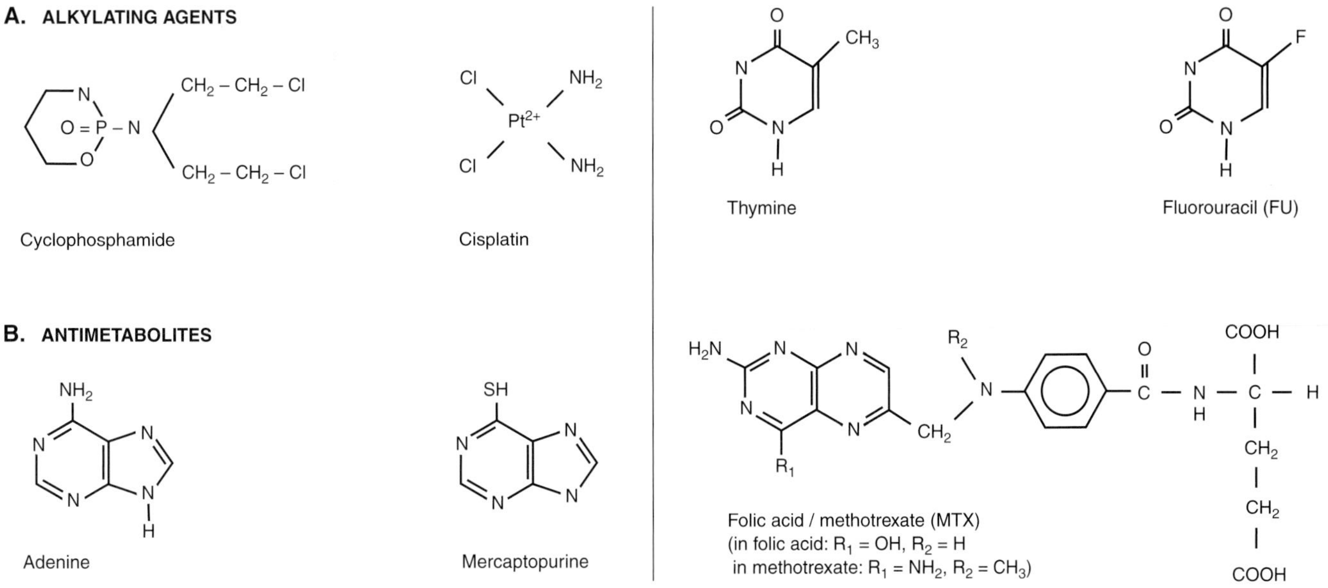

A. ALKYLATING AGENTS

Cyclophosphamide

Cisplatin

Thymine

Fluorouracil (FU)

B. ANTIMETABOLITES

Adenine

Mercaptopurine

Folic acid / methotrexate (MTX)
(in folic acid: R_1 = OH, R_2 = H
in methotrexate: R_1 = NH_2, R_2 = CH_3)

FIGURE 49-1 Chemical structures of representative antineoplastic agents. **A.** Alkylating agent (cyclophosphamide) and cisplatin. **B.** Antimetabolites: mercaptopurine, FU and MTX; compare with normal compounds adenine, thymine and folate.

Antimetabolite drugs

The **antimetabolites** group contains drugs that are analogues of folic acid or of the purine and pyrimidine bases. It is thought that these agents act by inhibiting enzymes involved in the pathways for macromolecular synthesis, or as false 'building blocks', causing impaired polymers of nucleic acids to be built up.

Groups of antimetabolites

The chemical structures of typical antimetabolites (*) are shown in Figure 49-1. The antimetabolites fall into three main groups:
- folic acid antagonists: **methotrexate**,* raltitrexed
- purine antagonists: thioguanine, fludarabine, cladribine, **mercaptopurine***
- pyrimidine antagonists: cytarabine, **fluorouracil**,* gemcitabine, capecitabine.

Folic acid is an essential co-factor in many biochemical reactions, particularly in one-carbon transfers, and is essential for the synthesis of purines and the methylation of uracil. The folic acid antagonists such as **methotrexate** (MTX; see Drug Monograph 49-2) mainly act by inhibition of the enzyme dihydrofolate reductase, which is required for the activation of folate to tetrahydrofolate. (The sulfonamide antibacterial drugs have a similar mechanism of action and are also classed as antifolate drugs, but are more specific for bacterial metabolic pathways than those in neoplastic cells.) Permetrexed, a new antifolate drug, inhibits folate-dependent enzymes.

The purine and pyrimidine base analogues can be incorporated into DNA strands in place of the true bases,

forming permanently modified DNA and leading to improper base pairing during replication of DNA, and improper transcription to RNA. They may also act as specific inhibitors of enzymes involved in DNA synthesis. Thus macromolecular synthesis and cell duplication are impaired. The antimetabolites are considered to be phase-specific agents, as they act particularly at the S phase of the cell cycle.

A cunning technique for making anticancer drugs more specific for neoplastic cells is exemplified in the new drug capecitabine, which is a prodrug for fluorouracil (FU). It has been rationally designed to be 'tumour-activated', in that after oral administration it is metabolised in three stages, the last of which involves the enzyme thymidine phosphorylase, which is more active in the liver and tumour cells than in normal cells. Hence higher levels (2.5 times) of active FU are reached in tumour cells than in adjacent tissue, which optimises therapeutic effects and minimises adverse effects. Capecitabine is proving particularly effective in breast and colorectal cancers.

Antibiotic antitumour drugs

The third main group of cytotoxic agents is the **antibiotic antitumour agents**, such as the anthracyclines and bleomycins. These drugs are defined as antibiotics because they are compounds that are isolated from one type of organism (usually fungi) and act against another type of organism, in this context against neoplastic cells (rather than bacterial cells, as with traditional antibiotics such as penicillins, aminoglycosides and macrolides). The early agents in this class (daunorubicin, doxorubicin) caused the clinically

DRUG MONOGRAPH 49-1 CYCLOPHOSPHAMIDE

Cyclophosphamide is a cell-cycle-non-specific agent that cross-links DNA strands and inhibits protein synthesis and DNA replication.

INDICATIONS Cyclophosphamide is indicated for acute and chronic leukaemias, lymphomas, multiple myeloma, carcinoma of the ovary, neuroblastomas, retinoblastoma and mycosis fungoides. It is also used as an immunosuppressant in autoimmune disorders, in immune disorders resistant to milder therapy, and to prevent transplant rejection.

PHARMACOKINETICS The drug is well absorbed after oral or parenteral administration, and the drug and its metabolites cross the blood–brain barrier. Cyclophosphamide undergoes hepatic metabolism to active and inactive metabolites. Excretion is primarily via the kidneys; accumulation of active metabolites in the bladder can cause nephrotoxicity and cystitis. The elimination half-life is about 4 hours.

DRUG INTERACTIONS The following effects can occur when cyclophosphamide is given with the drugs listed below:

Drug	Possible effect and management
Bone marrow depressants or radiation	Increased bone marrow depression may occur. Avoid, or a potentially serious drug interaction could occur. If necessary to use concurrently, a decrease in drug dosage is usually indicated
Aspirin and other NSAIDs	Enhance antiplatelet actions of cytotoxics
Drugs that induce CYP3A4 microsomal enzymes	Alter metabolism of cyclophosphamide, hence may enhance cytotoxic effects and toxic reactions
Immunosuppressant agents, including azathioprine, corticosteroids, cyclosporin and other cytotoxic agents	Increased risk of infections and possible development of secondary neoplasia. Avoid, or a potentially serious drug interaction could occur
Suxamethonium	Cyclophosphamide has significant anticholinesterase activity, hence potentiates depolarising neuromuscular blockade by suxamethonium and mivacurium
Vaccines, live viral	Cyclophosphamide-induced immunosuppression can lead to enhanced effects of viral vaccines

ADVERSE REACTIONS Severe bone marrow suppression occurs 1–2 weeks after treatment, with dose-limiting neutropenia and leucopenia; anaemia and thrombocytopenia also occur. Other adverse reactions include nephrotoxicity with haemorrhagic cystitis, severe nausea and vomiting, gastrointestinal (GI) tract dysfunction, hair loss and impaired wound healing, darkening of the skin, gonadal suppression or missed menstrual periods, cardiotoxicity, hyperuricaemia, and pneumonitis or interstitial pulmonary fibrosis.

The nephrotoxic effects in the renal tubular epithelium may be minimised by treatment with mesna, a thiol-donating compound that neutralises the effects of cyclophosphamide's toxic metabolite acrolein.

WARNINGS AND CONTRAINDICATIONS Baseline assessment before administration should include full blood cell count, tests of liver and kidney function and evaluation of disease course and progress. Patients must be closely monitored during therapy. Patients need to be hydrated before and during therapy, with 2–3 L fluid PO or infused. Staff are warned to observe safe handling procedures for cytotoxics.

Use with caution in patients with adrenalectomy (toxicity of cyclophosphamide increases), a history of gout or urate kidney stones, or cardiovascular disease. There is an increased risk of secondary neoplasia.

Avoid use in people with cyclophosphamide hypersensitivity, bone marrow suppression, chicken-pox, herpes zoster or other untreated infections, liver or kidney function impairment, urinary tract damage or infection, and in pregnancy (see Pregnancy Safety box).

DOSAGE AND ADMINISTRATION The usual adult antineoplastic loading dose is 40–49 mg/kg IV in divided doses over 2–5 days. A typical maintenance dosage is 1–5 mg/kg orally daily; however, oncology units have developed chemotherapy regimens depending on indication, other antineoplastics being administered concurrently, kidney function etc (see Table 48-2). The maximum tolerated dose is given, using total white cell count as a guide to toxicity. The immunosuppressive dose is markedly lower, starting at 1–3 mg/kg orally once daily, then reducing.

DRUG MONOGRAPH 49-2 METHOTREXATE

Methotrexate (MTX) is an antimetabolite that is cell-cycle-specific for the S phase. To synthesise DNA, folic acid must be reduced to tetrahydrofolate by the enzyme dihydrofolate reductase. Due to its close chemical similarity to folate (Figure 49-1), MTX competitively inhibits the enzyme, thus inhibiting the synthesis of DNA and RNA. Because cell proliferation is usually faster in malignant cells than in normal tissues, cancer growth may be impaired by MTX. The drug is also used for some other conditions marked by excessive proliferation, such as psoriasis, and its significant immunosuppressant actions make it useful in autoimmune conditions such as rheumatoid arthritis, in which MTX reduces the symptoms of inflammation.

INDICATIONS MTX is indicated for:
- treatment of breast, head and neck, and lung cancers; trophoblastic tumours; renal, ovarian, bladder and testicular carcinomas; acute lymphocytic leukaemia and non-Hodgkin's lymphomas; and mycosis fungoides and osteosarcoma
- prophylaxis and treatment of meningeal leukaemia
- treatment for some non-cancerous conditions such as cases of severe psoriasis, inflammatory bowel disease and rheumatoid arthritis unresponsive to standard therapies.

PHARMACOKINETICS MTX is administered orally or parenterally (IM, IV, intra-arterial and intrathecal routes). The oral preparation produces peak plasma concentrations within 1–2 hours. Only limited amounts of MTX can cross the blood–brain barrier; however, significant quantities may pass into the systemic circulation after intrathecal drug administration. It is bound about 50% to plasma proteins, and excreted largely unchanged by the kidneys.

DRUG INTERACTIONS There are many clinically significant drug interactions with MTX. Some of the more important are listed below; see also *Australian Medicines Handbook*, Appendix A.

Drug	Possible effect and management
Alcohol and other hepatotoxic drugs	Increased risk of hepatotoxicity; avoid and/or monitor liver enzymes
Calcium folinate	*NB*: Intentional drug interaction to 'rescue' cells by restoring intracellular folate levels
Colaspase (asparaginase)	Cell replication is inhibited by asparaginase, thus impairing the therapeutic effects of MTX

Drug	Possible effect and management
Bone marrow depressants or radiation	Bone marrow-depressant effects may be increased. Avoid or reduce drug dosage
Aspirin and other non-steroidal anti-inflammatory drugs (NSAIDs)	Concurrent administration can result in additive platelet inhibition; avoid. Low-dose aspirin may be used concurrently
Probenecid or salicylates	Can interfere with excretion of MTX, which results in elevated plasma concentrations and increased toxicity
Sulfonamides	Additive antifolate actions, hence enhanced toxicity
Vaccines, live oral	Can result in a decreased immunological response along with an increase in adverse reactions. Avoid, or a potentially serious drug interaction could occur

ADVERSE REACTIONS Toxic effects are possible even with low doses, and fatalities have occurred. The major adverse effects are bone marrow suppression (leucopenia, infections, thrombocytopenia), immunosuppression (infections, acne, boils) and loss of hair. GI tract effects include nausea, vomiting, anorexia, GI ulcers and bleeding, and stomatitis. With prolonged daily therapy, liver toxicity, pneumonitis or pulmonary fibrosis can occur, and carcinogenic effects and impaired fertility. With high-dose drug therapy, renal failure, hyperuricaemia and cutaneous vasculitis are possible; these may be minimised with leucovorin rescue, effective hydration and urine alkalinisation to enhance excretion of MTX.

WARNINGS AND CONTRAINDICATIONS Because of its very low therapeutic index, MTX should be prescribed only by specialist physicians with experience in the clinical use of antimetabolites. Patients should be warned of the high risk of potentially dangerous adverse reactions, and monitored closely before, during and after courses of therapy.

Use with caution in patients with aciduria (urine pH below 7), gout, GI obstruction, a history of kidney stone formation, nausea or vomiting (which may increase the potential for dehydration) and in dehydrated patients. Health-care professionals dealing with MTX should observe safe handling guidelines.

Avoid use in people with MTX hypersensitivity, ascites, pleural effusions, liver or kidney function impairment, bone marrow suppression, chickenpox (recent or current),

DRUG MONOGRAPH 49-2
METHOTREXATE—CONT'D

herpes zoster, other infections, peptic ulcer or ulcerative colitis, or oral mucositis. MTX is contraindicated in pregnancy (Australian Category D) and breastfeeding.

DOSAGE AND ADMINISTRATION The adult and paediatric MTX dosages vary according to the indication and course of treatment. The antineoplastic adult dosage orally is generally 15–30 mg daily for 5 days, repeated 3–5 times with a 7–14-day interval between courses. The paediatric oral dosage is 20–40 mg/m² once a week. The paediatric intrathecal dose for prophylaxis against meningeal leukaemia depends on the age of the child and the estimated volume of cerebrospinal fluid.

The doses for immunosuppression in rheumatoid arthritis are much lower, e.g. oral adult dose 7.5 mg once weekly, on a nominated day (e.g. on Tuesdays), to avoid risk of inadvertent daily dosing.

limiting adverse effect of irreversible cardiomyopathy; newer agents are being sought that lack this cardiac toxicity.

These cytotoxic agents act by various mechanisms. Anthracyclines (daunorubicin, **doxorubicin** [previously called adriamycin], idarubicin, epirubicin and the related compound mitozantrone) directly bind to DNA, thus inhibiting DNA and RNA synthesis. They may also inhibit topoisomerase II in its reversible 'swivelling' actions during DNA synthesis, and intercalate (insert between adjacent base pairs in DNA chains) to impair DNA transcription. Cytotoxicty is enhanced by production of active free radicals. Dactinomycin (formerly known as actinomycin-D) is also an intercalating agent and topoisomerase II inhibitor. As the anthracyclines have actions at many sites in the cell cycle, and may also affect non-cycling cells, they are said to be cell-cycle-non-specific agents.

The bleomycins are glycopeptide antibiotics with a different mechanism of action: through chelation of metal ions and generation of reactive radicals, they degrade preformed DNA into fragmented chains, and block incorporation of thymidine into DNA. They are cell-cycle-non-specific agents, active in both G₂ and M phases of the cell cycle, and against cells in G₀. They cause little bone marrow suppression, but can potentially cause pulmonary fibrosis. Mitomycin has actions similar to those of both bleomycin and the alkylating agents. (See Table 49-1 for the drugs in this classification, primary indications and major toxicities.)

Mitotic inhibitors

Important antineoplastic agents that are natural products isolated from plants include the vinca alkaloids, the podophyllotoxin derivatives and the taxanes (see Clinical Interest Box 49-2). These agents are **mitotic inhibitors**. (See Table 49-1 for primary indications and major toxicities.)

Mechanisms of action

During the metaphase stage of mitotic division (see Figure 48-1), the replicated chromosomes line up on a spindle formed from microtubules. Binding by the above agents to the protein tubulin, a constituent of microtubules, inhibits its polymerisation into microtubules, disrupts spindle formation and arrests mitosis in metaphase. Thus they are said to be cell-cycle-phase-specific agents, inhibiting cell cycling during the late G₂ and M phases. (Inhibition of microtubule actions impairs other processes in cells, including chemotaxis, phagocytosis and axonal transport of neurotransmitters.) The drugs may also have other actions that contribute to their cytotoxic effects (e.g. the vinca alkaloids impair uridine incorporation into mRNA).

Drug groups
VINCA ALKALOIDS

The vinca alkaloids vinblastine and **vincristine** (from the plant *Catharanthus* or *Vinca rosea*; Clinical Interest Box 49-2) and the related semisynthetic alkaloid vinorelbine have different therapeutic indications and different adverse effects. They have been used in the treatment of various lymphomas, carcinoma of the breast and testes, leukaemias and Hodgkin's disease, and for non-small-cell lung cancer. They are relatively non toxic compared with other cytotoxic agents; they have mild bone marrow-suppressant and neurotoxic effects, and can cause hypersensitivity reactions. Vincristine is irritant and is potentially fatal if administered intrathecally.

TAXANES

The taxanes (paclitaxel and docetaxel, from yew trees; Clinical Interest Box 49-2) are agents with antimitotic and immunostimulatory effects; they appear to stabilise microtubule bundles and thus inhibit mitosis. Their effects in stimulating immune responses and regulating lymphocyte activation are also useful in cancer chemotherapy. They are used particularly in breast, lung and ovarian cancers.

Paclitaxel is marketed for the treatment of metastatic ovarian cancer refractory to other drug treatments. It is also used for the treatment of metastatic breast cancer, and some studies indicate that it should be used earlier, such as immediately after surgery, as it then produces better effects than hormone therapy alone. Adverse reactions include severe allergic reactions (prevented by pretreatment with a corticosteroid and an antihistamine), bone marrow suppression, peripheral neuropathy, muscle pain, alopecia and gastric distress.

Other cytotoxic agents
Platinum compounds

The platinum-containing compounds **cisplatin**, carboplatin and oxaliplatin are sometimes considered as alkylating agents, as they have a rather similar mechanism of action. In cisplatin, the platinum atom is bonded to two amine groups, which cross-link between DNA strands (see Figure 49-1). Cell division is inhibited, leading to apoptosis; these compounds are cell-cycle-non-specific. Cisplatin is particularly emetogenic, and most likely to cause nephro- and neurotoxicities. The three platinum compounds have diferent indications, contraindications, adverse drug reactions, and dosage and administration guidelines, so individual specialist oncology protocols should be consulted for these details.

Podophyllotoxins

The podophyllin-type compounds etoposide and teniposide are sometimes included with mitotic inhibitors as they can cause metaphase arrest; however, their mechanisms of action are not simple, as they also kill cells in the S and G_2 phases of the cell cycle and may inhibit topoisomerase II (see Clinical Interest Box 49-2). They are used mainly in leukaemias and lymphomas.

Topoisomerase I inhibitors

The topoisomerase type I enzymes are involved in the untwisting, nicking and resealing of DNA strands during the processes of DNA translation and duplication. Agents that inhibit these enzymes cause breaks in double-stranded DNA, blocking macromolecular synthesis in the cell cycle and leading to tumour cell death. Two new antineoplastic agents with this mechanism of action are derivatives of the plant *Camptotheca accuminata* and have been given the generic name camptothecins. They are S phase-specific.

Topotecan, a topoisomerase I inhibitor, is indicated for the treatment of relapsed or refractory metastatic carcinoma of the ovary after failure of other therapies, and also for small-cell lung cancer. Adverse reactions include neutropenia (a dose-limiting toxicity), leucopenia, thrombocytopenia, anaemia, headache, GI tract disturbances, alopecia, tiredness, dyspnoea and neuromuscular pain. The usual dose is 1.5 mg/m^2 by IV infusion over 30 minutes daily for 5 days.

Irinotecan, another topoisomerase I inhibitor, is indicated for the treatment of metastatic colorectal cancer that has occurred or progressed after FU chemotherapy. Irinotecan can cause severe diarrhoea, which requires immediate treatment with atropine or loperamide. Severe myelosuppression, nausea and vomiting may also occur.

Colaspase (formerly known as asparaginase)

The enzyme asparaginase hydrolyses the amino acid L-asparagine to L-aspartic acid and ammonia. Asparagine is necessary for cell survival and, because normal body cells are capable of synthesising adequate supplies of asparagine, they are not affected by an asparagine deficiency. Certain cancer cells, however, are unable to synthesise asparagine and depend on a circulating supply of asparagine within the blood; administration of asparaginase enhances the breakdown of asparagine, so the cancer cells will die. Colaspase is sometimes classed as an antimetabolite, as it exploits differences between metabolic pathways in normal and neoplastic cells.

Colaspase is a form of asparaginase produced from cultures of *Escherichia coli*; as it is a protein, it cannot be given orally, but is administered by IM injection or IV infusion to treat leukaemias and lymphoma. Adverse reactions include allergic reactions (including anaphylaxis), a decrease in the blood clotting factors, hyperammonaemia (headache, anorexia, nausea, vomiting and abdominal cramps), liver toxicity and nervous system dysfunction. The drug should be administered only in hospital settings because of the risk of anaphylaxis.

Altretamine

Altretamine is a cytotoxic agent for the palliative treatment of persistent or recurrent ovarian cancer. Its mechanism of action is unknown, although chemically it resembles the alkylating agents. Clinically, however, it is effective for ovarian tumours that are resistant to the previously marketed alkylating agents. Its main adverse reactions are bone marrow suppression, GIT dysfunction and neurotoxicity.

Hydroxyurea

Hydroxyurea inhibits DNA synthesis by interfering with the conversion of ribonucleotides to deoxyribonucleotides; it is sometimes classified with the antimetabolites. It is indicated for the treatment of ovarian carcinoma, chronic myelocytic leukaemia and malignant melanoma. Adverse reactions include bone marrow suppression and GI tract dysfunctions.

HORMONES

Hormonal agents are used in the treatment of neoplasias that are sensitive to hormonal growth controls in the body. Growth of prostate cancer, for example, is stimulated by the male sex hormones (androgens), breast cancers by oestrogens, and thyroid cancer by thyrotrophin. Thus there are several options for treatment of these cancers. For example, prostate cancer may be treated by:

• surgical removal of the prostate and/or testes

CLINICAL INTEREST BOX 49-2
ANTINEOPLASTIC AGENTS FROM NATURAL SOURCES

About two-thirds of commercially available anticancer drugs are derived from, or related to, natural products, including not only enzymes, hormones, interferons, oncogene proteins and antimetabolites but also plant and fungal extracts.

The autumn crocus plant, *Colchicum autumnale*, was prized in Roman times as a treatment for gout, and later for rheumatism also. Its major active ingredient, colchicine, is effective as an anti-inflammatory agent because of its ability to bind to tubulin, a structural protein in the microtubules in cells, and hence to interfere with the migration of neutrophils into a joint. This mechanism also accounts for the antitumour activity of colchicine, as inhibition of tubulin action inhibits mitosis and has cytotoxic effects. Colchicine is, however, too toxic for regular use.

An extract of wild chervil was mentioned in a medical book written in about 950 AD as being useful as a salve (ointment) against tumours. This may have been due to a cytotoxic agent now known as podophyllotoxin, also present in *Podophyllum* species plants. Native Americans used the root extracts as a purgative, emetic, poison and treatment for warts. Because of the similarity between viral warts and viral tumours, the extract was tested for antitumour activity and found to be effective but toxic. Synthesis of compounds related to the natural lignans produced two potent cytotoxic agents effective against leukaemia and lung cancers: etoposide and teniposide. These act by inhibition of topoisomerase II.

Extracts of the rosy periwinkle plant, *Catharanthus rosea* (formerly called *Vinca rosea*), were used in several cultures to treat diabetes. When tested in animals (in

the 1950s), the extracts showed not antidiabetic effects but immunosuppressant effects, with severe depletion of white cells. As this is a common adverse effect of cytotoxic agents, the extracts were tested against animal tumours, with excellent results, leading to the development of the drugs vincristine and vinblastine. The 5-year survival rate for patients with Hodgkin's disease rose from 5% in 1970 to more than 98% with the combination chemotherapy regimen of vincristine, MTX, mercaptopurine and prednisolone.

Antibiotics with antitumour activity include the anthracyclines, such as doxorubicin and daunorubicin; dactinomycin; and the bleomycins, mainly extracted from *Streptomyces* species of fungi (see earlier section on antitumour antibiotics).

More recent natural products with anticancer activities include the taxanes (paclitaxel and docetaxel), agents that have antimitotic and immunostimulatory effects and are derived from bark of the yew tree *Taxus baccata*; and the camptothecins (topotecan and irinotecan), a group of drugs with topoisomerase inhibitory actions derived from *Camptotheca accuminata*.

It is recognised by scientists in research institutions and drug companies that the millions of diverse species in tropical rain forests and marine environments potentially contain novel compounds with important antineoplastic (and other useful medical) actions. Screening programs with fast throughputs test millions of new compounds annually for potentially useful actions against human neoplastic cell lines (see Clinical Interest Box 4-2). Compounds isolated from marine molluscs and sponges are currently being trialled for their anticancer properties.

- radiation
- administration of antiandrogenic drugs
- oestrogenic hormones (as the female hormones have antiandrogenic effects)
- gonadotrophin-releasing hormone (GnRH) analogues (given continuously, to suppress gonadotrophin release)
- cytotoxic agents.

In the early stages, 'watchful waiting' is also an option, while monitoring levels of prostate-specific antigen (PSA) as an indicator of disease progression, and considering benefits and risks of the various treatment modalities. The decision as to which type of therapy will be used is usually based on the preference of the patient as well as the clinical expertise of the oncologist, and judgement as to the progress and prognosis of the cancer and the relative adverse effects of the treatments.

The hormones are not specifically antiproliferative or cytotoxic in neoplastic cells, but have their usual hormonal actions. Hormonal agents are more selective and less toxic than

other antineoplastic medications, and include corticosteroids, androgens and antiandrogens, oestrogens and anti-oestrogens, progestogens, and analogues of GnRH (see Table 49-2 for a summary of hormonal agents used in neoplastic conditions, their indications and major adverse effects).

Corticosteroids

Glucocorticoids retard lymphocytic proliferation by their effects in suppressing white cell production; therefore their greatest value lies in the treatment of lymphocytic leukaemias and lymphomas. Prednisone and dexamethasone are also used in conjunction with radiation therapy to decrease the occurrence of radiation oedema in critical areas such as the superior mediastinum, brain and spinal cord. In addition, they are often used in conjunction with antiemetic drugs and as supportive therapy for their general metabolic, anti-inflammatory and euphoric effects (see Chapter 40).

Androgens and antiandrogens
Androgens

Androgens such as testosterone and fluoxymesterone (see Chapter 47) are used to treat advanced breast carcinoma if surgery, radiation and other therapies are inappropriate or ineffective.

Antiandrogens

The group of antiandrogenic agents includes flutamide, bicalutamide, nilutamide and cyproterone (a partial agonist). These drugs inhibit the uptake or the binding of androgens at their target cells or receptors. The result is suppression of ovarian and testicular steroidogenesis, thus inducing a 'medical castration'. They are indicated in combination with surgery and a GnRH analogue (see below) for treatment of advanced prostate cancer. This combination has been reported to prolong survival by at least 25% compared with GnRH therapy alone. Adverse reactions include diarrhoea, impotence and other symptoms of low testosterone levels, and hepatotoxicity.

Gonadotrophin-releasing hormone analogues

GnRH (also known as LHRH) analogues such as goserelin and leuprorelin, when administered on a continuous basis, effectively suppress production of gonadotrophins from the pituitary gland, and thus have indirect antiandrogenic and anti-oestrogenic effects (see Figure 43-3). They are used for gonadal suppression in precocious puberty, endometriosis,

TABLE 49-2 Summary of hormonal agents used in neoplastic conditions

HORMONES	CLINICAL INDICATIONS	COMMON ADVERSE EFFECTS
Antiandrogens		
Bicalutamide, cyproterone, flutamide, nilutamide	Advanced prostatic cancer, metastatic prostatic cancer, suppression of GnRH 'flare'	Impotence, impaired libido, decreased spermatogenesis, gynaecomastia, nausea, dizziness, alcohol intolerance, dyspnoea, hepatotoxicity, impaired dark–light adaptation
Anti-oestrogens		
Tamoxifen, toremifene	Breast cancer	Hot flushes, dizziness, nausea and vomiting, oedema, vaginal bleeding, musculoskeletal pain
Aromatase inhibitors		
Aminoglutethimide, anastrozole, exemestane, letrozole	Postmenopausal breast cancer (ER receptor-positive)	Hot flushes, vaginal bleeding, hair thinning, nausea, GIT disturbances, joint pain, rash, fatigue, oedema, headache
Progestogens		
Megestrol, medroxyprogesterone acetate	Palliative therapy of metastatic breast, endometrial and renal cell cancers	Hypersensitivity, nausea and vomiting, CNS disturbances, breast tenderness, menstrual irregularities, weight gain
GnRH analogues (= LHRH agonists)		
Goserelin, leuprorelin	Palliative treatment of prostate cancer, advanced breast cancer (premenopausal)	Males: 'flare-up' of prostate cancer (bone pain, ureter obstruction, spinal cord compression), oedema, hot flushes, testicular atrophy, GIT disorders, reduced libido. Females: decreased libido, hot flushes, headache, abdominal pain, hypertension, dysmenorrhoea
Others		
Octreotide (somatostatin analogue)	Carcinoid tumours of GIT and pancreas secreting 5-hydroxytryptamine (serotonin) or VIP	GIT disorders (pain, bloating, diarrhoea)

ER = (o)estrogen receptors; GIT = gastrointestinal tract; GnRH = gonadotrophin-releasing hormone; LHRH = luteinising hormone-releasing hormone; VIP = vasoactive intestinal polypeptide.

polycystic ovary syndrome, and prostatic and premenopausal breast cancer (see Table 43-1).

Goserelin is used as a palliative agent in the treatment of advanced prostate carcinoma. With chronic administration, there is an initial surge in gonadotrophin release (causing a 'flare' in prostatic cancer growth), then the plasma concentrations of testosterone usually drop to the range seen in surgically castrated men within 2–4 weeks after initiation of drug therapy. A 3.6 mg dose as a prolonged-release formulation is implanted subcutaneously in the upper abdominal wall every 28 days, or 10.8 mg into the anterior abdominal wall every 3 months. Adverse reactions reported generally are related to the lowered testosterone levels and may include sexual dysfunction, hot flushes and decreased erections, and cardiovascular dysfunction.

Oestrogens and anti-oestrogens
Oestrogens

Oestrogens may be used to treat androgen-sensitive prostatic carcinomas or advanced breast carcinoma in postmenopausal women. Oestrogens such as diethylstilboestrol and ethinyloestradiol, for example, have been used to treat advanced prostatic carcinoma; however, they are rarely used for this indication now due to adverse cardiovascular effects (see Chapter 44 for typical oestrogenic actions).

Oestrogens may occasionally be used in breast cancer to 'recruit' resting cells from the G_0 phase into active cell cycling again (G_1 phase), so the cells will be sensitive to cytotoxic agents.

Anti-oestrogens

Anti-oestrogens are useful in treatment of postmenopausal breast cancers that are oestrogen receptor (ER)-positive, i.e. tumours that contain high concentrations of oestrogen receptors. They have replaced both androgens and oestrogens as the initial approach in breast cancer therapy. (Anti-oestrogens are less useful in premenopausal women because their effects would be swamped by the high levels of oestrogens produced by the ovaries.)

Tamoxifen (Drug Monograph 49-3) is a synthetic non-steroidal anti-oestrogen preparation with both agonist and antagonist effects; it can be considered a partial agonist at oestrogen receptors. It is believed to bind to ERs in breast cancer cells, where it acts as a competitive inhibitor of

---

DRUG MONOGRAPH 49-3 TAMOXIFEN

Tamoxifen is a non-steroidal compound with a range of both agonist and antagonist activities at oestrogen receptors (ER) in various tissues. In patients with oestrogen receptor-positive breast tumours, it acts primarily as an anti-oestrogen, binding to the receptors and inhibiting growth of the tumour.

INDICATIONS Tamoxifen is indicated for treatment of breast cancer, especially postmenopausal ER-positive cancers.

PHARMACOKINETICS Tamoxifen is administered PO and absorbed from the GIT; peak plasma levels are reached 3–6 hours after a single dose, and concentration at steady-state is achieved about 4 weeks after commencement of once-daily dosing. The drug is distributed widely to many organs and tissues, including uterus and ovary. It is highly bound to plasma albumin (>99%), also to ERs in target tissues. Tamoxifen is extensively metabolised in the liver; the major metabolite has actions similar to those of the parent drug. Slow elimination via the faeces accounts for the accumulation and long half-life of the drug and its major metabolite.

DRUG INTERACTIONS Tamoxifen is metabolised by CYP3A4, so its level and activities can be affected by the many other drugs that affect or are affected by this enzyme; CYP3A4 inducers that can reduce tamoxifen

effects include rifampicin, corticosteroids, pioglitazone, many anticonvulsants and St John's wort; while CYP3A4 inhibitors that can enhance the effects of tamoxifen include cimetidine, ciprofloxacin, erythromycin, many -conazole antifungals, many antivirals and grapefruit juice (see Australian Medicines Handbook, Appendix A, Table A-1). Tamoxifen increases the anticoagulant effects of warfarin, and bleeding is likely; bleeding time should be monitored by INR and the dose of warfarin may need to be reduced.

ADVERSE REACTIONS Abnormal gynaecological reactions are common, such as vaginal bleeding and hot flushes; endometrial changes such as polyps and cancer can also develop. Other adverse reactions include nausea and vomiting, visual disturbances and leucopenia.

WARNINGS AND CONTRAINDICATIONS Tamoxifen is contraindicated in pregnancy, breastfeeding women, and children; also in those who have shown hypersensitivity reactions to it. If a woman patient is of childbearing age and sexually active, effective non-hormonal contraception must be practised.

DOSAGE AND ADMINISTRATION The usual daily dose is 20 mg; in advanced stages of breast cancer, the dose may be raised to 40 mg/day.

oestrogen. It is an oestrogen agonist in the liver, which has desirable effects on plasma lipids in postmenopausal women. It also helps to preserve bone mineral density, which may decrease the osteoporosis risk in these women. The adverse effects are mainly those of low oestrogen levels, i.e. hot flushes, vaginal disorders, and nausea and vomiting.

Toremifene is a newer anti-oestrogen product for the treatment of metastatic breast cancer in postmenopausal women; the actions and adverse effects profile are similar to those of tamoxifen.

Raloxifene

Raloxifene is a selective ER modulator (SERM) currently used to prevent postmenopausal osteoporosis, as it has oestrogenic effects in bone, but anti-oestrogenic effects in uterus and breast tissues (see Chapter 44). It is also being studied for the treatment of breast cancer, with results showing a significant decrease in invasive breast cancer in women at increased risk of breast cancer (Vogel et al 2006).

Aromatase inhibitors

In the biochemical pathways for the synthesis of oestrogens, a critical stage is the 'aromatisation' of the steroid A ring, from testosterone to oestradiol (see Figures 37-2 and 40-1); this step was difficult in the early attempts to synthesise oestrogens in the laboratory. In postmenopausal women, the main source of oestrogens in the body is from androgens via the aromatase enzyme actions in peripheral (non-ovary) tissues. Various compounds that inhibit the aromatase enzyme have been synthesised, including anastrozole, letrozole and exemestane. They are indicated for use in women with natural or induced postmenopausal status, whose breast cancer has progressed despite anti-oestrogen therapy. Aromatase inhibitors do not block the synthesis of glucocorticoids or mineralocorticoids.

A related compound, aminoglutethimide (Drug Monograph 40-3), inhibits not only aromatase but also the first stage in the pathway, i.e. conversion of cholesterol to pregnenolone (Figure 40-1); thus it inhibits synthesis of corticosteroids as well as sex hormones. It is used to suppress adrenal gland function in Cushing's disease, in treatment of adrenal gland cancers, and in postmenopausal (and male) breast cancer. In the latter case, replacement with corticosteroids (gluco- and mineralocorticoids) is required. Common adverse reactions include lethargy, rash and dizziness.

Progestogens

Progestogens such as medroxyprogesterone (Drug Monograph 44-2) and megestrol are used to treat advanced endometrial cancer, and breast cancer unresponsive to anti-oestrogens or aromatase inhibitors, because they suppress gonadotrophin release. This is primarily a palliative approach that seeks tumour regression and an increase in the patient's survival time. Megestrol is also indicated for advanced carcinoma of the breast, and medroxyprogesterone is used in patients with advanced renal carcinoma.

Somatostatin analogues

Analogues of somatostatin (= growth hormone release-inhibiting factor; see Table 38-1 and Drug Monograph 38-2) are used to treat cancers of the pituitary gland that produce excess growth hormone (causing acromegaly), and in carcinoid tumours of the GIT that secrete excess 5-hydroxytryptamine. The analogues are octreotide and lanreotide; adverse reactions in the GIT are common (see Table 49-2).

MISCELLANEOUS ANTINEOPLASTIC AGENTS

Miscellaneous agents include those that cannot readily be classified by their mechanism of action into any of the previous groups. As these drugs are not cytotoxic agents, they are unlikely to cause severe bone marrow depression, nausea and vomiting, or hair loss.

Antineoplastic monoclonal antibodies

Monoclonal antibodies (Ab) are immunoglobulins produced synthetically from a single clone (genetically identical cells) of B lymphocytes; all will be identical proteins with specificity against the same antigen. The binding of the antibody to the antigen usually inactivates the antigen and/or causes cell lysis. The suffix -mab is being adopted to indicate a monoclonal antibody. Monoclonal antibodies are most effective when administered in combination with chemotherapeutic regimens. As they are large proteins, antibodies must be administered parenterally (see Ward 2003).

Trastuzumab

Trastuzumab targets a growth factor receptor. It is a monoclonal antibody against the receptor for epidermal growth factor (EGF), a protein encoded by an oncogene (known as HER-2) overexpressed in about 30% of women with breast cancer.* By

---

* An interesting example of how drug trade names can be derived is shown by the drug Herceptin, a brand name for trastuzumab, which is a **h**uman epid**er**mal growth factor re**cept**or 2 **in**hibitor.

blocking the EGF receptor, trastuzumab slows breast cancer progression and increases tumour reduction in women with this altered gene. It is used as monotherapy, or has synergistic effects when used in combination with paclitaxel or with an antitumour antibiotic and cyclophosphamide.

The antibody is administered by IV infusion. It has a very long half-life (about 6 days), but steady state is not reached for 4–8 months as the pharmacokinetics are non-linear. Hypersensitivity reactions and cardiotoxicity can occur.

Rituximab

Rituximab is another genetically engineered monoclonal antibody, this one specific against an antigen (CD20) located on the surface of both normal and malignant B lymphocytes. The CD20 antigen governs the early steps in cell cycle initiation and differentiation, and it is found on more than 90% of B cell non-Hodgkin's lymphomas. Rituximab is indicated in treatment of B cell non-Hodgkin's lymphoma, and is usually administered with the CHOP regimen: cyclophosphamide/hydroxydaunomycin/Oncovin (vincristine)/prednisone.

Others

Other new monoclonal antibodies include bevacizumab, specific against a vascular endothelial growth factor, hence useful in slowing growth of new blood vessels supplying a tumour (angiogenesis); and cetuximab, against an epidermal growth factor receptor overexpressed in many patients with colorectal cancer.

Tyrosine kinase inhibitors

As described in Chapter 48 and Figure 48-2, the cell cycle is regulated by many growth factors, some of which act by binding to specific transmembrane receptors, which 'switches on' the receptor's kinase (phosphorylating) enzyme activity to cause phosphorylation of the tyrosine residues in proteins that induce cell growth or differentiation. Drugs designed to inhibit specific protein kinase enzymes can thus act as inhibitors of particular metabolic reactions in cell growth or differentiation pathways, and hence act as antineoplastic agents.

Two such tyrosine kinase inhibitors (-tinibs) are imatinib and gefitinib. They are relatively new drugs, so clinical experience with their use is still accumulating. Imatinib inhibits the tyrosine kinase in the receptor for Philadelphia chromosomal platelet-derived growth factor, and is indicated for use in chronic myelocytic leukaemia and gastrointestinal tumours. Adverse reactions, bone marrow suppression, gastrointestinal disorders and fluid retention are common. Gefitinib inhibits the tyrosine kinase associated with the receptor for epidermal growth factor, which occurs

particularly in solid tumours derived from epithelial tissues, such as non-small-cell lung cancers. Its major adverse reactions are interstitial pneumonitis, and gastrointestinal and skin disorders.

Other miscellaneous antineoplastics
Tretinoin

Retinoids (vitamin A derivatives) such as tretinoin have wide-ranging actions in many tissues and at high concentrations are toxic and teratogenic. They have useful effects in cancer cells because of their antiproliferative and prodifferentiation actions, especially in leukaemic cells, and are being used to treat acute promyelocytic leukaemia (as well as acne; see Drug Monograph 56-2). Adverse effects occur particularly in the skin and mucous membranes. Retinoids are known to be teratogenic (Pregnancy Category D or X), and are contraindicated in pregnancy or in women of childbearing age unless using effective contraception.

Anagrelide

Anagrelide is a different type of agent; it has specific actions in reducing the platelet count and so is useful in essential thrombocytopenia, a condition in which platelets proliferate.

Arsenic trioxide

Arsenic has long been known as a toxic chemical, blocking the tricarboxylic acid cycle, and causing kidney damage, psychotomimetic effects and skin cancers. It has been used to treat psoriasis and various infections including syphilis, and as a weed-killer, insecticide and rodenticide. Recent research has shown that arsenic trioxide activates cysteine proteases, and thus promotes cell differentiation and enhances apoptosis; hence it may have useful antineoplastic actions. It is administered by IV infusion in treatment of acute promyelocytic leukaemia refractory to other treatments. Cardiovascular adverse effects are common.

Methyl aminolevulinate

This unusual drug is a photosensitising agent that is applied as a cream to skin lesions (actinic keratoses or basal cell carcinomas) for 3 hours, then the area is exposed to red light, which activates the chemical to produce reactive oxygen radicals that selectively destroy tumour cells. Common adverse reactions include burning pain and ulceration at the site of application. The drug is a porphyrin precursor, and is related to verteporfin, used in a similar way as a photosensitiser to treat ocular macular degeneration (see Chapter 35).

Radioactive isotopes

As described in Chapter 48 under Treatment modalities, radioactive isotopes may be used in cancer therapy; radiopharmaceuticals used include iodine-131 (see Drug Monograph 39-2), phophorus-32 and strontium-89. Preparing and administering these isotopes is a highly specialised area of hospital pharmacy practice.

SUPPORTIVE THERAPY IN THE TREATMENT OF CANCER

Treatment of adverse drug reactions

As discussed in Chapter 48, adverse drug reactions to antineoplastic drugs most commonly impair rapidly dividing cells, such as those in the hair, skin, GIT mucosa and bone marrow. As the drugs are usually excreted via the kidneys, the kidney tubules are also very vulnerable. These adverse effects may be sufficiently severe as to require treatment, often prophylactically. In addition, particular drugs may have other specific adverse drug reactions, e.g. anthracycline antibiotics cause cardiomyopthy, and sex hormone inhibitors cause reduced libido.

Treatment of nausea and vomiting

As described in chapters 34 and 48, the commonest and most distressing adverse reactions to cytotoxic drugs include nausea and vomiting. The chemoreceptor trigger zone in the medulla oblongata is sensitive to chemical stimuli, including emetogenic substances produced by cytotoxics, and to endogenous substances produced in radiation sickness and in the tumour lysis syndrome. Cytotoxics can be classified in terms of their emetogenic potential (see Table 48-3).

Nausea and vomiting are treated with antiemetic drugs, preferably prophylactically (see Chapter 34, and Drug Monographs 34-2 and 34-3); for low-risk agents, metoclopramide when necessary; for intermediate-risk agents, metoclopramide 20 mg IV or orally plus dexamethasone 20 mg IV or orally. For drugs with high emetic risk, a stronger antiemetic is required, such as an oral 5-hydroxytryptamine (5-HT$_3$) antagonist (e.g. ondansetron) plus dexamethasone before chemotherapy. Other similar antiemetics are dolasetron, tropisetron and granisetron. Phenothiazine antiemetic drugs (e.g. prochlorperazine) and antianxiety agents may also be helpful. For severe delayed emesis (>24 hours after chemotherapy), regular administration of IV antiemetics for 2–4 days may be necessary.

Aprepitant is a new antiemetic acting by a different mechanism: it inhibits substance P-mediated vomiting by selectively antagonising the neurokinin-1 receptor. Currently, it is recommended for use only with highly emetogenic cytotoxics such as high-dose cisplatin.

DRUG MONOGRAPH 49-4   CALCIUM FOLINATE (FOLINIC ACID, LEUCOVORIN)

Calcium folinate (or folinic acid, or Leucovorin) is a precursor to tetrahydrofolate, the conversion to which does not require dihydrofolate reductase. It enters and 'rescues' normal cells preferentially to cancer cells owing to differences in the uptake mechanisms. It is therefore used to prevent or treat toxicity induced by folic acid antagonists, especially methotrexate (MTX), and to enhance the cytotoxicity and therapeutic efficacy of fluorouracil.

INDICATIONS Calcium folinate is indicated as an antidote (prophylaxis and treatment) for folic acid antagonists, such as MTX, pyrimethamine and trimethoprim, and in treating megaloblastic anaemias caused by folic acid deficiencies, sprue, or pregnancy, and whenever oral folic acid therapy is not appropriate.

PHARMACOKINETICS Calcium folinate is rapidly absorbed orally and converted by the intestinal mucous membrane and liver to 5-methyltetrahydrofolate, an active metabolite. The onset of action is 20–30 minutes orally, 10–20 minutes IM, and <5 minutes IV. The duration of action by all routes is 3–6 hours. Metabolites are primarily excreted by the kidneys.

DRUG INTERACTIONS Calcium folinate may enhance the toxicity of fluorouracil. The antagonism between calcium folinate and folic acid antagonists such as MTX or raltitrexed is intentional.

ADVERSE REACTIONS These include allergic reactions (rash, hives, itching and wheezing) and convulsions.

WARNINGS AND CONTRAINDICATIONS Use with caution in patients with aciduria (urine pH below 7), ascites, gastrointestinal obstruction, pleural effusion or nausea and vomiting (decreased hydration may result in an increase in MTX toxicity) and in dehydrated patients. Avoid use in persons with calcium folinate hypersensitivity and kidney function impairment. Calcium folinate is not effective in treating anaemias associated with a deficiency of vitamin B$_{12}$.

DOSAGE AND ADMINISTRATION The dosage and duration of 'rescue' with calcium folinate depends on the MTX dose, concentration of MTX in serum and serum creatinine levels. A typical regimen is 15 mg orally, IM or IV every 6 hours for 60 hours (10 doses starting 24 hours after start of MTX infusion), plus hydration and urinary alkalinisation.

Treatment of myelosuppression (bone marrow depression)

Bone marrow depression is usually the limiting factor in the clinical use of cytotoxics, causing treatment delays and dose reductions. White cells and platelets are the first affected, leading to immunosuppression, infections, bruising and bleeding. Neutrophil counts and platelet counts are monitored to indicate when levels have risen high enough for another cycle of chemotherapy to commence. The main risk from thrombocytopenia (low platelet count) is haemorrhage; this may be treated or prevented with infusions of platelets or with haemostatic agents.

Myelosuppression from the antifolate agent methotrexate may be minimised with folinic acid rescue, in which **calcium folinate** (Leucovorin, folinic acid, an analogue of tetrahydrofolate [Drug Monograph 49-4]) is administered a few hours after high-dose methotrexate. In normal cells, calcium folinate bypasses the enzyme blocked by methotrexate and helps prevent much of the bone marrow toxicity without reversing the antineoplastic effects in cancer cells.

Bone marrow suppression may also be overcome by administration of recombinant versions of granulocyte colony-stimulating factor, G-CSF (filgrastim or lenograstim) (see below under immunomodulatory agents). These cytokines stimulate neutrophil precursor cells, reducing the duration of neutropenia and risk of infections after cytotoxic chemotherapy or bone marrow transplant. A related growth factor for haemopoietic stem cells is ancestim.

Hydration therapy and treatment of tumour lysis syndrome

Rehydration, to prevent renal tubular damage or hyperuricaemia, requires vigorous IV fluid infusion. During therapy with high-dose cisplatin, for example, about 2.5 litres of fluids (saline, mannitol and/or glucose) are infused before chemotherapy over 2–3 hours, with frusemide to encourage diuresis if necessary; then, after the chemotherapy, 2 litres of fluids are given over the next 10 hours.

The phosphamide alkylating agents (cyclophosphamide, ifosfamide) are specifically toxic in the kidney epithelium, causing haemorrhagic cystitis. This toxicity may be prevented or reduced by prior administration of a sulfur-donating compound such as mesna or amifostine. These release thiol groups in the kidneys, which detoxify metabolites of the alkylating agents and protect against toxicity from alkylating agents or platinum-containing cytotoxic agents. Two specific examples of effective cytoprotective combinations are described here.

Ifosfamide, an alkylating agent, is used for the treatment of germ cell testicular tumours, but its adverse effect of haemorrhagic cystitis (urotoxicity) has limited its usefulness. Mesna, a thiol donor in the kidneys, acts as a specific antidote for this type of toxicity. Using the drugs in combination therefore allows more aggressive therapy while reducing the dose-limiting adverse effects of ifosfamide.

Amifostine is a cytoprotective agent administered before cisplatin to reduce its potential for renal toxicity. It is a prodrug activated to free thiol groups that protect normal cells against radiation and DNA-binding agents.

TUMOUR LYSIS SYNDROME

This condition is due to massive release of cell breakdown products from large tumour masses (especially leukaemias and lymphomas) treated with chemotherapy; it is manifested by excessive levels of potassium, phosphate and uric acid in the bloodstream (see description in Chapter 48).

Allopurinol is a drug primarily used in treatment of gout. It is a xanthine oxidase inhibitor that reduces the synthesis of uric acid and hence the load of urate to be excreted, thus relieving nephropathy, kidney stone formation and gouty arthritis. In neoplastic disease and myeloproliferative disease, there is also a build-up of urates in the body, due both to the high turnover rates of neoplastic cells and to the cell death induced by cytotoxic agents. Hyperuricaemia is therefore often a clinical feature of cancers, so allopurinol is given to reduce the manifestations of urate deposition.

Rasburicase is a new drug, an enzyme that catalyses the conversion of uric acid to a more soluble metabolite. It is given for prophylaxis and treatment of hyperuricaemia associated with cytotoxic chemotherapy.

Immunomodulatory agents

Immunodeficiency is a serious problem in many cancer patients, partly because cancer itself is immunosuppressant and especially because cytotoxic antineoplastic agents cause T-cell depletion. Alkylating agents, purine antimetabolites and corticosteroids all have major immunosuppressant actions. Some subsets of T cells recover relatively quickly postchemotherapy, especially in children, but there can be prolonged T-cell depletion in adults.

Immunosuppression commonly predisposes to increased incidence of infections. When white cell counts become very low, patients may require antibiotics, antifungal agents and/or antiviral therapy. If a patient has an acute infection, chemotherapy is usually deferred until the patient has recovered from the infection.

Clinical management of patients with iatrogenic T-cell depletion involves monitoring and effective antimicrobial treatment of opportunistic infections, irradiation of blood products for infusion, prophylaxis and possibly reimmunisation against viral infections, and administration of **immunostimulatory agents**.

Interferons

Interferons are naturally occurring small protein molecules that have antiviral, antiproliferative and immunostimulating actions. They can be produced by recombinant technology, resulting in highly purified proteins that have effects similar to the interferon subtypes produced by human leucocytes. Interferons are expensive, however, and the cost of treatment courses is often prohibitive.

Immunomodulatory properties include enhanced phagocyte activity and increased cytotoxic properties of lymphocytes for target cells. Their mechanism of action as antineoplastic agents is unknown, but may be the result of one or more of the three properties identified above. In some types of cancer, for example, interferon appears to have a dual effect of both cytotoxicity and immune stimulation. Some patients demonstrate an increase in haematological factors, granulocytes, platelets and haemoglobin plasma levels.

Interferons alfa-2a and alfa-2b are indicated for the treatment of some leukaemias and lymphomas, genital warts, AIDS-related Kaposi's sarcoma, bladder cancer, osteosarcoma and chronic active hepatitis. Toxicities reported include a flu-like syndrome with fever, chills, muscle pain, loss of appetite and lethargy. At higher doses, myelosuppression, nausea, vomiting, neurotoxicity and cardiotoxicity can occur. (Other interferons are more selective in actions against multiple sclerosis or viral infections.)

Levamisole

Levamisole was initially used clinically as a treatment for intestinal worm infestations. It was also found to have useful immunostimulant effects, enhancing T cell-mediated immunity and macrophage actions. Levamisole is used in combination with FU to treat colorectal carcinoma. This combination has resulted in a lengthened survival time (decreased mortality) and lowered risk of cancer recurrence. Levamisole can be administered orally, and adverse effects are usually mild; however, reversible bone marrow suppression and a flu-like syndrome can occur.

Aldesleukin

Aldesleukin is another immunoregulatory lymphokine that stimulates immune function and is a recombinant version of human interleukin-2 (IL-2). This substance appears to stimulate T-cell proliferation and is a co-factor in enhancing growth of the body's natural killer cells and the lymphokine-activated killer cells; it also increases production of interferons. Aldesleukin is indicated for the treatment of metastatic renal cell carcinoma, melanoma and thymoma, and after bone marrow transplant. Adverse effects of aldesleukin include oedema, anaemia, thrombocytopenia and hypotension.

Colony-stimulating factors

Granulocyte colony-stimulating factors (G-CSFs: filgrastim, lenograstim, pegfilgrastim) are recombinant versions of bone marrow-stimulating factors with immunomodulatory actions. G-CSFs are used to mobilise stem cells and decrease the potential for infection in people receiving myelosuppressant agents that are associated with severe neutropenia and fever. Neutrophil counts are closely monitored after the nadir (lowest level) induced by bone marrow transplant or chemotherapy. G-CSFs should be discontinued when the absolute neutrophil count reaches $10,000/mm^3$ or higher. The major adverse reactions include splenomegaly, hair loss, diarrhoea, fevers, mucositis, anorexia and fatigue. Bone pain has been reported about 2–3 days before the increase in neutrophil count. This pain is usually controlled with non-opioid analgesics. The usual doses are in the range 1–20 mcg/kg per day by SC injection.

BCG (non-vaccine)

BCG stands for bacille Calmette–Guérin, or the *Mycobacterium bovis* bacillus. The BCG vaccine is a live bacterial vaccine for immunisation against tuberculosis. The non-vaccine formulation is also a preparation of an attenuated strain of the bacterium; however, it is administered for its immunostimulatory effects rather than to produce immunity against the particular organism. The mechanism whereby BCG reduces cancerous lesions of the urinary bladder is unknown; it promotes a local inflammatory response and white cell infiltration of tissue.

It is administered not intradermally (as is the vaccine) but instilled by urethral catheter into the urinary bladder of patients with carcinoma of the urinary bladder, to reduce tumour recurrence. Patients who are immunocompromised are at risk of systemic tuberculosis infection; other adverse effects include urinary tract pain and dysfunction, and fever and malaise.

Other immunostimulating therapy

Imiquimod is a new drug that enhances the immune response to tumours and viruses. It is indicated in treatment of some warts, and of basal cell carcinomas where surgery is inappropriate.

Thalidomide is the drug infamous for having caused thousands of congenital malformations during the late 1950s and 1960s in babies whose mothers took it as a supposedly safe sedative in early pregnancy. After having been banned from use for many years, it is undergoing re-evaluation for limited specific uses, such as in treatment of leprosy and as adjunctive therapy in some AIDS-associated infections and tumours (see Clinical Interest Box 4-1). It has immunostimulatory actions and inhibits tumour necrosis factor, and is being trialled as an antiangiogenic agent in several cancers, including multiple myeloma, renal cell carcinoma and glioblastoma. In Australia, it is tightly controlled because of its teratogenicity (Pregnancy Category X); patients must give written informed consent

CLINICAL INTEREST BOX 49-3
COMPLEMENTARY AND ALTERNATIVE THERAPIES IN CANCER

Many CAM modalities have been tried in prevention and treatment of cancer.

Dietary modification

- High intake of fish oils (ω-3-polyunsaturated fatty acids): may be preventive.
- Antioxidants (vitamin A, β-carotene and other retinoids in fruit and vegetables; turmeric, copper, zinc): most studies show no reduction in cancer risk.
- High intake of folic acid, selenium, garlic, onions to prevent GI tract cancers: no proven benefit in colon cancer; reduced occurrence of gastric cancer. Garlic has been shown to block experimentally induced cancers in many organs, especially stomach and colorectal cancers; however, excess garlic can be toxic, leading to allergic reactions, gastrointestinal disorders, asthma, anaemia, impaired spermatogenesis and reduced serum calcium, as well as garlic odour on the breath and skin.
- Keyhole limpet haemocyanin: increases natural killer cell activity.
- Hydrazine sulfate, amygdalin (cyanide in apricot kernels), melatonin, shark cartilage: no evidence of clinical benefit.
- Coffee enemas as part of a 'detoxification' program and pain management: no evidence of efficacy.

Physical techniques

- Chiropractic in cancer pain: contraindicated; paraplegia has resulted.

Herbal 'remedies'

- Polysaccharide Krestin from mushrooms: increases phagocytic activity of leucocytes, suppresses growth of some tumours.
- Chlorella (green algae) polysaccharides and glycolipids, and phyto-oestrogens in some Chinese herbal mixtures: some immunostimulatory and antitumour actions.
- Capsaicin (from peppers, capsicums): chemoprotective or carcinogenic? No convincing evidence either way.
- Evening primrose oil, garlic, ginseng, mistletoe: antineoplastic activity in some tests, no improvement in others.
- The Australian prickly fanflower shrub (*Scaevola spinescens*) contains triterpenoids with reported antiviral immunostimulant activities; it has been used to treat terminally ill cancer patients.

Mind–body techniques

- Prayer, hypnotherapy, meditation, biofeedback, yoga: anecdotal evidence for some success in people with ability to concentrate intently.

Adapted from: Spencer & Jacobs 1999; see also Braun & Cohen 2005.

---

before treatment. Thalidomide was listed on the Australian Pharmaceutical Benefits Scheme (PBS) in February 2006, with strong warnings that even one dose can cause birth defects.

Treament of problems due to bony metastases
Bisphosphonates

The bisphosphonates (including pamidronate, zoledronic acid and sodium clodronate; see Chapter 42) bind to hydroxyapatite in bone and specifically inhibit osteoclast-mediated bone resorption. They are used to improve bone mineral density in osteoporosis and Paget's disease of bone, and to prevent corticosteroid-induced osteoporosis (see Drug Monograph 42-4). In cancers, they are used to reduce the skeletal morbidity that occurs with bony metastases; zoledronic acid is a potent injectable bisphosphonate specifically for tumour-induced hypercalcaemia.

Radioactive isotopes

The radioisotopes strontium-89 and samarium-153 are used for palliation of bone pain in osteoblastic skeletal metastases (secondary cancers in the bone).

Palliative care

Palliative care provides integrated and comprehensive care for all the medical and nursing needs to improve the quality of life of a patient for whom cure is not possible. Palliative care aims to treat all aspects of a patient's suffering—physical, psychological, social, cultural and spiritual—and to include the patient's family and close friends in the care. Traditionally, palliative care was employed when anticancer treatment had failed and active medical treatment of related medical problems had ceased. It is now recognised that palliative care is most successful when introduced at an earlier stage, in conjunction with other therapeutic modalities, and is also usefully employed in the end-stage of neurological diseases such as multiple sclerosis and motor neuron disease, and in severe renal or hepatic failure and AIDS.

Optimal care acknowledges that suffering includes many aspects and that a multidisciplinary approach is needed. Aspects to be considered include the patient's responses to diagnosis of a life-threatening illness; the patient's choice to transfer from curative to palliative care; the deterioration to a terminal stage; discussion (or not) of death and dying; optimal ways to answer questions put by patients and their families (see Clinical Interest Box 49-4); ethical isses related to withdrawal of treatment and life-support; support for

---

CLINICAL INTEREST BOX 49-4 FREQUENTLY ASKED QUESTIONS ABOUT PALLIATIVE CARE (RELEVANT TO PHARMACOLOGY)

Questions asked by providers:

When is it appropriate to introduce palliative care?
When the goal of care is comfort rather than cure; disease-modifying treatments may be continued if they benefit the patient.

How can I introduce the idea of palliative care?
With the idea that a team of medical, nursing, allied health and support staff can work together with the general practitioner to improve the quality of life for the patient and family.

Questions asked by patients:

Do I have to take morphine/opioids?
These medications provide the best pain relief, and are safe and predictable; however, there is a range of pain relief medicines and other techniques available.

Does taking morphine/opioids mean that I am going to die soon?
No, these medications can be taken for long periods to improve quality of life and allow more activities.

Will I become addicted to them? Should I 'save them for later'?
No, people taking opioids for pain relief rarely become addicted. Controlling pain early is important.

Will opioids make me 'woozy' or unsafe to drive?
They will help you sleep better at night. They may make you drowsy, especially on long trips; be especially careful if you have taken 'top-up' doses.

Can I keep taking my herbal medicines (or using other CAM)?
If they are not dangerous or too expensive for you; please tell us what you are taking so we can check for any interactions with prescribed medicines.

Questions asked by family and carers:

Why does (s)he need painkillers if (s)he is unconscious?
The patient may regain consciousness, and deserves ongoing pain relief.

Shouldn't the patient be 'on a drip' (IV fluids)?
Only if dehydrated; as the body 'closes down', less fluid is required or tolerated.

Adapted from: Palliative Care Expert Group 2005.

---

completing essential life-tasks; and the later bereavement and grief of family and friends.

Palliative care may be carried out in a variety of settings, including general practice, the home, aged-care facilities, hospitals and hospices. Large hospitals with oncology units usually have a palliative care service and a multidisciplinary team of health-care professionals to whom patients can be referred (see Palliative Care Expert Group 2005). The team aims to provide specialist palliative care services coordinated by one member; the team may include the patient's general practitioner, a palliative care nurse, palliative medicine specialist, other specialist physicians (e.g. oncologist, radiologist, neurologist), clinical pharmacist, social worker, counsellor, chaplain, dietitian, other allied health professionals, volunteer carer, and patient support group representative. Team members themselves need support and care, as this is a very demanding area of medicine.

Pharmacological aspects of palliative care

As well as the drugs used to treat the disease for which the patient is receiving care, many other drugs may be useful in providing improved quality of life and comfort, such as analgesics for pain, and drugs to treat side-effects of the primary drugs (e.g. antiemetics or immunostimulants). Decisions may also need to be made as to whether or for how long to continue with drugs being administered for other

concurrent chronic conditions, such as diabetes mellitus, hypertension, arthritis or asthma.

Drugs commonly administered in palliative care situations include:

- analgesics: paracetamol, non-steroidal anti-inflammatory drugs, opioids (see Ch. 16)
- analgesic adjuvants: anaesthetics (Ch. 15), antiepileptic agents (Ch. 18), antidepressants (Ch. 19), antianxiety drugs and sedatives (Ch. 17), corticosteroids (Ch. 40)
- laxatives and antiemetics (Ch. 34)
- skeletal and/or smooth muscle relaxants (Chs 11, 13, 15).

Analgesics in palliative care

Pain is one of the commonest symptoms in advanced cancer and the most feared; it is often not adequately treated. Apart from physical signs and symptoms, pain may exacerbate anxiety and depression, social problems, and cultural and spiritual problems. Patients need reassurance that there are effective analgesic drugs to treat pain, that they are unlikely to become dependent on opioid analgesics, and that satisfactory pain control can be achieved for more than 90% of cancer patients. Analgesics are used in the stepwise 'ladder' approach: non-opioids first (aspirin), then mild opioids (codeine), then strong opioids (morphine or fentanyl); see Chapter 16.

Analgesic drugs need to be chosen appropriately and given in adequate doses and frequently enough to keep the patient pain-free, with instructions for extra dosing for 'breakthrough' pain, and warning of and treatments for adverse effects such as constipation.

Adequate control of **breakthrough pain** is an important issue in palliative care, for example in patients with bony metastases from cancer. It is defined as pain that occurs between regular doses of an analgesic that normally controls the patient's pain. It is important for the patient's quality of life that this pain be controlled effectively, usually with an extra dose of the patient's regular opioid. The breakthrough dose is determined by consideration of the current 24-hour analgesic dose equivalent, one-sixth of which is given every 4 hours (for immediate-release formulations). The breakthrough dose may be 50%–100% of the regular 4-hourly dose, at intervals not less than 30 minutes, for up to three doses. The normal dose should then be given at the regular time. The number of breakthrough doses required over a 24-hour period is an indication of the need to consider increasing the regular dose.

Particularly careful dosing of opioids is required in elderly patients, those with renal or severe liver impairment, and when changing between formulations (oral to parenteral, or immediate- to sustained-release) or between opioids (morphine to fentanyl).

CANCER CHEMOTHERAPY RESEARCH

Research into the cell biology and pathology of cancer and into new agents for cancer chemotherapy is a priority area of study in medical science. Many new drugs are being developed and trialled with the hope of improving the treatment and survival of cancer patients. Some of the new 'targets' for anticancer drugs are discussed in Chapter 48.

Clinical trials of anticancer drugs

Because of their potential toxicity, antineoplastic agents are usually not tested on healthy volunteers but are fast-tracked through to phase II of clinical trials. Their first use in humans is in a small number of patients with the condition to be treated, starting with low doses, and with regular monitoring for safety and efficacy. Patients are often invited to participate in multicentre clinical trials, as cooperation between medical scientists and physicians in several oncology units will increase the numbers of patients with a particular condition able to be recruited and thus will reduce the time taken for trials to be completed and results published and implemented.

Special Access Scheme

The Special Access Scheme (SAS) is a process administered in Australia by the Therapeutic Goods Administration of the Commonwealth Department of Health and Ageing (see www.tga.gov.au/index.htm). It refers to arrangements whereby an unapproved therapeutic good (e.g. drug or device) can be imported or supplied for a single patient on a case-by-case basis. The medical practitioner must provide details of the patient, the product and the prescriber, and give clinical justification for the requirement for the product. The SAS may be applied in the case of seriously ill patients who may benefit from a new anticancer agent that is being used overseas but has not yet been approved for general use in Australia.

Liposomes

Another promising area of study is the use of liposomes as a drug delivery system for lipid-soluble drugs. Liposomes are synthetic spherical vesicles consisting of one or more lipid bilayers. They are used as artificial membrane models and diagnostic agents, and as carriers to deliver drugs, vaccines, genes or imaging agents. Drugs encapsulated in a liposome capsule can be distributed differently in the body from free drugs. Liposomes accumulate at sites of inflammation and infection, as well as in some solid tumours, and can be 'triggered' to release their drug contents in specific cell types, by light, heat or enzymes.

Liposomes are under study for the drugs used in treatment of systemic fungal infections (amphotericin B) and for the treatment of specific cancers. Doxorubicin, cisplatin and MTX are antineoplastic agents currently undergoing clinical testing in liposome formulations. Doxorubicin in liposomes has been reported to deliver the drug more directly to the site of action, resulting in fewer cardiac and other adverse reactions. Cisplatin in liposomes has been reported to cause much less kidney damage than other formulations. The potential exists for liposomes to be an exciting new avenue of drug delivery.

Complementary and alternative medicine modalities

Many people search for relief from symptoms of cancer in treatment modalities other than scientific medicine (although, as described earlier, a large proportion of anticancer agents do in fact come from or are based on natural products from plants, fungi and mammalian cells; see Clinical Interest Box 49-2). This is a worldwide phenomenon, especially in people in developed countries who are wealthy, well educated and under 50 years old.

The types of complementary and alternative medicine modalities that are popular include 'metabolic' therapies, diets, megadoses of vitamins, acupuncture, electrotherapy, herbal remedies, imagery, homeopathy, spiritual methods and 'immune' treatments. Although some of the methods may be useful, inexpensive or harmless, many are costly and potentially toxic, and have never been subjected to the rigorous scientific testing that is required of drugs before approval and marketing. Sadly, many people also rely on unproven 'natural remedies' until a tumour has grown so large that it is too late for conventional anticancer treatments (surgery, radiation, drugs) to be effective.

With respect to prevention of cancer, it is worth recalling that up to 80% of cancers are initiated by or exacerbated by natural causes, including carcinogens in the environment (e.g. tars and other hydrocarbons, UV radiation) or dietary or lifestyle factors (high-fat/low-fibre diets, nitrosamines, aflatoxins, cigarettes). We cannot alter our genotype, which

may endow us with oncogenes or predisposition to particular cancers, but some of the environmental factors are avoidable.

Patients often use both prescribed medical therapies and complementary and alternative therapies concurrently. It is becoming apparent that drug interactions between conventional medical treatments and complementary and alternative medicines do occur and that the latter can have adverse effects, so it is important that patients discuss with their physicians what other remedies they are using. Some unorthodox methods tried in treatment of cancer are listed in Clinical Interest Box 49-3. Complementary and alternative techniques have also been used to treat the symptoms of cancer and the adverse effects of conventional treatments, such as pain, breathlessness, nausea and vomiting, and mucositis. Relaxation training and hypnosis have been shown to improve patients' coping skills.

PREGNANCY SAFETY

ADEC Category	Drug
A	Calcium folinate (Leucovorin), metoclopramide
B1	Dolasetron, imiquimod, mesna, ondansetron
B2	allopurinol, BCG (non-vaccine), rasburicase, trastuzumab
B3	Amifostine, anagrelide, filgrastim, interferon alfa-2a, interferon alfa-2b, lenograstim, levamisole, tamoxifen, toremifene, zoledronic acid
C	Anastrozole, exemestane, gefitinib, octreotide, rituximab
D	Bleomycin, capecitabine, carboplatin, carmustine, chlorambucil, cisplatin, cladribine, colaspase, cyclophosphamide, cytarabine, dacarbazine, dactinomycin, daunorubicin, docetaxel, doxorubicin, etoposide, fluorouracil, flutamide, gemcitabine, goserelin, ifosfamide, leuprorelin, medroxyprogesterone, megestrol, mercaptopurine, methotrexate, paclitaxel, procarbazine, samarium-153, teniposide, thioguanine, topotecan, vinblastine, vincristine
X	Isotretinoin (oral), raloxifene, thalidomide

Note: Due to the large number of drugs discussed in this chapter, sample drugs only have been included in this Pregnancy Safety listing. In general, it should be noted that:
- because of their inherent toxicity and potential mutagenicity and carcinogenicity, cytotoxic agents (alkylating agents, antimetabolites, antitumour antibiotics, mitotic inhibitors and topoisomerase I inhibitors) and radioactive isotopes are all in Category D (suspected or expected to cause human fetal malformations)
- hormones tend to be in Categories B3 or D
- supportive therapy, including thiol donors, colony-stimulating factors, immunostimulants, bisphosphonates and antiemetics, are less toxic and hence fall in Categories A, B and C.

DRUGS AT A GLANCE 49: Antineoplastic agents

Note: Tables 49-1 and 49-2 contain extensive summaries of the main categories of cytotoxic and hormonal drugs, including clinical indications for use and major adverse drug reactions and toxicities; below is an abbreviated overview.

Therapeutic group	Pharmacological group	Key examples	Key pages
Cytotoxic agents (see also Table 49-1)	Alkylating agents	cyclophosphamide dacarbazine	770–4 770
	Antimetabolites	methotrexate fluorouracil	773, 5, 6 773
	Antibiotics	bleomycin } doxorubicin }	773, 6
	Mitotic inhibitors	vincristine } paclitaxel }	776
	Topoisomerase I inhibitors Topoisomerase II inhibitors	topotecan } teniposide }	777
	Platinum compounds	cisplatin	773, 7
	Asparaginase enzyme	colaspase	777
Hormonal antineoplastic agents (see also Table 49-2)	Androgens	fluoxymesterone	779
	Antiandrogens	cyproterone } flutamide }	779
	Gonadotrophin-releasing hormone analogues	goserelin } leuprorelin }	779, 80
	Anti-oestrogens	tamoxifen } toremifene }	780, 1
	Progestogens	megestrol	781
	Somatostatin analogues	octreotide	781
Miscellaneous antineoplastic agents	Monoclonal antibodies	trastuzumab } rituximab }	781, 2
	Tyrosine kinase inhibitors	imatinib } gefitinib }	782
	Retinoids	tretinoin	782
	Radioactive isotopes	iodine-131	783
Supportive therapy	Antiemetics	metoclopramide } ondansetron }	783
	Folinic acid rescue	calcium folinate	783, 4
	Granulocyte colony-stimulating factors	filgrastim	784
	Sulfur-donating compounds	mesna	784
Treatment of hyperuricaemia	Xanthine oxidase inhibitor Uric oxidase enzyme	allopurinol } rasburicase }	784
	Immunostimulating agents	interferons levamisole BCG (non-vaccine) imiquimod thalidomide	784, 5
	Bisphosphonates	alendronate	786

DRUGS AT A GLANCE 49: Antineoplastic agents

| **Palliative care** (analgesics; breakthrough pain) | Non-steroidal anti-inflammatory drugs Opioids | paracetamol morphine } | 786–8 |

BCG = bacille Calmette–Guérin.

KEY POINTS

- Drugs used to treat cancers, i.e. antineoplastic agents, include cytotoxic agents, hormones and antihormones, immunostimulating agents and agents acting by miscellaneous mechanisms.

- The use of cytotoxic agents in the treatment of cancer is based on the individual drug's effects in inhibiting macromolecular synthesis and thus interfering with cell division or replication at some point in the cell cycle. These drugs are classified according to their potential mechanisms of action: alkylating agents, antimetabolites, antibiotic antitumour agents and mitotic inhibitors.

- Alkylating agents such as cyclophosphamide contain reactive alkyl groups that can bind strongly to bases in DNA, thus impairing DNA replication and transcription of RNA.

- Antimetabolites are chemically related to folic acid (e.g. methotrexate) or to a purine or pyrimidine base (mercaptopurine, fluorouracil). They inhibit macromolecular synthesis by causing copying errors during DNA synthesis, or by inhibiting enzymes in pathways to the macromolecules DNA, RNA and proteins.

- Antibiotic antitumour agents include the anthracycline, bleomycin and actinomycin groups. These may bind to DNA, intercalate between DNA strands or inhibit topoisomerase II enzymes.

- Mitotic inhibitors such as the vinca alkaloids and taxanes are phase-specific agents, inhibiting the cell cycle during the mitosis stage.

- Cytotoxic drugs are usually non-selective, with antiproliferative actions on all rapidly dividing cells. They can therefore impair normal body cells that have high rates of growth, such as those in the GI tract, bone marrow and hair follicles, commonly causing mouth ulceration and GI tract dysfunction, bone marrow suppression and alopecia.

- Growth of hormone-dependent tumours can be inhibited by depriving the tumour of its hormone (by surgery, radiation, or suppression of synthesis or release) or by use of an antagonistic hormone. Prostate tumours may be treated pharmacologically with antiandrogens (flutamide), and breast cancers with anti-oestrogens (tamoxifen) or aromatase inhibitors (exemestane).

- Other antineoplastic agents include topoisomerase I inhibitors (the camptothecins), the enzyme colaspase, specific tyrosine kinase inhibitors, and monoclonal antibodies against specific oncogene proteins.

- Serious adverse drug reactions to antineoplastic agents are treated with specific methods or drugs, e.g. with powerful antiemetics or bone marrow-supportive drugs.

- Immune responses against neoplastic cells can be enhanced by administration of immunostimulating agents such as interferons, other cytokines, colony-stimulating factors and BCG (non-vaccine). Other adjunctive and supportive therapies include drugs to reduce uric acid load or minimise bone resorption in metastatic cancers.

- Palliative care involves attention to all the medical and nursing needs of the cancer patient, including physical, psychological, social and spiritual aspects; this usually requires a multidisciplinary approach.

- Research into new methods and agents useful in treating cancers is targeting chemicals in transduction pathways; natural products from plants, microorganisms and marine organisms; and methods to deliver drugs to or activate them in cancer cells.

- CAM modalities applied in preventing, treating or palliating cancer include dietary modifications, herbal remedies and mind–body techniques.

REVIEW EXERCISES

1 Describe the proposed mechanisms of action and pharmacological effects of the four main groups of cytotoxic agents.

2 Discuss the various therapeutic modalities and drug groups useful in treating hormone-dependent cancers, taking prostate cancer or breast cancer as an example.

3 Explain how adjunctive therapy can be used to modify bone marrow suppression, immunosuppression, hyperuricaemia, and bone resorption occurring during cancer treatment.

4   Describe the reasons why live virus vaccines should not be administered to patients receiving antineoplastic drug therapy.

5   Name the specific dose-limiting adverse effects for methotrexate, cyclophosphamide, vincristine and doxorubicin. Discuss methods of managing these toxicities.

6   Explain the causes and describe possible treatments of severe nausea and vomiting during cancer chemotherapy.

7   Define the term palliative care and describe important aspects of it.

REFERENCES AND FURTHER READING

Ackland SP. Drug treatment of breast cancer. *Australian Prescriber* 1998; 21: 15–19.

Adlard JW. Thalidomide in the treatment of cancer. *Anti-Cancer Drugs* 2000; 11: 787–91.

Andresen TL, Jensen SS, Jorgensen K. Advanced strategies in liposomal cancer therapy: problems and prospects of active and tumor specific drug release. *Progress in Lipid Research* 2005; 44(1): 68–97.

Australian Drug Evaluation Committee. *Prescribing Medicines in Pregnancy: An Australian Categorisation of Risk of Drug Use in Pregnancy*. 4th edn. Canberra: Therapeutic Goods Administration, 1999.

Australian Medicines Handbook 2006. Adelaide: AMH, 2006.

Bowman WC, Rand MJ. *Textbook of Pharmacology*. 2nd edn. Oxford: Blackwell, 1980 [ch. 38].

Boyer MJ. Drug therapy of lung cancer. *Australian Prescriber* 2003; 26(5): 103–5.

Braun L, Cohen M. *Herbs and Natural Supplements: An Evidence-Based Guide*. Sydney: Elsevier Mosby; 2005.

Caswell A (ed.). *MIMS Annual 2005*. Sydney: CMPMedica Australia, 2005.

Chan OT, Yang LX. The immunological effects of taxanes. *Cancer Immunology, Immunotherapy* 2000; 49: 181–5.

Clarke S. New treatments for advanced and metastatic colorectal cancer: clinical applications. *Australian Prescriber* 2002; 25(5): 111–13.

Clarke S, Sharma R. Angiogenesis inhibitors in cancer: mechanisms of action. *Australian Prescriber* 2006; 29(1) 9–12.

Cragg GM, Newman DJ. Discovery and development of antineoplastic agents from natural sources. *Cancer Investigation* 1999; 17: 153–63.

Dagher R, Johnson J, Williams G, Keegan P, Pazdur R. Accelerated approval of oncology products: a decade of experience. *Journal of the National Cancer Institute* 2004; 96(20): 1500–9.

Glare PA, Virik K. Can we do better in end-of-life care? The mixed management model and palliative care. *Medical Journal of Australia* 2001; 175: 530–3.

Mackall CL. T-cell immunodeficiency following cytotoxic antineoplastic therapy: a review. *Stem Cells* 2000; 18: 10–18.

Mainwaring P. Angiogenesis inhibitors in cancer: clinical applications. *Australian Prescriber* 2006; 29(1): 13–15.

Mann J. *Murder, Magic and Medicine*. Oxford: Oxford University Press, 1992.

Medical Journal of Australia 2001; 175 [whole issue devoted to death and dying].

Newell DR. How to develop a successful cancer drug: molecules to medicines or targets to treatments? *European Journal of Cancer* 2005; 41(5): 676–82.

Palliative Care Expert Group. *Therapeutic Guidelines: Palliative Care, version 2*. Melbourne: Therapeutic Guidelines, 2005.

Patel GB, Sprott GD. Archaeabacterial ether lipid liposomes (archaeosomes) as novel vaccine and drug delivery systems. *Critical Reviews in Biotechnology* 1999; 19: 317–57.

Peter MacCallum Cancer Institute. *Standard Treatment Guidelines (Draft)*. Melbourne: Medical Oncology Unit, Peter MacCallum Cancer Institute, 2000.

Rang HP, Dale MM, Ritter JM, Moore PK. *Pharmacology*. 5th edn. Edinburgh: Churchill Livingstone, 2003 [chs 5, 50].

Rivlin RS. Historical perspective on the use of garlic. *Journal of Nutrition* 2001; 131(Suppl): 951S–54S (and following papers on effects of garlic supplements).

Rivory LP. New drugs for colorectal cancer: mechanisms of action. *Australian Prescriber* 2002; 25(5): 108–10.

Rothenberg ML, Carbone DP, Johnson DH. Improving the evaluation of new cancer treatments: challenges and opportunities. *Nature Reviews. Cancer* 2003; 3(4): 303–9.

Segelov E. The emperor's new clothes: can chemotherapy survive? *Australian Prescriber* 2006; 29(1): 2–3.

Speight TM, Holford NHG (eds). *Avery's Drug Treatment*. 4th edn. Auckland: Adis International, 1997.

Spencer JW, Jacobs JJ. *Complementary/Alternative Medicine: An Evidence-Based Approach*. St. Louis: Mosby, 1999.

Torchilin VP. Recent advances with liposomes as pharmaceutical carriers. *Nature Reviews. Drug Discovery* 2005; 4(2): 145–60.

Vogel VG, Costantino JP, Wickerham DL et al. Effects of tamoxifen vs raloxifene on the risk of developing invasive breast cancer and other disease outcomes: the NSABP Study of Tamoxifen and Raloxifene (STAR) P-2 trial. *Journal of the American Medical Association* 2006; 295: 2727–41.

Tuckwell K (ed.). *MIMS Disease Index*. 2nd edn. Sydney: MediMedia Australia, 1996.

Ward R. Antineoplastic antibodies: clinical applications. *Australian Prescriber* 2003; 26(6): 141–3.

Watson MS, Lucas CF, Hoy AM, Back IN. *Oxford Handbook of Palliative Care*. Oxford: Oxford University Press, 2005.

ON-LINE RESOURCES

New Zealand medicines and medical devices safety authority: www.medsafe.govt.nz

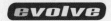 More weblinks at http://evolve.elsevier.com/AU/Bryant/pharmacology/

CHAPTER 50

Overview of Antimicrobial Chemotherapy and Antibiotic Resistance

CHAPTER FOCUS

Infections have always been a concern to those caring for the ill and injured. There is no doubt that the development of antimicrobial drugs throughout the 20th century has had an enormous effect on the health and wellbeing of the global population. Since the mass production of penicillin in 1943, the number of antibiotics has continued to grow. Unfortunately, along with the use of antimicrobial drugs has been the emergence of resistant microorganisms. The problems facing health-care professionals now include not only the prudent use of antimicrobial drugs but the need to develop new agents and to curtail the continued emergence of resistant 'superbugs'.

OBJECTIVES

- To discuss the goals of antimicrobial therapy.
- To differentiate bacteriostatic and bactericidal actions.
- To explain how microorganisms develop drug resistance.
- To discuss strategies for combating antimicrobial drug resistance.
- To discuss the general guidelines for the use of antibiotics.

KEY TERMS

antibiotics
bacteraemia
bactericidal agents
bacteriostatic agents
colonisation
Gram stain
infection

inflammation
microorganisms
resistance
sepsis
septicaemia
superinfection

INFECTIONS

INFECTIOUS diseases comprise a wide spectrum of illnesses caused by pathogenic microorganisms. Some common pathogens and their most likely sites of infection in the body are listed in Table 50-1. These pathogens can cause pneumonia, urinary tract infections, upper respiratory tract infections, gastroenteritis, venereal disease, vaginitis, tuberculosis and candidiasis, to name but a few.

Infection, the invasion and multiplication of pathogenic microorganisms in body tissues, causing disease by local cellular injury, secretion of a toxin or by antigen–antibody reaction in the host, is classified primarily as local or systemic. A localised infection involving the skin or internal organs may progress to a systemic infection. A systemic infection involves the whole body rather than a localised area of the body. Several terms describe the degree of local or systemic infection.

Colonisation is the localised presence of microorganisms in body tissues or organs; these microorganisms can be pathogenic or part of the normal flora. Colonisation alone is not necessarily an infection: it signifies the potential for infection, depending on the multiplication of the microorganisms or an alteration in the individual's host defence mechanisms. When flora at their normal colonisation site are altered (e.g. by the administration of an antibiotic that affects pathogens and some but not all of the normal microorganisms), the unaffected microorganisms within that environment may grow in an uninhibited manner, causing a secondary infection.

Inflammation is a protective mechanism of body tissues in response to invasion or toxins produced by colonising microorganisms (see Chapter 54). This reaction consists of cytological and histological tissue responses for the localisation of phagocytic activity and destruction or removal of injurious material, leading to repair and healing.

Bacteraemia is the presence of viable bacteria in the circulatory system. **Septicaemia** refers to a systemic infection caused by microorganism multiplication in the circulation. Although bacteraemia can lead to septicaemia in an immunocompromised host, it is (depending on the pathogen) usually a short-lived, self-limited process. In an immunocompromised host, bacteraemia can rapidly produce an overwhelming systemic disease. **Sepsis** is a syndrome with multiple organ involvement that is a result of microorganisms or their toxins circulating in the blood.

For non-pathogenic organisms colonising humans or causing transient bacteraemia without tissue invasion, antibiotic therapy is rarely required in immunocompetent people, whereas prophylactic antibiotic therapy might be required in immunocompromised individuals. In most cases of localised inflammation, such as wound infections, pneumonia or urinary tract infections, antimicrobial drugs reduce the number of viable pathogens. This permits the immune system to eliminate microorganisms. Antimicrobial drugs are also an essential part of the treatment of septicaemia and sepsis.

Microorganisms are divided into several groups: bacteria, mycoplasma, spirochaetes, fungi and viruses. Bacteria are classified according to their shape, such as bacilli, spirilla and cocci, and their capacity to be stained. Specific identification of bacteria requires a Gram stain and culture with chemical testing. A **Gram stain** is a sequential procedure involving crystal violet and iodine solutions followed by alcohol, and allows the rapid classification of organisms into groups such as Gram-positive or Gram-negative rods or cocci. The culture procedures identify specific organisms, but they require 24–48 hours for completion.

Often, antibiotic selection is empirical and is based on the prescriber's clinical impression. Once culture and sensitivity results are available, the antibiotic might be changed. This is referred to as directed therapy.

ANTIMICROBIAL THERAPY

The treatment of an infectious disease depends on the microorganism responsible, and different groups of antimicrobial drugs are used to treat different groups of microorganisms. Antimicrobial drugs can help cure or control most infections caused by microorganisms but they alone do not necessarily produce the cure. They are often adjuncts to methods such as surgical incision and drainage, and wound debridement for removal of non-viable infected tissue.

The first major antimicrobial drug group was the sulfonamides, which were introduced into clinical practice in 1933. So successful were these drugs in treating staphylococcal septicaemia that Gerhard Domagk was awarded the Nobel Prize for Medicine in 1939 for his discovery of the antibacterial effects of the sulfonamide drug prontosil. The authorities in Germany at that time forced him to decline the award but he later received the diploma and the medal. The second major group of antimicrobial drugs was the penicillins (introduced in the 1940s).

Antibiotics are natural substances derived from certain organisms (bacteria, fungi and others) that can suppress growth or destroy microorganisms. There are now thousands of natural, synthetic and semisynthetic antibacterial drugs that are all commonly referred to as antibiotics. Other antimicrobial agents include the antimycobacterial, antifungal and antiviral agents. These drugs differ markedly in their physicochemical characteristics, mechanisms of action, pharmacological properties and antibacterial spectra.

Mechanism of action

The goal of antimicrobial therapy is to destroy or suppress the growth of infecting microorganisms so that normal host defences and other supporting mechanisms can control the infection, resulting in its cure. To exert its effects, an antimicrobial agent

TABLE 50-1 Primary organisms and common sites of infection

ORGANISM	INFECTION SITE
Gram-positive cocci	

Staphylococcus aureus
  Non-penicillinase-producing
  Penicillinase-producing
Staphylococcus epidermidis
  Non-penicillinase-producing
  Penicillinase-producing
  Methicillin-resistant
	Burns, skin infections, decubital and surgical wounds, paranasal sinus and middle ear (chronic sinusitis and otitis), lungs, lung abscess, pleura, endocardium, bone (osteomyelitis), joints

Streptococcus pneumoniae	Paranasal sinus and middle ear, lungs, pleura
Streptococcus pyogenes (group A β-haemolytic)	Burns, skin infections, decubital and surgical wounds, paranasal sinus and middle ear, throat, bone (osteomyelitis), joints
Streptococcus, viridans group	Endocardium
Gram-positive bacilli	
Clostridium tetani (anaerobe)	Puncture wounds, lacerations and crush injuries; toxins affecting nervous system
Corynebacterium diphtheriae	Throat, upper part of the respiratory tract
Gram-negative cocci	
Neisseria gonorrhoeae	Urethra, prostate, epididymis and testes, joints
Neisseria meningitidis	Meninges
Enteric Gram-negative bacilli	
As a group (*Bacteroides, Enterobacter, Escherichia coli, Klebsiella pneumoniae, Proteus mirabilis*, other *Proteus, Salmonella, Serratia, Shigella*)	Peritoneum, biliary tract, kidney and bladder, prostate, decubital and surgical wounds, bone
Bacteroides	Brain abscess, lung abscess, throat, peritoneum
Enterobacter	Peritoneum, biliary tract, kidney and bladder, endocardium
Escherichia coli	Peritoneum, biliary tract, kidney and bladder
Klebsiella pneumoniae	Lungs, lung abscess
Other Gram-negative bacilli	
Haemophilus influenzae	Meninges, paranasal sinus and middle ear, lungs, pleura
Pseudomonas aeruginosa	Burns, paranasal sinus and middle ear (chronic otitis media), decubital and surgical wounds, lungs, joints
Acid-fast bacilli	
Mycobacterium tuberculosis, Mycobacterium avium	Lungs, pleura, peritoneum, meninges, kidney and bladder, testes, bone, joints
Mycoplasma	
Mycoplasma pneumoniae	Lungs
Spirochaetes	
Treponema pallidum (syphilis)	Any tissue or vascular organ of the body

TABLE 50-1 Primary organisms and common sites of infection—cont'd

ORGANISM	INFECTION SITE
Fungi	
Aspergillus	Paranasal sinus and middle ear, lungs
Candida species	Skin infections, throat, lungs, endocardium, kidney and bladder, vagina
Cryptococcus	Lungs
Viruses	
Herpes virus or varicella-zoster virus	Skin infections (herpes simplex or zoster)
Enterovirus, mumps virus, and others	Meninges, epididymis, testes
Respiratory viruses (including Epstein–Barr virus)	Throat, lungs
Anaerobes	
Gram-positive	
Clostridium difficile	
Clostridium perfringens	
Peptococcus species	
Peptostreptococcus species	Deep wounds, gut
Gram-negative	
Bacteroides fragilis	
Fusobacterium species	

must first gain access to the target site. This is influenced by the drug's pharmacokinetic profile, which includes absorption and distribution of the drug into and by way of the circulatory system, metabolism and elimination. Specific antibiotics or antimicrobial agents in certain circumstances (e.g. changes in permeability of the blood–brain barrier with meningitis) are capable of penetrating the site of infection and having an affinity for the bacterial target proteins. Sometimes, as in the case of infections of the skin and eyes, local application to the infected area is necessary. Once the drug has reached its site of action, it can exert either bactericidal or bacteriostatic effects, depending on its mechanisms of action.

Bacteriostatic agents inhibit bacterial growth, allowing host defence mechanisms additional time to remove the invading microorganisms. **Bactericidal agents**, on the other hand, cause bacterial cell death and lysis. Antimicrobial agents can be divided into bacteriostatic and bactericidal categories; the sulfonamides are an example of the former and the penicillins the latter. Such categorisation is not always valid or reliable because the same antimicrobial agent might have either effect depending on the dose administered and the concentration achieved at its site of action. Tetracycline, for example, is generally bacteriostatic but may be bactericidal in high concentrations. Chloramphenicol, which is often listed as a bacteriostatic drug, has bactericidal effects against

Streptococcus pneumoniae and *Haemophilus influenzae* in the cerebrospinal fluid.

Antimicrobial agents exert their bacteriostatic or bactericidal effects in one of four major ways (see Chapter 51):
• inhibiting bacterial cell wall synthesis: unlike host cells, bacteria are not isotonic with body fluids, so their contents are under high osmotic pressure and their viability depends on the integrity of their cell walls. Any compound that inhibits any step in the synthesis of the cell wall weakens it and causes the cell to lyse. Antimicrobial agents with this mechanism of action are bactericidal
• disrupting or altering membrane permeability: this results in leakage of essential bacterial metabolic substrates. Agents causing these effects can be either bacteriostatic or bactericidal
• inhibiting protein synthesis: some antimicrobial agents induce the formation of defective protein molecules; such agents are bactericidal in their action. Antimicrobial agents that inhibit specific steps in protein synthesis are bacteriostatic
• inhibiting synthesis of essential metabolites: antimicrobial agents that work in this manner structurally resemble normal intracellular chemicals and act as competitive inhibitors in a metabolic pathway. Generally, they are bacteriostatic agents.

CLINICAL INTEREST BOX 50-1 AUSTRALIAN MEDICINAL PLANTS

It has been suggested that more than 100 species of Australian plants are used by Aborigines to treat sores, cuts and wounds. Many exhibit promising properties for treating bacterial and fungal infections. Plants exhibiting astringent properties can be used to staunch bleeding and to provide a natural protective bandage. Tinctures of the inner bark of river red gum (*Eucalyptus camaldulensis*) and cocky apple (*Planchonia careya*) have been applied to sores for this reason. The stalks of the caustic bush, or caustic vine (*Sarcostemma australe*), and milkwood tree (*Alstonia actinophylla*) ooze a milky sap that also provides a protective bandage. This sap might possess antibacterial activity, as the proteolytic enzymes are reported to digest bacteria in infected tissue. Antibacterial activity has also been reported in root decoctions of hopwood (*Dodonea viscosa*). These have been used for cuts and open wounds and the leaves chewed as a remedy for toothache. This plant is widespread throughout eastern Australia and the presence of numerous active constituents (perhaps flavonoids) might provide the noted antibacterial and anti-inflammatory effects.

Wounds can be disinfected by infusions from plants of the Myrtaceae families known for their essential or volatile oils (tea tree and eucalypt). The active ingredients are thought to be cineoles. The yellow box (*Eucalyptus melliodora*) is one of the few eucalypts containing greater than 70% cineoles and which exhibits antibacterial activity. Studies at the University of Western Sydney have determined moderate antibacterial activity against *Staphylococcus aureus*, *Escherichia coli* and *Candida albicans*. Extracts of the lemon-scented gum (*Eucalyptus citriodora*) exhibit bacteriostatic activity; the active ingredients are thought to be citronellal, citriodorol and kinos. A well-known antiseptic available for sale is tea-tree oil, obtained from distillation of the leaves of *Melaleuca alterniflora*. It contains the substance terpinen-4-ol, which is thought to be bacteriostatic.

Bathing the eyes in an infusion of sneezeweeds (*Centipeda minima* or *Centipeda thespidioides*) may treat ocular infections such as sandy blight. Although the active ingredient is unknown, the leaves, stems and flowers may contain alkaloids. Similarly the inner bark and sapwood of the green plum (*Buchanania obovata*) is used for treating oral and eye infections.

ANTIBIOTIC RESISTANCE

Resistance refers to the ability of a particular microorganism to resist the effects of a specific antibiotic. From a historical perspective, with each cycle of introduction of new antibiotics, there has been an accompanying cycle of emerging resistance to the drugs. This is a worldwide problem but it is not a new one. Resistant microorganisms were present in our environment before the introduction of antibiotics into clinical medicine. In terms of 'bacterial warfare', many bacteria produce antibiotics to protect themselves against the inhibitory effects of antibiotics produced by a neighbouring bacterial species. This "strong selective pressure consistently resulted in the survival and spread of resistant bacteria" (Barbosa & Levy 2000). Within 2 years of the introduction of penicillin, resistance began to be noted. The emergence of microorganisms resistant to antibiotics has continued (Table 50-2).

Mechanisms of antimicrobial drug resistance

Resistance can occur in one of several ways (Figure 50-1), for example:

- the antimicrobial drug is unable to reach the potential target site of its action. Some organisms, such as *Pseudomonas*, form a protective membrane (a glycocalyx or slime) that prevents the antibiotic from reaching the cell wall

- the microorganism produces an enzyme that acts to reduce or eliminate the toxic effect of the antibiotic on the cell wall. Examples of these enzymes are the β-lactamases, which cleave the β-lactam ring on penicillins and cephalosporins, forming inactive compounds

- the target site for the drug is altered so the drug can no longer bind to the target (e.g. the low-affinity penicillin-binding proteins)

- the drug is pumped out by an efflux pump (this mechanism confers tetracycline resistance)

- the development of bypass pathways that compensate for the loss of function due to the antimicrobial drug (e.g. resistance to sulfonamides).

Combating antimicrobial drug resistance

Many resistant strains of bacteria exist in Australasia, and there are ongoing problems with methicillin-resistant *Staphylococcus aureus* in outpatients and inpatients in Australia. In 1994, the first case of vancomycin-resistant *Enterococcus faecium* was reported in Melbourne. The appearance and spread of antimicrobial resistance is, however, not limited to bacteria. Resistance has now been reported among fungi, for example *Candida albicans*, and helminths (Geerts & Gryseels 2000). Of increasing importance worldwide is the emergence and spread of multi-drug-resistant HIV-1 (Omrani & Pillay 2000) and *Mycobacterium tuberculosis* (Schluger 2000).

TABLE 50-2 Examples of emergence of antibiotic resistance

YEAR	ANTIBIOTIC RESISTANCE
1947	Resistance to penicillin
1960s	Streptomycin-resistant *Enterococcus*
1968	Multi-drug resistant *Shigella*
1960–1970s	Methicillin-resistant *Staphylococcus aureus*
1970s	Ampicillin-resistant *Neisseria gonorrhoeae*, *Haemophilus influenzae* and *Escherichia coli*
1970s	Penicillin-resistant *Streptococcus pneumoniae*
1979	Gentamicin-resistant *Enterococcus faecalis*
1980s	Cephalosporin-resistant *Klebsiella pneumoniae*
1980s	Vancomycin-resistant *Staphylococcus aureus*
1986	Vancomycin-resistant *Enterococcus faecium*
1987	Ciprofloxacin-resistant *Escherichia coli*
1994	Vancomycin-resistant *Enterococcus faecium*, reported in Melbourne
1997	Vancomycin-resistant *Staphylococcus aureus*, reported in Japan

Source: Swartz 2000.

The adverse consequences of increasing antimicrobial drug resistance will inevitably be increases in rates of hospitalisation, duration of hospital stay and rates of mortality.

Strategies to combat antimicrobial drug resistance include:

- encouraging optimal use of antimicrobials
- selective control, restriction or removal of antimicrobial agents or classes
- use of antimicrobial drugs in rotation or cyclical patterns
- use of combinations of antimicrobial drugs to prevent the emergence of resistance (Walsh 2000).

SUPERINFECTION

Superinfection is an infection that occurs during antimicrobial therapy delivered for therapeutic or prophylactic reasons. Most antibiotics reduce or eradicate the normal microbial flora of the body, which are then replaced by resistant exogenous or endogenous bacteria. If the number of these replacement organisms is large and the host conditions favourable, clinical superinfection can occur.

Around 2% of people treated with antibiotics contract superinfections. The risk is greater when large doses of antibiotics are given, when more than one antibiotic is administered concurrently and when broad-spectrum drugs are used. Some specific antimicrobials are more commonly associated with superinfection than others. For example,

Pseudomonas organisms frequently colonise and infect individuals taking cephalosporins. In a similar manner, people taking tetracyclines may become infected with *Candida albicans*. Generally, superinfections are caused by microorganisms that are resistant to the drug the individual is receiving. In the past, penicillinase-producing staphylococci were the most common cause of superinfection. *Staphylococcus aureus* and *Staphylococcus epidermidis* superinfections, especially with methicillin-resistant strains, are again on the rise. Gram-negative enteric bacilli and fungi are the most common offenders. The proper management of superinfections includes discontinuing the drug being given or replacing it with another drug to which the organism is sensitive, culturing the suspected infected area, and administering an antimicrobial agent effective against the new offending organism.

GENERAL GUIDELINES FOR USE OF ANTIBIOTICS

Perhaps the first question that should be posed is whether an antimicrobial drug is needed. Several important principles, however, guide the judicious and optimal use of the antibiotics (Antibiotic Expert Group 2006). These include:

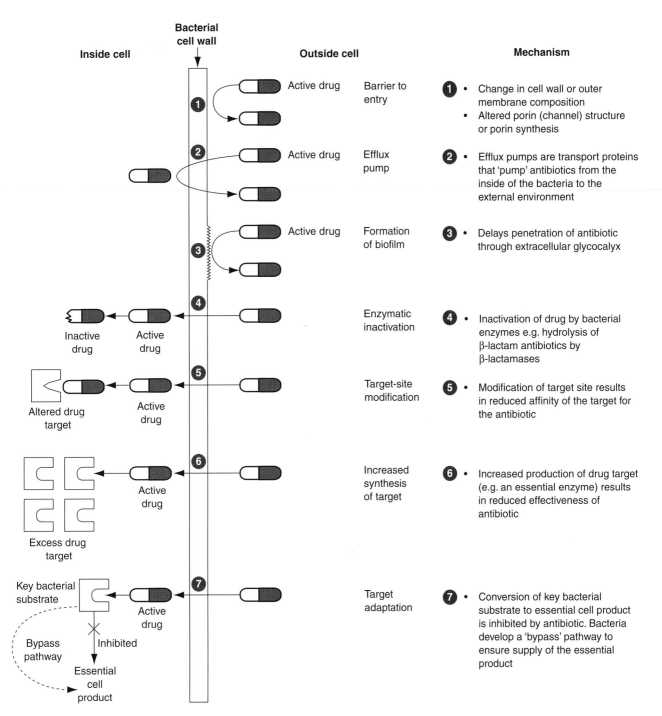

FIGURE 50-1 Seven mechanisms of antibiotic resistance.

- using an antibacterial drug only when indicated
- identifying the infecting microorganism
- determining susceptibility of the microorganism
- using a drug with the narrowest spectrum of activity for the known or likely organism
- using a single drug unless combination therapy is specifically indicated to ensure efficacy or reduce the emergence of resistance

- using a dose of drug that is high enough to ensure efficacy with minimal toxicity and reduces the likelihood of resistance
- using a short duration of treatment (e.g. 1 week) unless evidence indicates that a longer duration is required.

Because most antimicrobial agents have a specific effect on a limited range of microorganisms, the prescriber must formulate a specific diagnosis about the potential pathogens or organisms most likely causing the infection. The drug most likely to be specifically effective against the suspected microorganism can then be selected (empirical therapy). It is known, for example, that microorganisms commonly isolated in acute adult infections of the lung include pneumococci, *Haemophilus*-strain streptococci, and staphylococci. Antimicrobial agents specifically toxic to those organisms may be administered temporarily. The drugs can then be changed, if necessary, after laboratory reports have been received.

Identification of the microorganism is most reliably accomplished by obtaining specimens from the infected area if possible (e.g. urine, sputum or wound drainage) or by obtaining venous blood specimens and sending them to the laboratory for culture and identification of the causative organism. It is desirable to receive culture and sensitivity reports before initiating antimicrobial therapy. Once the organism has been identified, the appropriate drug can be administered (directed therapy).

In some situations, however, it is not practical to wait for laboratory results. For example, antimicrobial therapy must be initiated without delay in acute, life-threatening situations, such as peritonitis, septicaemia or pneumonia. In such situations, the choice of antimicrobial agent for initial use may be based on a tentative identification of the pathogen.

Some infections are most effectively treated with only one antibiotic. In other situations, combined antimicrobial drug therapy may be indicated. Indications for the simultaneous use of two or more antimicrobial agents include:

- the treatment of mixed infections, in which each drug acts on a separate portion of a complex microbial flora
- the need to delay the rapid emergence of bacteria resistant to one drug
- the need to reduce the incidence or intensity of adverse reactions by decreasing the dose of a potentially toxic drug.

Indiscriminate use of combined antimicrobial drug therapy should be avoided because of expense, toxicity and higher incidence of superinfections and resistance.

ROLE OF HOST DEFENCE MECHANISMS

No antimicrobial agent will cure an infectious process if host defence mechanisms are inadequate. Such drugs act only on the causative organisms of infectious disease, and have no effect on the defence mechanisms of the body, which need to be assessed and supported. Many infections do not require drug therapy and are adequately combated by the individual's defence mechanisms, including antibody production, phagocytosis, interferon production, fibrosis or gastrointestinal rejection (vomiting and diarrhoea). Host defence mechanisms

may, however, be diminished, for example in people with diabetes mellitus or neoplastic disease and in immunocompromised individuals (e.g. those with HIV).

The status of the host's defence mechanisms will also influence the choice of therapy, route of administration and dosage. If an infection is fulminating, for example, parenteral (preferably intravenous) administration of a bactericidal drug will be selected rather than oral administration of a bacteriostatic drug. Large loading doses of antimicrobial agents are often administered at the beginning of treatment of severe infections to achieve maximum blood concentrations rapidly. Factors influencing drug dosage are, however, often related to the status of a patient's renal function. Because many antimicrobial agents are excreted by the kidneys, a major management problem exists with individuals who have compromised renal function. Drug dosages are then generally reduced in parallel with the person's creatinine clearance levels. Haemodialysis can further alter the therapeutic regimen. In some disease states (such as burns), antibiotic dosage may need to be increased to achieve therapeutic levels. In short, the administration of an antimicrobial agent specifically toxic to the isolated microorganism is not the only important measure in antimicrobial therapy. An additional and very important determinant of the effectiveness of an antimicrobial agent is the functional state of the host's defence mechanisms.

DOSAGE AND DURATION OF THERAPY

Administering antimicrobial drugs for therapeutic purposes in adequate dosage and for long enough periods is an important principle of infectious disease therapy. Fortunately, plasma concentrations of some of the more potent antibiotics (e.g. aminoglycosides) can be monitored to prevent or minimise the risk of toxicity. Failure of antimicrobial therapy is frequently the result of drug doses being too small or being given for too short a period. Follow-up cultures should be obtained to assess the effectiveness of therapy.

Inadequate drug therapy may lead to remissions and exacerbations of the infectious process, and can contribute to the development of resistance. When antibiotics are used prophylactically, they are usually given for short periods to enhance host defence mechanisms. For example,

with perioperative antibiotics, a loading dose is given immediately before surgery and continued for 48 hours after surgery.

Many antimicrobial agents are currently in use, and health-care professionals should be familiar with the general characteristics of each drug group or category and with one or two prototype drugs in each group. Because the dosage for any given antibiotic varies with the type of infection, the site of infection and the age and health status of the individual, only general dosages or dose ranges are given in this text. The manufacturer's package insert or a hospital formulary or pharmacy should be consulted for specific dosages.

KEY POINTS

- Infectious diseases comprise a wide spectrum of illnesses caused by pathogenic microorganisms.
- Pathogenic microorganisms include bacteria, mycoplasma, spirochaetes, fungi and viruses.
- Antimicrobial therapy may include either bacteriostatic (inhibiting bacterial growth) or bactericidal (causing bacterial cell death and lysis) drugs or drugs that have both effects, depending on the concentration at the site of action.
- The goal of antimicrobial therapy is to destroy or to suppress the growth of infecting microorganisms so that normal host defences and other supporting mechanisms can control the infection, resulting in its cure.
- Resistance refers to the ability of a particular microorganism to resist the effects of a specific antibiotic. From a historical perspective, with each cycle of introduction of new antibiotics, there has been an accompanying cycle of emerging resistance to the drugs.
- Resistance is a worldwide problem but it is not a new one, as resistant microorganisms were present in our environment before the introduction of antibiotics into clinical medicine.
- Resistance can occur in one of several ways: (1) inability of the antimicrobial drug to reach the potential target site of its action, (2) the production of an enzyme that reduces or eliminates the effect of the antibiotic on the cell wall, (3) alteration of the target site for the drug so it can no longer bind to the target, (4) the drug being pumped out by an efflux pump, or (5) the development of bypass pathways that compensate for the loss of function due to the antimicrobial drug.
- Strategies to combat antimicrobial drug resistance include encouraging optimal use of antimicrobials; selective control, restriction or removal of antimicrobial agents or classes; use of antimicrobial drugs in rotation or cyclic patterns; and use of combinations of antimicrobial drugs to prevent emergence of resistance.
- Superinfection is an infection that occurs during antimicrobial therapy delivered for therapeutic or prophylactic reasons.
- Guidelines have been developed for the prudent use of antibiotics; these include using an antibacterial drug only when indicated, identifying the infecting microorganism, determining susceptibility of the microorganism, using a drug with the narrowest spectrum of activity for the known or likely organism, using a single drug unless combination therapy is specifically indicated to ensure efficacy or reduce the emergence of resistance, using a dose of drug that is high enough to ensure efficacy with minimal toxicity and reduces the likelihood of resistance, and using a short duration of treatment (e.g. 1 week) unless evidence indicates that a longer duration is required.

REVIEW EXERCISES

1 Describe the ways that bacteriostatic or bactericidal drugs produce their effects against infecting microorganisms. Name a drug from each category.

2 Discuss the term superinfection.

3 Discuss three mechanisms postulated for the development of drug resistance.

4 What are the general guidelines for the prudent use of antibiotics?

REFERENCES AND FURTHER READING

Antibiotic Expert Group. *Therapeutic Guidelines: Antibiotic, version 13.* Melbourne: Therapeutic Guidelines, 2006.

Barbosa TM, Levy SB. The impact of antibiotic use on resistance development and persistence. *Drug Resistance Update* 2000; 3: 303–11.

Chambers HF. Antimicrobial agents: general considerations. In: Hardman JG, Limbird LE, Gilman AG (eds.). *Goodman & Gilman's The Pharmacological Basis of Therapeutics.* 10th edn. New York: McGraw-Hill, 1996 [ch. 43].

Geerts S, Gryseels B. Drug resistance in human helminths: current situation and lessons from livestock. *Clinical Microbiology Reviews* 2000; 13: 207–22.

Omrani AS, Pillay D. Multi-drug resistant HIV-1. *Journal of Infection* 2000; 41: 5–11.

Schluger NW. The impact of drug resistance on the global tuberculosis epidemic. *International Journal of Tuberculosis and Lung Disease* 2000; 4: 571–5.

Swartz MN. Impact of antimicrobial agents and chemotherapy from 1972 to 1998. *Antimicrobial Agents and Chemotherapy* 2000; 44: 2009–16.

Walsh C. Molecular mechanisms that confer antibacterial drug resistance. *Nature* 2000; 406: 775–81.

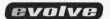 More weblinks at http://evolve.elsevier.com/AU/Bryant/pharmacology/

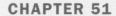

CHAPTER 51

Antibacterial drugs

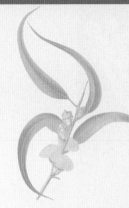

CHAPTER FOCUS

The discovery of sulfonamides and penicillin in the 1940s revolutionised the treatment of infectious diseases. Since then, numerous antibiotics or antimicrobial agents have been discovered and released for use. Of the top 10 prescription drugs distributed through community pharmacies in Australia during 2003, amoxycillin was fifth on the list, with about 4.3 million prescriptions (AIHW 2005). Although many infections have been controlled with antimicrobial drugs, during the past 10–15 years drug-resistant strains of microorganisms have steadily increased, and now threaten effective disease management. The challenge facing health-care professionals is the continued and prudent use of antimicrobial drugs in the face of increasing antibiotic resistance.

OBJECTIVES

- To list the mechanisms of action of penicillins, cephalosporins, macrolides, lincosamides, aminoglycosides, tetracyclines and quinolones.

- To discuss the broad categories of penicillins, listing one drug example from each.

- To compare the effectiveness of penicillins and cephalosporins.

- To name three aminoglycosides and present their mechanisms of action and primary indications.

- To discuss the mechanisms of action of and indications for the tetracyclines.

- To discuss the common adverse drug reactions associated with different classes of antibiotics.

- To compare and contrast the roles of antibiotics in the treatment of urinary tract infections.

KEY DRUGS

amoxycillin
amoxycillin–potassium clavulanate
ampicillin
aztreonam
benzylpenicillin
cefaclor
ciprofloxacin
clindamycin
doxycycline
erythromycin
gentamicin
imipenem
linezolid
metronidazole
tetracycline
trimethoprim–sulfamethoxazole
vancomycin

KEY TERMS

aminoglycosides
antibiotics
bactericidal
bacteriostatic
carbapenems
cephalosporins
quinolones
lincosamides
macrolide antibiotics
penicillins
superinfection
tetracyclines

KEY ABBREVIATIONS

MRSA methicillin-resistant
      Staphylococcus aureus
MRSE methicillin-resistant
      Staphylococcus epidermis
UTI   urinary tract infection

ANTIBIOTICS are chemical substances produced from various microorganisms (bacteria and fungi) that kill or suppress the growth of other microorganisms. This term is commonly used also to describe synthetic antimicrobial agents such as sulfonamides and quinolones that are not products of microorganisms. Hundreds of antibiotics are available that vary in antibacterial spectrum, mechanism of action, potency, toxicity and pharmacokinetic properties. For ease of understanding, this chapter is divided into:

- Inhibitors of bacterial cell wall synthesis
  — penicillins, e.g. penicillin
  — cephalosporins, e.g. cefaclor
  — carbapenems, e.g. imipenem
  — glycopeptides, e.g. vancomycin
  — aztreonam;
- Inhibitors of bacterial protein synthesis
  — macrolides, e.g. erythromycin
  — lincosamides, e.g. lincomycin
  — aminoglycosides, e.g. gentamicin
  — tetracyclines, e.g. tetracycline
  — chloramphenicol
  — oxazolidinones, e.g. linezolid
  — stretogramins, e.g. quinupristin with dalfopristin
  — spectinomycin;
- Inhibitors of DNA synthesis
  — quinolones, e.g. ciprofloxacin;
- Miscellaneous antimicrobials and urinary tract antimicrobials
  — e.g. metronidazole
  — e.g. trimethoprim—sulfamethoxazole.

INHIBITORS OF BACTERIAL CELL WALL SYNTHESIS

Penicillins

Penicillins are antibiotics derived from several strains of common moulds often seen on bread or fruit (Figure 51-1). Introduced into clinical practice in the 1940s, penicillin and related antibiotics constitute a large group of antimicrobial agents that remain the most effective and least toxic of all available antimicrobial drugs. The common chemical feature of penicillins, cephalosporins, monobactams and carbapenems is a β-lactam ring that is essential to activity of the drug but is also the site of attack by resistant bacteria that possess β-lactamase enzymes that render the antibiotic useless.

Mechanism of action

The bacterial cell wall is a rigid cross-linked structure composed of peptidoglycan, which is essential to the normal

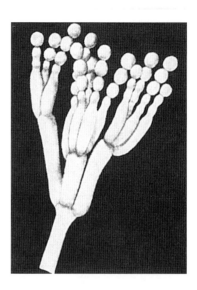

FIGURE 51-1 Typical penicillus of *Penicillium notatum*, Fleming's strain (from Raper & Alexander 1945).

growth and development of bacteria. The thickness of the cell wall varies: in gram-positive bacteria it is 50–100 molecules thick, whereas in gram-negative bacteria it is 1–2 molecules thick. Penicillins weaken the cell wall by inhibiting the transpeptidase enzymes responsible for cross-linking the cell wall strands; this results in cell lysis and death (Figure 51-2). Penicillins are considered to be **bactericidal** agents because they kill susceptible bacteria, but they are ineffective in the presence of β-lactamase enzymes.

To a limited extent, certain antibiotics are combined with β-lactamase inhibitors such as clavulanate or tazobactam. This extends the spectra of their antibacterial activity and improves their effectiveness but increases the cost. Although most penicillins are much more active against gram-positive than gram-negative bacteria, ticarcillin, aztreonam, imipenem, and the combination of penicillins with β-lactamase inhibitors are more effective against gram-negative bacteria (*Escherichia coli*, *Klebsiella pneumoniae* and others). Penicillins are divided into the following categories.

NARROW-SPECTRUM PENICILLINS

These include **benzylpenicillin** (also known as penicillin G), phenoxymethylpenicillin (also called penicillin V) and procaine penicillin. Penicillin G and penicillin V are comparable therapeutically but penicillin V is more stable in stomach acid and is available as an oral preparation. Penicillin G is available in various IM and IV salt formulations—benzylpenicillin sodium, procaine penicillin and benzathine benzylpenicillin. The active substance in all formulations is benzylpenicillin. Examples of susceptible and resistant bacteria are shown in Table 51-1.

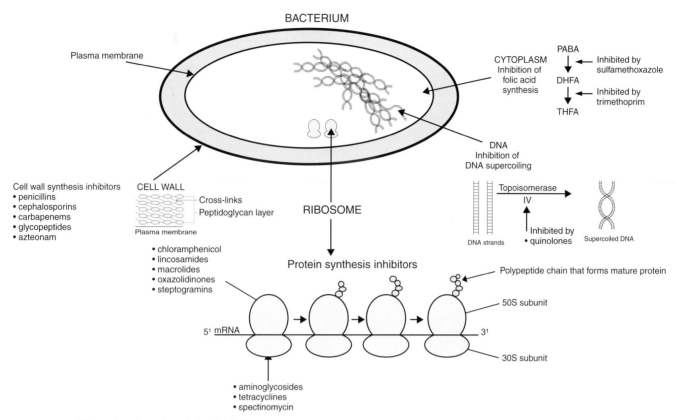

FIGURE 51-2 Sites of action of antimicrobial drugs.

TABLE 51-1 Susceptibility and resistance of bacteria to narrow-spectrum penicillins

	DRUG		
ORGANISM	Benzylpenicillin	Phenoxymethylpenicillin	Procaine penicillin
Gram-negative			
Escherichia coli	R	R	R
Haemophilus influenzae	S	R	R
Klebsiella spp.	R	R	R
Neisseria meningitidis	S	S	S
Pseudomonas aeruginosa	R	R	R
Gram-positive			
Enterococcus faecalis	S*	R	R
Staphylococcus aureus	R	R	R
Streptococcus pneumoniae	S	S	S
Anaerobes			
Clostridium perfringens	S	S	S
Clostridium difficile	R	R	R

R = resistant; S = susceptible; *must be used with synergistic drug (e.g. gentamicin).
Source: AMH 2006.

NARROW-SPECTRUM PENICILLINASE-RESISTANT PENICILLINS

These are resistant penicillins with antistaphylococcal activity, and include dicloxacillin and flucloxacillin. A chemical alteration of the penicillin structure resulted in penicillins resistant to β-lactamase inactivation; thus they are used against penicillinase-producing staphylococci. These antibiotics are not, however, effective against methicillin-resistant bacteria.

MODERATE-SPECTRUM β-LACTAMASE-SENSITIVE AMINOPENICILLINS

These include amoxycillin and ampicillin. Although these antibiotics have a similar spectrum of activity to that of penicillin, they have greater efficacy against selected gram-negative bacteria (e.g. *Haemophilus influenzae*) but are usually not very effective against *Staphylococcus aureus* and *Escherichia coli* (β-lactamase-producing bacteria) unless combined with clavulanic acid (e.g. amoxycillin with clavulanic acid).

BROAD- AND EXTENDED-SPECTRUM (ANTIPSEUDOMONAL) PENICILLINS

This group includes piperacillin, piperacillin–tazobactam and ticarcillin–potassium clavulanate. These antibiotics have a broader spectrum of antimicrobial activity, but only piperacillin (as the single drug) is effective against *Pseudomonas aeruginosa*.

Health-care professionals should be aware that antibiotic therapy may provide an environment that is conducive to the unrestrained growth of undesirable microorganisms, such as bacteria or fungi that would ordinarily have been controlled by the normal body flora. This is a condition known as **superinfection** and may present as diarrhoea from altered gastrointestinal (GI) flora or a *Candida* infection vaginally. Table 51-2 lists penicillin pharmacokinetics and usual adult dosages.

CLINICAL INTEREST BOX 51-1 DON'T TAKE THE BITE OUT OF ANTIBIOTIC

Doctors around New Zealand are urging people to make sure antibiotics don't lose their effectiveness. The Wise Use of Antibiotics Campaign launched in May 2001 aimed to educate people to use antibiotics only when required because of rising concern over the number of cases of methicillin-resistant *Staphylococcus aureus*.

In 2000, only 20% of New Zealanders understood that antibiotics were not an effective way to treat colds and flu. By the end of winter 2003, research showed that nearly half the people who visited their doctor understood this role of antibiotics. Chicken soup, fluids, simple analgesics and rest were promoted as suitable management for uncomplicated viral respiratory conditions. PHARMAC (the Pharmaceutical Management Agency) announced an almost 15% drop in antibiotic prescribing in the year after the campaign had been launched. However, the 2003 PHARMAC annual report noted that antibiotics continued to be a significant source of expenditure, and accounted for NZ$13 million of the annual pharmaceutical budget. *Adapted from*: www.pharmac.govt.nz, accessed 20 January 2006.

DRUG INTERACTIONS 51-1 Penicillins

Drug	Possible effect and management
Allopurinol	Combination of allopurinol with either amoxicillin or ampicillin increases the risk of a rash occurring. Monitor carefully
Aminoglycosides	May result in enhanced bactericidal activity from greater penetration of aminoglycosides. These drugs are incompatible and should not be mixed in the same syringe
Anticoagulants	High IV doses of penicillin increase the risk of bleeding by inhibiting platelet aggregation. Monitor closely for signs of bleeding. Avoid, or a potentially serious drug interaction may occur
Combined oral contraceptives	When used concurrently with ampicillin, amoxicillin or penicillin V, the effectiveness of the oral contraceptives may be decreased. Advise patients to use an alternative method of contraception while taking these antibiotics
Non-steroidal anti-inflammatory drugs (NSAIDs), valproic acid, platelet aggregation inhibitors (e.g. salicylates and dipyridamole)	With high doses of ticarcillin (parenteral dosage forms), an increased risk of bleeding or haemorrhage exists. These drugs inhibit platelet function, and large doses of salicylates may induce hypoprothrombinaemia and also GI ulcers (from NSAIDs or salicylates), all adding to the potential risk of haemorrhage. Avoid, or a potentially serious drug interaction may occur
Probenecid	Decreased renal tubular secretion of penicillins, resulting in elevated plasma concentration and an increase in half-life. Prolongs penicillin activity

TABLE 51-2 Pharmacokinetics and usual adult dosage of penicillins

CLASSIFICATION	PHARMACOKINETICS			USUAL ADULT DOSAGE
	Oral absorption (%)	Peak plasma conc. (h)	Renal excretion* (%)	
Narrow-spectrum				
Benzylpenicillin (penicillin G) (IM/IV)	–	0.5–1	60–90	0.6–1.2 g IV/IM 4–6-hourly (max. 18 g IV daily)
Phenoxymethylpenicillin (penicillin V) (oral)	60–73	0.5–1	20–40	250–500 mg 6–8-hourly (max. 3 g daily)
Procaine penicillin (IM)	–	1–3	60–90	1–1.5 g once daily (max. 4.5 g IM daily)
Narrow-spectrum penicillinase-resistant				
Dicloxacillin (oral)	37–50	0.5–1	50–70	250–500 mg 6-hourly (max. 4 g daily)
Flucloxacillin (oral)	>80	0.5–1	40–70	250–500 mg 6-hourly (max. 4 g daily)
Moderate-spectrum β-lactamase-sensitive aminopenicillins				
Amoxycillin (oral) (IM/IV)	75–90	1–2	60–75	250–500 mg 8-hourly (max. 4 g daily)
	–	1	60–75	1 g 6-hourly (max. 12 g daily)
Ampicillin (oral) (IM/IV)	35–50	1–1.5	75–90	250–500 mg 6-hourly (max. 4 g daily)
	–	1	75–90	0.5–1 g 4–6 hourly (max. 14 g daily)
Broad- and extended-spectrum (antipseudomonal activity)				
Amoxycillin–clavulanate (oral)	90	1–2	50–78	500–875 mg 12-hourly
Piperacillin (IV)	–	E of I	60–80	3–4 g 4–6-hourly (max. 24 g IV daily)
Piperacillin–tazobactam (IV)	–	E of I	68	2–4 g 6–8-hourly (max. 24 g IV daily)
Ticarcillin–clavulanate (IV)	–	E of I	60–70	3 g IV 4–6-hourly (max. 18 g IV daily)

*Renal excretion = % excreted unchanged; E of I = end of infusion; max. = maximum.
Sources: United States Pharmacopeial Convention 1998; AMH 2006.

Drug interactions

Examples of interactions with penicillins are given in the table Drug Interactions 51-1.

Adverse reactions

For penicillins these include diarrhoea, nausea, vomiting, headache, sore mouth or tongue, oral and vaginal candidiasis, allergic reactions, anaphylaxis, serum sickness-type reaction (rash, joint pain and fever), hives and pruritus. Rare adverse reactions include cholestatic hepatitis with some penicillins, especially dicloxacillin, flucloxacillin, amoxycillin–potassium clavulanate, and ticarcillin–potassium clavulanate; leucopenia or neutropenia; mental disturbances (with large dosages of procaine penicillin); convulsions (with high dosages of penicillin and/or in people with advanced renal function impairment); and interstitial nephritis. Platelet dysfunction has been reported with piperacillin and ticarcillin, especially in people with renal impairment.

Warnings and contraindications

Use penicillins with caution in people with general allergies or on salt-restricted diets, and in those with poor cardiac reserve or renal or hepatic impairment. Many parenteral formulations of penicillins (e.g. benzylpenicillin) contain a high concentration of sodium that may precipitate or worsen heart failure in patients with cardiac reserve. Avoid use in people with penicillin hypersensitivity (see Figure 51-3, Clinical Interest Box 51-2), bleeding disorders, congestive heart failure, cystic fibrosis, GI disease (especially antibiotic-associated colitis, as penicillins may cause pseudomembranous colitis) and mononucleosis.

TABLE 51-3 Effect of food on oral penicillin absorption*

DRUG	FOOD EFFECT	DRUG	FOOD EFFECT
Amoxycillin	None	Dicloxacillin	Decreased
Amoxycillin–clavulanate	None	Flucloxacillin	Decreased
Ampicillin	Decreased	Phenoxymethylpenicillin potassium	Decreased slightly

*Penicillins whose absorption decreases after food intake are generally acid-labile; therefore administer with a full glass of water on an empty stomach 1 hour before or 2 hours after meals.

See the Pregnancy Safety box for classification of all drugs in this chapter and the Paediatric Implications box for appropriate antibiotic therapy in children (both at the end of this chapter) and Table 51-3 for the effect of food on oral penicillin absorption.

Cephalosporins

Penicillins were discovered as a result of someone leaving a window open in Fleming's laboratory (or so the story goes!), while **cephalosporins** were isolated from sea fungus found near a sewerage outlet off the Sardinian coast in 1948. Since then, chemical modification of the central active component, 7-aminocephalosporanic acid, and the addition of side-chains have created compounds with different and greater microbiological and pharmacological activities. To classify easily the differences in antimicrobial activity, cephalosporins are divided into first, second, third and fourth generations.

Mechanism of action

Like penicillin, cephalosporins inhibit bacterial cell wall synthesis and are also bactericidal (Figure 51-2). Because

they inhibit cell division and growth, rapidly dividing bacteria are affected most. They are effective in numerous situations, but with only a few exceptions they are rarely the drugs of first choice. The first-generation cephalosporins are primarily active against gram-positive bacteria, whereas the second-generation drugs (cephamandole and others) had increased activity against gram-negative microorganisms. The third-generation drugs are more active against gram-negative bacteria (ceftazidime is also effective against *P. aeruginosa*) and β-lactamase-producing microbial strains but less effective against gram-positive cocci. Cefepime is a fourth-generation cephalosporin with antimicrobial effects comparable to those of third-generation cephalosporins and is also more resistant to some β-lactamases.

Initially, the advantage of cephalosporins over penicillins was their resistance to degradation by β-lactamase, but widespread use of cephalosporins has been linked to the emergence of resistant strains of *K. pneumoniae*, methicillin-

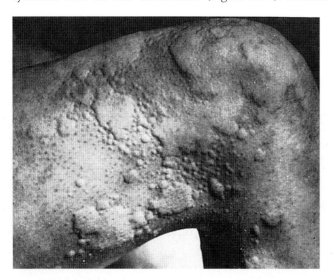

FIGURE 51-3 Urticaria, as seen in individuals sensitive to penicillin.

CLINICAL INTEREST BOX 51-2 PENICILLIN RASH AND ANAPHYLAXIS

A hypersensitivity reaction to penicillin is perhaps the one adverse drug reaction most people seem to have an awareness of, either through personal experience or through knowledge of someone who has experienced a reaction. In fact, a hypersensitivity reaction is the commonest adverse effect noted with penicillins (varying from 1% to 10% of people), and it appears that no one penicillin is the sole culprit. Manifestations of penicillin allergy range from the most common maculopapular or urticarial rash through to bronchospasm and the least common reaction anaphylaxis. A reaction can occur with any dosage and in the absence of prior knowledge of exposure, which often occurs as a result of ingestion of food of animal origin where antibiotics may have been used in animal feed, or through ingestion of fungi-producing penicillin. Anaphylaxis occurs in approximately 0.004%–0.04% of exposed people, and about 0.001% will die as a result. This reaction most often occurs after injection, but has been reported after ingestion of small doses and even after minute intradermal injection to test for penicillin sensitivity.

TABLE 51-4 Cephalosporin-susceptible and -resistant bacteria

ORGANISM	DRUG			
	cephalexin	cefaclor, cefuroxime	cefoxitin	ceftriaxone
Gram-negative				
Escherichia coli	S	S	S	S
Haemophilus influenzae	R	S	S	S
Klebsiella spp.	S	S	S	S
Neisseria meningitidis	R	S	S	S
Pseudomonas aeruginosa	R	R	R	R
Gram-positive				
Enterococcus faecalis	R	R	R	R
Staphylococcus aureus	S	S	*	*
Streptococcus pneumoniae	S	S	S	S
Anaerobes				
Clostridium perfringens	S	S	S	S
Clostridium difficile	R	R	R	R

R = resistant; S = susceptible, *no data or drug not recommended.
Source: AMH 2006.

resistant *S. aureus* (MRSA) and *Clostridium difficile*. Examples of susceptible and resistant bacteria are shown in Table 51-4.

Indications

Cephalosporin antibiotics may be prescribed for patients allergic to penicillins. However, the possibility of a cross-reaction is 5%–15%, and cephalosporins should not be used if a person reports a history of a serious reaction or anaphylaxis to penicillin. If use is critical, specialist advice should always be sought prior to administration. Drugs in this group are indicated for the treatment of a variety of infections and are also used as prophylaxis in bowel and gynaecological surgery. Combinations of third-generation cephalosporins and aminoglycosides are used synergistically to treat *P. aeruginosa*, *Serratia marcescens* and other susceptible organisms.

Table 51-5 lists cephalosporin pharmacokinetics and the usual adult dosages.

Drug interactions

Drug interactions are summarised in the table Drug Interactions 51-2.

Adverse reactions

These include diarrhoea, abdominal cramps or distress, oral and/or vaginal candidiasis, rash, pruritus, redness, oedema, allergic reaction, anaphylaxis, Stevens–Johnson syndrome, haemolytic anaemia, renal toxicity, convulsions, thrombophlebitis, hypoprothrombinaemia (mostly with cephamandole) and pseudomembranous colitis. In addition, an increase in bleeding episodes and bruising due to hypoprothrombinaemia is reported with cephamandole.

Warnings and contraindications

Use cephalosporins with caution in individuals with impaired/low vitamin K synthesis because of increased risk of bleeding. Monitoring of the international normalised ratio (INR [see Chapter 30]) is recommended. Because parenteral cephalosporins have high sodium contents, their use should be avoided in sodium-restricted individuals. Avoid use in people with reports of anaphylaxis to penicillin, penicillin derivatives, penicillamine or cephalosporins; bleeding disorders; GI disease or kidney function impairment.

DRUG INTERACTIONS 51-2 Cephalosporins

Drug	Possible effect and management
Anticoagulants	Risk of bleeding and haemorrhage increases when given concurrently with IV cephamandole, cephazolin or ceftriaxone. These cephalosporins interfere with vitamin K metabolism in the liver, resulting in hypoprothrombinaemia. Dosage adjustments of the anticoagulants may be necessary during and after administration of these drugs
NSAIDs, especially aspirin	When given with cephamandole, cephazolin or ceftriaxone, an increased risk of haemorrhage exists because of the additive effect on platelet inhibition. High dosages of salicylates and the specified antibiotics may induce hypoprothrombinaemia, and the potential for GI ulcers or haemorrhage with NSAIDs or salicylates may increase when used with the previously mentioned cephalosporins. Avoid, or a potentially serious drug interaction may occur
Probenecid	Probenecid decreases renal tubular secretion of the cephalosporins excreted by this mechanism, which can result in increased cephalosporin plasma concentration, extended half-life, and increased potential for toxicity. Probenecid does not affect the secretion of ceftazidime or ceftriaxone. Cephalosporins and probenecid are also used concurrently to treat specific infections such as sexually transmitted diseases, in which a high plasma concentration and prolonged effect are desirable

Carbapenems

Ertapenem, imipenem and meropenem are members of a class of antibiotics called **carbapenems**, which are related to the β-lactam antibiotics but differ from them in having another 5-membered ring in their chemical structure. They bind to penicillin-binding proteins, thus inhibiting bacterial cell wall synthesis. Carbapenems have the broadest spectrum of activity of all the antimicrobials against gram-positive and gram-negative aerobic and anaerobic organisms. All of these drugs are inactive against MRSA and *Enterococcus faecium*, and ertapenem is inactive against *P. aeruginosa* and *Acinetobacter*. Imipenem is degraded by renal dipeptidase and is combined with the dipeptidase inhibitor cilastatin, which inhibits renal dihydropeptidase and blocks the tubular secretion of imipenem, thus preventing renal metabolism of this drug. Meropenem and ertapenem are more resistant to renal dipeptidase degradation and are given alone. These drugs are expensive and are generally reserved (with the exception of ertapenem) for nosocomial and life-threatening infections when other antibiotics are contraindicated or inappropriate. Meropenem is used for treating meningitis, whereas imipenem is contraindicted because of the high incidence of seizures (this is likely to apply also to ertapenem, which is likewise associated with seizures, but there are currently no data on ertapenem use in meningitis).

When carbapenems are administered intravenously, peak plasma concentration is achieved rapidly. The half-life of imipenem is 2–3 hours, about 1 hour for meropenem and about 4 hours for ertapenem. These drugs are excreted unchanged to varying degrees in urine within 10 hours. Dosage adjustment is required in people with significant renal impairment. Imipenem and meropenem should not be given with probenecid, as renal secretion of the carbapenems is inhibited, increasing the risk of toxicity. Seizures have been reported in combination with ganciclovir, so this combination should be avoided.

Adverse reactions include gastric distress, diarrhoea, nausea, vomiting, allergic-type reactions, confusion, psychiatric disturbances, insomnia and raised liver enzyme levels. Pseudomembranous colitis has also been reported with these drugs. The risk of seizures is high in people with pre-existing central nervous system (CNS) disturbances and in renal impairment if the plasma concentration increases substantially. Avoid use in people with hypersensitivity to imipenem, cilastatin or other β lactams (e.g. penicillin and cephalosporin), and in kidney impairment and CNS disorders. Renal and hepatic function, and haematological parameters should be monitored during prolonged treatment.

Glycopeptides

Vancomycin and teicoplanin are both complex glycopeptide antibiotics. Vancomycin was isolated from the soil actinomycete *Streptococcus orientalis*, while teicoplanin was isolated from *Actinoplanes teichomyceticus*. Both drugs inhibit bacterial wall synthesis and are primarily active against gram-positive bacteria. Due to increasing problems with vancomycin resistance, Australia has adopted the guidelines recommended for vancomycin use by the US Centers for Disease Control Hospital Infection Control Practices Advisory Committee. These guidelines are as follows (AMH 2006):

- treatment of serious infections caused by susceptible organisms resistant to penicillins (MRSA and multi-resistant *S. epidermidis*, MRSE) or in people with serious allergy to penicillins
- pseudomembranous colitis (relapse or unresponsive to metronidazole treatment)

TABLE 51-5 Pharmacokinetics and usual adult dosage of cephalosporins

DRUG	PHARMACOKINETICS			USUAL ADULT DOSE
	Oral absorption (%)	Peak plasma conc. (h)	Renal excretion % (per number of hours)*	
First-generation				
Cephazolin	–†	IM: 1–2	56–89 (6)	0.5–1 g IV 6–8-hourly (max. 6 g daily); avoid IM route (painful)
	–	IV: E of I	80–100 (24)	
Cephalexin	95	PO: 1	80 (6)	250–500 mg 6-hourly (max. 4 g daily)
Cephalothin	–	IV: 0.5	60–70 (6)	0.5–1 g IV 4–6-hourly (max. 12 g daily); avoid IM route (painful)
Second-generation				
Cefaclor	95	PO: 0.5–1	60–85 (8)	250–500 mg 8-hourly or 375–750 mg 12-hourly of controlled-release tablet
Cephamandole	–	IM: 0.5–2 IV: E of I	65–85 (8)	0.5–1 g IM/IV 4–8-hourly (max. 12 g daily)
Cefoxitin	–	IM: 0.3–0.5 IV: E of I	85 (6)	1–2 g IV/IM 8-hourly (max. 12 g daily)
Cefuroxime	52	PO: 2–3.6	32–48 (12)	250–500 mg 12-hourly
Third-generation				
Cefotaxime	–	IM: 0.5 IV: E of I	60 (6)	1–2 g IV 8–12-hourly (max. 6 g IV daily); avoid IM route (painful)
Ceftazidime	–	IM: 1 IV: E of I	80–90 (24)	1–2 g IM/IV 8–12-hourly (max. 6 g daily)
Ceftriaxone	–	IM: 2–3 IV: E of I	33–67 (24)	1–2 g IM/IV once daily or in 2 divided doses (max. 2 g daily)
Fourth-generation				
Cefepime	–	IM: 1–2 IV: E of I	80 (24)	1–2 g IM/IV 12-hourly (max. 6 g daily)
Cefpirome	–	IV: E of I	80–90 (24)	1–2 g IV 12-hourly (max. 4 g daily)

*Renal excretion = % excreted unchanged per stated period of time (h); E of I = end of infusion; † i.e. not given orally.
Source: AMH 2006.

- antibacterial prophylaxis for endocarditis following certain procedures (e.g. some genitourinary and GI procedures) in penicillin-hypersensitive people at high risk of endocarditis
- surgical prophylaxis for major procedures involving implantation of prostheses (e.g. cardiac and vascular procedures) in institutions with a high rate of MRSA or MRSE.

Vancomycin's absorption from the intestinal tract is poor, hence it is usually administered intravenously and never intramuscularly. In contrast, teicoplanin can be administered IM. An oral formualtion of vancomycin is available but is only ever used for the treatment of pseudomembranous colitis. The elimination half-life varies between the two drugs: parenteral vancomycin has an elimination half-life of 4–6 hours in adults and about 2–3 hours in children, whereas it is close to 100 hours for teicoplanin. Both are excreted primarily by the kidneys, and dosage adjustment is crucial in persons with compromised renal function. Routine therapeutic plasma drug concentration monitoring is undertaken for vancomycin in circumstances such as during concomitant aminoglycoside administration, in patients on haemodialysis, and during high-dose prolonged treatment in patients with unstable or impaired renal function. Therapeutic plasma drug concentration monitoring is usually unnecessary with teicoplanin unless treating severe infections such as endocarditis. With both drugs the intention is to allow individualisation of dose to ensure effective plasma drug concentrations.

See the Drug Interactions table 51-3 for the drug interactions with vancomycin or teicoplanin.

Adverse reactions are more common with rapid IV infusions and include rash, itching, chills and fever. Rarely, the 'red-neck' or 'red-man' syndrome is reported after bolus or too rapid drug injection with vancomycin (less often with teicoplanin), which results in histamine release and chills, fever, tachycardia, pruritus, rash, or red face, neck, upper body, back and arms (AMH 2006). In combination with aminoglycosides, there is an increased risk of nephrotoxicity and ototoxicity, particularly in people with renal impairment. Avoid use in people with glycopeptide hypersensitivity (allergic cross-reactions occur between teicoplanin and vancomycin), deafness, history of hearing loss or kidney disease. The dosage of either drug depends on age, renal function and indication, and relevant drug information sources should be consulted prior to administration.

DRUG INTERACTIONS 51-3 Glycopeptides (vancomycin or teicoplanin)

Drug	Possible effect and management
Aminoglycosides	Increased potential for ototoxicity and nephrotoxicity with vancomycin and teicoplanin. Monitor renal function and plasma drug concentrations, adjust dose if necessary
Bile acid-binding resins (cholestyramine or colestipol)	When given concurrently with the oral dosage form, a reduction in vancomycin antibacterial activity is reported. Avoid this combination if possible. If not, give oral vancomycin several hours apart from the other medications
Muscle relaxants and general anaesthetics	Vancomycin may potentiate the neuromuscular blockade produced by non-depolarising muscle relaxants and suxamethonium. Vancomycin infusion should be completed before induction of general anaesthesia because of increased risk of vancomycin-related adverse reactions (e.g. hypotension)

Aztreonam

Aztreonam, the first drug in the monobactam class of antibiotics, is a synthetic bactericidal antibiotic with activity similar to that of penicillin. It binds to penicillin-binding proteins, resulting in inhibition of bacterial cell wall synthesis, cell lysis and death. It is active only against gram-negative aerobic organisms (e.g. *P. aeruginosa*). It is reserved for treatment of infections when other antibacterial drugs are contraindicated and for urinary tract, bronchitis, intra-abdominal, gynaecological and skin infections. Aztreonam is highly resistant to most β-lactamase enzymes.

Aztreonam is not given orally, as it is not absorbed from the GI tract. After IM injection, peak plasma concentration occurs in 0.6–1.3 hours. The half-life in adults with normal renal function is 1.4–2.2 hours, and 60%–70% of the drug is eliminated in the urine within 8 hours. Concomitant administration of probenecid or frusemide results in a clinically insignificant increase in the plasma concentration of aztreonam. No significant drug interaction has been reported at this stage.

Adverse reactions include gastric distress, diarrhoea, nausea, vomiting, hypersensitivity, and thrombophlebitis at the site of injection. Rarely, anaphylaxis, hepatitis, jaundice, thrombocytopenia and prolonged bleeding time have been reported. Use aztreonam with caution in people receiving anticoagulant therapy. A low risk of allergic reaction exists in those allergic to penicillins or cephalosporins. The drug is contraindicated in people with aztreonam hypersensitivity. Administered by IV infusion, the dose in adults with normal renal function is 0.5–2 g every 6–8 hours. The maximum dose is 8 g IV daily. Dose reduction is required in moderate and severe renal impairment.

BACTERIAL PROTEIN SYNTHESIS INHIBITORS
Macrolide antibiotics

The **macrolide antibiotics** are so named because they contain a many-membered lactone ring that has one or more sugar molecules attached. They inhibit bacterial RNA-dependent protein synthesis by binding to the 50S ribosomal subunit (Figure 51-2). Macrolides are **bacteriostatic**: that is, they inhibit growth of microorganisms and, in high concentrations with selected organisms, may be bactericidal. The macrolide antibiotics include azithromycin, clarithromycin, erythromycin and roxithromycin. Erythromycin was the first macrolide and is the key drug from this classification.

These agents have similar antimicrobial action (against gram-positive and some gram-negative microorganisms) and are used for respiratory, GI tract, skin and soft tissue infections when β-lactam antibiotics are contraindicated because of

TABLE 51-6 Pharmacokinetics and usual adult dose of macrolide antibiotics

| DRUG | PHARMACOKINETICS | | | USUAL ADULT DOSE |
	Oral Absorption (%)	Peak plasma conc. (h)	Excretion	
Azithromycin	Good	2–4	Biliary (72%)	Varies depending on infecting organism
Clarithromycin	Good	2–3	Urine (20%–30%)	Oral 250–500 mg 12-hourly (max. 2 g daily)
Erythromycin	30–65	2–4	Biliary (high)	Oral 250–500 mg 6–8-hourly (max. 4 g orally/ IV daily)
Roxithromycin	50	1–2	Faecal (about 53%)	Oral 300 mg daily in 1 or 2 doses

Source: AMH 2006.

allergy. Clarithromycin is used in conjunction with the proton pump inhibitor omeprazole for the eradication of *Helicobacter pylori* (see Chapter 34). For macrolide pharmacokinetics and usual adult dosages, see Table 51-6.

Macrolides inhibit hepatic CYP3A4 and as a consequence are subject to numerous drug interactions. In general, they inhibit the metabolism of other drugs, leading to increased plasma concentration and the risk of toxicity. The potential for drug interactions is greatest with erythromycin > clarithromycin > roxithromycin > azithromycin. The table Drug Interactions 51-4 lists some of the more significant drug interactions but is not complete, and reference should be made to appropriate sources if uncertain about a specific drug.

Adverse reactions to these drugs are as follows:
- *azithromycin:* stomach pain, nausea, vomiting, diarrhoea, dizziness, headache; rarely, allergic reactions, acute interstitial nephritis
- *clarithromycin:* anorexia, headache, nausea, vomiting, lethargy, severe anaemia, fever, infection, rash, headache, abnormal taste sensations; rarely, *C. difficile* colitis, hepatotoxicity, hypersensitivity, thrombocytopenia

DRUG INTERACTIONS 51-4 Macrolide antibiotics

Drug	Possible outcome	Management
Benzodiazepines (triazolam, midazolam)	Increased/prolonged sedation	Avoid combined use with erythromycin. Exercise caution with other macrolides
Bromocriptine	Increased adverse reactions	Avoid combined use
Buspirone	Increased adverse reactions	Avoid combined use with erythromycin. Exercise caution with other macrolides
Carbamazepine	Neurotoxicity	Decrease dose of carbamazepine if necessary
Cisapride	Cardiotoxicity	Combination contraindicated
Cyclosporin, tacrolimus	Nephrotoxicity, neurotoxicity	Adjust doses of cyclosporin and tacrolimus if necessary
Digoxin	May cause digoxin toxicity	Monitor plasma digoxin concentration
Ergot alkaloids	Ergotism	Adjust dose of ergot alkaloid or stop administration
Pimozide	Cardiac arrhythmias	Combination contraindicated
Theophylline	Theophylline toxicity	Monitor plasma theophylline concentration. Use alternative agent
Warfarin	Increased risk of bleeding	Monitor INR, decrease or cease warfarin. Use alternative antibiotic

INR = international normalised ratio.
Source: AMH 2006.

- *erythromycin:* abdominal cramps, diarrhoea, nausea, vomiting, oral and/or vaginal candidiasis; rarely, hypersensitivity, hearing loss, pancreatitis, hepatotoxicity. Rapid IV administration may cause serious ventricular arrhythmias
- *roxithromycin:* nausea, vomiting, epigastric pain, diarrhoea; hypersensitivity reactions, including rash, angio-oedema, asthma, bronchospasm and anaphylactic-type reactions. Rises in hepatic enzyme levels have been reported but acute hepatocellular damage is rare.

Use macrolide antibiotics with caution in people with severe liver function impairment. In addition, use erythromycin cautiously in patients with hearing loss, and clarithromycin cautiously in persons with severe kidney function impairment. Avoid these drugs in people with individual drug hypersensitivity and avoid use of erythromycin in those with cardiac arrhythmias.

Lincosamides

The **lincosamides** include lincomycin and **clindamycin**. Lincomycin inhibits protein synthesis by binding to the bacterial 50S ribosomal subunit and preventing peptide bond formation. It is primarily bacteriostatic, although it may be bactericidal in high doses with selected organisms. It is used to treat serious streptococcal and staphylococcal infections but clindamycin is preferred, as it is has better oral absorption and is more potent than lincomycin.

Clindamycin, which is a semisynthetic derivative of linco-mycin, has a similar mechanism of action to that of lincomycin but is more effective. It is indicated for the treatment of bone and joint, pelvic (female), intra-abdominal and skin and soft tissue infections, bacterial septicaemia, and pneumonia caused by susceptible bacteria.

Oral clindamycin is well absorbed and should be administered with food or with a full glass of water. It is rapidly distributed to most body fluids and tissues, with the exception of cerebrospinal fluid; the highest concentrations are noted in bone, bile and urine. The half-life of clindamycin in adults is 2–3 hours. It reaches peak blood concentrations within 0.75–1 hour of oral administration in adults, within 1 hour in children, and within 3 hours of intramuscular injection. It is metabolised in the liver and excreted primarily in bile, with only a small proportion (6%–10%) excreted as unchanged drug in urine.

The effects shown in the table Drug Interactions 51-5 may occur when clindamycin is given with the drugs listed.

Adverse reactions include GI distress (stomach pain, diarrhoea, nausea, vomiting) oral and/or vaginal candidiasis, hypersensitivity, neutropenia and thrombocytopenia. A significant adverse and limiting effect for both drugs is antibiotic-associated pseudomembranous colitis. Use with caution in people with GI disorders, especially ulcerative colitis, antibiotic-induced colitis and regional enteritis. Avoid use in those with clindamycin or lincomycin hypersensitivity.

The usual adult oral dose of clindamycin is 150–450 mg 6–8-hourly; by IV infusion, it is 600–2700 mg daily to a maximum of 4.8 g IV daily. In children, the IM/IV infusion dose is 5–10 mg/kg every 6–8 hours.

Aminoglycosides

Aminoglycosides are potent bactericidal antibiotics usually reserved for serious or life-threatening infections. They are very effective against many bacteria (gram-positive and gram-negative) but are generally reserved for gram-negative infections. (Safer and less toxic agents are available to treat most gram-positive infections.) Currently available are the parenteral aminoglycosides, including amikacin, **gentamicin** and tobramycin; and the oral aminoglycoside neomycin (available through the Special Access Scheme).

The mechanism of action for aminoglycosides involves irreversible binding to the 30S ribosomal subunit of susceptible bacteria, thus inhibiting protein synthesis (interferes with the mRNA–ribosome complex), leading to eventual cell death (bactericidal). They are indicated for the treatment of serious or life-threatening infections when other agents are ineffective or contraindicated. They are used with penicillins, cephalosporins or vancomycin for their synergistic effects and are especially useful for the treatment of gram-negative infections such as those caused by *Pseudomonas* spp., *E. coli*, *Proteus* spp., *Klebsiella* spp., *Serratia* spp. and others. These drugs exhibit a significant postantibiotic effect, inhibiting the growth of organisms after the plasma concentration has fallen below the minimal inhibitory concentration.

Aminoglycosides are poorly absorbed (<1%) from the intestinal tract but are rapidly absorbed intramuscularly, with peak plasma concentrations occurring 30–90 minutes after injection. As the aminoglycosides are strongly polar

DRUG INTERACTIONS 51-5 Clindamycin	
Drug	**Possible effect and management**
Antidiarrhoeals, adsorbent-type (kaolins, attapulgite)	Decreases absorption of oral lincosamides. Avoid concurrent use or advise the patient to take the antidiarrhoeal 2 hours before or 3–4 hours after the oral lincosamides
Chloramphenicol or erythromycin	May antagonise the therapeutic effect of lincomycins. Avoid concurrent administration
Neuromuscular blocking agents	May result in enhanced neuromuscular blockade, skeletal muscle weakness, respiratory depression or paralysis. Avoid, or a potentially serious drug interaction may occur

molecules, they do not distribute to the CNS, and tissue concentrations are low. They are almost entirely eliminated by the kidneys, and in people with normal renal function the plasma half-life is in the range of 2–3 hours.

Determining the plasma concentration of aminoglycosides is essential to ensuring that therapeutic concentrations are achieved without the risk of adverse reactions due to high plasma concentrations. Although aminoglycosides have in the main been administered 2–3 times daily, there is a body of evidence to indicate that once-daily dosing in adults and children is as effective and no more toxic than the 2–3 times daily dosing regimens. In the absence of any contraindications, dosing once daily is recommended in people with normal renal function. Monitoring the plasma concentration is generally not undertaken if the course of treatment is shorter than 48 hours. If it is longer, monitoring of plasma concentration and renal function determines the dosage regimen. Methods used for drug concentration monitoring vary among facilities and may rely on interpreting either the trough plasma concentration from a special graph or

the area under the plasma concentration–time curve (AUC). Local diagnostic laboratory services should be contacted for specialist information.

The effects shown in the table Drug Interactions 51-6 may occur when aminoglycosides are given with the drugs listed.

Adverse reactions include nausea, vomiting, tinnitus, increase or decrease in urinary frequency, ataxia, dizziness, nephrotoxicity, neurotoxicity, ototoxicity (auditory and vestibular), hypersensitivity, peripheral neuritis and, rarely, neuromuscular blockade (difficulty breathing, increased sedation, weakness). Use these drugs with extreme caution in dehydrated individuals (increased risk of toxicity) and in people with myasthenia gravis, parkinsonism and hearing impairment. Aminoglycosides are contraindicated in people with a known allergic reaction or hypersensitivity to these drugs.

The usual adult doses of aminoglycosides in adults with normal renal function are: for amikacin, 15 mg/kg IM/IV daily in 2–3 divided doses; and for gentamicin or tobramycin, 3–5 mg/kg IM/IV daily in 3 divided doses. For additional dosing recommendations, refer to current recommendations. For neomycin, the oral dose is 1 g hourly for 4 hours, then 1 g every 4 hours up to a maximum daily dose of 8 g.

Tetracyclines

Tetracyclines were the first broad-spectrum antibiotics developed after a systematic search for antibiotic-producing microorganisms in soil. The first drug produced was chlortetracycline, which was released in 1948. This group now includes a large number of drugs that have a common basic structure and similar chemical activity: **doxycycline**, minocycline and **tetracycline**. Minocycline is not as well tolerated as the other tetracyclines.

Tetracyclines are bacteriostatic for many gram-negative and gram-positive organisms; they exhibit cross-sensitivity and cross-resistance. Tetracyclines inhibit protein synthesis by reversibly blocking the 30S subunit of the ribosome and preventing access of tRNA to the mRNA–ribosome complex.

DRUG INTERACTIONS 51-6 Aminoglycosides

Drug	Possible effect and management
Aminoglycosides (two or more concurrently)	Potential for ototoxicity, nephrotoxicity and neuromuscular blockade is enhanced. Hearing loss may progress to deafness even after the drug is stopped. In some cases, hearing loss may be reversed. Avoid, or a potentially serious drug interaction may occur
Loop diuretics	Increased risk of irreversible hearing loss. Avoid prolonged use of high doses of aminoglycosides
Muscle relaxants	Aminoglycosides may potentiate the neuromuscular-blocking effect of non-depolarising muscle relaxants and suxamethonium
NSAIDs	NSAID-induced reduction in renal function may lead to increased plasma concentration of aminoglycoside. Monitor drug concentration and renal function and adjust dose if necessary
Penicillins and cephalosporins	Antibacterial action of aminoglycoside may be enhanced as a result of greater penetration. Do not mix aminoglycosides with penicillins and cephalosporins, as the parenteral solutions are incompatible

Source: AMH 2006.

TABLE 51-7 Half-life and usual adult dosage of tetracyclines

DRUG	HALF-LIFE (h) NORMAL	USUAL ADULT DOSAGE
Doxycycline	12–22	200 mg on day 1, then 100 mg daily (max. 200 mg daily)
Minocycline	11–23	200 mg on day 1, then 100 mg twice daily (max. 200 mg daily)
Tetracycline	6–11	250–500 mg 6-hourly (max. 2 g daily)

These drugs have been commonly used to treat many infections, such as acne vulgaris, actinomycosis, anthrax, bacterial urinary tract infections, bronchitis, and numerous systemic bacterial infections sensitive to this class of drug.

Oral tetracyclines are fairly well absorbed and are distributed in most body fluids. Concentration in cerebrospinal fluid varies and can range from 10% to 25% of the plasma drug concentration after parenteral administration. Tetracyclines localise in teeth, liver, spleen, tumours and bone. Doxycycline can reach clinical concentrations in the eye and prostate, whereas minocycline reaches high levels in saliva, sputum and tears. Doxycycline and minocycline are metabolised in the liver, but most tetracyclines are excreted via the kidneys. Table 51-7 lists the tetracycline half-lives and usual adult dosages.

Examples of drug interactions with tetracycline are shown in the table Drug Interactions 51-7

Adverse reactions include dizziness (minocycline), oesophagitis (doxycycline and minocycline, see Clinical Interest Box 51-3), ataxia, GI distress, photosensitivity (depends on dose and extent of sun exposure), discoloration of infants' or children's teeth (do not give to children under 8 years), skin and mucous membrane pigmentation (minocycline), dark or discoloured tongue, and oral, rectal or genital fungal overgrowth; rarely, hepatotoxicity, pancreatitis and benign intracranial hypertension. Tetracyclines are not recommended in people with renal impairment, but doxycycline and minocycline may be used. These drugs are

**CLINICAL INTEREST BOX 51-3
MORE THAN A LUMP
IN THE THROAT**

The New Zealand Centre for Adverse Reactions Monitoring (CARM) has received 56 case reports of oesophagitis with antibiotics, of which 46 were associated with doxycycline. Damage to the oesophagus may occur as a result of poor swallowing technique (not enough fluid) where the passage of the drug through the oesophagus is slow, or from reflux if the person lies down after taking the drug. The symptoms include pain on swallowing and a searing and burning chest pain within minutes of ingestion, and may be described as 'something stuck in the throat'. In severe cases recovery took more than 2 weeks.

All individuals prescribed doxycycline should be advised by their prescribers and pharmacists of the need to take the drug with a meal or a large glass of water, and to remain sitting upright or standing for at least 30 minutes and up to 2 hours after administration.
Source: Prescriber Update 2003; 24(2): 30, www.medsafe.govt.nz

DRUG INTERACTIONS 51-7 Tetracyclines

Drug	Possible effect and management
Antacids, calcium supplements, iron supplements, magnesium or magnesium laxatives, foods containing milk and milk products	May result in non-absorbable complex, reducing the absorption and plasma levels of the antibiotic. Also, antacids may raise gastric pH, which decreases the absorption of tetracyclines and reduces antibacterial effectiveness. If given concurrently, separate medications by 2–3 hours from the oral tetracyclines
Bile acid-binding resins (colestipol and cholestyramine)	May bind oral tetracyclines, decreasing their absorption. Separate drugs by at least 2 hours
Oestrogen-containing oral contraceptives	Concurrent long-term therapy may reduce contraceptive effectiveness and may also result in breakthrough bleeding. Avoid concurrent drug usage or increase contraceptive cover

contraindicated in pregnant women after week 18 and in children under 8 years of age, as they cause discoloration of teeth and enamel dysplasia.

Chloramphenicol

Chloramphenicol, a broad-spectrum antibiotic, potently inhibits bacterial protein synthesis by binding to the 50S subunit of the bacterial ribosome. It is a bacteriostatic agent used for a wide variety of gram-negative and gram-positive organisms and anaerobes; however, because it has the potential to be seriously toxic to bone marrow (aplasia, leading to aplastic anaemia and possibly death), its use has declined. It is indicated for the treatment of *Haemophilus influenzae*, *Streptococcus pneumoniae* and *Neisseria meningitidis*, as it may be bactericidal to these organisms.

Chloramphenicol has good oral and parenteral bioavailability, with the highest concentrations reported in the liver and kidneys. Concentrations up to 50% of those in plasma have been noted in cerebrospinal fluid. Chloramphenicol is metabolised in the liver to an inactive glucuronide, 75%–90% of which is excreted in the urine over a 24-hour period. In neonates, chloramphenicol causes 'grey baby syndrome': a blue–grey skin discoloration, hypothermia, irregular breathing, coma and cardiovascular collapse (see Clinical Interest Box 8-3). This occurs because of lack of maturation of glucuronide-conjugating enzymes in the liver during the first 3–4 weeks of life, and inadequate renal capacity to excrete unchanged drug. The half-life of chloramphenicol in an adult is 1.5–3.5 hours; in neonates 24–48 hours old it is 1–2 days or more; in those 10–16 days

---

DRUG INTERACTIONS 51-8 Chloramphenicol

Drug	Possible effect and management
Barbiturates	Increased metabolism of chloramphenicol and reduced antibacterial activity. Increase chloramphenicol dose if necessary
Phenytoin	Impaired phenytoin metabolism and increased risk of toxicity. Monitor phenytoin concentration and reduce dose if required
Tacrolimus	Increased plasma concentration of tacrolimus when administered concurrently with chloramphenicol. Monitor plasma concentration of tacrolimus and decrease tacrolimus dose if necessary to avoid toxicity
Warfarin	Inhibition of warfarin metabolism may lead to bleeding. Monitor INR and reduce warfarin dose if necessary

INR = international normalised ratio.

---

of age it is approximately 10 hours. Peak plasma concentration is reached in 1–1.5 hours via the IV route.

The effects shown in the table Drug Interactions 51-8 may occur when chloramphenicol is given with the drugs listed.

Adverse reactions include diarrhoea, nausea, vomiting, blood dyscrasias, grey baby syndrome in neonates, hypersensitivity, neurotoxic reactions (delirium, confusion and headaches), peripheral neuritis, optic neuritis and, possibly, irreversible bone marrow depression that may result in aplastic anaemia. Use chloramphenicol with extreme caution in people who have had antineoplastic chemotherapy or radiation therapy. Chloramphenicol is contraindicated in people with a history of hypersensitivity to the drug, and in those with pre-existing bone marrow suppression and/or blood dyscrasias. Specialist advice should be sought before prescribing to infants and children.

Oxazolidinones

The only drug available in this class is linezolid, a novel compound with a broad spectrum of activity against community and nosocomial gram-positive organisms (e.g. vancomycin-resistant enterococci and MRSA). Unlike chloramphenicol, which binds to the 50S ribosomal subunit, inhibiting bacterial protein synthesis, linezolid's site of action is proximal to the 50S subunit. At that specific site, linezolid inhibits protein synthesis by interfering with the formation of a complex that is essential for protein translation. The site and mechanism of action of linezolid were thought to reduce the likelihood of cross-resistance between gram-positive bacterial strains; however, enterococci resistant to linezolid and MRSA resistant to linezolid have now been isolated.

Linezolid is indicated for the treatment of serious infections due to gram-positive organisms where other drugs are either contraindicated or not appropriate. It is available in both oral and IV formulations. After oral administration, linezolid is well absorbed (~100% bioavailability) and peak plasma concentrations occur in 1–1.5 hours. It is metabolised by the liver to inactive metabolites, and approximately 30% of the drug is excreted unchanged in urine. The half-life is in the order of 4.5–5.5 hours and dose adjustment is generally not necessary in the elderly or in the presence of renal or hepatic dysfunction.

The predominant adverse reactions include nausea, diarrhoea and headache. As linezolid may cause thrombocytopenia, leucopenia, eosinophilia and neutropenia, full blood count should be monitored before treatment and weekly during therapy. Linezolid is a weak inhibitor of monoamine oxidase and hence has the potential to interact with adrenergic drugs (e.g. adrenaline, dopamine, ephedrine), serotonergic drugs (e.g. SSRIs) and tyramine-rich foods or drinks. Stop linezolid for at least 7 days before commencing any drugs that interact with MAOIs (to avoid hypertension due to accumulation of endogenous catecholamines) or to avoid serotonin syndrome. Counselling should be provided on foods to be avoided during linezolid treatment.

Streptogramins

Quinupristin with dalfopristin is a combination of 30 parts streptogramin B (quinupristin) with 70 parts streptogramin A (dalfopristin). These compounds are semisynthetic derivatives of a naturally occurring antibiotic produced by *Streptomyces pristinaespiralis*. The combination acts synergistically to inhibit bacterial protein synthesis through binding to the 50S ribosomal subunit. Quinupristin with dalfopristin is active against gram-positive cocci and is indicated for the treatment of vancomycin-resistant *Enterococcus faecium* and severe MRSA when other antibiotics are inappropriate.

Quinupristin with dalfopristin is administered only via the IV route, and after reconstitution is further diluted with 5% glucose and infused over 60 minutes. This drug combination should never be given in sodium chloride solutions, nor the line flushed with sodium chloride or heparin solutions, because of incompatibility. The half-life is <1 hour for both drugs, and metabolism via conjugation is the main route of clearance. Approximately 80% of the administered dose is excreted in bile and hence no dosage adjustment is necessary in renal failure. Quinupristin with dalfopristin is an inhibitor of CYP3A4, and toxicity resulting from higher plasma concentrations of the interacting drugs may occur with drugs that are metabolised by CYP3A4. These include indinavir, midazolam, nifedipine and other calcium channel blockers, and the immunosuppressant cyclosporin.

As would be anticipated, the commonest adverse reactions are infusion-related (e.g. pain and thrombophlebitis at the injection site). Nausea, vomiting and diarrhoea are also commonly observed, and arthalgias and myalgia may be related to accumulation of metabolites, particularly in people with hepatic dysfunction. Specialist advice should be sought prior to using this drug and it is extremely expensive.

Spectinomycin

Spectinomycin's therapeutic indication is the treatment of infections caused by multi-resistant *Neisseria gonorrhoeae*. It is bacteriostatic and inhibits protein synthesis in gram-negative bacteria by binding to the 30S ribosomal subunit. It is for intramuscular use only, and generally is recommended as an alternative regimen for individuals with gonorrhoea who are allergic to quinolones or cephalosporins. It is not effective for treating syphilis and should not be used for mixed infections (gonorrhoea and syphilis), as it can mask the symptoms of syphilis.

Spectinomycin is rapidly absorbed after IM injection and reaches peak plasma concentration in 1–2 hours (after a 2–4 g IM dose). The half-life is 1–3 hours, with elimination via the kidneys. Spectinomycin enhances the neuromuscular blockade induced by botulinum toxin; the combination should be avoided. Adverse reactions include hypersensitivity (chills and fever), nausea, dizziness, urticaria, and pain at the site of injection.

The usual adult dose for gonorrhoea is 2 g IM as a single dose. Combination with doxycycline or azithromycin may be used to cover other non-gonococcal infection.

Inhibitors of DNA synthesis
Fluoroquinolones

The **quinolones** (including fluoroquinolones) are synthetic, broad-spectrum agents with bactericidal activity. They interfere with bacterial topoisomerase II (DNA gyrase) and topoisomerase IV, the enzymes involved in the supercoiling of DNA that is necessary for the duplication, transcription and repair of bacterial DNA (see Figure 51-2). An equivalent topoisomerase II enzyme exists in eukaryotic cells, but this enzyme is inhibited by fluoroquinolones only at much higher concentrations. Examples of fluoroquinolones include **ciprofloxacin**, gatifloxacin, moxifloxacin, norfloxacin and ofloxacin (available through the Special Access Scheme). The

quinolones are reserved for infections when alternative drugs are either contraindicated or ineffective. These include bone and joint infection, gastroenteritis, enteric fever, gonorrhoea, pneumonia, complicated urinary tract infections, and many other infections caused by susceptible microorganisms. Individual quinolones may vary in their spectrum of activity. Unfortunately, bacterial resistance to the quinolones is increasing worldwide, and appropriate use is needed to extend their clinical life.

The oral bioavailability of quinolones is 70%, with the exception of norfloxacin (30%–40%). They are widely distributed in the body with the following half-lives: ciprofloxacin, 4 hours; norfloxacin, 3–4 hours; and ofloxacin, 4–7 hours. Ciprofloxacin, gatifloxacin and moxifloxacin are the only quinolones available for parenteral use. Qinolones are metabolised in the liver (minimally for ofloxacin) and excreted primarily by the kidneys.

Quinolones inhibit the metabolism of some other drugs listed in the table Drug Interactions 51-9 and the effects shown may occur when quinolones are given with the drugs listed.

Adverse reactions include dizziness, drowsiness, restlessness, stomach distress, diarrhoea, nausea, vomiting and photosensitivity; rarely, CNS stimulation (psychosis, confusion, hallucinations, tremors), hypersensitivity (skin rash, redness, Stevens–Johnson syndrome, face or neck

DRUG INTERACTIONS 51-9 Quinolones	
Drug	**Possible effect and management**
Antacids, ferrous sulfate or sucralfate	May decrease absorption of ciprofloxacin, reducing drug effectiveness. Administer quinolone at least 2 hours before these medications
Nitrofurantoin	Antibacterial effect of quinolones is antagonised. Avoid combination
Theophylline and other xanthines	Ciprofloxacin and norfloxacin may inhibit theophylline metabolism, resulting in increased theophylline plasma concentration and toxicity. Monitor theophylline plasma concentration closely, as dosage adjustments may be necessary
Warfarin	May result in increased anticoagulant effect and potential for bleeding. While not currently reported with all quinolones, it is recommended that the INR be monitored closely whenever these drugs are administered concurrently. Reduce warfarin dose if necessary

INR = international normalised ratio.

swelling, shortness of breath) and interstitial nephritis. In addition, Achilles tendinitis and tendon rupture injuries have been reported. Use quinolones with caution in people with CNS disorders, including epilepsy and seizures. Avoid use in those with quinolone hypersensitivity.

MISCELLANEOUS ANTIBIOTICS

Metronidazole

Metronidazole is reduced intracellularly in anaerobic microorganisms or anoxic or hypoxic cells to a short-acting cytotoxic agent that interacts with DNA, inhibiting bacterial synthesis and causing cell death. It is selectively toxic to many anaerobic bacteria and protozoa. Metronidazole is indicated for the treatment of amoebiasis (intestinal and extraintestinal), bone infections, brain abscesses, CNS infections, bacterial endocarditis, genitourinary tract infections, septicaemia, trichomoniasis, and other infections caused by organisms susceptible to metronidazole's action.

Oral metronidazole is well absorbed and distributed throughout the body, penetrating many tissues, including vaginal secretions, seminal fluid, saliva and breast milk. It reaches peak plasma concentration within 1–2 hours and has a half-life of 8 hours. It is metabolised in the liver (about 50%), and both unchanged metronidazole and metabolites are excreted by the kidneys.

The effects shown in the table Drug Interactions 51-10 may occur when metronidazole is given with the drugs listed.

Adverse reactions include dizziness, headache, gastric distress, diarrhoea, anorexia, nausea, vomiting, dry mouth, taste alterations, dark urine, peripheral neuropathy, CNS toxicity, hypersensitivity, leucopenia, thrombophlebitis, vaginal candidiasis and convulsions (with high drug doses). Use with caution in people with renal disease and hepatic impairment. Avoid use in those with metronidazole hypersensitivity, blood dyscrasias, severe liver disease or active organic CNS disease.

Dosage regimens vary according to the infection being treated, and relevant sources should be consulted for information.

Trimethoprim–sulfamethoxazole (co-trimoxazole)

The use of sulfonamides has declined substantially because of widespread bacterial resistance. These agents are primarily bacteriostatic, rather than bactericidal, in concentrations that are normally useful in controlling infections in humans. All the sulfonamides used therapeutically are synthetically produced and, because they are structurally similar to para-aminobenzoic acid (PABA), they competitively inhibit the bacterial enzyme dihydropteroate synthetase, necessary for incorporating PABA into dihydrofolic acid (see Figure 51-2). The blocking of dihydrofolic acid synthesis results in a decrease in tetrahydrofolic acid, which interferes with the synthesis of purines, thymidine, and DNA in the microorganism. Susceptible bacteria are particularly sensitive to sulfonamides because bacteria need to synthesise their own folic acid. The combination with trimethoprim (trimethoprim–sulfamethoxazole) is synergistic, as this agent blocks a further step in the synthesis of folic acid. The combination often has no advantage over the use of trimethoprim as monotherapy but is associated with a greater incidence of adverse reactions. Trimethoprim alone is indicated for urinary tract infections.

After oral administration of trimethoprim–sulfamethoxazole the absorption of trimethoprim is more rapid than that of sulfamethoxazole. Peak concentration occurs within 2 hours for trimethoprim and 4 hours for sulfamethoxazole. Trimethoprim distributes into tissues while sulfamethoxazole distributes in extracellular fluids. About 60% of the trimethoprim and 25%–50% of the sulfamethoxazole is excreted by the kidneys in 24 hours.

The effects shown in the table Drug Interactions 51-11

DRUG INTERACTIONS 51-10 Metronidazole	
Drug	**Possible effect and management**
Alcohol	Metronidazole interferes with the metabolism of alcohol, leading to an accumulation of acetaldehyde. This may result in disulfiram-type effects: flushing, headaches, nausea, vomiting and abdominal distress. Avoid, or a potentially serious drug interaction may occur
Anticoagulants (warfarin)	May enhance anticoagulant effects by inhibiting warfarin metabolism. Monitor INR closely, as dosage adjustments may be necessary. Consider using an alternative drug
Barbiturates	Induce metabolism of metronidazole, reducing its effectiveness. To avoid treatment failure an increased dose of metronidazole may be necessary
Disulfiram	Avoid concurrent use or use within 14 days of disulfiram administration in alcoholic patients. Adverse reactions such as confusion and psychosis have been reported
INR = international normalised ratio.	

DRUG INTERACTIONS 51-11 Sulfonamides/ trimethoprim

Drug	Possible effect and management
Cyclosporin, tacrolimus	Sulfonamides may increase the risk of nephrotoxicity. Monitor cyclosporin/tacrolimus concentration and adjust dose if necessary
Methotrexate	Sulfonamides may reduce renal clearance of methotrexate, increasing the risk of bone marrow suppression. Use alternative antibacterial agent
Phenytoin	Metabolism of phenytoin is inhibited, increasing the risk of toxic effects of phenytoin. Monitor plasma concentration and adjust phenytoin dose if necessary
Warfarin	Warfarin metabolism is inhibited, increasing the risk of bleeding. Monitor INR and adjust dose of warfarin if necessary

INR = international normalised ratio.

TABLE 51-8 Predisposing risk factors for UTIs

RISK FACTORS	FREQUENCY REPORTED
Urinary tract instrumentation (urethral and ureteral catheterisation)*	Up to 67%
Pregnant women	4%–10%
Non-pregnant women	2%–5%

*After a week of indwelling catheterisation, up to 100% colonisation and bacteriuria (Ahronheim 1992).

may occur when sulfonamides and/or trimethoprim are given with the drugs listed.

Adverse reactions include sore mouth, fever, nausea, vomiting and, in severe cases, phototoxicity, interstitial nephritis, hypoglycaemia and lowered mental acuity. Use with caution in HIV-infected people, because of the increased risk of allergic reactions, and in renal impairment, as dose may need to be reduced. The combination is contraindicated in those with a history of previous allergic reaction to a sulfonamide (or related drugs, e.g. thiazide diuretics) or trimethoprim, and in severe renal or hepatic impairment.

The ratio of trimethoprim to sulfamethoxazole is 1:5 (i.e. 160/800 mg means 160 mg trimethoprim with 800 mg sulfamethoxazole). The usual adult oral dose is 80/400–160/800 mg every 12 hours and, in children, 4/20 mg/kg 12-hourly.

URINARY TRACT ANTIMICROBIALS

Urinary tract infections (UTIs) rank as the 16th most commonly reported problem to general practitioners in Australia (AIHW 2000). Between 10% and 20% of women will experience at least one urinary tract infection in their lifetime. The incidence of UTIs increases in institutional settings, up to as much as 35%–40% of the population in extended-stay hospitals (Sahai 1995). See Table 51-8 for predisposing risk factors for UTIs.

UTIs are primarily caused by bacteria. In community-acquired infections, most UTIs are caused by gram-negative aerobic bacilli from the intestinal tract, such as *E. coli*. It has been reported that *E. coli* may cause up to 90% of all community-acquired uncomplicated UTIs (Sahai 1995). Hospital-acquired infections are often complicated and difficult to treat. Organisms involved include *P. aeruginosa*, *Serratia* spp., *Enterobacter* spp. and other gram-negative microorganisms.

Drug therapies for lower UTIs are often started before culture and sensitivity reports are available. Treatment guidelines for urinary tract infections can be found in the *Therapeutic Guidelines: Antibiotic* (Antibiotic Expert Group 2006); depending on the circumstances, drug regimens may include amoxycillin–clavulanate, ampicillin, cephalexin, ciprofloxacin, gentamicin, nitrofurantoin, norfloxacin or trimethoprim. Many of these drugs have been covered in preceding sections; the remaining drugs indicated for treatment of UTIs are discussed below.

Hexamine hippurate

Hexamine hippurate, which is used to treat UTIs, combines the action of hexamine with hippurate. Its effectiveness depends on the release of formaldehyde, which requires

DRUG INTERACTIONS 51-12 Hexamine

Drug	Possible effect and management
Urinary alkalisers, e.g. potassium citrates and sodium bicarbonate	May result in an alkaline urine, which inhibits hexamine's conversion to formaldehyde and renders it ineffective. Avoid concurrent drug administration
Sulfonamides	In acid urine, the formaldehyde produced may precipitate with certain sulfonamides, which increases the potential for crystalluria. Avoid, or a potentially serious drug interaction may occur

an acid medium. The acids released from hippurate salts contribute to this acidity. Formaldehyde may be bactericidal or bacteriostatic and its effects are believed to be the result of denaturation of bacterial protein. It is ineffective in alkaline urine. Because of its fairly wide bacterial spectrum, low toxicity and low incidence of resistance, hexamine has often been the drug of choice in the long-term suppression of infections.

Hexamine is absorbed orally and takes 0.5–2 hours to reach peak urinary formaldehyde concentration at a urinary pH of 5.6. Excretion is via the kidneys. The effects shown in the table Drug Interactions 51-12 may occur when hexamine is given with the drugs listed.

Use hexamine with caution in severely dehydrated patients. Avoid use in people with severe kidney impairment, as renal tubule concentration will be inadequate to achieve a response. For prophylaxis of recurrent UTIs, the adult oral dose is 1 g 12-hourly, and that for children aged 6–12 years is 500–1000 mg every 12 hours.

Nitrofurantoin

Nitrofurantoin is a broad-spectrum bactericidal agent. Its mechanism of action is not fully understood but it is reduced by bacteria to reactive substances that inactivate or alter cell wall synthesis, bacterial ribosomal proteins and DNA and RNA function. It is indicated for the treatment of acute UTIs caused by organisms such as *E. coli*, *S. aureus* and *Klebsiella* species, and for prophylaxis of recurrent UTIs.

After oral administration, nitrofurantoin is well absorbed and has a half-life of 20–60 minutes. About 65% of the drug is excreted, mainly as unchanged drug in the urine. Use nitrofurantoin with caution in people with G6PD deficiency.

PREGNANCY SAFETY

ADEC Category	Drug
A	Amoxycillin, ampicillin, benzylpenicillin, cephalexin, cephalothin, chloramphenicol, clindamycin, erythromycin, hexamine hippurate, lincomycin, phenoxymethylpenicillin, procaine penicillin
B1	Amoxycillin–clavulanate, aztreonam, azithromycin, cefaclor, cefepime, cefotaxime, cefoxitin, ceftazidime, ceftriaxone, cefuroxime, cephamandole, cephazolin, flucloxacillin, piperacillin, piperacillin–tazobactam, roxithromycin, spectinomycin
B2	Cefpirome, dicloxacillin, meropenem, metronidazole, ticarcillin–clavulanate, vancomycin
B3	Clarithromycin, ertapenem, imipenem, linezolid, quinolones, quinupristin with dalfopristin, teicoplanin
C	Trimethoprim–sulfamethoxazole
D	Amikacin, doxycycline, gentamicin, minocycline, neomycin, paromomycin, streptomycin, tetracycline, tobramycin

Avoid use in those with nitrofurantoin hypersensitivity, peripheral neuropathy, lung disease or moderate to severe renal impairment.

The effects shown in the table Drug Interactions 51-13 may occur when nitrofurantoin is given with the drugs listed.

PAEDIATRIC IMPLICATIONS

Antibiotic therapy
In assessing the appropriateness of antibiotic therapy in children, the following criteria are generally accepted:
- In choosing empirical therapy, the selected antimicrobial should have documentation of both adequate penetration at the site and proven effectiveness against the common organisms usually isolated from that specific site.
- If a broad range of possible microorganisms is suspected or if multiple organisms have been isolated from an infection site, then multiple drug therapy may be indicated. Whenever possible, though, the minimum number of drugs necessary to treat the infection should be used. If no contraindication is present, the drug of first choice should be selected.
- Young children have larger volumes of distribution than adults, so dosing based on body weight is recommended. Doses are generally expressed in mg/kg, and the dose calculated should not exceed the recommended adult dose. Manufacturers' instructions should be consulted for details of administration, dosage, duration etc.
- Unless the benefit completely outweighs the risk, no antibiotic should be used in patients with prior documentation of an allergic or adverse reaction to the specific medication.
- Children receiving potent and potentially dangerous drugs, such as gentamicin, amikacin, tobramycin or vancomycin, for more than 2 days should have plasma drug concentrations monitored at the appropriate times.
- Whenever possible, samples for culture should be taken before initiating antibiotic therapy. Usual sites cultured include sputum, urine, blood, wound or non-healing topical sites.
- Antibiotic therapy should be continued until infection is no longer present; however, the duration should not exceed the usual treatment time established for the suspected infection. Prophylactic antibiotic therapy given after uncomplicated surgery is usually discontinued within 48 hours, with few exceptions, such as cardiac surgery.

DRUG INTERACTIONS 51-13 Nitrofurantoin

Drug	Possible effect and management
Antacids	Decrease extent and rate of absorption of nitrofurantoin. Separate administration by at least 2 hours
Probenecid or sulfinpyrazone	Tubular secretion of nitrofurantoin will be inhibited, leading to increased plasma concentration and possible toxicity. A decrease in urinary concentration and effectiveness may also result. Dosage adjustment of probenecid may be required
Quinolones	Antibacterial action antagonised by nitrofurantoin. Avoid combination

DRUGS AT A GLANCE 51: Antibacterial drugs

Therapeutic group	Pharmacological group	Key examples	Key pages
Antibiotics	Inhibitors of bacterial cell wall synthesis	penicillins	
		ampicillin	806, 7
		benzylpenicillin	804, 7
		flucloxacillin	806, 7
		cephalosporins	
		cephalexin	808, 9
		cefaclor	808, 9
		ceftriaxone	808, 9
		carbapenems	
		imipenem	810
		meropenem	810
		glycopeptides	
		vancomycin	810–12
		teicoplanin	810–12
		monobactams	
		aztreonam	812
	Bacterial protein synthesis inhibitors	macrolides	
		azithromycin	812
		erythromycin	812–4
		roxithromycin	812–4
		lincosamides	
		clindamycin	814
		lincomycin	814
		aminoglycosides	
		gentamicin	814, 5
		neomycin	814, 5
		tobramycin	814, 5
		tetracyclines	
		doxycycline	815, 6
		tetracycline	815, 6
	Inhibitors of DNA synthesis	fluoroquinolones	
		ciprofloxacin	818
		gatifloxacin	818
		nalidixic acid	818
		norfloxacin	818

KEY POINTS

● Antibiotics are chemical substances, produced by microorganisms, that kill or suppress the growth of other microorganisms. The term antibiotic is now commonly used also to describe synthetically produced antimicrobial drugs.

● Penicillin was originally discovered in moulds and then found to be bactericidal by inhibiting the synthesis of the bacterial cell wall.

● Penicillins can be broadly divided into the following groups: narrow-spectrum penicillins; narrow-spectrum penicillinase-resistant penicillins with antistaphylococcal activity; moderate-spectrum β-lactamase-sensitive aminopenicillins; and the broad- and extended-spectrum (antipseudomonal activity) penicillins.

● There are now four generations of cephalosporins. Modification of the central β-lactam ring has resulted in many drugs with different microbiological and pharmacological activities.

● Ertapenem, imipenem and meropenem are members of the class of antibiotics called carbapenems, which are related to the β-lactam antibiotics. They have a wide spectrum of activity against gram-positive and gram-negative aerobic and anaerobic organisms.

● Vancomycin is reserved for treatment of serious infections that are resistant to penicillins—methicillin-resistant *Staphylococcus aureus* (MRSA) and multi-resistant *Staphylococcus epidermis* (MRSE).

● The macrolide antibiotics, typified by erythromycin, are bacteriostatic agents that inhibit protein synthesis and, at high concentrations, are bactericidal for selected microorganisms.

● The lincosamides, such as clindamycin, are primarily bacteriostatic and are used to treat serious streptococcal and staphylococcal infections.

● The aminoglycosides are very potent bactericidal antibiotics that are primarily indicated for serious or life-threatening infections. Therapeutic drug monitoring plays a major role in ensuring that a therapeutic plasma concentration is achieved and the risk of toxicity is minimised.

● Tetracyclines are bacteriostatic; the fluoroquinolones inhibit bacterial DNA synthesis and are bactericidal.

● Metronidazole is a short-acting cytotoxic agent that is selectively toxic to protozoa as well as anaerobic bacteria.

● Drug therapy for urinary tract infections may include the use of trimethoprim, ampicillin, cephalexin, nitrofurantoin and other agents.

● Although many antibiotic products are available, the health-care professional should be alert to the problems of antibiotic resistance and superinfection.

REVIEW EXERCISES

1 Discuss the mechanism of action of penicillins.
2 Discuss the four generations of cephalosporins in relation to their indications.
3 Discuss the alcohol–cephamandole drug interaction. How can this reaction be avoided?
4 Name and describe the major drug interactions reported with vancomycin and the aminoglycosides.
5 Describe the drug interaction between tetracycline and oestrogen-containing oral contraceptives.
6 Discuss the 'red-neck syndrome' reported with vancomycin. How can it be avoided?

REFERENCES AND FURTHER READING

Ahronheim JC. *Handbook of Prescribing Medications for Geriatric Patients*. Boston: Little Brown, 1992.

Antibiotic Expert Group. *Therapeutic Guidelines: Antibiotic, version 13*. Melbourne: Therapeutic Guidelines, 2006.

Australian Institute of Health and Welfare. *Australia's Health 2000: The Seventh Biennial Health Report of the Australian Institute of Health and Welfare*. Canberra: AIHW, 2000.

Australian Institute of Health and Welfare 2005. *Statistics on Drug Use in Australia 2004*. AIHW cat. no. PHE 62. Canberra: AIHW (Drug Statistics Series no. 15), 2005.

Australian Medicines Handbook 2006. Adelaide: AMH, 2006.

Chambers HF. Antimicrobial agents: the aminoglycosides. In: Hardman JG, Limbird LE, Gilman AG (eds). *Goodman & Gilman's The Pharmacological Basis of Therapeutics*. 10th edn. New York: McGraw-Hill, 2001 [ch. 46].

Chambers HF. Antimicrobial agents: protein synthesis inhibitors and miscellaneous antibacterial agents. In: Hardman JG, Limbird LE, Gilman AG (eds). *Goodman & Gilman's The Pharmacological Basis of Therapeutics*. 10th edn. New York: McGraw-Hill, 2001 [ch. 47].

Petri WA Jr. Antimicrobial agents: penicillins, cephalosporins, and other β-lactam antibiotics. In: Hardman JG, Limbird LE, Gilman AG (eds). *Goodman & Gilman's The Pharmacological Basis of Therapeutics*. 10th edn. New York: McGraw-Hill, 2001 [ch. 45].

Raper KB, Alexander DF. Penicillin. V. Mycological aspects of penicillin production. *Journal of the Elisha Mitchell Scientific Society* 1945; 61: 74.

Sahai JV. Urinary tract infections. In: Young LY, Koda-Kimble MA (eds). *Applied Therapeutics: The Clinical Use of Drugs*. 6th edn. Vancouver: Applied Therapeutics, 1995.

United States Pharmacopeial Convention. *USP DI: Drug Information for the Health Care Professional*. 18th edn. Rockville, MD: USPDI, 1998.

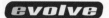 More weblinks at http://evolve.elsevier.com/AU/Bryant/pharmacology/

CHAPTER 52

Antifungal and Antiviral Drugs

CHAPTER FOCUS

Over the past 20 years, the number of immunocompromised individuals has risen dramatically as a result of the spread of HIV and the use of immunosuppressant drugs in organ transplant recipients and chemotherapy for neoplastic diseases. These factors have contributed to a substantial rise in the incidence of severe fungal infections and the use of antifungal drugs. Similarly, viral infections (e.g influenza and hepatitis), continue to exist globally, necessitating the continued development of effective antiviral drugs. The development of antiretroviral drugs has evolved in concert with our knowledge of HIV and the need for multiple drug therapy to combat the devastating consequences of AIDS.

OBJECTIVES

- To describe four major adverse reactions with the use of amphotericin B and the azole antifungals.
- To discuss four other commonly used antifungal agents, including their mechanisms of action and indications.
- To explain why effective antiviral drug therapy is limited compared with antibacterial therapies.
- To compare the actions of antiretroviral drugs, including mechanisms of action, indications and significant drug interactions.

KEY DRUGS

aciclovir
amantadine
amphotericin B
amprenavir
delavirdine
didanosine
ganciclovir
indinavir
ketoconazole
nystatin
oseltamivir
ribavirin
zidovudine

KEY TERMS

azole antifungals
candidiasis
chemoprophylactic
DNA polymerase
fungi
fungistatic agent
mycoses
neuraminidase
non-nucleoside reverse transcriptase
  inhibitors
nucleoside reverse transcriptase
  inhibitors
protease inhibitors

KEY ABBREVIATIONS

AIDS	acquired immunodeficiency syndrome
CMV	cytomegalovirus
HIV	human immunodeficiency virus
HSV	herpes simplex virus
NRTI	nucleoside reverse transcriptase inhibitor
NNRTI	non-nucleoside reverse transcriptase inhibitor
PI	protease inhibitor
VZV	varicella zoster virus

ANTIFUNGAL DRUGS

HUMAN infections by **fungi** can be caused by any of about 50 species of plant-like, parasitic microorganisms. These simple organisms, lacking chlorophyll, are unable to make their own food and so are dependent on other life forms. Infections by fungi, termed **mycoses**, can range from mild and superficial to severe and life-threatening. Infecting organisms can be ingested orally, become implanted under the skin after injury, or be inhaled if the fungal spores are airborne. One species of fungi, *Candida albicans*, is usually part of the normal flora of the skin, mouth, intestines and vagina, and overgrowth and systemic infection from it can result from antibiotic, antineoplastic and corticosteroid drug therapy. This is often referred to as an opportunistic infection. Oral **candidiasis** (thrush) is common in newborn infants and immunocompromised individuals, whereas vaginal candidiasis is more common in pregnant women, women with diabetes mellitus and women who take oral contraceptives. The prevalence of mycoses as opportunistic infections in people with HIV is growing, whereas non-opportunistic fungal infections such as blastomycosis and histoplasmosis are usually rare.

The first antifungal agent was introduced in 1939, with others following throughout the 1940s. A lag in the further development of antifungal agents then occurred, primarily because after the discovery of penicillin the emphasis was on the development of antibiotics. With the increasing number of individuals with HIV and the use of immunosuppressant therapy during the 1980s and 1990s, severe fungal infections have again become a problem. This has resulted in renewed searches for antifungal agents with reduced toxicity to humans. Only a few antifungal compounds (e.g. amphotericin [Drug Monograph 52-1], azole antifungals, nystatin) are available for systemic use, and these are discussed below. The topical antifungal preparations are discussed in Chapter 56.

Azole antifungals

The **azole antifungals** in clinical use are fluconazole, itraconazole, **ketoconazole**, miconazole and voriconazole. Those that contain two nitrogens in the azole ring are called imidazoles (e.g. ketoconazole and miconazole) and those with three nitrogens are called triazoles (e.g. itraconazole, fluconazole and voriconazole). These agents are fungistatic and affect the biosynthesis of fungal ergosterols by interfering with the cytochrome P450 enzyme system that catalyses ergosterol formation (Figure 52-1). The result is impaired or depleted ergosterol biosynthesis, which inhibits fungal growth and causes cell leakage and death. Fluconazole and itraconazole have a greater affinity for fungal cytochrome P450 enzyme than for the human liver cytochrome P450 system, and this improves their safety profile.

INDICATIONS

Fluconazole has good penetration in cerebrospinal fluid (CSF) and is used for treating cryptococcal meningitis, whereas itraconazole has poor CSF penetration but is widely distributed in the body and is indicated for treatment of aspergillosis, blastomycosis and histoplasmosis.

Ketoconazole is well distributed in body fluids (saliva, bile, urine, breast milk and inflamed joint fluid), tendons and other body tissues. It is indicated for the treatment of disseminated and mucocutaneous candidiasis, paracoccidioidomycosis and recalcitrant tinea infections. Miconazole is also widely distributed in body tissues, but neither ketoconazole nor miconazole adequately crosses the blood–brain barrier.

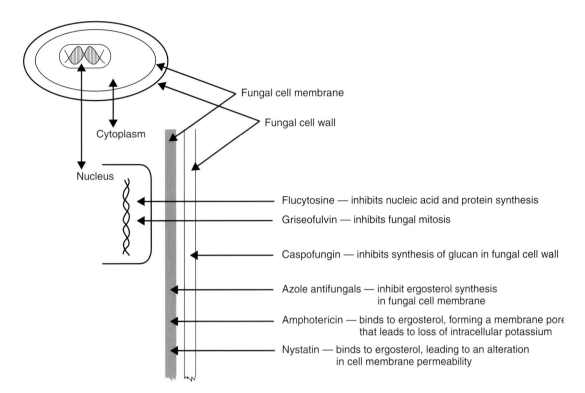

FIGURE 52-1 Sites of action of antifungal drugs.

Miconazole is primarily indicated for the treatment of disseminated and chronic mucocutaneous candidiasis. Voriconazole, the newest of the triazoles, is indicated for serious fungal infections, including invasive aspergillosis, and *Candida*, *Scedosporium* and *Fusarium* spp. infections. Fluconazole, itraconazole and voriconazole have replaced ketoconazole to a large extent because they have broader spectra of activity, fewer adverse reactions, and reduced risk of drug interactions, compared with ketoconazole.

PHARMACOKINETICS
All of the azoles are administered orally; fluconazole and voriconazole may also be administered intravenously. Absorption rates are good if fluconazole is administered to a fasting person, while itraconazole and ketoconazole should be administered with food, and voriconazole at least 1 hour before or 1 hour after a meal. Ketoconazole requires an acid medium for dissolution and absorption; therefore achlorhydria, hypochlorhydria or a rise in stomach pH caused by medications will impair its absorption.

For pharmacokinetics and the usual adult dosages of azole antifungals, see Table 52-1.

DRUG INTERACTIONS
Ketoconazole inhibits human CYP3A4 and is subject to many drug interactions. The same interactions rarely occur with miconazole. The triazoles fluconazole and itraconazole inhibit a range of cytochrome P450 isoenzymes and are also subject to many drug interactions. Voriconazole is metabolised by CYP2C9 and CYP3A4 and is also an inhibitor of the metabolism of other drugs metabolised by CYP3A4 (e.g. vincristine). Drug Interactions 52-1 lists the drugs that can interact with an azole antifungal agent, and the possible outcomes and management.

ADVERSE REACTIONS
For azole antifungals, adverse reactions include nausea, vomiting, stomach distress, diarrhoea, flushing, drowsiness, dizziness, headache and hypersensitivity (fever, chills and rash). Miconazole has caused redness, swelling or pain at the injection site. Rarely, ketoconazole may cause photophobia, menstrual irregularities, and gynaecomastia and impotence due to inhibition of adrenal steroid and testosterone synthesis. Other rare effects include liver toxicity, anaemia, agranulocytosis, and exfoliative skin disorders such as Stevens–Johnson syndrome (for fluconazole) and thrombocytopenia (for fluconazole and miconazole). Voriconazole is associated with visual abnormalities including altered visual perception, blurred vision and colour changes. These effects are dose-related and are in general reversible.

WARNINGS AND CONTRAINDICATIONS
Avoid use in people with azole antifungal hypersensitivity, achlorhydria or hypochlorhydria (reduces drug absorption, especially of itraconazole and ketoconazole), alcoholism, and liver or kidney function impairment.

DRUG MONOGRAPH 52-1 AMPHOTERICIN B

Amphotericin B was introduced in 1960 and is the premier drug for the treatment of severe systemic mycoses. It binds to ergosterol in the fungal cell membrane; this binding alters cell permeability and results in a loss of potassium and other elements from the cell (Figure 52-1). Ergosterol is a major component of fungal cell membranes and not only provides the structure but is also involved in nutrient transport. Amphotericin B is effective for treating aspergillosis, blastomycosis, candidiasis (moniliasis), coccidioidomycosis, cryptococcosis, fungal endocarditis, histoplasmosis, cryptococcal meningitis, fungal septicaemia and many other severe systemic fungal infections.

PHARMACOKINETICS Amphotericin B is widely distributed in the body. After oral administration, little or no absorption occurs from the gastrointestinal tract. It has an initial half-life in adults of 24 hours and a terminal half-life of about 15 days. The routes of elimination are unknown, but excretion is via the kidneys. Around 40% of the drug is excreted over 7 days, but it can still be detected in the urine for at least 7 weeks after the drug is discontinued.

DRUG INTERACTIONS The following effects can occur when amphotericin B is given with the drugs listed below:

Drug	Possible effect and management
Adrenocorticoids, glucocorticoids and mineralocorticoids (ACTH)	Can result in severe hypokalaemia; if given concurrently, frequent plasma potassium determinations should be performed. Can decrease adrenal cortex response to corticotrophin (ACTH)
Bone marrow depressants and radiation therapy	Can produce increased bone marrow-depressant effects; monitor blood cell counts closely because dosage adjustments may be necessary if anaemia, leucopenia or thrombocytopenia occurs
Digitalis glycosides	Amphotericin B-induced hypokalaemia can increase the potential for digitalis toxicity. Monitor closely for dysrhythmias, anorexia, nausea, vomiting or other indications of possible toxicity

Drug	Possible effect and management
Flucytosine	Increased cellular uptake or decreased renal excretion of flucytosine increases the risk of bone marrow suppression. Monitor blood count
Nephrotoxic medications and potassium-depleting diuretics	Increased risk of nephrotoxicity; monitor closely for oedema or decrease in urination, as drug dosage adjustments may be necessary

ADVERSE REACTIONS Adverse reactions with the IV infusion of amphotericin B include headache, gastrointestinal (GI) distress, anaemia, hypokalaemia, infusion reaction (fever, chills, nausea, vomiting and hypotension), renal impairment, thrombophlebitis at the infusion site, blurred vision, cardiac dysrhythmias, rash, leucopenia, peripheral neuropathy, convulsions and thrombocytopenia. With oral administration, mild nausea and vomiting may be observed.

WARNINGS AND CONTRAINDICATIONS Caution should be exercised in people with renal impairment, as IV amphotericin alters renal function. The drug is contraindicated in people with amphotericin B hypersensitivity unless no alternative exists.

DOSAGE AND ADMINISTRATION Amphotericin is available as a conventional IV formulation, as a cholesteryl sulfate complex, as a lipid complex and in a liposomal form. The lipid complex injection is a liposomal encapsulation of amphotericin used to treat aspergillosis and cryptococcosis in people who have infections that are refractory to, or who are unable to tolerate, standard amphotericin B therapy. The liposome formulation is effective but has significantly less nephrotoxicity than amphotericin B. The dosage of each formulation varies according to the infection, and specialist advice should be sought. In general, to avoid infusion-related reactions, the initial dose is either infused slowly over 2–6 hours, or a test dose of 1 mg is infused over the first 30 minutes, with the remainder infused over the next 2–4 hours. The commonest adverse reactions include fever, chills, nausea, hypotension, vomiting, dyspnoea and respiratory failure.

Caspofungin

Caspofungin is the first drug in a new class of antifungals, called the echiocandins, which have significant activity against *Candida* spp. and *Aspergillus* spp. It acts by inhibiting synthesis of glucan, a vital component of the fungal cell wall. Available only for intravenous administration, caspofungin is highly protein-bound (97%) and is slowly metabolised by hydrolysis and N-acetylation, with less than 2% excreted as unchanged drug in urine. Dosage adjustment is not necessary in patients with mild renal or mild hepatic impairment but dose reduction is required in those individuals who have moderate hepatic impairment, and this drug should not be used in the presence of severe hepatic impairment.

TABLE 52-1 Azole antifungals: pharmacokinetics and usual adult dosage

DRUG	PHARMACOKINETICS Time to peak plasma concentration (H)	Half-life (H)*	USUAL ADULT DOSAGE
Fluconazole	1–2	Adults: 30 Children: 14–20	50–200 mg orally/IV daily
Itraconazole	3–4	Single dose: 21 Steady state: 64	100–200 mg orally daily
Ketoconazole	1–4	8	200–400 mg orally daily (max. 800 mg daily)
Miconazole	2–4	20–25	62 mg (gel) 6 hourly for 7–14 days
Voriconazole	1–2	~6†	Consult relevant sources for IV/oral loading and maintenance doses

*Half-life for normal renal function. †Varies depending on dose because of non-linear (saturable) metabolism.

DRUG INTERACTIONS 52-1 Azole antifungals

Drug	Possible outcome	Management
Interaction with imidazoles		
Amphotericin	Antagonistic effect, reduced antifungal activity	Avoid concurrent use
Cyclosporin, tacrolimus*	Increased plasma concentrations	Monitor renal function and cyclosporin/tacrolimus plasma concentrations
H$_2$ antagonists, proton pump inhibitors, antacids	Reduced absorption, reduced antifungal effect	Avoid combination with H$_2$ antagonists and proton pump inhibitors. Give 2 hours apart from antacids
Indinavir	Decreased metabolism leads to increased concentration	Reduce dose of indinavir
Phenytoin*	Voriconazole increases phenytoin concentration and risk of toxicity. Phenytoin increases metabolism of voriconazole, decreasing its efficacy	Monitor plasma concentration of phenytoin and reduce dose if necessary. Increase voriconazole dose
Rifamycins, isoniazid*	Increased metabolism, reduced antifungal effect	Avoid combination
Thiazolidinediones*	Reduced metabolism increases risk of hypoglycaemia	Monitor blood glucose, reduce dose of thiazolidinediones if necessary
Triazolam*	Decreased metabolism increases risk of sedation	Avoid combination or reduce dose of triazolam
Warfarin*	Reduced metabolism increases risk of bleeding	Monitor INR and reduce warfarin dose if necessary
Interaction with triazoles		
Carbamazepine	Decreased metabolism of carbamazepine and increased risk of adverse reactions	Reduce dose of carbamazepine if required
Zidovudine	Increased concentration of zidovudine	Monitor for haematological toxicity. Adjust dose if necessary

* These drugs have interactions with triazoles similar to their interactions with imidazoles.
Source: AMH 2006.

Although caspofungin does not induce or inhibit CYP, a number of drug interactions have been reported. The exact mechanisms are unclear, but when caspofungin is coadministered with known inducers (e.g. carbamazepine, dexamethasone, phenytoin and rifampicin), the plasma concentration of caspofungin is reduced substantially and an increase in dose is usually necessary. Cyclosporin increases caspofungin concentration, thereby increasing the risk of toxicity, and a reduction in the dose of caspofungin may be required. In contrast, caspofungin reduces tacrolimus concentration, and an increased dose of tacrolimus may be necessary.

As the site of action of caspofungin is unique to fungi, the drug is reasonably well tolerated. Adverse reactions include phlebitis at the injection site, rash, itch, fever, flushing, chills, nausea, vomiting and diarrhoea. Some elevations in liver enzymes have been reported and, rarely, resulting from possible histamine-mediated effects, facial swelling, bronchospasm and anaphylaxis. Hence, this drug is contraindicated in individuals allergic to caspofungin.

Flucytosine

Flucytosine enters fungal cells, where it is converted to fluorouracil, an antimetabolite (Figure 52-1). It interferes with pyrimidine metabolism, thus preventing nucleic acid and protein synthesis. It has selective toxicity against susceptible strains of fungi because human cells do not convert significant quantities of this drug into fluorouracil. Flucytosine is indicated for the treatment of fungal endocarditis (caused by *Candida* spp.), fungal meningitis (caused by *Cryptococcus* spp.), and fungal pneumonia, septicaemia or urinary infections caused by *Candida* or *Cryptococcus* spp. As resistance develops rapidly, combined use with another antifungal is recommended.

Flucytosine is administered IV and is widely distributed in the body, including CSF, concentration in the latter being about 60%–90% of the plasma concentration. Flucytosine, with a half-life of 2.5–6 hours in individuals with normal renal function, is not significantly metabolised but is excreted via the kidneys, mostly as unchanged drug (80%). Capsules are not marketed but are available through the SAS.

Concurrent use in individuals who are receiving bone marrow suppressants or radiation therapy can result in an increased bone marrow-depressant effect. Monitor closely, as drug dosage reduction may be necessary. Antacids delay absorption, so administration should be separated by at least 2 hours. Adverse reactions include confusion, hallucinations, photosensitivity, headache, dizziness, sedation, gastric distress, anaemia, hepatitis, hypersensitivity and bone marrow suppression (leucopenia and thrombocytopenia).

The adult oral/IV infusion is 37.5–50 mg/kg every 6 hours.

Griseofulvin

Griseofulvin is a **fungistatic agent** that inhibits fungal cell mitosis during metaphase. It is also deposited in the keratin precursor cells in skin, hair and nails, thus inhibiting fungal invasion of the keratin. When infested keratin is shed, healthy keratin will replace it. Griseofulvin is indicated for the treatment of susceptible organisms for onychomycosis (nail fungus), tinea barbae (fungal infection of the bearded section of face and neck), tinea capitis (fungal infection of the scalp; ringworm), tinea corporis (fungal infection of non-hairy skin), tinea cruris (fungal infection in the groin) and tinea pedis (fungal infection of the foot; athlete's foot).

The oral absorption of griseofulvin varies from 25% to 70%. If griseofulvin is administered with or after a fatty meal, absorption is significantly enhanced. Griseofulvin is distributed in keratin layers in the skin, hair and nails, with very little being distributed in body tissues and fluids. It has a half-life of 24 hours and reaches peak plasma concentration in about 4 hours. The drug is metabolised by the liver, and metabolites are excreted in urine (about 50%) and in faeces (about 30%).

The table Drug Interactions 52-2 shows what can occur when griseofulvin is given with the drugs listed.

Adverse reactions include headache, dizziness, gastric distress, insomnia, weakness, confusion, hypersensitivity (rash or hives), photosensitivity and, rarely, leucopenia, hepatitis and peripheral neuritis. Use griseofulvin with caution in individuals with lupus erythematosus or lupus-like syndromes. Avoid use in people with griseofulvin hypersensitivity, liver disease or porphyria.

DRUG INTERACTIONS 52-2 Griseofulvin

Drug	Possible effect and management
Alcohol	Potentiated effects of alcohol (e.g. flushing). Avoid combination
Anticoagulants (warfarin)	Decreased anticoagulant effect may be noted. Consider alternative antifungal drug or monitor INR and increase warfarin dose if necessary
Contraceptives, oestrogen-containing, oral	Chronic, long-term use of griseofulvin can decrease the effectiveness of oral contraceptives. Intercycle menstrual bleeding and pregnancy can occur. Advise the patient to use an alternative method of contraception when taking griseofulvin and for 4 weeks after treatment
Phenobarbitone	Increased metabolism of griseofulvin and reduced antifungal effect. Avoid combination

The usual adult oral dose for tinea of the skin, hair and groin is 500 mg/day, and 1 g daily for tinea of the feet and nails. The duration of therapy depends on the infection site and severity of infection.

Nystatin

Nystatin is an antibiotic with antifungal activity and is used to treat cutaneous or mucocutaneous infections caused by the monilial organism *Candida albicans*. It has both fungistatic and fungicidal effects and is also used to suppress intestinal candidiasis. Nystatin adheres to sterols in the fungal cell membrane, altering cell membrane permeability, which results in loss of essential intercellular contents. Nystatin is poorly absorbed from the GI tract and is not absorbed when applied topically to skin or mucous membranes. It produces a local antifungal effect. Nystatin is not metabolised, and most of the unabsorbed nystatin is excreted in the faeces. No drug interaction has been documented.

Adverse reactions are uncommon and the drug is well tolerated by all ages. Large doses may cause gastric distress. Nystatin is contraindicated in people with nystatin hypersensitivity. The usual oral dose (tablet/capsule) for intestinal candidiasis in adults or children is 500,000–1,000,000 units every 8 hours. The dose of the oral liquid or lozenge for oral candidiasis is 100,000 units four times daily.

ANTIVIRAL DRUGS

Chemotherapy for viral diseases has been more limited than chemotherapy for bacterial diseases because the development and clinical application of antiviral drugs is more difficult. In many viral infections the replication of the virus in the body reaches its peak before any clinical symptoms appear. By the time signs and symptoms of illness appear, the multiplication of the virus is maximal and the subsequent course of the illness has been determined. To be clinically effective, antiviral drugs must be administered in a **chemoprophylactic** manner as preventive agents before disease appears. Development of antiviral drugs has also been impeded by the fact that viruses are simply either double-stranded DNA or single-stranded RNA contained within a capsid (viral protein coat), and they lack any metabolic capacity. Hence, viruses are true parasites; they replicate within the mammalian cell and use the host cells' enzyme systems. Thus drugs that inhibit virus replication often disturb the host cells and in many instances are too toxic for use.

The antiviral drugs reviewed in this chapter are separated into two groups:
1. antiviral (non-retroviral) drugs
2. antiretroviral drugs used in the treatment of HIV.

Antiviral (non-retroviral) drugs

The following drugs are used in the treatment of viral infections due to DNA and RNA viruses (excluding retroviruses, e.g HIV):
- DNA polymerase inhibitors—aciclovir, famciclovir, ganciclovir, valaciclovir and valganciclovir
- neuraminidase inhibitors—oseltamivir and zanamivir
- miscellaneous antiviral drugs—adefovir, amantadine, cidofovir, foscarnet, palivizumab and ribavirin.

DNA polymerase Inhibitors

Aciclovir (see Drug Monograph 52-2) is the prototypical drug and was the first to be approved (1982) for use in the treatment of herpes simplex virus (HSV) and varicella zoster virus (VZV). Other drugs similar to aciclovir (an acyclic guanine nucleoside analogue) include famciclovir, an oral prodrug that is metabolised to penciclovir; ganciclovir, structurally similar to aciclovir; valaciclovir, a prodrug of aciclovir; and valganciclovir, a prodrug of ganciclovir.

FAMCICLOVIR

Famciclovir has inhibitory actions against HSV (types 1 and 2) and VZV. It is indicated for the treatment of acute herpes zoster (shingles) infections and recurrent genital herpes. Administered orally, famciclovir is well absorbed and converted in the intestinal wall to the active antiviral metabolite penciclovir. Peak plasma concentration is achieved in about 1 hour; its half-life is 2–3 hours and it is excreted unchanged primarily in urine and faeces.

Adverse reactions include headaches, weakness, gastric distress (nausea, vomiting and diarrhoea) and fatigue. Exercise caution in people with kidney function impairment, as dosage reduction is required. Avoid use in lactating women. For recurrent genital herpes, the usual adult dose is 125 mg orally 12 hourly for 5 days, and as a prophylactic, 250 mg twice daily for up to 12 months.

CLINICAL INTEREST BOX 52-3
HIV–AIDS IN AUSTRALIA

The cumulative number of HIV-infected people in Australia at the end of 2002 was estimated at 13,120 (AIHW 2004). New diagnoses of HIV infection declined from a high of 1077 in 1993 to 657 in 1998 and then rose to 808 in 2002. The majority of newly diagnosed cases of HIV were predominantly through homosexual contact, with relatively few new cases among injecting drug users or heterosexuals. By the end of December 2002, a total of 9083 cases of AIDS and 6272 AIDS-related deaths had been notified. AIDS incidence remained stable between 1999 and 2002 at 200–250 cases per year.
Source: AIHW 2004.

DRUG MONOGRAPH 52-2 ACICLOVIR

Aciclovir is selectively taken up by herpes simplex virus (HSV)-infected cells and is eventually converted via several cellular enzymes, including thymidine kinase, to an active triphosphate form. This active form (acyclo-GTP) inhibits viral DNA synthesis by two actions: it inhibits the incorporation of the normal deoxyguanosine into viral DNA by the viral DNA polymerase, and in its place acyclo-GTP is incorporated into the growing DNA chain; this then causes termination of synthesis of the viral DNA.

INDICATIONS Aciclovir is used in the prophylaxis and treatment of genital herpes infections and for the treatment of varicella (chickenpox) infections and HSV encephalitis. It is also used in people with AIDS.

PHARMACOKINETICS The oral dose form is poorly absorbed (15%–30%), but plasma concentrations achieved are therapeutic. It is widely disseminated to various body fluids and tissues, including CSF and herpetic vesicular fluid. Concentrations in CSF are around 50% of the plasma drug concentration. The half-life is about 2.5 hours in individuals with normal renal function, and about 20 hours in anuric patients. The drug is minimally metabolised by the liver (about 15%) and is excreted primarily as unchanged drug in urine.

DRUG INTERACTIONS Concurrent use of aciclovir with probenecid will result in high plasma concentration of

aciclovir and the risk of adverse neurological effects. During concomitant administration with theophylline, the plasma concentration of theophylline may increase and a decrease in theophylline dose may be necessary.

ADVERSE REACTIONS Adverse reactions with the oral dosage form include gastric distress, headache, dizziness, nausea, diarrhoea and vomiting. With the parenteral form, phlebitis at the injection site, acute renal failure with rapid injection or, rarely, encephalopathic alterations such as confusion, hallucinations, convulsions, tremors and coma can occur.

WARNINGS AND CONTRAINDICATIONS Use with caution in individuals with neurological abnormalities or kidney function impairment, or in dehydrated people (risk of precipitation of aciclovir crystals in the kidneys). Avoid use in people with aciclovir hypersensitivity.

DOSAGE AND ADMINISTRATION Aciclovir is available as oral, topical and IV formulations. The usual oral adult dose for herpes genital infection is 400 mg orally every 8 hours during waking hours (three times daily) for 5–10 days. For prophylaxis of recurrent infection, the dose is 200 mg orally 2–3 times a day for up to 6 months. The parenteral adult dosage for HSV encephalitis and varicella zoster in immuno-compromised individuals is 10 mg/kg IV 8-hourly. For other dosage recommendations, see a current package insert.

GANCICLOVIR AND VALGANCICLOVIR

Ganciclovir is converted intracellularly to the triphosphate form, which is the active, antiviral agent. In the presence of the cytomegalovirus, ganciclovir is rapidly phosphorylated to ganciclovir triphosphate, which inhibits viral DNA polymerase, suppressing viral DNA synthesis. If ganciclovir is discontinued, viral replication will resume.

Ganciclovir is considered to be carcinogenic, and appropriate cytotoxic handling procedures should be adopted. It is used for cytomegalovirus (CMV) pneumonitis in bone marrow and renal transplant recipients, and for sight-threatening CMV retinitis in severely immunocompromised individuals (AMH 2006). Valganciclovir is a prodrug of ganciclovir: the indications for its use include prophylaxis of CMV disease after organ transplant. As valganciclovir is quickly metabolised to the active component ganciclovir, the pharmacodynamics and pharmacokinetics of valganciclovir are the same as those of ganciclovir.

Ganciclovir is administered orally, by IV infusion or by ocular implant. The plasma half-life is 2.5–3.6 hours and the vitreous fluid half-life is about 13 hours. This drug is excreted unchanged, primarily by the kidneys, and the half-life is substantially prolonged in people with renal impairment.

Oral ganciclovir is indicated only for maintenance of CMV retinitis in people who have had resolution of active retinitis after induction therapy with parenteral ganciclovir. The plasma half-life following oral administration is 3–5.5 hours and peak plasma concentration occurs in 3 hours if administered with food. An ocular ganciclovir implant is used to treat sight-threatening CMV retinitis.

The table Drug Interactions 52-3 shows what can occur when ganciclovir or valganciclovir is given with the drugs listed.

Adverse reactions with ganciclovir after IV or oral administration include granulocytopenia, thrombocytopenia, anaemia, gastric distress, central nervous system (CNS) effects (e.g. anxiety and tremors), hypersensitivity, and phlebitis or pain at the injection site. After ocular implantation, a variety of ophthalmic disorders may result, such as retinal detachment, scleral induration, subconjunctival haemorrhage, conjunctival scarring and bacterial endophthalmitis. Use with caution in people with moderate to severe renal impairment, as dosage reduction will be required. Avoid use in people with aciclovir or ganciclovir hypersensitivity, an absolute neutrophil count <500 × 10⁶ cells/L, a platelet count <25 × 10⁹/L, and in people with bone marrow suppression. Ganciclovir and

DRUG INTERACTIONS 52-3 Ganciclovir/valganciclovir

Drug	Possible effect and management
Bone marrow-depressant drugs	Concurrent use can result in increased bone marrow-suppressant effects. Monitor blood closely for neutropenia and thrombocytopenia
Foscarnet	Synergistic antiviral effects but increased haematological and renal toxicity. Monitor blood count and electrolytes
Imipenem with cilastin	Avoid combined use because of increased risk of seizures
Probenecid	Inhibits renal secretion of ganciclovir, increasing the concentration and risk of toxicity. Avoid combination
Zidovudine (AZT)	Can result in severe haematological toxicity. Withhold zidovudine or change to another antiretroviral drug

valganciclovir are contraindicated in pregnancy and lactation because of potential embryotoxic and teratogenic effects. The adverse reactions of valganciclovir are similar to those of ganciclovir.

The usual adult dose of ganciclovir for CMV retinitis is 5 mg/kg by IV infusion every 12 hours for 1–2 weeks. The maintenance dosage is 5 mg/kg IV daily or 1000 mg orally three times daily with food. For valganciclovir, the oral dose is 900 mg 12 hourly for 21 days, with a maintenance dose of 900 mg daily.

VALACICLOVIR

Valaciclovir is a prodrug that is converted to aciclovir by first-pass intestinal and liver metabolism. It is indicated for the treatment of varicella zoster infections and for primary and recurring genital HSV. Administered orally, valaciclovir is well absorbed and is converted to aciclovir, the active substance. It reaches peak plasma concentration in 1.6–2 hours; its half-life is 2.5–3.3 hours. Valaciclovir is converted to inactive metabolites by alcohol and aldehyde dehydrogenase, and excreted primarily in urine.

Adverse reactions include nausea, headache, weakness, gastric distress (constipation, diarrhoea, anorexia, abdominal pain and vomiting), dizziness, agitation and renal impairment. Rarely, valaciclovir can cause haematological toxicity, including neutropenia, leucopenia and thrombocytopenia. Use valaciclovir with caution in people with liver or renal function dysfunction. Avoid use in people with valaciclovir or aciclovir hypersensitivity, bone marrow or kidney transplant, advanced HIV infections or kidney function impairment. The usual adult dose for genital herpes simplex is 500 mg 12 hourly for 5–10 days.

Neuraminidase inhibitors

OSELTAMIVIR

Neuraminidase is an essential enzyme for replication of both influenza A and B strains because it plays an important role

in releasing the virus from infected cells, enabling it to spread to other cells. **Oseltamivir** is a prodrug that is metabolised in the liver to the active metabolite, which inhibits the action of neuraminidase on the surface of the viral cell and prevents release of the viral particles (Robinson 2001). It is indicated for the treatment of influenza A and B in adults and children over 1 year.

Oseltamivir is well absorbed after oral administration and is metabolised (about 75%) by esterases in the liver to its active metabolite. Peak plasma concentration is reached 2–3 hours after dosing. The half-life is 6–10 hours in normal individuals but may be prolonged in people with renal impairment. Drug interactions are unlikely because oseltamivir is not metabolised by the hepatic cytochrome P450 system.

Adverse reactions include vomiting, nausea, headache, dizziness and vertigo. Use with caution in people with underlying respiratory or cardiac conditions and complicated influenza (e.g. pneumonia). The usual dose is 75 mg twice daily for 5 days. Oseltamivir should be started within 48 hours of the onset of symptoms and taken with food to reduce stomach discomfort.

ZANAMIVIR

Similar to osteltamivir, zanamivir is a potent and selective inhibitor of the viral neuraminidase enzyme. It is indicated for the treatment of influenza A and B in adults and children >5 years old within 48 hours of the onset of symptoms. Administration is via oral inhalation, and approximately 10%–20% of the dose is systemically available. After inhalation, zanamivir is widely deposited within the respiratory tract. It is not metabolised and is excreted as unchanged drug in the urine.

Zanamivir is generally well tolerated and in clinical trials the frequency of adverse reactions is similar to that for placebo. Rarely, an allergic reaction has been reported (facial and oropharyngeal oedema), as have bronchospasm and dyspnoea.

Miscellaneous antiviral drugs

ADEFOVIR

Adefovir dipivoxil is a new oral prodrug that is effective in the treatment of chronic hepatitis B in adults. In the host cell, enzymes phosphorylate adefovir (an analogue of adenosine) to adefovir diphosphate, which then inhibits viral polymerase, resulting in termination of viral DNA synthesis.

Adefovir dipivoxil is rapidly absorbed and metabolised by esterases to the active drug adefovir. The half-life after oral administration is 5–7 hours, and approximately 60% of the drug is eliminated unchanged by the kidney. To date, dose-related nephrotoxicity has been reported but other adverse reactions may not yet be fully known. Concomitant administration with other nephrotoxic drugs (e.g. NSAIDs) may increase the risk of nephrotoxicity. The dosage is 10 mg once daily, but in the presence of renal impairment a reduction in dose is necessary.

AMANTADINE

Amantadine appears to block the uncoating of the influenza A virus and the release of viral nucleic acid into host respiratory epithelial cells. It also increases dopamine release and inhibits the reuptake of dopamine and noradrenaline centrally. Amantadine is indicated for the prevention and treatment of influenza A, for treatment of Parkinson's disease and for the treatment of drug-induced extrapyramidal reactions.

Amantadine is rapidly absorbed orally; it is distributed to saliva and nasal secretions and crosses the blood–brain barrier. It has a half-life of 11–15 hours, reaching peak plasma concentration within 2–4 hours. It is excreted mostly unchanged by the kidneys, and the half-life is prolonged in people with renal impairment.

Adverse reactions include CNS toxicity, gastric distress and, with chronic therapy, livedo reticularis (a vasospastic disorder, worsened by exposure to cold, that is evidenced by a reddish-blue mottling of the legs and sometimes arms), anticholinergic effects (dry mouth, constipation, blurred vision, confusion and difficult urination), vomiting and orthostatic hypotension. Use amantadine with caution in patients with (or a history of) eczema rash or psychosis, and in individuals with severe psychoneurosis. Avoid use in people with amantadine hypersensitivity, peripheral oedema, congestive heart failure, kidney impairment, or epilepsy or other convulsive disorders.

The table Drug Interactions 52-4 shows the effects that can occur when amantadine is given with the drugs listed.

The adult oral antiviral dose is 200 mg daily or 100 mg every 12 hours for 5–7 days. For those aged <10 years or >65 years, the once-daily dose is 100 mg for 5–7 days. Antiviral effects diminish within two days following the cessation of treatment.

CIDOFOVIR

Cidofovir is used for treating CMV retinitis in AIDS. It

DRUG INTERACTIONS 52-4 Amantadine

Drug	Possible effect and management
Alcohol	Increased risk of CNS adverse reactions such as dizziness, fainting episodes, confusion or circulatory problems. Avoid, or a potentially serious drug interaction could occur
Anticholinergics	Can result in an increase in anticholinergic adverse reactions, such as hallucinations, dry mouth, blurred vision, confusion and nightmares. Monitor closely, as dosage adjustment of amantadine may be required
Dopamine antagonists	Opposing effects on dopamine receptors. Avoid combination

selectively inhibits viral DNA polymerase and prevents DNA synthesis. It is administered IV with oral probenecid, which blocks active renal tubule secretion and hence the renal clearance of the drug. The drug is not metabolised, and 70%–85% of the dose is excreted unchanged in urine within 24 hours. Additive nephrotoxicity is observed with the aminoglycosides, amphotericin, foscarnet, vancomycin and NSAIDs. Reduction in dosage of drugs that undergo renal secretion (e.g. zidovudine) is required.

Adverse reactions include weakness, GI distress, alopecia, headache, nephrotoxicity, elevated plasma concentrations of liver enzymes, neutropenia, fever and, rarely, ocular hypotony. Cidofovir is contraindicated in individuals with cidofovir or probenecid hypersensitivity or severe kidney function impairment. Pretreatment with probenecid is used to reduce the nephrotoxicity. Administer 2 g probenecid orally 3 hours before cidofovir infusion and 1 g at 2 and 8 hours after completing the infusion. The induction dose of cidofovir is 5 mg/kg IV once weekly for 2 weeks and 5 mg/kg IV once every 2 weeks as maintenance therapy.

FOSCARNET

Foscarnet is a virustatic agent that inhibits viral replication of all known herpes viruses in vitro, including CMV, HSV types 1 and 2, Epstein–Barr virus and varicella zoster virus. It acts by selective inhibition at the pyrophosphate binding site of viral DNA polymerase. If the drug is discontinued, viral replication will resume. It is currently used to treat CMV retinitis in patients with AIDS.

This drug is administered by intravenous infusion, has an elimination half-life of 3.3–6.8 hours, reaches peak plasma concentration at the end of the infusion, is not metabolised and is excreted primarily unchanged in the urine.

The table Drug Interactions 52-5 shows the effects that can occur when foscarnet is given with the drugs listed.

Adverse reactions include nephrotoxicity, gastric distress, neurotoxicity, anaemia, leucopenia, and phlebitis or pain at injection site. Use with caution in people with anaemia, hypomagnesaemia, hypocalcaemia or a history of seizures. Avoid use in people with foscarnet hypersensitivity or kidney impairment, and in dehydrated people. For CMV retinitis, the usual adult dose by IV infusion is 60 mg/kg administered over a minimum of 1 hour by infusion pump, every 8 hours for 2–3 weeks. The maintenance dosage is 90–120 mg/kg IV daily over 2 hours.

PALIVIZUMAB

Palivizumab is a humanised monoclonal antibody directed against a protein of the surface of respiratory syncytial virus (RSV). Once bound to the virus, palivizumab inhibits RSV replication. It is indicated for serious lower respiratory tract diseases caused by RSV in infants and children at high risk of RSV disease. These include infants born at 32–35 weeks' gestation, or with bronchopulmonary dysplasia or with significant congenital heart disease (AMH 2006). Determination of the pharmacokinetics of monoclonal antibodies is difficult, and considerable individual variation in palivizumab plasma concentration has been reported. To date, the metabolism of palivizumab has not been determined and drug interactions have not been described.

Adverse reactions include fever, rash, wheeze, cough and, rarely, hypersensitivity including anaphylaxis. This drug is contraindicated in those with known sensitivity to palivizumab or any other humanised monoclonal antibody. Consult relevant sources for dosages for IM administration in infants.

RIBAVIRIN AEROSOL

Ribavirin is virustatic, with a mechanism of action that is diverse and not completely understood. It rapidly penetrates virus-infected cells and is believed to reduce intracellular guanosine triphosphate (GTP) storage. It inhibits viral RNA and protein synthesis, thus inhibiting viral duplication, spread to other cells, or both. It is indicated for serious viral pneumonia caused by respiratory syncytial virus in children <2 years of age.

After oral inhalation, ribavirin is well absorbed and rapidly distributed to plasma, respiratory tract secretions and erythrocytes. Its half-life is 9.5 hours after oral inhalation and around 40 days in erythrocytes. Ribavirin is metabolised in the liver and excreted primarily by the kidneys. In-vitro studies indicate that ribavirin and zidovudine are antagonistic and should not be administered concurrently.

Adverse reactions are uncommon and can include skin rash or irritation (inhalation product), CNS effects (insomnia, headache and lethargy) with IV and oral dosages, and gastric distress (anorexia and nausea) and anaemia (usually with higher doses). The health-care professional or provider should use caution in administering this medication, as headache, itching, swelling and red eyes have been reported. Use with caution in individuals with severe anaemia and avoid use in people with ribavirin hypersensitivity. In addition, worsening of lung function may occur in asthmatics, and ribavirin should be stopped if deterioration occurs.

The adult dose for ribavirin as an inhalation aerosol has not been established. For viral pneumonia in children, administer by oral inhalation via a small-particle aerosol generator, using a 20 mg/mL ribavirin concentration in the reservoir. Inhale for 12–18 hours/day for 3–7 days.

Ribavirin combined with peginterferon alfa (refer to Chapter 55) is used in the treatment of chronic hepatitis C (see Clinical Interest Box 52-4) in individuals over the age of 18 years with compensated liver complications (e.g. cirrhosis).

DRUG INTERACTIONS 52-5 Foscarnet

Drug	Possible effect and management
Ciprofloxacin	Avoid combination because of increased risk of seizures
Nephrotoxic medications	Can result in increased risk of renal toxicity. Monitor renal status closely if drugs such as aciclovir, aminoglycosides, amphotericin B or other nephrotoxic medications are administered concurrently
Pentamidine	Concurrent administration of IV pentamidine with foscarnet can result in severe hypocalcaemia, hypomagnesaemia and nephrotoxicity. Avoid, or a potentially serious drug interaction could occur

CLINICAL INTEREST BOX 52-4 HEPATITIS C

There are approximately 30,000 people in NZ with hepatitis C, and this number is expected to double by 2010. It is estimated that there are 19,000 injecting drug users, and approximately 16,000 of these people have hepatitis C. Few patients are receiving treatment for the virus. Although hepatitis C medication is expensive, the courses are short and can prevent future health costs. For some of types of the disease, combination therapy has been shown to cure 80% of cases. Without adequate treatment and control, hepatitis C will spread among drug users and the wider NZ society. Costs have been predicted to rise by between $166 million and $400 million in the next 30 years. Hepatitis C has major effects on the liver and can be fatal.
Adapted from: I. Sheerin: www.otago.ac.nz/news/2005/01-04.05pressrelease.html/ accessed 19 January 2006.

Peginterferon alfa is administered SC once weekly combined with twice daily oral ribavirin dosed according to weight. This treatment is less effective in people who also have HIV.

Antiretroviral drugs

The following drugs are used in the treatment of the human immunodeficiency virus (HIV):

- **nucleoside reverse transcriptase inhibitors** (NRTIs)—abacavir, didanosine, emtricitabine, lamivudine, stavudine, zalcitabine, zidovudine (see Drug Monograph 52-3)
- **non-nucleoside reverse transcriptase inhibitors** (NNRTIs)—delavirdine, efavirenz, nevirapine
- **protease inhibitors** (PIs)—amprenavir, atazanavir, fosamprenavir, indinavir (see Drug Monograph 52-4), lopinavir with ritonavir, nelfinavir, ritonavir, saquinavir
- other antiretrovirals—enfuvirtide, tenofovir.

Nucleoside reverse transcriptase inhibitors (NRTIs)

These drugs are indicated for the treatment of HIV infection (in adults and children) in combination with other retroviral drugs, for prophylaxis during pregnancy to prevent transmission to the fetus, and for prophylaxis post-exposure to HIV. NRTIs are used in combination therapy with NNRTIs and PIs in HIV-infected patients. The most effective regimens continue to be combinations of three or more drugs that include at least two different classes of antiretrovirals. Unfortunately, the problems faced in the treatment of HIV continue to be rebound viral replication, development of resistance and inadequate drug potency.

**CLINICAL INTEREST BOX 52-5
AN AIDS VACCINE**

The development of a vaccine often proceeds not long after an infectious disease emerges. The search for an AIDS vaccine began in the early 1980s. There was considerable optimism that one would be found and that the problem could be controlled, as had smallpox. Progress on development of a vaccine has not been easy and the hurdles encountered have included identification of immunogens that will produce broad and long-lasting immunity, defining of structures and immunisation strategies that will elicit antibody production, and development of strategies to deal with the different HIV strains and viral coats (Nable 2001). According to Nable (2001), "The search for an HIV vaccine has been slow and at times frustrating, but the resolve of the biomedical research community to address this problem has grown. Although the solution is not yet at hand, progress is tangible and encouraging results now develop on a regular basis".

All of these drugs are substrates for the viral reverse transcriptase enzyme (Figure 52-2), which converts viral RNA into proviral DNA before it becomes incorporated in the host cell chromosome. In order to do this, the drugs must first be phosphorylated in the cytoplasm to enable them to effectively compete with the normal host cell triphosphates. The phosphorylated drug, once incorporated in the growing viral DNA chain, causes chain termination. These drugs are thus effective only in susceptible cells, but are ineffective in cells already infected with HIV.

Significant adverse reactions of the NRTIs include lipodystrophy (changes in cutaneous fat distribution: loss in the face, limbs and buttocks but accumulation in the abdominal, breast and dorsocervical region). Metabolic abnormalities may also occur, and these include insulin resistance and hyperlipidaemia. Many of the NRTIs are subject to numerous drug interactions, and current drug information sources should be consulted before commencing therapy.

ABACAVIR

Abacavir is selective against HIV-1 and HIV-2 and is indicated for the treatment of HIV infection. It is administered orally, bioavailability is ~83%, half-life 1.5 hours, and the drug is widely distributed, including good penetration of the CSF. Abacavir is extensively metabolised by the liver, and less than 2% is excreted as unchanged drug in urine.

Adverse reactions include a hypersensitivity reaction in at least 5% of people within 6 weeks. The severity of this reaction is such that the drug should be stopped immediately and never reintroduced as therapy, as fatalities have occurred on rechallenge. Other adverse reactions include the whole range of GI symptoms, muscle problems (e.g. fatigue, myalgia, arthralgia) and respiratory symptoms (e.g. dyspnoea, sore throat, cough). The usual adult dose is 300 mg 12-hourly or 600 mg once daily.

DIDANOSINE

Didanosine (also known as ddI) is converted intracellularly to its active form, ddA-triphosphate, which inhibits HIV DNA reverse transcriptase. This inhibition suppresses HIV replication.

This product, which is available in oral dosage forms, is acid-labile. The oral formulations are buffered to increase gastric pH to protect didanosine from gastric acid destruction. Didanosine crosses the blood–brain barrier, has a half-life of 1.5 hours in adults and reaches peak plasma concentration in 30–60 minutes. Excretion is primarily via the kidneys.

The table Drug Interactions 52-6 shows the effects that can occur when didanosine is given with the drugs listed.

Adverse reactions include peripheral neuropathy, CNS toxicity (e.g. headache, anxiety, increased irritability and insomnia), gastric distress (stomach pain, nausea and diarrhoea) and dry mouth. Less frequent and rare adverse reactions include pancreatitis, cardiomyopathy, blood disorders (anaemia,

DRUG MONOGRAPH 52-3   ZIDOVUDINE

Zidovudine (azidothymidine [AZT]) was the first antiretroviral drug developed to target HIV infection. It was first used in 1987 and by the early 1990s it was evident that zidovudine slowed the rate of progression of AIDS. Survival rates, however, did not improve and it became apparent that resistant HIV strains had developed. By 1996, the use of combination therapy had emerged, with better results in retarding disease progression and decreasing mortality (Hovanessian 1999).

Zidovudine is an antiviral agent (virustatic) that intracellularly is converted by cellular enzymes to monophosphate, diphosphate and then to zidovudine triphosphate. The triphosphate form competitively inhibits the reverse transcriptase with respect to the incorporation of natural thymidine triphosphate in growing chains of viral DNA, thus inhibiting viral replication. It has a greater affinity for retroviral reverse transcriptase than for the human alpha-DNA polymerase; thus it selectively inhibits viral replication.

INDICATIONS Zidovudine is indicated for the treatment of HIV infection and AIDS in adults with CD4+ lymphocyte counts of 500/μL or less. Zalcitabine may be used in combination with zidovudine, especially when the CD4+ count is 300/μL or less. This drug is also used to prevent vertical transmission of HIV during pregnancy (2nd and 3rd trimesters) and to the neonate.

PHARMACOKINETICS Administered orally, zidovudine is rapidly absorbed and distributed in plasma and CSF, reaches peak plasma concentration in 0.5–1.5 hours and has a half-life of around 1 hour in plasma (3.3 hours intracellularly). It is metabolised in the liver, and the major metabolite does not have antiviral activity. Both unchanged zidovudine (about 15%) and the main metabolite (about 75%) are excreted in urine.

DRUG INTERACTIONS The following effects can occur when zidovudine is given with the drugs listed below:

Drug	Possible effect and management
Bone marrow depressants, radiation therapy	Can exacerbate bone marrow depression and toxicity. Dosage reductions may be necessary. Monitor full blood counts closely for leucopenia and anaemia
Ganciclovir	Concurrent use has been reported to result in synergistic myelosuppressive toxicity. As this is a serious adverse reaction, avoid or a potentially serious drug interaction could occur
NSAIDS, probenecid	Can cause decreased glucuronidation of zidovudine, resulting in increased plasma concentrations and an increased risk of toxicity. Probenecid can also decrease renal excretion. Dosage reduction of zidovudine may be possible
Ribavirin and stavudine	These drugs antagonise the antiviral action of zidovudine, and the combination should be avoided

ADVERSE REACTIONS These include nausea, myalgia, insomnia, severe headaches, bone marrow depression (anaemia and neutropenia), hepatotoxicity, myopathy, neurotoxicity and hyperpigmentation of nails.

WARNINGS AND CONTRAINDICATIONS Use with caution in individuals with folic acid or vitamin B_{12} deficiency; such deficiencies increase the risk of anaemia. Avoid use in people with zidovudine hypersensitivity, bone marrow depression, or liver or kidney function impairment.

DOSAGE AND ADMINISTRATION The adult oral dose for treatment of symptomatic HIV infection is 500–600 mg daily in two divided doses, but a range of drug regimens has been used, including 500 mg every 12 hours.

---

leucopenia or thrombocytopenia), hepatitis, convulsions, hypersensitivity and retinal depigmentation. Use with caution in individuals with gout, liver dysfunction, phenylketonuria (tablets contain phenylalanine) or impaired kidney function. Avoid use in people with hypertriglyceridaemia, pancreatitis, alcoholism or peripheral neuropathy. Didanosine tablets contain magnesium, which may present an unacceptable load in individuals with renal impairment, so dose reduction may be necessary.

The usual adult dose for patients weighing <60 kg is 250 mg once daily; for patients weighing >60 kg the dose is 400 mg daily. For dosing schedules in children, check a current package insert or drug reference such as the *Australian*

Medicines Handbook. Capsules should be taken on an empty stomach at least half an hour before or 2 hours after food.

EMTRICITABINE

Emtricitabine is an analogue of cytosine and is effective against HIV-1, HIV-2 and hepatitis B. It is rapidly absorbed after oral administration, with peak plasma concentrations occurring at 1–2 hours post-dose. Emtricitabine is excreted predominantly by the kidneys (86%) and in faeces (14%). Only 13% of the dose is hepatically metabolised, hence renal impairment significantly influences the plasma drug concentration and dose reduction may be necessary. The potential for drug interactions is low, and no clinically

DRUG INTERACTIONS 52-6 Didanosine

Drug	Possible effect and management
Alcohol, azathioprine, oestrogens, frusemide, nitrofurantoin, pentamidine IV, sulfonamides, sulindac, stavudine, tetracyclines, thiazide diuretics, valproic acid, or other drugs associated with pancreatitis	Concurrent drug use can result in pancreatitis. Avoid, or a potentially serious drug interaction could occur. If combination therapy is necessary, use extreme caution
Chloramphenicol, cisplatin, hydralazine, isoniazid, lithium, metronidazole, nitrofurantoin, nitrous oxide, phenytoin, stavudine, vincristine, zalcitabine, or other drugs associated with peripheral neuropathy	Can increase the potential for peripheral neuropathy. Avoid, or a potentially serious drug interaction could occur. If one of these drugs must be used, monitor closely for numbness and tingling in the fingers and toes
Dapsone, itraconazole, ketoconazole, quinolone antibiotics, tetracyclines and indinavir	Buffered formulation of didanosine can result in decreased absorption of these drugs because they require an acidic medium. Administer these drugs at least 2 hours before didanosine

significant drug interactions have been noted with indinavir, zidovudine, stavudine and famciclovir.

Common adverse reactions include headache, diarrhoea, nausea and a rash. Predominantly in females, emtricitabine causes hyperpigmentation of the palms and/or soles of the feet. The dose in adults is 200 mg daily.

LAMIVUDINE

Lamivudine (also known as 3TC) is converted in the body to an active metabolite, lamivudine triphosphate (L-TP), which inhibits HIV reverse transcription by terminating the viral DNA chain. It also inhibits RNA- and DNA-dependent DNA polymerase functions of reverse transcriptase. Synergism of antiviral activity is achieved with a combination dosage form containing 150 mg lamivudine and 300 mg zidovudine.

Rapidly absorbed after oral administration, lamivudine reaches peak plasma concentration in 1 hour (fasting state) or 3.2 hours (with food). L-TP has an intracellular half-life of 10–15 hours and is excreted unchanged by the kidneys. The potential for drug interactions exists with IV pentamidine, which increases the risk of pancreatitis, and trimethoprim, which competes with lamivudine for renal excretion. This latter combination can result in increased lamivudine concentration, and the combination should be avoided in people with renal impairment.

Adverse reactions with lamivudine include headaches, dizziness, fatigue, fever, nausea, vomiting, diarrhoea, gastric pain or distress, anorexia, neuropathy, insomnia, depression, cough, skeletal muscle pain, pancreatitis, paraesthesias, peripheral neuropathy and, rarely, anaemia, rash and neutropenia. Use lamivudine with caution in individuals with pancreatitis or peripheral neuropathy, including people with a history of these conditions, and in diabetics, as 5 mL of oral solution contains 1 g sucrose. Avoid use in people with lamivudine hypersensitivity and kidney function impairment.

For the treatment of HIV, the usual dose of lamivudine for children <12 years is 4 mg/kg 12-hourly to a maximum of 300 mg daily, and for adults 150 mg orally twice a day or 300 mg once daily.

STAVUDINE

Stavudine is converted to stavudine triphosphate, which competes with deoxythymidine triphosphate, resulting in inhibition of HIV replication and DNA synthesis. Oral stavudine is rapidly absorbed and reaches peak plasma concentration in 0.5–1.5 hours. It has a half-life of 1–1.6 hours and is excreted unchanged, primarily by the kidneys.

The table Drug Interactions 52-7 shows the effects that can occur when stavudine is given with the drugs listed.

Adverse reactions include dose-related peripheral neuropathy, increased liver enzymes and anaemia. Other

DRUG INTERACTIONS 52-7 Stavudine

Drug	Possible effect and management
Drugs that cause peripheral neuropathy, such as chloramphenicol, cisplatin, dapsone, didanosine, hydralazine, isoniazid, lithium, metronidazole, nitrofurantoin, phenytoin, vincristine or zalcitabine	Stavudine can cause peripheral neuropathy; whenever possible, avoid combination with other drugs that can cause peripheral neuropathy
Ganciclovir, pentamidine (IV)	Increased risk of pancreatitis. Avoid combination
Zidovudine	Combination is antagonistic but the clinical relevance is unknown. Avoid combination

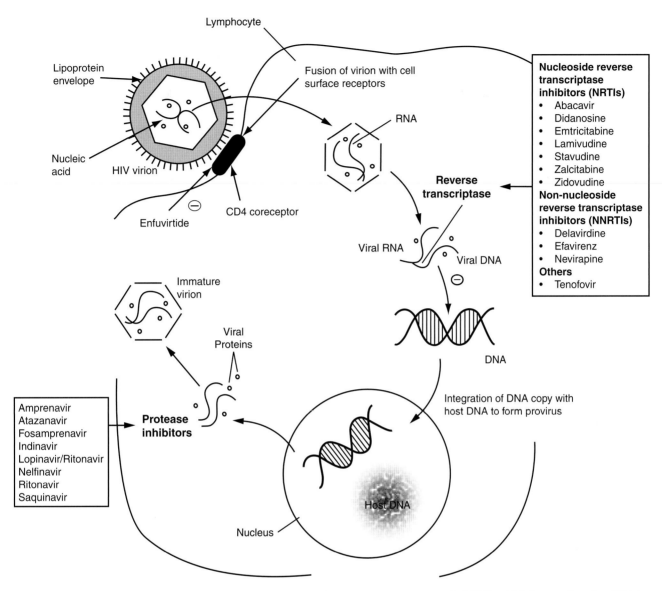

FIGURE 52-2 Inhibition sites for HIV replication. The HIV redundant genes are composed of RNA, which is translated to DNA by reverse transcriptase (RT) for viral reproduction. The RT inhibitors interfere with virus production at this site. When integrated DNA becomes part of the cell, the cell produces viral proteins requiring the protease enzyme for the production of new HIVs. The protease inhibitors block this enzyme to prevent the release of new viruses into the bloodstream. As a result, combination therapies can reduce the viral load of new HIV produced in the body. ⊖ = inhibition.

adverse reactions include arthralgia, hypersensitivity, myalgia, pancreatitis, weakness, GI distress, headache and insomnia. Use with caution in individuals with liver function impairment or alcoholism. Avoid use in people with peripheral neuropathy or kidney function impairment.

The usual adult oral dose of stavudine is 30 mg every 12 hours for people weighing <60 kg, or 40 mg every 12 hours for people weighing >60 kg.

ZALCITABINE

The antiviral agent zalcitabine is converted by cellular enzymes to its active form, ddC-triphosphate, which inhibits viral

reverse transcriptase, inhibiting viral replication. Administered orally, zalcitabine reaches peak plasma concentration in 1–2 hours and has a half-life of 1–3 hours. It is excreted primarily via the kidneys.

The table Drug Interactions 52-8 shows the effects that can occur when zalcitabine is given with the drugs listed.

Adverse reactions include peripheral neuropathy, arthralgia, hypersensitivity, myalgia, mouth and throat ulcers, gastric distress (stomach pain, diarrhoea and nausea), headache and, rarely, hepatotoxicity, leucopenia and pancreatitis. Use with caution in people with kidney function impairment. Avoid use in people with hypertriglyceridaemia or pancreatitis

DRUG INTERACTIONS 52-8 Zalcitabine	
Drug	**Possible effect and management**
Alcohol, azathioprine, frusemide, methyldopa, pentamidine IV, sulfonamides, sulindac, tetracyclines, thiazide diuretics or valproic acid	Concurrent use increases the potential risk of pancreatitis. Avoid, or a potentially serious drug interaction could occur. Monitor for symptoms and rising amylase or lipase concentrations
Aminoglycosides (parenteral), amphotericin B and foscarnet	Can decrease renal excretion of zalcitabine, which may result in toxicity. Reduce dose of zalcitabine
Chloramphenicol, cisplatin, didanosine, hydralazine, isoniazid, lithium, metronidazole, nitrofurantoin, nitrous oxide, phenytoin or vincristine	Concurrent drug administration can result in increased potential for peripheral neuropathy. Avoid, or a potentially serious drug interaction could occur. If given, monitor patient closely for numbness and tingling in the fingers and toes

or a history of these conditions, alcoholism, liver function impairment or peripheral neuropathy.

The usual adult oral dosage for zalcitabine is 0.75 mg every 8 hours at least 1 hour before or 4 hours after food. Dosage reduction is required with moderate to severe renal impairment.

Non-nucleoside reverse transcriptase inhibitors (NNRTIs)

The **non-nucleoside reverse transcriptase inhibitors** (NNRTIs) delavirdine, efavirenz and nevirapine block RNA-dependent and DNA-dependent DNA polymerases (Figure 52-2). These drugs are usually combined with two or more drugs to suppress HIV viral replication because use as sole agents results in rapid emergence of viral resistance (can occur within 1 week). Many interactions occur with these drugs because of the involvement of specific isoforms of the cytochrome P450 system. Relevant drug information sources should be consulted for specific drug interactions, as some are life-threatening.

DELAVIRDINE

Delavirdine is rapidly absorbed following oral administration, and peak plasma concentration occurs within 1 hour. The drug is extensively bound to plasma proteins and is metabolised in the liver by CYP3A4 and CYP2D6 to several inactive metabolites. The involvement of these cytochrome P450 enzymes makes delavirdine subject to drug interactions.

Many significant drug interactions have been reported with drugs inhibiting metabolism (e.g. erythromycin, ketoconazole) and inducing metabolism (e.g. phenytoin, carbamazepine). Check a current reference source for full information on potential drug interactions. A decrease in gastric acidity due to H_2-receptor antagonists (cimetidine and others) or concurrent antacids will decrease absorption of delavirdine. Avoid chronic use of these medications and separate antacid dosing by at least 1 hour.

Adverse reactions include diarrhoea, weakness, headache, nausea, vomiting, severe skin rash, conjunctivitis, fever, joint and muscle aches, oral lesions in mouth and, rarely, dyspnoea. Use with caution in people with renal impairment, as the metabolites are eliminated via the kidneys. Avoid use in individuals with known hypersensitivity to delavirdine and in people with hepatic impairment. Limited data are available on use during pregnancy, and specialist advice should be sought. The usual adult dose is 400 mg every 8 hours.

EFAVIRENZ

Peak plasma concentration of efavirenz occurs 3–5 hours after oral administration. Metabolism of the drug is complex, as it both induces its own metabolism and inhibits the metabolism of other drugs by the hepatic cytochrome P450 system. Involvement of CYP3A4 in the metabolism of efavirenz increases the likelihood of drug interactions. The half-life is 52–76 hours, and less than 1% appears in urine as unchanged drug.

Many drug interactions occur and current information sources should be consulted. Drugs that should not be administered concurrently with efavirenz include the benzodiazepines midazolam and triazolam, and cisapride. Other potentially significant drug interactions occur with warfarin, alcohol and protease inhibitors.

Individuals commonly complain of dizziness, drowsiness, insomnia, headache and abnormal dreaming. Allergic-type reactions and cardiovascular effects such as palpitations and tachycardia have been reported. Use with extreme caution in people with renal or hepatic impairment. Efavirenz is contraindicated in pregnancy, as it is embryotoxic and teratogenic in animals (ADEC Category D). The adult dose (capsule) is 600 mg daily and 720 mg (24 mL) of the oral liquid once daily. Refer to the manufacturer's literature for other dosing information.

NEVIRAPINE

Administered orally, nevirapine is well absorbed. It reaches peak plasma concentration in 4 hours and is distributed in

CSF (45% of plasma concentration). Nevirapine is metabolised in the liver and is also an inducer of hepatic cytochrome P450 enzymes; thus autoinduction, or an increased clearance and a decrease in drug half-life, occurs within 2–4 weeks of therapy.

The effects that can occur when nevirapine is given with other drugs are listed in the table Drug Interactions 52-9.

Adverse reactions include nausea, headache, diarrhoea, fever, hepatitis, ulcerative stomatitis and life-threatening skin reactions such as Stevens–Johnson syndrome. Nevirapine should be discontinued in individuals who develop a severe rash or a rash accompanied by symptoms such as fever, myalgia, fatigue, oral lesions and conjunctivitis. The rash usually occurs in the first 6 weeks, and women are at greater risk. Use with caution in individuals with kidney function impairment. Avoid use in people with nevirapine hypersensitivity or liver function impairment.

Initial therapy is 200 mg orally daily for 2 weeks. The maintenance dose is 200 mg twice daily in combination with another antiretroviral agent.

Protease inhibitors

The HIV protease, which is essential for viral infectivity, cleaves the viral precursor polypeptide into active viral enzymes and structural proteins. The protease inhibitors (PIs) prevent the protease from cleaving the polypeptide and hence block the subsequent maturation of the virus (Figure 52-2). The PIs include amprenavir, atazanavir, fosamprenavir, indinavir (see Drug Monograph 52-4), lopinavir with ritonavir, nelfinavir, ritonavir and saquinavir. These drugs are the most potent antiviral agents available and have suppressed viral replication for up to a year in clinical trials. Administering them in combination therapies has decreased viral loads and increased CD4 counts. Various combinations of these agents and their effects on HIV infection and AIDS complications and disease progression are continually under investigation.

Adverse reactions are common and include headache, diarrhoea, nausea, vomiting, elevated liver enzymes and a variety of metabolic disorders (e.g. diabetes, hypertriglyceridaemia and hypercholesterolaemia). Like many of the other antiretroviral drugs, PIs are subject to multiple drug interactions, and in particular their use is contraindicated with cisapride, ergot alkaloids, pimozide, midazolam and triazolam.

Comparative data for amprenavir, atazanavir and fosamprenavir (the prodrug of amprenavir) are shown in Table 52-2.

LOPINAVIR WITH RITONAVIR

This drug is a combination of lopinavir, which is an inhibitor of HIV-1 and HIV-2 proteases, and ritonavir, which is also a protease inhibitor but also an inhibitor of the metabolism of lopinavir by CYP3A. The drug is formulated as soft capsules and as an oral liquid, and enhanced bioavailability occurs when both formulations are taken with food. Lopinavir is metabolised by hepatic CYP3A, and after multiple dosing <3% is excreted as unchanged drug in urine. Ritonavir is also metabolised by CYP3A, and although this was initially viewed as undesirable, it was later realised that this inhibitory action could be useful in allowing a lower dose of a PI to be given, as inhibition of metabolism by ritonavir would effectively increase the plasma concentration of the PI. This combination is now being investigated in numerous clinical trials.

Drug interactions are to some extent predictable, and include interactions with rifampicin, corticosteroids, statins, St John's wort, azole antifungals, methadone, efavirenz and nevirapine. Adverse reactions include exacerbation of diabetes mellitus, increased bleeding, lipodystrophy (redistribution of fat including central obesity and 'buffalo hump'), hyperlipidaemia and, rarely, pancreatitis.

NELFINAVIR

Nelfinavir is well absorbed in the presence of food, and peak plasma concentration occurs within 2–4 hours. The half-life is 3–5 hours, and most of the dose is recovered in faeces as oxidative metabolites. Like the other protease inhibitors, nelfinavir is metabolised by CYP3A4 and is subject to numerous drug interactions. Check a current reference for an extensive list of drug interactions. Nelfinavir also reduces the efficacy of oral contraceptives, so alternative approaches are recommended.

DRUG INTERACTIONS 52-9 Nevirapine	
Drug	**Possible effect and management**
Oral contraceptives containing oestrogen; protease inhibitors such as indinavir, ritonavir and saquinavir	Nevirapine increases CYP3A activity, which will decrease the plasma concentrations of the oral contraceptives and the protease inhibitors. Concurrent use is not recommended
Methadone	Increased metabolism can cause methadone withdrawal or ineffective pain relief. Adjust dose if required
Rifabutin or rifampicin	Nevirapine induction of CYP3A can decrease plasma concentrations of these drugs. Monitor closely if used concurrently

DRUG MONOGRAPH 52-4 INDINAVIR

The complete mechanism of action of indinavir is unknown. It appears to inhibit the replication of retroviruses (HIV types 1 and 2) by interfering with HIV protease, which cleaves inactive viral protein precursors into active proteins that make the HIV particle infectious. Indinavir affects the replication cycle of HIV. It is active both in acute infection and in chronically infected cells, which are generally not affected by the nucleoside analogue reverse transcriptase inhibitors, such as didanosine, lamivudine, stavudine, zalcitabine and zidovudine. Thus this product has a virustatic effect due to its HIV protease inhibitor effects.

PHARMACOKINETICS Administered orally, indinavir reaches peak plasma concentration in about 1 hour. It is extensively metabolised in the liver by CYP3A4 and excreted primarily in faeces.

DRUG INTERACTIONS The following effects can occur when indinavir is given with the drugs listed below:

Drug	Possible effect and management
Cisapride, midazolam or triazolam	Indinavir and these drugs are metabolised in the liver by CYP3A4. Concurrent use can result in a decreased metabolism of these drugs and toxicity. Avoid, or a potentially serious drug interaction could occur
Didanosine	When given concurrently, space drugs at least 2 hours apart and take indinavir on an empty stomach. Indinavir needs an acidic pH for absorption, and didanosine needs a buffer to raise pH to prevent acid from destroying it

Drug	Possible effect and management
Ketoconazole	Concurrent use results in an increased plasma concentration of indinavir. Reduce the dose of indinavir to 600 mg every 8 hours if administered with ketoconazole
Rifabutin	Concurrent use results in an increased plasma concentration of rifabutin. Reduce the dose of rifabutin to 400 mg every 8 hours if administered concurrently with indinavir
Rifampicin	Rifampicin is a potent inducer of CYP3A4, which can decrease the plasma concentration of indinavir. Avoid concurrent use

ADVERSE REACTIONS These include gastric distress, nausea, vomiting, diarrhoea, headache, dizziness, fatigue, insomnia, changes in taste sensation, kidney stones, fever, flu-like syndrome and, rarely, diabetes or hyperglycaemia and ketoacidosis.

WARNINGS AND CONTRAINDICATIONS Use with caution in individuals with hyperbilirubinaemia or hyperglycaemia. The risk of nephrolithiasis is increased in dehydrated people. Avoid use in people with indinavir hypersensitivity or liver function impairment.

DOSAGE AND ADMINISTRATION The usual adult dose is 800 mg every 8 hours on an empty stomach.

TABLE 52-2 Comparative information on protease inhibitors

DRUG	HALF-LIFE (H)	METABOLISM	DRUG INTERACTIONS*	ADVERSE REACTIONS
Amprenavir	7–10.5	Hepatic (~97%) (CYP3A4)	St John's wort, antacids, rifampicin, midazolam, triazolam, cisapride, pimozide, phenobarbitone, phenytoin, statins	Paraesthesia, rash, headache, fatigue, GI disturbances; rarely, severe or life-threatening skin reactions
Atazanavir	~6	Hepatic (CYP3A4)	Antimycobacterials, antineoplastics, benzodiazepines, calcium channel blockers, statins, pimozide, indinavir, proton pump inhibitors, St John's wort	Hyperbilirubinaemia, heart block, rash, depression, abdominal pain, fatigue, dizziness, insomnia, GI disturbances, worsening cough
Fosamprenavir	~7	Hepatic† (CYP3A4)	Ritonavir, statins, amiodarone, tricyclic antidepressants, quinidine, warfarin, rifabutin, St John's wort	Same as amprenavir

*Examples of drug interactions with PIs; relevant drug information sources should be consulted, as drug interactions are numerous and often not predictable.
†Fosamprenavir is hydrolysed to amprenavir, which is the active drug.

Adverse reactions include diarrhoea, flatulence, nausea, skin rash, diabetes or hyperglycaemia, and ketoacidosis. Use with caution in people with phenylketonuria, as the oral formulation contains phenylalanine. Nelfinavir is contraindicated in individuals with nelfinavir hypersensitivity or liver impairment. The adult dose is 750 mg every 8 hours or 1250 mg twice daily. For optimal absorption, nelfinavir should be taken with a light meal.

RITONAVIR

Administered orally, ritonavir reaches peak plasma concentration within 2 or 4 hours (fasting or non-fasting). Five metabolites have been identified with ritonavir, but only the M-2 metabolite has antiviral activity. It has a half-life of 3–5 hours and is excreted primarily in faeces.

The effects that can occur when ritonavir is given with the drugs listed are shown in the table Drug Interactions 52-10.

Adverse reactions include weakness, nausea, vomiting, diarrhoea, stomach distress, allergic reactions, back or chest pain, chills, facial oedema, dizziness, headache, drowsiness, alterations in taste perception, numbness or tingling around mouth (circumoral paraesthesia), peripheral paraesthesia, flu symptoms and, rarely, diabetes, hyperglycaemia and ketoacidosis. Use with caution in patients with haemophilia and liver function impairment. Avoid use in people with ritonavir hypersensitivity. The usual dose is 600 mg twice a day, with meals. A lower starting dose (300 mg 12-hourly) may reduce the incidence of nausea, but the desirable dose of 600 mg 12-hourly should be achieved within 2 weeks.

SAQUINAVIR

Administered orally, saquinavir has extensive first-pass metabolism, is highly protein-bound, is metabolised in the liver and is excreted primarily in the faeces.

DRUG INTERACTIONS 52-10 Ritonavir

Drug	Possible effect and management
Zolpidem, midazolam or triazolam	Ritonavir's inhibition of various cytochrome P450 isoforms can also produce a large increase in plasma concentrations of some medications, which may result in excessive sedation and respiratory depression. Do not administer these drugs concurrently with ritonavir, as a potentially serious drug interaction could occur
Antiarrhythmics, antidepressants and ergot alkaloids	Do not administer these medications concurrently with ritonavir, as large increases in the plasma concentrations of these medications can occur. This increases the potential for dysrhythmias, haematological disorders, convulsions and other serious adverse reactions. Avoid, or a potentially serious drug interaction could occur
Oral contraceptives containing oestrogen	When contraceptives containing ethinyloestradiol are given concurrently with ritonavir, the oestrogen plasma concentration is lower. An oral contraceptive with a higher oestrogen content or an alternative contraception method should be used
Theophylline	Concurrent use reduces theophylline plasma concentration by up to 40%. Monitor theophylline plasma concentration closely, as drug dosage adjustment may be necessary

DRUG INTERACTIONS 52-11 Saquinavir

Drug	Possible effect and management
Calcium channel blockers, clindamycin, dapsone, quinidine, triazolam, midazolam or amiodarone, atorvastatin*, simvastatin* or pimozide*	Saquinavir can increase plasma concentrations of these drugs because the drugs are substrates of CYP3A4. Monitor patients closely if concurrent drug therapy is used
Ergot alkaloids	Reduced metabolism of ergot alkaloids increases likelihood of peripheral ischaemia. Avoid concurrent administration
Nelfinavir	Concentration is significantly increased by saquinavir and a dosage reduction may be required
Rifampicin, rifabutin, carbamazepine, dexamethasone, phenobarbitone or phenytoin	These drugs are potent inducers of cytochrome P450 enzymes; concurrent use may reduce plasma concentrations of the drugs and possibly of saquinavir. Avoid concurrent drug administration

*Combination not recommended

The effects that can occur when saquinavir is given with the drugs listed are shown in the table Drug Interactions 52-11.

Adverse reactions are usually mild and include diarrhoea, abdominal distress, headache, weakness and, rarely, paraesthesia, skin rash, confusion, ataxia, Stevens–Johnson syndrome, seizures, thrombocytopenia, anaemia and hepatotoxicity. Avoid use in people with saquinavir hypersensitivity. Dosage reduction may be required in individuals with hepatic dysfunction. The usual dose in combination with a nucleoside analogue (e.g. zalcitabine or zidovudine) is 600 mg three times a day, administered within 2 hours of a full meal.

Other antiretrovirals
ENFUVIRTIDE
Enfuvirtide is a new and novel antiretroviral drug termed a fusion inhibitor. It is a synthetic 36-amino-acid peptide that binds to the gp41 subunit of a glycoprotein found in the viral envelope. This blocks viral fusion with the CD4 receptor of the host cell and prevents the conformational changes required to allow fusion. Currently, this drug is indicated for HIV-1 infection in people where other treatments have failed.

The half-life is approximately 4 hours and pathways of elimination have not yet been determined. It is administered SC, and because it is a peptide, it is likely that it is catabolised to its constituent amino acids. Unlike many other antiretrovirals, enfuvirtide is not an inhibitor of CYP450 enzymes. Adverse reactions are common and include injection site reactions (e.g. pain, erythema, itch), which result in discontinuation in about 3% of people; peripheral neuropathy; insomnia; depression; respiratory symptoms (e.g. cough, dyspnoea) and loss of weight and appetite. The adult dose is 90 mg SC twice daily.

TENOFOVIR
Tenofovir disoproxil fumarate is a prodrug that is converted to tenofovir, an analogue of adenosine. Similar to the NRTIs, tenofovir competitively inhibits the HIV reverse transcriptase and causes chain termination after its incorporation in DNA. Currently it is indicated for use in combination with other antiretrovirals. Administered orally, the bioavailability of tenofovir is enhanced if taken with a high-fat meal.

Similar to enfuvirtide, tenofovir is not an inhibitor of CYP and, as it is excreted predominantly by the kidney (70%–80%), clinical CYP drug interactions are unlikely. However, tenofovir can cause nephrotoxicity, which may be exacerbated if administered concomitantly with other nephrotoxic drugs (e.g. lopinavir with ritonavir increases tenofovir concentration, increasing the risk of nephrotoxicity). Adverse reactions include GI disturbances, headache and hypophosphataemia. The usual adult dose is 300 mg daily of tenofovir disoproxil fumarate, which is equivalent to 136 mg of the active constituent tenofovir.

ADEC Category	Drug
	PREGNANCY SAFETY*
A	Miconazole, nystatin
B1	Emtricitabine, famciclovir, oseltamivir, saquinavir, zanamivir
B2	Amphotericin, atazanavir, didanosine, enfuvirtide, nelfinavir
B3	Abacavir, aciclovir, adefovir, amantadine, amprenavir, caspofungin, delavirdine, flucytosine, fosamprenavir, foscarnet, griseofulvin, indinavir, itraconazole, ketoconazole, lamivudine, lopinavir/ritonavir, nevirapine, ritonavir, stavudine, tenofovir, valaciclovir, voriconazole, zidovudine
D	Cidofovir, efavirenz, fluconazole, ganciclovir, valganciclovir, zalcitabine
X	Ribavirin

* Unknown for palivizumab, as studies have not been conducted.

DRUGS AT A GLANCE 52: Antifungal and antiviral drugs

Therapeutic group	Pharmacological group	Key examples	Key pages
Antifungal drugs	Systemic/topical antifungals	amphotericin B	828
		azoles	
		fluconazole	826–7, 9
		itraconazole	826–7, 9
		ketoconazole	826–7, 9
		caspofungin	828
		griseofulvin	830
		nystatin	831
Antiviral (non-retroviral) drugs	DNA polymerase inhibitors	aciclovir	832
		ganciclovir	832
	Neuraminidase inhibitors	oseltamivir	833
		zanamivir	833
	Miscellaneous drugs	amantadine	834
		ribavirin	835
Antiretroviral drugs	Nucleoside reverse transcriptase inhibitors (NRTIs)	didanosine	836
		stavudine	838
		zidovudine	837
	Non-nucleoside reverse transcriptase inhibitors (NNRTIs)	delavirdine	840
		efavirenz	840
	Protease inhibitors (PIs)	amprenavir	842
		indinavir	842
		ritonavir	843

KEY POINTS

- Systemic fungal and viral infections can be serious (even life-threatening).
- The systemic antifungal agents are potent and potentially toxic medications. They include amphotericin B, fluconazole, flucytosine, griseofulvin, itraconazole, ketoconazole, miconazole and nystatin.
- Drugs that are systemic fungistatic or fungicidal agents are used to treat a wide variety of mycotic infections.
- Chemotherapy for viral diseases has tended to be more limited than chemotherapy for bacterial diseases because the development and clinical application of antiviral drugs is more difficult.
- The antiviral and antiretroviral drugs discussed in this chapter include the DNA polymerase inhibitors (aciclovir, famciclovir, ganciclovir, valaciclovir, valganciclovir); the nucleoside analogue reverse transcriptase inhibitors (abacavir, didanosine, emtricitabine, lamivudine, stavudine, zalcitabine and zidovudine); the non-nucleoside reverse transcriptase inhibitors (delavirdine, efavirenz and nevirapine); the protease inhibitors (amprenavir, atazanavir, fosamprenavir, indinavir, lopinavir with ritonavir, nelfinavir, ritonavir and saquinavir); the neuraminidase inhibitors (oseltamivir and zanamivir); and miscellaneous antiviral drugs (adefovir, amantadine, cidofovir, foscarnet, palivizumab and ribavirin).
- Many antiviral drugs are subject to various drug–drug interactions, and relevant sources should be consulted in relation to specific drugs.

REVIEW EXERCISES

1. Describe the differences in absorption rates among the oral azole antifungal agents. Which agents require an acid medium, a fasting state, or food for absorption?

2. Discuss the mechanism of action of griseofulvin in the treatment of onychomycosis, or nail fungus.

3. What is the action of aciclovir in the treatment of herpes simplex virus? Name the primary drug interactions, adverse reactions and contraindications with the use of this product.

4. Name two antiviral drugs that should not be used in individuals with peripheral neuropathy. Name five other drugs that can also cause peripheral neuropathy.

5. Why are antiviral drugs often used in combination for the treatment of HIV?

6. Explain why the protease inhibitors are in general subject to many drug interactions.

REFERENCES AND FURTHER READING

Australian Medicines Handbook 2006. Adelaide: AMH, 2006.

Australian Institute of Health and Welfare 2004. *Australia's Health 2004.* Canberra: AIHW, 2004.

Bennett JE. Antimicrobial agents: antifungal agents. In: Hardman JG, Limbird LE, Gilman AG (eds). *Goodman & Gilman's The Pharmacological Basis of Therapeutics.* 10th edn. New York: McGraw-Hill, 2001 [ch. 49].

Hayden FG. Antimicrobial agents: antiviral agents (nonretroviral). In: Hardman JG, Limbird LE, Gilman AG (eds). *Goodman & Gilman's The Pharmacological Basis of Therapeutics.* 10th edn. New York: McGraw-Hill, 2001 [ch. 50].

Hovanessian HC. New developments in the treatment of HIV disease: an overview. *Annals of Emergency Medicine* 1999; 33: 546–55.

MacDonald L, Kazanjian P. Antiretroviral therapy in HIV infection: an update. *Hospital Formulary* 1996; 31:780–804.

Nabel GJ. Challenges and opportunities for development of an AIDS vaccine. *Nature* 2001; 410: 1002–7.

Raffanti SP, Haas DW. Antimicrobial agents: antiretroviral agents. In: Hardman JG, Limbird LE, Gilman AG (eds). *Goodman & Gilman's The Pharmacological Basis of Therapeutics.* 10th edn. New York: McGraw-Hill, 2001 [ch. 51].

Robinson M. Reining in influenza: the benefits of early treatment with oseltamivir. *Australian Pharmacy Trade* 2001; 19 April: 17–22.

Sheehan DJ, Hitchcock CA, Sibley CM. Current and emerging azole antifungal agents. *Clinical Microbiology Reviews* 1999; 12: 40–79.

evolve   More weblinks at http://evolve.elsevier.com/AU/Bryant/pharmacology/

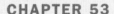

CHAPTER 53

Antiprotozoal, Antimycobacterial and Anthelmintic Drugs

CHAPTER FOCUS

This chapter reviews the various drugs used to treat protozoal diseases such as malaria and amoebiasis, mycobacterial infections such as tuberculosis and leprosy, and helminth (worm) infections. These diseases are prevalent throughout the world and their control peaks and wanes, often due to factors such as availability of drugs, patient compliance with specific drug therapies, and the development of drug-resistant strains. Control of these infections is important and challenging to the health-care professional, and in some instances a global approach to eradication (as with malaria, tuberculosis and leprosy) has been adopted.

OBJECTIVES

- To describe the life cycle of the malarial parasite and amoeba in the human body.
- To describe the mechanism of action of chloroquine and mefloquine.
- To discuss the epidemiology, pathogenesis and treatment of tuberculosis.
- To discuss the drugs used to treat leprosy and helminthiasis.

KEY DRUGS

albendazole
chloroquine
clofazimine
dapsone
isoniazid
ivermectin
paromomycin
pyrantel
pyrazinamide
quinine
rifampicin

KEY TERMS

amoebiasis
cestodes
helminths
leprosy
malaria
toxoplasmosis
trichomoniasis
tuberculosis

MALARIA

Malaria has been and still is a prevalent disease despite efforts to control the causative parasite and insect vector. Each year 300–500 million cases of clinical malaria occur, with a further 10,000–30,000 people contracting the disease after visiting endemic areas (Croft 2000). The majority of cases reported within Australia in recent years have been in people returning from endemic areas (AIHW 2004). However, in 2002, 10 local cases of malaria were diagnosed and these were the first reports of malaria in Australia since 1986. Four species of the genus *Plasmodium* are responsible for human malaria: *P. vivax*, *P. malariae*, *P. ovale* and *P. falciparum*. *P. ovale* malaria, which is found in West Africa, is considered rare. *P. falciparum* malaria is the most lethal form of malaria and is usually resistant to chloroquine.

Malaria is transmitted to humans by the bite of an infected female *Anopheles* mosquito, as well as by blood transfusion (usually *P. malariae*).

Life cycle of the malarial parasite

To understand the chemotherapy of malaria, it is essential to review the life cycle of the malarial parasite, the plasmodium. Figure 53-1 presents the cycle in seven basic steps. Plasmodia have two interdependent life cycles: the sexual cycle, which takes place in the mosquito; and the asexual cycle, which occurs in the human body.

Sexual cycle

The sexual cycle is noted in step 7 of Figure 53-1. The female *Anopheles* mosquito becomes the carrier of the parasite by drawing blood containing male and female gametocytes (sexual forms of the parasite) from an infected person. In the stomach of the mosquito, the female gametocytes are fertilised by the male gametocytes to form zygotes, which undergo numerous cell divisions to develop into sporozoites. The formation of sporozoites in the mosquito completes the sexual cycle. Sporozoites then migrate to the salivary glands of the infected mosquito and are injected into the bloodstream of the human by the bite of the female insect (step 1, Figure 53-1).

Asexual cycle

In humans, the asexual cycle of the plasmodium consists of the exoerythrocytic phase and the erythrocytic phase.

EXOERYTHROCYTIC PHASE

Shortly after the introduction of the sporozoites into the circulation of the human, they leave the blood and enter fixed tissue cells (reticuloendothelial cells) of the liver, where multiplication and maturation take place (step 2). For a period of time that varies with different plasmodia (8–42 days), the individual exhibits no symptoms, no parasites are found in erythrocytes, and the blood is non-infective. This phase is known as the pre-erythrocytic stage. The parasites are called primary tissue schizonts, or pre-erythrocytic forms. After this stage, the young parasites burst from the liver cells as merozoites.

ERYTHROCYTIC PHASE

When merozoites enter the bloodstream, they penetrate the erythrocytes and begin the erythrocytic phase of their existence (step 3a). In the case of *P. vivax* (but not *P. falciparum*), some of the merozoites invade other tissue cells to form secondary exoerythrocytic forms (step 3b). The relapses seen in *P. vivax* and other forms of malaria are believed to be caused by the successive formations of merozoites produced by various secondary exoerythrocytic forms of the parasite. Drugs affecting malarial parasites in the bloodstream do not always destroy those in the exoerythrocytic, or tissue, stage.

After the merozoites bore into red blood cells, they again multiply, but this time asexually, forming erythrocytic schizonts (Figure 53-2). The erythrocytic phase is completed when the parasitised red blood cells rupture, setting free many more merozoites that have formed from the schizonts. Pyrogenic substances are also liberated, causing a rapid rise in body temperature (step 4, Figure 53-1). Some of the merozoites may be destroyed in the plasma of the blood by leucocytes and other agents, but some enter other erythrocytes to repeat the cycle (step 5). The recurring chills, fever and prostration that are prominent clinical symptoms of malaria occur when the red blood cells rupture and release the young parasites with foreign protein and cell products. The erythrocytic phase lasts 48–72 hours, depending on the plasmodium involved. After a few cycles, some of the asexual forms of the malarial parasites develop into sexual forms called gametocytes (step 6). When the mosquito bites a person infected with malarial parasites and ingests the sexual forms, the cycle begins again.

P. vivax is the most common form of malaria; this infestation is usually mild, drug resistance is uncommon, and it can easily be suppressed with antimalarial medications. The *P. falciparum* strain of malaria is less common but much more severe than the *P. vivax* form. Drug-resistant strains of *P. falciparum* exist, and the symptoms with this infestation occur at irregular intervals and can cause very serious complications. If untreated or if treatment is delayed, the disease may progress to irreversible cardiovascular shock and death. Although relapses are reported with *P. vivax* malaria, once the *P. falciparum* form is eliminated, no dormant forms remain in the liver, therefore no relapses are reported with *P. falciparum*.

People who harbour the sexual forms of plasmodia are called carriers, as it is from carriers that mosquitoes receive

HUMAN ASEXUAL CYCLE OF THE MALARIAL PARASITE

Exoerythrocyte phase (may continue several months or years)	Erythrocytic phase

Exoerythrocyte phase
(may continue several months or years)

Primary tissue phase
(primarily liver)

Pre-erythrocytic stage (8–42 days [varies with species of *Plasmodium*]); asymptomatic

Erythrocytic phase

Red blood cells
(erythrocytes)

48–72 hours; symptoms coincide with discharge of merozoites from the erythrocytes

Female mosquito

1 *Anopheles* mosquito inoculates human with sporozoites, which localise in liver tissue

2 Sporozoites penetrate tissue cells and grow

Mature merozoites

Secondary tissue phase
(primarily liver)

3b Merozoites are released into the bloodstream, invade body tissue and penetrate cells, where they grow and divide; this may cause relapse of the disease after several months or years of remission

Bloodstream

3a Merozoites are released from tissue cells into the bloodstream and invade red blood cells

Red blood cell

Merozoites, foreign protein cell products (symptoms: chills, fever, profound sweating)

4 Merozoites grow and divide, red blood cell ruptures

5 Merozoites invade and penetrate other red blood cells

6 Some merozoites grow and divide and produce gametocytes within red blood cell

Sporozoites in saliva of mosquito

Oocysts

Zygotes

Anopheles female mosquito bites human and acquires gametocytes from red blood cells

7 Mosquito: sexual cycle of malaria parasite

FIGURE 53-1 Life cycle of the malarial parasite.

the parasite forms that perpetuate the disease. The asexual forms cause the clinical symptoms of malaria. Carriers should avoid giving blood because the recipient of this blood could contract malaria or become a carrier. A large number of malaria cases (some fatal) have arisen from transfusions of infected blood.

Antimalarial drugs

The choice of a drug for treatment of malaria is based on the particular malarial strain involved and the stage of the *Plasmodium* life cycle. Drugs (schizonticides) are therefore classified according to the type of therapy they provide, which is as follows.

Travellers to endemic areas should receive malaria chemoprophylaxis, beginning 1–3 weeks before entering the area. Current information on this can be obtained from several sources in Australasia (see Box 53-1). **Chloroquine**, which suppresses the asexual erythrocytic forms, is effective against all species of malaria except drug-resistant *P. falciparum* (see Drug Monograph 53-1). In chloroquine-resistant *P. falciparum* areas, mefloquine is used for prophylaxis,

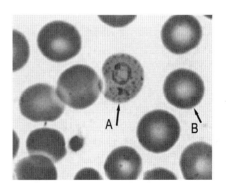

FIGURE 53-2 Peripheral blood film (magnification ×100) showing a normal red cell (**B**) and a red cell with a trophozoite of *P. vivax* displaying the typical signet ring form and Schüffners stippling (**A**). With kind permission of John Rumpff and Ros Biebrick, Haematology, *SouthPath*, Flinders Medical Centre, Adelaide, Australia.

or if the person cannot take mefloquine, doxycycline is recommended.

Clinical cure of an acute malaria attack occurs when multiplication of the parasites within the erythrocyte is interrupted, thereby terminating the malarial symptoms of the attack. If chloroquine-resistant *P. falciparum* is present, then combination therapies such as pyrimethamine and a sulfonamide (sulfadoxine) may be necessary.

To eradicate latent forms of *P. vivax* that persist and may cause infection relapse, primaquine therapy may be recommended. This drug is usually started after an acute attack or during the last few weeks of chloroquine prophylaxis. Inducing a radical cure requires medications that destroy both the exoerythrocytic and erythrocytic parasites to prevent relapsing malaria; therefore primaquine is given with chloroquine, which suppresses the erythrocytic cycle.

The emergence of drug-resistant strains of malaria, particularly that caused by *P. falciparum*, poses a major public health problem throughout the world. Despite the combined efforts of many countries to eradicate malaria, it remains the most devastating infectious disease in the world because of the many lives lost and the economic burden it imposes.

It is essential that travellers contemplating a trip to areas of the world where malaria is endemic be aware of the need to obtain information about measures for reducing exposure to the disease. Malaria exists in New Guinea, Indonesia, Asia, Central and South America, the Middle East and many other countries.

Mefloquine

Mefloquine is a blood schizonticide; it prevents the replication of asexual erythrocytic parasites but has no effect on the gametocytes of *P. falciparum*. Its exact mechanism of action is unknown but it is believed to inhibit protein synthesis (by binding plasmodial DNA), inhibit plasmodial haem polymerase and raise the intravascular pH of the acidic food vacuoles in the parasite. It is not effective in eliminating the

exoerythrocytic or intrahepatic stages of *P. vivax* or *P. ovale* infections.

Mefloquine is indicated for the prevention and treatment of chloroquine-resistant malaria and multiple-drug-resistant strains of *P. falciparum*, and to prevent malaria caused by *P. vivax*, *P. ovale* and *P. malariae*. It is a potent and fast-acting antimalarial drug that is well absorbed orally, widely distributed in the body and reaches peak plasma concentration in 2–12 hours. It has a long elimination half-life of 13–33 days and is extensively metabolised by the liver, with <10% of the drug excreted unchanged in the urine. Most of the drug is excreted through bile in faeces. See the Drug Interactions table 53-1 for mefloquine.

Adverse reactions are generally dose-related and occur more commonly in therapeutic than in prophylactic drug regimens. Adverse effects include nausea, vomiting, headache, dizziness, insomnia, gastric distress, diarrhoea, visual disturbances and,

DRUG INTERACTIONS 53-1 Mefloquine

Drug	Possible effect and management
Anticonvulsants	The effect of anticonvulsants is antagonised by mefloquine and it is contraindicated in epilepsy
β-blockers, calcium channel blockers, amiodarone or quinine	Concurrent use may result in higher risk of arrhythmias, cardiac arrest and seizures (the latter especially with quinine). Avoid or a potentially serious drug interaction may occur. If concurrent use cannot be avoided, monitor closely
Chloroquine	May increase seizure activity. Monitor closely
Valproic acid	Decreased plasma concentration of valproic acid, with loss of seizure control. Avoid this combination

rarely, bradycardia and central nervous system (CNS) toxicity (depression, hallucinations, convulsions, psychosis, anxiety and confusion). Use mefloquine with caution in people with cardiac disease or hepatic impairment. Avoid use in people with epilepsy, heart block (first- or second-degree) and a history of psychiatric problems (psychosis, hallucinations, anxiety and depression). Mefloquine may impair the performance of skilled tasks for 2–3 weeks after dosing.

The usual adult dosage for prophylaxis is 250 mg each week, commencing 1 week before departure, then on the same day of each week during and for 2 weeks after the visit to the malarious area.

Primaquine

Primaquine's mechanism of action is unknown but it can bind to and alter plasmodial DNA. It is very effective in the exoerythrocytic stages of *P. vivax* and *P. ovale* malaria and against the primary phase (exoerythrocytic stage) of *P. falciparum* malaria. It is also effective against the sexual forms (gametocytes) of plasmodia (especially *P. falciparum*). Indications include the prevention of malaria relapses (radical cure) caused by *P. vivax* and *P. ovale*, and it is also effective against gametocytes of *P. falciparum*.

Primaquine is absorbed rapidly from the gastrointestinal tract (GIT) and reaches peak plasma concentrations within 2–3 hours. The drug undergoes extensive presystemic metabolism to the main metabolite, carboxyprimaquine, which is further metabolised to unidentified compounds. It has a half-life of about 6 hours, and the amount of unchanged drug excreted in urine is <4%.

Adverse reactions include gastric distress (stomach cramps or pain, nausea and vomiting), haemolytic anaemia (anorexia; back, leg or abdominal pain; dark urine; pale skin; weakness, fever), methaemoglobinaemia (cyanosis, dizziness, respiratory difficulty, weakness) and, rarely, leucopenia. The use of mefloquine concurrently with other myelosuppressive drugs should be avoided because of the higher risk of myelosuppression. Use primaquine with caution in people with a history (personal or family) of acute haemolytic anaemia or a nicotinamide adenine dinucleotide (NADH) methaemoglobin reductase deficiency. Avoid use in people with primaquine hypersensitivity or G6PD deficiency (primaquine may cause haemolytic anaemia, especially in people deficient in G6PD) and in children under 12 months old because of increased risk of methaemoglobinaemia.

When used for prophylaxis (third-line drug) of malaria (susceptible organisms) the adult dose (base) is 30 mg daily starting 7 days before entering a malaria-endemic area and continuing for 1 week after leaving the area.

Quinine

Quinine was the first drug used to treat malaria (see Clinical Interest Box 53-2). As a schizonticidal agent, it concentrates

DRUG MONOGRAPH 53–1 CHLOROQUINE

The mechanism of action of **chloroquine** as an antimalarial agent is not fully known, but it is a potent schizonticidal drug acting against the erythrocytic form of all four plasmodial species. It causes accumulation of haem, which is toxic to the parasite, in infected erythrocytes by inhibiting haem polymerase. It also inhibits plasmodial DNA/RNA synthesis and raises the pH of the acidic food vacuoles in sensitive parasites, thus interfering with its functions. During suppressive therapy, chloroquine inhibits the erythrocytic stage of development of plasmodia, whereas in acute malarial attacks it interferes with erythrocytic schizogony (asexual fission) of parasites. Because it selectively accumulates in parasitised erythrocytes, it has a selective toxicity in the erythrocytic stages of plasmodial infestation.

INDICATIONS Chloroquine (and hydroxychloroquine, which is used if chloroquine is not available) is indicated for the prevention and treatment of malaria for the four strains of *Plasmodium*; however, widespread resistance to chloroquine exists. Curing *P. vivax* and *P. ovale* malaria requires concurrent administration of primaquine. Chloroquine and hydroxychloroquine are also used for the treatment of rheumatoid arthritis and for discoid and systemic lupus erythematosus (see Chapter 55). Chloroquine is further used to treat amoebic liver abscess, usually in combination with a primary intestinal amoebicide.

PHARMACOKINETICS Chloroquine and hydroxychloroquine are fairly well absorbed orally, are widely distributed in body tissues and reach peak plasma concentrations in around 1–3.5 hours. Erythrocytes containing the parasites accumulate 100–600 times more chloroquine than uninfected cells. The terminal half-life of chloroquine is 1–2 months, while the terminal half-life for hydroxychloroquine in blood is about 50 days, and in plasma 32 days. Both drugs are partly metabolised in the liver (about 50%) and in each case both metabolites and unchanged drug are excreted by the kidneys.

DRUG INTERACTIONS Antacids reduce the bioavailability of chloroquine, which reduces its effectiveness as an antimalarial. Administration of these drugs should be separated by at least 4 hours.

ADVERSE REACTIONS These are usually dose-related and reversible, and include gastric distress, headaches, pruritus, blurred vision, difficulty in reading, headache, itching (reported mostly in black patients), hair loss or bleaching of hair, rash, corneal opacities, keratopathy, retinopathy and a blue–black discoloration of skin, nails or the inside of the mouth. Rarely, blood disorders (agranulocytosis, neutropenia or thrombocytopenia), hypotension, cardiac dysrhythmia, mood alterations,

(Continued)

DRUG MONOGRAPH 53-1 CHLOROQUINE

(continued)

psychosis, ototoxicity, muscle weakness and convulsions have been reported for both drugs.

WARNINGS AND CONTRAINDICATIONS These drugs should be used with caution in patients with severe gastrointestinal (GI) disorders, porphyria, or glucose-6-phosphate dehydrogenase (G6PD) deficiency. About 5%–10% of Sephardic Jews, Greeks, Iranians, Chinese, Filipinos and Indonesians have G6PD deficiency, so it is particularly important to check this in people descended from these ethnic groups. This deficiency is transmitted as an X-linked trait, and in G6PD deficiency, red blood cell metabolism is impaired by chloroquine and other antimalarials.

Avoid use in people with psoriasis, retinal damage, severe blood dyscrasias, liver function impairment, severe neurological disorders or retinal or visual field changes (both drugs may cause ototoxicity, polyneuritis, convulsions or neuromyopathy). These drugs are contraindicated in people with chloroquine or hydroxychloroquine hypersensitivity.

DOSAGE AND ADMINISTRATION The usual adult oral chloroquine dosage for malaria prophylaxis is 310 mg (base) once weekly; for children 4–8 years, half the adult dose (155 mg) weekly; and, for children 1–4 years, 77.5 mg weekly. For hydroxychloroquine prophylaxis the adult oral dose is 400 mg once weekly and, for children, 6.5 mg/kg (maximum 400 mg) once weekly.

ADDITIONAL COMMENTS Both drugs should be taken at the same time and on the same day each week, beginning 1 week before entering the malarial endemic area and continuing for 4 weeks after leaving the area.

DRUG INTERACTIONS 53-2 Quinine

Drug	Possible effect and management
Digoxin	Increased plasma concentration of digoxin due to decreased clearance. Halve digoxin dose and monitor plasma concentration
Mefloquine	When used concurrently, an increased incidence of convulsions and electrocardiogram (ECG) abnormalities have been reported. This predisposes the persons to cardiac arrhythmias. If possible, avoid this combination. If not, then administer mefloquine at least 12 hours after the last dose of quinine. If both drugs must be given concurrently, the patient should be hospitalised and closely monitored for cardiac arrhythmias and seizure activity
Warfarin	Increased risk of bleeding due to inhibition of synthesis of clotting factors. Monitor international normalised ratio (INR) and adjust dose of warfarin if necessary

cardiac arrhythmias, G6PD deficiency or myasthenia gravis. Avoid use in people with quinine or quinidine hypersensitivity or a history of haemoglobinuria or optic neuritis.

The adult dosage (i.e. for persons >50 kg) for chloroquine-resistant *P. falciparum* malaria is 600 mg orally every 8 hours for 7 days, plus either pyrimethamine with sulfadoxine, or doxycycline.

Combination antimalarials

A number of combination antimalarials are available. These include:

- artemether with lumefantrine
- atovaquone with proguanil
- pyrimethamine with sulfadoxine.

Artemether with lumefantrine

Artemether is a synthesised derivative of a natural antimalarial (artemisinin) extracted from a Chinese weed called qing hao. It acts rapidly on the asexual erythrocytic stages of *P. vivax* and chloroquine-sensitive/resistant and multi-drug-resistant *P. falciparum*. Artemether is not suitable for prophylaxis as it does not affect either primary or latent tissue-stage parasites. Lumefantrine is structurally related to quinine and is very effective against *P. falciparum*. A combination with an artemisinin derivative such as artemether gives effectiveness greater than that of either drug alone. The currently available drug combination is a fixed ratio of 1 part artemether to 6 parts lumefantrine. Both drugs are thought to interfere with

in parasitised erythrocytes, which may be why it has selective toxicity during the erythrocytic stages of plasmodial infections. It can also bind to plasmodial DNA, thus inhibiting RNA synthesis and DNA replication.

Quinine sulfate is indicated in combination with other drugs (doxycycline, or pyrimethamine plus sulfadoxine) for the treatment of chloroquine-resistant malaria caused by chloroquine-resistant *P. falciparum*. See the Drug Interactions table 53-2 for quinine.

Adverse reactions include cinchonism (changes in colour vision or blurred vision, headache, very severe nausea and vomiting, tinnitus and transient hearing loss), GI distress (stomach pain or cramps, diarrhoea, nausea and vomiting) and, rarely, haemolytic uraemic syndrome (haemolytic anaemia, thrombocytopenia, disseminated intravascular coagulation and acute renal failure), hypoglycaemia, hypersensitivity and hepatotoxicity. Use with caution in people with a history of

CLINICAL INTEREST BOX 53-2 QUININE, GIN AND TONIC, AND BITTER LEMON FOR MALARIA

Malaria is one of the most important infectious diseases in the world, especially in tropical areas. Epidemics ('the ague') have been described since the first century AD. It is due to an infection with parasites of the *Plasmodium* species, and involves bouts of severe fevers at regular 2- or 4-day intervals; severe damage to the brain, liver and spleen is likely if untreated. Among the early herbalist cures was St John's wort.

The first specific effective treatment was found in the 17th century, with bark of the cinchona trees (called 'quin' by the Incas) found in South America. This remedy was brought from Ecuador to Europe by returning Jesuit missionaries, so the powder was called 'Jesuit's powder'. It quickly proved to be effective in Italy, Europe and England, and was highly prized.

The active principal was isolated in pure form in 1820 and named quinine; much effort went into procuring seeds and growing high-yield strains of the trees in Europe. Pharmacological studies on quinine led to the development of related drugs: chloroquine, mepacrine, primaquine and other aminoquinolines. Many strains of the *Plasmodium* parasites, however, have developed resistance to these drugs, and chloroquine-resistant malaria is now a major problem world-wide. Quinine also proved to have useful skeletal muscle-relaxant properties, and has been used in the past to treat muscle spasms.

Quinine has a very bitter taste, so a tradition was instituted by the British Raj rulers in India and the Far East of putting gin into their quinine mixtures ('tonic water') to disguise the taste. This became a habit and nowadays tonic water (containing quinine) is taken to enhance the flavour of gin! Bitter lemon drinks also have added quinine to enhance the bitter flavours. Tonic water now contains about 83 mg quinine per litre, and bitter lemon about 44 mg quinine per litre.

the conversion of haem to the malaria pigment haemozoin in the food vacuole of the malarial parasite. Additionally, both inhibit nucleic acid synthesis within the malarial parasite.

Very little is known about the pharmacokinetics of this combination due to the lack of an intravenous formulation for pharmacokinetic studies, and because large intersubject and intrasubject variability occurs in the plasma drug concentrations. Administered orally, artemether is rapidly absorbed and peak plasma concentration is reached in approximately 2 hours. In contrast, lumefantrine is highly lipophilic and absorption is slow, with peak plasma concentration reached at about 6–8 hours after dosing. Absorption is improved if the tablets are taken with food. Both drugs are extensively bound to plasma proteins (>97%), artemether being extensively metabolised to the active metabolite dihydroartemisinin,

predominantly by CYP3A4/5, and lumefantrine to the active debutylated metabolite by CYP3A4. Of clinical significance is the fact that lumefantrine is an inhibitor of CYP2D6; hence drug interactions occur with other drugs (e.g. flecainide, metoprolol, clomipramine) metabolised by CYP2D6, resulting in increased plasma concentration of the coadministered drug. Relevant drug information sources should be consulted for potential drug interactions, prior to administration of artemether with lumefantrine. Although the drugs are cleared from plasma with an elimination half-life of 2 hours for artemether and a terminal half-life of 2–3 days for lumefantrine, no urinary excretion data are available.

Common adverse effects include nausea, vomiting, diarrhoea, headache, dizziness, fatigue and muscle problems (e.g. myalgia, weakness). Rarely, an increase in Q-T interval occurs and hence this combination should be avoided in persons with coexisting prolongation of the Q-T interval or in persons with a family history of sudden death. Serious birth defects have been observed in animal studies, and this combination is contraindicated in the first trimester of pregnancy (ADEC Category D).

Atovaquone with proguanil

Atovaquone is a hydroxynaphthoquinone drug that is used in combination with proguanil. Together they cause a synergistic antimalarial effect as a result of interference with the synthesis of pyrimidines, which are required for nucleic acid synthesis. Atovaquone inhibits mitochondrial electron transport in *P. falciparum*. In contrast, proguanil, through its active metabolite cycloguanil, inhibits dihydrofolate reductase (like pyrimethamine) and potentiates the ability of atovaquone to collapse the mitochondrial membrane potential. The currently available drug combination is a fixed ratio of 2.5 parts atovaquone to 1 part proguanil (e.g. 250 mg atovaquone/100 mg proguanil tablet) and it is used for the treatment of uncomplicated *P. falciparum* malaria.

Atovaquone is poorly and erratically absorbed (affected by dose and diet), while proguanil is rapidly and extensively absorbed regardless of diet. It is recommended that the drug be taken with food or a milky drink, as dietary fat enhances absorption of atovaquone. Unlike proguanil, atovaquone is not metabolised and >90% is excreted as unchanged drug in faeces, with very little excretion via urine. Proguanil is metabolised to polar metabolites, which along with unchanged drug (~40%) are excreted in urine. The elimination half-life of atovaquone is 2–3 days in adults (1–2 days in children), whereas the elimination half-life of proguanil is 12–15 hours.

At the doses used, adverse effects are mild (e.g. abdominal pain, nausea and vomiting) and of limited duration. The safety of the combination in human pregnancy has not been fully established (ADEC Category B2), and breastfeeding is not recommended as atovaquone is excreted in breast milk.

Pyrimethamine with sulfadoxine

Pyrimethamine is an antiprotozoal agent used to treat malaria and toxoplasmosis. It binds to and inhibits the protozoal enzyme dihydrofolate reductase, thus inhibiting the conversion of dihydrofolic acid to tetrahydrofolic acid. This results in a depletion of folate, which is essential for nucleic acid synthesis and protein production. A synergistic effect is achieved in combination with sulfadoxine, which inhibits the utilisation of para-aminobenzoic acid (PABA) in the synthesis of dihydropteroic acid (see Chapter 51). Pyrimethamine with sulfadoxine is administered with oral quinine for the treatment of chloroquine-resistant *P. falciparum* malaria.

Pyrimethamine is orally absorbed and widely distributed in the body, although it concentrates mainly in blood cells, kidneys, liver and spleen. It reaches peak plasma concentrations in 2–6 hours and has a half-life of 35–175 hours. It is extensively metabolised in the liver to unknown metabolites and about 30% is excreted in the urine over 40 days.

Adverse reactions are usually rare, but in high doses, gastric distress (anorexia, nausea, vomiting, diarrhoea), atrophic glossitis (pain, burning or inflamed tongue, changes or a loss in taste sensation) and blood dyscrasias (e.g. agranulocytosis, megaloblastic anaemia, thrombocytopenia) may be seen. When pyrimethamine is administered concurrently with other bone marrow depressants, an increase in leucopenia and/or thrombocytopenia may result. Monitor full blood counts closely. Use this combination with caution in people with liver function impairment. Avoid use in people with pyrimethamine hypersensitivity, anaemia, bone marrow suppression or a history of convulsive disorders. Pyrimethamine and sulfadoxine are both excreted in breast milk.

The adult oral dosage for the treatment of chloroquine-resistant malaria is three tablets (75 mg/1500 mg) or 7.5 mL IM as a single dose on the third and fourth days of oral quinine treatment.

AMOEBIASIS

Amoebiasis is an infection of the large intestine produced by a protozoan parasite, *Entamoeba histolytica*. This infestation is found worldwide but is prevalent and severe in tropical areas. Transmission is usually through ingestion of cysts (faecal to oral route) from contaminated food or water, or from person-to-person contact. Poor personal hygiene can increase the spread of this parasite.

Life cycle of amoebae

This protozoan has two stages in its life cycle: the trophozoite (vegetative amoeba), which is the active, motile form; and the cyst, or inactive, drug-resistant form that appears in intestinal excretion. The trophozoite stage is capable of amoeboid motion and sexual activity. Because of its susceptibility to injury, it generally succumbs to an unfavourable environment. However, in certain circumstances, the trophozoite protects itself by entering the cystic stage. During this phase, the protozoan becomes inactive by surrounding itself with a resistant cell wall within which it can survive for a long time, even in an unsuitable environment.

The complete life cycle of the amoeba occurs in humans, the main host. It begins with ingestion of cysts that are present on hands, food or water contaminated by faeces. In the stomach, the hydrochloric acid does not destroy the swallowed cysts, which pass unharmed into the small intestine. The digestive juices penetrate the cystic walls and the trophozoites are released. The motile amoebae later pass into the colon, where they live and multiply for a time, feeding on the bacterial flora of the gut.

The presence of bacteria is essential to their survival. Finally, before excretion, the trophozoites move towards the terminal end of the bowel and again become encysted. After the cysts are eliminated in the faeces, they remain viable and infective. The cycle may begin again when the cysts appearing in faecal excretion are ingested through contamination of food or water.

The parasite causing amoebiasis replicates in three major locations: the lumen of the bowel; the intestinal mucosa; and extraintestinal sites. Amoebiasis is thus classified according to its primary site of action: intestinal amoebiasis, where amoebic activity is restricted to the bowel lumen or intestinal mucosa; or extraintestinal amoebiasis, where parasitic invasion occurs outside the intestine.

Intestinal amoebiasis

Intestinal amoebiasis may be manifested as an asymptomatic intestinal infection or a symptomatic intestinal infection that may be mild, moderate or severe.

Asymptomatic intestinal amoebiasis

In asymptomatic intestinal amoebiasis, the action of the parasite is restricted to the lumen of the bowel. The individual is asymptomatic but becomes a carrier of the disease by passing mature cysts of the parasite in formed stools. Outside the body, the cysts can live for several weeks, surviving dry, freezing or high-temperature conditions. By this route the infection is transmitted from person to person by flies or contaminated food or water. Ordinary concentrations of chlorine used for purification do not destroy the cysts. If the carrier fails to follow any drug treatment, serious GI pathological problems eventually develop. Occasionally, mild symptoms occur, including vague abdominal pain, nausea, flatulence, fatigue and nervousness.

Symptomatic intestinal amoebiasis

Symptomatic amoebiasis occurs when the trophozoites in the lumen of the bowel penetrate the mucosal lining of the colon. After they multiply and thrive on bacterial flora, a large infestation occurs, producing diarrhoea and abdominal pain. The increased loss of fluid may cause prostration. In addition, ulcerative colitis may result. This state of the disease is called intestinal amoebiasis and is usually diagnosed as mild, moderate or severe, according to the intensity of the symptoms and the extent of the disease.

Extraintestinal amoebiasis

The term extraintestinal amoebiasis means the parasites have migrated to other parts of the body, such as the liver or, occasionally, the spleen, lungs or brain. When the parasites are in the liver, necrotic foci develop because of their destructive effect on tissues. When there is liver involvement, the terms liver abscess and hepatic amoebiasis are usually used.

Amoebicidal agents

Drugs for the treatment of amoebiasis are classified according to the site of the previously described amoebic action. Luminal amoebicides act primarily in the bowel lumen and are generally ineffective against parasites in the bowel wall or tissues. Tissue amoebicides are drugs that act primarily in the bowel wall, liver and other extraintestinal tissues. No single drug is effective for both types of amoebiasis; therefore a luminal and extraluminal (tissue) amoebicide or combination therapy is often prescribed. Drugs used for symptomatic intestinal or extraintestinal amoebiasis include metronidazole (Chapter 51) and tinidazole, and for the eradication of cysts, paromomycin.

Paromomycin

Paromomycin is both an amoebicidal and an antibacterial agent. The drug is an aminoglycoside antibiotic with antibacterial properties similar to those of neomycin. Paromomycin acts directly on intestinal amoebae and on bacteria such as *Salmonella* and *Shigella*. Because the drug is poorly absorbed from the GIT, it exerts no effect on systemic infections such as extraintestinal amoebiasis. It is indicated for the treatment of acute and chronic intestinal amoebiasis. (For drug interactions, warnings and contraindications, see aminoglycosides in Chapter 51.) Paromomycin is poorly absorbed from the GIT; thus most of the drug is excreted in the faeces.

Adverse reactions include nausea, diarrhoea and gastric distress. Paromomycin is an aminoglycoside, so the drug interactions possible with this family of medications may also occur with paromomycin. See the discussion of aminoglycoside antibiotics in Chapter 51.

The adult dosage for treating intestinal amoebiasis is 25–35 mg/kg daily in three divided doses given with meals for 7 days. Paromomycin is available only through the Special Access Scheme. (In Australia, the Special Access Scheme is one mechanism by which a non-marketed [unregistered] drug may be provided to an individual.)

TOXOPLASMOSIS

Toxoplasmosis is caused by an intracellular parasite *Toxoplasma gondii*. This parasite is found worldwide in raw vegetables and the soil, and infests a variety of animals, including humans. Cats and other feline species are the natural hosts, and it is often harboured in the host with no evidence of the disease. Toxoplasmosis is contracted by ingesting cysts in inadequately cooked or raw meat, fish or vegetables or by accidentally ingesting cysts from cat faeces.

Symptomatically, the individual may experience lymphadenopathy, fever and, occasionally, a rash on the palms and soles. The most serious complication of toxoplasmosis is meningoencephalitis, which is common in HIV patients. Acute infection is treated with a combination of sulfadiazine plus pyrimethamine orally, both of which alter the folic acid cycle of the *Toxoplasma* organism, resulting in its death. Lifelong suppressive therapy is essential to prevent relapse, and inclusion of calcium folinate reduces bone marrow suppression.

TRICHOMONIASIS

Trichomoniasis is a disease of the vagina caused by *Trichomonas vaginalis*. Its characteristic presentation consists of a wet, inflamed vagina, a 'strawberry' cervix and a thin, yellow, frothy malodorous discharge. Usually, both sexual partners are infected by this organism, which can be identified microscopically from semen, prostatic fluid or exudate from the vagina. Infections often recur, which indicates that the protozoans persist in extravaginal foci, the male urethra or the periurethral glands and ducts of both sexes.

Metronidazole is the drug of choice for treating trichomoniasis. Treatment must be given simultaneously to both partners involved in order to effect a cure.

MYCOBACTERIAL INFECTIONS

The two main mycobacterial infections in humans are tuberculosis and leprosy.

Tuberculosis

Tuberculosis (TB), a chronic granulomatous infection caused by the acid-fast bacillus *Mycobacterium tuberculosis*, is both a curable and a controllable infection that is transmitted from person to person. About 4 million cases of TB were registered worldwide in 2004, and on average over 2 million people die from this disease each year (World Health Organization [WHO] 2006).

The WHO's new 2006 'Stop TB Strategy' aims to have a TB-free world. The current goals are to reduce TB prevalence and death rates by 50% (relative to 1990) by 2015, and to eliminate TB as a public health problem (1 case per million population) by 2050. Within Australasia, TB remains a problem among Aboriginal people, the aged, immigrants from endemic countries and Maoris; in 2000–2005 4902 cases were recorded by the Communicable Diseases Australia–National Notifiable Diseases Surveillance System (www.health.gov.au).

The development of drug-resistant TB is a major concern. A recent study estimated the incidence of resistance to at least one antituberculosis drug among new cases of TB at about 10% in Australia, 11% in New Zealand, 2% in New Caledonia, 12% in the USA, and 7% in England and Wales. The highest incidences of multi-drug resistance were found in Estonia (14.1%) and Henan Province in China (10.8%). In contrast, multi-drug resistance rates were low in Australia (2%) and New Zealand (1.1%) (Espinal et al 2001).

The WHO recommends management under the Directly Observed Treatment—Short Course (DOTS) strategy as the approach to TB control and cure in 85% of all new cases. The DOTS strategy includes five steps and involves the health system in the steps to a cure:

- **D, directly**: community resources should be focused on identifying people with sputum-positive TB so that treatment can be started. In other words, identify and treat the people with the worse cases of TB first, to reduce the spread of the disease.
- **O, observed**: observe that individuals actually swallow each dose of medication prescribed, which is especially critical during the first 2 months of treatment. At this time, the person is usually more seriously ill and infectious to others and is also at a greater risk of acquiring a drug resistance. While it may not be possible to monitor each dose, the health-care professional can institute an individual plan concerning observation of treatment, and should follow up on patients who do not keep their appointments. The specified observer must be accountable to the health-care service and also be accessible to the individual.
- **T, treatment**: this is a two-step process that includes treatment and monitoring. People with contagious disease should have microscopic examination of their sputum for TB bacilli after 2 months and at the end of treatment. The goal is to achieve a TB bacilli-free result. Monitor and report on each individual with TB person so that a health-

care service can identify and intervene in communities that are not obtaining an 85% cure rate. Additional resources such as support and training may be necessary.
- **S, short-course**: the right drug combination and dosage should be used for the proper length of time to kill the TB bacilli. The drugs may include isoniazid, pyrazinamide, rifampicin, streptomycin and ethambutol. They are typically prescribed for 6 months of therapy.

The DOTS program needs government support and funding to achieve long-term TB control. The result of not instituting such a plan is obvious—increased numbers of cases of TB, multi-drug-resistant TB and deaths.

Pathogenesis

TB most commonly affects the lungs but other body areas can also be infected, such as bones, joints, skin, meninges or the genitourinary tract. *M. tuberculosis* is an aerobic bacillus that needs a highly oxygenated organ site for growth; thus the lungs, the growing ends of bones and the cerebral cortex are ideal sites. The bacilli can become inactive and be walled off by calcified and fibrous tissues, often for the lifetime of the person. If host defences break down, however, or if the individual receives an immunosuppressive drug, the bacilli may be reactivated.

Tubercle bacilli may be transmitted via airborne droplets when an infected person coughs or sneezes, but cannot be transmitted on objects such as dishes, clothing or sheets and bedding (Figure 53-3). Persons producing sputum generally have many bacilli and are more infectious than the infected person who does not cough. Sharing an enclosed environment with an infected person creates a high risk of developing this infection (Ebert 1993).

Drug treatment regimens

Effective drug regimens are available to treat TB. Drug selection is based on the development of drug-resistant organisms and drug toxicity. General guidelines include:

- to avoid the development of drug-resistant organisms, all people in whom TB is diagnosed (and *M. tuberculosis* isolated) should have drug susceptibility tests on their first isolation
- in most instances, the result of the in-vitro susceptibility test is unknown when drug therapy is started. It is recommended that a four-drug regimen be instituted (especially in areas where primary isoniazid resistance occurs) because this regimen provides an adequate drug regimen that will be at least 95% effective, even in the presence of drug-resistant organisms. The recommended first-line drugs are **isoniazid** (see Drug Monograph 53-2), **rifampicin** (see Drug Monograph 53-3), **pyrazinamide**, and ethambutol or streptomycin (Mandell & Petri 1996; Antibiotic Expert Group 2006; AMH 2006).

DRUG INTERACTIONS 53-3 Capreomycin	
Drug	**Possible effect and management**
Aminoglycosides	Increased risk of developing ototoxicity, nephrotoxicity and neuromuscular blockade. Hearing loss may progress to deafness, even after the drug is stopped. This can be a very dangerous combination. Avoid concurrent drug administration
Amphotericin B cisplatin, cyclosporin, ethacrynic acid, frusemide (parenteral), paromomycin, streptomycin or vancomycin	Concurrent or even sequential use of capreomycin with any of these drugs can increase the risk of ototoxicity and nephrotoxicity. Hearing loss may occur and progress to deafness, even if drugs are stopped. Avoid if at all possible
Neuromuscular-blocking agents	May result in increased neuromuscular-blocking effects, causing respiratory depression or paralysis. Monitor closely, especially during surgery or in the postoperative period. If possible, avoid this combination

- when drug susceptibility results are available, the drug regimen can be adjusted
- monitor the prescribed therapy regimen closely to support compliance, detect adverse reactions and register progress of the treatment program.

Antituberculous agents
Capreomycin

Capreomycin is an antimycobacterial agent with an unknown mechanism of action. It is indicated in combination therapy for the treatment of pulmonary TB after primary medications (streptomycin, isoniazid, rifampicin, pyrazinamide and ethambutol) fail, or when these medications cannot be used because of resistant bacilli or drug toxicity. Administered parenterally, capreomycin has a half-life of 3–6 hours and reaches peak plasma concentration in 1–2 hours after IM administration. It is excreted by the kidneys primarily unchanged.

When capreomycin is given with any of the drugs in the Drug Interactions table 53-3, very serious reactions may result. Avoid concurrent use if possible. Adverse reactions include nephrotoxicity, hypokalaemia, neuromuscular blockade,

ototoxicity (auditory: hearing loss, ringing or buzzing noise; vestibular: ataxia, dizziness, nausea, vomiting), hypersensitivity, and pain, soreness or hardness at the injection site. Use capreomycin with caution in people with dehydration. Avoid use in persons with capreomycin hypersensitivity, eighth cranial nerve damage, myasthenia gravis or Parkinson's disease. Dosage reduction is required in people with renal impairment.

The adult dosage in combination with other antitubercular drugs is 1 g IM daily (max. 20 mg/kg/day) for 1–2 years.

Cycloserine

This is a second-line broad-spectrum antibiotic that can be bacteriostatic or bactericidal, depending on drug concentration at the infection site and on organism susceptibility. It is an antimycobacterial agent that interferes with bacterial cell wall synthesis. In combination with other drugs, it is indicated for the treatment of TB or *Mycobacterium avium* complex (MAC) after failure of first-line antitubercular medications.

Cycloserine is well absorbed orally and is widely distributed in body tissues and fluids. The peak plasma concentration occurs in 3–4 hours and the drug has a half-life of 10 hours. About 35% of cycloserine is metabolised, with excretion primarily via the kidneys. See the Drug Interactions table 53-4 for cycloserine.

Adverse reactions include headache, dose-related CNS toxicity (confusion, dizziness, sedation, irritability, restlessness, depression, tremors, nightmares, mood alterations, speech problems, anxiety, thoughts of suicide), hypersensitivity, peripheral neuropathy and convulsions. Use this drug with caution in people with severe anxiety, depression or psychosis. Avoid use in people with cycloserine hypersensitivity, a history of epilepsy and in alcoholics. Dosage reduction is required in people with renal impairment.

The adult oral dosage used in combination with other drugs is 250–500 mg every 12 hours to a maximum daily dose of 1 g. The paediatric dosage is 5 mg/kg twice daily to a maximum of 500 mg daily. If gastric distress occurs, administer medications after meals. Be aware that CNS toxicity increases with drug dosages greater than 500 mg/day.

DRUG INTERACTIONS 53-4 Cycloserine	
Drug	**Possible effect and management**
Alcohol	In chronic alcohol abusers, cycloserine may increase the risk of seizures. Avoid or a potentially serious drug interaction may occur
Isoniazid	May increase CNS adverse effects such as seizures. Monitor closely, as dosage adjustments may be necessary

DRUG MONOGRAPH 53–2 ISONIAZID

Isoniazid is an antimycobacterial (bactericidal) agent that affects mycobacteria in the dividing phase. Its exact mechanism of action is unknown but it is believed to inhibit mycolic acid synthesis and cause cell wall disruption in susceptible organisms. Isoniazid is indicated for the primary treatment, retreatment and prophylaxis of TB.

PHARMACOKINETICS Isoniazid is well absorbed orally and is widely distributed throughout the body. It is metabolised in the liver by acetylation, a characteristic that displays a genetic polymorphism in humans. In people who metabolise the drug quickly, often referred to as 'fast acetylators', peak plasma concentrations occur in 1–2 hours, while this takes 4–6 hours for those classed as 'slow acetylators'. The half-life in fast acetylators is 0.5–1.6 hours, and in slow acetylators 2–5 hours. Slow acetylators have a decrease in hepatic N-acetyltransferase, the enzyme that carries out the reaction. Excretion is primarily via the urine, partly as unchanged drug and as the inactive acetylated form.

Slow acetylators may need lower drug dosages and are more apt to develop adverse reactions, particularly peripheral neuritis. The incidence of slow acetylators is highest in Egyptian, Israeli, Scandinavian, other Caucasian, and black populations, while the lowest incidence is in Eskimo, Oriental and native American populations.

DRUG INTERACTIONS Various effects may occur when isoniazid is given with the drugs listed to the right.

ADVERSE REACTIONS These include gastric distress, anorexia, nausea, vomiting, weakness, hepatitis, peripheral neuritis and, rarely, blood dyscrasias, hypersensitivity and optic neuritis. Increases in plasma transaminases may occur in the first few months of treatment.

WARNINGS AND CONTRAINDICATIONS Use with caution in people with severe kidney disease and convulsive disorders. Avoid use in people with isoniazid, ethionamide, pyrazinamide, niacin or nicotinic acid hypersensitivity, or liver function impairment, and in alcoholics.

DOSAGE* AND ADMINISTRATION The adult oral dose (daily regimen) of isoniazid is 5 mg/kg (max. 300 mg daily). When a twice-weekly regimen is used the dose is 15 mg/kg (max. 900 mg) twice weekly. For children, the daily regimen is 10 mg/kg up to a maximum of 300 mg daily.

ADDITIONAL COMMENTS If gastric distress occurs, this drug may be taken with meals or an antacid, although aluminium antacids should be separated by at least 1 hour from isoniazid, as absorption is decreased when food or antacids are given concurrently. Pyridoxine

may be prescribed concurrently to prevent peripheral neuritis in at-risk individuals.

Drug	Possible effect and management
Alcohol	Daily use of alcohol may result in increased isoniazid metabolism and higher risk of hepatotoxicity. Monitor patients, as a drug dose adjustment may be necessary
Carbamazepine	Isoniazid may inhibit metabolism, resulting in increased carbamazepine plasma concentration and toxicity. Monitor plasma concentration closely and adjust dose if indicated
Disulfiram	May increase the incidence of CNS adverse effects such as ataxia, irritability, dizziness or insomnia. Monitor closely for these symptoms, as dosage reduction or even discontinuation of disulfiram may be required
Hepatotoxic drugs	May increase potential for hepatotoxicity. Avoid, or a potentially serious drug interaction may occur
Ketoconazole, miconazole or rifampicin	Isoniazid with ketoconazole may decrease plasma concentration of ketoconazole; if both isoniazid and rifampicin are given with ketoconazole, the plasma levels of ketoconazole or rifampicin have been reported to be undetectable. The combination of isoniazid or rifampicin together or individually with ketoconazole or parenteral miconazole is not recommended. Rifampicin with isoniazid may increase the potential for hepatotoxicity, especially in patients with liver impairment and in fast acetylators of isoniazid. Monitor closely for hepatotoxicity, especially during the first 90 days of therapy
Phenytoin	May result in impaired phenytoin metabolism, leading to increased plasma concentration and toxicity. The phenytoin dose may need to be adjusted. Monitor plasma phenytoin concentration closely

* Dosage regimens differ slightly between various authorities.

DRUG MONOGRAPH 53–3 RIFAMPICIN

Rifampicin is a broad-spectrum bactericidal antibiotic (antimycobacterial) that blocks mycobacterial RNA transcription. It is indicated for the treatment of TB and for asymptomatic carriers of *Neisseria meningitidis*. It is well absorbed orally and widely distributed in the body.

PHARMACOKINETICS Rifampicin is lipid-soluble, so it may reach and kill intracellular and extracellular susceptible bacteria. Therapeutic plasma concentrations occur in 1.5–4 hours, and the elimination half-life is up to 5 hours. Rifampicin is metabolised in the liver to a range of metabolites, including an active metabolite (25-O-desacetylrifampicin), and excreted primarily in the faeces.

DRUG INTERACTIONS Rifampicin induces hepatic cytochrome P450 enzymes, which results in increased clearance of drugs metabolised by the liver. The effects in the table below may occur when rifampicin is given with the drugs listed.

ADVERSE REACTIONS These include gastric distress, hypersensitivity, a flu-like syndrome, red–orange discoloration of urine, faeces, saliva, sputum, sweat and tears (soft contact lenses can be discoloured by rifampicin), fungal overgrowth and, rarely, blood dyscrasias, hepatitis and interstitial nephritis.

CONTRAINDICATIONS Avoid use in people with liver function impairment or previous allergic reaction to rifampicin or rifabutin, and in alcoholics.

DOSAGE AND ADMINISTRATION The oral dosage of rifampicin for adults and children in combination with other agents (for TB) is 10 mg/kg to a maximum of 600 mg daily, or 15 mg/kg (max. 600 mg) three times a week.

ADDITIONAL COMMENTS To obtain the maximum absorption, rifampicin should be taken with a full glass of water on an empty stomach, i.e. 1 hour before or 2 hours after a meal. If gastric distress is a problem, it may be taken with food. Concurrent alcohol consumption should be avoided. Blood counts should be monitored and dental procedures deferred until blood counts are normal.

Drug	Possible effect and management
Alcohol	Daily use of alcohol may increase the risk of rifampicin-induced hepatotoxicity and increase the rate of rifampicin metabolism. Monitor hepatic function closely, as dosage adjustment may be necessary
Antidiabetic agents (oral)	Concurrent use enhances the metabolism of antidiabetic drugs, so dosage adjustment may be indicated
Corticosteroids, glucocorticoids, mineralocorticoids, anticoagulants, (warfarin), digitalis glycosides, disopyramide, mexiletine, quinidine, azole antifungals, phenytoin, or chloramphenicol	Rifampicin induces hepatic metabolism and therefore may decrease the effectiveness of these medications, which are metabolised by the liver. Monitor plasma concentrations of these drugs for clinical effect and adjust dosage if necessary
Hepatotoxic drugs	Increases the risk of hepatotoxicity. Avoid, or a potentially serious drug interaction may occur
Ketoconazole, fluconazole, itraconazole	Increased risk of hepatotoxicity of rifampicin and reduced effectiveness of antifungal drugs. Avoid concurrent drug administration
Methadone	May decrease the effectiveness of methadone and may induce methadone withdrawal in dependent patients. Monitor closely, as dosage adjustments may be necessary during and after rifampicin therapy
Oral contraceptives	Decreased effectiveness due to increased liver metabolism of oestrogen. May result in menstrual irregularities, spotting and unplanned pregnancies. Advise person of the possible effects when these drugs are combined and suggest alternative contraception
Verapamil	Metabolism of verapamil is accelerated, decreasing blood concentration and reducing its cardiovascular effects
Xanthines, aminophylline and theophylline	Increases the metabolism of these drugs, thus increasing drug clearance. Monitor plasma concentration of xanthines and adjust dose if necessary

Ethambutol

This antitubercular agent is bacteriostatic; it is believed to diffuse into the mycobacteria bacilli and suppress RNA synthesis. It is effective only against actively dividing mycobacteria. It is indicated in combination with other drugs for the treatment and retreatment of TB. There is an increased risk of neurotoxicity, such as optic and peripheral neuritis, when ethambutol is administered concurrently with other neurotoxic medications. Monitor closely if concurrent therapy is instituted.

Ethambutol is absorbed orally and distributed to most body tissues and fluids, with the exception of cerebrospinal fluid. High concentrations are found in the kidneys, lungs, saliva, urine and erythrocytes. Therapeutic plasma concentrations occur within 4 hours and the half-life is 3–4 hours. Ethambutol is partly metabolised (15%) in the liver, and 75% of the oral dose is excreted unchanged in urine and 10% in faeces.

Adverse reactions include gastric distress, confusion, disorientation, headache, optic neuritis, peripheral neuritis, hypersensitivity and acute gouty arthritis.

Use ethambutol with caution in people with acute gouty arthritis, as ethambutol may raise uric acid levels. Avoid use in patients with ethambutol hypersensitivity, optic neuritis or kidney function impairment.

The adult oral dosage in combination with other agents is 15–20 mg/kg daily for 8 weeks and 15 mg/kg daily if the duration of treatment continues beyond 2 months. The maximum dosage is 1.6 g daily. Take medication with food if gastric distress occurs. Instruct individuals to report any visual changes to the doctor as soon as possible.

Pyrazinamide

Pyrazinamide is an antimycobacterial agent with an unknown mechanism of action. Depending on concentration at the

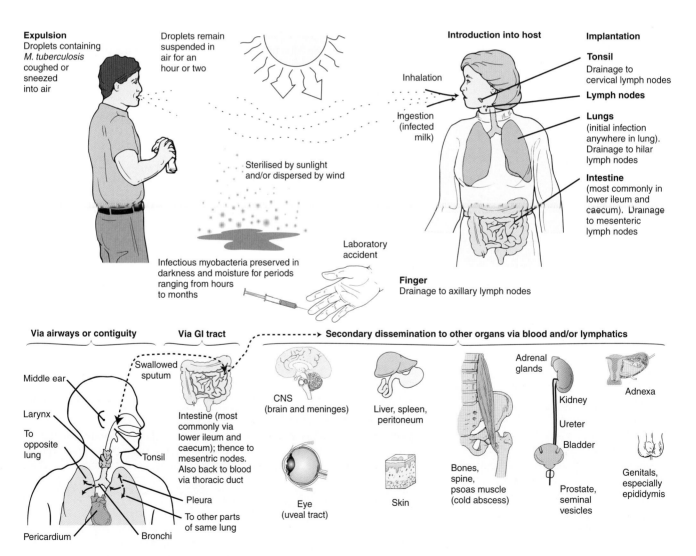

FIGURE 53-3 Dissemination of tuberculosis.

site of action and susceptibility of the mycobacteria, this drug can be bacteriostatic or bactericidal. It is indicated in combination with other agents for the treatment of tuberculosis. Pyrazinamide is well absorbed orally and is widely distributed in the body. The time to peak plasma concentration is 1–2 hours and the elimination half-life is 9–10 hours. Pyrazinamide is primarily metabolised in the liver and excreted by the kidneys.

Adverse reactions include arthralgia related to hyperuricaemia, pruritus, rash and, rarely, gouty arthritis and hepatotoxicity. Use this drug with caution in patients with gout and type 1 diabetes, as control may become more difficult. Avoid use in people with hypersensitivity to pyrazinamide, ethionamide, isoniazid, niacin or nicotinic acid, or severe liver disease. Use in patients with renal impairment may result in accumulation of uric acid crystals that can worsen renal impairment.

The adult oral dosage when given in combination with other agents is 20–25 mg/kg daily, up to a maximum of 2 g daily. Significant weight gain may occur during treatment, necessitating dose reduction.

Rifabutin

Rifabutin is an antimycobacterial agent indicated for the prophylaxis of disseminated MAC in people with advanced HIV infection. It inhibits DNA-dependent RNA polymerase in susceptible *Escherichia coli* and *Bacillus subtilis*, and has in-vitro activity against many strains of *M. tuberculosis*. It is used in combination with isoniazid for the prophylaxis of tuberculosis and MAC.

Rifabutin is absorbed from the GIT, reaches peak plasma concentration in 2–4 hours and has a terminal half-life of 45 hours. It is highly lipophilic and crosses the blood–brain barrier; cerebrospinal fluid levels are about 50% of the corresponding plasma concentration. It is metabolised in the liver (five metabolites have been identified) and excreted primarily by the kidneys. When rifabutin is administered concurrently with zidovudine (AZT), some studies indicate that the mean zidovudine plasma concentration may decrease. Monitor closely if combination therapy is used.

Adverse reactions include nausea, vomiting, skin rash and, rarely, joint pain, a change in taste sensations, myalgia, neutropenia, pseudojaundice (yellow-tinged skin) and uveitis. Avoid use in people with rifabutin or rifampicin hypersensitivity and active tuberculosis. Dosage reduction by about 50% is required in patients with renal impairment.

The usual adult dosage for prophylaxis of MAC is 300 mg daily, preferably on an empty stomach. For treatment of MAC, the dosage is 10 mg/kg orally to a maximum of 600 mg daily. Rifabutin colours sweat, tears, urine and faeces orange–red, so patients should be advised of this reaction.

Streptomycin injection

Streptomycin is an aminoglycoside antibiotic that is poorly absorbed from the GIT; it is therefore given intramuscularly. It was one of the first effective agents used in the late 1940s to treat TB and it is still an important agent in managing severe TB. Like the other aminoglycosides, its major toxicities include ototoxicity and nephrotoxicity, especially when given to patients with impaired renal function or with other medications with the same toxicities. (See Chapter 51 for detailed information on the aminoglycosides.)

The adult dosage for streptomycin is 0.75–1 g IM daily. Reduce this to 1 g 2–3 times weekly as soon as possible. For elderly patients, the dosage is 500–750 mg daily in combination with other antitubercular agents. For children, the dosage is 15 mg/kg daily in combination with other antitubercular agents. The maximum daily dose for children is 1 g.

Leprosy

Leprosy, or Hansen's disease, is caused by *Mycobacterium leprae* in humans. It was first reported in 600 BC and today the estimated number of infected people is nearly 15 million worldwide. Recent data indicate that leprosy is prevalent in many countries, including India (260,063 new cases in 2004) and Brazil (49,384 new cases in 2004). The South East Asian region ranked the highest for the number of new cases reported (298,603) in 2004 (WHO 2006). By the end of 1999 10 million patients had been cured of leprosy by using multi-drug therapy. In Australia during the period 1991–2005, 141 cases of leprosy were reported. Of these, 33 were from Western Australia, 25 from Victoria, 36 from New South Wales, 20 from the Northern Territory, 22 from Queensland, 4 from South Australia and 1 from the Australian Capital Territory. Tasmania was the only state free of leprosy over this period (Communicable Diseases Australia—National Notifiable Diseases Surveillance System, www.health.gov.au).

Although the precise mode of transmission is unknown, the incubation period for leprosy is a few months to decades. Large numbers of leprosy bacilli are generally shed from skin ulcers, nasal secretions, the GIT and, perhaps, biting insects.

M. leprae is a bacillus that in humans first presents as a skin lesion: a large plaque or macule that is erythematous or hypopigmented in the centre. More numerous lesions, peripheral nerve trunk involvement and the common complications of plantar ulceration of the feet, footdrop, loss of hand function and corneal abrasions may follow.

Drug therapy can cure leprosy, stop transmission of the disease and prevent the disfigurement that results in social exclusion and stigmatisation. Since 1982, the WHO has recommended the use of multi-drug therapy comprising dapsone, rifampicin and clofazimine. This combination is bactericidal and prevents the occurrence of drug resistance. For individuals not tolerating clofazimine, an alternative regimen of monthly rifampicin, ofloxacin and minocycline for 2 years has been recommended. For individuals not tolerating rifampicin, the WHO has recommended daily administration of a combination of clofazimine, ofloxacin and minocycline for 6 months, followed by daily administration of clofazimine with either minocycline or ofloxacin for an additional 18 months (WHO 1998). These WHO guidelines are followed in Australia.

Drugs used to treat leprosy
Dapsone

Dapsone is an antibacterial (antileprosy) agent that is bacteriostatic, with an action similar to that of the sulfonamides. It may also be a dihydrofolate reductase inhibitor. Dapsone is effective against *M. leprae* and is indicated for the treatment of all types of leprosy and for dermatitis herpetiformis. Dapsone is absorbed orally, distributed throughout the body

DRUG INTERACTIONS 53-5 Dapsone

Drug	Possible effect and management
Didanosine (ddl)	Concurrent drug administration may reduce absorption of dapsone. Dapsone requires an acid medium for absorption, while ddl is given with a buffer to neutralise stomach acid to increase absorption. Administer dapsone a minimum of 2 hours before ddl
Trimethoprim, trimethoprim–sulfamethoxazole	Decreased elimination of both dapsone and trimethoprim may occur. Monitor for increased incidence of adverse effects

and found in fluids and in all body tissues. Therapeutic plasma concentrations are achieved in 2–6 hours and the half-life is around 30 hours. The drug is acetylated by *N*-acetyltransferase in the liver; thus slow acetylators are more apt than fast acetylators to develop higher plasma concentrations and adverse reactions. Excretion is via the kidneys.

See the Drug Interactions table 53-5 for dapsone.

Adverse reactions include hypersensitivity, haemolytic anaemia, methaemoglobinaemia and, rarely, CNS adverse effects, gastric distress, blood disorders, exfoliative dermatitis, hepatic damage, mood alterations, peripheral neuritis and the sulfone syndrome (fever, tiredness, exfoliative dermatitis, jaundice, lympadenopathy, anaemia and methaemoglobinaemia). Use dapsone with caution in people with liver function impairment. Avoid use in patients with dapsone or sulfonamide hypersensitivity, severe anaemia, severe G6PD deficiency or methaemoglobin reductase deficiency.

The adult dapsone antileprosy dosage (given in combination with other antileprosy drugs) is 100 mg orally daily. As a suppressant for dermatitis herpetiformis, the adult dosage is 50 mg orally daily initially, increased as necessary to 300 mg daily. The dosage for children as an antileprosy agent is 1–2 mg/kg orally to a maximum of 100 mg daily.

Clofazimine

Clofazimine's antileprosy mechanism of action is unknown; it has a slow bactericidal effect on *M. leprae*, inhibits mycobacterial growth and tends to bind preferentially to mycobacterial DNA. Oral absorption of clofazimine is variable and it is distributed primarily in fatty tissues and cells. Macrophages accumulate the drug and further distribute it throughout the body. Its half-life is about 2–3 months with chronic therapy, and peak plasma concentrations occur 1–6 hours after dosing. It is excreted primarily in faeces.

Adverse reactions include gastric distress; ichthyosis; discoloration (red and brown–black) of skin, faeces, sweat, tears and urine; a change in taste sensations; dry, burning, itching or irritated eyes; photosensitivity; and, rarely, GI bleeding, hepatitis and depression. Use clofazimine with caution in people with liver function impairment. Avoid use in patients with clofazimine hypersensitivity or a history of GI disorders.

The adult dosage in combination therapy for leprosy is 50 mg orally daily and 300 mg once monthly in multi-drug regimens for 12 months.

HELMINTHIASIS

The disease-producing **helminths** (worms) are classified as metazoa, or multicellular animal parasites. Unlike the protozoa, they are large organisms with complex cellular structures and feed on host tissue. They may be present in the GIT but several types also penetrate tissues and some undergo developmental changes, during which they wander extensively in the host. Because most anthelmintics used today are highly effective against specific parasites, the organism must be accurately identified before treatment is started, usually by finding the parasite ova or larvae in the faeces, urine, blood, sputum or tissues of the host.

Parasitic infestations do not necessarily cause clinical manifestations although they may be injurious for a variety of reasons:

- worms may cause mechanical injury to the tissues and organs. Roundworms in large numbers may cause obstruction in the intestine, filariae may block lymphatic channels and cause massive oedema, and hookworms often cause extensive damage to the wall of the intestine and considerable loss of blood
- toxic substances produced by the parasite may be absorbed by the host
- the tissues of the host may be traumatised by the presence of the parasite and made more susceptible to bacterial infections
- heavy infestation with worms will rob the host of food. This is particularly significant in children.

Helminths parasitic to humans are classified as platyhelminths (flatworms), which include two subclasses; cestodes (tapeworms) and trematodes (flukes); or nematodes (roundworms).

Platyhelminths (flatworms)
Cestodes

Cestodes are tapeworms, of which there are four varieties: *Taenia saginata* (beef tapeworm), *Taenia solium* (pork tapeworm), *Diphyllobothrium latum* (fish tapeworm) and *Hymenolepis nana* (dwarf tapeworm). As indicated by the common name of the worm, the parasite enters the intestine by way of improperly cooked beef, pork or fish, or from contaminated food, as in the case of the dwarf tapeworm.

The cestodes are segmented flatworms with a head, or scolex, that has hooks or suckers used to attach to tissues, and a number of segments, or proglottids, which in some cases may extend for 6–9 metres in the bowel. Drugs affecting the scolex allow expulsion of the organisms from the intestine. Each of the proglottids contains both male and female reproductive units. When filled with fertilised eggs, they are expelled from the worm into the environment. On ingestion, the infected larvae develop into adults in the small intestine of the human. The larvae may travel to extraintestinal sites and enter other tissues, such as the liver, muscle and eye. The tapeworms, with the exception of the dwarf tapeworm, spend part of their life cycle in a host other than humans (pigs, fish

or cattle). The dwarf tapeworm does not require any such intermediate host.

The tapeworm has no digestive tract; it depends on the nutrients that are intended for the host. Subsequently, the victim suffers by eventually developing nutritional deficiency.

Trematodes

Trematodes, or flukes, are flat, non-segmented parasites with suckers that attach to and feed on host tissue. The life cycle begins with the egg, which is passed into fresh water after faecal excretion from the body of the human host. The egg containing the embryo forms into a ciliated organism, the miracidium. In the presence of water, the miracidium escapes from the egg and enters the intermediate host, the freshwater snail, which exists extensively in rice paddies and irrigation ditches. After entry, the fluke forms a cyst in the lungs of the snail. In the cyst, many organisms develop. They can penetrate other parts of the snail and grow into worms called cercariae. Eventually, the cercariae are released from the snail into the water, attaching themselves to blades of grass to encyst.

When encysted organisms in snails or fish and crabs are swallowed by humans, they develop into adult flukes in different structures of the body. The flukes are therefore classified according to the type of tissue they invade. After ingestion, the eggs of *Schistosoma haematobium* appear in the urinary bladder and cause inflammation of the urogenital system. This can result in chronic cystitis and haematuria. Infestations with *Schistosoma japonicum* and *Schistosoma mansoni* produce intestinal disturbance with resultant ulceration and necrosis of the rectum. *S. japonicum* is more concentrated in the veins of the small intestine. If the liver and spleen become infected, the disease is usually fatal. *S. mansoni* prefers the portal veins that drain the large intestine, particularly the sigmoid colon and rectum. Unlike the other parasites, the cercariae of *S. mansoni* are not ingested but burrow through the skin, especially between the toes of the human host who is standing in contaminated water. They then make their way to the portal system, where they mature into adult flukes.

Schistosomiasis (bilharziasis) is endemic to Africa, Asia, South America and Caribbean islands. The disease can be controlled largely by eliminating the intermediate host, the snail. Travellers to these areas must avoid contact with contaminated water for drinking, bathing or swimming.

Nematodes (roundworms)

Nematodes are non-segmented cylindrical worms that consist of a mouth and complete digestive tract. The adults reside in the human intestinal tract; there is no intermediate host. Two types of nematode infection exist in the human: the egg form and the larval form.

Egg infective form

Ascaris lumbricoides is a large nematode (about 30 cm in length) and is known as the 'roundworm of humans'. The adult *Ascaris* usually resides in the upper end of the small intestine of the human, where it feeds on semidigested foods. The fertilised egg, when excreted with faeces, can survive in the soil for a long time. When inadvertently ingested by another host, the embryos escape from the eggs and mature into adults in the host. To prevent the disease, proper sanitary conditions and meticulous personal habits must be observed.

Infection with *Enterobius vermicularis*, or pinworm, is highly prevalent among children and adults. Adult pinworms reside in the large intestine but the female migrates to the anus, depositing her eggs around the skin of the anal region. This causes intense itching and can be noted especially in children. Ingestion of excreted eggs can infect an individual. Eggs that contaminate clothing, bedding, furniture and other items may be responsible for continuing the reinfection of an individual and initiating the infection of others.

Larval infective form

Necator americanus (New World) or *Ancylostoma duodenale* (Old World) hookworms are somewhat similar in action. They reside in the small intestine of humans. When the eggs are excreted in the faeces, the larvae hatch in the soil. The larvae can penetrate the skin of humans, particularly through the soles of the feet, producing dermatitis (ground itch). On entry into the small intestine, they develop into adult worms. During the process, they extravasate blood from the intestinal vessels and cause a profound anaemia in the victim. The presence of eggs in the faeces indicates a positive test for hookworm disease. This infection can be avoided by wearing shoes.

Trichinella spiralis is a small pork roundworm that causes trichinosis. In humans, the disease begins by ingestion of insufficiently cooked pork meat. On entry of encysted meat into the small intestine, the larvae are released from the cysts. After maturation, the females develop eggs that later form into larvae. They then migrate via the bloodstream and lymphatic system to the skeletal muscles and encyst. Encapsulation and eventually calcification of the cysts occur. Diagnosis of trichinosis is made by muscle biopsy, whereby microscopic examination reveals the presence of larvae. The disease is prevented by thoroughly cooking pork meat before eating.

ANTHELMINTIC DRUGS

Anthelmintic drugs are used to rid the body of worms (helminths). Anthelmintics are among the most basic forms of chemotherapy. It has been estimated that one-third of the world's population is infested with these parasites. The main class of anthelmintic drugs are the benzimidazoles including albendazole and mebendazole. The other anthelmintics are ivermectin, praziquantel and pyrantel.

Benzimidazoles

The benzimidazoles are vermicidal and may also be ovicidal for most helminths. They cause degeneration of a parasite's cytoplasmic microtubules, which leads to blocking of glucose uptake in the helminth, and hence death of the parasite. They are indicated for the treatment of *Trichuris* (whipworm), *Enterobius* (pinworm), *Ascaris* (roundworm), *Ancylostoma* (common hookworm), and some tapeworms and liver flukes.

Albendazole

Albendazole is poorly absorbed and essentially remains within the GIT. Absorption is significantly increased by consumption of a fatty meal; the small amount of drug absorbed is rapidly metabolised by the liver to an active sulfoxide metabolite that is thought to be the active drug against tissue infestation. The plasma half-life of albendazole sulfoxide is 8–9 hours but, after release from cysts, low concentrations can be detected in plasma for several weeks. Elimination is principally via bile, with only small quantities detected in urine.

Adverse reactions occur with higher doses and extended dosing, and include headache, nausea, vomiting and diarrhoea. Rarely, allergic reactions, liver toxicity and haematological reactions occur.

In patients with hepatic impairment, dosage reduction may be necessary. Albendazole is contraindicated in pregnancy because of evidence of teratogenic effects in several animal species, and in lactation because it is excreted in breast milk (ADEC Category D).

Dosage varies according to the infecting species but in general, for adults a single dose of 400 mg is given before food in the case of roundworm, threadworm or hookworm infections. Consult current drug information sources for dosing schedules relevant to other helminth species and for dosing in children.

**CLINICAL INTEREST BOX 53-4
WORM TREATMENTS**

According to the latest data, the market in Australia for anthelmintic drugs grew by 5% from August 1999 to August 2000. This amounted to an annual turnover of around $7.5 million. The market continues to grow, with the introduction of flavoured formulations (e.g. orange-flavoured tablets, banana-flavoured suspensions and chocolate squares). Effective advertising and promotion have increased awareness of infections with worms, particularly threadworms.
Source: Martin 2000.

Ivermectin is a semisynthetic compound isolated from a fermented broth of *Streptomyces avermitilis*. It has a wide range of activity against helminths and is also used in veterinary medicine. It is thought to exert an effect on nematodes by stimulating the release of the inhibitory neurotransmitter γ-aminobutyric acid (GABA), which disrupts neuronal transmission. Opening of chloride channels, with subsequent increasing chloride conductance, paralyses the nematode. The sites of action in nematodes differ from those in mammals.

INDICATIONS This drug is indicated for treating infection with *Strongyloides stercoralis* (a threadworm found in northern Australia) and with the immature microfilariae of *Onchocerca volvulus*, reducing the incidence of 'river blindness' by up to 80%.

PHARMACOKINETICS Ivermectin is incompletely absorbed after oral administration, and peak plasma concentrations occur about 4 hours after administration. The drug is metabolised and both unchanged ivermectin and the metabolites are excreted in faeces, with less than 1% appearing in urine. The plasma half-life of ivermectin is 9–15 hours, and 3 days for the metabolites.

ADVERSE REACTIONS Those commonly encountered include nausea, diarrhoea, dizziness and pruritus. Rarely, ivermectin causes tachycardia, postural hypotension, uveitis, facial and peripheral oedema, or elevated liver enzymes.

WARNINGS AND CONTRAINDICATIONS Use with caution in people with hepatic impairment, as studies in this patient group have not been reported. Avoid use in pregnancy (ADEC Category B3) and lactation and in children under 5 years, as there are insufficient safety data.

DOSAGE AND ADMINISTRATION The dosage for adults and children >5 years of age is 150 mcg/kg as a single dose for onchocerciasis, and 200 mcg/kg as a single dose for strongyloidiasis, threadworm, whipworm and roundworm.

Mebendazole

Mebendazole's oral absorption is increased if given with fatty foods. It is distributed to plasma, cyst fluid, liver, hepatic cysts and muscle tissues, with a half-life of 2.5–5.5 hours. It is metabolised in the liver and excreted primarily in faeces.

Adverse reactions are uncommon and include gastric distress, diarrhoea, nausea, vomiting, alopecia, dizziness, headache and, rarely, hypersensitivity and neutropenia. Use this drug with caution in patients with Crohn's ileitis and ulcerative colitis. Avoid use in people with mebendazole hypersensitivity and liver function impairment.

The adult and paediatric dosage (children 2 years of age and over) is 100 mg orally as a single dose for threadworm, and 100 mg twice daily for 3 days for hookworm, roundworm and whipworm. If necessary, this dosage may be repeated in 2–3 weeks.

Other anthelmintics
Praziquantel

Praziquantel is an anthelmintic agent that penetrates cell membranes and increases cell permeability in susceptible worms. This results in an increased loss of intracellular calcium, contractions, and muscle paralysis of the worm. The drug also disintegrates the schistosome tegument (covering). Subsequently, phagocytes are attracted to the worm and ultimately kill it. Praziquantel is indicated for the treatment of schistosomiasis due to various blood flukes, and for tapeworms but is ineffective against roundworms.

Praziquantel is absorbed orally and reaches a peak plasma concentration in 1–3 hours. Half-life is 0.8–1.5 hours for praziquantel and 4–6 hours for its metabolites. It is excreted by the kidneys and is generally well tolerated.

See the Drug Interactions table 53-6 for praziquantel.

Adverse reactions include headache, light-headedness, gastric distress, sweating, rash, pruritus, dizziness, drowsiness, fever, increased sweating and GI distress, including bloody diarrhoea. Use this drug with caution in patients with severe liver disease. Avoid use in people with praziquantel hypersensitivity and ocular cysticercosis.

For intestinal tapeworms the adult dose is 20 mg/kg as a single dose. Swallow tablets whole with food and plenty of water to help disguise the bitter taste. Do not chew.

DRUG INTERACTIONS 53-6 Praziquantel	
Drug	**Possible effect and management**
Alcohol	CNS effects of praziquantel may be potentiated. Avoid this combination
Carbamazepine, phenytoin, dexamethasone and chloroquine	These drugs increase metabolism of praziquantel, reducing its effectiveness. A higher dose of praziquantel may be required
Cimetidine	Inhibition of metabolism of praziquantel, leading to an increased plasma concentration and effect. Use an alternative H$_2$ antagonist

Source: AMH 2006.

Pyrantel

Pyrantel is a depolarising neuromuscular-blocking anthelmintic agent; it causes contraction and then paralysis of the helminth's muscles. The helminths are dislodged and then expelled from the body by peristalsis. Pyrantel is indicated for the treatment of *Ascaris lumbricoides* (roundworm), *Enterobius vermicularis* (threadworm) and hookworm, but is ineffective against whipworm. This product is poorly absorbed from the GIT. Pyrantel reaches peak plasma concentration in 1–3 hours and is primarily excreted in the faeces.

Adverse reactions include diarrhoea, vomiting, nausea, headache and abdominal cramps. Rarely, pyrantel causes anorexia, dizziness, drowsiness and an increase in liver enzymes. Exercise caution in people with dehydration or malnourishment. Avoid use in patients with pyrantel hypersensitivity.

The dosage in adults and children for threadworm and roundworm is 10 mg/kg (maximum 750 mg) as a single oral dose. If necessary, it may be repeated in 1 week.

PREGNANCY SAFETY

ADEC Category	Drug
A	Chloroquine,* ethambutol, isoniazid
B1	Praziquantel
B2	Atovaquone with proguanil, dapsone, pyrantel, pyrazinamide
B3	Ivermectin, mebendazole, mefloquine
C	Capreomycin, clofazimine, pyrimethamine with sulfadoxine, rifabutin, rifampicin
D	Albendazole, artemether with lumefantrine, hydroxychloroquine, paromomycin, primaquine, quinine
Unclassified	Cycloserine should be avoided in pregnancy

*Chloroquine is classed as Category D when used for the treatment of malaria; specialist information services should be contacted.

DRUGS AT A GLANCE 53: Antiprotozoal, antimycobacterial and anthelmintic drugs

Therapeutic group	Pharmacological group	Key examples	Key pages
Antiprotozoals	Antimalarials	artemether with lumefantrine	852, 3
		ativaquone with proguanil	853
		chloroquine	851, 2
		mefloquine	850
		quinine	851, 2
	Amoebicidal drug	paromomycin	855
Antimycobacterials	Antituberculous drugs	capreomycin	857
		cycloserine	857
		isoniazid	858
		pyrazinamide	860, 1
		rifampicin	859
	Antileprotic drugs	clofazimine	862
		dapsone	862
Anthelmintics	Benzimidazoles	albendazole	864
		mebendazole	865
	Others	ivermectin	865
		praziquantel	865
		pyrantel	866

KEY POINTS

- Malaria and tuberculosis are still prevalent diseases throughout the world.
- Malaria is endemic in more than 100 countries and it has been reported that worldwide between 300 and 500 million individuals have clinical malaria.
- The choice of antimalarial drugs is based on the particular malarial strain involved and the stage of the plasmodium life cycle.
- Travellers to endemic areas should receive malaria chemoprophylaxis starting 1–3 weeks before entering the area.
- Amoebiasis is an infection of the large intestine produced by a protozoan parasite, *Entamoeba histolytica*. This infestation is found worldwide but is prevalent and severe in tropical areas.
- Amoebicidal drugs include paromomycin.
- The two main mycobacterial infections in humans are tuberculosis and leprosy.
- More than 2 million people die from tuberculosis annually.
- The World Health Organization (WHO) aims to reduce TB prevalence and death rates by 50% (relative to 1990) by 2015, and to eliminate TB as a public health problem (1 case per million population) by 2050.
- The incidence of tuberculosis in Australasia has remained relatively stable.
- The WHO has recommended the Directly Observed Treatment—Short Course (DOTS) approach for the control of tuberculosis and has projected that the use of this system would result in cure of 85% of all new cases.
- The recommended first-line drugs for tuberculosis are isoniazid, rifampicin, pyrazinamide and ethambutol. In developing countries streptomycin is also a first-line drug.
- Leprosy, or Hansen's disease, is caused by *Mycobacterium leprae* in humans. Today, the estimated number of infected people is nearly 15 million worldwide.
- Drug treatment of leprosy includes the use of dapsone and clofazimine.
- Anthelmintic drugs are used to rid the body of worms (helminths). It has been estimated that one-third of the world's population is infested with these parasites.
- The main class of anthelmintic drugs are the benzimidazoles, which include albendazole and mebendazole. Other anthelmintics include ivermectin, praziquantel and pyrantel.
- Knowledge of the various drugs available alone and in combination (when applicable) to treat malaria, tuberculosis, leprosy, amoebiasis and helminthiasis is vital information for the health-care professional.

REVIEW EXERCISES

1 How is a drug selected for the treatment of malaria? Name the four types of therapy, according to drug classification.
2 Discuss the luminal and tissue amoebicides and name one drug from each category.
3 Present the World Health Organization DOTS five-step plan for the treatment of tuberculosis. If properly implemented, what is the expected outcome?
4 Discuss drug selection for tuberculosis. What are the general guidelines for the drug regimens?
5 List four reasons why parasitic infestations are dangerous to the individual. Name the main human parasitic helminths and the drugs that are usually used to treat these infestations.

REFERENCES AND FURTHER READING

Antibiotic Expert Group. *Therapeutic Guidelines: Antibiotic, version 13*. Melbourne: Therapeutic Guidelines, 2006.
Australian Institute of Health and Welfare. *Australia's Health 2004*. Canberra: AIHW, 2004.
Australian Medicines Handbook 2006. Adelaide: Australian Medicines Handbook, 2006.
Croft A. Malaria: prevention in travellers. *British Medical Journal* 2000; 321: 154–60.
Ebert SC. Tuberculosis. In: DiPiro JT, Talber R et al (eds). *Pharmacotherapy: A Pathophysiologic Approach*. 2nd edn. Norwalk: Appleton & Lange, 1993.
Espinal MA, Laslo A, Simonsen L et al. Global trends in resistance to antituberculosis drugs. *New England Journal of Medicine* 2001; 344: 1294–303.

Mandell GL, Petri AW Jr. Drugs used in chemotherapy of tuberculosis, *Mycobacterium avium* complex disease, and leprosy. Ch 48 in: Hardman JG, Limbird LE, Molinoff PB et al (eds). *Goodman & Gilman's the Pharmacological Basis of Therapeutics*. 9th edn. New York: McGraw-Hill, 1996.

Martin K. The early bird catches the worm. *Australian Pharmacy Trade* 2000; November 16.

Skull SA, Tallis G. Epidemiology of malaria in Victoria 1999-2000: East Timor emerges as a new source of disease. *Communicable Diseases Intelligence* 2001; 25: 149–51.

United States Pharmacopeial Convention 1998. *USP DI: Drug Information for the Health Care Professional*. 18th edn. Rockville, MD: USPDI, 1998.

WHO. Expert Committee on Leprosy. TRS 874. Geneva: WHO, 1998.

WHO. Global leprosy situation, 2006. Available: www.who.int/wer/2006/wer8132.pdf, accessed 31 May 2006.

WHO. The global plan to stop TB 2006–2015. Available: www.who.int/tb/features_archive/global_plan_to_stop_tb/en/index.html, accessed 31 May 2006.

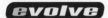 More weblinks at http://evolve.elsevier.com/AU/Bryant/pharmacology/

CHAPTER 54

Overview of Mediators of Inflammation, Allergy and the Immune Response

CHAPTER FOCUS

The body's resistance to disease is both non-specific, e.g. physical and chemical barriers that offer immediate protection, such as the skin, mucous membranes and gastric acidity; and specific, i.e. an acquired specific resistance or immunity that develops more slowly. When a chemical, foreign body or microorganism penetrates a barrier such as the skin, the body will try to contain the invader by eliciting an inflammatory response, and try to eliminate it by provoking a specific immune response. In some individuals who are sensitised to a particular antigen, further exposure can precipitate an allergic reaction. In humans, the immune system consists of lymph, lymphatic vessels, lymph nodes, red bone marrow, the spleen, tonsils, the thymus gland and billions of circulating cells, mainly lymphocytes and antibody-secreting plasma cells. During a lifetime, an individual may acquire immune capabilities through both natural and artificial means. A thorough knowledge of the immune system is essential for the health-care professional.

OBJECTIVES

- To describe the main components and functions of the immune system.
- To describe the four characteristic signs of inflammation.
- To describe and contrast the functions of T cells and B cells.
- To define humoral and cell-mediated immunity.
- To explain the functions of the five classes of antibodies.
- To describe natural and acquired immunity, and active and passive immunity.

KEY TERMS

acquired immunity
allergic, or hypersensitivity, reactions
antibodies
cell-mediated immunity
complement system
humoral immunity
immunocompetent cells
natural immunity
non-specific resistance
passive immunity
specific resistance

KEY ABBREVIATIONS

AIDS	acquired immune deficiency syndrome
Ig	immunoglobulin
IL	interleukin
NK	natural killer (cells)

THE immune system is composed of cells and organs that mount defensive responses against pathogens (e.g. microbes, toxins and chemicals) and cancer cells and in some cases, unfortunately, against normal body tissues (autoimmune diseases). The body's resistance to disease is both **non-specific**, e.g. physical and chemical barriers that offer immediate protection, such as the skin and gastric acidity; and **specific**, i.e. an acquired specific resistance or immunity that develops more slowly.

THE IMMUNE SYSTEM

The lymphatic system is responsible for eliciting highly specific immune responses, and comprises lymph, lymphatic vessels, lymph nodes, red bone marrow (see Chapter 29) and the thymus gland, spleen and tonsils. These organs and tissues are collectively responsible for the production and maturation of the immunocompetent cells and for facilitating the immune response. Figure 54-1 identifies the organs and tissues of the immune system.

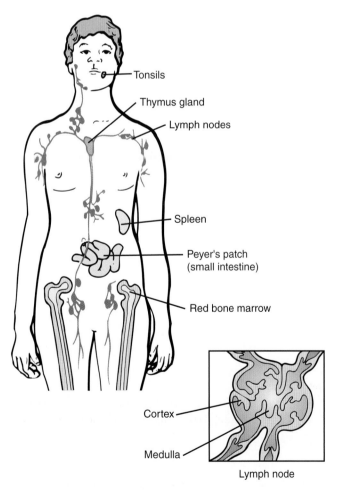

Tonsils

Thymus gland

Lymph nodes

Spleen

Peyer's patch
(small intestine)

Red bone marrow

Cortex

Medulla

Lymph node

FIGURE 54–1 Location of organs and tissues of the immune system. The inset shows a cross-section of a lymph node.

Thymus gland

The thymus gland has two lobes and is located in the mediastinal area. The thymus gland is larger at birth than it is in an adult. By the time a person reaches puberty, the thymus has grown to nearly six times its original size. After puberty, this gland undergoes involution, and in the elderly it is usually a small mass (about 3 g) of reticular fibres with some lymphocytes and connective tissue. Although its importance was largely discounted over the years, there are many unanswered questions about the thymus gland and its relation to the other tissues and organs in the immune system.

The immune system develops when lymphoid stem cells produced in the red bone marrow migrate to the thymus, spleen and other lymphoid tissues and organs in the body. Thymic hormones produced in the thymus are thought to aid in the maturation of the prothymocytes, which ultimately develop into T lymphocytes (see following section on Specific resistance).

Spleen

The spleen, the largest lymphatic organ in the body, is located on the left side of the body in the extreme superior, posterior corner of the abdominal cavity. Its main functions are to act as a storage site or reservoir for blood and a processing station for time-expired blood cells and platelets. Resident macrophages lining the white pulp (lymphatic tissue) and central arteries of the spleen remove pathogens from the blood, while the venous sinuses of the red pulp area of the spleen process worn-out blood cells and store platelets. The white pulp area of the spleen also contains lymphocytes and plasma cells that are involved in the immune process.

Tonsils

The tonsils are accumulations of lymphoid tissue (lymphatic nodules) named according to their location: lingual, palatine and pharyngeal tonsils. They intercept foreign substances that enter the body by way of the respiratory or gastrointestinal tracts. Similar lymphoid tissue located in the submucosal areas of the gastrointestinal tract (Peyer's patches) mount immune responses against bacteria and viruses entering from the gut. Other lymphatic nodules are located in the urinary and reproductive tracts and help to intercept antigens in the blood and in the lymph nodes.

Lymph nodes

The lymph nodes are capsulated organs located throughout the body and are involved with lymph circulation. They are essentially a row of unidirectional in-line filters, which screen the lymph flowing through them. Foreign material is either engulfed by the resident macrophages or destroyed by immune responses elicited by the lymphocytes located throughout the lymph nodes. Lymph nodes are common secondary malignant tumour sites.

The outer portion of the lymph node is called the cortex and contains B lymphocytes (B cells), which become antibody-secreting plasma cells. The thymus-dependent zone exists in the deep area or inner cortex and contains mainly T lymphocytes (T cells), formed or seeded from the thymus gland, which, when exposed to an antigen, divide rapidly and produce large numbers of new T cells sensitised to that antigen. The inner portion is the medulla, which contains B lymphocytes and plasma cells.

RESISTANCE TO DISEASE

Non-specific resistance
Inflammation

The initial and immediate lines of defence for the body are the skin, the mucous membranes of the respiratory and gastrointestinal tracts, and chemical secretions such as saliva and gastric acid. Penetration of these barriers by pathogens results in the mobilisation of internal defence mechanisms. These include natural killer (NK) cells, which are lymphocytes that are of neither B nor T cell type, and phagocytic neutrophils and macrophages. Phagocytosis involves several phases, including digestion and in some cases killing of the pathogen. If cells are damaged by bacteria or viruses, physical trauma (e.g. a cut), foreign bodies, chemical substances, surgery, radiation or electricity, the body will elicit an inflammatory response. The area affected will undergo a series of changes as the body processes attempt to wall off, heal and replace the injured tissue.

The four characteristic signs of inflammation are swelling (oedema), redness (erythema), pain and heat, which are accounted for by three basic events: (1) blood vessel vasodilation and increased capillary permeability, (2) cellular infiltration, and (3) tissue repair. These processes involve a variety of chemical mediators that modify and contribute to the inflammatory response. After an injury occurs, for example, the body will release chemical substances such as histamine, prostaglandins, leukotrienes, kinins and complement into the tissue, forming a chemotactic gradient, and fluids and cells will begin to accumulate in the area. Blood vessels dilate (primarily because of the action of histamine and kinins) within 30 minutes of the insult, and this allows an increase in blood flow and exudation of fluid due to increased capillary permeability in the injured tissues. The exudate includes protein-rich fluids high in fibrinogen that will attract other substances to the area, such as complement, antibodies and leucocytes. Fluid collection in the area results in oedema, which generally occurs within 4 hours of the injury.

During the cellular phase, neutrophils and monocytes attracted by chemotactic agents such as kinins, leukotrienes and complement will migrate into the area from the dilated blood vessels. If the injury is due to a foreign substance or bacteria, the monocytes will transform into wandering macrophages, which are more powerful phagocytes than the neutrophils and engulf and destroy the foreign material (phagocytosis). The phagocytosis process tends to localise, or wall off, the foreign material to prevent its spread through the tissues. Large numbers of phagocytes can lead to pus accumulation and the eventual destruction and removal of the foreign material. The resulting debris is removed by the macrophages and neutrophils, thus resolving the inflammatory reaction.

Mediators of inflammation
THE COMPLEMENT SYSTEM

The **complement system** is composed of plasma proteins (at least 18 distinct proteins and their cleavage products) present in the blood in the form of inactive proteases. Activation of the protein called complement 1 (C1) by proteolytic cleavage is the initial step in this cascading pathway that mediates destruction of invading pathogens. The system is divided into two pathways: the 'classical pathway', which is activated by an antigen–antibody complex, and the 'alternative pathway', which is antibody-independent and involves protein factors B, D and P (properidin) and activation of the complement cascade at C3 (Figure 54-2). Complement is essential in the response to an acute inflammatory reaction caused by bacteria, some viruses and immune complex diseases. Complement enhances chemotaxis, increases blood vessel permeability and eventually causes cell lysis.

LOCAL HORMONES

Histamine, a product of mast cells and basophils; prostaglandins generated from arachidonic acid (see Chapter 55); and cytokines released from inflammatory tissue are some of the mediators capable of producing local reactions, smooth muscle contraction, increased chemotaxis, blood vessel vasodilation and other inflammatory effects.

Specific resistance

Provocation of an immune response against specific pathogens or transplanted tissue is called specific resistance, or immunity. The primary types of immunity are **humoral (antibody-mediated) immunity** and **cell-mediated immunity**. The key features that differentiate immunity from non-specific resistance are the specificity of recognition of the antigen (e.g. pollen, bacteria and transplanted tissue) and memory evocation, i.e. a second encounter with the same antigen provokes an immediate and more substantial immune response. The part of an antigen that triggers an immune

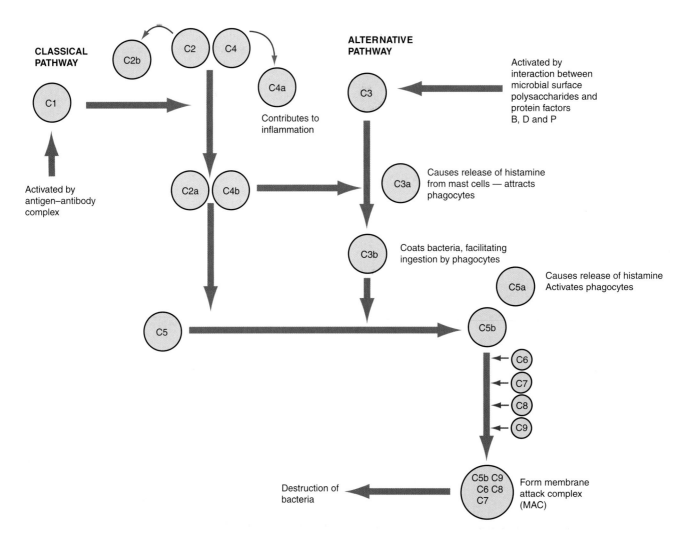

FIGURE 54–2 The complement system. Complement protein C1, activated by an antigen–antibody complex, initiates the classical pathway. The alternative pathway is initiated at C3 by an interaction between the microbe and factors B, D and P.

response, such as antibody production, or activates specific T cells is called the epitope. Sometimes the body's ability to differentiate between true antigenic proteins and self-proteins fails and the immune system attacks the normal body cells, producing autoimmune disorders. The cells that carry out the immune responses are described as **immunocompetent cells**. T and B cells and the polymorphonuclear leucocytes (PMLs) are involved in the immune response, although only mononuclear T and B cells are immunocompetent cells. The PMLs are non-specific cells that interact with lymphocytes to produce an inflammatory response, whereas B and T cells are capable of recognising specific antigens and initiating the immune response.

Cell-mediated immunity

In humans, stem cells from the bone marrow are transformed into T cells in the thymus gland and B cells in red bone marrow (see Chapter 29). Before migrating to lymphoid

tissue and organs, T and B cells acquire cell surface antigen receptors that are capable of recognising specific antigens. When in contact with an antigen, T cells proliferate to form specialised 'killer' T cells, thus providing cell-mediated immunity. The B cells transform into plasma cells, which form antibodies (immunoglobulins) that search out, identify and bind with specific antigens to provide humoral (antibody-mediated) immunity.

T lymphocytes

T cells are generally long-lived. When they are not in their special areas, they circulate continuously through the body by way of the bloodstream and lymphatic system. When the T cells first recognise the foreign substance (antigen), they are stimulated and become activated. The activated lympho-cytes then proliferate and differentiate into highly specialised cells that have the capacity to recognise and respond to the antigen. These specialised cells, or clones, constitute an identical population of lymphocytes that are capable of recognising one specific antigen.

Three major groups of T cells identified are cytotoxic (killer) T cells, helper T cells and memory T cells.

CYTOTOXIC (KILLER) T CELLS

These cells display a protein called CD8+ on their membranes and can bind tightly to organisms or cells that contain their binding-specific antigen. Following stimulation by cytokines produced by helper T cells, the killer cells become cytolytic, i.e. capable of lysing (killing) cancer cells, tissue transplant cells and other cells that are foreign to the person's body. Body tissue that contains viruses or foreign cells may also be attacked by the killer T cells.

HELPER T CELLS

These make up the majority of the T cells that have the plasma membrane protein CD4+. They increase the activation of B cells, T cells and NK cells. Helper T cells are activated by antigen-presenting cells; once activated, they secrete various cytokines, which comprise a large group of molecules that are involved in signal pathways between cells during immune responses. These cytokines include interleukin-2 (IL-2, the major stimulus for T-cell proliferation), IL-4 and IL-5 (which stimulate B cells and cause plasma cells to secrete antibodies)

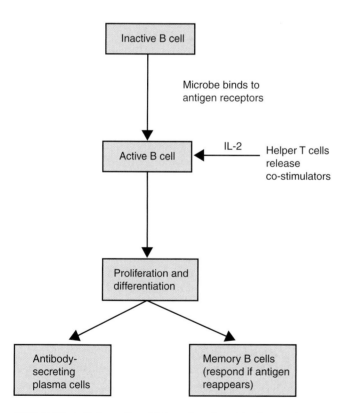

FIGURE 54–3 Schematic of B lymphocyte activation and differentiation into plasma cells (antibody-secreting) and memory B cells.

and gamma interferon (which stimulates phagocytosis and enhances immune responses). Helper T cells also secrete macrophage migration inhibition factor, which slows or stops the migration of macrophages away from the affected area. The activated macrophages can attack and destroy a vastly increased number of the invading organism.

AIDS is the final outcome of an infection with HIV. This virus binds to protein on the cell membranes of the helper T cells (T4 cells) and over the course of many years the T4 cells are destroyed by the virus. This ultimately leads to the immunodeficiency syndrome known as AIDS. Additional information on this disease and treatment is in Chapter 52.

MEMORY T CELLS

Cells remaining from a population of clones after a cell-mediated immune response are called memory T cells. The function of these cells is immediate recognition and vigorous handling of the same foreign antigen on presentation at a later date. In essence, they are the 'memory' of a previous response to a specific antigen.

Humoral (antibody-mediated) immunity

Humoral immunity is a response effective in the extracellular environment, in contrast to cell-mediated immunity, which deals with intracellular organisms. Humans possess B cells, which can produce an array of antibodies that recognise different antigens. Antibody response can be elicited by various antigenic proteins, such as the protein coat of a bacterium, or by intentional vaccination.

B lymphocytes

The body contains millions of B cells that reside in various parts of the body, e.g. lymph nodes, the spleen and gastro-intestinal tract. Following antigen recognition, B cells, assisted by helper T cells that secrete IL-2, become activated. Some of the activated B cells specific for the antigen will enlarge and differentiate to form plasmablasts, which are plasma cell precursors, and some will remain undifferentiated and become memory B cells (Figure 54-3). The plasma cells secrete an antibody specific to the antigen for around 4–5 days or until the plasma cell dies (primary response). Different antigens stimulate different B cells, and the respective clonal populations each produce only one type of antibody. Initially, the immunoglobulin is IgM (see following section), which increases in quantity for up to 2 weeks; production then declines so that very little IgM is present after a few weeks. After the initial IgM production, IgG antibodies start to appear at around day 10, peak in several weeks and maintain high levels for a much longer period (Figure 54-4).

The first (primary) response to an antigen may be slow, weak and of short duration, but the memory B cells on second

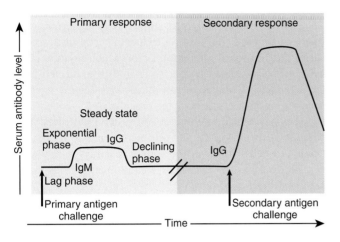

FIGURE 54–4 Primary and secondary immune responses. *Source*: Mudge-Grout 1992.

exposure to the same antigen will cause a more rapid and potent antibody response, and antibodies will be formed for months rather than for only a few weeks (secondary response). This is why vaccination using several doses given at periods of weeks or months apart is so effective (Figure 54-4).

Antibodies

Antibodies are gamma globulins (a type of protein), called immunoglobulins, that are specific for particular antigens. They are produced by lymphoid tissue in response to antigens, and consist of four polypeptide chains: two heavy (H) and two light (L) chains that can form either a T or a Y shape. Differences in the constant region of the H chains provide the basis for the five classes of antibodies that have been identified: IgG, IgM, IgA, IgD and IgE. ('Ig' stands for immunoglobulin; the other letters designate the classes.)

IgG is the major immunoglobulin in the blood (about 75%–80% of the total antibodies in the normal person) and is capable of entering tissue spaces, coating microorganisms and activating the complement system, thus accelerating phagocytosis. It is the only immunoglobulin capable of crossing the placenta to provide the fetus with passive immunity until the infant can produce its own immune defence system.

IgM is the first immunoglobulin produced during an immune response. It is located primarily in the bloodstream and develops in response to an invasion of bacteria or viruses. IgM activates complement and can destroy foreign invaders during the initial antigen exposure. Its level decreases in about 2 weeks, while IgG levels are progressively increasing.

IgA is located primarily in external body secretions—saliva, sweat, tears, mucus, bile and colostrums—and it is found in respiratory tract mucosa and in plasma. It helps to provide a defence against antigens on exposed surfaces and antigens that enter the respiratory and gastrointestinal tracts. The plasma cells in the intestinal area secrete IgA and secretory component to defend the body against bacteria and viruses.

IgD is located in blood and on lymphocyte surfaces together with IgM. IgD is involved in activation of B cells. Levels are elevated in chronic infections.

IgE binds to histamine-containing mast cells and basophils. It is involved in allergic and hypersensitivity reactions, and can mediate the release of histamine in immune response to parasites (helminths). Concentrations of it are low in the plasma because the antibody is firmly fixed on tissue surfaces. Once activated by an antigen, it will trigger the release of the mast cell granules, resulting in the signs and symptoms of allergy and anaphylaxis.

Allergic (hypersensitivity) reactions

Substances foreign to the body act as antigens to stimulate the production of antibodies or immunoglobulins (IgE, IgG, IgM). When a previously sensitised individual is again exposed to the foreign substance, the antigen reacts with the antibodies to release substances such as histamine, which then provoke allergic symptoms. There are four different types of **allergic**, or **hypersensitivity**, **reactions**.

Type I: Immediate, or anaphylactic, reaction is a reaction that occurs within minutes of exposure to the antigenic material (e.g. pollen, dust, animal dander, some drugs or food) in a previously sensitised person. This reaction is mediated by IgE antibodies that fix to the surfaces of mast cells and basophils, releasing histamine and cytokines. An immediate, severe reaction results, which may be fatal if not recognised and treated quickly. The most dramatic form of anaphylaxis is sudden, severe bronchospasm, vasospasm, severe hypotension and rapid death. Signs and symptoms are largely caused by contraction of smooth muscles, mucosal oedema and increased vascular permeability, and may begin with irritability, extreme weakness, nausea and vomiting, and then proceed to dyspnoea, cyanosis, convulsions and cardiac arrest. Some drugs are associated with this type of reaction, e.g. penicillin.

Type II: Antibody-dependent cytotoxic reaction involves IgG- or IgM-directed complement activation and lysis of normal cells; it has sometimes been called an autoimmune response. This reaction may manifest as systemic lupus erythematosus and other autoimmune diseases, as haemolytic anaemia after incompatible blood transfusion, or as agranulocytosis.

Type III: Arthus, or complex-mediated, reaction is sometimes called serum sickness. With this reaction, the antigen forms a complex with IgG antibodies, often in small blood vessels, resulting in fever, swollen lymph nodes (lymphadenopathy) and splenomegaly in about 1–3 weeks.

Type IV: Cell-mediated, or delayed hypersensitivity, reaction is the basis for most skin rashes, such as contact dermatitis from poison ivy and reactions to insect bites. Direct skin contact between sensitised cells results in an inflammatory reaction and cell-mediated immune response involving sensitised T lymphocytes (CD4+ cells).

NATURAL AND ACQUIRED IMMUNITY

The body has certain inherited and innate abilities to resist antigens. This ability is known as natural resistance, or **natural immunity**, which is different from **acquired immunity**. Some general defences inherent in natural resistance come from factors familiar to the focus of health care: for example, adequate rest, nutrition, exercise and freedom from undue stress. Physiological factors, which discourage proliferation of microbes, include the acidity of gastric secretions, respiratory tract cilia and bactericidal lysozyme in tears. During a lifetime, an individual may also acquire further immune capabilities through both natural and artificial means. This type of acquired immunity is acquired either actively or passively (Figure 54-5).

Antibodies activate cellular defences to engulf antigens. Custom-made immunoglobulins, or antibodies, provide acquired immunity to the specific type of antigen for varying lengths of time. Those antibodies gradually disappear from the plasma but the potential for their rapid replication in response to a repeat challenge by that specific antigen continues to exist after the initial exposure. The result, known as **naturally acquired immunity**, is a process of active immunity because of the body's active involvement in creating the antibodies. Naturally acquired immunity can also result from a process of **passive immunity**, when antibodies made by the mother's body are passively transferred by means of the placenta or by breast milk (especially colostrum, the breast milk produced shortly after delivery) to the fetus or infant.

On the other hand, artificial induction of the immune state, or **artificially acquired immunity**, is initiated purposefully for the protection of an individual (see Clinical Interest Box 54-1). It can also be induced either actively or passively. Artificially acquired active immunity is evoked by the deliberate administration of antigens, which may be live, partly modified organisms; killed organisms; or their toxins. The parenteral route is the predominant mode of administration. Periodic reactivation of actively acquired

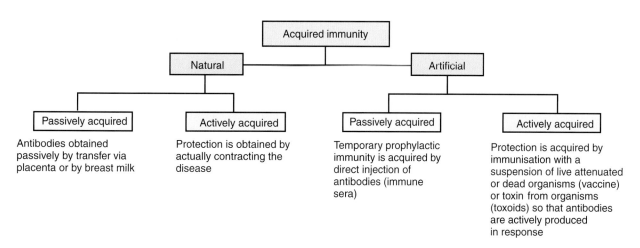

FIGURE 54–5 The process of acquired immunity.

TABLE 54-1 Comparison of active and passive immunity

Characteristic	Active immunity	Passive immunity
Source	Individual	Other human or animal
Efficacy	High	Low to moderate
Method	Contracting disease Immunisation with vaccines or toxoids	Administer preformed antibody by injection, maternal transplacental transfer or in breast milk
Time to develop	5–21 days	Immediate effect
Duration	Long, up to years	Usually shorter than active immunity
Ease of reactivation	Easy with booster dose	Can be dangerous; anaphylaxis may occur, especially if animal sources are used
Purpose	Prophylaxis	Prophylaxis and therapeutic

CLINICAL INTEREST BOX 54-1 MENINGOCOCCAL DISEASE IN NEW ZEALAND

New Zealand has been experiencing a meningococcal disease epidemic. Prior to the start of the epidemic in 1991, around 60 cases were reported each year. The average number of cases per year for the past 5 years is 463. The highest annual total recorded in the epidemic was in 2001, when the total number of cases of meningococcal disease was 650 (a rate of 17.4 per 100,000), including 26 deaths (a case-fatality rate of 4.0%).

The Meningococcal B Immunisation Programme was launched in Counties Manakau on 19 July 2004. Not all of the cases reported in 2005 were due to the same strain that the vaccine is designed to protect against. In 2004, 73.0% of laboratory-confirmed cases were caused by the strain that the vaccine is designed for. By 18 December

2005, a total of 2,884,996 doses of MeNZB had been administered. A fourth dose of MeNZB was licensed on 12 January 2006 for babies, who received their first dose aged under 6 months.

Information on possible adverse events is being collected from the following sources:
- hospital-based monitoring in Middlemore, Auckland and Whangarei hospitals
- health professional reporting of adverse events to the Centre for Adverse Event Monitoring (CARM)
- the Intensive Vaccine Monitoring Programme (IVMP) at sentinel GP practices with reporting to CARM.

Adapted from: www.moh.govt.nz, accessed 20 January 2006.

artificial immunity to certain organisms by booster doses (e.g. tetanus) is sometimes necessary. Artificially acquired passive immunity is conferred by the parenteral administration of antibody-containing immune plasma from immune humans or animals (Figure 54-5).

Artificially acquired active immunity generally secures protection for a longer duration than any kind of passive immunity, and is usually the prophylactic treatment of choice for populations at potential risk. Adverse effects include local pain at the injection site, and headache with mild to moderate

fever. Artificially acquired passive immunity is often chosen for susceptible individuals after a known exposure. A combination of active and passive approaches is also used occasionally. Various products used in artificial passive immunisation have caused adverse reactions because of individual hypersensitivities to animal products, especially horse plasma or eggs; to the preservative used in a medication; or to an antibiotic. The products of bacterial metabolism are the agents responsible for other adverse reactions. Table 54-1 compares the processes of active and passive immunity.

KEY POINTS

- The body's resistance to disease is both non-specific, which offers immediate protection, and specific, i.e. an acquired specific resistance or immunity that develops more slowly.
- The lymphatic system, which is responsible for eliciting highly specific immune responses, comprises lymph, lymphatic vessels, lymph nodes, red bone marrow and the thymus gland, spleen and tonsils.
- The initial and immediate lines of defence for the body are the skin, the mucous membranes of the respiratory and gastrointestinal tracts, and chemical secretions such as saliva and gastric acid.
- Damage to cells by bacteria or viruses, physical trauma (e.g. a cut), foreign bodies, chemical substances, surgery, radiation or electricity will elicit an inflammatory response.
- The four characteristic signs of inflammation are swelling (oedema), redness (erythema), pain and heat, which are accounted for by three basic events: (1) blood vessel vasodilation and increased capillary permeability, (2) cellular infiltration, and (3) tissue repair.
- Mediators of inflammation include the complement system and local hormones such as histamine, prostaglandins and cytokines.
- Provocation of an immune response against specific pathogens or transplanted tissue is called specific resistance or immunity.
- The primary types of immunity are humoral (antibody-mediated) immunity and cell-mediated immunity.
- Humoral immunity is a response effective in the extracellular environment, in contrast to cell-mediated immunity, which deals with intracellular organisms.
- The cells that carry out the immune responses are described as being immunocompetent.
- T and B lymphocytes and the polymorphonuclear leucocytes (PMLs) are involved in the immune response, although only mononuclear T and B lymphocytes are immunocompetent cells.

- Antibodies are gamma globulins (a type of protein), called immunoglobulins, that are specific for particular antigens. Five classes of antibodies have been identified: IgG, IgM, IgA, IgD and IgE.
- The four different types of allergic or hypersensitivity reactions are Type I (immediate or anaphylactic), Type II (antibody-dependent), Type III (complex-mediated), and Type IV (delayed hypersensitivity).
- An individual can acquire further immune capabilities through both natural and artificial means. This type of immunity is acquired either actively or passively.

REVIEW EXERCISES

1   Discuss the biochemical and physiological processes that contribute to the signs of inflammation.
2   Name and describe the three major groups of T cells. Which type of cell is compromised in acquired immunodeficiency syndrome (AIDS)?
3   Describe the functions of the B lymphocytes.
4   What effect does the complement system have in the human body?
5   Describe the functions of the five classes of antibodies.
6   Describe the four different types of allergic (hypersensitivity) reactions.
7   Present the contrasting features of active immunity and passive immunity.

REFERENCES AND FURTHER READING

Mudge-Grout CL. *Immunologic Disorders*. St Louis: Mosby, 1992.
Tortora GJ, Grabowski SR. The lymphatic system, nonspecific resistance to disease, and immunity. In: Tortora GJ, Grabowski SR (eds). *Principles of Anatomy and Physiology*. 9th edn. New York: John Wiley, 2000 [ch. 22].

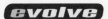 More weblinks at http://evolve.elsevier.com/AU/Bryant/pharmacology/

CHAPTER 55

Anti-inflammatory and Immunomodulating Drugs

CHAPTER FOCUS

This chapter reviews the uses of anti-inflammatory and immunomodulating drugs. These include the non-steroidal anti-inflammatory drugs (NSAIDs), which are among the most widely prescribed drugs in Australia; disease-modifying antirheumatic drugs (DMARDs), used as first-line treatment for rheumatoid arthritis; drugs used to treat gout, a disorder of uric acid metabolism; immunosuppressant drugs, crucial to the success of organ transplantation; and antihistamines, which are widely used for motion sickness, vertigo, and skin and allergic disorders.

OBJECTIVES

- To discuss the mechanisms of action of NSAIDs and DMARDs.
- To explain why drugs have been targeted to selectively inhibit cyclo-oxygenase.
- To describe the main drug interactions occurring with NSAIDs.
- To explain the rationale behind the use of DMARDs and discuss the sites of action of the main drugs in this class.
- To describe the cause and manifestation of gout.
- To list the four treatment goals for gout.
- To discuss the mechanisms of action and significant drug interactions for colchicine, allopurinol and probenecid.
- To list the four main classes of immunosuppressant drugs.
- To discuss the main adverse reactions of the immunosuppressant drugs azathioprine, cyclosporin, daclizumab and tacrolimus.
- To discuss the various actions of histamine and the main use of antihistamine drugs.

KEY DRUGS

allopurinol
azathioprine
basiliximab
colchicine
cyclosporin
etanercept
fexofenadine
ibuprofen
infliximab
interferon
loratadine
meloxicam
muromonab-CD3
mycophenolate
probenecid
promethazine
sulfasalazine
tacrolimus

KEY TERMS

cyclo-oxygenase
disease-modifying
  antirheumatic drugs
gout
hyperuricaemia
immunostimulating drugs
immunosuppressant drugs
non-steroidal anti-
  inflammatory drugs

KEY ABBREVIATIONS

COX	cyclo-oxygenase
DMARDs	disease-modifying antirheumatic drugs
NSAIDs	non-steroidal anti-inflammatory drugs
PG	prostaglandin

NON-STEROIDAL ANTI-INFLAMMATORY DRUGS (NSAIDS)

NSAIDs are one of the most commonly administered groups of drugs worldwide, and new formulations and new NSAIDs (e.g. coxibs) continue to enter the market place. Generally, NSAIDs are either prescribed or purchased over-the counter (OTC) for their analgesic, anti-inflammatory and antipyretic properties. In 2001, more than 6 million Australians were reported to have arthritis or other musculoskeletal disorders. These conditions now cause more disability than any other medical condition. Prescriptions for non-steroidal anti-inflammatory drugs in Australia exceeded 10 million in 2003/04, and the costs to the health system of musculoskeletal disorders over the period 2000/01 exceeded $4,600,000,000 (Australian Institute of Health and Welfare 2005).

Around 14 different NSAIDs are available in Australia and, although aspirin is also an NSAID, this term commonly refers to the aspirin-like substitutes on the market. Despite diversity in their chemical structures (Table 55-1), all the NSAIDs possess the same therapeutic properties—analgesic, antipyretic and anti-inflammatory effects. Unfortunately, they share to varying degrees the same adverse reactions. This is because inhibition of prostaglandin synthesis, which accounts for all the therapeutic effects, also causes renal and gastrointestinal (GI) toxicity (Figure 55-1).

Mechanism of action: inhibition of prostaglandin synthesis

Although aspirin was first introduced into clinical medicine in 1899, it was not until 1971 that Sir John Vane and his associates identified that the anti-inflammatory action of aspirin and indomethacin (introduced in 1965) was related to the inhibition of the enzyme cyclo-oxygenase (COX). COX catalyses the oxygenation of arachidonic acid, which is a 20-carbon fatty acid esterified to phospholipids of cell membranes. Arachidonic acid is released from the cell membrane by a

variety of physical, chemical and hormonal stimuli through the action of acylhydrolases, principally phospholipase A_2. Once released, arachidonic acid is metabolised principally to prostaglandins (PGs) and leukotrienes (LTs) (Figure 51-1). At the time, this single enzyme was thought to be responsible for the synthesis of all the prostaglandins, which fall into several main classes, designated by letters and distinguished by substitutions on the cyclopentane ring (e.g. PGE_1, PGE_2, PGI_2) (Figure 55-1).

It had been recognised in 1967 that the formation of cytoprotective prostaglandins by the stomach and the intestine was necessary to maintain the integrity of the GI mucosa. With the discovery that NSAIDs inhibited PG synthesis, the link between the common occurrence of gastric ulcers with NSAID use was established. With the knowledge of a relationship between COX inhibition and GI toxicity, the following decades (1970s–1990s) saw the development of drugs intended specifically to have fewer GI and renal adverse effects. Unfortunately, the newer NSAIDs were not an advance in terms of toxicity, and the increasing popularity of these drugs was paralleled by increasing incidences of adverse reactions. Risks of serious GI tract reactions were shown to be very high with indomethacin; high with piroxicam, naproxen and most others, including aspirin; and lower with ibuprofen.

By 1990, a second COX enzyme (COX-2) had been identified. It was soon established that COX-1 (the original enzyme identified) is expressed in most tissues and in particular catalyses the synthesis of protective mucosal prostaglandins in the GI tract, while COX-2 is expressed in synovial cells and macrophages and is induced by inflammation. As the older NSAIDs (e.g. the -profens) inhibit both COX-1 and COX-2, it was thought that inhibition of COX-2 accounted for the anti-inflammatory actions of NSAIDs, whereas inhibition of COX-1 explained the GI toxicity. This led to the search for drugs that would inhibit selectively COX-2. Celecoxib was the first COX-2 selective drug (-coxib) released (in 1998), and was followed soon after by rofecoxib, which was marketed in 1999. Clinical trials of celecoxib and rofecoxib showed they have some advantages over the older, non-selective NSAIDs in terms of gastrointestinal tolerability. This (and an intense marketing campaign) led to an unexpectedly high use of COX-2 inhibitors when they were made readily available in

TABLE 55–1 The main chemical classes of NSAIDs

ACETIC ACIDS	FENAMATES	PROPIONIC ACIDS	OXICAMS	SALICYLATES	COXIBS
Diclofenac	Mefenamic acid	Ibuprofen	Meloxicam	Aspirin	Celecoxib
Indomethacin		Ketoprofen	Piroxicam		Parecoxib
Ketorolac		Naproxen			
Sulindac		Tiaprofenic acid			

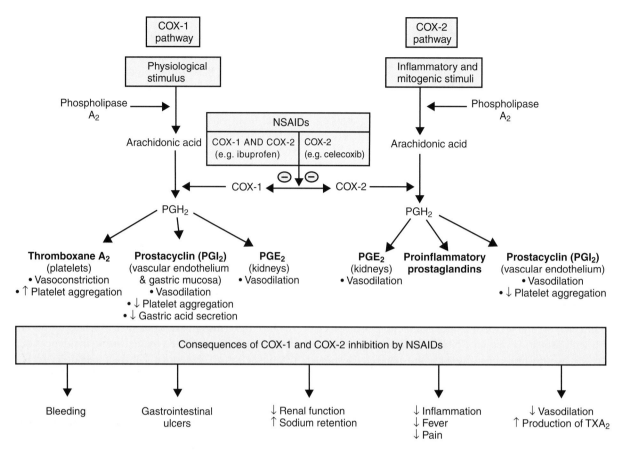

FIGURE 55-1 Simplified diagram of sites of action of NSAIDs and synthesis of thromboxane A_2, prostacyclin, prostaglandin E_2 (PGE_2) and proinflammatory prostaglandins from arachidonic acid, which is released from phospholipid membranes by the action of phospholipase A_2. The cyclo-oxygenase isoforms (COX-1 and COX-2) then catalyse the metabolism of arachidonic acid to prostaglandin H_2. Subsequent metabolism to the eicosanoids (e.g. thromboxane, and prostaglandins) differs in different cells. ⊖ = inhibition.

2001 in Australia. With the exception of the coxibs, which inhibit COX-2, and meloxicam, which inhibits COX-2 at normal doses and at higher doses also COX-1, all of the other NSAIDs in current clinical use inhibit both COX-1 and COX-2.

In general, by interfering with prostaglandin synthesis, NSAIDs tend to reduce the inflammatory process and ultimately provide pain relief. Hence NSAIDs are indicated for the treatment of acute or chronic rheumatoid arthritis, osteoarthritis, ankylosing spondylitis and other rheumatic diseases; mild to moderate pain, especially when the anti-inflammatory effect is also desirable (e.g. after dental procedures, obstetric and orthopaedic surgery, and soft-tissue athletic injuries); gout; fever; non-rheumatic inflammation; and dysmenorrhoea. The choice between the various drugs in the group comes down to a clinical decision based on pharmacokinetic properties (especially short versus long half-life) and pharmacodynamic properties. Table 55-2 lists most of the commonly used NSAIDs, grouped together under chemical class where possible, and shows important properties. Some of the newer' NSAIDs are available over

the counter, as are aspirin and paracetamol. The differences between the prescription and OTC NSAIDs are usually in the strengths of the products and the indications for which they are recommended. Prescription strengths of naproxen (base), for example, for treatment of inflammatory pain are 250 mg and 500 mg tablets and controlled-release tablets of 750 mg and 1000 mg. In contrast, the OTC product specifically for dysmenorrhoea is marketed as 275 mg tablets.

Pharmacokinetics

For specific NSAID pharmacokinetics, usual adult dose and comments, see Table 55-2. Oral absorption of these drugs is very good. Food may delay absorption but it has not been proven to significantly change the total amount of drug absorbed. Protein binding is high (greater than 90%). Most of these drugs are metabolised to varying degrees by the liver and excreted by the kidneys. Sulindac is an inactive substance (prodrug) that is converted by the liver to an active sulfide metabolite. Similarly, parecoxib is converted to the active metabolite valdecoxib.

TABLE 55-2 Pharmacokinetics and dosing of NSAIDs

NSAID	HALF-LIFE (H)	USUAL ADULT ORAL DOSE (MG/DAY)	DOSES/ DAY	COMMENTS
Acetic acids				
Diclofenac	1.2–2	75–150 (max. 200)*	2–3	Used to treat arthritis, pain, primary dysmenorrhoea, and acute gout attacks
Indomethacin	4.5–6	50–200	2–4	Higher risk for GI effects and renal function impairment than other agents. Used for acute gout attacks
Ketorolac	4–6	10 (max 40)	4–6	Should not be given by any route for longer than 5 days. Risks of GI bleeding and other severe effects increase with duration of treatment. Do not give preoperatively or intraoperatively if bleeding control is necessary. Severe allergic reactions or anaphylaxis may occur with first dose
Sulindac	7 (16#)	200–400	1–2	Renal calculi containing sulindac metabolites have been reported, although it is less likely than most NSAIDs to cause renal toxicity
Coxibs				
Celecoxib	4–15	100 (max. 200)	1–2	Ulcer-related complications can occur. Similar to conventional NSAIDs, causes adverse renal effects in some individuals
Parecoxib	3.5–4 (6.5–7#)	IM/IV route only	1	Indicated for postoperative pain in adults (single dose only)
Fenamates				
Mefenamic acid	3–4	500	3	Can prolong prothrombin time. Used for short-term treatment of pain and dysmenorrhoea; also for acute gout attacks and vascular headaches
Oxicams				
Piroxicam	30–50	10–20	1	Contraindicated in people with renal impairment. May cause flu-like syndrome. May accumulate in the elderly
Meloxicam	20	7.5–15	1	COX-2 selectivity is dose-dependent. Higher frequency of adverse GI effects with 15 mg dose
Propionic acids				
Ibuprofen	2–2.5	600–1600 (max. 2400)	34	Available in tablets, liquid and OTC. May decrease blood glucose concentration
Ketoprofen	1.5–2	100–200	2–4(1†)	Can cause fluid retention and rise in creatinine levels, especially in patients receiving diuretics and in the elderly. Monitor renal function closely
Naproxen	12–15	250–500	2 (1†)	Available as tablets and controlled-release tablets. Gluten-free formulations are available
Tiaprofenic acid	2–3	300–600	2–3	Non-bacterial cystitis has been reported. Observe for signs and discontinue drug immediately

*'max.' refers to maximum daily dose. †Controlled-release form. #Active metabolite. *Source*: AMH 2006.

Adverse reactions

Although NSAIDs are commonly used and readily available, there has been a long history of adverse reactions. Indeed, it has been said that if aspirin had not been discovered until after the thalidomide disaster in the 1960s, when controls on drug testing were tightened, it would never have been approved for marketing. NSAIDs are responsible for almost one-quarter of all adverse drug reactions officially reported in the UK, and feature worldwide in reports of drug-related deaths.

Adverse reactions of greatest concern are gastrointestinal (gastric pain, distress and/or ulceration, GI bleeding and perforation) and renal (nephrotoxicity, dysuria and haematuria). The risk of GIT effects appears to be higher with ketoprofen and piroxicam, and lower with ibuprofen and diclofenac. The beneficial effect of the latter two drugs is lost when the dose is increased. Virtually every person taking NSAIDs has some gastric damage, which may be unnoticeable or can develop into frank ulceration and haemorrhage. In attempts to lessen the risk, NSAIDs, including aspirin, have been formulated in enteric-coated forms to minimise the presence of drug in the stomach. This has been unsuccessful, however, because the effect is not only a local one but occurs also due to suppression of mucoprotective PGs by systemically absorbed NSAIDs. Treatment of NSAID-induced peptic ulcers is with misoprostol (a PG analogue) and proton pump inhibitors (see Chapter 34). The incidence of gastroduodenal ulceration appears to be lower with the COX-2-selective drugs, but ulcer healing rates may be impaired in individuals with pre-existing ulceration.

Recently, serious cardiovascular toxicity has been reported with the COX-2 inhibitors (see Clinical Interest Box 55-1). Unlike aspirin, the COX-2 inhibitors do not reduce platelet aggregation, and in many studies prothrombotic activity manifests, leading to a higher risk of myocardial infarction and stroke.

The availability of COX-2 inhibitors differs between Australia (only celecoxib and parecoxib are marketed) and New Zealand. In Australia, the Therapeutic Goods Administration (TGA) advised health professionals (doctors and pharmacists) in February 2005 that any individual taking more than 200 mg a day of celecoxib or more than 15 mg a day of meloxicam should have their drug therapy reviewed. Athough the magnitude of the cardiovascular risk and the exact duration of therapy associated with increased risk are still unknown, it was recommended that COX-2 inhibitors be prescribed only when other treatments could not be tolerated or had caused serious adverse effects. It is currently recommended that celecoxib and meloxicam not be prescribed for those individuals with increased risks of cardiovascular events, such as heart attacks. In addition, treatment should be limited to the shortest possible time, and the dose during long-term therapy of celcoxib should not exceed 200 mg daily. Similar recommendations have

---

been made by Medsafe in New Zealand (see Clinical Interest Box 55-2).

Other common adverse reactions to NSAIDs include skin reactions (rashes, urticaria), sodium retention and renal damage (due to inhibition of vasodilator PGs, particularly a problem in elderly patients on long-acting NSAIDs), and consequent heart failure and hypertension in predisposed individuals. The adverse renal effects appear to be comparable for the selective and non-selective NSAIDs. All NSAIDs, especially aspirin, can precipitate asthma attacks in sensitive persons, and some individual NSAIDs may cause specific adverse reactions, e.g. salicylates generally can cause tinnitus, impaired haemostasis and acid–base imbalances.

Use NSAIDs with caution in the elderly, in debilitated patients and in people with compromised cardiac function and/or hypertension. Avoid use in persons with a history of hypersensitivity or a severe allergic reaction to aspirin (or to other NSAIDs), asthma, severe renal or liver disease, active ulcer disease or GI bleeding.

Drug interactions with NSAIDs

In view of the widespread use of NSAIDs, both prescribed and OTC preparations, it is important to know the most common and serious drug interactions that can occur with this drug

CLINICAL INTEREST BOX 55-2 UPDATE ON COX-2 INHIBITORS IN NEW ZEALAND

Medsafe has recently concluded the updating of the data sheets for the following COX-2 inhibitors: Arcoxia (etoricoxib), Celebrex (celecoxib), Dynastat (parecoxib), Mobic (meloxicam) and Prexige (lumiracoxib). These changes were recommended by the Medicines Adverse Reactions Committee (MARC), and are intended to best manage the cardiovascular risks of the COX-2 inhibitors and to identify those select patients in whom appropriate use may be warranted.

Key points for prescribers are:
- The decision to prescribe a selective COX-2 inhibitor should only be made if non-pharmacological interventions and simple analgesic therapies have been tried and found to lack analgesic efficacy or have unacceptable adverse effects in the individual patient; and after assessment of the individual patient's overall risks.
- As the cardiovascular risks of the selective COX-2 inhibitors may increase with dose and duration of exposure, the shortest duration possible and the lowest effective daily dose should be used.
- Patients on long-term treatment should be reviewed regularly, such as every 3 months, with regard to efficacy, risk factors and ongoing need for treatment.
- Use in the perioperative period is contraindicated in patients undergoing cardiac or major vascular surgery; and contraindicated in patients who have previously had a myocardial infarction or stroke.
- A patient with significant risk factors for cardiovascular events should be treated with a COX-2 inhibitor only after careful consideration of the patient's overall risk and the potential risks and benefits of alternative analgesic therapies.

Prescribers should inform individual patients of the possibly increased risks when prescribing COX-2 inhibitors for patients at high risk of cardiovascular adverse events.

Prescribers are additionally encouraged to continue reporting any suspect adverse reaction of clinical concern relating to the use of COX-2 inhibitors. These reports will assist Medsafe and MARC in the ongoing safety monitoring of these medicines.

Source: Prescriber Update 2005; 26(2); available: www.medsafe.govt.nz/PUArticlesPage.htm, accessed 31 May 2006.

group. Generally speaking, NSAIDs have the potential to interact with other drugs that affect inflammatory responses, kidney or liver functions, blood pressure, blood coagulation mechanisms, acid–base balance and hearing. Important effects are detailed in the table Drug Interactions 55-1.

DRUG INTERACTIONS 55-1 NSAIDs

Drug	Possible effect and management
Antihypertensives, diuretics	Monitor blood pressure closely whenever an NSAID is used concurrently, as reduction in renal function may reduce the antihypertensive effect
Cyclosporin and other nephrotoxic drugs	Concurrent use with NSAIDs may result in higher plasma concentration of cyclosporin, resulting in an increased potential for nephrotoxicity. Concurrent use of nephrotoxic drugs and NSAIDs may also increase the risk for nephrotoxicity. Monitor closely during concurrent drug use
Lithium	NSAIDs may decrease excretion of lithium, which may result in higher plasma lithium concentration and toxicity. Monitor lithium plasma concentration and clinical symptoms
Methotrexate	Concurrent use of methotrexate with low to moderate doses of an NSAID may result in methotrexate toxicity due to reduced renal excretion of methotrexate. Avoid combination
Probenecid	May result in higher plasma concentration of the NSAIDs and increased risk of toxicity. Concurrent use with ketoprofen is not recommended. If probenecid is given with an NSAID, monitor closely, as a decrease in NSAID dosage may be indicated
Warfarin	May increase the risk of GI ulcers or haemorrhage. Monitor closely for signs of these effects. Warfarin may be displaced from protein-binding sites, resulting in a higher risk of bleeding episodes. Monitor international normalised ratio closely. Platelet inhibition may be dangerous in patients receiving anticoagulant or thrombolytic agents. Avoid concurrent drug administration if possible
Zidovudine	NSAIDs may reduce zidovudine elimination, increasing the risk of toxicity. Avoid combination or monitor for signs of toxicity, as dose reduction of zidovudine may be necessary

DISEASE-MODIFYING ANTIRHEUMATIC DRUGS (DMARDS)

Rheumatoid arthritis affects millions of people worldwide, and women are three times more likely to have the disease than men. The onset and clinical course of rheumatoid arthritis varies and the incidence increases with age. The traditional approach for many years involved the prescribing of NSAIDs as first-line therapy but this option has been superseded, and **disease-modifying antirheumatic drugs** (DMARDs) are now prescribed much earlier. Use of DMARDs has substantially improved the control of rheumatoid arthritis and the long-term quality of life of the individual. In many instances, combinations of DMARDs may be used.

DMARDs comprise a group of drugs with diverse chemical structures, and their mechanisms of action in many cases are largely unknown. The main drugs in this category are methotrexate (discussed in Chapter 49), auranofin, penicillamine, sulfasalazine, chloroquine and hydroxychloroquine. Other, newer agents include leflunomide, etanercept and infliximab.

Gold salts

Gold as a pharmaceutical agent has been in use for centuries to relieve 'the itching palm'. In more recent times, formulations in which gold is attached to sulfur (to increase solubility) have been used in the treatment of rheumatoid arthritis. Although the exact anti-inflammatory mechanism of action is unknown, these drugs appear to suppress the synovitis of the acute stage of rheumatoid disease. Proposed mechanisms of action include inhibition of sulfhydryl systems and various enzyme systems, suppression of phagocytic action of macrophages and leucocytes, and alteration of the immune response. Gold products (auranofin and aurothiomalate) are indicated for the treatment of rheumatoid arthritis; aurothiomalate is also used to treat juvenile arthritis.

The onset of action after oral administration of auranofin occurs in 3–4 months, while for parenteral aurothiomalate it is 6–8 weeks. The plasma half-life of the gold in these preparations is highly variable and may be as short as 1 week with a low dose, increasing to weeks and months with chronic therapy. In some people, gold can still be found in the liver and skin years after therapy has ceased. Auranofin is predominantly excreted in faeces, whereas aurothiomalate is mainly excreted by the kidneys, with a low percentage (10%–40%) found in faeces. These drugs are used with caution in people with inflammatory bowel disease, skin rash, diabetes or heart failure. In individuals with known gold drug hypersensitivity, blood dyscrasias, severe haematological disease, a history of bone marrow toxicity, renal or hepatic impairment, chronic skin disorders or systemic lupus erythematosus, these drugs should be avoided. Concurrent use of gold compounds with penicillamine (see below) will increase the risk of serious blood dyscrasias and/or renal toxicity.

It has long been recognised that efficacy and toxicity are positively related when it comes to the use of gold compounds. Not surprisingly, a significant number of individuals manifest adverse drug reactions, most commonly involving the skin (allergic reactions) and mucous membranes (sore, irritated tongue or gums; mouth ulcers or fungal infections). For auranofin, additional adverse drug reactions include abdominal distress or pain, gas, diarrhoea, nausea and vomiting. Those particular effects are less common with aurothiomalate, which instead may cause flushing, fainting, dizziness, palpitations and dyspnoea.

Penicillamine

Penicillamine is a chelating agent for heavy metals, such as mercury, lead, copper and iron. Knowledge of its metal-chelating properties has led to its use in Wilson's disease (characterised by an excess of copper) and heavy-metal intoxications. After chelation by penicillamine, the metals are made more soluble so that they can be readily excreted by the kidneys. The mechanism of action of penicillamine as an antirheumatic agent is unknown, although lymphocyte function is improved and levels of IgM rheumatoid factor and immune complexes located in blood and synovial fluids are reduced. The relationship of these effects to rheumatoid arthritis is unknown.

Penicillamine is indicated for the prophylaxis and treatment of Wilson's disease and for treating rheumatoid arthritis (especially for patients with moderate to severe arthritis who have not responded to other therapies), juvenile chronic arthritis and cystinuria. The onset of action in Wilson's disease is 1–3 months, and in rheumatoid arthritis 2–3 months. Penicillamine is metabolised extensively in the liver, and the metabolites are excreted in both urine and faeces.

Penicillamine may impair renal and haematological function; hence its concurrent use with gold compounds or phenylbutazone may result in serious blood dyscrasias and/or renal toxicity. Also, use in patients with renal impairment or blood dyscrasias should be avoided. Adverse reactions include anorexia, diarrhoea, loss of taste senses, nausea, vomiting, abdominal pain, allergic reactions and stomatitis. Use penicillamine with caution in people with Goodpasture's syndrome or myasthenia gravis, and avoid use in pregnancy, with the exception of patients with Wilson's disease and certain patients with cystinuria. Women receiving penicillamine should not breastfeed.

Sulfasalazine

The use of gold salts and penicillamine is limited by their toxicity, and sulfasalazine may be chosen as the first-line drug. Sulfasalazine consists of the sulfonamide antibiotic sulfapyridine linked to the anti-inflammatory salicylate mesalazine. Sulfasalazine is poorly absorbed, and in the colon it is split by bacteria into sulfapyridine and mesalazine, which is the active component. This drug is indicated for treating rheumatoid arthritis and is also used in treating inflammatory bowel disorders (see Chapter 34).

Most adverse reactions are dose-dependent and related to the drug being a sulfonamide. Common adverse reactions include nausea, anorexia, rashes, tinnitus, dizziness and headache. Of a more serious nature are the haematological effects, which include haemolytic anaemia, agranulocytosis and thrombocytopenia. Sulfasalazine is contraindicated in people with haematological disorders or with a known sensitivity to sulfonamide derivatives. Close monitoring is required in patients with renal or hepatic impairment.

Chloroquine and hydroxychloroquine

The quinoline drugs, which include chloroquine and hydroxychloroquine, were originally developed as antimalarial drugs during World War II. Although primarily used as antimalarials (see Chapter 53), these drugs also possess anti-inflammatory activity and are used for the treatment of mild rheumatoid arthritis. The mechanism of action is not well understood but chloroquine inhibits the action of phospholipase A_2 and thus decreases the formation of inflammatory mediators (see Figure 55-1). The onset of action is delayed; it takes several weeks to a month or more before a reduction in joint swelling is observed. The quinolines are considered to be less effective than other DMARDs but are better tolerated, with a lower incidence of toxicity.

People commonly experience nausea, diarrhoea, abdominal cramps and anorexia. Hydroxychloroquine has a lower incidence of ocular toxicity (retinopathy) than chloroquine (these drugs are contraindicated in patients with retinopathy) but both drugs can cause severe haematological reactions, including agranulocytosis, aplastic anaemia and thrombocytopenia. In people with haematological disorders the quinolines may cause further myelosuppression and exacerbate porphyria. The quinolones may exacerbate the symptoms of myasthenia gravis and psoriasis, and are not used in pregnant women (ADEC Category D) because of the risk of neurological disturbances in the fetus.

Newer DMARDs
Leflunomide

Leflunomide is an oral DMARD that inhibits pyrimidine synthesis, thus limiting the available pool of pyrimidine precursors needed for proliferation of cells, including T cells in the inflammatory response (Figure 55-2). It is highly protein-bound and undergoes continuous enterohepatic recirculation. In the liver, leflunomide is converted (95%) to the primary active metabolite, called A77 1726. This metabolite is excreted slowly in urine (about 30%) and faeces (about 70%) and has a long half-life of 2–3 weeks. As the active metabolite undergoes extensive enterohepatic recirculation, it may take up to 2 years for the drug concentration to decrease to an undectable level in plasma.

Common adverse reactions with this drug include diarrhoea, nausea, rashes and alopecia. Serious reactions such as pancytopenia and skin reactions of the toxic epidermal necrolysis type have been reported. Collection of long-term safety data for leflunomide is continuing.

Etanercept

Etanercept is a bioengineered fusion protein comprising two tumour necrosis factor (TNF) receptors coupled with a portion of human IgG, which binds to TNF and blocks its activity (Figure 55-2). Tumour necrosis factor is a cytokine that plays an important role in normal inflammatory and immune responses. It is also a proinflammatory mediator that plays a complex role in rheumatoid arthritis.

Etanercept has been shown to be effective when used as monotherapy in rheumatoid arthritis but has the disadvantage that it is administered subcutaneously twice a week. It is absorbed slowly, and peak plasma concentrations occur at approximately 50 hours; the half-life is in the order of 4–5 days. It is administered as 25 mg twice a week, but there is some evidence that 50 mg SC once a week may be as effective. In view of suppression of the activity of TNF, oral vaccines (e.g. polio vaccine) should not be administered to people receiving etanercept, and medical advice should be sought if a person is exposed to chickenpox or shingles during therapy. Contraindications to its use include hypersensitivity to etanercept, and sepsis. Adverse reactions have included fatal pancytopenia and aplastic anaemia. As with leflunomide, long-term safety data are not available.

Infliximab and adalimumab

Infliximab is an antibody against TNF-α and comprises the antigen-binding region of the mouse antibody and the constant region of human IgG_1 (Figure 55-2). It binds to soluble and membrane-bound TNF-α, preventing TNF-α from binding to its receptor and hence initiating inflammatory cell actions in chronic conditions such as rheumatoid arthritis. In addition to rheumatoid arthritis, infliximab is indicated for the treatment of Crohn's disease and ankylosing spondylitis. Like etanercept, infliximab should be used with great caution as it may reactivate latent tuberculosis, worsen heart failure,

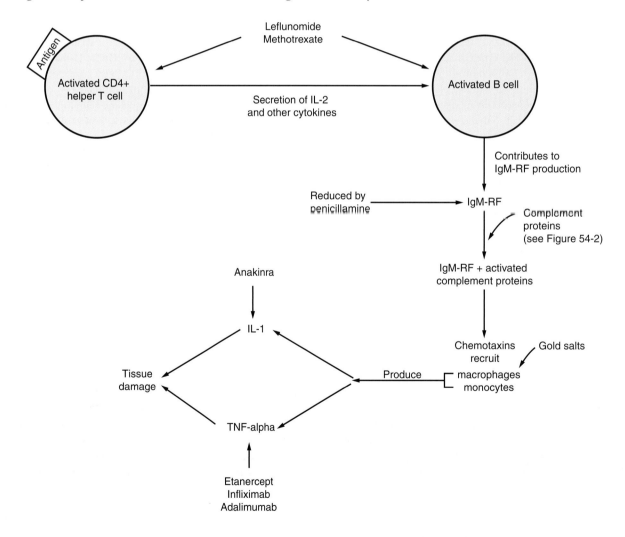

FIGURE 55-2 Likely sites of action of DMARDs. It is probable that for some DMARDs there are multiple sites of action within the inflammatory cascade. RF = rheumatoid factor.

exacerbate or induce a lupus-like syndrome and worsen multiple sclerosis. It is administered IV at a dose of 3–5 mg/kg, repeated every 2–6 weeks and then at 6–8-week intervals. Common adverse reactions include but are not limited to abdominal pain, cough, dizziness, headache, itching, fatigue and nausea.

Adalimumab, a relatively new drug, is a recombinant human monoclonal antibody that, like infliximab, binds to TNF-α, preventing its actions. Contraindications for use are similar to those of etanercept and infliximab. It is administered SC (40 mg) once every 2 weeks. In view of the predisposition to infection with this drug, signs of infection such as persistent fever should be reported immediately to the treating health professional.

Anakinra

Multiple mediators are involved in inflammatory processes, and one such mediator is interleukin-1 (IL-1). IL-1 is produced in a variety of cells, including monocytes, macrophages and specialised cells in the synovial lining of joints. It is a proinflammatory cytokine, and suppression of its activity by antagonists that bind to the IL-1 receptor tend to reduce the inflammatory response.

Anakinra is a recombinant form of the endogenous IL-1 receptor antagonist, and because of its relatively short half-life (6 hours), it is administered daily by the SC route. Contraindications, adverse reactions and predisposition to infection are similar to those of the other cytokine blockers. As there are no data, the use of anakinra should be avoided in pregnancy.

DRUGS USED FOR THE TREATMENT OF GOUT

Gout is a disease associated with a genetically determined error of uric acid metabolism that increases its production. The hallmark of gout is **hyperuricaemia**, or high concentration of uric acid in the blood. It predominantly affects men in Australasian society, and the onset of gout is usually during middle age. In some people, hyperuricaemia may occur as a result of underexcretion by the kidneys. Recurrent gouty arthritis is painful, and uric acid crystal deposits can occur throughout the body, including the kidneys, which results in an inflammatory response.

Gout is characterised by defective purine metabolism and manifests itself by attacks of acute pain, swelling and tenderness of joints, such as those of the big toe, ankle, instep, knee and elbow. The amount of uric acid in the blood becomes elevated and tophi (deposits of uric acid or urates) form in the cartilage of various parts of the body. These deposits tend to grow in size. Chronic arthritis, nephritis, and

premature sclerosis of blood vessels may develop if gout is uncontrolled.

Before treatment, causes of hyperuricaemia should be excluded. These include secondary hyperuricaemia as a result of increased cell breakdown in neoplastic diseases or cancer, psoriasis, Paget's disease or renal disease. Lifestyle factors that may also cause hyperuricaemia include obesity, hypertension, excess alcohol consumption and lead exposure. Many drugs have also been reported to increase uric acid levels, including cancer chemotherapeutic drugs and thiazide diuretics. Asymptomatic hyperuricaemia in an elderly person may or may not be drug-induced and often is not treated because of potential adverse drug reactions.

Treatment goals for gout include:
- ending an acute gout attack as soon as possible
- preventing a recurrence of acute gouty arthritis
- preventing the formation of uric acid stones in the kidneys
- reducing or preventing disease complications that result from sodium urate deposits in joints and kidneys.

Management strategies include the initial use of specific drugs for the acute attack, lifestyle modifications, and drugs for preventing recurrent gout. Drugs used to treat an acute gout attack include NSAIDs, intra-articular corticosteroids and, when indicated, colchicine. NSAIDs are primarily used to treat the acute inflammation and associated pain (all appear to be equally effective) but they have no effect on the underlying metabolic problem. They are often prescribed to relieve an acute gout attack, while colchicine, because of its potentially toxic effects, is reserved for people who are not responsive to these agents or those who cannot tolerate them.

To treat chronic gouty arthritis or to prevent recurrent gout attacks, **allopurinol** (Drug Monograph 55-1) and **probenecid** are used (Figure 55-3).

Colchicine

Colchicine is a plant alkaloid from the autumn crocus (*Colchicum autumnale*) and was introduced for the treatment of gout in 1763. It is remarkably effective during an acute attack but is of little benefit when used as prophylactic drug. The mechanism of action of colchicine in gout is unknown, although it is reported to have anti-inflammatory effects. It also decreases the release of a glycoprotein produced during phagocytosis of urate crystals. Additional actions include blocking the release of chemotactic factors and inflammatory mediators (Figure 55-3). These actions result in a decrease in urate deposits and inflammation, even though the drug does not affect uric acid production or excretion. Colchicine is used in low doses for the treatment of acute gout when NSAIDs or corticosteroids are inappropriate (see Clinical Interest Box 55-4).

Colchicine is rapidly but poorly absorbed after oral administration, and concentrates in white blood cells. In

DRUG MONOGRAPH 55-1 ALLOPURINOL

Allopurinol decreases the production of uric acid by inhibiting xanthine oxidase, the enzyme necessary to convert hypoxanthine to xanthine, and xanthine to uric acid (Figure 55-3). It also increases the reuse of both hypoxanthine and xanthine for nucleic acid synthesis, thus resulting in a feedback inhibition of purine synthesis. The result is a decrease in uric acid concentration in both the plasma and urine.

This decrease will prevent or decrease urate deposits, preventing or reducing both gouty arthritis and urate nephropathy. The reduction in urinary urate concentration prevents the formation of uric acid or calcium oxalate calculi in the kidneys.

INDICATIONS About one million prescriptions are written in Australia each year for allopurinol. This drug is indicated for treating chronic gout, urate nephrolithiasis and acute uric acid nephropathy. It is also used for treating hyperuricaemia (due to high levels of cell breakdown) secondary to disease, chemotherapy and radiotherapy.

PHARMACOKINETICS Allopurinol is well absorbed orally and about 70% of a dose is metabolised in the liver to an active metabolite, oxypurinol. The onset of action in reducing plasma uric acid concentration is 2–3 days, and a fall in uric acid concentration to within the normal range occurs in 1–3 weeks. In contrast, a decrease in frequency of acute gout attacks may require several months of drug therapy. Excretion is via the kidneys.

WARNINGS AND CONTRAINDICATIONS Avoid use in people with renal disease, as accumulation of the active metabolite (oxypurinol) may cause toxicity. Dosage reduction may be necessary in persons with hepatic or renal impairment. Avoid use in individuals with known allopurinol hypersensitivity.

DRUG INTERACTIONS The following effects may occur when allopurinol is given with the drugs listed:

Drug	Possible effect and management
Azathioprine or mercaptopurine	Inhibition of xanthine oxidase by allopurinol decreases metabolism of these drugs, leading to an increased risk of severe bone marrow toxicity. The dose of azathioprine or mercaptopurine should be reduced by 75%
Warfarin	Allopurinol may inhibit the metabolism of warfarin, resulting in an enhanced anticoagulant effect. Monitor international normalised ratio, as dosage adjustment may be necessary

ADVERSE REACTIONS These include pruritus, allergic reaction, rash, hives, diarrhoea, abdominal distress, vomiting, alopecia, dermatitis and, rarely, bone marrow depression, liver toxicity, a hypersensitivity reaction, peripheral neuritis, renal failure and nosebleeds.

DOSAGE AND ADMINISTRATION The adult dose is 100 mg daily initially, increased by 100 mg/day at monthly intervals if necessary. The maintenance dosage is 100–300 mg daily. For treatment of hyperuricaemia (from antineoplastic therapy), initially administer 600–800 mg orally daily beginning 2–3 days before chemotherapy or radiation therapy. For maintenance therapy, adjust the dose according to plasma uric acid concentration, which is analysed about 2 days after the initiation of allopurinol and periodically thereafter.

Patients should also be advised to increase their fluid intake, if not contraindicated, to 2.5–3 L/day, to reduce their risk of forming kidney stones. In addition, a neutral or slightly alkaline urine is recommended, which can be accomplished by dietary means such as by consuming milk, fruits (except plums, prunes and cranberries) and vegetables (except for corn and lentils), and other dietary alterations as recommended.

acute gouty arthritis, it has an onset of action within 18 hours of oral administration. The peak effect for relief of pain and inflammation is reached in 1–2 days but reduced swelling may require 3 days or more. Colchicine is partly metabolised in the liver, and undergoes extensive enterohepatic recirculation, with most of the inactive metabolites eliminated in the faeces. Only 10%–20% of unchanged drug is excreted in urine. As colchicine raises plasma cyclosporin concentration, monitoring is recommended; reduction of cyclosporin dosage may be necessary.

Common adverse reactions to colchicine include diarrhoea, nausea, vomiting, abdominal pain, anorexia and,

with chronic therapy, alopecia. Rare adverse reactions include hypersensitivity reactions, blood dyscrasias, neuropathy, myopathy and bone marrow suppression. Due to the inherent toxicity of colchine, it is used with caution in people with moderate to severe liver and kidney impairment and GI disorders, and avoided in individuals with known colchicine hypersensitivity, a history of blood dyscrasias and pregnancy.

Probenecid

Probenecid is indicated for treating hyperuricaemia and chronic gouty arthritis, and as an adjunct to antibiotic

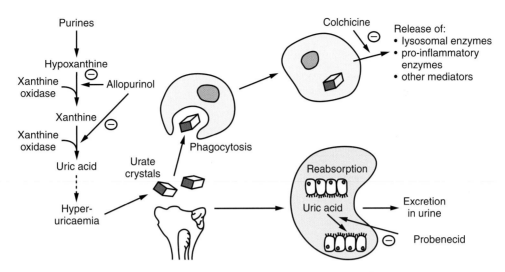

FIGURE 55-3 Uric acid production and the sites of action of drugs used for the treatment of hyperuricaemia. ⊖ = inhibition. (Reproduced with kind permission of Karen Lillywhite, Computer Assisted Learning Unit, School of Medicine, Flinders University, Adelaide, Australia.)

CLINICAL INTEREST BOX 55-4
COLCHICINE: LOWER DOSES FOR GREATER SAFETY

Coinciding with the marketing of a 0.5 mg strength tablet (Colgout), the dosage advice for colchicine in New Zealand has been revised. Colchicine is now indicated as second-line therapy for acute gout where treatment with an NSAID is either contraindicated, or has been found to lack analgesic efficacy, or has resulted in unacceptable adverse reactions. For healthy adults, the dosing interval has been increased from 2–3-hourly to 6-hourly, with a maximum dose of 2.5 mg in the first 24 hours and a maximum cumulative dose of 6 mg over 4 days. In elderly patients, patients with severe renal dysfunction (creatinine clearance <10 ml/min) or hepatic impairment, and patients weighing under 50 kg, other treatments should be considered (e.g. corticosteroids) or lower doses of colchicine used (a maximum cumulative dose of 3 mg over 4 days should be observed). Intensive dosing should not be repeated for at least 3 days in order to avoid the risk of toxicity due to colchicine accumulation. Individuals prescribed colchicine should be warned of the symptoms of colchicine toxicity, and advised to discontinue therapy immediately they occur. The revised dosage advice is consistent with the New Zealand Rheumatology Association's 2005 *Consensus Statement on the Use of Colchicine in the Treatment of Gout* (New Zealand Rheumatology Association, NZRA, November 2005, www.rheumatology.org.nz/colchicine.html).
Adapted from: Prescriber Update 2005; 26(2): www.medsafe.govt.nz, accessed 9 May 2006.

therapy. It lowers the serum concentration of uric acid by competitively inhibiting the reabsorption of urate at the proximal renal tubule, thus increasing the urinary excretion of uric acid. It has no anti-inflammatory action or analgesic effect.

Probenecid was developed during the late 1940s specifically to retard the renal elimination of penicillin, as this was expensive and in short supply during World War II. It competitively inhibits the secretion of weak organic acids, such as penicillin and some of the cephalosporins, at both the proximal and distal renal tubules. The result is an increase in blood concentration and duration of action of these antibiotics. This combination is used to treat sexually transmitted diseases (e.g. gonorrhoea, acute pelvic inflammatory disease and neurosyphilis).

Probenecid is well absorbed orally and is highly bound to plasma proteins, especially to albumin. The peak uricosuric effect is reached within 30 minutes, whereas peak suppression of penicillin excretion is noted in 2 hours and lasts nearly 8 hours. Probenecid is metabolised in the liver and excreted by the kidneys. Important interactions are detailed in the table Drug Interactions 55-2.

Adverse reactions to probenecid include headaches, anorexia, mild nausea or vomiting, sore gums, pain and/or blood on urination, lower back pain, frequent urge to urinate, renal stones, dermatitis and, rarely, anaphylaxis, anaemia, leucopenia and nephrotic syndrome. This drug should be avoided in people with probenecid hypersensitivity; in those with any conditions that may increase uric acid formation, such as a history of renal stones; in moderate to severe kidney function impairment; or in anyone undergoing treatment that may increase uric acid formation, such as cancer chemotherapy or radiation therapy. Also avoid use in persons with a history of blood disorders.

DRUG INTERACTIONS 55-2 Probenecid	
Drug	**Possible effect and management**
Aspirin or salicylates	Not recommended, because aspirin or salicylates in moderate to high doses given chronically will inhibit the effectiveness of probenecid
Cephalosporins, penicillins	Probenecid decreases the renal tubular secretion of penicillin and selected cephalosporins, which may result in higher plasma concentration and prolonged duration of action of the antibiotic
Methotrexate	Probenecid may decrease the tubular secretion of methotrexate, which may increase the risk of serious toxicity with methotrexate. Avoid combination or, if used concurrently, administer a lower dose of methotrexate and monitor closely for toxicity
NSAIDs: indomethacin, ketoprofen and naproxen	Probenecid decreases excretion of weak acids such as NSAIDs, which leads to higher plasma concentrations and increased potential for NSAID toxicity. The daily dose of NSAID may need to be adjusted
Nitrofurantoin	Probenecid may decrease the renal tubular secretion of nitrofurantoin, resulting in higher plasma concentration and possibly toxicity. This may reduce the urinary concentration and effectiveness of nitrofurantoin in urinary tract infections. Monitor effectiveness closely
Zidovudine	Concurrent drug administration may lead to inhibition of zidovudine metabolism and secretion, resulting in elevated plasma concentration and an increased risk of zidovudine toxicity. Avoid combination or monitor for adverse effects

The adult dosage is 250 mg twice daily for 7 days, and a maintenance dose of 500 mg twice a day. The dose may be adjusted if necessary every 4 weeks up to a maximum of 2 g daily in divided doses. As an adjunct to penicillin or cephalosporin drug therapy, the dose in adults is 500 mg four times daily. For infants and children, check a current drug reference for recommended dosing schedules. In addition, patients should be instructed to maintain a high fluid intake to reduce the risk of uric acid kidney stone formation.

IMMUNOSUPPRESSANT DRUGS

In Australia each year about 1000 people receive organ transplants and a range of drugs is used to prevent rejection of the transplanted kidney, liver or heart. The rejection of allogenic transplants led to the development of **immunosuppressant drugs**, or agents that decrease or prevent an immune response. These agents are crucial to the success of organ transplantation. A foreign substance or organ transplant in the body activates an immune response by the release of macrophages to phagocytose and process the foreign substance. In addition, interleukin-1 (IL-1) production increases, which activates helper T lymphocytes that have a surface CD3 receptor. The activated T cells stimulate production of killer, or cytotoxic, T lymphocytes, and B lymphocytes, in part by producing interleukin-2 (IL-2).

T cells are necessary for cellular immunity, while B cells are responsible for humoral immunity (production of antibodies). The primary sites of action of the immunosuppressant drugs are illustrated in Figure 55-4.

Immunodeficiency or immunosuppression may also occur from a genetic or an acquired disorder of the immune system. Acquired immune deficiency may be induced by a variety of drugs such as chemotherapeutic and immunosuppressant agents, by radiation therapy or through viral infection. Because AIDS often has devastating complications and a fatal outcome, much research interest has been directed towards developing immunomodulating or immunostimulating medications. There are four main classes of **immunosuppressant drugs**:
1. corticosteroids (discussed in Chapter 40)
2. calcineurin inhibitors: cyclosporin and tacrolimus
3. cytotoxic immunosuppressants: azathioprine, methotrexate, cyclophosphamide and 6-mercaptopurine (discussed in Chapter 49)
4. immunosuppressant antibodies: antithymocyte globulins, basiliximab, daclizumab and muromonab-CD3.

Other immunosuppressant drugs include everolimus, sirolimus and mycophenolate.

Calcineurin inhibitors

Complete T-cell activation involves translocation of the nuclear factor of activated T cells (NFAT) to the nucleus, where transactivation of genes that control synthesis of cytokines such as IL-2 occurs. IL-2 stimulates T-cell proliferation and generation of cytotoxic T lymphocytes. Calcineurin is

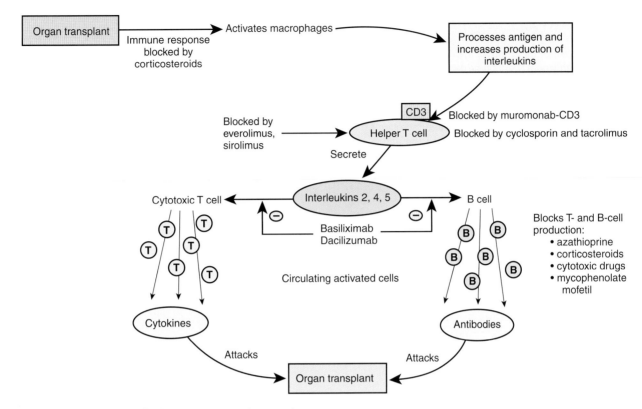

FIGURE 55-4 Sites of action for immunosuppressive agents.

the enzyme that removes phosphate groups from NFAT, which then allows its nuclear translocation. If calcineurin is inhibited, NFAT does not enter the nucleus, gene transcription does not proceed, and the T lymphocyte does not respond to specific antigenic stimulation. The two calcineurin inhibitors in clinical use are cyclosporin and tacrolimus.

Cyclosporin

See Drug Monograph 55-2 for the pharmacology of cyclosporin.

Tacrolimus

Tacrolimus, in conjunction with corticosteroids, is indicated for the prophylaxis of organ (liver and kidney) rejection. It inhibits activation of T lymphocytes and is believed to bind to cyclophilin or FKBP-12 protein, forming a complex with calcineurin that prevents T-cell activation.

Oral and parenteral formulations of tacrolimus are available. Oral absorption is variable, blood concentrations are reached in 0.5–4 hours and the elimination half-life is 11–40 hours. Tacrolimus is metabolised in the liver (primarily by cytochrome P450 3A) to a range of metabolites, including several active ones. Less than 1% is excreted in the urine. In view of its metabolism by CYP3A4, plasma

tacrolimus concentration may be reduced by inducers and increased by inhibitors of the enzyme. Drug interactions with tacrolimus have not been so fully investigated but are similar to those of cyclosporin. The absorption of tacrolimus is reduced by aluminium hydroxide gel, resulting in decreased bioavailability. Administration of the aluminium gel should be avoided for at least 3 hours either side of dosing with tacrolimus.

Adverse reactions are numerous and commonly dose-related. They include opportunistic infections, blood disorders, diabetes, GI distress, anorexia, hyperglycaemia, hyperkalaemia, hypomagnesaemia, nephrotoxicity, neurotoxicity, headaches, insomnia, tremors, convulsions, paraesthesia, pleural effusion, peripheral oedema, pruritus, rash, cardiac disorders (e.g. cardiomyopathy and hypertension), neuropathy, muscle cramps, sweating, tinnitus, blurred vision and, rarely, anaphylaxis and hepatotoxicity.

In view of the range of adverse reactions, tacrolimus is used with caution in patients with diabetes mellitus, liver or neurological dysfunction, hepatitis B or C infection, or hyperkalaemia. Its use is avoided in people with hypersensitivity to tacrolimus or polyoxyl 60 hydrogenated castor oil (the solubiliser in the IV preparation), current cancer, chickenpox, herpes zoster, infection, or kidney function impairment. The last is particularly important, as tacrolimus may cause permanent renal damage.

DRUG MONOGRAPH 55-2 CYCLOSPORIN

Cyclosporin is a potent immunosuppressant drug used to prevent organ (renal, hepatic or cardiac allograft) transplant rejection and to induce or maintain remission in people with immune or inflammatory disorders. It is usually administered in combination with corticosteroids. Both calcineurin inhibitors (cyclosporin and tacrolimus) form a complex with cyclophilin that blocks the action of calcineurin in activated T cells. This prevents cytokine production and subsequent cell proliferation and differentiation. Calcineurin inhibitors do not cause significant myelosuppression or bone marrow depression.

PHARMACOKINETICS Cyclosporin is available in oral and parenteral dosage forms. After oral administration, its bioavailability is variable (about 30%), and may improve with increasing doses and chronic administration. Absorption may decrease after a liver transplant or in patients with liver impairment or GI dysfunction, such as diarrhoea or vomiting. It has a half-life of about 7 hours in children and 19 hours in adults; orally, it reaches peak plasma concentration in 3.5 hours. Cyclosporin is extensively metabolised (99.9%) in the liver by the cytochrome P450 3A enzyme and is subject to many drug interactions. The metabolites are eliminated principally via the faeces, with approximately 6% excreted in urine.

ADVERSE REACTIONS These are dose-related and include hirsutism, tremors, acne or oily skin, headache, leg cramps, nausea, vomiting, gingival hyperplasia (swollen, bleeding gums), seizures, nephrotoxicity, hepatotoxicity, severe hypertension and, rarely, anaphylaxis, haemolytic–uraemic syndrome, hyperkalaemia and pancreatitis. The incidence of lymphomas, skin malignancies and other lymphoproliferative-type disorders increases as the extent and duration of immunosuppression increases. Gingival hyperplasia, a common problem with the use of this drug, is generally reversible about 6 months after cyclosporin is discontinued.

DRUG INTERACTIONS Therapeutic drug monitoring plays a major role in preventing both cyclosporin toxicity and subtherapeutic dosing, both of which can be potentially catastrophic situations. The effect on the plasma cyclosporin concentration of adding, removing or changing any drug should be monitored. Multiple drug interactions have been described and the effects in the following table may occur when cyclosporin is given with the drugs listed:

Drug	Possible effect and management
Cimetidine, danazol, calcium channel blockers (e.g. diltiazem), macrolide antibiotics (e.g. erythromycin), azole antifungals (e.g. ketoconazole or fluconazole)	May result in higher plasma concentration of cyclosporin due to decreased hepatic metabolism, increasing the potential risk for hepatotoxicity and nephrotoxicity. If drugs must be administered concurrently, use extreme caution and monitor closely. (Note: Diltiazem is commonly used with cyclosporin to reduce the dose of cyclosporin required.)
Diuretics (potassium-sparing [amiloride, spironolactone, triamterene]), potassium supplements, ACE inhibitors	May increase the risk of hyperkalaemia. Use with caution and monitor plasma concentrations and signs and symptoms of hyperkalaemia
Grapefruit juice	Inhibits prehepatic metabolism of cyclosporin by CYP3A in the GI tract, leading to increased bioavailability. Grapefruit juice should be avoided
HMG-CoA reductase inhibitors, e.g. simvastatin	May increase the risk of developing rhabdomyolysis and acute renal failure. Monitor closely if concurrent therapy is necessary
Nephrotoxic drugs, e.g. NSAIDs, aminoglycosides	Risk of additive renal toxicity. Avoid combinations
St John's wort (Hypericum perforatum)	Induces metabolism of cyclosporin, leading to lower cyclosporin drug concentration. Avoid combination

WARNINGS AND CONTRAINDICATIONS Use with caution in people with renal impairment or recent surgery. Avoid use in patients with cyclosporin hypersensitivity, recent chickenpox, herpes zoster or measles infections, and in severe liver or kidney function impairment.

DOSAGE AND ADMINISTRATION Regimens may vary in different transplant centres. The adult oral dosage is 8–15 mg/kg daily as two doses. Children may require a higher dose per kg, as they metabolise this drug rapidly. The IV dose is one-third of the oral dose.

Cytotoxic immunosuppressant drugs

The cytotoxic immunosuppressant drugs include azathioprine, and methotrexate, cyclophosphamide and 6-mercaptopurine; the last three are discussed in Chapter 49.

Azathioprine

Azathioprine is indicated as an adjunct medication to prevent rejection in renal organ transplant recipients, and for severe active rheumatoid arthritis in patients who have not responded to other therapies. The mechanism of action involves alterations in purine synthesis that primarily suppress

T- and B-cell production, cell-mediated hypersensitivity and antibody production. In combination with steroids, azathioprine appears to have a steroid-conserving effect, and a lower dose of steroid may be used to treat chronic inflammatory processes when given with azathioprine.

Azathioprine is available in oral and parenteral dosage forms. When given orally, it is well absorbed from the intestinal tract. It has a half-life of 5 hours, with an onset of action of 6–8 weeks in rheumatoid arthritis and perhaps 4–8 weeks in other inflammatory disease states. It is metabolised in the liver to active metabolites (6-mercaptopurine and 6-thioinosinic acid), with further metabolism by xanthine oxidase. It is primarily excreted via the biliary system.

A number of significant effects are detailed in the table Drug Interactions 55-3.

DRUG INTERACTIONS 55-3 Azathioprine	
Drug	**Possible effect and management**
Allopurinol	Allopurinol inhibits xanthine oxidase, which results in higher concentration of 6-mercaptopurine and potential bone marrow toxicity. Avoid, or a potentially serious drug interaction may occur. If it is absolutely necessary to give both drugs concurrently, reduce the dose of azathioprine to 1/4 to 1/3 the usually prescribed dose; monitor closely and adjust dosage as needed
Other immunosuppressant agents (glucocorticoids, cyclophosphamide, cyclosporin)	May increase the risk of developing infections and/or neoplasms. Avoid, or a potentially serious drug interaction may occur
Vaccines, live virus	Immunisation with live vaccines should be postponed in people receiving azathioprine, and in close family members. The use of a live virus vaccine in immunosuppressed patients may result in increased replication of the vaccine virus, may increase adverse reactions to the vaccine virus, and may cause a decrease in antibody response to the vaccine. Avoid, or a potentially serious drug interaction may occur

Adverse reactions are often observed and include anorexia, nausea, vomiting, leucopenia or infection, megaloblastic anaemia (the patient may be asymptomatic but may also have fever, chills, cough, low-back or side pain, pain on urination, or increased weakness), hepatitis (infrequent), thrombocytopenia, hypersensitivity, pancreatitis, pneumonitis, sores in the mouth and on the lips, and skin rash. The risk of hepatotoxicity is greater when the dosage of azathioprine exceeds 2.5 mg/kg daily.

Due to its immunosuppressant actions, azathioprine is used with caution in patients with pancreatitis or hepatic, renal or bone marrow impairment. It is also contraindicated in people with neoplastic disorders, uncontrolled infection or recent exposure to varicella virus infections.

Immunosuppressant antibodies

Antibodies directed against cell-surface antigens on T lymphocytes have been in clinical practice for decades and are widely used for preventing organ transplant rejection. Currently available immunosuppressant antibodies include antithymocyte globulins, basiliximab, daclizumab and muromonab-CD3.

Antithymocyte globulins

The available polyclonal antithymocyte globulins include a horse antibody directed against human thymocyte cell surface markers, and a rabbit antibody raised against human T lymphoblast cell surface markers. Both of these antibodies bind to cell-surface receptors (e.g. CD2–CD4 antigens, HLA class I and II molecules) on the surface of human T lymphocytes. Once bound, these antibodies are cytotoxic and hence deplete the number of circulating lymphocytes and block lymphocyte function. Both products (horse and rabbit) contain small concentrations of antibodies that will cross-react with other blood components, and are thus not interchangeable. It is usual to perform a skin test for allergy before administration, so these globulins are contraindicted in people who manifest an allergic response to the test dose.

Antithymocyte globulins are used for the prevention and treatment of organ (kidney, heart, lung and liver) transplant rejection. They are administered IV (infusion) and the dosage is calculated on a per-kg basis. Common adverse reactions include fever, chills, dyspnoea, chest pain, hypotension, diarrhoea, nausea and vomiting, and a variety of haematological complications (e.g. leucopenia and thrombocytopenia), which are all related to a cytokine release syndrome. As many people develop anti-antibodies (e.g. anti-rabbit antibodies), this limits the possibility of repeated doses. As would be expected with chronic immunosuppression, these antithymocyte globulins are associated with the development of lymphoproliferative disorders.

Basiliximab and daclizumab

Basiliximab and daclizumab are both purified monoclonal antibody immunosuppressants that are used in combination with cyclosporin and corticosteroids to prevent acute rejection of transplanted kidneys. These drugs are interleukin-2 (IL-2)-receptor antagonists, binding to the IL-2 receptor complex, and thus inhibiting IL-2 binding. This inhibition results in a decreased activation of lymphocytes and an impaired immune system response to antigens. Both drugs are administered parenterally; daclizumab has an elimination half-life of 11–38 days, while that of basiliximab is approximately 7–10 days.

Unlike the antithymocyte globulins, which produce a number of adverse reactions related to a cytokine release syndrome, basiliximab and daclizumab appear to be relatively free of adverse reactions other than those that would be expected to be observed in transplant patients on multiple therapies. Long-term adverse effects are unknown, but currently neither drug appears to increase the incidence of opportunistic infections or lymphoproliferative disorders (compared to baseline) in immunosuppressed patients.

Pregnancy should be prevented when using either of these drugs (ADEC Category D), and contraception continued for at least 2 months in the case of basiliximab and 4 months for daclizumab after the last dose.

Muromonab-CD3

Muromonab-CD3 is a purified mouse monoclonal antibody that reacts with CD3 receptors on the surface of T lymphocytes. It blocks the activation and functions of the T cells in response to an antigenic challenge; thus it functions as an immunosuppressant and does not cause myelosuppression.

Muromonab-CD3 is indicated for the treatment of acute renal organ transplant rejection and is usually given in combination with azathioprine, cyclosporin or corticosteroids. It is also administered to treat acute rejection (steroid-resistant) in cardiac and hepatic transplant patients. Available parenterally, it acts to reduce activated T cells within minutes of administration. It reaches steady-state plasma concentration in about 3 days and has a duration of action of about 7 days. The number of circulating CD3-positive T cells returns to baseline levels within a week of discontinuation of muromonab-CD3.

The most frequent adverse reactions with muromonab-CD3 occur with the first dose. The first-dose effect (cytokine release syndrome) consists of light-headedness, elevated temperature, chills, nausea, vomiting, diarrhoea, headache, dyspnoea, chest pain, tremors and trembling. These effects may be repeated to a lesser degree after the second dose but are rarely encountered with later doses. Fever and chills that occur later may be caused by infection. Anaphylaxis, hypersensitivity, encephalopathy, convulsions, cerebral oedema and aseptic meningitis syndrome are reported less often. Concurrent use with other immunosuppressant agents may increase the risk of infection and the development of lymphoproliferative diseases. A reduced dose of corticosteroids and azathioprine is recommended when muromonab-CD3 is started. (For interactions with live viral vaccines, see azathioprine above.)

Other immunosuppressant drugs

These include sirolimus and its derivative everolimus, and mycophenolate.

Sirolimus and everolimus

Both of these drugs act by complexing with cyclophilin of FKBP-12 in the same manner as cyclosporin and tacrolimus. Unlike the cyclosporin–FKBP-12 complex, which then inhibits calcineurin, the sirolimus/everolimus–FKBP-12 complex inhibits a kinase enzyme, which is crucial to cell cycle progression and cytokine-induced B- and T-cell proliferation. Everolimus is indicated for the prevention of kidney and heart transplant rejection, while sirolimus tends to be used in cases of renal transplant rejection.

Both drugs are administered orally, and peak blood concentrations occur within 1–2 hours. A high-fat meal decreases the peak concentration of both drugs, and it is recommended that these drugs be taken at the same time each day with the same type of food or fluid. This is important, because the plasma concentrations of these drugs are routinely monitored, and dosage adjustments may be made based on the result obtained.

Everolimus and sirolimus are metabolised by CYP3A4 and are substrates for P-glycoprotein. Not surprisingly, both are subject to many drug interactions, and concomitant administration of an inhibitor of CYP3A4 will increase plasma concentration, while administration of an inducer of CYP3A4 will decrease the plasma drug concentration.

Multiple drug interactions (see Drug Interactions 55-4) may occur with either everolimus or sirolimus. In addition, due to the involvement of CYP3A4, consumption of grapefruit should be avoided, as it may increase the risk of toxicity with either of these drugs.

The use of everolimus and sirolimus is associated with a dose-dependent rise in triglycerides and cholesterol. This may warrant either a dose reduction or treatment with a statin. Limited data are available and use should be avoided in pregnancy. Contraception is recommended during treatment and for 2–3 months after the last dose.

Common adverse reactions include hypertriglyceridaemia, hypercholesterolaemia and various haematological disorders, e.g. leucopenia, neutropenia, thrombocytopenia and raised plasma creatinine (with cyclosporin).

DRUG INTERACTIONS 55-4 Everolimus/Sirolimus

Drug	Possible effect and management
Cyclosporin	Increases the plasma concentration of everolimus, and plasma monitoring of everolimus concentration is necessary when adjusting cyclosporin dose
Erythromycin	May inhibit the metabolism of both drugs, leading to increased plasma concentrations and possible toxicity. Monitor and decrease dose if necessary
Itraconazole/ketoconazole	May inhibit metabolism of both drugs, increasing plasma concentrations and risk of toxicity. Avoid combination or monitor plasma concentration of everolimus and sirolimus
Rifampicin	May increase metabolism of everolimus and sirolimus, reducing plasma drug concentration and therapeutic effect. Monitor closely if this combination is used

DRUG INTERACTIONS 55-5 Mycophenolate mofetil

Drug	Possible effect and management
Aciclovir or ganciclovir	These drugs compete with mycophenolate mofetil for renal excretion and may increase each other's toxicity. Avoid, or a potentially serious drug interaction may occur. If used concurrently, monitor closely
Antacids (magnesium and aluminium hydroxide), cholestyramine, colestipol	These drugs decrease the absorption of mycophenolate mofetil. Administer mycophenolate mofetil 1 hour before or 2 hours after antacids and bile acid sequestrants
Immunosuppressant agents, e.g. azathioprine, glucocorticoids, cyclophosphamide, cyclosporin	Enhanced immunosuppression. May increase the risk of developing infections and neoplasms

Mycophenolate

Mycophenolate mofetil and mycophenolate sodium, used in conjunction with cyclosporin and corticosteroids, are indicated for the prophylaxis of renal transplant rejection. Both drugs are metabolised to mycophenolic acid, an active metabolite that inhibits the responses of T and B lymphocytes to mitogenic and allospecific stimulation. It also suppresses antibody formation by B cells and may inhibit the influx of leucocytes into inflammatory and graft rejection sites.

Available orally, mycophenolate is rapidly metabolised to the active metabolite mycophenolic acid and an inactive metabolite, a phenolic glucuronide. The half-life of mycophenolic acid is 18 hours, with excretion primarily as the phenolic glucuronide in urine (~85%).

Potential interactions with other drugs used commonly in transplant patients have been investigated (see Drug Interactions 55-5).

Adverse reactions are dose-related and include abdominal pain, constipation or diarrhoea, nausea, vomiting, dizziness, acne, insomnia, rash, anaemia, chest pain, cough, dyspnoea, haematuria, hypertension, leucopenia, peripheral oedema, arrhythmia, arthralgia, colitis, GI bleeding, gingival hyperplasia, gingivitis, myalgia, oral moniliasis, pancreatitis, thrombocytopenia and tremors.

Mycophenolate is used with caution in patients with delayed post-transplant renal graft function, and dose reduction may be necessary. This drug should be avoided in people with mycophenolate mofetil hypersensitivity, active GI system disease or severe kidney function impairment.

IMMUNOSTIMULANT DRUGS

Advances in biotechnology have allowed the development of new agents that can either activate the body's immune defences or modify a response to an unwanted stimulus, such as an antitumour response. These agents are called biological response modifiers; when the immune system is activated, they are commonly referred to as **immunostimulants**. With the advent of recombinant deoxyribonucleic acid (DNA) technology in the early 1980s, new agents were made available in larger quantities for clinical trials and investigations. Although still in its infancy, this area of study has the potential for solving some of the mysteries about disease that have eluded researchers for centuries. Research may also provide future drugs that will control the devastation, pain and suffering induced by many viral diseases (e.g. AIDS) and cancer. Common immunostimulants include vaccines, colony-stimulating factors and the interferons. **Interferons** (alpha, beta, gamma) bind to specific cell-surface receptors that are linked through to the inner networks of the cell that control functions such as enzyme activity, cell proliferation and enhancement of immune activity.

Lymphokines (IL-1 and IL-2), interferons (primarily alpha-interferon), and granulocyte or granulocyte–macrophage colony-stimulating factors (G-CSF or GM-CSF-leukine) are under investigation as immunostimulants. Lymphokines are protein substances released by sensitised lymphocytes when in contact with specific antigens. They activate macrophages to stimulate humoral and cellular immunity for the host. Interleukins have been called the chemical messengers of immune cell communication. Interleukin-2 is believed to be a T-cell growth factor that promotes the long-term survival and growth of T lymphocytes, which is necessary for the continuation of the immune response and is also involved in the rejection of transplanted organs. Aldesleukin is a recombinant variant of IL-2 that binds to the IL-2 receptor and stimulates cell proliferation and the production of interferon gamma. Although some patients have been helped with these therapies, major problems are limited effectiveness or extreme systemic toxicity. The currently available immune stimulants are listed in Table 55-3.

HISTAMINE AND HISTAMINE-RECEPTOR ANTAGONISTS (ANTIHISTAMINES)
Distribution of histamine

Histamine is a chemical mediator that occurs naturally in almost all body tissues. It is present in highest concentration in the skin, lung and GI tract and, when liberated from cells, plays an early transient role in the inflammatory process.

In many tissues, the chief site of production and storage of histamine is the cytoplasmic granules of the mast cell or, in the case of blood, the basophil, which closely resembles the mast cell in function. Mast cells are small ovoid structures widely distributed in the loose connective tissue. They are especially abundant in small blood vessels and in bronchial smooth muscle, which appears to have the highest concentration of mast cells of any organ in the body. The mast cells and basophils make up the mast-cell histamine pool. A second major site of histamine production is known as the non-mast-cell pool, where the histamine is stored in the cells of the epidermis, GI mucosa and the CNS. Although histamine is present in various foods and is synthesised by intestinal flora, the amount absorbed does not contribute to the body's stores of this amine.

Actions

The reactions mediated by histamine are attributed to receptor activity, which involves two distinct populations of receptors, called H_1 and H_2 receptors. A third histamine receptor has been identified (H_3), but research is ongoing to define its role. The principal actions of histamine are listed in Table 55-4.

Vascular effects

In the microcirculatory component of the cardiovascular system (arterioles, capillaries, venules), the liberation of histamine has been shown to involve both the H_1 and H_2 receptors. Stimulation of these receptors dilates the capillaries and venules, producing increased localised blood flow, increased capillary permeability, erythema and oedema. By activating the H_1 and H_2 receptors on the smooth muscles of the arterioles, histamine is also capable of eliciting a systemic response, that is, vasodilation of the arterioles, which can result in a profound fall in blood pressure.

TABLE 55-3 Immunostimulants

DRUG	USE(S)	COMMON ADVERSE REACTIONS	ADEC PREGNANCY CATEGORY
Interferon alpha-2a Interferon alpha-2b	Chronic hepatitis B & C, hairy cell leukaemia, Kaposi's sarcoma, malignant melanoma (2b only), multiple myeloma (2b only), cutaneous T cell lymphoma (2a only)	Flu-like symptoms (dose-related), anaemia, anorexia, abdominal pain, alopecia, nausea, diarrhoea, weight loss, palpitations, muscle aches	B3
Interferon gamma	Reduce infections in chronic granulomatous disease	Flu-like symptoms; less commonly, nausea and vomiting	B3
Aldesleukin	Bone marrow transplant, HIV, melanoma, thymoma	Adverse reactions are dose-related and include pulmonary oedema, neurological effects (e.g. headache, confusion, ataxia), flu-like symptoms, thyroid dysfunction	C

Smooth muscle effects

Although histamine exerts a powerful relaxing effect on the smooth muscle of the arterioles, it produces a contractile action on the smooth muscles of many non-vascular organs, such as the bronchi and GI tract. In sensitised individuals, activation of the H_1 receptors of the lungs can cause marked bronchial muscle contraction that often progresses to dyspnoea and airway obstruction.

Exocrine glandular effects

While histamine stimulates the gastric, salivary, pancreatic and lacrimal glands, the main effect is seen in the gastric glands. Stimulation of H_2 receptors in the exocrine glands of the stomach increases production of gastric acid secretions. The high hydrochloric acid concentration is attributed to the activity of the parietal cells of the stomach and is implicated in the development of peptic ulcers (see Chapters 33 and 34).

Central nervous system effect

Histamine is known to be present throughout the tissues of the brain. Its effects seem to involve both H_1 and H_2 receptor mediation. The activation of H_1 receptors of the semicircular canals is associated with motion sickness.

Inflammatory effects

Histamine as a chemical mediator is implicated in many pathological disorders. Although four different types of hypersensitivity responses to immunological injury exist, the type I anaphylactic reaction is the one associated with the release of histamine.

People with type I-mediated hypersensitivity develop allergies as a result of sensitisation to a foreign agent that may be ingested, inhaled or injected. An incalculable number of these allergenic agents exist. They vary widely in that different forms of allergy can develop in response to seasonal exposure to pollens, grasses and weeds, or to non-seasonal agents such as house dust, feathers, moulds and other similar substances. Hypersensitivity to a variety of foods such as shellfish or strawberries requires ingestion of the antigen. Insects such as bees or wasps, and even drugs, particularly penicillin, also possess allergenic properties that may induce a severe response in hypersensitive individuals.

Type I anaphylactic hypersensitivity accounts for a substantial number of allergic disorders, and involves a complex series of anomalies ranging from mild urticaria to anaphylactic shock. The mechanism of type I anaphylactic reaction involves the attachment of an antigen (Ag) to an antibody (Ab), specifically immunoglobulin E (IgE), and this complex in turn becomes fixed to the mast cell. The pathological manifestations of Ag–IgE interaction are caused by mast cell degranulation, resulting in the release of histamine and other mediators responsible for producing the allergic symptoms. The type I anaphylactic reaction is responsible for various disorders, such as urticaria, atopy (allergic rhinitis and hay fever), food allergies, bronchial asthma and systemic anaphylaxis.

URTICARIA

Urticaria is a vascular reaction of the skin characterised by immediate formation of a wheal and flare accompanied by severe itching. Contact with an external irritant such as drugs or foods produces the Ag–IgE-mediated response,

STRUCTURE	HISTAMINE RECEPTORS	EFFECTS
Vascular system		
Capillary (microcirculation)	H_1 and H_2	Dilation, increased permeability
Arteriole (smooth muscle)	H_1 and H_2	Dilation
Smooth muscle		
Bronchial, bronchiolar	H_1	Contraction
Gastrointestinal	H_1	Contraction
Exocrine glands		
Gastric	H_2	Gastric acid secretion (HCl)
Epidermis	H_1	Triple response (flush, flare, wheal)
Adrenal medulla	H_1	Adrenaline and noradrenaline release
Central nervous system	H_1	Motion sickness

TABLE 55-4 Histamine receptor-mediating effects

with resultant release of histamine from the mast cell into the skin. The local vasodilation produces the red flare, and the increased permeability of the capillaries leads to tissue swelling. These swellings are often called hives; when giant hives occur, the condition is known as angioneurotic oedema. Antihistaminic drugs administered before exposure to the antigen will prevent this response.

ATOPY

Atopy occurs in genetically susceptible individuals and is usually caused by seasonal pollen. This condition is manifested as an upper respiratory tract disorder known as allergic rhinitis (hay fever). After the interaction of Ag–IgE antibody on the surface of the bronchial mast cells, histamine is released, producing local vascular dilation and increased capillary permeability. This change produces a rapid fluid leakage into the tissues of the nose, resulting in swelling of the nasal linings. In certain people, antihistaminic therapy can prevent the oedematous reaction if the drug is administered before antigen exposure.

FOOD ALLERGIES

Food allergies involve an intestinal IgE–mast cell response to ingested antigens. If the upper GI tract is affected, vomiting results; if the lower GI tract is invaded, cramps and diarrhoea occur. This condition also has been known to produce systemic anaphylaxis after ingestion of a large amount of antigen.

BRONCHIAL ASTHMA

When an inhaled antigen combines with IgE, stimulation of the mast cells triggers the release of mediators in the lower respiratory tract, usually in the bronchi and bronchioles. Histamine plays a role in the early asthma response, but administration of antihistaminic drugs actually does not help to relieve bronchoconstriction because more potent chemical mediators than histamine are responsible for causing the reaction (see Chapter 32).

SYSTEMIC ANAPHYLAXIS

Systemic anaphylaxis is a generalised reaction manifested as a life-threatening systemic condition. The Ag–IgE mediator response involves the basophils of the blood and the mast cells in the connective tissue. The commonest precipitating causes of this response are drugs (particularly penicillin), insect stings (wasps and bees) and, occasionally, certain foods. The release of massive amounts of histamine into the circulation causes widespread vasodilation, resulting in a profound fall in blood pressure. The excessive dilation also allows plasma to leave the capillaries and a loss of circulatory volume ensues. When the reaction is fatal, death is usually caused not only by shock but also by laryngeal oedema. The symptoms of the latter condition include smooth muscle contraction of the bronchi and pharyngeal oedema, which usually leads to asphyxiation.

Drug allergies often develop in susceptible individuals who show no adverse effect after the first dose of a drug. A second or subsequent exposure to even a minute amount of this same antigen may elicit an exaggerated IgE response, either locally or systemically. People who exhibit such reactions are said to be allergic to the drug. The IgE-mediated response, particularly with penicillin, may occur in either the skin, producing severe urticaria, or the respiratory tract, causing bronchial asthma. Even limited contact in certain sensitised individuals can produce a fatal systemic anaphylaxis. Some of the drugs that elicit an allergic response include penicillin, chloramphenicol, streptomycin, sulfonamides and aspirin.

Antihistamines

Many histamine receptor antagonists are available over the counter and are widely used for motion sickness, vertigo and skin and allergic disorders. In general, these drugs antagonise the action of histamine at H_1 receptors and are conventionally referred to as antihistamines.

With the discovery of two histamine receptors, H_1 and H_2, the antihistamines were divided into the H_1-receptor antagonists and the H_2-receptor antagonists. The H_2-receptor-blocking agents, which include cimetidine and ranitidine and others, are discussed in Chapter 34. This section reviews the sedating and newer, less sedating antihistamines.

H_1-receptor antagonists

The H_1 antihistamines have the greatest therapeutic effect on nasal allergies. These drugs are more effective if given before histamine is released. They relieve symptoms better at the beginning of the hay fever season than during its height but fail to relieve the asthma that often accompanies hay fever. These preparations are palliative and do not immunise the individual or protect against allergic reactions. Dozens of antihistamine drugs are available. They generally differ from one another in potency, duration of action and incidence of adverse reactions, particularly sedation. In general, they fall into two categories: the older, sedating drugs and the newer, less sedating antihistamines.

INDICATIONS

The sedating antihistamines are indicated for the treatment of allergies, skin disorders, vertigo, motion sickness and nausea, and for sedation. Generally, their oral absorption pattern is good, with onset of action within 15–60 minutes for most of them. The newer, less sedating antihistamines are primarily used for allergic disorders. They have a reduced incidence of anticholinergic effects and sedation, and are generally better tolerated. Individual response to antihistamines varies, and nearly all of these drugs are recommended for short-term treatment. Antihistamines are primarily metabolised in the liver and excreted by the kidneys.

Potential interactions with other drugs are shown in the table Drug Interactions 55-6.

ADVERSE REACTIONS/WARNINGS AND CONTRAINDICATIONS

The commonest adverse reactions are sedation (with older-type antihistamines), dizziness, dry mouth, tinnitus, fatigue, headache, nausea and vomiting. The anticholinergic effect of antihistamines will exacerbate closed-angle glaucoma, pyloroduodenal obstruction, bladder neck obstruction and hyperthyroidism. Avoid using these drugs in people with specific antihistamine hypersensitivity, hypokalaemia, liver function impairment (phenothiazine-type), prostatic hypertrophy or urinary retention. The elderly may be more sensitive to adverse effects such as hypotension and dizziness; lower doses are preferable in this group.

DRUG INTERACTIONS 55-6 Antihistamines

Drug	Possible effect and management
Alcohol, CNS depressants	Concurrent use may enhance CNS-depressant effects. If the CNS depressant also has anticholinergic adverse effects, enhanced effects may be seen. Avoid combined use
Anticholinergic medications, psychotropics, others	Enhanced CNS-depressant and anticholinergic adverse effects may be noted. Avoid combined use
Levodopa	Phenothiazine antihistamines antagonise the action of levodopa. Avoid combined use

TABLE 55-5 Antihistamines: available dosage forms and ADEC pregnancy category

DRUG	FORMULATION	COMMENT	PREGNANCY CATEGORY
Sedating antihistamines			
Azatadine	Tablet, oral liquid	Least sedating	B2
Cyproheptadine	Tablet	Least sedating	A
Dexchlorpheniramine	Tablet, CR tablet, oral liquid	Sedating	A
Dimenhydrinate	Tablet, oral liquid	Significant sedation	A
Diphenhydramine	Capsule	Significant sedation	A
Methdilazine	Tablet	Significant sedation	B2
Pheniramine	Tablet, CR tablet, oral liquid	Sedating	A
Promethazine hydrochloride	Tablet, oral liquid, injection	Significant sedation	C
Trimeprazine	Tablet, oral liquid	Significant sedation	C
Less-sedating antihistamines			
Cetirizine	Tablet, oral liquid, oral drops	Increased risk of sedation in elderly	B2
Desloratadine	Tablet	Metabolite of loratadine; similar effects	B1
Fexofenadine	Tablet	Least likely to cause sedation in elderly	B2
Loratadine	Tablet, oral liquid	Increased risk of sedation in elderly	B1

Source: AMH 2006. ADEC = Australian Drug Evaluation Committee; CR = controlled-release.

DOSAGE AND ADMINISTRATION

The dosage varies for each drug and among adults, children and infants. The newer agents released are generally longer-acting drugs with fewer sedative effects. **Loratadine**, for example, is taken once a day and has few, if any, sedative and anticholinergic effects. The available dosage forms and ADEC

PREGNANCY SAFETY	
ADEC Category	**Drug**
A	Sulfasalazine
B2	Allopurinol, etanercept, probenecid, sodium aurothiomalate
B3	Auranofin
C	Adalimumab, cyclosporin, everolimus, infliximab, tacrolimus
D	Azathioprine, basiliximab, chloroquine, colchicine, daclizumab, hydroxychloroquine, mycophenolate, penicillamine
X	Leflunomide
Unclassified but contraindicated	Muromonab-CD3

DRUGS AT A GLANCE 55: Anti-inflammatory and immunomodulating drugs

Therapeutic group	Pharmacological group	Key examples	Key pages
Non-steroidal anti-inflammatory drugs (NSAIDs)	Non selective cyclo-oxygenase (COX) inhibitors	diclofenac	879, 81
		ibuprofen	879, 81
		naproxen	879, 81
	Selective COX-2 inhibitors	celecoxib	879, 81
Disease-modifying antirheumatic drugs (DMARDs)	Gold salts	auranofin	884
	Cytokine blockers	etanercept	886
		infliximab	886
	Pyrimidine synthesis inhibitor	leflunomide	885
Drugs for gout	Xanthine oxidase inhibitor	allopurinol	888
	Miscellaneous	colchicine	887
Immunosuppressant drugs	Calcineurin inhibitors	cyclosporin	892
		tacrolimus	891
	Cytotoxic immunosuppressant	azathioprine	892
	Immunosuppressant antibodies	basiliximab	894
		muromonab-CD3	894
Immunostimulant drugs	Interferons	interferon alpha-2a	895, 6
Antihistamines	Histamine receptor (H_1) antagonists	azatadine	898, 9
		diphenhydramine	898, 9
		fexofenadine	898, 9
		loratadine	898, 9

pregnancy category are noted in Table 55-5.

Fexofenadine, an antihistamine approved in 1996, is a metabolite of terfenadine. Manufacture of terfenadine has ceased because of the serious and potentially fatal cardiovascular drug interactions associated with its use. The likelihood of serious cardiac arrhythmias with fexofenadine is low but care should still be exercised in persons with prolonged QT interval.

KEY POINTS

- Inflammatory disorders such as rheumatoid arthritis require lifelong therapy, and the choice of drugs is often weighed against the risk of adverse effects.
- Despite diversity in their chemical structures, all the non-steroidal anti-inflammatory drugs (NSAIDs) possess the same therapeutic properties—analgesic, antipyretic and anti-inflammatory effects.
- NSAIDs also share, to varying degrees, the same adverse reactions because inhibition of prostaglandins, which accounts for all the therapeutic effects, also causes the renal and gastrointestinal toxicity.
- NSAIDs are indicated for the treatment of acute or chronic rheumatoid arthritis, osteoarthritis, ankylosing spondylitis and other rheumatic diseases, and mild to moderate pain.
- Disease-modifying antirheumatic drugs (DMARDs) comprise a group of drugs with diverse chemical structures, and their mechanisms of action in many cases are largely unknown.
- Use of DMARDs has substantially improved the control of rheumatoid arthritis and the long-term quality of life of the individual. In many instances, combinations of DMARDs may be used.
- Gout is a metabolic disorder of uric acid metabolism that is characterised by hyperuricaemia.
- The primary goals of therapy for gout are to end the acute attack as soon as possible, to prevent a recurrence, to prevent the formation of uric acid stones in the kidneys and to prevent or minimise the complications of sodium urate deposits in the joints.
- The primary medications used for these purposes are colchicine, allopurinol and probenecid.
- The rejection of kidney, liver and heart allogeneic transplants has led to the development of immunosuppressant drugs, or agents that decrease or prevent an immune response.
- There are four main classes of immunosuppressant drugs: corticosteroids, calcineurin inhibitors, cytotoxic immunosuppressants and immunosuppressant antibodies.
- Histamine is a natural chemical found in most body tissues and has been implicated in a range of conditions such as urticaria, atopy, food allergies, bronchial asthma and systemic anaphylaxis.
- Histamine receptor antagonists, principally of the H_1 receptor, are called antihistamines. The older drugs tend to produce a greater degree of sedation; the newer agents, such as loratadine, have reduced sedating effects.
- Antihistamines block the action of histamine at its receptors and are primarily used for allergic disorders.

REVIEW EXERCISES

1. Why do non-steroidal anti-inflammatory drugs cause gastric ulceration and acute renal failure?
2. Why is asymptomatic hyperuricaemia generally not treated, especially in the elderly?
3. Why are colchicine and allopurinol effective drugs for treating gout?
4. Why is probenecid used as an adjunct to antibiotic therapy, such as penicillin and some cephalosporins? Describe the site of action and ultimate effect of probenecid.
5. Explain why live virus vaccines should be avoided in people receiving an immunosuppressant drug.
6. Name four indications for the use of histamine receptor antagonists. Why do these drugs cause a dry mouth?

REFERENCES AND FURTHER READING

Australian Institute of Health and Welfare (AIHW). *Health Expenditure Australia 2003–04.* AIHW cat. no. HWE 32 (Health and Welfare Expenditure Series no. 25). Canberra: AIHW, 2005.
Australian Medicines Handbook 2006. Adelaide: AMH, 2006.
Bombardier C, Laine L, Reicin A et al. Comparison of upper gastrointestinal toxicity of rofecoxib and naproxen in patients with rheumatoid arthritis. *New England Journal of Medicine* 2000; 343: 1520–8.

Brater DC, Harris C, Redfern JS, Gertz BJ. Renal effects of COX-2 selective inhibitors. *American Journal of Nephrology* 2001; 21: 1–15.

Bresalier RS, Sandler RS, Quan H et al. Cardiovascular events associated with rofecoxib in a colorectal adenoma chemoprevention trial. *New England Journal of Medicine* 2005; 352: 1092–1102.

Cribb AB, Cribb JW. *Wild Medicine in Australia*. Sydney: Collins Publishers, 1981.

Halpern GM. Anti-inflammatory effects of a stabilised lipid extract of *Perna canaliculus* (Lyprinol). *Allergie et Immunologie* 2000; 32: 272–8.

Krensky AM, Strom TB, Bluestone JA. Immunomodulators: immunosuppressive agents, tolerogens, and immunostimulants. In: Hardman JG, Limbird E, Gilman AG (eds). *Goodman & Gilman's The Pharmacological Basis of Therapeutics*. 10th edn. New York: McGraw Hill, 2001 [ch. 53].

Lassak EV, McCarthy T. *Australian Medicinal Plants*. Sydney: Reed-New Holland, 2001.

Low T. *Bush Medicine: A Pharmacopoeia of Natural Remedies*. Sydney: Angus & Robertson, 1990.

New drugs. *Australian Prescriber* 2000; 23: 21–2.

Olsen NJ, Stein CM. New drugs for arthritis. *New England Journal of Medicine* 2004; 350: 2167–79.

Perazella M, Tray K. Selective cyclo-oxygenase-2 inhibitors: a pattern of nephrotoxicity similar to traditional nonsteroidal anti-inflammatory drugs. *American Journal of Medicine* 2000; 111: 64–7.

Reginster JY, Deroisy R, Rovati LC, Lee RL et al. Long-term effects of glucosamine sulphate on osteoarthritis progression: a randomised, placebo controlled clinical trial. *Lancet* 2001; 357: 251–6.

Silverstein FE, Faich G, Goldstein JL, Simon LS et al. Gastrointestinal toxicity with celecoxib vs nonsteroidal anti-inflammatory drugs for osteoarthritis and rheumatoid arthritis. The CLASS Study: a randomized controlled trial. *Journal of the American Medical Association* 2000; 284: 1247–55.

Vane J. Towards a better aspirin. *Nature* 1994; 367: 215–16.

Zola N, Gott B. *Koorie Plants, Koorie People: Traditional Aboriginal Food, Fibre and Healing Plants of Victoria*. Melbourne: Koorie Heritage Trust, 1992.

evolve More weblinks at http://evolve.elsevier.com/AU/Bryant/pharmacology/

CHAPTER 56

Drugs Affecting the Skin

CHAPTER FOCUS

The skin is the largest organ of the body; it is combined with hair, nails and glands to form the integumentary system. It serves as a barrier against the environment, protects underlying tissues, helps regulate body temperature and produces vitamin D. The health-care professional must know the structure, function and pathophysiology of the skin to understand the topical and systemic agents used in treatment of skin conditions, and the application to the skin of drugs intended for transcutaneous absorption and systemic action. This chapter reviews the various formulations and topical products available, such as sunscreen preparations and therapeutic agents used to treat specific skin problems. It also includes discussion of the treatment of burns, and prevention, cleansing and debridement of pressure sores.

OBJECTIVES

- To describe the structure and functions of the skin.

- To discuss the application of drugs to the skin for local or systemic effects, and the principles of percutaneous absorption of drugs.

- To list groups of drugs that commonly cause adverse reactions in the skin.

- To describe the general properties of dermatological formulations and indications for their use.

- To list the types of drugs commonly applied to the skin and describe their pharmacological actions.

- To describe the damage that sun exposure can cause to the skin and discuss the mechanisms of action and use of sunscreens.

- To discuss the properties and dermatological uses of antimicrobials and anti-inflammatory and immunosuppressant agents, and the treatment of acne, burns and pressure sores.

KEY DRUGS

aciclovir
amorolofine
antibiotics
bacitracin
betamethasone
corticosteroids
imidazoles
permethrin
retinoids
silver sulfadiazine
sunscreens
terbinafine
tretinoin

KEY TERMS

acne vulgaris
antifungal
antimicrobial
antipruritic
astringent
burns
cream
debridement
dermis
dermatitis
ectoparasites
eczema
epidermis
eschar
formulation
granulation tissue

keratolytic
lotion
melanin
occlusive dressing
ointment
phototoxicity
pressure sore
psoriasis
skin
sun protection factor
sunscreen
transcutaneous
  absorption
urticaria
ultraviolet radiation
vehicle

KEY ABBREVIATIONS

SPF   sun protection factor
UVR   ultraviolet radiation
UVA, UVR of wavelengths
UVB   in the A, B or C region
UVC

THE SKIN (or integument) has been described as the largest organ in the body. Medications for most diseases are administered at a site distant from the target organ, but in dermatology, medications can readily be applied directly to the target site. In addition, lipid-soluble drugs can be applied to the skin with the intention that they be absorbed into the systemic circulation to act at distant sites, and drugs can be administered systemically to treat skin disorders. Because skin functions are vital to an individual's survival and are also quite diverse, this chapter reviews the structure and functions of the skin and skin appendages.

The chapter also covers debriding agents, which are used to remove dirt, foreign objects, damaged tissue and cellular debris from a wound or burn to prevent infection and promote healing. In treatment of a wound, debridement is the first step in cleansing it; debridement also allows examination of the extent of the injury.

STRUCTURE AND FUNCTIONS OF THE SKIN

Structure of the skin

The **skin** is made up of two main layers, the **epidermis** and the **dermis**. The epidermis, or thin outer skin layer, consists of four strata, or layers, of epithelial cells (see Figure 56-1). The epidermis has no direct blood supply of its own; it is nourished only by diffusion.

The *stratum corneum*, or horny layer, consists of outer dead cells that have been filled with keratin, a water-repellent protein, and forms a protective cover for the body. It desquamates, or sheds, and is replaced by new cells from the lower layers.

The *stratum lucidum*, or clear layer, is present in the palms and soles and contains translucent flat cells. Keratin is formed here.

The *stratum granulosum*, or granular layer, is composed of cells that contain granules in their cytoplasm. Cells die in this layer of skin.

The *stratum germinativum* contains the stratum spinosum and the innermost layer, the stratum basale. The cells in the stratum basale undergo cellular mitosis to generate new cells for the skin.

Melanocytes, which are responsible for synthesising **melanin**, a pigment that occurs naturally in the hair and skin, are also located deep in the stratum germinativum. The more melanin that is present, the deeper brown the skin colour. Melanin is a protective agent; it blocks ultraviolet rays, thus preventing injury to underlying dermis and tissues.

The dermis lies between the epidermis and subcutaneous fat. It is about 40 times thicker than the epidermis and contains elastic and connective tissues that provide support for its blood vessels, nerves, lymphatic tissue, sweat glands, sebaceous glands and hair follicles.

Below the dermis is the hypodermis, or subcutaneous layer, which contributes flexibility to the skin. Subcutaneous fat tissue is an area for thermal insulation, nutrition, and cushioning or padding.

The skin contains three types of exocrine glands: sebaceous, eccrine and apocrine. These exocrine glands are multicellular glands that open on the surface of the skin through ducts in the epithelium. Sebaceous glands are large, lipid-containing cells that produce sebum, the oil or film layer that covers the epidermis, especially abundant in the scalp, face, anus and external ear. This protects and lubricates the skin, is water-repellent and has some antiseptic effects. The eccrine glands, or sweat glands, are also widely distributed on the skin surface, including the soles and palms. These glands help to regulate body temperature by promoting cooling via evaporation of their secretion. They also help to prevent excessive skin dryness. The apocrine glands are located mainly in the axillae, genital organs and breast areas. They are odoriferous and are believed to represent scent or sex glands.

Normal skin pH is 4.5–5.5, which is weakly acidic. This acid mantle is a protective mechanism because most microorganisms grow best at pH 6–7.5. Infected areas of the skin usually have a higher pH.

The appendages of the skin are the hair, nails and skin glands, which basically carry out protective and lubricating functions. These areas are discussed when drug therapy is relevant to these sites.

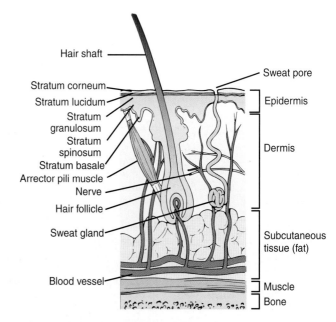

FIGURE 56-1 Structures of the skin.
Note: Details of nerves (autonomic and sensory) and sensory nerve endings are not shown.

Functions of the skin

The skin serves many functions in the body; some of the major functions are listed here.

Protection

The skin forms a protective covering for the entire body. It protects the internal organs and their environment from external forces. As the old song puts it, 'Skin's what keeps your insides in' and, more importantly, keeps the outsides out. Thus it is a barrier against microorganism invasion, chemicals, loss of water and heat, and physical abrasion.

Sensation

Nerve endings permit the transfer of sensations, such as heat, cold, touch, pressure and pain.

Body temperature regulation

Skin helps maintain body temperature homeostasis by regulating heat loss or heat conservation. Blood vessels in the dermis area can dilate, and perspiration increases when the body temperature is elevated. If the body temperature is below normal, the skin blood vessels constrict and perspiration is decreased.

Blood reservoir

The dermal blood vessels contain 8%–10% of the blood volume in adults.

CLINICAL INTEREST BOX 56-1
POISONED THROUGH THE SKIN!

Some of the most toxic agents liable to be absorbed through the skin are the organophosphorus anticholinesterases, such as dyflos and malathion (now known as maldison). These were intended to be highly lipid-soluble, as they were developed to be absorbed through the lungs and skin of humans (as war gases) or the cuticle of insects (as insecticides). Cases of toxicity occurring after transdermal absorption of these agents are quite common, e.g. in chemical workers, pest controllers and gardeners.

A case was reported in Melbourne in 1997 of an ambulance transporting an elderly man who had accidentally ingested insecticide solution (metasystox), mistaking it for a cough mixture. One of the ambulance officers became dizzy, disoriented and nauseous from the fumes in the ambulance; he was poisoned indirectly both by handling the clothing and by inhaling fumes escaping through the skin of the patient. Both patient and 'ambo' were successfully treated.

Source: The Age, Melbourne, 11 April 1997.

Absorption, metabolism and excretion

Skin excretes fluid and electrolytes (via sweat glands), stores fat, synthesises vitamin D (when skin is exposed to sunlight or ultraviolet rays, the steroid 7-dehydrocholesterol, which is normally present in the skin, is converted to vitamin D_3) and provides a site for drug absorption. Fat-soluble vitamins (A, D, E and K), oestrogens, corticosteroid hormones and some drugs and chemicals can be absorbed through skin (see Clinical Interest Box 56-1).

Body image

Skin contributes to the concept of body image and a feeling of wellbeing. A disfiguring skin condition can lead to emotional problems and a chronic skin condition can lead to depression.

SKIN DISORDERS
Signs and symptoms

Reactions or disorders of the skin are manifested by symptoms such as itching, pain or tingling, and by signs such as swelling, redness, papules, pustules, blisters and hives. Some common dermatological disorders include acne vulgaris (cystic acne and acne scars), atopic dermatitis, eczema, folliculitis, fungal infections, herpes simplex, lichen simplex chronicus, psoriasis, seborrhoeic dermatitis, skin cancers, verrucae (warts) and vitiligo.

Dermatological diagnosis may require physical assessment; personal and family medical history; drug history; including over-the-counter (OTC) medications; and laboratory tests, cytodiagnosis and biopsy. When the nature of the lesion has been established, its characteristics should be defined according to size, shape, surface and colour (Figure 56-2).

The next step is to discover the distribution of the condition, because a diagnosis can at times be made from the distribution. Psoriasis, for example, is commonly found on the extensor surfaces of the elbows, but occasionally it will be seen as a solitary lesion in the external ear. A basal cell carcinoma is most common on the face, but occasionally it occurs on the trunk. On the other hand, rosacea affects only those areas of the face that flush.

Skin conditions vary over time. Acute conditions tend to show red, burning, blistered or weeping skin (such as from burns); thick ointments cannot be applied to these lesions, which are best treated with lotions that cool by evaporation. Subacute conditions may be oedematous, hot and chapped; creams and gels can be applied. Chronic skin conditions tend to be scaling, lichenified, crusting and dry; moisturising creams and ointments may soften such skin.

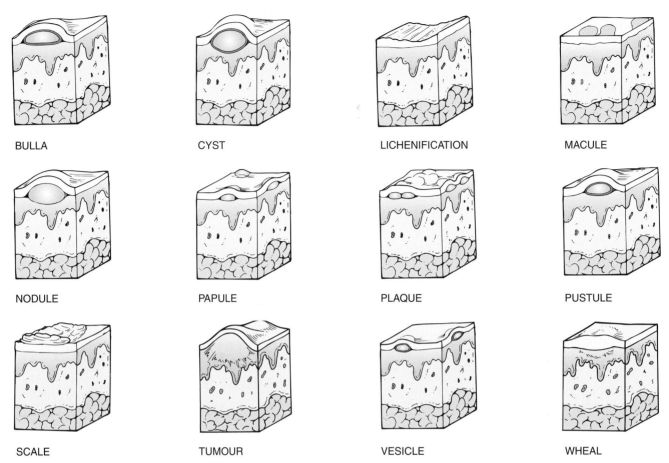

BULLA CYST LICHENIFICATION MACULE

NODULE PAPULE PLAQUE PUSTULE

SCALE TUMOUR VESICLE WHEAL

FIGURE 56-2 Different types of skin lesions and some conditions associated with them. **BULLA:** vesicle greater than 1 cm in diameter (examples: blister; pemphigus vulgaris). **CYST:** elevated; circumscribed; palpable; encapsulated; filled with liquid or semisolid material (example: sebaceous cyst). **LICHENIFICATION:** rough, thickened epidermis; accentuated skin markings due to rubbing or irritation; often involves flexor aspect of extremities (example: chronic dermatitis). **MACULE:** flat; non-palpable; circumscribed; less than 1 cm in diameter; brown, red, purple, white or tan in colour (examples: freckles; flat moles; rubella; rubeola; drug eruptions). **NODULE:** elevated; firm; circumscribed; palpable; deeper in dermis than papule; 1–2 cm in diameter (examples: erythema nodosum; lipomas). **PAPULE:** elevated; palpable; firm; circumscribed; less than 1 cm in diameter; brown, red, pink, tan or bluish-red in colour (examples: warts; drug-related eruptions; pigmented naevi; eczema). **PLAQUE:** elevated; flat-topped; firm; rough; superficial papule greater than 1 cm in diameter, may be coalesced papules (examples: psoriasis; seborrhoeic and actinic keratoses; eczema). **PUSTULE:** elevated; superficial; similar to vesicle but filled with purulent fluid (examples: impetigo; acne; variola; herpes zoster). **SCALE:** heaped-up keratinised cells; flaky exfoliation; irregular; thick or thin; dry or oily; varied size; silver, white, or tan in colour (examples: psoriasis; exfoliative dermatitis). **TUMOUR:** elevated; solid; may or may not be clearly demarcated; greater than 2 cm in diameter; may or may not differ in skin colour (examples: basal cell carcinoma; malignant melanoma). **VESICLE:** elevated; circumscribed; superficial; filled with serous fluid; less than 1 cm in diameter (examples: blister; varicella). **WHEAL:** elevated, irregular-shaped area of cutaneous oedema; solid, transient, changing variable diameter; pale pink in colour (examples: urticaria; insect bites). *Source*: Beare & Myers 1998.

Causes of skin disorders

A reaction of the skin that makes the individual uncomfortable or unsightly may be due to allergy, infection, sensitivity to drugs or other chemicals, emotional stress, genetic predisposition (e.g. atopic eczema or psoriasis), hormonal imbalance or degenerative disease. Sometimes the cause of the skin disorder is unknown and the treatment is empirical, in the hope that the right remedy will be found; corticosteroids are often used in skin disorders for their anti-inflammatory and immunosuppressant actions.

Table 56-1 is a summary of the vast range of dermatological reactions caused by chemicals; some of these can be life-threatening (see Table 56-2 for characteristic lesions and sequelae of serious skin eruptions). The health-care professional always needs to be aware of the patient's drug history and current therapy in order to relate such lesions

TABLE 56-1 Chemicals commonly inducing dermatological conditions

Chemicals causing an acneiform reaction

ACTH, androgenic hormones, corticosteroids, cyanocobalamin, hydantoins, iodides, oral contraceptives

Chemicals causing purpura

ACTH, allopurinol, amitriptyline, anticoagulants, corticosteroids, digoxin, fluoxymesterone, gold salts, griseofulvin, iodides, nifedipine, paracetamol, penicillins, phenothiazines, quinidine, sulfonamides, thiazides

Chemicals causing urticaria

Aciclovir, amitriptyline, cephalosporins, chloramphenicol, chlorhexidine, enzymes, erythromycin, gold salts, griseofulvin, hydantoins, insulins, iodides, nitrofurantoin, opioids, penicillins, phenothiazines, salicylates, streptomycin, sulfonamides, tetracyclines, vaccines

Chemicals causing alopecia

Alkylating agents, anticoagulants, antimetabolites, antitumour antibiotics, lithium, norethisterone, spironolactone

Chemicals causing lichenoid reactions

Chloroquine, gold salts, nifedipine, quinidine, thiazides

Chemicals causing fixed eruptions

Antihistamines, atropine, barbiturates, bismuth salts, chloral hydrate, chlorpromazine, digoxin, disulfiram with alcohol, ergot alkaloids, eucalyptus oil, gold compounds, griseofulvin, iodine, opioids, penicillins, phenytoin, quinidine, quinines, salicylates, saccharin, streptomycin, sulfonamides, tetracyclines, vaccines and immunising agents

Chemicals causing contact dermatitis or eczema

Antihistamines, antiseptics, aspirin, bleomycin, captopril, cephalosporins, chloramphenicol, chlorpromazine, cosmetics, formaldehyde, glyceryl trinitrate, gold salts, iodine, lanolin, local anaesthetics, miconazole, neomycin, paraben preservatives, penicillins, peru balsam, phenol, quinines, streptomycin, sulfonamides, tetracyclines, transdermal patches

Photosensitisers

Amiodarone, anaesthetics (procaine group), antihistamines, antimalarials, barbiturates, benzene, bergamot (perfume), carbamazepine, carrots (wild), celery, chlorhexidine, chlorophyll, citrus fruits, clover, coal tar, corticosteroids (topical), desipramine, dill, disopyramide, dyes (fluorescein, methylene blue, toluidine blue), fennel, 5-fluorouracil, gold salts, grass (meadow), griseofulvin, haloperidol, mercaptopurine, methoxsalen, methoxypsoralen, mustards, naphthalene, oils (cedar, lavender, lime, sandalwood, vanillin), oral contraceptives, p-aminobenzoic acid, parsley, parsnips, phenolic compounds, phenothiazines, phenytoin, porphyrins, quinines, salicylates, silver salts, sulfasalazine, sulfonamides, sulfonylureas (antidiabetics), sunscreens, tetracyclines, thiazide diuretics, toluene, tricyclic antidepressants, xylene

TABLE 56-2 Life-threatening drug-induced skin eruptions

SKIN ERUPTION	DESCRIPTION	DRUGS INVOLVED
Exfoliative dermatitis	Entire surface of skin is red and scaly and will eventually slough off. Hair and nails may also be affected. Eruption may take weeks or months to resolve after causative agent is stopped; if not resolved, it can be fatal	Amiodarone, barbiturates, carbamazepine, frusemide, gold salts, griseofulvin, nifedipine, penicillin, phenothiazines, phenytoin, sulfonamides, tetracyclines
Stevens–Johnson syndrome (erythema multiforme)	Severe form that involves widespread eruptions or lesions usually on face, neck, arms, legs, hands and feet. May also involve mucosa and may produce fever and malaise. Syndrome can last months and is life-threatening	Many drugs, especially carbamazepine, penicillins and cephalosporins, phenytoin, sulfonamides, tetracyclines
Lupus erythematosus	Erythematous rash that may be flat or elevated (butterfly) on cheek (malar), and across nose. Joint swelling and pain, rash, oral ulcers, serositis; renal, haematological, pulmonary and other systems may be affected. Reversible when drug is stopped	Hydantoins, hydralazine, isoniazid, procainamide, quinidine

and sequelae to the appropriate cause, because simply discontinuing a particular drug often resolves a complicated dermatological problem of unknown origin.

APPLICATION OF DRUGS TO THE SKIN

The general principles of treatment of skin disorders are to:
- identify and remove the cause of the skin disorder, if possible
- institute measures to restore and maintain the structure and normal function of the skin
- relieve symptoms that are produced by the disorder, such as itching, dryness, pain and inflammation.

Topical administration of drugs

Drugs may be administered to the skin for a topical or local effect, or with the intention that the drug be absorbed and have systemic actions elsewhere in the body. Even drugs that are applied for local actions may be absorbed, and systemic effects and toxicity can occur.

How much of a topical preparation should be prescribed? This is less easy to estimate than the quantity of tablets or other solid dose forms. Current guidelines suggest that for a cream or ointment to cover the area of the face and neck it would require about 1.25 g for one application, so twice-daily application for 10 days would require a 25–30 g tube of cream. Another way to calculate is to follow the guidelines of the *Australian Medicines Handbook*, where it is suggested, for example, that for a 3–5-year-old child, twice-a-day application of a topical ointment for 1 week would require 10 g for the face and neck, 15 g for arm and hand, 20 g for leg and foot etc.

Keratin in the outer skin layer provides a waterproof barrier. To enhance drug absorption, the epidermis, or keratin skin layer, needs to be hydrated. Some medications are therefore placed under an **occlusive dressing** (such as plastic wrap, rubber gloves or shower cap; see Figure 56-3 later) or administered in an occlusive type of ointment (e.g. zinc cream or petroleum jelly) because both will trap and prevent water loss (sweat) from the skin, thus increasing epidermis hydration.

Transcutaneous absorption of drugs
Skin layers to be crossed

For **transcutaneous absorption** of drugs, the layers of skin cells and membranes through which drugs must pass before being absorbed into the systemic circulation are:

- the surface layer of epidermis: most drugs are very water-soluble (as they must be to dissolve readily in aqueous fluids such as the blood plasma and extracellular fluids), and so do not readily penetrate unbroken skin. Drugs such as sunscreens, insect repellents and antimicrobials may be applied to enhance the barrier functions of the skin and to protect the surface layer
- the stratum corneum: this is the thickest layer and provides the strongest barrier, and passage across it is the rate-limiting step. Emollients, moisturisers and keratolytics may soften and moisten this layer and remove dead cells
- skin appendages can be affected by drugs: antiperspirants, depilatory agents and antimicrobials alter the functions of skin glands and hairs
- the epidermis and dermis layers: for a drug to be readily absorbed through the skin its lipid solubility must be high. Anti-inflammatory agents, topical local anaesthetics and antipruritic (anti-itching) drugs act in these layers on viable skin cells and structures
- endothelial cells of skin blood vessels: very lipid-soluble drugs will pass through into the circulation. Drugs such as nicotine, hyoscine, oestrogens, fentanyl and glyceryl trinitrate are formulated in ointments or patches for transdermal absorption. Chemicals can also be absorbed unintentionally across the skin, with unexpected consequences (see Clinical Interest Box 56-1).

Factors affecting transcutaneous absorption

Absorption through the skin (except with very lipid-soluble agents) is slow, incomplete and variable. The extent of absorption depends on:
- the person's age: the skin of infants is very thin and delicate, and elderly people may also have thin, fragile skin; this can be both dangerous (e.g. fatalities have occurred after absorption of boric acid from dusting powders) and advantageous (useful levels of zinc can be absorbed from zinc cream to assist healing)
- lipid solubility: lipid-soluble drugs are better absorbed through skin than water-soluble drugs
- alcohol content: products with alcohol content may be administered for drying effects after evaporation
- the condition and site of the skin: the stratum corneum layers of the palms and soles are usually toughened and thickened, so are less permeable to drugs; diseased or damaged skin is more permeable
- metabolism and circulation: wound healing is compromised and ulcers may develop readily in people with poor peripheral circulation; 'rubbing in' a drug with a cream or ointment may enhance circulation to the area and penetration of the drug

- hydration of the skin: moist 'washerwoman's hands' skin is more permeable, so moisturisers, moist dressings and occlusive wrapping of skin are used to enhance drug absorption.
- the **vehicle** in which the drug is administered: the drug needs to leave the vehicle to be available for absorption.

Formulations and medications for topical application

Dermatological preparations are available in many **formulations** to treat the numerous common skin disorders. Often, particular ointments, creams, lotions or specific vehicles provide a desired effect without an active ingredient. For a person with dry, scaly skin as found in psoriasis or dry eczema, an ointment with an occlusive emollient (softening) effect is desired, such as lanolin or zinc cream. A person with an acute inflammation that is weeping or oozing often needs a drying and soothing lotion, such as a saline solution, aluminium acetate solution or calamine lotion. If the skin lesion is painful, wet and located on an area rubbed by clothing, then a dusting powder such as talcum or starch may be appropriate to reduce friction and help dry the area. The old saying in dermatology 'If it's wet, dry it; if it's dry, wet it' is still valid.

Pharmaceutical formulations for topical administration may include a wide range of ingredients, such as ointment or cream bases, water, suspending agents, emulsifying agents, preservatives, antioxidants, thickening agents, long-chain fatty acid esters and alcohols, colouring agents and perfumes, as well as the active drug. For example, one commercial 'lip revitalizer' contains 38 listed ingredients plus flavours! Some of the different types of formulations or agents suitable for application to the skin are listed below.

Antipruritic agents

Antipruritics (preparations that relieve itching) include dilute solutions containing phenol, menthol, pine tar, potassium permanganate, aluminium subacetate, boric acid or physiological saline solution. Lotions such as calamine or calamine with phenol (phenolated calamine), cornstarch or oatmeal baths, and hydrocortisone lotion or ointment may also be used. Local anaesthetics such as benzocaine can decrease pruritus, but they readily induce allergic reactions. Antihistamines are poorly absorbed topically, so are less useful than might be expected in relieving allergic and itchy conditions.

Astringents

Astringents are solutions that, when applied topically, cause precipitation of proteins, vasoconstriction and reduced cell permeability; examples are aluminium acetate or calcium hydroxide solutions, calamine lotion, hamamelis (witch hazel), potassium permanganate and the alcohol vehicle in aftershave lotions.

Baths and soaks

Baths and soaks are used to cleanse or medicate the skin, or to reduce temperature, usually with soap and water or with oils that have a moistening and soothing effect. Water generally has an antipruritic (anti-itch) effect, as well as cooling and drying by evaporation. Soaps have a detergent and drying action, and are alkaline.

Cleansers

These are usually free of soap or are modified soap products that are recommended for people with sensitive, dry or irritated skin, or for those who have had a previous reaction to a soap product. These cleansers are less irritating, may contain an emollient substance and may also have been adjusted to a slightly acidic or neutral pH.

Creams and ointments

Creams and **ointments** are thick semisolid preparations to be smoothed onto the skin; they may consist of one phase (usually oily, as in ointments), or may be emulsions, i.e. two-phase preparations (creams). Water-in-oil (W/O) creams, such as lanolin, zinc cream and cold cream, feel greasy, are occlusive and help retard water loss through the skin; they effectively deliver lipid-soluble drugs to the skin. Oil-in-water (O/W) preparations, such as aqueous cream and vanishing creams, have cooling and moisturising effects, are good vehicles for water-soluble drugs, and are more easily washed off. Creams and ointments have emollient and protective properties and may be used as the vehicle for active drugs, e.g. eye ointments containing antibiotics or anti-inflammatory agents, and aqueous cream.

Emollients

Emollients are fatty or oily substances that are used to soften or soothe irritated skin and mucous membrane. An emollient is often used as a vehicle for other medicinal substances. Examples of emollients include lanolin, petroleum jelly (Vaseline), soft paraffins, silicones, oils, vitamin A and D ointments and aqueous cream.

Gels

Gels are viscous, non-oily, water-miscible, semisolid preparations that contain gelling agents; they have a cooling effect as the solvent evaporates and leave a film on the skin.

Keratolytics

Keratolytics (keratin dissolvers) are drugs that soften skin squames (scales) and loosen the outer horny layer of the skin; salicylic acid (5%–20%) and resorcinol are drugs of choice. Their action makes the penetration of other medicinal substances possible by cleaning the lesions. Agents used in treatment of psoriasis, eczema and dandruff may be keratolytics. Salicylic acid is particularly important for its keratolytic effect in local treatment of scalp conditions, warts, corns, fungal infections, acne and chronic types of dermatitis. It is used at concentrations up to 20% in ointments, plasters or collodion for this purpose. In treatment of dandruff, a type of seborrhoeic dermatitis of the scalp, shampoos may contain active ingredients such as coal tar, pyrithione zinc, aloe vera, selenium sulfide and/or an imidazole antifungal agent.

Keratoplastics

These are agents that stimulate the epidermis and thus cause thickening of the cornified layer; examples are coal tar and sulfur preparations and low concentrations (1%–2%) of salicylic acid.

Liniments and rubs

These are indicated for pain relief for intact skin; pain caused by muscle aches, neuralgia, rheumatism, arthritis and sprains usually responds to these products. Simply massaging an oily substance into the skin has a rubefacient (reddening) effect and the dilation of skin blood vessels may assist healing. The ingredients in the preparations may include a counterirritant (e.g. camphor or oil of cloves), an antiseptic (chloroxylenol, eugenol, thymol), a local anaesthetic (benzocaine) or analgesic (salicylate-containing substances such as methyl salicylate [Oil of Wintergreen]).

Lotions and solutions

Liquid preparations have soothing and cooling effects due to their evaporation. They may be suspensions of an insoluble powder that is left behind on the skin, such as calamine **lotion**, or they may be mild acidic or alkaline solutions, such as boric acid solution, limewater or aluminium acetate, used as wet dressings and soaks.

Aluminium acetate solution (Burow's solution) is a mild astringent that coagulates bacterial and serum protein. It is diluted with 10–40 parts water before application.

Calamine lotion contains calamine (a powdered mixture of zinc carbonate and ferric oxide), zinc oxide, bentonite (a suspending agent), phenol and glycerol in a sodium citrate solution. It is a soothing and mildly astringent lotion used for the dermatitis caused by plant secretions, insect bites, sunburn and prickly heat. (It has been said that calamine lotion may make a lot of mess without doing a lot of good. This could be said of many old-fashioned topical preparations, which remain in the pharmacopoeia without ever having been subjected to controlled clinical trials of safety and efficacy.)

Pastes

These are very thick mixtures of solids in cream or ointment bases; for example, Magnoplasm is a magnesium sulfate and glycerin paste with very high osmotic pressure, used to withdraw fluid from lesions, such as boils.

Patches

A transdermal patch is rather like an adhesive dressing that has a reservoir of active drug incorporated in the dressing behind a rate-controlling polymer membrane designed to deliver the drug to the skin at a specified rate (see Figure 25-2). Patches are useful for delivery of potent lipid-soluble drugs, such as glyceryl trinitrate, oestradiol or nicotine, and have the advantage that they eliminate many variables affecting oral absorption, including gastric emptying time, stomach acidity, presence of food and the first-pass effect.

Powders

Powders are mixtures of finely divided drugs in a dry form. Dusting powders such as talcum, zinc oxide or starch are intended for external application. They are useful in body fold areas, where they reduce friction and promote drying.

Preservatives

These are chemicals added to aqueous formulations to retard oxidation or microbial growth. Common preservatives are hydroxybenzoates, alcohols, chlorocresol and benzalkonium chloride. Preservatives can frequently cause contact dermatitis. Preparations such as ointments with very little or no water usually do not pose a problem with respect to microbial growth (because of their high osmotic pressure) and hence do not require preservatives.

Protectants

Skin protectants are soothing, cooling preparations that form a film on the skin. They are used to coat minor skin irritations or to protect the person's skin from chemical irritants. They can also help healing by preventing crusting and trauma.

Examples are Compound Benzoin Tincture (see below), and Collodion, a 5% solution of pyroxylin in a mixture of ether and alcohol, which evaporate to leave a transparent, protective film that adheres to the skin. Non-absorbable powders (including zinc stearate, zinc oxide, certain bismuth preparations, talcum powder and aluminium silicate) are also protectants; however, they adhere to wet surfaces and have to be scraped off.

Psoralens

These are plant constituents that have been known for centuries to induce pigmentation in skin, and are used for treatment of vitiligo, a condition in which there is patchy whitening of the skin and hair. They are photosensitising agents that absorb ultraviolet A radiation (UVA), so are also used in conjunction with exposure to ultraviolet radiation in treatment of psoriasis; an example is methoxsalen.

Soaps

Ordinary soap, the sodium salt of palmitic, oleic or stearic acids alone or in a mixture, is made by saponifying fats or oils with alkalis. The consistency of the soap depends on the acid and alkali used. All soaps are relatively alkaline and are potential sources of skin irritation, as are perfumes or antiseptics added to soaps. Soaps are irritating to mucous membranes and they are used in enemas mainly because of this action.

Sprays

Sprays are fine mists or aerosols of drug in solution, often with a propellant gas. The vehicle evaporates and deposits the drug on the skin or mucous membrane.

Tars

Extracts of coal tar or of bitumen are mild irritants to the skin, reduce epidermal thickness, suppress DNA synthesis and have antipruritic and antiseptic properties. They are used in treatment of dermatoses, including eczema, psoriasis and dandruff; examples are coal tar solution and ichthammol.

Tinctures

Tinctures are alcoholic solutions of chemicals or extracts of plant products. When the tincture is applied to the skin, the alcohol evaporates, leaving the ingredient on the skin. Alcohol has an astringent effect and can cause stinging of raw or damaged surfaces.

Compound Tincture of Benzoin (also known as Tinct. Benz. Co. and Friar's Balsam) is an alcoholic solution of three balsams (i.e. dried exudates from the cut stems of plants) and of aloes. It is administered as a paint or spray for its antiseptic, protective and styptic properties, and as an inhalation for upper respiratory tract infections.

Wet Dressings

These liquids include some of the preparations discussed under solutions and lotions, and are either a wet or an astringent type of dressing used to treat inflammatory skin conditions, e.g. due to insect bites and plant secretions.

Types of drugs affecting the skin

So many dermatological products are available, both OTC and by prescription, that it would be difficult to discuss them all in this chapter. For the sake of simplicity, we discuss only a few selected groups of dermatological products: sunscreens, topical antimicrobials and anti-inflammatories, retinoids and other drugs used to treat acne, and agents used specifically for burns and pressure ulcers. (The detailed pharmacology of most of these drugs has been discussed in previous chapters, e.g. under hormones, anti-inflammatories and antimicrobial agents.)

Other general dermatological products include the astringents, cleansers, liniments, antiseptics and keratolytics described earlier, and antiperspirants, antidandruff shampoos, face washes for acne, freezing sprays for warts, skin lighteners, medicated toothpastes, mouth-washes, mosquito repellents, hair removers and hair restorers. (Strictly speaking, topical agents acting on mucous membranes could also be included, such as eye-drops and ointments, nasal drops and sprays, and even suppositories and enemas.) Natural plant extracts and oils with some proven or claimed antiseptic properties include oils of melaleuca (tea-tree), lemon, lemongrass, eucalyptus, clove leaf, thyme, pine, citronella and peppermint flowers, and extract of aloe vera. Most of these products are available OTC in pharmacies and supermarkets.

SUNSCREEN PREPARATIONS

Skin damage from the sun
Phototoxicity and photoallergy reactions

Certain chemicals and drugs (e.g. dyes, suntanning preparations, tetracyclines, oestrogens, sulfonamides, thiazides and phenothiazines), plants, cosmetics and soaps can cause a phototoxic reaction—an excessive response to solar radiation occurring in the presence of a photosensitising agent. Photosensitivity, or **phototoxicity**, occurs when the inducing agent is present in the skin in sufficient amounts and is exposed to a particular sunlight wavelength. The substance absorbs the radiation and energy is transferred, producing a reactive molecule or free radical, which is destructive to cell membranes or lysosomes. The exposed skin rapidly becomes red, painful, prickling or burning, with peak skin reaction reached within 24–48 hours of exposure. This reaction does not involve the immune system but resembles excessive sunburn.

A photoallergy reaction is different from a phototoxic reaction; it is less common and requires prior exposure to a photosensitising agent, which is activated to an allergen or hapten by radiation. The immune system is involved and when the photosensitisers react with UVR, a delayed hypersensitivity reaction occurs, presenting as severe pruritus and a rash that can spread to skin areas that were not exposed to sunlight.

Ultraviolet radiation damage

Extended exposure to the sun, whether from sunbathing or as a normal consequence of an outdoor occupation, can lead to sunburn and premature ageing of the skin (photoageing). The damage is caused by solar **ultraviolet radiation** (UVR), which comprises the part of the spectrum of electromagnetic radiation with wavelengths shorter than those of visible light (at the violet end of the colour spectrum) and longer than those of X-rays.

UVR has useful effects in activating sterols to vitamin D compounds and has been used to treat acne and neonatal jaundice (and prevent kernicterus and permanent brain damage). UVR can also damage DNA strands by causing thymine bases to link in dimers, and may inactivate viruses. Excessive exposure to UVR can result in skin damage that progresses from minor irritations, blistering, skin darkening (tanning) and thickening, through severe sunburn to a precancerous skin condition and possibly to skin cancer later in life. Cutaneous malignant melanoma has been associated with excessive sun exposure, especially during childhood, whereas large cumulative UVR doses over a lifetime appear to increase the incidence of non-melanoma skin cancers (see Clinical Interest Box 56-2).

The spectrum for UVR has been subdivided into UVA, UVB and UVC.

UVA, or long-wave radiation, has wavelengths in the range 400–320 nm and is the closest to visible light. It produces darkening of preformed melanin in the basal layer of the epidermis and results in a light suntan. UVA is responsible for many photosensitivity reactions.

UVB has wavelengths of 320–290 nm. It causes erythema, sunburn and photoageing and is associated with vitamin D_3 synthesis. UVB has also been determined to be responsible for

CLINICAL INTEREST BOX 56-2 SUNBURN, SKIN CANCER AND SPF

Incidence
Skin cancers essentially comprise malignant melanomas and non-melanocytic cancers (basal [BCC] and squamous cell [SCC] carcinomas). The incidence of skin cancers in Australia is now more than three times the incidence of all other cancers combined. Two out of three people who live their lives in Australia will require treatment for at least one skin cancer, and about 1000 Australians die each year from skin cancer, mainly melanomas. Because of excessive sun exposure, Australia and New Zealand have by far the highest rates of both incidence and mortality of melanoma in the world.

Statistics on the incidence of non-melanocytic cancers are not easy to ascertain, as the cancers are very common and may be treated by general practitioners without numbers being notified to a central cancer registry. BCCs make up around 80% of skin cancers, SCCs 15%, and melanomas about 5%. BCC and SCC are almost twice as common in men as in women, as they are closely related to sun exposure. In the 15–24 age group in Australia, melanomas are the most common cancers. The annual incidence of melanomas in Australia in 2001 was about 55 per 100,000 for males, and 37 per 100,000 for females.

Preventive measures
Sun protection is necessary, as sunlight is the major external cause of skin cancer. Childhood exposure to sunlight is important in development of all types of skin cancers, with episodic high exposure causing burning a significant factor in melanomas. There is a 10–20-year delay between the

UVR exposure (especially UVB) and the appearance of skin cancer.

The primary means of protection is avoiding sunburns, especially in childhood and adolescence. If possible, avoid outdoor activities when the sun is strongest (11 am to 3 pm), wear protective clothing (hat and long sleeves) and use a broad-spectrum sunscreen that blocks exposure to UVA and UVB light (sun protection factor [SPF] 15 or 30). Reapply every 1–2 hours and after swimming.

UVR can also affect the eyes, increasing the risk for cataracts and other eye disorders, and it can suppress the immune system. It is recommended that sunglasses that block 99%–100% of UVR be worn, especially by people with light-coloured eyes.

Treatment measures
Choice of treatment is based on assessment of type of tumour, site, size and stage; age and condition of the patient; and facilities and skills of the physician. Surgical excision is most common for all skin cancers and the only treatment for melanomas. Non-melanocytic cancers, if inaccessible by surgery, may be treated with radiotherapy, curettage and cryotherapy. Topical treatment with retinoids, antibiotics and cytotoxic agents is being trialled. Lifelong follow-up is required for all patients who have been treated for a skin cancer, as they are at greater than normal risk of recurrence and of developing another primary tumour.
Sources: Speight 1996; Anti-Cancer Council of Victoria 1999; AIHW 2004.

skin cancer induction, although the carcinogenic properties of UVB appear to be augmented by UVA. Around 90% of UVB has in the past been blocked by the Earth's ozone layer, hence the worldwide concern that 'holes' in the ozone layer (caused mainly by environmental pollutants and 'greenhouse gases' such as chlorofluorocarbons) will allow passage of greater proportions of solar UVB and increase the incidence of skin cancers.

Most of the UVC from the sun (wavelength 290–200 nm) does not reach the earth's surface. Exposure to this type of radiation is usually from artificial sources such as mercury lamps and arc-welding. UVC can cause some erythema but will not stimulate tanning; it is very damaging to the retina.

Very little UVR is blocked by cloud cover, although infrared radiation that contributes to the sensation of heat is usually reduced, which can give a person a false sense of security against sunburn. The sun's rays can be reflected onto skin from water, concrete, snow and sand, but are deflected by the Earth's atmosphere and by sweat; hence sunburn is worse at high altitudes and in dry desert conditions.

Sunscreens
Absorbers or reflectors

Sunscreen preparations are applied either to absorb or to reflect UVR.

Absorbing chemicals absorb and block at least 85% of the UVB. Absorbing agents are chemicals such as *p*-aminobenzoic acid (PABA) derivatives, benzophenones (which absorb both UVA and UVB), cinnamates, some salicylates and anthranilates (see Table 56-3).

Physical or opaque sunblocks contain agents that reflect and scatter UVB and UVA but do not absorb it. Reflectors include chemicals such as titanium dioxide and zinc oxide. These agents are opaque (e.g. zinc creams, which look like thick white paste) and must be applied heavily to physically block out the UVR, thus they are not cosmetically acceptable to most people.

It should be noted that sunscreens may be more effective at preventing sunburn than skin cancers.

Sun protection factors

The **sun protection factor** (SPF) is a value given to a sunscreen preparation to indicate its effectiveness. It is largely determined by the sunscreening agents (whether chemical or physical) present in the preparation. The SPF for a product is the ratio between the exposures to UVB required to cause erythema (reddening) with and without the sunscreen. This is expressed as the MED, or the minimal erythemal dose: if a person experiences 1 MED with 25 units of UVR (in an unprotected state) and if after application of a sunscreen the person requires 250 units of radiation to produce 1 MED, then this product will be given an SPF rating of 10. The higher the SPF, the longer it takes to burn or develop a tan. If a person

TABLE 56-3 Selected sunscreen preparations

SUNSCREEN PRODUCT	CHEMICAL SCREENING AGENT	PHYSICAL SCREENING AGENT	SPF RATING	WR RATING
Aquasun SPF4 Lotion	Octyl methoxycinnamate 3%, butyl methoxydibenzoylmethane 1.5%		SPF 4	WR 40 mins
Aquababy SPF 30+ with Zinc Oxide Lotion	Octyl methoxycinnamate 7.5%	Zinc oxide 5%	SPF 30+	WR 4 hours
Sunsense 30+ Cream	Octyl methoxycinnamate 7.5%, oxybenzone 3%	Titanium dioxide 3%	SPF 30+	
Sunsense 30+ Sport Cream	Octyl methoxycinnamate 7.5%, oxybenzone 3%, 4-methylbenzylidene camphor 2.5%	Titanium dioxide 2.6%	SPF 30+	WR 4 hours
Blistex Lip Balm	Padimate-O 6.6%, oxybenzone 2.5%		SPF 16	
Blistex Ultra Lip Balm	Octyl methoxycinnamate 7.4%, oxybenzone 5.2%, octyl salicylate 5%, methyl anthranilate 4.8%, homosalate 4.5%		SPF 30+	
Hamilton's Family Cream	Octyl methoxycinnamate 7.5%, octyl salicylate 4%, butyl methoxydibenzoylmethane 1.5%		SPF 15	
Hamilton's Quadblock Stick	Octyl methoxycinnamate 7.5%, butyl methoxydibenzoylmethane 2.5%, octocrylene 0.9%, 4-methylbenzylidene camphor 4%	Titanium dioxide 1.85%	SPF 30+	WR 4 hours

SPF = sun protection factor, the ratio of the time taken to burn with and without the sunscreen; WR = water resistance (hours).

normally burns with 1 MED within 30 minutes, then applying a sunscreen with an SPF of 6 theoretically allows that person to stay in the sun six times longer, or for nearly 3 hours, before reaching 1 MED; however, 'SPF numbers should not be translated into burn times for individuals' (Dermatology Expert Group 2004).

The SPF scale is a logarithmic scale rather than an arithmetic one, thus a sunscreen with SPF 2 gives a 50% reduction in UVB passage (50% penetration), SPF 4 gives 75% reduction (25% penetration) etc. Hence it can be calculated that SPF 16 (i.e. 15+) reduces UVB passage by about 94% of UVB, whereas a screen with SPF 32 (30+) reduces it by 97%. In practice, there is little useful difference between preparations with very high SPF values. A more important consideration is the water-resistance time of the product, because this period may be much shorter than the 'SPF-allowed' time.

The best way to choose a sunscreen is according to skin type (see Table 56-4), the length of time spent in the sun, whether water resistance is important, the usual intensity of the sun's rays in the geographic area, and the type of preparation or formulation preferred. An SPF 30 sunscreen is recommended for use in tropical areas.

Water resistance of sunscreens

The efficacy of a sunscreen agent depends on its ability to remain effective during vigorous exercise, sweating and swimming. Two categories established are 'water-resistant' and 'very water-resistant' (waterproof). Water-resistant products maintain sun protection for at least 40 minutes in water; very water-resistant products maintain sun protection for at least 80 minutes in water. Water resistance is largely dependent on the vehicle used in the product, in particular how water-soluble it is; thus oil-based lotions and creams are likely to remain on the skin longer while swimming than are O/W creams or lotions.

TABLE 56-4 Recommended SPF for various skin types

TYPE	DESCRIPTION	SPF RECOMMENDED
1	Always burns very easily, never tans	20–30
2	Always burns easily, tans minimally	12–20
3	Moderate burn, tans gradually	8–12
4	Minimal burn, always tans well	4–8
5	Burns rarely, tans profusely	2–4

Source: DeSimone 1996.

Application of sunscreens

Sunscreens should be liberally applied to all exposed body areas (except eyelids) and reapplied frequently to achieve the maximum effectiveness. It has been recommended that sunblock be applied 30 minutes before exposure to allow adequate skin penetration. Reapplication depends on factors such as the product used (the SPF and water resistance category), the planned activity of the individual, the time of day, cloud cover and reflections. It is recommended that individuals stay out of the sun when the UVR is at the highest intensity, usually between 11 am and 3 pm, when two-thirds of the daily solar radiation occurs ('from 11 to 3, stay under a tree').

Logically, it can be seen that reapplication does not 'allow' another number of hours of sun—if a person has already had enough UVR to reach the MED, then any further exposure will cause more erythema, i.e. burning. Because the amount of sunscreen applied is often only one-third to half of what is necessary, the theoretical SPF is rarely achieved, which explains why people burn despite applying sunscreen. Generally, Australians do not use enough sunscreen—a family of four on a beach holiday should use a bottle of sunscreen every couple of days, but many families make a bottle last a couple of years! Sunscreens are dated products and may lose efficacy if kept after their use-by date.

Infants should be kept out of the sun; children older than 6 months should always wear protective clothing, hats and sunscreens, with SPF 15 to SPF 30. It has been projected that consistent use of SPF 15 products from 6 months through to 18 years of age will result in about 80% reduction in the risk of skin cancer over a person's lifetime.

TOPICAL ANTIMICROBIAL AGENTS

General principle of antimicrobial chemotherapy of skin infections

Antimicrobial agents used on the skin or to treat skin infections include antibacterial, antiviral, antifungal and antiparasitic agents. There is an increasing problem worldwide with the spread of organisms developing resistance to antimicrobials, hence concerted efforts are being made to rationalise the prescribing of broad-spectrum antibiotics and use drugs specific to organisms that are sensitive to them. Antimicrobials used topically are preferably not the same as those used systemically, both to minimise the risk of development of resistance and to use drugs that may be toxic systemically but not topically. Whenever possible, skin or nail infections are treated with topical antimicrobials; however, in some severe infections, e.g. fungal nail infections or acne resistant to topical treatment, systemic chemotherapy may be required with antimicrobial agents administered orally.

Antiseptics are solutions or creams of antimicrobial agents applied topically to the skin; they usually contain chemicals that are very effective but too toxic to be administered internally. Many have simple detergent, solubilising actions. Examples include benzalkonium chloride, triclosan, chlorhexidine, cetrimide, povidone-iodine and hypochlorite solutions (see Appendix 2).

Antibacterial agents

The most frequent causative organisms of skin infections are the common body flora bacteria *Streptococcus pyogenes* and *Staphylococcus aureus*. Folliculitis, impetigo, furuncles (boils), carbuncles (multi-headed boils of several adjacent hair follicles) and cellulitis often result from infection by these organisms. These common skin disorders are infections for which topical antibiotics, including **bacitracin**, neomycin, sodium fusidate, polymyxin B, silver sulfadiazine, framycetin, gramicidin, mupirocin and metronidazole, may be applied. (The detailed pharmacology of these agents and their mechanisms of action are discussed in Chapters 50–53.) Antimicrobial agents are sometimes formulated in combination with a corticosteroid, for treatment of inflammatory conditions in which there is a major component of infection as well.

Sensitisation to many topical antibiotics can occur. Prolonged use can produce superinfection as an overgrowth of non-susceptible organisms such as fungi. Photosensitivity is reported with topical gentamicin. Chloramphenicol used topically can cause systemic adverse effects, including bone marrow hypoplasia and blood dyscrasias, as well as local effects such as itching, burning, urticaria, and vesicular and maculopapular dermatitis.

Many topical preparations are available OTC, labelled as first-aid products to help prevent infection in minor cuts, burns or injuries. These generally contain simple antiseptic or disinfectant-type products and are effective for first-aid treatment but not for specific bacterial infections.

Neomycin

Neomycin is a broad-spectrum aminoglycoside antibiotic, indicated for topical application in the treatment of infections of the skin and mucous membranes by organisms susceptible to neomycin's actions, such as impetigo ('school sores') and boils. It is also used in an anti-acne lotion and in preparations for topical application to eye or ear infections. Overgrowth of resistant organisms can occur with prolonged use.

Applied topically, neomycin occasionally irritates the skin, and allergic contact dermatitis has been reported, especially

when neomycin is used on stasis ulcers. For conditions where absorption of neomycin can occur (including burns and trophic ulceration), there is the potential for nephrotoxicity, ototoxicity and neomycin hypersensitivity reactions. This risk is seen more frequently in people with compromised renal function, in people with extensive burns and in patients using other aminoglycoside antibiotics. Use in pregnancy can lead to ototoxicity and renal toxicity in the fetus (Pregnancy Safety Category D).

An ointment that combines neomycin, bacitracin and polymyxin B ('triple antibiotic') may be more efficacious in mixed infections than when these agents are used singly.

Bacitracin

Bacitracin is useful in the local treatment of infectious lesions. The ointment form is most commonly used, although bacitracin has also been used in solution to moisten wet dressings or as a dusting powder. It is odourless and non-staining and its use seldom results in sensitisation; however, allergic contact dermatitis has occurred.

Mupirocin

Mupirocin is a topical antibacterial preparation indicated for the treatment of impetigo caused by *S. aureus* and beta-haemolytic streptococci, and in eradicating the carrier status for *S. aureus*. It is usually applied to affected areas three times daily.

Antiviral agents
Aciclovir and idoxuridine

Aciclovir and idoxuridine are used for treatment of cutaneous herpes simplex infections of the lips ('cold sores') or genital areas. Aciclovir is activated in herpes-infected cells to a metabolite that inhibits viral DNA polymerase, thus inhibiting further viral replication. Idoxuridine is an antimetabolite with a mechanism of action analogous to those of the antitumour antimetabolites: its structure is very similar to that of the nucleic acid base thymidine, and it inhibits the incorporation of thymidine into viral DNA and hence blocks viral replication, analogous to the antimetabolites used in cancer chemotherapy (see Figure 49-1).

Topical aciclovir is used for the treatment of herpes simplex (non-life-threatening) in immunocompromised patients. In many instances, however, systemic aciclovir is much more effective and may be the preferred formulation.

Adverse reactions from topical application of aciclovir or idoxuridine include hypersensitivity reactions, pruritus and stinging. The dosage is adequate covering of the lesions with ointment, from as early as possible in the infection, every 4 hours daily for 5 days.

Treatment of warts

Although warts are caused by a virus (human papillomavirus), they are not treated with specific antiviral drugs. Warts usually resolve without treatment, as they are overcome by the body's immune defences. In immunocompromised patients, however, they can become extensive. Anogenital warts are predominantly transmitted in young people by sexual intercourse. The condition can undergo malignant transformation, and in women there is a strong association with cervical cancer.

Treatment for warts depends largely on the site involved and extent of spread. Topical application of keratolytics, such as salicylic acid and trichloracetic acid, and topical antimicrobials, including podophyllotoxin and glutaraldehyde, have been used. A new drug, imiquimod, is used for treating external genital and perianal warts; it acts by enhancing the body's immune response. Non-pharmacological treatments include curettage, electrosurgery, and cryotherapy with liquid nitrogen or solid carbon dioxide.

Treatment of fungal skin infections

Three pathogenic fungi (dermatophytes) that can cause superficial fungal infections (dermatophytoses) without systemic infection are *Microsporum*, *Trichophyton* and *Epidermophyton*; there can also be mixed infections. Systemic mycoses usually occur only in severely immunocompromised patients.

Fungi exist in moist, warm environments, such as skin areas covered by shoes and socks (tinea pedis, or athlete's foot), or in the groin, scalp or trunk. The fungi invade the stratum cornea (see section on Structure of the skin above) and cause inflammation and induce sensitivity when they penetrate the epidermis and dermis.

Because the stratum corneum is shed daily, the spread or transmission of the fungi occurs by contact, commonly around swimming pools or in bathrooms. General hygiene measures such as wearing sandals in communal change-rooms and showers, and drying skin well, especially between the toes, help reduce infection. Before starting treatment, skin or nail scrapings should be taken for microscopic identification of the causative organism.

Antifungal agents

The primary topical **antifungal** agents include the **imidazole** group (clotrimazole, ketoconazole, bifonazole, miconazole etc.), **terbinafine** and **amorolfine**, and miscellaneous antifungal agents, including undecylenic acid and propionic acid products, tolnaftate, the antibiotics nystatin and griseofulvin, povidone-iodine, and a variety of antifungal combination creams, ointments, powders, sprays, liquids and paints (see Chapter 52).

If topical antifungal agents prove ineffective despite prolonged treatment, then systemic antifungals are required. Fungal infections of the nails (onychomycoses) are particularly resistant to treatment by usual topical or oral formulations, so a medicated nail varnish has been developed (Drug Monograph 56-1). See Table 56-5 for the generic names, and availability status (OTC or prescription) and comments on selected antifungal products.

Adverse reactions with the use of the topical antifungals are generally mild, and include local irritation, pruritus, erythema and stinging.

Topical ectoparasiticidal drugs

Ectoparasites are insects that live on the outer surface of the body; ectoparasiticides are drugs used against those parasites. For human use, these drugs are more frequently referred to as pediculicides and scabicides (miticides), reflecting the type of parasite treated with each group.

Treatment of pediculosis (lice infestation)

Pediculosis is a parasite infestation of lice on the skin of a human. Lice are transmitted from one person to the next by close contact with infested people, clothing, combs and towels. There are three different varieties of infestations: (1) pediculosis pubis, caused by *Phthirus pubis* (pubic or crab louse); (2) pediculosis corporis, caused by *Pediculus humanus corporis* (body louse); and (3) pediculosis capitis, caused by *Pediculus humanus capitis* (head louse). In pediculosis corporis, except in heavily infested individuals, the parasite is often absent from the body but inhabits seams of clothing in the axillae, beltline or collar.

Common findings in a person who is infested include pruritus (itching), nits (eggs of lice) on hair shafts, lice on skin or clothes and, occasionally with pubic lice, sky-blue macules on the inner thighs or lower abdomen. The drugs of choice are the pediculicides permethrin and maldison (malathion) in lotions or shampoos; local public health officers usually recommend the optimal current treatment regimen, including use of medicated shampoo and combing of hair to remove nits. Affected family members may also require treatment, and hairbrushes, hats, clothing, bedding etc. require cleaning.

Permethrin acts on the nerve cell membranes of lice, ticks, mites and fleas. It disrupts the sodium channel depolarisation, thus paralysing the parasites. It has a high cure rate (up to 99%) in treating head lice after only a single application. The most common adverse reactions include pruritus, mild burning on application and transient erythema.

DRUG MONOGRAPH 56-1   AMOROLFINE NAIL VARNISH

Amorolfine is one of a pair of antifungal agents (the other is terbinafine) that have selective fungistatic and fungicidal actions against a broad spectrum of yeasts, dermatophytes and other fungi, and moulds. They impair sterol synthesis in fungal cell membranes and, because the sterols are different from those in mammalian cells, there are few adverse effects. They are active both orally and topically. Amorolfine is the only antifungal agent that is sufficiently well absorbed through fingernails and toenails to be effective topically in treating fungal nail infections (onychomycoses).

INDICATIONS Amorolfine nail varnish is indicated for topical treatment of onychomycoses; it alleviates or cures 70%–80% of cases.

PHARMACOKINETICS Amorolfine is very lipophilic but is virtually insoluble in intestinal fluids. After application to the nail, it permeates and diffuses through the nail plate and can reach measurable levels in the blood.

ADVERSE REACTIONS Occasionally a slight burning sensation is felt after application; allergic reactions are rare. (In animal tests, oral administration led to some cataract formation; the relevance of these findings to human use is not known.)

DRUG INTERACTIONS There are no known drug interactions; however, patients are advised not to use any other nail preparations (polishes, artificial nails) during treatment. If the fungal infection is too severe to be treated by amorolfine nail varnish as monotherapy, PO antifungals such as griseofulvin may be required concurrently.

WARNINGS AND CONTRAINDICATIONS Amorolfine is contraindicated if a previous hypersensitivity to it has occurred. Users are warned not to apply the varnish to the skin beside the nails.

There is little information on the use of this product in pregnant or lactating women or in children, so its use in these people is not recommended.

DOSAGE AND ADMINISTRATION Amorolfine is supplied as a 5% solution in a nail lacquer base; also included in the kit are cleaning pads, nail files and spatulas to be used in applying the varnish. The varnish is applied 1–2 times weekly after first cleaning the nail and filing it down (including the nail surface) to remove as much as possible of the affected nail. Before the next application, the nail is cleaned to remove the remaining varnish and filed down again. Because nail infections are so difficult to eradicate, the process needs to be continued for about 6 months for fingernails and longer for toenails.

Maldison (also known as malathion) is an organophosphate cholinesterase inhibitor available for treating head lice and nits. This product is usually effective in lice-infested individuals within 24 hours and is well tolerated. Malathion lotion is rubbed into the scalp and left to air-dry. Because the drug is flammable, the individual must be warned to avoid open flames and smoking, and not to use a hairdryer. The hair should be shampooed 8–12 hours after application; dead lice and nits are combed out.

Treatment of scabies (mite infestation)

Scabies is a parasitic infestation caused by the itch mite *Sarcoptes scabiei*. It is transmitted by close contact with an infested individual. It bores into the horny layers of the skin in cracks and folds (almost exclusively at night), causing irritation and pruritus. The infestation in adults is usually generalised over the body, especially in web spaces between fingers, wrists, elbows and buttocks.

The drug of choice is **permethrin** cream or lotion, two applications 1 week apart. This is considered more effective than crotamiton or benzyl benzoate. Family members and close contacts should also be treated, and items such as bedding, clothes and soft toys should be sprayed.

ANTI-INFLAMMATORY AND IMMUNOMODULATING AGENTS

As many conditions manifested in the skin involve inflammatory or autoimmune pathological processes, drugs that modify the immune response are widely used in dermatology to target mediators such as cytokines, receptors and inflammatory cells. Most commonly used are the corticosteroids; other immunosuppressants include drugs such as cyclosporin and methotrexate, and newer 'immunobiological agents' such as pimecrolimus, infliximab and etanercept (see Chapters 54 and 55).

Corticosteroids
Actions and uses

Topical **corticosteroids** are generally indicated for relief of inflammatory and pruritic dermatoses. They offer the benefit of allowing direct contact with the localised lesion, with fewer systemic effects than from oral or parenteral administration.

TABLE 56-5 Some topical antifungal agents

NAME	STRENGTH	AVAILABILITY	FORMULATION*	SPECIAL COMMENTS
Imidazoles				
Bifonazole	1%	OTC	C	Broad-spectrum antifungal agent
Clotrimazole	1%	OTC	C, L	Broad-spectrum antifungal agent
Clotrimazole with hydrocortisone	1%/1%	OTC/Rx	C	Inflamed fungal skin infections
Econazole nitrate	1%	OTC	C, L, P	Broad-spectrum antifungal agent
Ketoconazole	2%	OTC	C	Broad-spectrum antifungal agent
Miconazole	0.25%, 2%	OTC	C, L, O, P, S, T	Used for tinea pedis (athlete's foot), tinea cruris, tinea corporis and tinea versicolor
Miconazole with hydrocortisone	2%/0.5%, 1%	OTC	C	Inflamed fungal skin infections
Other antifungals				
Amorolfine	5%	OTC	NV	Onychomycoses (fungal nail infections)
Nystatin	100,000 U/g	OTC	C, O	Antifungal antibiotic with both fungicidal and fungistatic effects; *Candida* infections
Sodium propionate	0.2%	OTC	P	Fungal skin infections
Terbinafine	1%	OTC	C, G	Tinea, *Candida* infections
Tolnaftate	0.07%, 1%	OTC	C, L, O, P, S	Used for fungal skin infections, including tinea
Undecenoic acid/ zinc undecenoate	1%, 5%/25%	OTC	C, L, P	Antifungal and antibacterial agent for athlete's foot and ringworm, with exception of nails and hairy sites; also used for nappy rash, prickly heat, minor skin irritations, jock itch, excessive perspiration and skin irritation in the groin area

OTC = over-the-counter (mainly Schedules 2 [PHARMACY ONLY] and 3 [PHARMACIST ONLY]); Rx = prescription only.
*Formulations: C = cream; G = gel; L = lotion; NV = nail varnish; O = ointment; P = powder; S = spray; T = tincture.

They are very often used in a multitude of skin conditions in which inflammation or immune responses play roles, including various types of dermatitis (eczema) and psoriasis, and in skin reactions to insect bites and sunburn.

The effectiveness of the topical corticosteroids is a result of their anti-inflammatory, antipruritic, vasoconstrictor and immunosuppressant actions. These drugs are discussed in greater detail in Chapter 40 (see Drug Monograph 40-1) and Chapter 55. Topical corticosteroids may also stabilise epidermal lysosomes in the skin, and fluorinated steroids are antiproliferative (antimitotic). Corticosteroids have the advantages of being available in a wide range of topical formulations that are stable, compatible and easy to apply; causing no pain, discoloration or odour on application; and having a broad range of applicability with rapid actions.

Inhalation of corticosteroids (see Drug Monograph 32-4) in treatment and prevention of asthma is a specialised topical application, in this case to the mucous membranes and thence to the smooth muscle of the airways.

Adverse reactions for topical corticosteroids include skin atrophy and striae, acneiform eruptions, contact dermatitis, burning sensations, dryness, itching, hypopigmentation, purpura and haemorrhage, hirsutism (usually facial), folliculitis, alopecia (usually of scalp) and masking or aggravation of fungal infections. If a significant amount of the corticosteroid is absorbed, systemic adverse effects can occur, with the classical cushingoid effects of moon face, fluid retention, skin striae, weak skin and bones, hypertension, immunosuppression, overgrowth of microorganisms leading to secondary infections, glaucoma and poor wound healing.

Vehicle and penetration

Corticosteroids available in topical formulations include betamethasone, methylprednisolone, triamcinolone, hydrocortisone, desonide and mometasone. Fluorinated corticosteroids are particularly recommended for topical application to thickened skin because of their potency, lipid solubility (hence topical actions) and low tendency to cause sodium retention. In decreasing order of potency, some topical corticosteroids are: **betamethasone** dipropionate[f] > betamethasone valerate[f], mometasone, methylprednisolone, triamcinolone[f] > flumethasone[f], desonide[f] > hydrocortisone. (Those marked [f] are fluorinated compounds.)

Acute inflammatory eruptions usually respond to the medium- and low-potency steroids, whereas chronic hyperkeratotic lesions require potent or highly potent drugs.

Types of formulations for topical application of corticosteroids include creams, ointments, lotions and scalp lotions, at various strengths. Combination preparations with antifungal or antibacterial antibiotics are also available for use in inflammatory dermatitis with a large component of infection.

The **vehicle** (aerosol, cream, gel, lotion, ointment, solution or tape) in which the corticosteroid is placed can alter the therapeutic efficacy. Corticosteroid penetration of the skin is enhanced by (in decreasing order of effectiveness) ointments, gels, creams and lotions. As a result of their occlusive nature, ointments hydrate the stratum corneum, enhancing steroid penetration. Lotions, sprays and gels are well suited to hairy areas or for lesions that are oozing and wet. Creams and ointments are well suited to dry, scaling, thickened and pruritic areas.

The rate of transcutaneous penetration after application also influences therapeutic efficacy. It is limited by three factors: the rate of dissolution of the drug in the vehicle, the rate of passive diffusion of the drug across membranes, and the drug penetration rate through the stratum corneum. Inflamed or moist skin absorbs topical steroids to a greater degree than thick or lichenified skin. Occlusive dressings (e.g. using an occlusive ointment base or wrapping in plastic cling-wrap, see Figure 56-3) increase the hydration of the skin and penetration of the drug up to 100-fold, hence systemic adverse effects are possible.

For most topical formulations, the adult dosage is one or two applications daily as directed. Application frequency depends on the site, response of the cutaneous eruption to medication, and application technique.

In some conditions resistant to milder treatment, intralesional injection of corticosteroids is used. Triamcinolone is most often used, injected for example into the lesions of keloid scars, acne cysts or alopecia areata.

Newer immunomodulators

Pimecrolimus is a new calcineurin inhibitor, related to tacrolimus and sirolimus, which are used mainly to prevent

A.
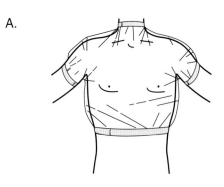

B.
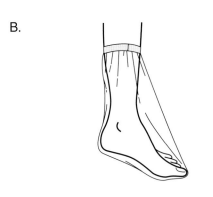

C.
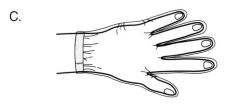

FIGURE 56-3 Examples of occlusive dressing to enhance hydration of particular areas of skin.
A. Plastic wrap applied to upper trunk. **B.** Plastic wrap applied to foot. **C.** Rubber glove applied to hand.

transplant rejection. These agents block T-cell activation and thus prevent release of inflammatory mediators. Pimecrolimus is indicated for short-term or intermittent use in treatment of psoriasis and eczema, applied twice daily as a cream. It can be used safely in children over 3 months, which is a benefit in childhood. Main adverse reactions are local irritation and erythema, and secondary infections.

Two new drugs that bind to lymphocyte receptors and thus interfere with T-lymphocyte activation are the monoclonal antibody efalizumab and the receptor antagonist alefacept. They are immunosuppressants especially indicated in psoriasis. As they are both proteins, they are themselves potentially antigenic and can cause allergic reactions; general suppression of the immune response can lead to secondary infections and possible cancers. Their overall position in the treatment of psoriasis is not yet fully determined

Uses in eczema, psoriasis and urticaria

In treatment of inflammatory dermatoses, many other drugs are used as well as corticosteroids. In **eczema** (also known as **dermatitis**, an inflammatory condition in which skin becomes red, itchy, scaly, moist and blistered), moisturisers are indicated to maintain skin hydration, and tar preparations (coal tar, ichthammol) are used for their antipruritic effects. The potent new immunosuppressant pimecrolimus is second-line therapy after corticosteroids. Antibiotics may be required for infected patches of skin, and antihistamines for relief from itching. UVR therapy and avoidance of triggering factors such as soaps, perfumes and preservatives are also useful.

Psoriasis is a common skin disease characterised by epidermal proliferation and pink–red thickened patches of skin covered with silvery scales, with pain, itching and bleeding. The elbows, knees, buttocks and scalp are most frequently affected. The cause is unknown, although trigger factors include stress, injury, smoking, alcohol, infections and drugs such as some angiotensin-converting enzyme inhibitors, β-blockers, non-steroidal anti-inflammatory drugs (NSAIDs), quinine derivatives and lithium. Drugs used in treatment include those administered for eczema (see above), the psoralens, vitamin D analogues (calcipotriol, calcitriol), a retinoid (acitretin) and, in severe cases, the immunosuppressants cyclosporin and methotrexate (in considerably lower dose than that used in anticancer chemotherapy). The new immunomodulators (see above) are also tried.

Urticaria, or hives, is a common skin condition in which there is transient itchiness, reddening and swelling of the dermis or subcutaneous tissue; angio-oedema may be associated. In about 20% of cases, some precipitating factor may be identifiable, e.g. heat, cold, sun exposure, emotion, drugs or infection. Although a skin condition, urticaria is treated not with topical agents but with systemic antihistamines, corticosteroids, NSAIDs, tricyclic antidepressants or various other drugs. Acute severe angio-oedema is a medical emergency, as airways can become obstructed, and requires treatment with parenteral adrenaline, hydrocortisone, antihistamine and fluids, together with airways support and oxygen.

RETINOIDS AND TREATMENT OF ACNE

Acne vulgaris is a skin disease that involves increased sebum production, abnormal keratinisation leading to the formation of a keratin plug at the base of the pilosebaceous follicle,

proliferation of the bacterium *Propionibacterium acnes*, and inflammation. It affects up to 90% of adolescents and is associated with high androgen levels. Mild acne involves skin comedones ('blackheads'), papules and pustules, and severe acne involves extension of pustules to abscesses, cysts and widespread scarring. There may be significant psychological and emotional trauma associated with the disfigurement caused.

The reduction and removal of sebum and bacteria, specifically *P. acnes*, are the targets of acne vulgaris therapy, along with improvement of the complexion, reduction in scarring and effectively improving the appearance of the individual for psychosocial benefits. Treatment of acne may include (1) removal of keratin plugs, (2) treatment and prevention of infection by *P. acnes*, and (3) decreasing sebum production. There is no clinical evidence of links between diet and acne, although some people note increased skin oiliness after eating particular foods. Excessive skin washing can in fact exacerbate acne by causing skin irritation, as can some cosmetics. There is no 'quick fix' for acne and most treatments need to be continued for many months for significant benefits to be achieved.

Retinoids (vitamin A analogues)

Vitamin A has long been known to be involved in skin physiology, as it has roles in shedding and repair of epithelial tissues, stability of membranes and maintenance of normal growth (see Clinical Interest Box 56-3). Retinoids (analogues of vitamin A) are now drugs of choice in treatment of acne because of their actions modifying cell proliferation and differentiation. They facilitate the extrusion of material from existing comedones and prevent the formation of new lesions.

Topical retinoids

Topical retinoids are used for treating mild acne vulgaris; examples of topical preparations are isotretinoin gel, **tretinoin** gel and cream (Drug Monograph 56-2), and adapalene cream and gel. These medications are contraindicated in pregnancy because of the possibility of birth defects if absorbed. In severe cases of acne, retinoids may be prescribed for oral administration.

Oral retinoids

For treatment of severe cystic acne resistant to milder therapies, systemic drugs may be required. Isotretinoin and acitretin are available in oral formulations (capsules). These products inhibit sebaceous gland activity and thus decrease sebum formation

CLINICAL INTEREST BOX 56-3 VITAMIN A, ACNE AND ANTARCTICA

Vitamin A, or retinol, is a carotenoid substance formed from β-carotene pigments in fruit and vegetables, and also present in some fish oils and animal foods. It is a fat-soluble vitamin required for normal growth, bone formation, retinal function, skin and membrane functions and reproduction.

The recommended daily intake in adults is about 0.75 mg/day, with higher amounts needed by lactating women. Deficiency of vitamin A occurs during malnutrition, in food faddists and people on diets deficient in fats, and in people with disorders of fat absorption and storage. Signs of deficiency include night blindness, corneal opacity and damaged epithelium, with skin becoming dry and infected.

Overdosage and toxicity can occur, particularly in children and elderly people being given herbal remedies laced with vitamin A or taking 'mega-doses' of vitamin supplements. Chronic overdose causes irritability, itchiness, hypertrophy of bone, increased incidence of metaplasia and neoplasia, and cardiotoxicity, whereas acute toxicity causes vomiting, peeling of skin and raised intracranial pressure; deaths have occurred. High doses of retinoids are mutagenic and teratogenic and are contraindicated in pregnancy (Category X).

During the Australian Antarctic expeditions (1911–1914), Sir Douglas Mawson and his companion, Xavier Mertz, suffered from severe malnutrition after their sledge and supplies (and a third member of the team) were lost down a crevasse. Mawson and Mertz were forced to eat the meat from their husky dogs that had died. They became very ill, with layers of skin peeling off, severe diarrhoea, convulsions and headaches; Mertz succumbed but Mawson survived after months of illness. It is thought that they suffered from vitamin A toxicity from eating the livers and fat of the dogs, which would have been fed fish and seal meat that had accumulated vitamin A from plankton in seawater. At the top of the food chain, the men received toxic overdoses of retinoids. Eskimos and Arctic explorers in the northern hemisphere knew from folklore that eating the livers of polar bears or seals was taboo; 100 g has been shown to contain toxic doses of vitamin A.

The acid form, retinoic acid (RA), acts via activation of RA receptors and retinoid X receptors. RA is involved in many biochemical pathways, including liberation of proteolytic enzymes, breakdown of cartilage, synthesis of mucopoly-saccharides and steroids, morphogenesis, differentiation and proliferation of epithelial tissues, induction of neural growth factors and development of the kidneys.

Retinoids have found two important new uses: in acne and psoriasis, and in cancer. Given orally or topically, retinoids act as keratolytics, enhance discharge and drainage of acne pustules, and reduce epithelial proliferation in psoriasis. Retinoids have been shown to have effective anticancer actions in some leukaemias and renal cancers, and are being studied to determine the mechanism of their antineoplastic action, thought to be via inhibition of telomerase enzymes.

Tretinoin emollient cream has been released in the USA to treat facial wrinkles and photoageing caused by the sun. This product contains 0.05% tretinoin and is the first prescription with this indication.
Information on Mawson's expedition from: Howell & Ford 1985.

and secretion, and have keratolytic and anti-inflammatory effects. They are reserved to treat severe acne and have induced prolonged remissions in severe cystic acne.

Women who are pregnant or are planning to become pregnant should not use these preparations. Many spontaneous abortions have been reported, as well as major abnormalities (hydrocephalus, microcephalus and external ear and cardiovascular problems) in the fetus at birth in women who have taken retinoids during pregnancy (see the Pregnancy Safety box). Because of this risk, prescription of oral retinoids is restricted to specialist dermatologists and authorised physicians. Women who are prescribed these drugs must use efficient contraceptive methods for 1 month before starting the treatment, continuously during treatment, and for 1 month (isotretinoin) or 2 years (acitretin) after cessation of treatment. The latter requirement is due to the long half-lives of acitretin (>2 days) and its active metabolite etretinate (>3 months). The use of oral retinoids with topical retinoids is not recommended because additive toxicity may result.

Adverse reactions are as described in Clinical Interest Box 56-3 for overdose and toxicity of vitamin A.

Other acne products
Keratolytics and antiseptics

In mild acne, topical **keratolytics** and antibacterials are the treatments of first choice. Creams and lotions containing benzoyl peroxide and azelaic acid are recommended. Benzoyl peroxide slowly and continuously liberates active oxygen, producing an antibacterial, keratolytic and drying effect. The release of oxygen into the pilosebaceous and comedone area creates unfavourable growth conditions for *P. acnes* and reduces the release of the fatty acids from sebum. The drying vehicle also aids in shrinking the papules or pustules.

Azelaic acid, a straight-chain 9-carbon dicarboxylic acid, is a relatively new topical agent useful in acne. It has antibacterial activity against *P. acnes* and reduces keratinisation. It has also been tried in hyperpigmentary skin disorders and in malignant melanoma. As an acid, it can cause skin irritation (burning, stinging or pruritus) if it is applied on broken skin.

Other measures include avoidance of oil- or alcohol-based cleansers and avoidance of vigorous scrubbing of the skin, as these tend to increase oiliness of the skin. Older medications include formulations with sulfur and resorcinol as keratolytics and mild antimicrobial agents, and antiseptic washes.

DRUG MONOGRAPH 56-2 TRETINOIN ACNE CREAM

Tretinoin, all-trans retinoic acid, is the active metabolite of vitamin A. It is an irritant that stimulates epidermal cell turnover, which causes skin peeling; this reduces the free fatty acids and horny cell adherence within the comedone. It also causes changes in cellular differentiation and reduces keratinisation.

INDICATIONS Tretinoin cream is used in the treatment of acne vulgaris in which comedones, pustules and papules predominate.

PHARMACOKINETICS Topical application of the tretinoin cream to normal skin does not lead to significant absorption of tretinoin. Repeated application over a prolonged period to inflamed skin may cause some transcutaneous absorption.

ADVERSE REACTIONS Adverse reactions of tretinoin are all reversible. They include red and oedematous blisters; crusted, stinging or peeling skin; temporary alterations in skin pigmentation; and increased sensitivity to sunlight.

DRUG INTERACTIONS Concomitant topical use with drying or peeling agents such as benzoyl peroxide, resorcinol, salicylic acid, sulfur, strong soaps and astringents can result in excessive keratolytic and peeling effects. There are additive adverse effects if used with oral

retinoids or with other photosensitising agents, so these combinations should be avoided.

WARNINGS AND CONTRAINDICATIONS Use of tretinoin cream is contraindicated in eczematous skin or if there have been previous hypersensitivity reactions. Because of the risk of birth defects (see above), it rates Pregnancy Safety Classification D. In women of childbearing age, a negative pregnancy test must be confirmed in the 2 weeks before starting treatment. Patients using the cream should be warned about the risk of excessive sunburning effects and advised to use a sunscreen and protective clothing. Contact of the cream with mucous membranes and skin around the eyes and mouth should be avoided.

DOSAGE AND ADMINISTRATION The cream is available in strength 0.05%; an amount of 0.5 g is estimated to contain the equivalent of 250 mcg vitamin A. The cream is applied to the affected areas before retiring at night. A slight exacerbation of the condition may occur at first, but improvement should be noted within 2–3 weeks. Treatment is prolonged for several months to achieve remission of acne.

Tretinoin is also available as 0.025% and 0.1% creams, as a 0.01% gel, and as 10 mg capsules (Pregnancy Safety Category X) for treating promyelocytic leukaemia.

Antibiotics

Topical and systemic **antibiotics** used in the treatment of acne have an unknown mechanism of action. Acne is not an infection nor is it contagious, but *P. acnes* appears to convert comedones to inflamed pustules or papules. Antibiotics may decrease the colonisation of *P. acnes,* thus decreasing the formation of sebaceous fatty acid byproducts and preventing the formation of new acne lesions. The antibiotics used include clindamycin, erythromycin and tetracycline. Topical erythromycin and clindamycin are most commonly prescribed for mild to moderate acne, whereas oral antibiotics (tetracyclines) are generally reserved for individuals with severe acne, and for those who are intolerant or whose acne did not respond to topical agents. Treatment failures have been associated with antibiotic resistance.

Hormones

Because acne is associated with excess androgen production, women with acne can be treated with antiandrogen agents, which reduce sebum secretion. Drugs with antiandrogenic activity include cyproterone acetate and spironolactone (see Chapter 46) and oestrogens, usually prescribed in a combined contraceptive pill type of formulation. It is important

that the preparation not contain an oestrogen with significant androgenic activity.

TREATMENT OF BURNS
Pathophysiology of burns

Burn injuries range from mild and superficial to very severe, with extensive skin loss associated with systemic and metabolic complications. **Burns** can be caused by heat, chemical agents (strong acids or bases) or electricity. The types of burns that result from various sources are relatively specific and diagnostic. Burns cause lesions of the skin accompanied by pain; however, the chief cause of death after burning is shock, which must be anticipated in any effective plan of treatment.

At first, capillary permeability is altered in the injured area: permeability is increased, resulting in a loss of plasma and weeping of the surface tissues. If the burn is extensive, considerable amounts of plasma fluid can be lost in a relatively short time. This depletes the blood volume and causes decreased cardiac output and diminished blood flow. Unless the situation is rapidly brought under control, irreversible shock can result from rapidly developing tissue anoxia, with damage extending to tissues remote from those

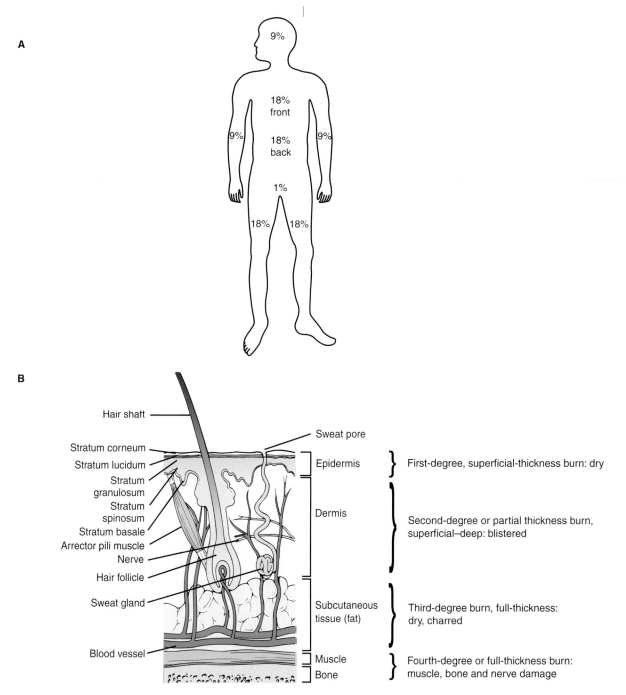

FIGURE 56-4 Extent of body burns: percentage and thickness. **A.** The 'rule of nines' in describing percentage of adult body burned: the head (front and back) and the arms each count as 9%, the front and back of the trunk each count as 18%, each leg as 18%, and the groin area as the remaining 1% of body surface area. **B.** Diagram of layers of skin and subcutaneous tissue, showing definition of burn depth. Thus second-degree burns are those in which the superficial or deep layers of the dermis are damaged, causing blistering.

suffering the initial injury. One of the aims of the treatment of burns is therefore to stop the loss of plasma and to replenish that which is lost as quickly as possible.

The proportion of body surface area affected is estimated by the 'rule of nines' for adults (see Figure 56-4A). If large areas of skin are burnt, there is great danger of infection to the patient; it is estimated that about 75% of people suffering 30% burns or more are likely to die of infection and its consequences.

Burns are classified by degree, which is determined by

the depth of skin involved within a geographic designation (see Figure 56-4B). First-degree or superficial-thickness burns involve only the epidermis, causing erythema with characteristic dry, painful reddening and inflammation (e.g. overexposure to sun or flash burn). Second-degree or partial-thickness burns involve the epidermis extending into the dermis and may be superficial or involve deep dermal necrosis. Epithelial regeneration may extend from the deep skin appendages, such as hair follicles and sebaceous glands, which penetrate the dermis. This burn is characterised by a moist, blistered, very painful surface (e.g. flash or scald burns from non-viscous liquids). Third-degree or full-thickness burns involve destruction of the entire epidermis and dermis and adnexal structures, and are characterised by white, opaque, dry, leathery skin or coagulated, charred skin without sensation as a result of the destruction of nerve endings (e.g. flame burns or hot viscous liquids). Fourth-degree burns extend into subcutaneous fat, muscle or bone, appear black and dry in appearance and cause scarring.

Partial- or full-thickness burns must be thought of as open wounds with the accompanying danger of infection. Normal body flora organisms including *Staphylococcus*, *Candida* and *Pseudomonas* become pathogenic. If the tissue becomes anoxic and necrotic, anaerobic organisms such as *Clostridium tetani* and *C. perfringens* can grow. Mixed infections with multiple organisms occur frequently. The immune system can become suppressed because of injury and shock, with resulting poor defence mechanisms.

Infection must be prevented or treated. The treatment, however, must not cause any further destruction of tissue or of the areas of remaining epithelium from which growth and regeneration can take place or skin grafts be harvested.

The severity of electrical burns depends on the current received, the condition of the skin (e.g. cuts, abrasions and moisture, which lower resistance) and duration of contact, which can be affected by flexor muscles contracting and so inhibiting release from the power source. Electrical burns result in necrosis of more tissue than thermal burns. Chemical burns occur after contact with strong acid or alkali; the initial treatment is water irrigation of the affected area followed by neutralisation.

Management of burns
First-aid treatment of burns

An important first-aid treatment for minor and major burns regardless of cause (chemical, electrical or thermal) is to cool the wound immediately to remove irritants, decrease inflammation and constrict blood vessels; this reduces the permeability of the blood vessels and reduces oedema formation. Cold tap water can be used to flush the wound thoroughly and to cool hot clothing. The more quickly the wound is cooled, the less tissue damage there is likely to be and the more rapid will be the recovery. No greasy ointments, butter or dressings should be applied, because these agents inhibit loss of heat from the burn, which increases both discomfort and tissue damage. The burn can be cleaned and covered with cling wrap or sterile sheet until the person can be transported for medical attention. Major burns need referral to a burns unit (see Clinical Interest Box 56-4).

Drugs used in management of burns patients

Burned patients treated in an emergency room or burns unit are stabilised with intravenous fluids, given analgesics for pain and sedated if necessary; they may require immunisation against tetanus. Catheterisation may be necessary to measure urinary output, depending on the patient's status. After stabilisation, the burn wound is cleaned with a mild soap and water, and a sterile, non-adherent dressing is applied to the wound.

Small, uncontaminated burns that can be adequately dressed do not require topical or oral antimicrobials. **Silver sulfadiazine** was usually preferred because of its broad-spectrum activity and because it is easy and painless to apply and remove from the burn (see Drug Monograph

---

CLINICAL INTEREST BOX 56-4 SPRAY-ON SKIN, A GREAT WESTERN AUSTRALIAN INVENTION

Dr Fiona Wood, Clinical Professor in the School of Paediatrics and Child Health at the University of Western Australia, and plastic surgeon and Head of Royal Perth Hospital's Burns Unit, came to prominence when a large proportion of the survivors of the 2002 Bali bombings arrived at Royal Perth Hospital. Professor Wood led a courageous and committed team to save 28 patients suffering severe burns (from 2% to 92% of body surface area), life-threatening infections and delayed shock.

In her research, Dr Wood had discovered that scarring after burns is markedly reduced if replacement skin can be provided within 10 days; however, previous techniques of skin culturing took 21 days to produce enough cells. With her colleague Dr Marie Stoner, Dr Wood extended the technique from growing sheets of skin cells to culturing a suspension of cells that could be sprayed onto the damaged area, after only 5 days.

Her vision in having developed a plan to cope with large-scale disasters 5 years before the first Bali tragedy, and her exceptional leadership, research and surgical skills, led to Dr Wood being honoured as Australian of the Year for 2005.

Source: www.australianoftheyear.gov.au/bioFW-8678.asp/ accessed 27 January 2006.

DRUG MONOGRAPH 56-3 SILVER SULFADIAZINE

Silver sulfadiazine is the antimicrobial agent of choice in treatment of burns, leg ulcers and pressure sores: it has broad antimicrobial activity against many gram-negative and gram-positive bacteria, and some yeasts and anaerobic bacteria. It combines the antibacterial actions of silver nitrate with those of sulfonamides. It has bacteriostatic actions through inhibition of enzymes involved in folic acid synthesis. Silver sulfadiazine is formulated in an O/W cream, combined with the antiseptic chlorhexidine.

INDICATIONS Silver sulfadiazine is used for prophylaxis and treatment of infections associated with second- and third-degree burns, leg ulcers, pressure sores and extensive denuded areas of skin. It softens eschar, facilitating its removal and preparation of the wound for grafting.

PHARMACOKINETICS When silver sulfadiazine is applied to extensive areas of the body, significant amounts of the drug may be absorbed, reaching therapeutic plasma concentrations and producing adverse reactions characteristic of the sulfonamides. Renal function in these patients should be monitored.

ADVERSE REACTIONS Pain, burning and itching occur infrequently after application of the silver sulfadiazine cream. Hypersensitivity to sulfonamides can occur; if so, the drug should be discontinued.

WARNINGS AND CONTRAINDICATIONS Caution should be observed with extensive use in patients with renal or liver impairment. The cream (initially white) darkens on exposure to light. Sulfonamides can cause kernicterus in babies if used extensively by pregnant women, so silver sulfadiazine is in Pregnancy Category C. It retards re-epithelialisation, so should be discontinued once the wound starts healing.

DOSAGE AND ADMINISTRATION Silver sulfadiazine is available as a 1% cream to be applied topically to cleansed, debrided burn wounds once or twice daily. It should be applied with a spatula or gloved hand to a thickness of about 2–3 mm. Burn wounds should be continuously covered with the cream. Daily bathing and debriding are important and a dressing may or may not be used.

56-3). Povidone-iodine has been used in some centres, and it also penetrates eschar (the dead, separated, damaged skin). Povidone-iodine causes pain on application, however, and hardens the eschar area when dry.

MANAGEMENT OF PRESSURE SORES

Pressure sores

The **pressure sore** (bedsore or decubitus ulcer) is a break in the skin and underlying subcutaneous and muscle tissue caused by abnormal, sustained pressure or friction exerted over the bony prominences of the body by the object on which the body part rests. It results in vascular insufficiency and ischaemic necrosis, and most frequently affects debilitated, immunosuppressed, comatose, immobilised or paralysed patients. The prevalence of pressure ulcers ranges from about 9% in acute care facilities to 33% in critical care patients and those with spinal injuries, and up to 23% in skilled care facilities and nursing homes. In addition to the human suffering of patients and their families, the total cost to the health-care system of treating such wounds is enormous.

There are many causes contributing to this condition that must be addressed. Local and systemic causes include local circulatory impairment, obesity or malnutrition, debilitation, a pressure and shearing force on the lower body if the head of the bed is raised more than 30°, a loss of sensation of

pressure or pain, muscle atrophy and motor paralysis, a reduction in the amount of adipose tissue between skin and underlying bone, emaciation and dehydration, poor nutrition with inadequate intake of vitamins (especially vitamin C) and minerals (such as copper and zinc), friction or trauma, local anatomical defects, oedema or hypertension, infection and septicaemia, and heat and moisture (maceration), e.g. from incontinence.

Pressure sores are classified into four stages or grades (Figure 56-5):

- grade I: a red area of intact skin overlying a bony or tendinous site, which remains even when the pressure is relieved; this is a precursor of ulceration
- grade II: a partial-thickness skin loss involving epidermis and/or dermis
- grade III: full-thickness skin loss (skin ulcer) extending into exposed subcutaneous tissue
- grade IV: deep skin ulcer that exposes muscle and bone; usually the body enzymes separate the eschar and sloughing of tissue results in an ulcer; may include necrotic tissue, sinus tract formation (undermining of the ulcer edge), exudate or infection.

The bacterial flora of pressure sores (present in grades II, III and IV) are both gram-negative and gram-positive organisms, which include *Staphylococcus aureus*, *Streptococcus* groups A and D, *Escherichia coli*, *Clostridium tetani*, and *Bacteroides*, *Proteus*, *Pseudomonas*, *Klebsiella* and *Citrobacter* organisms. Systemic antibiotics are not usually indicated as adequate levels in granulating wounds are not reached, but may be

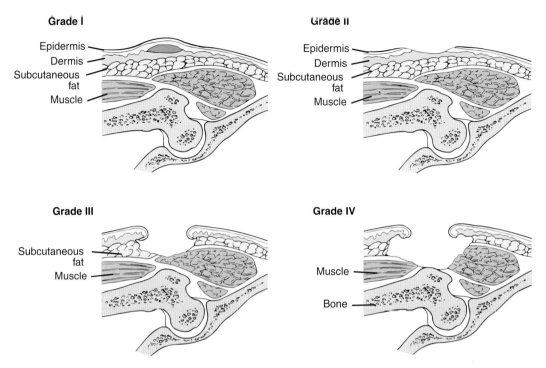

Grade I

Epidermis
Dermis
Subcutaneous
fat
Muscle

Grade II

Epidermis
Dermis
Subcutaneous
fat
Muscle

Grade III

Subcutaneous
fat
Muscle

Grade IV

Muscle

Bone

FIGURE 56-5 The four grades of pressure sore (decubitus ulcer or bedsore), and recommended treatments. In grade IV, the underlying muscle and bone are affected, with the consequent risk of osteomyelitis. The recommended treatment protocols for the four stages are as follows. Grade I or II: silicone or antiseptic spray; transparent or hydrocolloidal dressings. Grade III: wet to dry dressings, enzymatic debridement, hydrocolloidal dressing. Grade IV: wet to dry dressings, enzymatic debridement, surgical debridement.

needed in difficult-to-treat infected pressure sores; for sepsis, osteomyelitis, bacteraemia and advancing cellulitis; and as an adjunct to surgical management. Chronic ulcers may be complicated by increased risk of development of squamous cell carcinomas and of extension to bone, causing osteomyelitis. Wound management has become a specialised area of nursing and podiatry, with many techniques and dressings available (see Carville 2005; Dermatology Expert Group 2004).

Management of pressure sores

Pressure sores, like leg ulcers, are notoriously difficult to treat, and if possible should be prevented by watchful nursing care with frequent turning of bedridden patients and ambulation whenever possible. If ulcers do develop, maximum activity is even more essential to relieve pressure, optimise the muscle pump and venous return, and stimulate circulation.

A treatment plan for pressure sores should take into consideration four basic principles:

- assessment and interventions to improve the patient's general health, which may help to reduce factors contributing to the problem, such as diabetes and other vascular problems, incontinence, anaemia, oedema or nutritional deficiencies

- reduction of pressure sites by positioning or the use of padding, special beds and other supports, thus increasing blood flow to the site
- maintenance of a clean wound site, with dressings and topical antiseptics if necessary
- use of appropriate agents for debriding the wound or stimulation of **granulation tissue** (pink, healthy, soft new tissue).

A person with a full-thickness loss of skin may be a candidate for surgical intervention either to cover the ulcer area or to stabilise the wound. The decision to perform surgery includes the following considerations: the underlying disease, the ability of the patient to withstand surgery, and the condition or prognosis of the pressure sore (especially sores in which subcutaneous tissue is destroyed, exposing bone).

Physical therapies that have been tried include electrical stimulation, infrared and UV radiation, laser therapy and ultrasound. An ancient therapeutic technique gaining renewed interest is that referred to euphemistically as 'biosurgery': the use of living maggots (larvae of insects) as debriding agents. The larvae clean wounds by gently removing necrotic devitalised tissue, thus decreasing the risk of infection and improving healing. This technique is gaining acceptance around the world and is considered safe, efficacious and simple.

Pharmacological management
Topical cleaning of pressure sores

Saline solutions are safe and effective for cleaning most pressure sores. Less mild antiseptics such as povidone-iodine, other iodophors, potassium permanganate and hydrogen peroxide are usually contraindicated because they are reported to be cytotoxic to fibroblasts and thus interfere with the granulation process. Antimicrobials similar to those used in burns (silver sulfadiazine) and bacterial skin infections (mupirocin) may be required.

Dressings

Sterile, non-stick dressings are applied to the ulcer or wound to keep it moist, as moist wounds heal more effectively and faster than dry wounds. Antiseptic dressings include those impregnated with chlorhexidine, povidone-iodine, silver, honey or triclosan; there is also a dressing impregnated with the antibiotic framycetin. Finely powdered sterile gelatin is available for dusting into wounds, where it stimulates the growth of granulation tissue and healing of ulcers; the gelatin protein is gradually resorbed naturally. Packs of sterile calcium alginate fibres are used in bleeding or exuding wounds to act as haemostatics by releasing calcium, filling wounds and aiding coagulation. Unless pain or exudation occurs, dressings can be left on the wound for days or weeks, as constant removal of dressings delays healing. Bioengineered tissue substitutes such as epidermal cells or artificial fibres can help protect wounds and encourage healing.

Debriding agents

Debridement means the cleaning of wounds and removal of **eschar**, or slough, which may be retarding healing and providing a medium for bacterial infection. Before the application of debriding agents, the wound should be thoroughly but gently cleansed to flush away necrotic debris and exudates, with a solution that does not inactivate enzymes (preferably normal saline or sterile distilled water). All previously applied topical preparations should be removed before the new agent is applied. Slough may need to be removed surgically.

Dextranomers are hydrophilic beads placed in the wound to absorb exudate, bacteria and other matter. The preparation is used for cleansing a wet or secreting wound (not dry wounds) and the action continues until all the beads are saturated. The assumption of a greyish-yellow colour by the beads indicates that they are saturated and ready for removal. Therapy with dextranomer is continued until healthy granulation is evident. Patients who have diabetes mellitus or immunosuppression

need to be closely monitored as they are more susceptible to the development of severe infections.

Metronidazole is an antibacterial agent used systemically to treat stage III and IV decubitus ulcers infected with anaerobic bacteria. (A topical metronidazole gel is used to treat acne rosacea in adults.)

PREGNANCY SAFETY

Category	Drug
A	Chlorhexidine, clindamycin (topical), most corticosteroids (topical), erythromycin, nystatin
B1	Azelaic acid, calcipotriol, mupirocin
B2	Crotamiton, dithranol, maldison (malathion), methoxsalen, permethrin, pyrethrins
B3	Amorolfine and other imidazoles, pimecrolimus
C	Alefacept, efalizumab, minoxidil (topical), silver sulfadiazine
D	Adapalene, isotretinoin (topical), tetracyclines,# tretinoin
X	Acitretin, isotretinoin (systemic)
Unlisted	Aluminium solutions, benzoyl peroxide, calamine preparations, ichthammol and other tar products, pyrithione zinc, resorcinol, selenium sulfide, sulfur products, zinc oxide preparations

Tetracyclines are generally safe during the first 18 weeks of pregnancy; after this they may cause yellowish discoloration of the baby's teeth.

DRUGS AT A GLANCE 56: Drugs treating skin disorders

Therapeutic group	Pharmacological group	Key examples	Key pages
Sunscreens	UV absorbers	PABA derivatives, cinnamates	911–4
	UV reflectors	zinc oxide, titanium dioxide	
Antimicrobials (topical)			
Antibacterials	Aminoglycosides (bacterial protein synthesis imhibitors)	neomycin	914, 5
	Bacterial cell wall synthesis inhibitors	bacitracin	
Antivirals		aciclovir	915
Antifungals	Imidazoles	clotrimazole, ketoconazole	916
	Sterol synthesis inhibitors	amorolfine	916–8
		terbinafine	916, 8
Drugs treating lice or mite infestations	Pediculocides	permethrin, maldison	916, 7
	Scabicides	permethrin	917
Anti-inflammatory agents	Corticosteroids	betamethasone, triamcinolone	917–9
	Calcineurin inhibitors	pimecrolimus	919, 20
Acne treatments	Retinoids	isotretinoin	920, 1
		tretinoin	920–2
	Miscellaneous antiacne agents	benzoyl peroxide, azelaic acid	921, 2
Burns treatments	Antibacterials	silver sulfadiazine	924, 5
Pressure sore treatments	Antiseptics	chlorhexidine	927
	Debriding agents	dextranomers	

Note: Non-specific agents such as antipruritics, antiseptics, astringents, cleansers, keratolytics, tars and wart treatments are not included in this table.
PABA = p-aminobenzoic acid; UV = ultraviolet light.

KEY POINTS

- The skin, combined with its exocrine glands, hair and nails, forms the integumentary system; skin consists of two main layers (the epidermis and dermis) plus the subcutaneous tissue.

- The main function of the skin is defence: it serves as a barrier to the external environment. It also contains sensory nerve endings, synthesises vitamin D and helps in body temperature regulation.

- The skin serves as the site for topical drug application for the treatment of a variety of dermatological problems, and can be used as the site of administration of lipid-soluble drugs intended for transcutaneous absorption and systemic actions.

- Penetration of topical drugs into the skin, and absorption through the skin, are affected by the age, condition, hydration and site of skin; the metabolism and skin circulation; and the vehicle in which the drug is formulated.

- A wide variety of pathological conditions affect the skin; most are due to infection, excessive inflammatory or immune responses, or reactions to sun exposure. Examples are fungal and viral infections, acne vulgaris, eczema and dermatitis, psoriasis, urticaria, sunburn and skin cancers.

- Drugs, given either topically or systemically, can cause adverse reactions in the skin, in particular urticaria, purpura, fixed eruptions, dermatitis or eczema, and photosensitisation.

- There are numerous formulations available as vehicles for administration of drugs to the skin; such preparations include creams and ointments, lotions and solutions, skin protectants and emollients, wet dressings and soaks, rubs and liniments, pastes, patches, powders and sprays. Many are available over the counter, contain several ingredients and may have little clinically proven efficacy.

- Therapeutic agents applied topically for actions on or in the skin include sunscreens, antimicrobials (antibiotics, antivirals, antifungals and ectoparasiticidal drugs), corticosteroids and other immunosuppressants, keratolytics, acne products, burn products, antipruritics, and wound dressings and treatments for skin ulcers and pressure sores. Understanding the effects of topical agents is important in the care of patients with skin disorders.

- Exposure to the sun, in particular to ultraviolet radiation in the UVB wavelength range, causes major harm to the skin, ranging from sensitisation, allergies, ageing, reddening and burning through to benign and malignant skin cancers.

- Chemicals used in sunscreens may act by either absorbing particular UVR (e.g. aminobenzoates and benzophenones) or reflecting UVR (zinc cream). Sunscreens are given SPF numbers, indicating their protective capacities; people who burn easily should use a product with SPF15+ or 30+.

- Antimicrobials used topically for skin infections should be those that are not administered systemically; antibacterial antibiotics frequently prescribed for topical use include bacitracin, neomycin and mupirocin. For herpes simplex viral infections, aciclovir and idoxuridine are available topically.

- Fungal skin infections, particularly of moist areas of skin or of finger- and toenails, can be difficult to eradicate. Many topical preparations of antifungals are available; examples are the imidazoles, and terbinafine and amorolfine. Severe infections may require systemic antifungal therapy.

- Skin infections with insects (lice and mites) cause severe itching; permethrin can be applied as a shampoo, lotion or cream.

- Because many dermatological conditions such as dermatitis and urticaria have an inflammatory or immune component, the corticosteroids are commonly used topically for their anti-inflammatory and immunosuppressant effects, in ointments, creams and lotions. Fluorinated steroids such as betamethasone are particularly effective. Hydration of skin, e.g. by use of occlusive dressings or ointments, markedly enhances absorption of corticosteroids, which improves actions but increases the risk of systemic adverse effects.

- New immunomodulators such as pimecrolimus are being used in eczema and psoriasis.

- Psoriasis may require treatment with more potent immunosuppressants, including the cytotoxic agents cyclosporin and methotrexate.

- Acne vulgaris may be alleviated by topical treatment with skin cleansers, keratolytics, antibiotics and hormones, or topical retinoids such as isotretinoin. Severe cases of acne may require oral retinoids, which carry the risk of teratogenesis and must not be prescribed in women of childbearing age without adequate contraception being assured.

- When large areas of skin are burned, there is severe risk of infection and shock. Fluid replacement is critical, and topical silver sulfadiazine is the antibacterial agent of choice in early stages of treatment.

- The best treatment for pressure sores (decubitus ulcers) is prevention, as when they do occur they are painful, cause necrosis and osteomyelitis, and may require prolonged extensive care and hospitalisation. Wound dressings impregnated with antimicrobial agents or adsorbent particles are used, as are also proteolytic enzyme preparations or insect larvae.

REVIEW EXERCISES

1. Describe how the skin protects the individual from a high temperature on a hot summer day. What other protections are required? Explain their mechanisms of action.

2. What other protective functions are provided by the skin?

3. What is the pH of normal skin? How does this affect microbial growth?

4. Describe the structure of the layers of the skin, and how drugs applied to the skin are repelled or absorbed by these layers.

5. List commonly used types of formulations applied to the skin, with possible advantages and indications for different preparations.

6. List the types of drugs commonly used for treatment of dermatological conditions, and describe their pharmacological actions and mechanisms of action.

7. Define the sun protection factor (SPF) and how it is derived. What are the definitions of water-resistant and very water-resistant sunscreen products? What are the practical implications of these terms? What sunscreen SPF would you recommend for a person who burns easily and never tans?

8. Describe the main antibacterial, antiviral, antifungal and antiparasitic agents used in skin infections.

9. Discuss the pharmacology of corticosteroids administered topically.

10. List the main groups of drugs used in the treatment of psoriasis, urticaria, dermatitis (eczema) and acne, comparing their actions and uses.

11. Discuss first-aid treatment of minor and major burns, explaining the rationale. Name one important drug used to treat burns and describe its mechanism of action, directions and adverse effects.

12. Discuss the physiological and pharmacological actions of vitamin A derivatives, including their adverse effects and precautions required for clinical use.

13. Describe the four stages of classification for pressure sores, and the types of care and medications appropriate for the different stages.

14. Discuss and compare the various agents used for debridement of pressure ulcers.

REFERENCES AND FURTHER READING

Anti-Cancer Council of Victoria. *Cancer in Victoria 1996*. Canstat 28, Sept 1999. Melbourne: Anti-Cancer Council of Victoria, 1999.

Australian Drug Evaluation Committee. *Prescribing Medicines in Pregnancy: An Australian Categorisation of Risk of Drug Use in Pregnancy*. 4th edn. Canberra: Therapeutic Goods Administration, 1999.

Australian Institute of Health and Welfare & Australasian Association of Cancer Registries. *Cancer in Australia 2001*. Canberra: AIHW, 2004. Available: www.aihw.gov.au/publications/index.cfm/title/10083/ accessed 27 January 2006.

Australian Medicines Handbook 2005. Adelaide: AMH, 2005.

Beare PG, Myers JL. *Adult Health Nursing*. 3rd edn. St Louis: Mosby, 1998.

Bellamy D, Pfister A. *World Medicine: Plants, Patients and People*. Oxford: Blackwell, 1992.

Braun L, Cohen M. *Herbs and Natural Supplements: An Evidence-Based Guide*. Sydney: Elsevier Mosby, 2005.

Carville K. *Wound Care Manual*. Osborne Park, WA: Silver Chain Nursing Association, 2005.

Caswell A (ed.). *MIMS Annual June 2005*. Sydney: CMPMedica Australia, 2005.

Cervo FA, Cruz AC, Posillico JA. Pressure ulcers: analysis of guidelines for treatment and management. *Geriatrics* 2000; 55: 55–60.

Commens C. The treatment of scabies. *Australian Prescriber* 2000; 23: 33–5.

Dermatology Expert Group. *Therapeutic Guidelines: Dermatology, version 2*. Melbourne: Therapeutic Guidelines Limited, 2004.

DeSimone EM II. Sunscreen and suntan products. In: Covington TR (ed.). *Handbook of Nonprescription Drugs*. 11th edn. Washington, DC: American Pharmaceutical Association, 1996.

Duffull S. Facing up to acne. *Australian Pharmacy Trade* 2001; 8 March: 18–20.

Gies PH, Roy CR, Toomey S, McLennan A. Protection against solar ultraviolet radiation. *Mutation Research* 1998; 422: 15–22.

Habif TP, Campbell JL, Dinulos JGH, Chapman MS, Zug KA. *Skin Disease: Diagnosis and Treatment*, 2nd edn. Philadelphia: Elsevier Mosby, 2005.

Howell M, Ford P. *Medical Mysteries*. London: Viking, 1985.

Katelaris C. Treatment of urticaria. *Australian Prescriber* 2001; 24: 124–6.

Klasen HJ. A historical review of the use of silver in the treatment of burns. II. Renewed interest for silver. *Burns* 2000; 26: 131–8.

MacLellan DG. Chronic wound management. *Australian Prescriber* 2000; 23: 6–9.

Roth JJ. *The Essential Burn Unit Handbook*. St Louis: Quality Medical Publishers, 2004.

Sauder DN. Mechanism of action and emerging role of immune response modifier therapy in dermatologic conditions. *Journal of Cutaneous Medicine and Surgery* 2004; 8 Suppl. 3: 3–12.

Shargel L, Mutnick AH, Souney PF, Swanson LN, Block LH. *Comprehensive Pharmacy Review*. 3rd edn. Baltimore: Williams & Wilkins, 1997.

Sherman RA, Hall MJ, Thomas S. Medicinal maggots: an ancient remedy for some contemporary afflictions. *Annual Review of Entomology* 2000; 45: 55–81.

Speight TM. *MIMS Disease Index*. Sydney: IMS Publishing, 1996.

Stewart K. A case for counselling: treating atopic eczema. *Australian Pharmacy Trade* 2001; 8 March: 22–5.

Sullivan JR. Oral isotretinoin. *Australian Prescriber* 2005; 28(3): 59–91.

Tortora GJ, Grabowski SR. *Principles of Anatomy and Physiology*. 9th edn. New York: HarperCollins, 2000.

van de Kerkhof PC. New developments in the treatment of psoriasis. *Skin Pharmacology and Applied Skin Physiology* 2001; 14: 129–35.

Wargon O. Treating head lice. *Australian Prescriber* 2000; 23: 62–3.

Webster G. Combination azelaic acid therapy for acne vulgaris. *Journal of the American Academy of Dermatology* 2000; 43 (2 Pt 3): S47–50.

Youngson RM (ed.) *Collins Dictionary: Medicine*. 2nd edn. Glasgow: HarperCollins, 1998.

ON-LINE RESOURCES

Website for checking NZ drugs: http://www.medsafe.govt.nz/ accessed 31 January 2006.

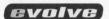 More weblinks at http://evolve.elsevier.com/AU/Bryant/pharmacology/

CHAPTER 57

Drugs in Sport

CHAPTER FOCUS

Competitors in sporting events often use drugs or other methods in attempts to enhance their performance; this is usually seen as unfair and potentially dangerous. Equally, competitors with medical conditions may require drugs to treat their condition and allow them to compete to their best ability. In this chapter, the use and abuse of drugs in sport is reviewed. The drug groups prohibited or restricted by the World Anti-Doping Agency (WADA) are considered, with their possible advantages and disadvantages. The procedures for testing for drugs in athletes' urine or blood samples are described briefly, and ethical issues related to the use of doping methods in sport are also discussed. (*Note:* For full details of drugs prohibited or restricted, and legal levels in bodily fluids, consult the latest WADA listing, available at: www.wada-ama.org/en/)

OBJECTIVES

- To discuss the use in sport of banned substances or methods to enhance performance, the rationales for their use, possible disadvantages and related ethical issues.

- To review the pharmacology of the main groups of drugs prohibited by the World Anti-Doping Agency: anabolic agents, anti-oestrogens, B_2 agonists, diuretics and masking agents, narcotic analgesics, hormones and analogues, cannabinoids and stimulants.

- To describe the blood doping and sample manipulation methods that are banned.

- To consider the clinical use and abuse in sport of erythropoietin (EPO) and the methods of testing for EPO use.

- To review the drugs (alcohol, beta-blockers), substances and methods that are restricted or permitted in particular situations in sport.

- To consider the use of ergogenic aids, dietary manipulation, and complementary and alternative therapies as possible performance-enhancing methods.

- To describe the WADA rules for the procedures for doping controls.

KEY DRUGS

amphetamines
anabolic steroids
B_2 agonists
clenbuterol
erythropoietin
growth hormone
stimulants
testosterone

KEY TERMS

blood doping
doping
drug testing
ergogenic aids
erythropoiesis
ethical issues
manipulation of samples
permitted drugs
prohibited methods
prohibited substances
restricted substances
specified substances
World Anti-Doping Agency

KEY ABBREVIATIONS

AAS	anabolic androgenic steroid
ASADA	Australian Sports Anti-Doping Authority
ASDA	Australian Sports Drug Agency
E	epitestosterone
EPO	erythropoietin
GH	growth hormone
IOC(MC)	International Olympic Committee (Medical Commission)
IU	International Unit
T	testosterone
TUE	Therapeutic Use Exemption
WADA	World Anti-Doping Agency

THE desire to excel in sport, and the pressure to win at all costs, may lead athletes to experiment with taking substances or using methods that are perceived to provide such advantages as improved strength, motor coordination, endurance or concentration.

It is not a recent phenomenon for athletes participating in sporting competitions to use drugs or magic potions in attempts to gain an advantage or improve performance. The Greek physician Galen, writing in the first century AD, reported athletes at the ancient Olympic Games using stimulants and special diets (including dried figs) to enhance performance. The ancient Egyptians used a drink made from ground and boiled hooves of asses (probably rich in gelatine and other proteins) and flavoured with roses, while in Roman times gladiators used stimulants to help recovery after injury.

In the 19th century, swimmers, cyclists and long-distance runners used stimulants, especially strychnine, caffeine and cocaine. Not surprisingly, many athletes died after taking such cocktails, which provided the impetus to control the abuse of drugs in sport. In the mid-20th century, the drugs most commonly abused were amphetamines, after their widespread use during World War II among military personnel to increase alertness and reduce fatigue. Cyclists on amphetamines died in the 1960 Olympic Games and the 1967 Tour de France. Abuse of anabolic steroids came to prominence in the 1950s in America among bodybuilders, weightlifters and footballers. Amphetamines and anabolic steroids are still widely abused despite more sophisticated detection methods.

There is in fact little hard scientific evidence of significant beneficial effects of many of the drugs or methods used; however, athletes and coaches often put great faith in the perceived efficacy of drugs while ignoring their proven adverse effects (see Clinical Interest Box 57-2). It is important that double-blind placebo-controlled clinical trials be run on the safety and efficacy of drugs in athletes, but there are major logistical and ethical problems—not least that athletes trialling banned drugs would be liable to sanctions and prohibition from sporting competition.

Doping is defined as the use in sport of substances and/or methods prohibited under that sport's rules, to enhance performance or mask banned behaviours. Doping practices are prohibited in sport because it is generally agreed that doping can artificially enhance sports performance, contravenes the ethics of both sport and medical science, and can be detrimental to the health of athletes.

The IOC and WADA codes

The International Olympic Committee (IOC) over the years promulgated a medical code that listed classes of prohibited substances and methods of doping, as the basis of its doping policy. Recently, the **World Anti-Doping Agency** (WADA) assumed responsibility for doping control at the international level from the IOC. The national sporting organisations of

> ### CLINICAL INTEREST BOX 57-1
> ### SOME RECENT DOPING-IN-SPORT CASES
>
> Many cases of doping in sport have become infamous:
> - Some female athletes from the former German Democratic Republic, whose swag of gold medals has never been equalled by a single nation, later admitted their success had been due to prescribing of anabolic steroids by official doctors.
> - Canadian Ben Johnson forfeited the Olympic gold medal for the 100 metres sprint after testing positive for the anabolic steroid stanozolol in Seoul, 1988.
> - Some members of the Chinese swimming team were apprehended at the World Championships in Perth in 1998 with unlicensed quantities of growth hormone.
> - The 1996 Olympic Irish triple-gold-medallist swimmer Michelle Smith was later disqualified for 4 years for manipulating urine samples.
> - The debacle of the 1998 Tour de France saw widespread drug taking detected, with seven cycling teams pulling out and one stage being cancelled.
> - An Australian pentathlete recorded excessive blood levels of caffeine in the 1988 Olympics, and was sent home. (Caffeine is no longer banned.)
> - A young 2000 Olympic gold-medal gymnast tested positive to pseudoephedrine and had her gold medal rescinded.
> - The Australian spin bowler Shane Warne was banned for 1 year for taking a combination diuretic tablet (amiloride plus hydrochlorothiazide); a simple check in MIMS or on the ASDA website would have shown it to contain two banned diuretics.

most countries adopt WADA's policies and classifications of 'Prohibited Substances and Methods in Doping'. The WADA code classifies drugs and methods into four main groups: those banned at all times (in- and out-of-competion), those banned only in-competition, those called restricted (banned only in particular sports), and those which are not banned but are 'specified' as being particularly likely to lead to inadvertent violations. WADA also regulates the approval of therapeutic use in sport of drugs that would otherwise be banned. The list is updated annually; the onus is always on the athlete to ensure that any substance taken is approved for use in sport; ignorance is no excuse for a violation.

The classes of drugs and methods that come under bans or restrictions include:
- anabolic agents (steroids, B$_2$ agonists)
- anti-oestrogens
- diuretics and other masking agents
- narcotics*
- some hormones and analogues
- glucocorticosteroids*
- stimulants*

- cannabinoids*
- blood doping (enhancement of oxygen transfer)
- sample manipulation
- gene doping
- alcohol and beta-blockers, prohibited only in certain sports.

(* These drugs are prohibited in-competition but allowed out-of-competition; other substances and methods are prohibited at all times.)

The presence of a prohibited substance or its metabolite or marker in a bodily specimen is a violation of the WADA rules, as are using, attempting to use, possessing or trafficking in a prohibited substance. Recommending, facilitating or authorising use of these doping drugs and methods are also prohibited. Refusing to submit to a test, unavailability for testing or interfering with testing procedures are also violations.

It is recognised that in some cases there may be a medical requirement for an athlete to take particular drugs; for example, people with diabetes cannot stop using insulin, nor can those with asthma be expected to go without bronchodilators. In these situations, athletes are strongly advised to check with their national sporting association for approval procedures (such as applying for a Therapeutic Use Exemption), to take only medications prescribed by a doctor familiar with the WADA rules, and to ensure that the preparations they take do not contain prohibited or restricted substances.† When an athlete is required to provide a sample (urine or blood) for doping control, it is essential that all medications administered in the previous three days be declared on the official record.

The sanctions (penalties) applied to athletes testing positive to banned substances range from an initial warning to a 4-year ban for a first offence, and a possible life ban for subsequent offences.

The Australian Sports Anti-Doping Authority

Australia's anti-doping program in relation to drugs in sport is administered by the Australian Sports Anti-Doping Authority (ASADA), which was established in 2006. ASADA is an integrated anti-doping organisation with functions outlined in the *Australian Sports Anti-Doping Authority Act 2006* (Cth) and the *Australian Sports Anti-Doping Authority Regulations 2006* (Cth).

On its creation, ASADA assumed the drug testing, education and advocacy roles that were previously the mandate of the

---

†There have been many cases of athletes testing positive for drugs, being banned from competition and even having Olympic gold medals removed after taking cough and cold cures or headache tablets given them by 'well-meaning' coaches, family or friends (see Clinical Interest Box 57-1).

Australian Sports Drug Agency (ASDA) and also the functions of the Australian Sports Drug Medical Advisory Committee. ASADA has the power to investigate suspected violations of the Anti-Doping Rules, make recommendations on its findings, and present cases against alleged offenders at sport tribunals. ASADA is also empowered to exchange sensitive information with the Australian Customs Service and the Australian Federal Police.

DRUGS AND METHODS BANNED IN SPORTS

International lists of banned and restricted substances and methods are published (see for example in Australia in the early pages of *MIMS Annual* under General Medical and Scientific Information). Because the lists cannot include every **prohibited substance** by every name used in every country, drugs are listed by class, and the term 'and related substances' or 'includes but is not limited to' is often added to embrace all substances having similar structures or actions. (The pharmacology of all these drugs is discussed in detail in earlier chapters.)

Substances prohibited at all times
Anabolic androgenic steroids

Examples of **anabolic androgenic steroids** (AASs) are testosterone, androstenedione, stanozolol, nandrolone, fluoxymesterone, 5-α-dihydrotestosterone, boldenone and dehydroepiandrosterone (DHEA). These are similar to the natural androgenic hormone testosterone (see Drug Monograph 46-1). The male sex hormones have physiological actions in promoting tissue growth and repair (anabolic effects) and in maintaining the male sex organs and characteristics (androgenic actions). Synthetic formulations are widely abused by both men and women, in conjunction with high-protein diets and intensive training, to increase muscle strength and body weight, to maximise the effects of training, to enhance appearance and to improve the chances of winning in sports. Use of AASs in the USA has been estimated to be as high as 80% in weightlifters and bodybuilders, while use overall by competitors in strength, power and endurance sports may be as high as 50%. Many users continue to abuse AASs despite knowing about and suffering from the adverse reactions (see Clinical Interest Box 57-2).

Athletes often use the drugs in amounts far in excess (10–100-fold) of the recommended dosages. 'Stacking' of drugs (taking multiple anabolic steroids at one time) is a practice used by some. 'Pyramiding' refers to starting with a low dose, increasing gradually to high doses, then dropping

Users (past, present and potential) of **anabolic androgenic steroids** (AASs) were invited to attend anonymously a clinic at an inner-city Sydney hospital, specifically to study their AAS use by questionnaire and physical examination. The 58 men reported:

- cyclical use of both human and veterinary AAS by oral and IM routes
- commonest sources of the drugs: friends (59%), gymnasia (25%), doctors (14%)
- commonest reported adverse drug reactions: altered libido (61%), changes in mood (48%), reduced testis volume (46%), acne (43%)
- physical examinations showing gynaecomastia in 49% of users and abnormal liver function tests in 68%.

The conclusions from the study were that the majority of AAS users experienced serious adverse effects; however, after discussion of the results, only 19% of the men reported that they would not use AASs in the future. (O'Sullivan et al 2000).

back to lower doses to avoid detection by doping control tests during competition. AASs are readily detectable in urine but, as androgens are natural body hormones, their levels vary. If levels of endogenous AAS hormones exceed those likely to occur naturally, further testing is required.

As **testosterone** (T) is convertible in the body to oestrogens, there may be adverse oestrogenic effects of T in men, including hypercalcaemia, infertility, gynaecomastia and decreased gonadotrophin production. Anti-oestrogens such as tamoxifen are sometimes taken in an attempt to reverse these effects; these are also banned (see below). The general public, and particularly those who work out at gymnasiums and are confronted with the abuse of steroids, should be informed of the potential serious health problems, especially for women and adolescent males, associated with short-term and long-term consumption of anabolic steroids (see Box 57-1).

Advocates of steroid use claim that AASs boost muscle bulk and strength, while antidrug campaigners believe that the steroids merely engender feelings of aggression that encourage the person to train harder, and have serious adverse effects. There is little objective scientific evidence of positive effects of AASs on performance in athletes. The disqualification of Olympic athletes for using steroids, along with the many undesirable and harmful effects reported from their use, has led to an increase in regulation of this category of drugs. The concentration in a urine sample of a natural but inactive male steroid epitestosterone (E) is used to monitor abuse of AAS: if the T/E ratio is greater than 4, this is taken as evidence that T levels have been artificially increased by administration of exogenous hormone.

Anti-oestrogens

Anti-oestrogens such as tamoxifen and toremifene, and aromatase inhibitors (anastrazole and exemestane), are used clinically in treatment of breast cancers. They may be abused in sport in attempts to overcome some of the adverse feminising effects of AAS, such as gynaecomastia. Previously banned only in men, they are now banned in both sexes. (The pharmacology of these drugs is discussed in Chapters 46, 47 and 49.)

B_2-adrenoceptor agonists

B2 agonists such as salbutamol (see Drug Monograph 32-2) and eformoterol are usually administered by inhalation for their bronchodilator effects in asthma. They also, however, have anabolic actions through stimulation of β receptors, including increased glycogenolysis, hyperglycaemia, lipolysis and heat production. They have therefore been abused in sport to increase lean body mass and decrease body fat. There is no evidence that β_2 agonists such as **clenbuterol** alter athletic performance or strength in healthy people; there are, however, reports of sudden deaths in bodybuilders taking the drugs.

These drugs are unusual in that they are classified as both stimulants and anabolics. The 'stimulant' effects are those due to stimulation of β_1-adrenoceptors in the heart, i.e. increased rate and force of contraction; there may also be effects in skeletal muscle, such as increased rate of contraction, but muscle tremor and cramps are unhelpful in many sports. Systemic β_2 agonists are prohibited in sports when administered by oral or parenteral routes.

It is recognised that β_2 agonists are essential therapy for asthma. Some (currently four: eformoterol, salbutamol, salmeterol, terbutaline) are therefore permitted for use by inhalation for registered asthmatics, after approval of a Therapeutic Use Exemption (TUE).* It has been shown that about 90% of a dose of inhaled aerosol is actually swallowed, then absorbed from the gastrointestinal tract, so the distinction here between inhaled and oral agents is probably very tenuous.

With respect to doping control testing, a urinary salbutamol concentration higher than 1000 ng/mL counts as a positive result for an anabolic agent even if a TUE has been granted. A standard 'puffer' delivers a 100 mcg dose of salbutamol; it can be calculated from salbutamol pharmacokinetic data that to record a positive test result for salbutamol from an inhaler, an athlete would have to administer about 12–14 puffs within a short space of time. This would certainly cause significant systemic adverse effects such as palpitations, tremor and hypokalaemia.

*The cynics would (and do) say that in some sports there are many more participants registered as asthmatics than would be predicted by epidemiological data.

BOX 57-1 MAJOR EFFECTS AND ADVERSE REACTIONS OF ANABOLIC STEROIDS

Androgenic effects
- Increased growth and development of the seminal vesicles and prostate gland
- Increased body and facial hair
- Increased production of oil from the sebaceous glands
- Deepening of the voice
- Increased sexual interest and desire

Anabolic effects
- Increased organ and skeletal muscle mass
- Increased calcium in bones
- Increased retention of total body nitrogen
- Increased haemoglobin concentration
- Increased protein synthesis

Adverse reactions
Females
- Oily skin, acne
- Decrease in breast size, ovulation, lactation or menstruation
- Hoarse and deep voice tone (usually irreversible)
- Clitoral enlargement
- Unusual hair growth and/or male-type baldness (usually irreversible)
- If pregnant: fetal damage

Males
- Increased penis size, and enhanced secondary male characteristics
- Baldness
- Priapism (continuing erections), difficult/increased urination
- Increase in breast size (gynaecomastia)
- Testicular atrophy, oligospermia, impotence, infertility

Both sexes
- Hypercalcaemia, urinary calculi
- Cardiovascular disease, oedema of feet or legs
- Jaundice, liver impairment; liver carcinoma (rare)
- Hypersensitivity
- Acne, tendon rupture
- Insomnia; mood swings: depression, paranoia, aggression ('roid rage')
- Iron-deficiency anaemia
- Nausea, vomiting, anorexia, stomach pains
- Increased risk of tumours

Hormones and related substances

Many peptide hormones and related substances have been abused in sport for their growth-promoting or anabolic effects. Some are banned only in men. Where relevant, the appropriate hypothalamic-releasing factor or its analogues are also banned; thus growth hormone (GH; somatotrophin), its analogues such as somatropin, and the GH-releasing factor somatorelin are all banned. Glucocorticosteroids are classified by WADA as a separate group.

The WADA rules stipulate that the detection in urine of an abnormal concentration of any of the banned hormones or their diagnostic markers constitutes an offence unless it can be conclusively proven to be solely due to a physiological or pathological condition (or, in the case of insulin, the person is registered as having insulin-dependent diabetes). Examples of banned hormones are:

- gonadotrophins, such as human chorionic gonadotrophin (hCG; Drug Monograph 43-1), banned in men because of their actions in increasing the rate of production of endogenous androgenic steroids and reducing the testicular damage from anabolics
- corticotrophin (ACTH) and the analogue tetracosactrin, used to raise blood levels of glucocorticoids and hence improve mood and induce the gluconeogenic, lipolytic and anti-inflammatory effects
- **growth hormone**, banned because its use in sport is considered unethical and dangerous (see discussion in Chapter 38 and Drug Monograph 38-1). The Atlanta Olympics in 1996 were nicknamed the 'growth hormone Games' because of suspicions of widespread abuse of GH there. At the time of the Sydney 2000 Olympic Games, there was no accepted test for GH abuse, despite many years and millions of dollars of research, and tall and large athletes had to defend themselves against innuendo.* By the 2004 Athens Olympics, testing methods had been developed such that abuse of GH in the previous 84 days could be identified.
- insulin-like growth factors (somatomedins, e.g. IGF-1), which are stimulated by GH and mediate many of its anabolic actions, hence are considered likely to be abused and are prohibited. Insulin (Drug Monograph 41-1) is the body's fuel-conserving hormone and so is likely to be abused for its anabolic actions, often in association with anabolic steroids. It is permitted in sport for use by those registered as having diabetes, after approval of a TUE.

Erythropoietin

Erythropoietin (EPO; epoetin) is a glycoprotein hormone produced naturally in the kidney and liver when tissue hypoxia occurs. Its main physiological function is to bind to receptors on red blood cell (RBC) precursors in the bone marrow and increase production of RBCs (**erythropoiesis**) and oxygen-carrying capacity. EPO and a long-acting derivative, darbepoetin, are indicated for pharmacological treatment of

---

*Champion Australian swimmer Ian Thorpe offered to donate a blood sample to be kept frozen until GH testing is accurate and accepted, to clear his name of suggestions of GH abuse due to his large 'flipper' feet.

DRUG MONOGRAPH 57-1 EPOETIN ALFA

Epoetin alfa (EPO) is the approved name for a form of human **erythropoietin** produced by recombinant technology from Chinese hamster cell lines. It is a glycoprotein hormone, normally produced by the kidneys, that acts as a colony-stimulating factor, stimulating erythropoiesis in anaemic patients with chronic renal failure in whom normal synthesis of EPO is impaired. The increase in number of mature RBCs takes several days to occur; the subsequent rise in haemoglobin levels may not be significant for 2–10 weeks. EPO improves energy levels and exercise performance, and reduces fatigue and the need for blood transfusions.

INDICATIONS The cause of anaemia should be investigated and other possible treatments tried before EPO therapy is initiated. The indications for therapeutic use of EPO are in prevention and treatment of anaemia associated with chronic renal failure, anaemia following chemotherapy in patients with non-myeloid malignancies, and anaemia in patients scheduled for elective surgery with an expected blood loss, to increase yield of autologous blood donations.

PHARMACOKINETICS Because EPO is a protein, it cannot be administered orally. After IV injection, about 10% of the EPO dose is eliminated by the kidneys, with a half-life of 4–6 hours in normal volunteers and 6–9 hours in patients with renal failure. Patients with liver impairment may show increased effects due to decreased metabolism of EPO. Bioavailability after SC injection is only 20%–30% of that after IV administration.

ADVERSE DRUG REACTIONS Early in treatment, flu-like symptoms, bone pain and chills occur. Hypersensitivity reactions may induce rashes, urticaria, respiratory symptoms and hypotension. Later reactions due to increased RBC mass include hypertension, seizures and thrombotic events.

DRUG INTERACTIONS The erythropoietic effects may be potentiated by other haematinic agents, including iron supplements. Blood levels of drugs that bind to RBCs, such as cyclosporin, may be altered and should be monitored.

WARNINGS AND CONTRAINDICATIONS EPO is contraindicated in patients with severe cardiovascular disease, including hypertension and vascular diseases. Hypertension develops during the first 3 months in about 30% of patients treated with EPO. Seizures and thrombotic events may also occur. The growth factor activity of EPO may stimulate growth of tumour cells.

DOSAGE AND ADMINISTRATION EPO is formulated in vials or prefilled syringes containing a range of strengths of solution, from 1000 IU/0.5 mL to 40,000 IU/mL. Dosage varies depending on indication and on response as monitored by RBC counts; for example, in chronic renal failure, during the correction phase, the dose is 50 IU/kg three times weekly for 1 month, increasing gradually until haemoglobin level is 10–11.5 g/dL.

renal failure and anaemias, and in AIDS-related conditions (see Drug Monograph 57-1). Prolonged administration of EPO has been shown to raise haemoglobin levels and aerobic performance in healthy men, so it has been widely abused in endurance sports such as cycling.

Raised levels of RBCs combined with dehydration during endurance sports are likely to raise the haematocrit and potentially cause hypertension, thrombosis, and thromboembolic events such as strokes and myocardial infarctions.

Detection of abuse of EPO proved a difficult problem for many years, as the hormone is endogenous and has a short half-life (5–6 hours) but long duration of action. Safety guidelines were developed to prevent athletes competing if their haematocrit exceeded 50%. Just in time for the Sydney 2000 Olympic Games, scientists at the Australian Sports Drug Testing Laboratory in Sydney announced the successful development of a blood test for EPO that could detect EPO use up to 4 weeks earlier. The test was approved by the IOC and in use at the Games. It involves a battery of tests including EPO levels, haematocrit and various markers of iron deficiency and transport.

Diuretics and other masking agents

Diuretics such as the thiazide, potassium-sparing and loop diuretics have been abused in sport to reduce body weight quickly in sports with strict weight classifications, to dilute urine in an attempt to mask the presence of banned substances, or to relieve oedema from AAS abuse. Potential adverse drug reactions include dehydration, muscle cramps and cardiovascular impairment.

Other masking agents are those used to impair the excretion of prohibited substances or to conceal their presence in bodily samples, whether urine or blood. Examples include epitestosterone to confuse T/E ratio values, probenecid (an antigout drug) to impair excretion of other drugs, or plasma expanders to dilute the banned drug in the bloodstream.

Substances banned in-competition only
Narcotic analgesics

Strong narcotic analgesics such as morphine (Drug Monograph 16-1), buprenorphine, pethidine and methadone (Drug

Monograph 22-2) are prohibited in sport; heroin is not a legal drug in Australia at any time. They are sometimes abused in sport to mask pain or for their euphoriant actions. Adverse effects include tissue damage from ignoring pain signals, sedation, constipation, nausea and vomiting, respiratory depression and addiction. Mild narcotic analgesics, including codeine (Drug Monograph 32-7), pholcodine and dextropropoxyphene, are permitted.

Stimulants

Various types of drugs that enhance alertness and aggressiveness and reduce fatigue are classified by WADA as **stimulants**. Such drugs are likely to be used during competition and may cause impairment of judgement, hyperthermia and cardiovascular collapse and heighten risk of accidents. Sports in which intense anaerobic exercise is required are those in which stimulants are abused, including cycling, ice hockey, football and baseball. Examples of stimulants are:

- a subgroup of the sympathomimetic amines including the **amphetamine** group (Drug Monograph 20-1) and 'designer drugs', which are notorious for producing problems in sport. Sympathetic stimulation may lead to hypertension, tachycardia, tremor and anxiety; deaths have occurred from excessive cardiovascular and central stimulation
- another subgroup of the sympathomimetic amines, the B$_2$ agonists, which are also classed as anabolic agents (described above)
- cocaine, abused for its CNS-stimulant effects in increasing alertness and reducing fatigue. It is not available medically in Australia. The high risk of excessive cardiovascular and CNS stimulation, and addiction, suggests that there is little potential benefit to athletes.*

In previous IOC lists, sympathomimetic amines such as ephedrine, pseudoephedrine and phenylpropanolamine (Drug Monograph 32-8), and the stimulants caffeine and bupropion, were banned. In the 2006 WADA code, these substances are 'specified' (see later).

Glucocorticosteroids

Glucocorticosteroids (also often referred to as glucocorticoids or corticosteroids) are powerful anti-inflammatory and immunosuppressant agents (see Chapters 40 and 55); they may be natural hormones secreted by the adrenal gland or

---

*It is interesting that nicotine, a proven stimulant, antidiuretic and lipolytic agent, is permitted, presumably because it is such a commonly used drug that there would be an outcry if it were to be banned. Possibly also the adverse respiratory and cardiovascular effects of smoking are considered sufficiently detrimental to performance and hazardous to health to deter elite athletes.

synthetic compounds with similar actions. They are likely to be abused in sport for their anti-inflammatory and euphoriant effects or to mask injury. Adverse reactions that limit the usefulness of corticosteroids in athletes include osteoporosis, mood changes, fluid retention and impaired healing.

The status of glucocorticosteroids in sport depends critically on the route by which they are administered. Dermatological administration, e.g. in creams, ointments or sprays applied to the skin, is permitted at all times. Systemic administration of corticosteroids, including via the oral, intravenous and rectal routes, is universally banned, and medical use requires an abbreviated Therapeutic Use Exemption (TUE). Glucocorticoids administered by other non-systemic routes, such as by inhalation for asthma, as eye- or ear-drops, and by intra-articular routes when medically necessary are permitted after approval of a full TUE.

Cannabinoids

All forms of ingested or inhaled cannabinoids (see Chapter 22), such as marijuana, THC and hashish, are prohibited during competition; it is considered that dermatological administration of cannabis is unlikely to lead to significant absorption. Adverse effects are impaired coordination, slowing of responses, and increased appetite; long-term effects include higher incidence of psychosis and impairment of respiration (from smoking 'joints').

Prohibited methods of doping

Prohibited methods include techniques for **blood doping** to enhance oxygen transfer, altering blood or urine parameters, or manipulating or interfering with samples; these are banned at all times. Gene doping, i.e. non-therapeutic use of genes or genetic material to enhance performance, is considered a potential method, and as such has already been prohibited.

Blood doping

Blood doping is the administration of blood, RBCs or blood products to an athlete. It usually involves transfusion of extra blood, either the athlete's own (autologous) or a compatible donor's (homologous), into the circulatory system to increase red cell mass to provide extra oxygen-carrying capacity and enhance aerobic performance. It creates a similar effect to training at high altitude (shown to be important in the Mexico Olympics) and so is useful in endurance events such as marathon-running, cycling and cross-country skiing. The risks involved are those of infections, mismatching of blood, blood or iron overload, increased viscosity (hence thrombosis or embolism), and cardiovascular problems such as heart attack, heart failure or stroke. The ready availability of EPO has now essentially made blood doping by transfusion obsolete.

Another type of blood doping is the administration of artificial oxygen carriers such as perfluorocarbons and haemoglobins, or plasma expanders; these methods are also prohibited. Plasma expanders are used to replace volume after dehydration, or to dilute the blood in attempts to mask prohibited substances.

Manipulation of samples

Sample manipulation is the use of pharmacological, chemical or physical means to alter or substitute the body fluid sample, usually urine or blood, taken in a doping control test. Whether or not the attempt at manipulation succeeds is immaterial; attempts are prohibited at all times. Examples of such techniques include:

- catheterisation to produce an altered or substituted sample
- sample substitution, dilution or adulteration
- use of drugs that affect renal excretion, e.g. diuretics, masking agents or bicarbonate
- interference with the safe custody of samples, methods of analysis or promulgation of results
- use of drugs or fluids that alter urine levels of other drugs or metabolites, e.g. excess water intake to dilute urine.

DRUGS RESTRICTED IN CERTAIN SPORTS OR COMPETITORS

Restricted substances

Some drugs are **restricted** in some sports, in some situations or by specified routes of administration, and are permitted in other cases. As described above, four β_2 agonists are permitted for inhalation by registered asthmatics, but systemic administration is prohibited. In international archery, many drugs with sedative actions are banned, including hypnotics, antipsychotics, anxiolytics and antihistamines.

Alcohol

Alcohol use would be detrimental to most sports, as it can cause impaired motor coordination, prolonged reaction time, sedation and mental confusion, and can become a safety hazard. Athletes are warned that blood alcohol levels may be tested in doping controls in some sports (e.g. archery, karate, billiards). Alcohol use by referees and umpires is prohibited by some sporting organisations.

Beta-blockers

Beta-blockers such as propranolol and metoprolol are banned in some sports, as they reduce excitability of the cardiovascular system, thereby reducing blood pressure, cardiac output, heart rate and tremor. In some sports, a steady action and reduced response to stress can be beneficial, so β-blockers are restricted in-competition in sports such as gymnastics, shooting, archery, ski-jumping, wrestling and modern pentathlon. In strenuous physical sports, however, reduced cardiovascular response to stress would be detrimental. Whether or not β-blockers are prohibited, and when, is determined by the international bodies regulating specific sports.

Specified substances

The new WADA category of **Specified Substances** includes drugs that may appear in commonly available and taken medicines, and hence are particularly likely to incur inadvertent violations. Provided that an athlete can prove that administration of the drug was not intended to enhance performance, the sanction for a violation may be less heavy than otherwise would be imposed.

Examples include alcohol and beta-blockers (except in sports in which they are banned), cannabinoids, some sympathomimetic amines, glucocorticoids, and inhaled B_2 agonists. Sympathomimetic amines such as ephedrine, pseudoephedrine (Drug Monograph 32-8) and phenylpropanolamine, previously banned, are usually taken as decongestants or appetite suppressants or to 'burn fat'. Many cases have occurred of athletes being banned (and medals removed) after testing positive to these substances taken in 'cold cures'.

Caffeine (Drug Monograph 20-2), being the most commonly taken psychoactive drug worldwide, is no longer prohibited or monitored; even very young athletes sometimes abuse caffeine to seek performance advantages from cardiovascular and CNS stimulation.

SUBSTANCES AND METHODS PERMITTED IN SPORTS

Permitted drugs

It is important for athletes to know not only what drugs are prohibited or restricted in their sports but also what drugs and substances are **permitted**. Athletes are advised to double-check that medications are permitted before taking them, including over-the-counter, complementary and alternative preparations, and drugs from overseas. Some drugs are permitted only in women (e.g. hCG, luteinising hormone) or only in people registered as having particular diseases (e.g. asthma or diabetes). Local anaesthetics (except cocaine) are permitted if medically justified; local anaesthetics mask pain, thus putting the person at risk of tissue damage.

Lists of permitted drugs are available from ASADA, particularly drugs used to treat common conditions such as allergies and hay fever, diarrhoea, pain and inflammation, nausea and vomiting, and coughs and colds. Interested persons are always advised to check in a current edition of the MIMS bimonthly or on the WADA website for the approval status of any questioned drug.

Ergogenic aids and nutrients

In attempts to enhance performance without contravening WADA prohibitions, athletes have tried to find other substances that improve energy utilisation (i.e. are **ergogenic**); nutritional supplements are often taken. Such substances, unlike drugs, do not have to go through extensive clinical trials of safety and efficacy before being marketed, and claims made as to their usefulness are rarely scientifically validated. Thus far, WADA has not banned any ergogenic aids, which in itself suggests that they do not significantly or unfairly enhance performance.

DIETARY MANIPULATION

Carbohydrates consumed immediately before or after performance boost glycogen stores and delay fatigue, thus enhancing performance. Protein and amino acid supplementation has anabolic effects, increasing protein synthesis. Some other complementary and alternative medicine therapies used in sport are described in Clinical Interest Box 57-3.

CREATINE

The amino acid creatine is an important constituent of muscle and is involved in energy utilisation and phosphate exchange. Short-term creatine loading may improve performance during high-intensity exercise such as sprinting, by overcoming creatine depletion.

BICARBONATE

During long intense exercise, adenosine triphosphate (ATP) is formed from anaerobic glycolysis, and lactic acid accumulates. In an attempt to overcome this acidosis, bicarbonate loading has been tried, with a dose of 300 mg/kg sodium bicarbonate (baking soda) taken 1–2 hours before high-intensity exercise. In some studies, performance has been enhanced by up to 30%. Adverse reactions such as gastrointestinal bloating and diarrhoea can occur, especially if overdoses or insufficient water are taken.

β-HYDROXY-β-METHYLBUTYRATE

β-hydroxy-β-methylbutyrate (HMB) has an inhibitory action on protein catabolism and is available as a nutritional supplement. In tests, it has been shown to have some effect in increasing strength and oxygen consumption.

ANTIOXIDANTS

Antioxidants such as carotenes (vitamin A, see Clinical Interest Box 56-3) and vitamins C and E may enhance performance indirectly by detoxifying free radicals (lipid peroxides) formed, thus enhancing recovery. It is accepted that nutritional supplementation with these vitamins may protect athletes from oxidative stress.

ANDROSTENEDIONE

Androstenedione is a natural precursor to the sex hormones and is produced naturally in the adrenal glands and gonads, and in plants. It has gained wide popularity as an ergogenic aid, assuming that it is converted to testosterone and will thus have anabolic effects. Some studies have demonstrated oestrogenic rather than androgenic effects in humans, and it is suggested that if useful anabolic actions are possible, then adverse androgenic effects will also occur.

CLINICAL INTEREST BOX 57-3
COMPLEMENTARY AND ALTERNATIVE THERAPIES IN SPORT

Complementary and alternative therapies are increasingly popular and marketed as sport performance enhancers, both as 'natural' aids and to circumvent WADA testing. As well as the ergogenic aids described in the text, various food supplements and natural compounds have been tried, including:

- herbs—ginseng, guarana, ephedra, yohimbine, saw palmetto
- natural substances—acetylcholine, amino acids, bee pollen, carnitine, eicosanoids, inosine, iron, oils, omega-3 fatty acids, royal jelly, spirulina (a blue–green alga)
- mega-doses of vitamins, especially vitamin C.

As with all herbal and natural products, there are potential problems with respect to knowing the actual constituents, the strengths of any active ingredients, and the presence of any contaminants. Cases are documented of 'natural' antiasthma products being proven to contain synthetic β_2 agonists, 'natural' antidiabetic remedies containing oral hypoglycaemic agents, and 'natural' remedies for inflammation containing synthetic glucocorticoids.

ASADA cannot provide information as to the status of complementary and alternative products, as information about the ingredients is usually sparse. ASADA warns athletes that 'natural remedies' may contain banned substances and/or may be toxic. Thus the onus is on the athlete to ensure that a product is safe and not prohibited.

DRUG TESTING PROCEDURES

Drug testing policies

The IOC, international sports federations and some national authorities have regulations to require athletes to undergo **drug testing** procedures to enforce anti-doping policies. Testing is intended to be a deterrent rather than sufficiently extensive to catch all incidences of use of banned drugs or methods. The first Olympic Games at which testing was carried out were the Mexico Games in 1968; the Australian runner Ron Clarke was the first athlete to be tested.

Testing is mainly carried out at competitions, which means that drugs taken long-term during training may be missed. Many drugs (especially anabolics and blood-doping drugs and methods) are abused chronically for their long-term effects, but if stopped before competition may not show up in samples taken immediately after events. Out-of-competition testing is logistically more difficult to implement. Athletes in a 'Registered Testing Pool' are required to provide information as to their whereabouts to enable effective no-notice testing.* For the Sydney Olympic Games, for the first time, many athletes were subjected to testing before competition and out-of-competition, as well as after their events. Summary statistics relating to testing over the period 1988–2004 are shown in Table 57-1.

The drug testing process

The doping control procedures carried out at the Sydney 2000 Olympic Games were under the control of the IOC Medical Commission (IOCMC). The Sydney Organising Committee for the Olympic Games (SOCOG) was responsible for setting up the Doping Control Program to ensure that all testing was done in accordance with the IOC code, in particular the safe chain of custody of the competitors and samples through the procedures. Normally, urine samples were collected, but after the last-minute accreditation of a blood EPO method, some blood samples were also taken. Breath-testing for alcohol was also implemented.

Doping controls were carried out in all sports, and all competitors had to agree to comply with the IOC Anti-Doping Code and provide samples as requested. The selection of competitors to be tested was made by IOCMC and SOCOG. Generally, the first four competitors or teams in a final were tested, plus other competitors selected randomly. Competitors were warned that they could be selected more than once and could be tested out of competition.

Important stages of the doping control procedures for urine samples include providing the urine sample and controlling it until sealed; splitting the sample into aliquots A and B; recording any medications, vitamins, herbal products or food supplements taken over the past 7 days; and safe transport of samples to the accredited laboratory where sample A is analysed for banned drugs or methods. The presence of a banned substance is sufficient to count as a positive test: the testing authority does not have to prove how the substance was taken. Positive results are further tested by the IOC, and the duplicate, sample B, may be tested in the presence of the competitor or a representative.

A report on the drug testing carried out at the Sydney 2000 Games was published, and is summarised in Clinical Interest Box 57-4.

---

*In the Athens Olympic Games in 2004, two Greek athletes who had successfully evaded out-of-competition testing for several years failed to appear for drug testing after claiming to have been involved in a motorcycle accident. At the subsequent court hearing, the athletes withdrew from the Games.

TABLE 57–1 Statistics for drug testing by IOC-accredited laboratories

YEAR	TOTAL NUMBER OF A-SAMPLES ANALYSED	% SAMPLES POSITIVE FOR STIMULANTS	% SAMPLES POSITIVE FOR ANABOLICS
1988	47,069	0.89	1.68
1993	89,166	0.37	1.05
1998	105,250	0.39	0.81

Similar more recent comparative data are hard to find. However, it can be noted that:
- In the financial year 2003/04, the Australian Sports Drug Agency (ASDA) conducted 6614 tests, 71% on a no-notice basis. There were 24 adverse test findings ('positives'), from 19 athletes, including one positive result for EPO (ASDA media release, 28 July 2004).
- In 2004, WADA conducted 2327 out-of-competition doping controls across 118 nationalities; 1848 were urine tests, 378 urine EPO tests, 59 tests for hGH and 42 blood screens. There were 19 adverse findings and 4 refusals (WADA 2004 Annual Report).

CLINICAL INTEREST BOX 57-4   DRUG TESTING AT THE SYDNEY OLYMPIC GAMES

The Post-Olympic Report on doping controls at the Sydney Olympics summarises the activity of the 'fight against doping'. A total of 2846 tests were performed, including some out-of-competition tests. In addition, positive controls to which the testing authorities were 'blind' were run through the tests, to validate the procedures. In summary:

- In-competition, 2052 tests were carried out, including at the football (soccer) matches played before the Olympic dates in other cities in Australia. The sports most commonly tested were swimming, athletics, rowing, shooting and wrestling.
- Out-of-competition testing was carried out on 404 urine samples of athletes from 99 countries.
- The IOCMC was notified by 607 athletes who were asthmatic and so allowed to use β_2 agonists; the most common was salbutamol (548), then terbutaline (39) and salmeterol (20).
- EPO was tested out-of-competition in 307 blood and urine samples of athletes from endurance sports such as athletics (>800 m), rowing, road cycling, kayak, swimming (>400 m), triathlon and modern pentathlon; both top athlete testing and random tests were done.

- Excluding notified asthmatics and 'blind' positive controls, 11 samples were detected as positive: four in weightlifting (three frusemide, one stanozolol), three in wrestling (one frusemide, two nandrolone), one in rowing (nandrolone), one in gymnastics (pseudoephedrine) and two in athletics out-of-competition (one nandrolone, one stanozolol). All were notified to the IOCMC Chairman and all required testing and confirmation in the B sample
- There were six 'blind' positive controls: these were in urine or blood samples from simulated male and female athletes (cycling, weightlifting, swimming, athletics) and contained EPO, clopamide (a diuretic), clostebol (an AAS), nikethamide (a stimulant), clenbuterol (a β_2 agonist) or epimetendiole (an AAS metabolite), some at the lower limit of detection. All were detected as positives and reported to the IOCMC Chairman.

Source: International Olympic Committee Medical Commission. Post-Olympic report on doping controls at the Games of the XXVII Olympiad in Sydney (Australia). 2000: www.olympic.org/ioc/e/org/medcom/medcom_post_olymp_report_e.html

Rights and responsibilities
Health professionals' rights and responsibilities

Health professionals, especially doctors, physiotherapists and podiatrists, are often consulted by athletes to treat medical conditions, including those arising from participation in sport; to advise on therapeutic and adverse effects from drug use; or to prescribe or provide drugs that may enhance performance. The main responsibility of such health professionals is the health of the athlete; they must also avoid prescribing any drugs banned in the particular sport.

The Royal Australasian College of Physicians (1997) has prepared a position paper on drugs in sport and discussed the ethical aspects of prescribing drugs such as anabolic steroids. The College opposes prescribing of drugs for performance enhancement or bodybuilding. In a recent paper (Orchard et al 2006), the essentials for the practice of sports medicine in Australia were summarised as: 'Doctors need to know if a patient is an athlete subject to drug testing, and to be aware of the legal situation surrounding drugs they prescribe such patients'.

ETHICAL ASPECTS OF DRUGS IN SPORT

There are many **ethical** and philosophical **issues** related to the use and abuse of drugs in the sporting arena. Some of these issues and controversial questions are summarised below:

- Drug abuse is widespread in society—why should stricter rules apply to sport?
- All competition involves risk-taking; adverse drug reactions are just another type of risk.
- What constitutes cheating? Why are ergogenic nutritional supplements allowed but anabolic drugs banned? Why is nicotine allowed but amphetamine banned?
- Can a 'level playing field' ever exist at the international level? How can developing 'Third World' countries compete equitably against wealthy countries supporting athletes at institutes of sport, or athletes living at sea level compete equitably at high altitude?
- Issues of autonomy: do athletes have the right to risk adverse effects if they wish to? Do they have the right to refuse to use agents encouraged by their coaches or sporting authorities?
- Gender issues: gonadotrophins, for example, are allowed for women but not men.
- If there is little evidence of the efficacy of drugs in enhancing performance, why are the substances banned?
- If unscrupulous athletes, coaches or sporting bodies will always stay ahead of anti-drug agencies, why not give up and allow any drugs or methods to be used?
- Why is it cheating to enhance performance by using drugs but not by using drag-reducing swimwear or costumes?
- Why is EPO banned but training at high altitude encouraged?

- Why should honest athletes be penalised by having to compete against drug cheats who are not caught (the 'women with beards' effect)?
- Why are adverse effects from drugs in sport considered differently from sporting injuries?
- What are appropriate health practitioners' roles? Should health practitioners be allowed to prescribe banned drugs in the interests of harm minimisation? Should they have to report illegal use of drugs?
- Major international sporting fixtures are no longer simply competitions to find the highest, fastest or strongest; they

are festivals to provide entertainment, create idols and make money; so performance enhancement is in the best interests of the event.

As they are ethical and philosophical questions rather than scientific hypotheses, these issues cannot readily be resolved; however, it is important that they be debated and not ignored. Meanwhile, the testing authorities continue to refine techniques to assay more drugs down to lower blood levels, and some competitors still manage to circumvent the anti-doping policies of sporting authorities.

DRUGS AT A GLANCE 57: Drugs in sport

Note: (1) The pharmacological mechanisms and therapeutic uses of these drugs are all covered in earlier chapters.
(2) Some of the prohibited substances are allowed in competitors registered as requiring them for therapeutic purposes; a valid Therapeutic Use Exemption certificate may be necessary.

WADA Group	Pharmacological group	Key examples	Key pages
Substances prohibited at all times	Anabolic androgenic steroids (AAS)	testosterone stanozolol	934–6
	Anti-oestrogens	tamoxifen	935
	β₂-adrenoceptor agonists	salbutamol eformoterol	935
	Hormones	human chorionic gonadotrophin (hCG) growth hormone (GH)	936
		erythropoietin (EPO)	936, 7
		insulin	936
	Diuretics	frusemide hydrochlorothiazide	937
	Other masking agents	probenecid	
Substances banned in-competition	Narcotic analgesics	morphine methadone	937, 8
	Stimulants	amphetamines	938
	Glucocorticosteroids (banned by some routes)	hydrocortisone	938
	Cannabinoids	marijuana	938
Substances restricted in certain sports	CNS depressants	alcohol	939
	β-blockers	metoprolol	
Specified substances (includes some substances restricted or banned in-competition)	Sympathomimetic amines	pseudoephedrine	939
	Stimulants	caffeine	

CNS = central nervous system.

KEY POINTS

- Doping is the use in sport of banned substances or methods to enhance performance; doping contravenes the ethics of sport and can be detrimental to the health of athletes. Doping is sometimes carried out out-of-competition (for long-term effects) or in-competition (for acute effects).

- The groups of drugs prohibited or restricted by the World Anti-Doping Agency are anabolic agents, anti-oestrogens, B_2 agonists, cannabinoids, diuretics and other masking agents, glucocorticosteroids, other hormones and related substances, narcotics and stimulants; blood doping and sample manipulation methods are also banned.

- Banned substances or methods are abused in attempts to enhance performance; there is little objective evidence for their efficacy. All substances have potential adverse effects.

- Erythropoietin is a natural hormone that increases red cell production; it is often abused in endurance sports and is detectable by blood and urine tests.

- Some drugs are restricted (banned only in specific sports), and others are specified as being likely to incur inadvertent violations. Some drugs may be permitted by specified routes or in patients with particular conditions.

- Other substances and methods that have been applied in attempts to enhance performance include dietary manipulation, various ergogenic aids and nutrients, and complementary and alternative therapies.

- Drug testing procedures are carried out in accredited laboratories and can screen samples for a battery of prohibited substances. The World Anti-Doping Agency (WADA) has strict rules for the procedures for doping controls.

- Many ethical issues impinge on the use and abuse of drugs and methods to enhance sporting performances.

REVIEW EXERCISES

1. Discuss the use and abuse of anabolic steroids in society today.
2. Describe the rights and responsibilities of health professionals relating to drug use and testing.
3. List the groups of drugs prohibited or restricted by the World Anti-Doping Agency, and summarise the reasons for abuse and potential adverse effects of each group of drugs.
4. Set up a debate (or list the arguments useful in such a debate) on the topic 'There is no such thing as a level playing field in international sporting competition'.

REFERENCES AND FURTHER READING

Ahrendt DM. Ergogenic aids: counselling the athlete. *American Family Physician* 2001; 63 (5): 913–22.
Applegate E. Effective nutritional ergogenic aids. *International Journal of Sport Nutrition* 1999; 9: 229–39.
Australian Sports Drug Agency. *Anti-Doping Information Handbook 2005*. Canberra: ASDA, 2005.
Bains A. EPO to finish last, in Aussie first. *Today's Life Science* 2000; Sept/Oct: 18.
Breymann C. Erythropoietin test methods. *Clinical Endocrinology & Metabolism* 2000; 14 (1): 135–45.
Bucci LR. Selected herbals and human exercise performance. *American Journal of Clinical Nutrition* 2000; 72 (2 Suppl): 624S–36S.
Carlyon, P. Vial bodies. *The Bulletin* 2000: Sep 19: 38–41.
Caswell A (ed.). Drugs in Sport–WADA Guide. *MIMS Annual 2005*. Sydney: CMPMedica Australia, 2005: G36–G38.
Clarkson PM, Thompson HS. Drugs and sport: research findings and limitations. *Sports Medicine* 1997; 24 (6): 366–84.
Corrigan B, Kazlauskas R. Drug testing at the Sydney Olympics. *Medical Journal of Australia* 2000; 173: 312–13.
Council on Scientific Affairs. Medical and nonmedical uses of anabolic-androgenic steroids. *Journal of the American Medical Association* 1990; 264 (22): 2923.
Dawson RT. Drugs in sport: the role of the physician. *Journal of Endocrinology* 2001; 170 (1): 55–61.
Dillon P, Cox G, O'Connor M. *What's the score? The Facts on Alcohol, Drugs and Sport*. Canberra: Australian Sports Commission, 2004.
Fricker P. The anti-doping code in sport: update for 2004. *Australian Prescriber* 2004; 27 (4): 84–7.
George AJ. Central nervous system stimulants. *Clinical Endocrinology & Metabolism* 2000; 14 (1): 79–88.
Gerrard D. The misuse of drugs in sport. *Today's Life Science* 2000; Sep/Oct: 22–6.
Gray P. Drug testing at the Sydney Olympics (letter). *Medical Journal of Australia* 2001; 174: 203–4.
Jelkmann W. Use of recombinant human erythropoietin as an antianaemic and performance enhancing drug. *Current Pharmaceutical Biotechnology* 2001; 1: 11–31.
Kennedy MC. Newer drugs used to enhance sporting performance. *Medical Journal of Australia* 2000; 173: 314–17.
Kennedy MCS. Drugs, sport and the Olympics 2000–20004. *Medical Journal of Australia* 2004; 181(4): 227.
Kennedy MC, Kennedy JR. Ethics of prescribing drugs to enhance sporting performance. *Medical Journal of Australia* 1999; 171: 204–5.
Kron J. Staying clear of steroids. *Australian Doctor* 2000; Oct 6: 51–2.
Laura RS, White SW. *Drug Controversy in Sport: The Socio-Ethical and Medical Issues*. Sydney: Allen & Unwin, 1991.

Martin M, Yates WN. *Therapeutic Medications in Sports Medicine*. Baltimore: Williams & Wilkins, 1998.

Maurer HH. Screening procedures for simultaneous detection of several drug classes used for high throughput toxicological analyses and doping control: a review. *Combinatorial Chemistry & High Throughput Screening* 2000; 3 (6): 467–80.

Mottram DR (ed.). *Drugs in Sport*. London: Spon Press, 1996.

Mottram DR. Banned drugs in sport: does the International Olympic Committee (IOC) list need updating? *Sports Medicine* 1999; 27(1): 1–10.

Mottram DR, George AJ. Anabolic steroids. *Clinical Endocrinology & Metabolism* 2000; 14 (1): 55–69.

Mullis PE (ed.). Doping in Sport. *Clinical Endocrinology & Metabolism* 2000; 14(1). [Special issue devoted to drugs in sport; including papers on anabolic steroids, growth hormone, CNS stimulants, blood boosting, EPO, and analytical testing.]

Orchard JW, Fricker PA, White SL, Burke LM, Healey DJ. The use and misuse of performance-enhancing substances in sport. *Medical Journal of Australia* 2006; 184(3): 132–6.

O'Sullivan AJ, Kennedy MC, Casey JH et al. Anabolic-androgenic steroids: medical assessment of present, past and potential users. *Medical Journal of Australia* 2000; 173: 323–7.

Reilly T, Orme M (eds). *The Clinical Pharmacology of Sport and Exercise*. Amsterdam: Elsevier, 1997.

Royal Australasian College of Physicians. Drugs in sport: a position paper. RACP Fellowship Affairs, 1997.

Rubinstein ML, Federman DG. Sports supplements: can dietary additives boost athletic performance and potential? *Postgraduate Medicine* 2000; 108 (4): 103–12.

Seidler R. Advice to a patient on steroids. *Australian Doctor* 2000; 6 Oct: 58–61.

Shaskey DJ, Green GA. Sports haematology. *Sports Medicine* 2000; 29 (1): 27–38.

Sinclair CJ, Geiger JD. Caffeine use in sports: a pharmacological review. *Journal of Sports Medicine & Physical Fitness* 2000; 40(1): 71–9.

Sonksen PH. Insulin, growth hormone and sport. *Journal of Endocrinology* 2001; 170 (1): 13–25.

Speight TM, Holford NHG (eds). *Avery's Drug Treatment*. 4th edn. Auckland: Adis International, 1997.

Stuart M. The war on drugs in sport: a perspective from the Athens Olympics. *Pharmaceutical Journal* 2004; 273(7315): 320–1.

Sydney Organising Committee for the Olympic Games (SOCOG). *Doping Control Guide, Sydney 2000*. Sydney: SOCOG, 2000.

Tokish JM, Kocher MS, Hawkins RJ. Ergogenic aids: a review of basic science, performance, side effects, and status in sports. *American Journal of Sports Medicine* 2004; 32(6): 1543–53.

Verroken M. Drug use and abuse in sport. *Clinical Endocrinology & Metabolism* 2000; 14 (1): 1–23.

Warren MP, Shantha S. The female athlete. *Clinical Endocrinology & Metabolism* 2000; 14 (1): 37–53.

Wilson W, Derse E (eds). *Doping in Elite Sport: The Politics of Drugs in the Olympic Movement*. Champaign, IL: Human Kinetics; 2001.

Yesalis CE, Bahrke MS. Doping among adolescent athletes. *Clinical Endocrinology & Metabolism* 2000; 14(1): 25–35.

ON-LINE RESOURCES

Australian Sports Anti-Doping Authority: www.asada.gov.au/index.html/

Australian Sports Drug Agency. Australia's drug testing results for 2003–04; media release 28 July 2004: www.asda.org.au

International Olympic Committee Medical Commission. Post-Olympic report on doping controls at the Games of the XXVII Olympiad in Sydney (Australia). 2000: www.olympic.org/ioc/e/org/medcom/medcom_post_olymp_report_e.html

New Zealand medicines and medical devices safety authority: www.medsafe.govt.nz

WADA: http://www.wada-ama.org/en/

World Anti-Doping Agency. *2004 Annual Report*. www.wada-ama.org

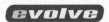 More weblinks at http://evolve.elsevier.com/AU/Bryant/pharmacology/

CHAPTER 58

Drugs in Obesity

CHAPTER FOCUS

Obesity is a common and costly nutritional problem affecting a significant proportion of the Australian and New Zealand populations. Overweight and obese individuals with body mass index >25 have a higher long-term risk of morbidity and mortality. A wide range of interacting biopsychological factors contribute to obesity, which in some cases may not be simply solved by reducing food intake and increasing energy expenditure. Although alterations in diet, increased physical activity and behavioural modification are central to the prevention and treatment of obesity, improving knowledge of the pathophysiology of obesity may lead to the development of safer and more effective antiobesity drugs.

OBJECTIVES

● To discuss the pathophysiology of obesity.

● To understand the relationship between body mass index, waist:hip ratio and the health risks associated with obesity.

● To appreciate the complexity of impinging factors that influence the balance between energy intake and energy expenditure.

● To discuss the mechanism of action of the currently available antiobesity drugs.

KEY DRUGS

diethylpropion
phentermine
orlistat
sibutramine

KEY TERMS

body mass index
cholecystokinin
energy balance
leptin
obesity
pancreatic lipase
waist:hip ratio

KEY ABBREVIATIONS

BMI   body mass index
WHR   waist:hip ratio

HOW often the headlines in the glossy magazines catch the eye: 'Ten ways to conquer your cravings', 'Is your fridge a health hazard?', 'Lose 15 kg in 15 days', 'From 100 kg blimp to size 8 cover girl', 'Fast fat-burning diet'. Self-interest in our weight and body shape maintains a billion-dollar industry that ranges from glossy magazines to the sale of diet food, fitness centre exercise packages and sojourns at health resorts: "Australians spend in excess of $500 million on commercial weight control measures" (Caterson 1999a). Without a doubt, Australians and New Zealanders are increasing in weight, and a proportion of each population is now considered either overweight or obese (see Clinical Interest Box 58-1). A key issue, however, is the measurement of body weight. How do we define underweight, normal weight, overweight and obesity?

It has long been recognised that simply weighing an individual does not provide an indication of weight distribution or of risk factors. The measurement now most frequently used is the **body mass index** (BMI). The BMI is highly correlated with body fat and is calculated by dividing an individual's body mass (kg) by the square of his or her height in metres (m^2); for example, a 100 kg person who is 1.7 metres tall has a BMI of 34.6 (100 divided by 1.7^2) and would, according to World Health Organization (WHO) guidelines, be considered obese (Table 58-1).

With the BMI used as the main indicator, the proportion of overweight and obese women in Australia increased from 27% in 1980 to 43% in 1995, and for men from 48% to 63% over the same period. This translates to 5 million Australians in 1995 being classified as overweight and 2.4 million (19% of the adult population) classed as obese (AIHW 2000). The situation among indigenous adults was even less favourable: 28% of women and 25% of men were classified as obese (AIHW 2000). Of more concern are recent data for 1999/2000, which indicate that of the Australian population 67% of adult males and 52% of adult females are classified as overweight or obese (Cameron et al 2003). Obesity is not unique to Australasia; it is common in industrialised countries throughout the world and is becoming a growing problem in developing countries.

HEALTH RISKS ASSOCIATED WITH OBESITY

Obesity is well recognised as a disease in its own right. Health risks associated with obesity are enormous, and overweight individuals have a higher mortality rate than people with a normal BMI. Worldwide, approximately 1 billion adults and 10% of children are now classified as overweight or obese. In terms of contribution to the overall global burden of disease

The results from the 2002/03 NZ Health Survey indicate that many adult New Zealanders are overweight. Using standard BMI cut-offs for 'overweight' (≥26 for Maori and Pacific; ≥25 for European, Asian and 'others'), one-third of NZ adults were classified as overweight. One in five adults was considered to be obese (BMI ≥32 for Maori and Pacific; ≥30 for European, Asian and 'others'). Over half of the adults had gained 10 kg or more since the age of 18, and obesity was significantly more prevalent in lower socioeconomic areas.

For both males and females, the prevalence of obesity was highest in the Pacific ethnic group, followed by Maori, European/other and Asian ethnic groups, and the prevalence of obesity increased with age until 55–64 years, then declined slightly.

Adapted from: Ministry of Health 2004.

TABLE 58-1 Body mass index: international standard (WHO 2000)

CLASSIFICATION	BMI (kg/m^2)
Underweight	<18.5
Normal weight	18.5–24.9
Overweight (pre-obese)	25–29.9
Obese	≥30
Class I	30–34.9
Class II	35–39.9
Class III	≥40.0

and disability, excessive weight (corpulence) is the sixth most important factor. Many studies have reported that obese individuals have a greater risk of:

- breast cancer
- cardiovascular disease
- colon cancer
- gallbladder cancer
- gallstones
- hirsutism
- hypercholesterolaemia
- hyperinsulinaemia
- hypertension
- hypertriglyceridaemia
- hyperuricaemia (gout)
- hypogonadism
- infertility
- insulin resistance
- ischaemic heart disease
- osteoarthritis
- ovarian and uterine cancer
- prostate cancer
- sleep apnoea
- type 2 diabetes mellitus
- varicose veins.

The distribution of fat is also very important in relation to disease risk. A high proportion of visceral (e.g. abdominal) fat carries a greater risk of morbidity and mortality than does a peripheral distribution. Although large studies that have measured concomitantly body weight and glucose and insulin concentrations are rare, a strong association exists between abdominal adiposity, blood glucose concentration, insulin resistance and the development of type 2 diabetes. Within Australia, the higher prevalence of obesity has been identified as a major contributing factor to the increasing incidence of diabetes, specifically type 2 diabetes (AIHW 2004).

A simple measurement of visceral fat is the **waist: hip ratio** (WHR)—waist circumference divided by hip circumference. The WHR should be <0.9 in men and <0.8 in women. Although there is no standard cut-off for waist circumference that provides an indication of greater risk, the WHO (2000) suggests that a waist measurement >94 cm in men and ≥80 cm in women indicates some risk, and a waist circumference >102 cm in men and >88 cm in women indicates a substantially increased risk of health problems. In 1995, waist measurements were >94 cm for 35% of Australian men and >102 cm for 19%. For women, waist measurements were >80 cm for 37% and >88 cm for 23% (AIHW 2000). These waist circumference measurement guidelines have been developed for Caucasians; similar guidelines have not yet been established for other populations.

The need for prevention and intervention to reduce obesity has been recognised in Australia. A range of strategies has been developed, including the Active Australia initiative that was launched in 1996. This is a national approach to encouraging Australians to participate in physical activity. Several reports were also published in response to the Active Australia campaign, e.g. *Developing an Active Australia: A Framework for Action for Physical Activity and Health* (June 1998) and *National Physical Activity Guidelines for Australians* (June 1999). In September 2003, the National Health and Medical Research Council of Australia developed *Clinical Practice Guidelines for the Management of Overweight and Obesity in Adults.* It was recommended that the guidelines be updated and revised by 2006.

The management of obesity is complex, however, and increasing physical activity is just one strategy for weight control. To understand the disorder of obesity and to develop management strategies, it is essential to appreciate the complexity of the disorder.

PATHOPHYSIOLOGY OF OBESITY

Obesity is a complex multifactorial disorder involving changes in **energy balance** (intake and expenditure), genetic factors, environmental factors (dietary and physical activity) and psychosocial factors (Figure 58-1). The complexity of these interacting forces has made the management of obesity difficult, and some individuals have resorted to surgical procedures such as gastric bypass and banded gastroplasty.

Primary obesity rarely results from endocrine disorders (e.g. Cushing's syndrome, hypothyroidism or hypogonadism) or from neurological disorders or drug treatment. From the simplest viewpoint, obesity, which is manifest by increased fat storage, is a consequence of an imbalance between increased energy (food) intake and decreased energy expenditure. Although on the surface this is a simple relationship, various factors can modify the balance between energy intake and expenditure.

Energy balance: integration involving the periphery and the hypothalamus

The control of food intake is not fully understood. It is regulated by a complex system of interacting monoamine

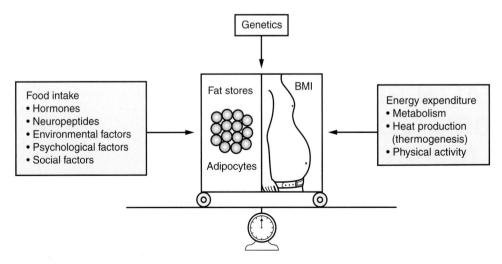

FIGURE 58-1 Energy balance: factors influencing energy intake and energy expenditure.

and peptide neurotransmitters, involving both peripheral and central hypothalamic pathways. The involvement of the sympathetic nervous system (and its neurotransmitter noradrenaline) in regulating energy expenditure has been well documented scientifically and is popularly accepted—obese individuals are often perceived as having 'slow metabolism' and lean people as having 'high metabolism'. Stimulation of α-adrenoceptors by noradrenaline decreases food intake via an action in the feeding centre in the hypothalamus, and increases energy expenditure via stimulation of peripheral β-adrenoceptors. Similarly, activation of central 5-hydroxytryptamine (5-HT, serotonin) receptors by an excess of 5-HT inhibits food intake (Figure 58-2).

In addition to these monoamine transmitters, many central and peripheral peptide neurotransmitters are involved. These are classed as orexigenic (increasing food intake, e.g. neuropeptide Y) or anorexigenic (decreasing food intake, e.g. cholecystokinin). Interest has focused more recently on the role of peripherally released leptin and cholecystokinin, and antiobesity drugs targeted at these sites are being developed.

Leptin

Leptin (derived from the Greek word *leptos*, meaning thin) is the protein product of the obesity (*ob*) gene identified in 1994 (Zhang et al 1994). This protein is released from adipocytes (fat cells) and signals the brain about the fat stores of the body. Generation of leptin is increased by oestrogen, glucocorticoids and possibly by insulin, and is reduced by β-adrenoceptor agonists. On reaching the brain, leptin reduces the production of neuropeptide Y, which normally stimulates food intake and causes a reduction in energy expenditure. Leptin also stimulates the production of corticotrophin-releasing hormone, which reduces food intake (Figure 58-2). Obese humans have higher levels of leptin that correlate with the amount of body fat, but the leptin in those individuals fails to normalise the fat stores. This has led some investigators to propose that obese individuals may have leptin resistance, analogous to the insulin resistance encountered in type 2 diabetes (Mertens & Van Gaal 2000).

Cholecystokinin

Cholecystokinin (CCK) is secreted from the duodenum in the presence of food. It inhibits gastric emptying, pyloric sphincter contraction and stimulation of pancreatic exocrine secretions, and significantly reduces feelings of hunger and increases satiety (feeling of fullness) (Figure 58-2). Stimulation of CCK-A receptors on the vagus nerve sends signals to the hypothalamus and an interaction appears to occur between

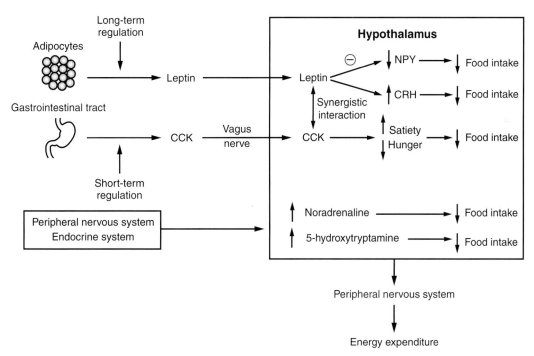

FIGURE 58-2 Schematic representation of food-regulating pathways. The long-term regulation of food intake involves the leptin system, which causes a reduction in food intake by decreasing hypothalamic neuropeptide Y (NPY) synthesis and release, and increasing the release of corticotrophin-releasing hormone (CRH). Short-term control involves cholecystokinin (CCK) released from the duodenum; CCK stimulates receptors on the vagus nerve to signal the hypothalamus of reduced feelings of hunger and satiety. Signals are also received by the hypothalamus from the peripheral nervous system and various hormonal stimuli. Specialised nuclei in the hypothalamus integrate the various signals and modulate the release of chemicals that affect food intake, and of impulses to the autonomic nervous system that regulate energy expenditure.

leptin and CCK (Mertens & Van Gaal 2000). This interaction may play a role in both the short- and long-term regulation of body weight. Other peripheral and central pathways may also be involved in the regulation of food intake and energy storage, but our knowledge is still incomplete.

Genetic factors

There is now widespread acceptance of a genetic component to obesity. Studies with adopted children have shown that their weight is related to that of their biological parents and not to that of their adopted parents. Estimates of a contribution of genetic effects to obesity range from 25% to 80%, and these findings have undoubtedly given credibility to the widely held perception that overweight parents have overweight kids.

It has long been recognised that many people with diabetes are obese, but a link between the two disorders has been difficult to establish. In a recent hallmark study using mice, a team of researchers has shown a link between diabetes and a protein called resistin, which is produced in adipocytes. Their studies established that diabetic mice have higher resistin levels, and these are linked to both diet-induced and genetic obesity (Steppan et al 2001). Determining associations between human obesity and genetic mutations is still in its infancy, but there is no doubt that obesity has a genetic basis in some individuals.

Environmental factors

The availability of 'fast foods' and foods high in fat is an ever-present problem, coupled with changing lifestyles and a tendency for more sedentary pursuits. In consequence, the average weight of Australian women has increased by 4.8 kg and that of men by 3.6 kg since 1980 (AIHW 2000). The tendency for us to obtain our daily energy from bread, milk and potatoes (mashed potato or hot chips) does not fit with the National Health and Medical Research Council's guidelines for weight reduction (NHMRC 2003). Strategies are aimed at increasing the consumption of vegetables, fruit, grains and cereals in an attempt to control the pandemic of obesity. Increased physical activity is also being encouraged, again attempting to redress the imbalance between high dietary fat intake and reduced energy expenditure.

MANAGEMENT OF OBESITY

Obesity is a complex disorder, and a complete understanding of all the interacting factors that lead to obesity is still to come. Management is difficult, and individuals' compliance with one or all aspects of a program may vary enormously. Regulation of weight and the adoption of a healthy lifestyle

are the main issues for many people, especially those whose genes predispose them to obesity: 'A man, for example, with a marked family history of obesity who has been obese since childhood will probably never be thin, despite his best efforts' (Wadden et al 1999). There is often initial difficulty in losing weight, and further difficulties in maintaining the weight reduction. Preferred strategies include dietary modification (low-fat diet), exercise programs and behavioural modification (Wadden et al 1999). Obesity is a lifelong problem for many people. Pharmacological agents could play an increasingly important role as knowledge of the biochemical and genetic factors contributing to obesity improves. Although drugs may produce an initial weight loss, maintaining the weight loss is still the key issue.

DRUG THERAPY

Truly safe and effective drugs for the treatment of obesity are not yet available, but several drugs targeted at specific sites are in development (Figure 58-3). Previously, and still to a limited extent, the main drugs used for the treatment of obesity were the centrally acting appetite suppressants that mimic the actions of noradrenaline.

Noradrenergic drugs

Dextroamphetamine was introduced during the 1930s for the treatment of narcolepsy (desire to sleep) and was found

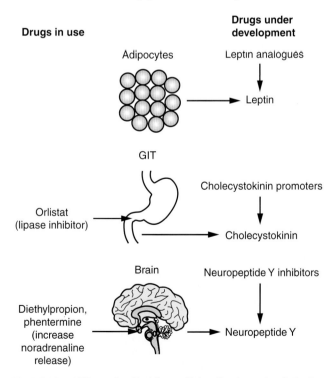

FIGURE 58-3 Sites of action for antiobesity drugs in clinical use and drugs under development.

to produce weight loss. It was later established that the anorectic effect of amphetamine is mediated via release of noradrenaline in the hypothalamus, which enhances sympathetic neurotransmission, resulting in appetite suppression and increased energy expenditure. Because of actions on central dopaminergic pathways producing central excitatory effects, amphetamine unfortunately had very high addictive and abuse potential.

Other noradrenergic amphetamine-like drugs with reduced potential for drug abuse were developed specifically as appetite suppressants. These included benzphetamine, diethylpropion, phentermine, methamphetamine and phendimetrazine. Diethylpropion and phentermine are the only ones currently available in Australia; a comparison of their pharmacological properties is shown in Table 58-2. The action of these drugs in increasing catecholamine concentrations makes them unsuitable for use in obese people with cardiovascular disease (see Chapter 12). Both drugs are indicated for short-term treatment (about 3 months) of obesity in conjunction with a management plan of caloric restriction, an exercise program and behavioural modification. Tolerance to the anorectic effect of these drugs develops at varying times, and this limits their long-term usefulness.

Drugs acting via 5-HT

Dexfenfluramine and fenfluramine were drugs that enhanced 5-HT release and inhibited neuronal reuptake of 5-HT. This led to an increase in 5-HT concentration in the hypothalamus and a subsequent decrease in food intake. Both drugs had minimal effect on sympathetic and dopaminergic neurotransmission. These agents were often used in combination with phentermine but were found to cause pulmonary hypertension and thickening of cardiac valves, requiring valve replacement in some women (see Clinical Interest Box 58-2). Both drugs have been withdrawn voluntarily from the market, leaving only the older noradrenergic drugs and the new drug, sibutramine.

Sibutramine

Like many drugs acting on central neurotransmitters, sibutramine was originally developed for the treatment of depression. Sibutramine increases the central concentrations of noradrenaline and 5-HT by inhibiting their reuptake mechanisms. This leads to weight loss via the induction of the sensation of satiety. In relation to other drugs (e.g. dexfenfluramine, orlistat), sibutramine produces significantly greater weight loss; however, weight is regained when the treatment is stopped. Currently, trials are limited to less than 2 years of sibutramine use, and long-term data on overall effectiveness are not available.

Beneficial changes following sibutramine-induced weight loss are observed in obesity-related risk factors such as hyperlipidaemia, serum uric acid concentration and control of blood glucose. In general, sibutramine is well tolerated; common adverse effects include elevated heart rate, raised BP, headache, anxiety, insomnia, nausea and constipation. In view of the adverse effects on the cardiovascular system, sibutramine is contraindicated in individuals with a history of hypertension, and is not recommended in persons with coronary artery disease, dysrhythmias, congestive heart failure and stroke. In view of the synergistic effects, sibutramine should not be used in combination with diethylpropion or phentermine. Concern continues to be expressed as to whether sibutramine will produce the same effects on cardiac valves as fenfluramine and likewise produce pulmonary hypertension. As with other drug therapy, sibutramine use should be accompanied by caloric restriction, increased exercising, and eating behaviour modification.

Inhibition of nutrient absorption
Orlistat

Orlistat is synthesised from lipstatin, a natural product of *Streptomyces toxytricini*, and was approved for use in Australia in 2000. It is a potent and irreversible inhibitor of gastric and **pancreatic lipase** (Figure 58-3). Inhibition of the lipases prevents the breakdown of dietary triglycerides (fat) and inhibits the absorption of cholesterol and lipid-soluble vitamins. Orlistat therefore decreases the absorption of dietary fat and promotes a reduction in body weight and plasma cholesterol (Carek & Dickerson 1999). In several clinical

---

CLINICAL INTEREST BOX 58-2
ANOREXIANTS AND VALVULAR DISORDERS

In June 1999, the New Zealand Ministry of Health issued an alert on valvular abnormalities with dexfenfluramine and fenfluramine. The alert advised that those who at any time had taken these drugs for 3 months or longer should be investigated for valvular abnormalities. The Accident Compensation Corporation received more than 400 claims for investigation; two claims of medical mishap have been accepted.

The NZ Centre for Adverse Reactions Monitoring (CARM) received eight reports of abnormalities possibly associated with the use of fenfluramine. In two cases, there were cardiac features consistent with those described in the literature; one patient required a valve replacement and the other had evidence of disease some 20 years after exposure to fenfluramine. These drugs are no longer available in New Zealand.
Source: Prescriber Update 2001; 20; available: www.medsafe.govt.nz, accessed 31 January 2006.

TABLE 58-2 Appetite-suppressing noradrenergic drugs

	DIETHYLPROPION	PHENTERMINE
Mechanism of action	Both drugs predominantly cause the release of noradrenaline and, to a variable extent, the release of dopamine from storage sites in the brain and periphery. The appetite-suppressant effect is generally considered to be due to enhanced catecholamine concentration in the hypothalamus	
Pharmacokinetics		
Absorption	>95%	About 100%
Metabolism/excretion	Undergoes extensive hepatic metabolism (about 12 metabolites have been identified). The metabolites and unchanged drug (about 5%) are excreted in the urine over 30–40 hours	About 15% is metabolised in the liver and most is excreted unchanged in urine over 72 hours
Plasma half-life	About 2 hours	About 25 hours (urinary acidification reduces half-life to 7–8 hours)
Drug interactions	Combination with monoamine oxidase inhibitors (MAOIs) is contraindicated because of the likelihood of a hypertensive crisis. Care should be exercised if concurrent general anaesthesia is anticipated, as arrhythmias can occur. Response to antidiabetic drugs (e.g. insulin) may be altered	Action of adrenergic neuron blockers (e.g. clonidine and methyldopa) may be antagonised, reducing their antihypertensive effect. Combination with MAOIs is contraindicated because of the likelihood of a hypertensive crisis. Alcohol potentiates central nervous system adverse effects such as dizziness and light-headedness. Response to antidiabetic drugs (e.g. insulin) may be altered
Adverse reactions		
Cardiovascular	Commonly reported adverse reactions with both drugs include palpitations, tachycardia and dysrhythmias. Rarely, angina and myocardial infarction have been reported with phentermine, and pulmonary hypertension and valvular heart disease with diethylpropion	
Central nervous system	These primarily occur as a result of overstimulation, and include nervousness, restlessness, jitteriness, insomnia, dizziness and headache. Rarely, euphoria may occur followed by depression and fatigue	
Gastrointestinal	These include nausea, vomiting, abdominal discomfort, dryness of the mouth, diarrhoea and constipation	
Warnings and contraindications	Manufacturers' current information and other reference sources should be consulted, as many warnings and contraindications exist. Both drugs, for example, are contraindicated in people with cardiovascular disease (e.g. pulmonary artery hypertension, arterial hypertension, valve abnormalities, arrhythmias, arteriosclerosis), cerebrovascular disease, hypersensitivity to sympathomimetic amines, hyperthyroidism, or history of psychiatric illness or drug abuse. Combined use with other anorectic agents is also contraindicated	
Dosage and administration	For adults and children over 12 years, the recommended dose is 25 mg 3–4 times daily 1 hour before meals. A sustained-release preparation of 75 mg may be used once daily, preferably swallowed whole midmorning. Use in children <12 years is not recommended. Treat for a maximum of 12 weeks	The recommended starting dose is 15 mg given once daily at breakfast. For maintenance a dose of 15–40 mg daily may be used 4–6 weeks, depending on responsiveness. Treat for a maximum of 12 weeks
ADEC Pregnancy Category	B2	B3*

*Weight reduction using appetite suppressant drugs is not recommended in pregnancy.

studies conducted over 1–2 years, the percentage of people losing weight with orlistat was 10%–20% higher than in the placebo-treated groups (Bray 1999). Further long-term clinical trials are continuing. Weight loss generally occurs within 2 weeks of commencement of drug therapy and is maintained with continued use.

PHARMACOKINETICS

Orlistat undergoes minimal systemic absorption and is essentially retained within the gastrointestinal tract. Metabolism occurs within the gastrointestinal wall, and two major metabolites have been identified. Less than 2% of orlistat is excreted in urine and most of the drug is eliminated in faeces (>96%), with unchanged drug accounting for 83% of the total dose excreted.

Drug interaction studies are limited with orlistat, and to date several studies have reported that coadministration of orlistat and cyclosporin may result in reduced plasma concentration of cyclosporin. As vitamin K absorption may also be decreased, people taking warfarin or phenindione should be monitored for changes in coagulation parameters. Additional contraceptive precautions are recommended when taking combined oral contraceptives and orlistat concurrently because of reports of breakthrough bleeding and contraceptive failure. In the absence of extensive drug interaction studies, concomitant administration of other antiobesity agents is not recommended (Caswell 2005).

The most commonly observed adverse reactions involve the gastrointestinal tract and include fatty or oily stools, oily spotting, flatulence, liquid stools, abdominal pain, and faecal incontinence and urgency. Other commonly reported adverse reactions from clinical trials with orlistat included headache, nausea and dyspepsia.

Current package insert information should be consulted with regard to warnings and contraindications, as data on this drug are limited. Orlistat should be used with caution in individuals with active peptic ulcer disease or significant cardiac, gastrointestinal, renal, hepatic or endocrine disorders. Use in people with cholestasis, chronic pancreatitis or pancreatic enzyme deficiency or chronic malabsorption syndrome is contraindicated. Although orlistat is classed in ADEC Pregnancy Category B1, its safety in pregnant women has not been established.

**CLINICAL INTEREST BOX 58-3
NON-PRESCRIPTION WEIGHT LOSS
SUPPLEMENTS**

Millions of dollars are spent each year on commercial weight loss products for which effectiveness has often never been established. A review of popular over-the-counter products available in Australia was conducted in 1999 (Egger et al 1999). The authors concluded that the weight loss benefits of most of the substances could not be supported. The products reviewed included ones containing brindelberry, capsaicin, caffeine/guarana, l-carnitine, chitosan, chromium picolinate, *Fucus vesiculosus* (seaweed), *Ginkgo biloba*, pectin, grapeseed extract, lecithin, horse chestnut, sweet clover/soy beans or St John's wort.

The authors concluded that "lack of positive evidence, while not necessarily disqualifying sale of a particular product (provided safety issues are satisfied), should certainly disqualify the use of unverified claims relating to these products".
From: Egger et al 1999.

THE FUTURE

Weight gain after discontinuation of drug therapy is common. Maintaining a desirable and realistic weight on a long-term basis is a difficult, soul-destroying task for many individuals. The current antiobesity drugs can cause problems, so long-term use is not recommended. Investigations of the effectiveness of leptin analogues, neuropeptide Y antagonists, B_3 adrenergic agonists and lipolytic growth hormone fragments are in progress. The search for safe and effective drugs continues but it is unlikely that there will ever be a drug that allows a person to lose weight despite increased food intake and reduced physical activity. Future drugs may help some individuals but until then "a supportive, knowledgeable medical environment in which individuals can be helped to understand what is necessary in the way of food intake and daily activity is vital . . . the aim is not to make everyone thin, but to prevent some becoming overweight or obese" (Caterson 1999b).

DRUGS AT A GLANCE 58: Drugs in obesity			
Therapeutic group	**Pharmacological group**	**Key examples**	**Key pages**
Antiobesity drugs	Lipase inhibitor	orlistat	951
	NA/5-HT reuptake inhibitor	sibutramine	951
	Sympathomimetic anorectics	diethylpropion	952
		phentermine	952

KEY POINTS

- Obesity is a complex multifactorial disorder involving changes in energy balance, genetic factors, environmental factors and psychosocial factors.
- The body mass index (BMI) is highly correlated with body fat and is calculated by dividing an individual's body mass (kg) by the square of his or her height in metres (m^2).
- People with a BMI >25 are considered overweight and those with a BMI >30 are considered obese.
- Overweight and obese individuals have a higher mortality than people with a normal BMI.
- A waist:hip ratio >0.9 for men and >0.8 for women indicates significant visceral fat distribution, which is associated with a greater risk of morbidity and mortality.
- The control of food intake is not fully understood. It is regulated by a complex system of interacting monoamine and peptide neurotransmitters involving both peripheral and central hypothalamic pathways.
- Interest has more recently focused on the role of peripheral modulators, which include leptin and cholecystokinin.
- There is widespread acceptance of a genetic component to obesity, and estimates of a genetic contribution range from 25% to 80%.
- Management of obesity is difficult because of the complexity of the disorder. Preferred strategies include dietary modification (low-fat diet), exercise programs and behavioural modification.
- Truly safe and effective drugs for the treatment of obesity are not yet available.
- Current drugs include the two centrally acting noradrenergic appetite suppressants diethylpropion and phentermine, the noradrenergic and 5-HT reuptake inhibitor sibutramine and the lipase inhibitor orlistat. Tolerance to the anorectic effect of the noradrenergic drugs has limited their usefulness. There are limited long-term data on the use of orlistat and sibutramine.
- Obesity is a lifelong problem for many people. Pharmacological agents could play an increasingly important role as knowledge of the biochemical and genetic factors contributing to obesity improves.

REVIEW EXERCISES

1. What factors contribute to a disturbance of energy balance in obese individuals?
2. What pharmacological strategies may be adopted to decrease food intake?

REFERENCES AND FURTHER READING

Australian Institute of Health and Welfare. A growing problem: trends and patterns in overweight and obesity among adults in Australia, 1980–2001. *AIHW Bulletin* 2003; Issue 8.

Australian Institute of Health and Welfare. *Australia's Health 2000: The Seventh Biennial Health Report of the Australian Institute of Health and Welfare*. Canberra: AIHW, 2000.

Australian Institute of Health and Welfare (AIHW) and National Heart Foundation of Australia. *The Relationship Between Overweight, Obesity and Cardiovascular Disease*. AIHW Cat. CVD 29. Canberra: AIHW (Cardiovascular Disease Series No. 23), 2004.

Bray GA. Drug treatment of obesity. *Best Practice and Research Clinical Endocrinology and Metabolism* 1999; 13: 131–48.

Cameron AJ, Welborn TA, Zimmet PZ et al. Overweight and obesity in Australia: the 1999–2000 Australian Diabetes, Obesity and Lifestyle Study (AusDiab). *Medical Journal of Australia* 2003; 178: 427–32.

Carek PJ, Dickerson LM. Current concepts in the pharmacological management of obesity. *Drugs* 1999; 57: 883–904.

Caswell A (ed.). *MIMS Annual 2005*. Sydney: CMPMedica Australia, 2005.

Caterson ID. Obesity and its management. *Australian Prescriber* 1999a; 22: 12–16.

Caterson ID. What should we do about overweight and obesity? *Medical Journal of Australia* 1999b; 171: 599–600.

Egger G, Cameron-Smith D, Stanton R. The effectiveness of popular, non-prescription weight loss supplements. *Medical Journal of Australia* 1999; 171: 604–8.

Mertens IL, Van Gaal LF. Promising new approaches to the management of obesity. *Drugs* 2000; 60: 1–9.

Ministry of Health. *A Portrait of Health: Key Results of the 2002/03 New Zealand Health Survey*. Wellington: Ministry of Health, 2004.

National Health and Medical Research Council of Australia. *Clinical Practice Guidelines for the Management of Overweight and Obesity in Adults*. Canberra: NHMRC, 2003.

National Health and Medical Research Council. *Acting on Australia's Weight: A Strategic Plan for the Prevention of Overweight and Obesity*. Canberra: NHMRC, 1997.

Steppan CM, Bailey ST, Bhat S, Brown EJ, Banerjee RR et al. The hormone resistin links obesity to diabetes. *Nature* 2001; 409: 307–12.

Wadden TA, Sarwer DB, Berkowitz RI. Behavioural treatment of the overweight patient. *Best Practice and Research Clinical Endocrinology and Metabolism* 1999; 13: 93–107.

World Health Organization. *Obesity: Preventing and Managing the Global Epidemic. Report of a WHO Technical Report Series 894 on Obesity.* Geneva: WHO, 2000.

Zhang Y, Proenca R, Maffei M, Barone M, Leopold L, Friedman JM. Positional cloning of the mouse *obese* gene and its human homologue. *Nature* 1994; 372: 425–32.

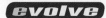 More weblinks at http://evolve.elsevier.com/AU/Bryant/pharmacology/

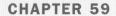

Envenomation and Antivenoms

CHAPTER FOCUS

Millions of people are bitten or stung annually, but the bite or injury usually causes little more than a local irritation. This is in contrast to the clinical manifestations that may arise from a bite by a venomous creature such as a snake or spider, or a sting from a venomous marine creature. Australia has a number of the world's most venomous species, although not all bites result in envenomation. In some instances, no deaths have occurred since the introduction of an antivenom.

OBJECTIVES

- To have an appreciation of the management of a snake bite.
- To understand the mechanisms of action of snake toxins and how these relate to the clinical manifestations.
- To discuss the advantages of monovalent antivenoms.
- To understand the risks associated with snake antivenom administration.
- To discuss the common adverse reactions arising from snake antivenom administration.
- To discuss the local effects of spider bites and to contrast these with the clinical manifestations of severe envenomation by either a funnel web or redback spider.
- To describe the local reactions observed with box jellyfish and stonefish stings.
- To have an awareness of the range of currently available antivenoms.

KEY TERMS

envenomation
coagulopathy
monovalent antivenom
myolysis
polyvalent antivenom
pressure-immobilisation
snakes
spiders
units of antivenom

KEY ABBREVIATIONS

CSL   Commonwealth Serum Laboratories
SVDK   Snake venom detection kit

THROUGHOUT history, snakes have been associated with sinister acts:

- as in the legend of Cleopatra and the famous poisonous asp bite
- mystical powers, such as those of the Greek god of healing, Asklepios (rendered in Latin as Aesculapius), son of Apollo, famous for his rod wound with a single 'serpent', which emerged in the 16th century as a printer's symbol in pharmacopoeias and later as the true symbol of medicine (termed either the Staff of Aesculapius or Rod of Asklepios)
- the gorgon (female monster) Medusa, famous for her hair writhing with snakes and hideous visage that turned all who looked on her to stone.

In contrast, the modern era has given horror status to spiders through movies such as *Tarantula* (1955), *Arachnophobia* (1990) and *Snakes on a Plane* (2006), and glamour status through the comic strip and movie character *Spiderman*. In reality, envenomation is neither sinister nor mystical; it can simply be fatal.

SNAKES

It is estimated that 3000 species of **snakes** exist globally, of which about 600 species are venomous. The two families of most medical relevance are the Elapidae (e.g. sea snakes, brown snakes and death adders), which inhabit all continents except Antarctica, and Viperidae (e.g. vipers and rattlesnakes), which inhabit all continents with the exception of Australia (and New Guinea) and Antarctica. The true incidence of snake bites is unknown. Figures from the 1940s show 50,000 deaths annually, while reasonably reliable data from the World Health Organization estimate 5 million snake bites, 2.5 million envenomations and 125,000 deaths annually (Chippaux 1998). In Australia, approximately 3000 snake bites occur each year, with 200–500 victims receiving antivenom and an average mortality of 1–2 persons. The commonest bites are from brown snakes, which also cause the majority of deaths. The remainder are from the tiger snake, taipan and death adder (White 1998).

Unlike past practice, the current initial management of snake bite does not involve 'sucking the venom out', excision of the bite or application of an arterial tourniquet. The emphasis is on '**pressure-immobilisation**' (see Clinical Interest Box 59-1).

Mechanisms of venom toxicity

The toxic constituents of snake venoms, which are mostly proteins, vary among snakes, and each toxin produces distinct clinical features. Not all snake venoms cause all effects (Table 59-1). The major clinical features of **envenomation** in humans are highly variable, but include:

- headache (within 1 hour), irritability, nausea, vomiting, diarrhoea, confusion, and occasionally sudden hypotension with loss of consciousness
- flaccid paralysis resulting from presynaptic and postsynaptic neurotoxins that cause a progressive neuromuscular flaccid paralysis (within 1–3 hours), affecting muscles supplying the eye and causing ptosis and/or diplopia, dysphagia and, in severe envenomation, respiratory muscle paralysis (3–18 hours) and muscle weakness in limbs
- **coagulopathy** resulting from activation of the coagulation system, which results in consumption of coagulation factors, leading to clinical anticoagulation. Australian elapids possess potent procoagulant molecules in their venom but not all species cause this effect. Spontaneous bleeding is uncommon but individuals with procoagulant coagulopathy may develop unexpected massive intracranial bleeding. Where available, haematology tests (INR, APTT, fibrinogen, platelets etc) should be done immediately and at regular intervals thereafter

---

CLINICAL INTEREST BOX 59-1 MANAGEMENT OF SNAKE BITE

Throughout the management process, ensure as little movement by the victim as possible, lay the victim down, don't allow the victim to walk or move the limb, and provide constant reassurance. Attempt to identify the snake!

1. Do not wash the area of the bite, as it is essential to retain traces of venom if the Snake Venom Detection Kit is to be used.
2. Reduce lymphatic spread of the venom by pressure-immobilisation; apply firm bandaging evenly over a pad placed over the bitten area. The bandaging should be firm but not stop blood flow or cause venous congestion. If the bite is on the head, neck or trunk, apply a firm pressure dressing.
3. To aid in later retrieval of a venom sample through a small window cut in the bandage, mark on the outside of the bandage the site of the bite.
4. A splint/sling should be applied (if possible) to immobilise the limb.
5. Withhold any drugs or alcohol, which may confound clinical assessment.
6. If possible, bring transport to the victim or move victim on a (makeshift) stretcher; try to prevent walking.
7. Transport the victim to the nearest medical facility and, ideally, do not remove the pressure-immobilisation until antivenom is available, an IV line is in place and venom detection and blood test results are available. If severe envenomation is suspected, leave pressure-immobilisation in place until antivenom therapy has commenced.

Source: AMH, 2006.

TABLE 59-1 Examples of venomous elapid snakes, venom toxins and clinical manifestations of envenomation

SNAKES (COMMON NAME)	GENUS		VENOM TOXINS*	LOCAL REACTIONS	MAJOR SYSTEMIC REACTIONS*
Black snakes			Procoagulants	Minor	Coagulopathy
Red-bellied black	*Pseudechis porphyriacus*		Myotoxins		Myolysis
King brown (Mulga)	*Pseudechis australis*		Neurotoxins		Neurotoxicity
Spotted black or blue-bellied black	*Pseudechis guttatus*				
Papuan black	*Pseudechis papuanus*				
Butler's black	*Pseudechis butleri*				
Collett's black	*Pseudechis colletti*				
False mulga	*Pseudechis weigeli*				
Brown snakes			Neurotoxins	Negligible	Neurotoxicity
Eastern (common) brown	*Pseudonaja textilis*		Procoagulants		Coagulopathy
Western brown (Gwardar)	*Pseudonaja nuchalis*				
Dugite	*Pseudonaja affinis*				
Peninsula	*Pseudonaja inframacula*				
Ingram's	*Pseudonaja ingrami*				
Spotted	*Pseudonaja guttata*				
Ringed	*Pseudonaja modesta*				
Death Adders			Neurotoxins	Minor	Neurotoxicity
Common	*Acanthopis antarcticus*				
Northern	*Acanthopis praelongus*				
Desert	*Acanthopis pyrrhus*				
Pilbara	*Acanthopis wellsi*				
Sea snakes			Neurotoxins	Minor	Neurotoxicity
(multiple genera)	e.g. *Enhydrina, Astrotia, Aipysurus, Disteira, Hydrophis, Lapemis*		Myotoxins		Myolysis
Taipans			Neurotoxins	Minor	Neurotoxicity
Coastal taipan	*Oxyuranus scutellatus*		Myotoxins		Myolysis
Inland taipan (Fierce snake)	*Oxyuranus microlepidotus*		Procoagulants		Coagulopathy
Tiger snakes			Neurotoxins	Minor	Coagulopathy
Eastern tiger	*Notechis scutatus*		Myotoxins		Myolysis
Black tiger	*Notechis ater* (Note expert advice: 'Recent studies have found that the Black tiger snake is not genetically different from the Eastern tiger snake— hence, at the moment, there is only one tiger snake, *Notechis scutatus*')		Procoagulants		Neurotoxicity

*It should be noted that envenoming by snakes causes many potential effects in humans, and key information sources should be consulted (e.g. Clinical Toxinology Resources website: www.toxinology.com).

- **myolysis** as a result of myotoxins that bind to muscle fibres, causing progressive destruction of muscle cells. This may manifest as muscle pain and weakness, red discoloration of urine (myoglobinuria) and a significant increase in creatine kinase
- nephrotoxicity, resulting most probably from a combination of hypotension, rhabdomyolysis and coagulopathy. Serum electrolytes, creatinine, fluid status and urine output should be carefully monitored
- local tissue injury, which is uncommon with snake bites in Australia; fang marks may also easily be missed. However, local swelling and redness may be observed and minor pain reported.

Antivenom production

Snake antivenoms are produced using age-old technology. In general, venoms are obtained by 'milking' snakes and then injecting minute quantities of the venom into horses over a long period of time (e.g. 10–12 months). Blood is then removed from the horse and the plasma containing the antibodies to the venom is extracted and purified. Snake antivenoms used in Australia are all refined preparations of F(ab′)$_2$ portions of IgG obtained from the plasma of immunised horses. F(ab′)$_2$ preparations are obtained by pepsin treatment of IgG, which removes the Fc (constant) fragment from the IgG molecule. Use of the F(ab′)$_2$ fragment reduces the incidence of hypersensitivity reactions compared to that with whole IgG (see Chapter 54).

Most laboratories produce monovalent or polyvalent antivenoms. **Monovalent antivenoms** are, in general, raised against venom from a single snake species; a smaller dose of antivenom is then used for treatment, which decreases the risk of adverse reactions. However, when administering monovalent antivenom it is essential to identify the species of snake involved, as the antivenom is active only against that single species or against a few closely related species whose venoms cross-react with the specific antivenom. **Polyvalent antivenoms** are produced using venom from a number of species; this broadens the usefulness of the antivenom, but a larger dose is usually required to neutralise the venom. When using a polyvalent antivenom, identification of the snake species is less important.

The vast majority of antivenoms are still produced in horses using traditional inoculation, serum collection and fractionation technology. As antivenoms are administered by intravenous infusion, an issue of concern globally is the quality, safety and efficacy of antivenoms. A report of a WHO workshop on the production and control of antivenom production was published in 2003 (Theakston et al 2003). A key emphasis is on quality control of antivenom production, in order to reduce:
- the incidence of human adverse reactions to horse proteins

- transmission of viruses to humans (e.g. equine infectious anaemia virus)
- bacterial toxin contamination.

Snake Venom Detection Kits

It is important to remember that a snake may bite, but it might not leave fang marks and envenomation might not occur. To aid in diagnosis, the Snake Venom Detection Kit (SVDK) has been developed by the Commonwealth Serum Laboratories (CSL). This kit is designed to detect venom in samples taken at the bite site and in urine from victims of snake bites in Australia and Papua New Guinea (testing blood is unreliable). Detailed instructions are provided with the kit and, if venom is present in the sample, it will usually cause a colour change in one or a number of wells on the kit plate. No colour change indicates that venom was not detected. The purpose of the kit is to assist in matching antivenom therapy to the type of venom. A positive SVDK result from the bite site does not necessarily indicate significant envenomation. However, it does provide an indication of the type of antivenom to administer if the clinical features or laboratory tests indicate the need for antivenom therapy. The SVDK will detect venom from tiger snakes, brown snakes, black snakes, death adders and taipans.

Snake Antivenoms

Snake antivenoms available in Australia are listed in Table 59-2; the choice of antivenom is guided by the species of snake involved. Refer to relevant drug information sources for instructions on intravenous administration of antivenoms. In all cases of snake bite, consideration must be given to whether the benefit of neutralising the toxin (local or circulating) outweighs the possibility of adverse reactions, particularly allergic reactions to the antivenom. As this is a real risk, ensure that adrenaline is available (drawn up in a syringe or ready as an IV infusion) for immediate use, before commencing antivenom therapy.

Administration of an antivenom is indicated when there are clear clinical signs of envenomation (e.g. neurotoxicity, coagulopathy, renal failure). The dosage used is then determined by the degree of envenomation as evident from the clinical situation. In general, the **units of antivenom** contained in each vial have been standardised to neutralise in vitro the average yield of venom from the particular snake. Children are often victims of snake bites, and because of their lower body mass and the likelihood of physical activity after the bite (e.g. a panic-stricken run to find an adult) are at greater risk of severe envenomation. The dosage of antivenom for a child is the *same* as that for an adult, as the basis of antivenom therapy is neutralising the venom, which is snake-dependent and independent of the body weight of the victim.

TABLE 59-2 Snake antivenoms

ANTIVENOMS	VENOM NEUTRALISED	UNITS OF ANTIVENOM/VIAL	DOSE RANGE
Monovalent antivenoms			
Black snake	King brown (Mulga) snakes, Papuan black snakes, Collett's snake, (red- and blue-bellied black snakes, see Tiger venom)	18,000	1 vial
Brown snake	All brown snake species (except the King brown), dugite, gwardar	1000	2–8 vials
Death adder	Death adder species	6000	1–4 vials
Sea snake		1000	1–5 vials
Taipan	Taipan, Fierce snake	12,000	1–6 vials
Tiger snake	Tiger snake, copperhead, red-bellied black, blue-bellied black,* rough-scaled snake	3000	2–8 vials
Polyvalent antivenom	King brown, taipan, death adder, tiger snake, brown snake	40,000[†]	1–8 vials

*Tiger snake antivenom is used in preference to black snake antivenom to treat envenomation by red-bellied black and blue-bellied black snakes.
[†]The polyvalent antivenom contains King brown antivenom 18,000 units, taipan antivenom 12,000 units, death adder antivenom 6000 units, tiger snake antivenom 3000 units, and brown snake antivenom 1000 units.

TABLE 59-3 Adverse reactions to antivenoms*

SYSTEM/REACTION TYPE	COMMON REACTIONS	UNCOMMON REACTIONS
General	Pyrexia	Pain at infusion site
Cardiovascular		Chest pain, cyanosis
Gastrointestinal		Abdominal pain, vomiting
Hypersensitivity/skin	Urticaria, rash, hypotension, bronchospasm, anaphylaxis, delayed serum sickness	Angio-oedema
Musculoskeletal		Arthralgia, myalgia
Neurological	Headache	

* The frequency of sea snake envenomation is low in comparison to that by land snakes, so the usage of the antivenom is low and the adverse reaction profile is not as comprehensive.
Source: Caswell 2005.

Adverse reactions to antivenoms

The adverse reaction of greatest concern is anaphylaxis, and the risk is greater in individuals allergic to horses, horse-based products or antivenom. The risk of adverse reactions rises with increasing dosage of antivenom, and the frequency of adverse reactions is lower with the monovalent antivenoms. A summary of adverse reactions to CSL antivenoms is presented in Table 59-3.

SPIDERS

Similar to snakes, **spiders** can evoke much horror in some individuals (arachnophobia). Although spider bites are associated with significant morbidity, they do not have the same mortality as snake bites. However, such is the concern about spider bites that they rank as the second commonest reason for calls to the NSW Poisons Information Centre in

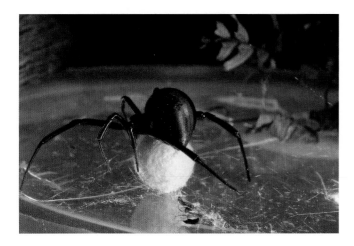

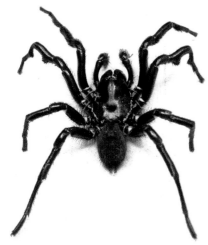

FIGURE 59-1 Female redback spider with egg sac (top) and male funnel-web spider (bottom).

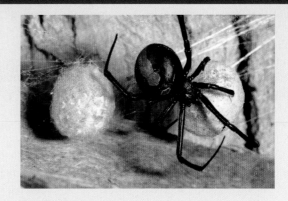
Australia, with about 4000–5000 calls a year. The majority of spider bites cause only minor effects, but the medically significant species that may require antivenom administration include the Australian funnel-web spiders (Hexathelidae, Atracinae: *Hadronyche* and *Atrax*) and the redback spider (*Latrodectus hasseltii*). More than 30 species of funnel-web spiders live on the eastern seaboard of Australia, in parts of South Australia and in Tasmania. It is the Sydney funnel-web spider (*Atrax robustus*), which inhabits a 160 km radius of the central business district of Sydney, that causes most concern, as the male funnel-web is considered to be the most venomous spider in the world (Figure 59-1). Prior to the introduction of the antivenom in 1981, 13 funnel-web fatalities had been recorded in Australia and attributed to the male funnel-web spider.

Redback spiders belong to the widow genus (*Latrodectus* spp.) of spiders, and a best guess is that more than 5000 redback spider bites occur each year in Australia. Redbacks live throughout Australia and prefer a drier habitat. In the redback family, it is the female that is the more venomous (Figure 59-1). The last recorded death attributed to *Latrodectus hasseltii* was in 1955, a year before the antivenom became available from CSL. Another member of the *Latrodectus* group is found in New Zealand (see Clinical Interest Box 59-2).

Mechanisms of toxicity

Spiders use their venom to immobilise their prey, to begin the digestive process, and as a defence against natural enemies. Unfortunately (from the spider's perspective!), humans appear in the latter category. Pain or discomfort is a universal feature of spider bites, and prolonged absence of pain after a bite is a good indication that the bite may not be from a spider. Local effects of spider bites include, but are not limited to:

- pain, which may vary in intensity, duration and extent of radiation, and which may be severe enough to prevent victims from sleeping
- fang marks or bleeding at bite site (common feature of funnel-web spider bites)
- redness or red marks (these vary in size but are a common feature in 60%–80% of spider bites)
- itchiness (immediate or delayed).

Swelling or inflammation is an uncommon finding with true spider bites (Isbister & White 2004).

The active component in the venom of the redback is a protein (molecular mass 130,000) called alpha-latrotoxin. It principally acts on nerve endings, causing the release of acetylcholine and other neurotransmitters including catecholamines, and structural changes to sensory nerve terminals. The clinical syndrome of lactrodectism has not been clearly characterised, but includes local pain, diaphoresis (local sweating), nausea, vomiting, headache, generalised sweating, dizziness and malaise. The actual frequency of hypertension, hyperthermia, neuromuscular effects (paralysis of voluntary muscles), abdominal rigidity and agitation/irritability has not been fully established (Isbister & White 2004).

The venom toxins identified with the funnel-web spider are principally neurotoxins; the most clinically relevant are δ-atracotoxins, which interfere with neuronal sodium current inactivation, leading to spontaneous repetitive firing of action potentials. This ultimately leads to depletion of the stores of neurotransmitters in nerves. Severe envenomation is characterised by neuromuscular excitation (e.g. paraesthesia, fasciculations); autonomic nervous system excitation (e.g. hypersalivation, hypertension, hyperlacrimation); pulmonary oedema; and generalised systemic effects (e.g. neuromuscular paralysis, secondary coagulopathy and multi-organ failure) (Isbister & White 2004).

Spider antivenoms
Funnel-web spider

An antivenom for the Sydney funnel-web spider was first developed for clinical use in 1981 by CSL, and no deaths have occurred since its introduction. Unfortunately, a kit for identification of funnel-web spider venom is not available. The antivenom is derived from rabbit IgG produced in response to inoculation of the rabbit with the venom from the Sydney funnel-web. Hypersensitivity reactions (e.g. anaphylaxis, serum sickness) are uncommon. As envenomation can result in death within 30 minutes, administration of the antivenom is not delayed. The initial dose is two vials (250 units) by slow intravenous injection, or four vials if there are systemic indications of severe envenomation. If the victim does not respond adequately, further antivenom therapy may be necessary (more than eight vials may be required).

Redback spider

The antivenom to the redback spider is raised in horses, and is an F(ab′)₂ portion of IgG. Adverse reactions to the antivenom are infrequent and minor, and in some cases have occurred as a result of using the antivenom undiluted. Unlike many of the other antivenoms, the redback antivenom is administered intramuscularly and the intravenous route is more often used for severe or refractory cases of envenomation. In general, the dose range is 1–3 vials, each containing 500 units of antivenom.

MARINE ENVENOMATION

Australian waters contain a number of venomous species, e.g. the blue-ringed octopus, jellyfish, sea snakes (see previous section on snakes), stingrays and stinging fish. It is estimated that more than 10,000 people suffer jellyfish stings annually (see Clinical Interest Box 59-3). Although a variety of marine creatures can bite (including sharks!) only two antivenoms are available, a box jellyfish antivenom and a stonefish antivenom.

Box jellyfish (*Chironex fleckeri*)

The box jellyfish (Figure 59-2) is venomous and dangerous, and 67 deaths from box jellyfish stings have occurred in the Indo-Pacific region. In Australia, the most recent fatalities were in 2000 (a 5-year-old boy) and 2003 (a 7-year-old boy). The box jellyfish can be found in coastal waters from Gladstone (Queensland) to Broome (Western Australia) but does not inhabit the Great Barrier Reef. It is a large jellyfish,

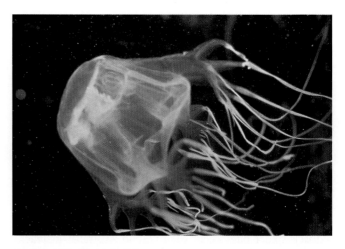

FIGURE 59-2 Box jellyfish.

CLINICAL INTEREST BOX 59-3 IRUKANDJI SYNDROME

The Irukandji syndrome is named after an Australian Aboriginal tribe located in northern Queensland around the Palm Cove region. Although it is believed that a number of jellyfish can cause Irukandji syndrome, the only jellyfish conclusively implicated is *Carukia barnesi*, a small (1.5–2 cm across the bell), transparent jellyfish that can be found both on- and offshore. Irukandji-like stings have been reported in northern Queensland, Western Australia, South Australia, offshore Florida and Hawaii. Although many people stung by *Carukia barnesi* present with non-life-threatening symptoms (e.g. anxiety, distress, generalised pain, nausea, vomiting and hypertension), others may require hospitalisation and, in severe cases, life support.

The clinical manifestations of Irukandji envenomation include (Nimorakiotakis & Winkel 2003a):
• generalised muscular pain, including acute chest and back pain
• effects due to catecholamine excess (anxiety, headache, nausea, sweating, vomiting, tachycardia, severe hypertension with supraventricular tachyarrhythmias)
• cardiopulmonary decompensation.

Due to the infrequency of Irukandji syndrome, treatment is based mainly on anecdotal reports. Analgesia is routinely required and the preference has often been a narcotic, used with caution because of myocardial depression. Antihypertensives may be used if appropriate, and glyceryl trinitrate has been used but again with caution in the

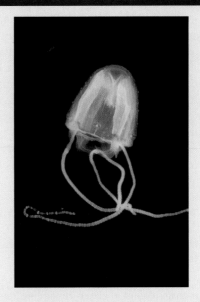

presence of pre-existing cardiac dysfunction. Pulmonary oedema is treated with supplemental oxygen, inotropic support and positive pressure ventilation (Bailey et al 2003). Magnesium reduces catecholamine release and receptor sensitivity and has been reported to be beneficial, with a loading dose of 10 mmol followed by an infusion of 5 mmol/hour (Corkeron 2003).

approximately 20–30 cm across the top, weighs up to 6 kg and has tentacles up to 3 metres in length. It is difficult to see in water as it is transparent, and contact with a single tentacle can result in the discharge of venom from millions of stinging cells (nematocysts) into the skin.

Most stings are minor, but entanglement in a large number of tentacles can result in massive envenomation and death. The mechanism of toxicity is unclear, but death results from respiratory failure or cardiotoxicity, and victims may be unconscious before they can leave the water. Wide erythematous weals are observed where a tentacle has been in contact with the skin, and pain intensifies over about 15 minutes. Immediate first aid involves dousing any attached tentacles with vinegar to inactivate the remaining stinging cells, providing respiratory support and getting immediate help. In Queensland, paramedics carry antivenom in endemic areas (Nimorakiotakis & Winkel 2003a).

The antivenom consists of the F(ab')₂ portion of a purified sheep IgG, and has been available since 1970. Adverse reactions are uncommon. The initial dose is one vial (20,000 units) diluted 1 in 10 (small children: 1 in 5) by slow IV infusion. If necessary, an alternative is to give three vials (60,000 units) undiluted IM at three separate sites.

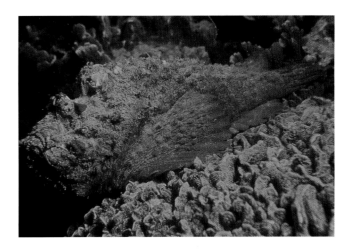

FIGURE 59-3: Stonefish.

Stonefish (*Synanceia trachynis* and *Synanceia verrucosa*)

The two Australian species of stonefish are found spread throughout tropical Indo-Pacific waters. These fish burrow (Figure 59-3) into sand or mud and are well camouflaged.

Accidentally standing on a stonefish results in expulsion of venom from its dorsal spines, which is purely a defence mechanism. No fatalities have been recorded in Australia.

The venom of a stonefish contains myotoxic, neurotoxic and cardiotoxic chemicals, and systemic manifestations of envenomation include muscle weakness, paralysis and shock. Depending on the number of spines penetrating the skin, the immediate reaction is an extremely painful sting, with pain radiating through the limb, accompanied by rapid local swelling (Nimorakiotakis & Winkel 2003b). The pain may be extreme and difficult to manage even with narcotic analgesics. Indications for antivenom use include multiple punctures, extreme pain, weakness and paralysis.

The antivenom consists of the $F(ab')_2$ portion of a purified horse IgG. Adverse reactions are uncommon. Intramuscular dosing is based on the number of puncture sites (AMH 2006):

- 1 vial (2000 units) for 1–2 spine puncture wounds
- 2 vials for 3–4 spine puncture wounds
- 3 vials for >4 spine puncture wounds.

KEY POINTS

- In Australia, approximately 3000 snake bites occur each year, with 200–500 victims receiving antivenom, and an average mortality of 1–2 persons.
- The commonest bites are from brown snakes, which also cause the majority of deaths. The remainder are from the tiger snake, taipan and death adder.
- Unlike past practice, the initial management of snake bite involves pressure-immobilisation.
- Common toxins found in snake venom include neurotoxins, myotoxins and procoagulant molecules.
- Clinical manifestations of snake envenomation include headache, flaccid paralysis, coagulopathy, myolysis and nephrotoxicity.
- Snake antivenoms used in Australia are all refined preparations of $F(ab')_2$ portions of IgG obtained from the plasma of immunised horses.
- Monovalent antivenoms are, in general, raised against venom from a single snake species, whereas polyvalent antivenoms are produced using venom from a number of species.
- Quality control of antivenom production is essential to reduce the incidence of human adverse reactions to horse proteins, transmission of viruses to humans (e.g. equine infectious anaemia virus) and bacterial toxin contamination.
- In all cases of snake bite, consideration must be given to whether the benefit of neutralising the toxin (local or circulating) outweighs the possibility of adverse reactions, particularly allergic reactions to the antivenom.
- The dosage of antivenom used is determined by the degree of envenomation as evident from the clinical situation.
- The units of antivenom contained in each vial have been standardised to neutralise in vitro the average yield of venom from the particular snake.
- The dosage of antivenom for a child is the *same* as for an adult, as the basis of antivenom therapy is neutralising the venom, which is snake-dependent and independent of the body weight of the victim.
- The majority of spider bites cause only minor effects; the medically significant species that may require antivenom administration include the Australian funnel-web spiders and redback spider and the New Zealand katipo spider.
- The venom toxins identified with the funnel-web spider are principally neurotoxins, the most clinically relevant being δ-atracotoxins; and with the redback spider, alpha-latrotoxin.
- The clinical syndrome of latrodectism following a bite from a redback spider has not been clearly characterised, but includes local pain, diaphoresis, nausea, vomiting, headache, generalised sweating, dizziness and malaise.
- Severe envenomation from a funnel-web spider bite is characterised by neuromuscular excitation (e.g. paraesthesia, fasciculations); autonomic nervous system excitation (e.g. hypersalivation, hypertension, hyperlacrimation); pulmonary oedema; and generalised systemic effects (e.g. neuromuscular paralysis, secondary coagulopathy and multi-organ failure).
- Funnel-web antivenoms are derived from rabbit IgG produced in response to inoculation of the rabbit with the venom from the Sydney funnel-web spider; for the redback spider the antivenom is raised in horses and is an $F(ab')_2$ portion of IgG.
- Most box jellyfish stings are minor, but entanglement in a large number of tentacles can result in massive envenomation and death. The mechanism of toxicity is unclear, but death results from respiratory failure or cardiotoxicity.
- The venom of a stonefish contains myotoxic, neurotoxic and cardiotoxic chemicals, and systemic manifestations of envenomation include muscle weakness, paralysis and shock.

REVIEW EXERCISES

1. Discuss the advantages of using monovalent snake antivenoms.
2. Discuss the adverse reaction profile of snake antivenoms.
3. What are the common local features of a spider bite?
4. In terms of antivenoms, what does the number of units in a vial represent?

REFERENCES AND FURTHER READING

Adams S. Bites and stings. *Journal of the Accident and Medical Practitioners Association* 2006; 3: 1–7.
Australian Medicines Handbook 2006. Adelaide: AMH, 2006.
Bailey PM, Little M, Jelinek GA, Wilce JA. Jellyfish envenoming syndromes: unknown toxic mechanisms and unproven therapies. *Medical Journal of Australia* 2003; 178: 34–7.
Caswell A (ed.). *MIMS Annual 2005.* Sydney: CMPMedica Australia, 2005.
Cheng AC, Currie BJ. Venomous snakebites worldwide with a focus on the Australia-Pacific region: current management and controversies. *Journal of Intensive Care Medicine* 2004; 19: 259–69.
Chippaux JP. Snake-bites: appraisal of the global situation. *Bulletin of the World Health Organization* 1998; 76: 515–24.
Corkeron MA. Magnesium infusion to treat Irukandji syndrome. *Medical Journal of Australia* 2003; 178: 411.
Duggin G, Kilham H, Kirby J. *NSW Poisons Information Centre Annual Report 2001.* Sydney, NSW.
Isbister GK, White J. Clinical consequences of spider bites: recent advances in our understanding. *Toxicon* 2004; 43: 477–92.
Nimorakiotakis B, Winkel KD. Marine envenomations. Part 1: Jellyfish. *Australian Family Physician* 2003a; 32: 969–74.
Nimorakiotakis B, Winkel KD. Marine envenomations. Part 2: Other marine envenomations. *Australian Family Physician* 2003b; 32: 975–9.
Nimorakiotakis B, Winkel KD. The funnel web and common spider bites. *Australian Family Physician* 2004; 33: 244–7.
Patrick B. Conservation status of the New Zealand red katipo spider (*Latrodectus katipo* Powell, 1871). *Science for Conservation* 2002; 33 p. Department of Conservation, Wellington, NZ.
Theakston RDG, Warrell DA, Griffiths E. Report of a WHO workshop on the standardization and control of antivenoms. *Toxicon* 2003; 41: 541–57.
White J. Envenoming and antivenom use in Australia. *Toxicon* 1998; 36: 1483–92.

evolve   More weblinks at http://evolve.elsevier.com/AU/Bryant/pharmacology/

APPENDIX 1
ABBREVIATIONS

5-HT	5-hydroxytryptamine (serotonin)
A	adrenaline
AAS	anabolic androgenic steroid
ACE	angiotensin-converting enzyme
ACh	acetylcholine
AChE	acetylcholinesterase
ACTH	adrenocorticotrophic hormone (corticotrophin)
ADE	adverse drug event
ADEC	Australian Drug Evaluation Committee
ADH	antidiuretic hormone (vasopressin)
ADHD	attention-deficit hyperactivity disorder
ADR	adverse drug reaction
ADRAC	Adverse Drug Reactions Advisory Committee
AED	antiepileptic drug
AIDS	virus-acquired immune deficiency syndrome
AMH	*Australian Medicines Handbook*
ANS	autonomic nervous system
APF	*Australian Pharmaceutical Formulary*
APTT	activated partial thromboplastin time
ASADA	Australian Sports Anti-Doping Authority
ASDA	Australian Sports Drug Agency
ATP	adenosine triphosphate
AV	atrioventricular
BAD	bipolar affective disorder
BCG	Bacille Calmette–Guérin, or the *Mycobacterium bovis* bacillus
BGL	blood glucose level
BMI	body mass index
BP	*British Pharmacopoeia*
BPH	benign prostatic hyperplasia (or hypertrophy)
BSA	body surface area
CA	carbonic anhydrase
CAD	coronary artery disease
CAM	complementary and alternative medicine
cAMP	cyclic 3,5-adenosine monophosphate
CBG	corticosteroid-binding globulin
CBT	cognitive behaviour therapy
CFC	chlorofluorocarbon
CIB	Clinical Interest Box
CL	systemic clearance
CMI	consumer medical information
CMV	cytomegalovirus
CNS	central nervous system
CO	cardiac output
COAD	chronic obstructive airways disease
COMT	catechol-*O*-methyltransferase
COPD	chronic obstructive pulmonary disease
COX	cyclo-oxygenase
CR	controlled release
CRF	corticotrophin-releasing factor
CSF	cerebrospinal fluid
CSFs	colony-stimulating factors
CSIRO	Commonwealth Scientific and Industrial Research Organisation
CSL	Commonwealth Serum Laboratories
C_{ss}	steady-state plasma drug concentration
CTN	Clinical Trial Notification
CTX	Clinical Trial Exemption
CTZ	chemoreceptor trigger zone
CYP	cytochrome P450
DA	dopamine
DCCT	Diabetes Control and Complications Trial
DDC	dopa decarboxylase
DHT	dihydrotestosterone
DIC	disseminated intravascular coagulation
DIT	di-iodotyrosine
DM	Drug Monograph
DMARDs	disease-modifying antirheumatic drugs
DNA	deoxyribonucleic acid
DOPA	dihydroxyphenylalanine
DTs	delirium tremens
DUE	drug usage evaluation
E	epitestosterone
EAA	excitatory amino acid
EBM	evidence-based medicine
EC	enteric-coated
ECG	electrocardiogram
ECL	enterochromaffin-like cells
ECT	electroconvulsive therapy
ED	erectile dysfunction
EE	ethinyloestradiol
EEG	electroencephalograph/-gram
EMLA	eutectic mixture for local anaesthesia
EPO	erythropoietin
ER	(o)estrogen receptor
ETS	environmental tobacco smoke
F	bioavailability
FAS	fetal alcohol syndrome
FDA	Food and Drugs Administration
FSH	follicle-stimulating hormone
FU	(5-)fluorouracil
G1, G2	gap or growth phase 1, 2
GA	general anaesthesia/anaesthetic
GABA	γ-aminobutyric acid
G-CSF	granulocyte colony-stimulating factor

GF	growth factor
GFR	glomerular filtration rate
GH	growth hormone (somatotropin)
GHRIF	growth hormone release-inhibiting factor
GI	gastrointestinal
GIT	gastrointestinal tract
Glu	glutamate
GMP	guanosine monophosphate
GnRH	gonadotrophin-releasing hormone
GORD	gastro-oesophageal reflux disease
GPCRs	G-protein-coupled receptors
H^+	hydrogen ion
hCG	human chorionic gonadotrophin
HCO_3^-	bicarbonate ion
HDL	high-density lipoproteins
HIV	human immunodeficiency virus
HMG-CoA	3-hydroxy-3-methylglutaryl coenzyme A
HPA	hypothalamic–pituitary–adrenal (axis)
HR	heart rate
HREC	Human Research Ethics Commitee
HRT	hormone replacement therapy
HSV	herpes simplex virus
HTS	high-throughput screening
IBD	inflammatory bowel disease
IBS	irritable bowel syndrome
ICP	intracranial pressure
ICSH	interstitial cell-stimulating hormone
IDDM	insulin-dependent diabetes mellitus
IDL	intermediate-density lipoproteins
IDUs	intravenous drug users
IEC	institutional ethics committee
Ig	immunoglobulin
IGF-1	insulin-like growth factor 1
IL	interleukin
IMMP	Intensive Medicines Monitoring Programme
INR	international normalised ratio
IOC(MC)	International Olympic Committee (Medical Commission)
IOP	intraocular pressure
IU	International Units
IUD	intrauterine device
IV	intravenous
IVF	in-vitro fertilisation
IVRA	intravenous regional anaesthesia
LA	local anaesthesia/anaesthetic
LDL	low-density lipoproteins
LH	luteinising hormone
LMWHs	low-molecular-weight heparins
LSD	lysergic acid diethylamide
LT	leukotriene
M	muscarinic
M	mitosis phase
M_3	muscarinic type 3 (receptors)
M6G	morphine-6-glucuronide
MAC	minimum alveolar concentration (for anaesthesia)
MAO	monoamine oxidase
MAOI	monoamine oxidase inhibitor
MDI	metered-dose inhaler
MDMA	3,4-methylenedioxymethamphetamine
MDR	maintenance dose rate
MIT	mono-iodotyrosine
MOPP	mustine, Oncovin, procarbazine, prednisone
MPA	medroxyprogesterone acetate
MRSA	methicillin-resistant *Staphylococcus aureus*
MRSE	multi-resistant *Staphylococcus epidermidis*
MTX	methotrexate
mV	millivolts
N	nicotinic
N_2O	nitrous oxide
NA	noradrenaline
NIDDM	non-insulin-dependent diabetes mellitus
NK	natural killer (cells)
NMDA	*N*-methyl-D-aspartate
NMJ	neuromuscular junction
NMP	National Medicines Policy
NNRTI	non-nucleoside reverse transcriptase inhibitor
NRTI	nucleoside reverse transcriptase inhibitor
NSAID	non-steroidal anti-inflammatory drug
OC	oral contraception/contraceptive
OHA	oral hypoglycaemic agent
OM	otitis media
OTC	over the counter
PABA	*p*-aminobenzoic acid
$PaCO_2$	partial pressure of carbon dioxide in arterial blood
PaO_2	partial pressure of oxygen in arterial blood
PBS	Pharmaceutical Benefits Scheme
PCA	patient-controlled analgesia
PCO_2	partial pressure of carbon dioxide
PCP	phencyclidine
PDE	phosphodiesterase
PEG	polyethylene glycol
PG	prostaglandin
PGE	prostaglandin E
PHARM	Pharmaceutical Health and Rational Use of Medicines
PI	protease inhibitor
PNMT	phenylethanolamine-*N*-methyltransferase
PNS	peripheral nervous system
PO_2	partial pressure of oxygen
POAG	primary open-angle glaucoma
PRIF	prolactin release-inhibiting factor
PTH	parathyroid hormone
QUM	quality use of medicines
RAS	reticular activating system
RBCs	red blood cells

RCCT	randomised controlled clinical trial
RDI	recommended daily intake
REM	rapid eye movement
RIMA	reversible inhibitor of MAO-A
RNA	ribonucleic acid
S	synthesis phase
S4	Schedule 4 (in Australian Poisons and Drug Regulations)
SA	sinoatrial
SC	subcutaneous
script	prescription
SERM	selective (o)estrogen receptor modulator
SI	Système International d'Unités (scientific units)
SMBG	self-monitored blood glucose
SPF	sun protection factor
SRS-A	slow-reacting substance of anaphylaxis
SSRI	selective serotonin reuptake inhibitor
STD	sexually transmissible disease
SUSDP	Standards for the Uniform Scheduling of Drugs and Poisons
SV	stroke volume
SVDK	Snake venom detection kit
SVR	systemic vascular resistance
T	testosterone
$t_{1/2}$	half-life
T3	tri-iodothyronine (liothyronine)
T4	tetra-iodothyronine (thyroxine)
TCAs	tricyclic antidepressants
TCM	traditional Chinese medicine
TDM	therapeutic drug monitoring
TENS	transcutaneous electrical nerve stimulation
TGA	Therapeutic Goods Administration
THC	tetrahydrocannabinol
TIVA	total intravenous anaesthesia
TM	tubular transport maximum
TPO	thrombopoietin
TPR	total peripheral resistance
TRH	thyrotrophin-releasing hormone
TSH	thyroid-stimulating hormone (thyrotrophin)
TUE	Therapeutic Use Exemption
UKPDS	United Kingdom Prospective Diabetes Study
USP	United States Pharmacopeia
UTI	urinary tract infection
UVA, UVB, UVC	UVR of wavelengths in the A, B or C region
UVR	ultraviolet radiation
V	volume of distribution
VLDL	very-low-density lipoproteins
W/V	weight in volume
WADA	World Anti-Doping Agency
WBCs	white blood cells
WHO	World Health Organization
WHR	waist:hip ratio

APPENDIX 2
ANTISEPTICS AND DISINFECTANTS

Antiseptics and disinfectants are distinguished on the basis of whether or not they are safe for application to living tissue.

Antiseptics are chemical agents that destroy or inhibit the growth of microorganisms in or on living tissue (e.g. surgical scrubs, handwashes and ointments).

Disinfectants are chemical agents used on inanimate objects or surfaces (e.g. contact lenses, floors, toilets).

CLASS	CHEMICAL	TYPICAL USE	PROPRIETARY PRODUCTS (containing constituent)
Alcohols	Ethyl alcohol (ethanol)	Antisepsis	Betadine alcoholic skin prep solution (30% ethanol) Microshield Tincture (70% ethanol)
	Isopropyl alcohol	Disinfection	Miraflow contact lens cleaner (20% isopropanol) Briemarpak alcohol wipes (70% isopropanol)
Biguanides	Chlorhexidine	Antisepsis	Savlon Antiseptic Liquid (0.3% chlorhexidine gluconate) Microshield Tincture (0.5% chlorhexidine gluconate) Hibiclens Skin Cleanser (4% chlorhexidine gluconate)
Bis-phenols	Triclosan	Antisepsis	Dettol Cream (3 mg/g triclosan) pHisoHex (solution) (10 mg/mL triclosan) Sapoderm Soap (10 mg/g triclosan) Oxy Skin Wash (50 mg/mL triclosan)
Diamidines	Propamidine	Antisepsis	Brolene Eye Drops (0.1% propamidine isethionate)
	Dibromopropamidine	Antisepsis	Brolene Eye Ointment (0.15% dibromopropamidine isethionate)
Halogen-releasing agents	Iodine compounds	Antisepsis	Betadine Antiseptic Ointment and Savlon Antiseptic Treatment (10% povidone-iodine) Betadine First Aid Cream (5% povidone-iodine) Betadine Surgical Scrub (7.5% povidone-iodine)
	Chlorine compounds	Antisepsis/ Disinfection	Cepacol antiseptic throat lozenge (0.7% cetylpyridinium chloride) Jasol lemon bleach (4% liquid chlorine) White King premium bleach (42 g/L sodium hypochlorite)
Halophenols	Chloroxylenol	Antisepsis	Dettol Liquid (48 mg/mL chloroxylenol) Dettol Cream (3 mg/g chloroxylenol)
Heavy metal derivatives	Silver compounds	Antisepsis	Silvazine Cream (1% silver sulfadiazine)
Herbal/plant origin	Eucalyptus oil	Antisepsis	Vicks VAPOsteam (27 mg eucalyptus oil) Eucanol Antiseptic Spray (40 mg/mL eucalyptus oil)
	Peppermint oil	Antisepsis	Vicks VAPOsteam (36 mg peppermint oil)
	Melaleuca (tea-tree) oil	Antisepsis	Goanna Tea-Tree Oil (lotion) (150 mg/mL *Melaleuca alternifolia* oil) Dettol Sting'n Graze Gel (30 mg/g *Melaleuca* oil)

(Continued)

CLASS	CHEMICAL	TYPICAL USE	PROPRIETARY PRODUCTS (containing constituent)
Peroxygens	Hydrogen peroxide	Disinfection	Omnicare 1 Step Disinfecting Solution (contact lens cleaner) (30 mg/mL hydrogen peroxide)
	Benzoyl peroxide	Antisepsis	Oxy 10 Vanishing Cream (10% benzoyl peroxide)
Quaternary ammonium compounds	Cetrimide	Antisepsis	Savlon Antiseptic Liquid (3% cetrimide) Microshield Antiseptic Concentrate (15% cetrimide)

Sources: McDonnell G, Russell AD. Antiseptics and disinfectants: activity, action, and resistance. *Clinical Microbiology Reviews* 1999; 12: 147–79)
MIMS Australia. eMIMS 2006, CMPMedica Australia, 2006.

APPENDIX 3
HERB–, NUTRIENT– AND FOOD–DRUG INTERACTIONS

The prescribing and administration of multiple drugs is commonplace throughout society. In addition to prescribed medications, people often add to their treatment regimens over-the-counter products that include vitamins, dietary supplements and herbal medicines. All substances ingested, including food, have the potential to interact with pharmaceutical drugs. There is a lack of experimental evidence in these fields, and in many instances the mechanistic bases of interactions have not been established. The following list of herb–, nutrient– and food–drug interactions is not definitive, as there are many possible and yet-to-be-reported interactions. (A comprehensive listing can be found in Braun & Cohen 2005.)

HERB/NUTRIENT/FOOD	DRUG	COMMENTS	CONSEQUENCES OF INTERACTION
Herb			
Chilli pepper (*Capsicum* spp.)	ACE inhibitors	Capsaicin depletes substance P	Cough
Dong quai (*Angelica sinensis*)	Warfarin	Dong quai contains coumarins	Increased INR and bruising
Garlic (*Allium sativum*)	Warfarin	Suggestion that garlic prolongs prothrombin time	Increased INR
Ginkgo (*Ginkgo biloba*)	Aspirin	Ginkogolides inhibit platelet-activation factor	Spontaneous hyphaema (bleeding in the eye)
	Warfarin		Intracerebral haemorrhage
Ginseng (*Panax* spp.)	Warfarin		Reduced anticoagulant effect, decreased INR
Liquorice (*Glycyrrhiza glabra*)	Prednisolone, hydrocortisone	Liquorice contains glycyrrhizin, which inhibits enzymes involved in steroid metabolism	Potentiation of steroid effects
St John's wort (*Hypericum perforatum*)	Cyclosporin	Induction of CYP3A4 and/or the P-glycoprotein transporter	Decreased plasma cyclosporin concentration, transplant rejection
	Digoxin	Induction of the P-glycoprotein transporter	Decreased plasma digoxin concentration
	Oral contraceptives	Induction of CYP3A4; increased metabolism of steroids	Breakthrough bleeding
	Selective serotonin reuptake inhibitors	Inhibits reuptake of 5-hydroxytryptamine, noradrenaline and dopramine	Mild serotonin syndrome
	Warfarin	Possible induction of CYPZC9; increased metabolism of warfarin	Reduced anticoagulant effect, decreased INR

(Continued)

HERB/NUTRIENT/FOOD	DRUG	COMMENTS	CONSEQUENCES OF INTERACTION
Nutrient/food			
Barbecued (charcoal-grilled) beef	Amitriptyline, codeine, erythromycin, felodipine, propranolol, theophylline	Contains polycyclic aromatic hydrocarbons that induce drug-metabolising enzymes	Decreased plasma drug concentration
Cruciferous vegetables (cauliflower, cabbage, Brussels sprouts and broccoli)	Caffeine and theophylline	Contain drug-metabolising enzyme-inducing chemicals	Decreased plasma drug concentration
Grapefruit juice	Cyclosporin, felodipine, saquinavir, verapamil	Specifically inhibits CYP3A4 in the wall of the small intestine	Increased bioavailability
Iron	Tetracycline, penicillamine, levodopa, ciprofloxacin	Formation of iron–drug complexes	Decreased bioavailability
Potassium	Triamterene, ACE inhibitors	Found in bananas, oranges and leafy green vegetables	Hyperkalaemia
Tyramine	Monoamine oxidase inhibitors	MAOIs inhibit inactivation of tyramine in foods: aged cheeses, Vegemite (yeast extracts), red wine, beer, pickled foods, broad beans	Hypertensive crisis
Vitamin E	Anticoagulants	May prolong clotting time	Increased risk of bleeding
Vitamin K	Warfarin	Found in beef liver, avocado, leafy green vegetables, cauliflower, soybeans and lentils	Antagonises the effect of coumarin anticoagulants

ACE = angiotensin-converting enzyme; INR = international normalised ratio.

Sources: Braun L, Cohen M. Herb and natural supplements: an evidence-based guide. Sydney: Elsevier Australia, 2005; Campbell NRC, Hasinoff BB. Iron supplements: a common cause of drug interactions. *British Journal of Clinical Pharmacology* 1991; 31: 251–5;
Ernst E. Second thoughts about safety of St John's wort, *Lancet* 1999; 354: 2014–16; Pugh-Berman A. Herb-drug interactions, *Lancet* 2000; 355: 134–8;
Lam YWF. New drug interactions reported with St John's wort. *Psychopharmacology Update* 2000; 11: 1, 7;
US Food and Drug Administration National Consumers League, 1998. Food and Drug Interactions. www.fda.gov;
Yue Q-V, Bergquist C, Gerden B. Safety of St John's wort (*Hypericum perforatum*). Lancet 2000; 355; 576–7.

APPENDIX 4
GLOSSARY

absorption   the process by which unchanged drug proceeds from the site of administration into the blood.

accommodation   the automatic process by which the eyes adjust the curvature of the lens to focus on distant or near objects.

acid-labile   describes a drug that is destroyed by acid.

acid-stable   describes a drug that is not affected by acid.

acquired immunity   any form of immunity that is not innate and is obtained during life.

action potential   an electrical signal produced by rapid changes in concentrations of sodium and potassium ions on either side of the cell membranes of neurons, and which results in a self-propagating wave of depolarisation and repolarisation.

adverse drug effect   an unwanted effect that occurs via a different mechanism from the pharmacological effect of the drug, and that may or may not be dose-related.

adverse drug event (ADE)   injury resulting from medical intervention related to a drug but not necessarily due to the drug. Examples of ADEs include under- or overmedication resulting from misuse or malfunction of infusion pumps or devices; aspiration pneumonia resulting from drug overdose; and errors in ordering, dispensing or administration.

adverse drug reaction   unintended and undesirable response to a drug.

   type A adverse drug reaction   predictable.

   type B adverse drug reaction   unpredictable.

   type C adverse drug reaction   a consequence of long-term use.

   type D adverse drug reaction   delayed effects.

afterload   the pressure that must be overcome before the ventricles can eject the blood; one of the factors that regulates stroke volume.

agonist   a drug that binds to (occupies) and activates the receptor, producing the same response as the endogenous ligand. Some drugs may be considered partial agonists, as they produce less than the maximal effect even when all receptors are occupied.

alkaloids   naturally occurring molecules that contain nitrogen, are alkaline and usually are bitter-tasting; drugs derived from plant alkaloids.

alkylating agents   agents that introduce an alkyl group into a molecule; they combine with DNA bases, altering their chemical structure, thus impairing synthesis of DNA and RNA; usually anticancer drugs.

aminoglycosides   potent bactericidal antibiotics that are usually reserved for serious or life-threatening infections.

anabolic agents   agents that promote build-up of tissues; drugs that treat debilitating states; they are abused to build muscle mass.

anaesthesia   the loss of the sensations of pain, pressure, temperature or touch, in a part or the whole of the body.

analgesic   a drug that relieves pain.

antacids   chemical compounds that buffer or neutralise hydrochloric acid in the stomach, thereby raising gastric pH.

antagonist   a drug that binds to the receptor and blocks access of the endogenous ligand, thus diminishing the normal response; drugs may act as competitive (reversible) or irreversible antagonists (drugs that are antagonists are commonly called 'blockers').

anterograde amnesic effect   a drug effect that decreases the patient's memory for a period following an event (anterograde amnesia).

antianxiety or anxiolytic agents   drugs that reduce anxiety.

antibiotic antitumour agents   cytotoxic agents from microbial sources; examples are the anthracyclines and bleomycins.

antibiotics   natural substances derived from certain organisms (bacteria, fungi and others) that can either suppress the growth of or destroy microorganisms.

anticoagulant drugs   drugs that prevent the blood from coagulating (see Figure 30-1); anticoagulation is primarily prophylactic because these agents act by preventing fibrin deposits, extension of a thrombus and thromboembolic complications.

antidiarrhoeal   relates to relief of symptoms of rapid passage of loose faeces, and the prevention of fluid and electrolyte loss.

antiemetics   substances that prevent or alleviate nausea or vomiting.

antifibrinolytic drugs   drugs that hasten clot formation and reduce bleeding.

antigen   any substance that is able to provoke an immune system response.

antimetabolites   drugs that are analogues of folic acid or of the purine and pyrimidine bases, and inhibit metabolic pathways in microorganisms or neoplastic cells.

antineoplastic agent   a substance, procedure or measure that prevents the proliferation of neoplastic (tumour) cells.

antiplatelet drugs   used in the treatment of arterial thrombosis, they include aspirin, dipyridamole, ticlopidine, and abciximab.

antiporters   secondary active-transport membrane proteins that transport two substances in opposite directions (those that move two substrates in the same direction are symporters).

antipruritic agents   preparations that relieve itching.

antipyretic drugs   drugs that decrease fever or high body temperature.

antitussive drugs   drugs that suppress cough.

aperient   a laxative.

apolipoproteins   proteins carried on the surface of lipoproteins; functions include serving as ligands for cell receptors, activating enzymes involved in lipoprotein metabolism and providing structure of the lipoprotein.

apoptosis   programmed cell death.

approved name   the name of a chemical approved by a drug-regulating authority, as distinct from the proprietary name (trade name, or brand name) under which a drug is marketed commercially.

area under the curve (AUC)   the total area under the plasma concentration versus time curve that describes the concentration of the drug in the systemic circulation as a function of time (from zero until infinity).

assay   the analysis of the purity, amount or effectiveness of a drug or other substance, including laboratory and clinical measurements.

astringent   a solution that, when applied topically, causes precipitation of proteins, vasoconstriction and reduced cell permeability.

automaticity   the ability to spontaneously initiate an electrical impulse; automaticity is a property of cells and fibres of the conduction system that normally controls heart rhythm.

azole antifungals   fungistatic drugs that affect the biosynthesis of fungal ergosterols by interfering with the cytochrome P450 enzyme system that catalyses ergosterol formation.

β-adrenoceptor agonist   a drug designed to directly stimulate beta (β) adrenoceptors, producing actions similar to those of β-sympathetic stimulation, such as increased cardiac output, dilation of coronary arterioles, bronchial dilation and a variety of other effects.

β-blockers   β-adrenoceptor antagonists; these drugs competitively block the actions of the catecholamines on β-adrenoceptors.

β-lactamase   some microorganisms produce this type of enzyme, which is able to destroy some penicillins and cephalosporins; it is also called penicillinase.

bacteraemia   the presence of viable bacteria in the circulatory system.

bacterial resistance   refers to the ability of a particular microorganism to resist the effects of a specific antibiotic.

bactericidal agents   agents that cause bacterial cell death and lysis.

bacteriostatic agents   agents that inhibit bacterial growth, allowing host defence mechanisms additional time to remove the invading microorganisms.

balanced anaesthesia   the use of a combination of agents to achieve unconsciousness, analgesia, muscle relaxation and amnesia. Premedication may include an antianxiety agent and atropine to suppress secretions. Antiemetics and opioids are used for postoperative nausea and pain.

bioassay   a biological test method to measure the amount of a pharmacologically active substance in a preparation (tissue extract or pharmaceutical formulation).

bioavailability   the proportion of the administered dose that reaches the systemic circulation intact.

bioequivalence   two formulations of the same drug that attain similar concentrations in blood and tissues at similar times, with no clinically important differences between their therapeutic or adverse effects.

blood doping   the administration of blood, red blood cells or blood products to an athlete; it usually involves transfusion of extra blood, either the athlete's own (autologous) or a compatible donor's (homologous) into the circulatory system, to provide extra oxygen-carrying capacity and enhance aerobic performance.

body mass index (BMI)   an individual's body mass in kg divided by the square of their height in metres; BMI is highly correlated with the proportion of body fat.

carcinogen   any agent that by either direct or indirect actions causes a normal cell to become a malignant neoplastic cell.

catecholamine   any one of a group of sympathomimetic compounds composed of a catechol moiety and the aliphatic portion of an amine There are three naturally occurring catecholamines in the body: dopamine, noradrenaline and adrenaline.

cell-kill fraction   the proportion of cancer cells killed by a chemotherapeutic drug given in adequate doses.

central nervous system (CNS)   one of the two main divisions of the nervous system, consisting of the brain and the spinal cord. The central nervous system processes information to and from the peripheral nervous system and is the main network of coordination and control for the entire body.

cephalosporins   antibacterial drugs that inhibit cell wall synthesis similarly to penicillin and are also bactericidal.

cestodes   tapeworms.

chemoreceptor trigger zone (CTZ)   an area of the brain that, in response to certain chemicals, causes vomiting.

chronotropic effect   a significant increase (positive chronotropic effect) or decrease (negative chronotropic effect) in cardiac rate occurring as a result of increased or decreased rate of membrane depolarisation in the pacemaker cells in the sinus node during diastole.

chylomicrons   large particles that transport dietary cholesterol and fatty acids absorbed from the gastrointestinal tract to the liver.

circadian rhythm   a pattern based on a 24-hour cycle, with the repetition of certain physiological processes; it is controlled by the dark–light and sleep–wakefulness cycles via the limbic system.

clearance   the rate at which a drug is removed from the blood; it determines the maintenance dose rate required to achieve the target plasma concentration at steady state.

clinical pharmacology   applies to the drug treatment of patients; the study of drugs 'at the bedside'.

coagulopathy   a condition in which the clotting ability of the blood is altered.

compliance   following all aspects of a treatment plan; in the context of drug therapy, it implies the patient receiving the right drug in the right dose at the right time for the right duration by the right route. In addition, all the other advice given related to therapy must be followed, including lifestyle aspects such as weight reduction, cessation of smoking, moderation in alcohol intake, etc.

conductivity   the ability of a cell (e.g. cardiac muscle, nerve) to transmit an action potential along its plasma membrane.

conjugation   union of a suitable functional group present in the drug molecule with the polar group of an endogenous substance in the body; combining of a drug with glucuronic acid in drug metabolism.

contamination   a condition of being soiled, stained, touched or otherwise exposed to harmful agents, making an object potentially unsafe for use as intended or without barrier techniques.

contraception   prevention of pregnancy after sexual intercourse.

contraindication   a factor that makes dangerous or undesirable the administration of a drug or the performance of an act or procedure in the care of a specific patient.

corticosteroids   (glucocorticoids and mineralocorticoids): steroidal hormones that are synthesised in and released from the adrenal cortex.

cortisone   a natural glucocorticoid, converted in the body to hydrocortisone.

cycloplegic drugs   drugs that paralyse the ciliary muscle, causing loss of accommodation.

cytoprotective agents   substances that protect cells from damage.

cytotoxic agents   agents that interfere with cell proliferation or replication; cytotoxic agents are divided into various classes based on their probable major mechanisms of action.

debridement   removal of dirt, foreign objects, damaged tissue and cellular debris from a wound or burn to prevent infection and to promote healing.

depolarisation   reduction of a membrane potential to a less negative value with respect to the cytosol.

depolarising drugs   nicotinic-receptor agonists that maintain the depolarised state of the motor end-plate, thus preventing transmission of another action potential.

desensitisation   a decrease in the response of the receptor–second messenger system; it is a common feature of many receptors.

dissolution   a process by which a solid drug goes into solution and becomes available for absorption.

distribution   the process of reversible transfer of a drug between one location and another (one of which is usually blood) in the body.

disulfiram–alcohol reaction   the reaction between disulfiram, a carbamate derivative used as an alcohol deterrent, and alcohol. When alcohol is ingested after administration of disulfiram, blood acetaldehyde concentrations are increased; this is followed by flushing.

diuretics   drugs that modify renal function and induce diuresis (increased rate of urine flow) and natriuresis (enhanced excretion of sodium chloride).

doping   the use in sport of substances and/or methods that are prohibited under that sport's rules, to enhance performance or mask banned behaviours.

dose form   the form in which the drug is administered, e.g. as a tablet, injection, eye-drop or ointment.

downregulation   a reduction in receptor numbers; it may contribute to desensitisation and loss of response.

dromotropic effect   effect of a drug in increasing (positive dromotropic effect) or decreasing (negative dromotropic effect) the rate of atrioventricular conduction; the effect may also occur in conduction abnormalities. Dromotropic drugs affect conduction velocity through specialised conducting tissues.

drug interaction   an effect on the responses of an individual to a drug with any other drug taken, including non-prescribed OTC drugs and complementary and alternative medicines, as well as other ingested compounds such as food and drinks.

elimination   the irreversible loss of drug from the body by the processes of metabolism and excretion.

emesis   vomiting.

emetic   a drug that induces emesis.

enema   a solution administered rectally.

enteral route   by mouth; the oral route.

enteric coating   a tablet coating that offers relative resistance to the digestive action of the stomach contents.

enteric nervous system   a collection of neural plexuses (networks) in the walls of the gastrointestinal tract that can function independently of the central nervous system.

enterohepatic cycle   excretion of a compound through bile and subsequent reabsorption from the intestine.

envenomation   the injection into the body of venom from a venomous snake, arachnid, insect or marine species.

epidural anaesthesia　an injection of local anaesthetic into the space between the dura mater and the ligamentum flavum, at spinal cord levels C7–T10. This 'space' is actually filled with loose adipose tissue and lymphatic and blood vessels; the solution tends to remain localised at the level where it is injected.

equianalgesic dose　a dose of one analgesic that is equivalent in pain-relieving effects to a dose of another analgesic. This equivalence permits substitution of medications to prevent possible adverse reactions to one of the drugs.

ergogenic aids　substances that improve energy utilisation; nutritional supplements are frequently used in this way.

ergot alkaloids　naturally occurring alkaloid compounds that have varied effects in the body due to their actions on several types of receptors; they are produced by the fungus *Claviceps* growing on cereal grains.

erythropoiesis　the process of erythocyte production in the bone marrow, involving the maturation of a nucleated precursor into a haemoglobin-filled nucleus-free erythrocyte; the process is regulated by erythropoietin, a hormone produced by the kidneys.

eschar　dead, separated, damaged skin.

euthyroid　pertaining to a normal thyroid gland and gland function.

excretion (of drug)　irreversible loss of chemically unchanged drug from the body e.g. in urine, bile, expired air or faeces.

exocytosis　discharge from a cell of particles that are too large to diffuse through the wall, by fusion of a vacuole to the cell membrane.

extrapyramidal symptoms　involuntary muscle movements induced by some drugs that inhibit normal dopaminergic function in the extrapyramidal tracts.

extrapyramidal system　a series of indirect motor pathways located in the CNS that are outside the main motor pathways that traverse the pyramids in the thalamus. The name embraces many pathways or tracts, which innervate mainly muscles in the limbs, head and eyes. This system is associated with coordination of muscle-group movements and posture.

first-pass effect　the amount of an orally administered drug that is 'extracted' by the liver before the drug reaches the systemic circulation (absorbed drugs travel first through the portal system and the liver before entering the systemic circulation). Often only a small fraction of the dose is available for distribution and to produce a pharmacological effect. For such medications, the oral drug dose is calculated to compensate for this variable first-pass effect.

formulary　similar to a pharmacopoeia but may include information on drug actions, adverse effects, general medical information, guidelines for pharmacists dispensing medicines, and the 'recipes' for formulation or production of different medicines.

formulation　the way the drug is presented, including dose form and active and inactive ingredients.

gate control theory　a theory that proposes that a mechanism in the dorsal horn of the spinal cord (the spinal 'gate') can modify the transmission of painful sensations from the peripheral nerve fibres to the thalamus and cortex of the brain, where the sensations are recognised as pain.

general anaesthesia/anaesthetic　a state of unconsciousness and general loss of sensation, with varying amounts of analgesia, muscle relaxation, and loss of reflexes; a drug used to achieve this state.

generic name　strictly speaking, this refers to a group name, e.g. the penicillins, the salicylates, or the β-blockers; however, it has come to be used interchangeably with the term 'approved name'.

globulins　globular proteins; they include the immuno-globulins (also called antibodies) that are important in the body's defence against viruses and bacteria.

glucocorticoid　an adrenocortical steroid hormone that affects carbohydrate, protein and fat metabolism, exerts an anti-inflammatory effect and influences many body functions.

gonadotrophins　glycoprotein hormones responsible for the development and maintenance of sex-gland functions.

haemostasis　the physiological process that stops bleeding. It involves blood vessel constriction, platelet plug formation and blood coagulation.

haemostatic agents　agents that enhance haemostasis, i.e. hasten clot formation and reduce bleeding. The purpose of these agents is to control rapid loss of blood.

half-life　the time taken for the blood or plasma concentration of a drug to fall by one-half (50%).

high-density lipoproteins (HDL)　one of three primary classes of lipoproteins found in the blood of fasting individuals.

homeopathy　a form of complementary/alternative treatment in which substances (minerals, plant extracts, chemicals or microorganisms), which in sufficient amounts would produce a set of symptoms in healthy persons, are given in minute amounts to produce a 'cure' of similar symptoms.

hypertonic　exerting a greater osmotic pressure than blood or 0.9% sodium chloride. Also, exhibiting increased muscle tension or tone.

hypnotics　drugs used to induce sleep.

hypothalamic factor　a factor from the hypothalamus that stimulates or inhibits the release of hormones from the anterior pituitary gland.

hypothalamic–pituitary–adrenal axis　linked functions of the hypothalamus, the anterior pituitary gland, and the adrenal cortex.

hypotonic　exerting a lower osmotic pressure than blood or 0.9% sodium chloride. Also, exhibiting decreased muscle tension or tone.

iatrogenic   pertaining to an illness caused by medical or surgical procedures.

immunomodulating drugs   new agents that can either activate the body's immune defences or modify a response to an unwanted stimulus, such as an antitumour response.

immunostimulating drug   an agent that activates the immune system.

immunosuppressant drug   an agent that decreases or prevents an immune response

indication   an illness or disorder for which a drug has a documented specific usefulness.

infertility   the absence of conception after more than one year of regular sexual intercourse without contraception.

infiltration anaesthesia   the use of local anaesthetics in an area that circles the operative field; it is produced by injecting dilute solutions of the agent into the skin and then subcutaneously into the region to be anaesthetised.

inhalation anaesthetic   inhalation, or volatile, anaesthetics are gases or volatile liquids that can be administered by inhalation when mixed with oxygen.

inotropic drugs   drugs that increase (positive inotropic effect) or decrease (negative inotropic effect) the force of myocardial contraction. Positive inotropes include digoxin, dobutamine, adrenaline and isoprenaline, while propranolol is a negative inotrope. Adrenaline produces a significant increase in myocardial contraction (positive inotropic effect) as a result of increased influx of calcium into cardiac fibres.

intravenous general anaesthesia   general anaesthesia induced and maintained by intravenous injection of a solution of anaesthetic agent.

intravenous local anaesthesia (Bier's block)   a specialised technique for anaesthesia of the upper limb. A tourniquet is applied to occlude the arterial flow, then the local anaesthetic is injected IV distal to the cuff (see Figure 15-5).

isotonic   exerting the same osmotic pressure as another solution, usually blood or 0.9% sodium chloride.

keratolytics   drugs that dissolve keratin, soften skin squames (scales) and loosen the outer horny layer of the skin.

ketoacidosis   acidosis accompanied by an accumulation of ketones in the body, resulting from extensive breakdown of fats because of faulty carbohydrate metabolism, as in diabetes or starvation.

ketone bodies   compounds (acetone, acetoacetic acid and β-hydroxybutyric acid) produced in the liver by acetyl coenzyme A and used for energy by cells. In disorders of carbohydrate metabolism, they can build up in the body and eventually cause serious illness and coma.

leptin   the protein product of the obesity (*ob*) gene (derived from the Greek word *leptos*, meaning thin).

ligand   a molecule that binds to a receptor.

lincosamides   agents used to treat serious streptococcal and staphylococcal infections.

lipodystrophy   a breakdown of subcutaneous fat occurring after repeated injections.

loading dose   the initial amount of drug required to 'fill up' the volume of distribution.

local anaesthesia/anaesthetic   absence of pain due to blocked sensory nerve conduction in a body region or localised area; an agent used to achieve this.

loop diuretics   one of three major classes of diuretics, so named because they inhibit resorption of sodium and chloride, and hence water, in the loop of Henle; an example is frusemide.

low-density lipoproteins (LDL)   one of three primary classes of lipoproteins found in the blood of fasting individuals

macrolide antibiotics   antibiotics that contain a many-membered lactone ring attached to deoxy sugars.

macromolecular synthesis   replication of macromolecules (DNA, RNA and proteins), which must be completed every cell cycle in order for cells to proliferate.

malignant hyperthermia   rare but potentially fatal condition of rapidly developing high body temperature occurring in susceptible patients with an inherited abnormality in muscle membranes. It appears to be precipitated by the combination of a depolarising neuromuscular-blocking agent (e.g. suxamethonium) with a general anaesthetic agent.

maximal drug efficacy   the maximal response that a drug can produce.

maximum safe concentration   the maximal concentration of a drug in the blood that does not cause toxicity.

medicine   drug(s) given for therapeutic purposes; possibly a mixture of drug plus other substances to provide stability in the formulation; also, the branch of science devoted to the study, prevention and treatment of disease.

membrane potential   the difference in voltage or charge between two sides of a membrane.

meta-analysis   a quantitative statistical procedure for combining the results of similar independent studies to better analyse the therapeutic effectiveness of specific treatments

mineralocorticoids   steroid hormones from the adrenal cortex that act in the kidneys to cause reabsorption sodium and water, and enhance the excretion of potassium and hydrogen.

miotic drugs   drugs that constrict the pupil, i.e. cause miosis. Their clinical uses are to reverse mydriatic effects and in the treatment of glaucoma.

mitotic inhibitors   important antineoplastic agents that are natural products isolated from plants, and disrupt mitosis in cells; they include the vinca alkaloids, the podophyllotoxin derivatives and the taxanes.

molecular target   with the exception of drugs that act on DNA, all drugs act by binding to proteins; such a protein is termed 'molecular target' or 'site of action'.

motor end-plate   the specialised region of synaptic contact between a skeletal muscle fibre and a presynaptic motor neuron.

mucolytic drugs   drugs that assist in the break-up of mucus.

mutagen   a physical or chemical agent that causes genetic material (DNA) to undergo a detectable and heritable structural change.

mydriatics   drugs that cause pupil dilation (mydriasis); they are primarily used to facilitate examination of the peripheral lens and retina in the diagnosis of ophthalmic disorders.

nebuliser   a pump that uses compressed air or oxygen or ultrasonic energy to produce a fine mist of drug in aerosol form from a solution, useful for delivering large doses to the airways for long periods.

nerve block   injection of a local anaesthetic into the vicinity of a nerve trunk, thus inhibiting the conduction of impulses to and from the area supplied by that nerve, the region of the operative site. The injection may be made at some distance from the surgical site.

neurogenic pain   pain arising from a primary lesion, alteration or dysfunction of tissues of the peripheral or central nervous system.

neuroleptanalgesia   an anaesthetic technique that induces a state of deep sedation, analgesia and amnesia, produced by a combination of a neuroleptic agent and an opioid analgesic.

neuromuscular junction (NMJ)   the junction between a lower motor (somatic) neuron and a skeletal muscle cell.

neuromuscular blocking agent   a chemical substance that interferes locally with the transmission or reception of impulses from motor nerves to skeletal muscles.

neuropathic pain   pain due to neurological disease that affects a sensory pathway.

neurotransmitter   any one of numerous chemicals that act as chemical messengers enabling the transmission of nerve impulses across synapses or neuromuscular junctions. Of the many chemicals proposed as neurotransmitters in the CNS, the most important are acetylcholine, the catecholamines (dopamine, noradrenaline and adrenaline), 5-hydroxytryptamine, some amino acids, and neuroactive peptides.

nociceptive pain   pain arising from stimulation of superficial or deep nociceptors by noxious stimuli such as tissue injury or inflammation.

non-depolarising drug   a drug that blocks the action of acetylcholine without first depolarising the cell.

non-nucleoside reverse transcriptase inhibitors (NNRTIs)   drugs that block RNA-dependent and DNA-dependent DNA polymerases (Figure 52-2).

non-steroidal anti-inflammatory drugs (NSAIDs)   a group of drugs having antipyretic, analgesic and anti-inflammatory effects; they bear no structural similarity to the corticosteroids.

nucleoside reverse transcriptase inhibitors (NRTIs)   substrates for the viral reverse transcriptase enzyme (Figure 52-2), which converts viral RNA into proviral DNA before it becomes incorporated in the host cell chromosome.

occlusive dressing   a treatment that closes off the pores of the skin, e.g. a type of ointment (such as petroleum jelly) or plastic wrapping, to trap and prevent water loss (sweat) from the skin, thus increasing hydration of the epidermis.

opioid   pertaining to natural and synthetic chemicals that have opium-like effects although they are not derived from opium.

orphan drug   drug used to treat, prevent or diagnose rare diseases. It is recognised that, although such drugs might not be commercially viable, patients with rare conditions have as much right as all others to access drugs that are safe and effective.

oxytocics   agents that stimulate contraction of the smooth muscle of the uterus, resulting in contractions and labour.

parasympathetic nervous system   one of the three divisions of the autonomic nervous system; it functions mainly to conserve energy and restore body resources.

parasympatholytic   pertaining to a blockade of acetylcholine receptors that results in the inhibition of the transmission of parasympathetic nerve impulses.

parasympathomimetic   pertaining to a substance producing effects similar to those caused by stimulation of a parasympathetic nerve.

parenteral administration   the administration of drugs by injection (literally: other than via the gastrointestinal tract).

penicillins   antibiotics related chemically to the original penicillin G, a product of the mould *Penicillium notatum*; they contain a β-lactam ring.

peptic ulcer disease   a broad term encompassing both gastric and duodenal ulcers.

perinatal period   the period around childbirth, defined as lasting from week 28 of pregnancy to the end of the first week of the infant's life.

pharmaceutics   the science of formulation of drugs into different types of preparation, e.g. tablets, ointments, injectable solutions or eye-drops; it also includes study of the ways in which various drug forms influence pharmacokinetic and pharmacodynamic activities of the active drug.

pharmacodynamics   the study of the interaction between a drug and its molecular target, and the pharmacological response; 'what the drug does to the body'.

pharmacoeconomics   the study of the cost effectiveness of drugs; decisions must be made to ration drugs and contain costs, if possible without compromising good health care.

pharmacokinetics   the study of how a drug is altered during the processes of absorption, distribution, metabolism, and excretion; 'what the body does to the drug'.

pharmacology   the study of the discovery, development, chemistry, use and effects of drugs.

pharmacopoeia   a reference book listing standards for drugs approved in a particular country; it may also include details of standard formulations and prescribing guidelines (a formulary).

pharmacy   the branch of science dealing with preparing and dispensing drugs; also the place where a pharmacist carries out these roles.

phocomelia   the absence or malformation of arms or legs.

phototoxicity   an adverse drug reaction that occurs when the inducing agent is present on the skin in sufficient amounts and is also exposed to particular sunlight wavelengths.

phytoestrogens   plant compounds with oestrogenic activity.

placebo   a Latin word literally meaning 'I will please'. In the pharmacological context, it refers to a harmless inactive preparation prescribed to satisfy a patient who does not require an active drug; in a clinical trial, it is formulated to look identical to the active drug under trial, to maintain 'double blinding', so that neither subject nor clinician knows which treatment group the subject is in.

polypharmacy   the concurrent use of multiple medications; in the clinical context, it has the connotation of implying over-prescription and use of too many or unnecessary drugs, often at frequencies greater than therapeutically essential.

potassium-sparing diuretics   one of three major classes of diuretics, so named because, unlike other diuretics, their use does not result in increased loss of potassium in urine; an example is amiloride.

potency   the amount of drug required to produce 50% of that drug's maximal effect; the more potent the drug, the lower the dose required for a given effect.

potentiation   an interaction between two drugs causing an enhanced effect of one or both of them.

pregnancy safety   a method of classifying drugs according to documented risks in pregnancy.

preload   the degree of stretch of heart fibres before contraction; the greater the preload, the greater the stretch.

premedication   any drug administered before anaesthesia to enhance the anaesthetic process, e.g. an antianxiety agent, an analgesic to reduce pain, or an anticholinergic agent to reduce secretions.

prodrug   a drug that is converted to its active form after absorption.

prophylactic   a treatment that prevents an illness.

proprietary name   when a drug company markets a particular drug product, it selects and copyrights a proprietary, or trade, name for the drug. This copyright restricts the use of the name to only the individual drug company and refers only to that formulation of the drug (cf. generic name).

proscribed drug   prohibited drug.

protease inhibitors   a group of substances that block the activity of proteases, such as in viruses.

psychogenic pain   pain with psychological, psychiatric or psychosocial causes as its primary aetiology; anxiety, depression and fear of dying have been known to cause severe pain.

psychotropic agents   drugs that affect the mind; may be used to treat neuroses and psychoses.

receptors   a large group of proteins that are the molecular targets for drugs; they are cellular macromolecules directly concerned with chemical signalling that initiates a change in cell function.

refractoriness   cardiac tissue is non-responsive to stimulation during the initial phase of systole (contraction). This is known as refractoriness, and it determines how closely together two action potentials can occur.

regional anaesthesia   the injecting of a local anaesthetic drug near a peripheral nerve trunk (nerve block) or around the spinal column to anaesthetise spinal nerve roots (epidural or subarachnoid techniques).

rhythmicity   the spontaneous excitation of pacemaker cells, which establishes the normal rhythm of the heart. The regularity of such pacemaking activity is termed rhythmicity.

sedatives   drugs that reduce alertness, consciousness, nervousness or excitability by producing a calming or soothing effect.

selective toxicity   a therapy designed to select for differences between healthy human cells and other cells such as cancer cells or microorganisms.

selectivity   the property of a drug that acts on a narrow range of receptors, cellular processes or tissues.

side effect   drug effect that is not necessarily the primary purpose for giving the drug in the particular condition. This term has been virtually superseded by the term adverse drug reaction.

specific resistance   provocation of an immune response against specific pathogens or transplanted tissue.

specificity   a term that is used loosely like 'selectivity' to refer to the narrowness of actions of a drug; the property of a drug that acts at one site, producing one effect.

spinal (subarachnoid) anaesthesia   in spinal anaesthesia (also called subarachnoid, intradural, or intrathecal block): injection of the local anaesthetic into the cerebrospinal fluid in the subarachnoid space, below the level of termination of the spinal cord, i.e. at L3–4 or L4–5; it affects the lower part of the spinal cord and nerve roots.

status epilepticus   the state of recurrent seizures for more than 30 minutes, without an intervening period of consciousness; status epilepticus is a clinical emergency.

steady state   the situation in which the rate of drug administration equals the rate of elimination and the plasma drug concentration remains constant. Clearance determines the maintenance dose rate required to achieve the target plasma concentration at steady state.

steroid   an organic molecule with a distinctive four-ringed chemical structure (see Figure 37-2); for example, one of a large number of hormones produced mainly in the adrenal cortex and gonads; see corticosteroids.

superinfection   an infection that occurs during the course of antimicrobial therapy delivered for either therapeutic or prophylactic reasons

surfactant   a surface-active agent that reduces surface tension and increases wettability in the airways; a phospholipid–glycoprotein lipoprotein mixture secreted in alveolar cells and present in the secretions lining the alveoli.

sustained release   release of active drug from a tablet or capsule, the rate of which is slowed by pharmaceutical processing, allowing prolonged drug actions.

sympathetic nervous system   one of the three divisions of the autonomic nervous system; it dominates the body during emergency and stress situations (the 'fight and flight' response).

sympathomimetic drug   a pharmacological agent that mimics the effects of stimulation of organs by the sympathetic nervous system.

symporters   secondary active-transport membrane proteins that move two substrates in the same direction (those that transport two substances in opposite directions are called antiporters).

tablets   solid disc-shaped compressed mixtures of active drug with various other chemicals, called excipients, which assist in the formulation.

tachyphylaxis   the term used clinically to describe rapidly developing loss of responsiveness after repeated exposure to a drug that stimulates the receptor.

teratogen   a substance that causes transient or permanent physical or functional disorders in the fetus, without causing toxicity in the mother.

teratogenesis   literally 'forming a monster'; in the medical context, it refers to abnormal embryonic development leading to congenital malformations.

tetracyclines   the first broad-spectrum antibiotics, developed after a systematic search for antibiotic-producing microorganisms in soil.

therapeutic index (TI)   a measure of safety of a drug, equal to the dose producing a particular toxic effect in 50% of a group of animals (TD_{50}) divided by the dose needed to generate an effective therapeutic response in 50% of the animals (ED_{50}): $TI = TD_{50} / ED_{50}$. In the clinical context, it is better defined as the maximum non-toxic dose divided by the minimum effective dose.

therapeutic range   generally considered to reflect the range of drug concentration having a high probability of producing the desired therapeutic effect and a low probability of producing adverse effects.

thiazide diuretics   one of three major classes of diuretics, e.g. hydrochlorothiazide.

threshold concentration   the plasma concentration at which a substance appears in the urine because of saturation of transporters, i.e. at a concentration exceeding the T_M.

thrombolytic (fibrinolytic) drugs   drugs used to treat acute thromboembolic disorders. Unlike anticoagulants, they dissolve clots.

tocolytics   drugs that relax the uterus and hence delay labour or inhibit threatened abortion.

tolerance   a phenomenon by which the body becomes increasingly resistant to a drug or other substance through continued exposure to the substance.

topical local anaesthesia   the administration of local anaesthetics to mucous membranes, skin surfaces, the cornea, wounds and burns.

toxicology   the study of the nature, properties, identification, effects and treatment of poisons, including the study of adverse drug reactions.

upregulation   an increase in receptor numbers; this situation can cause receptor supersensitivity.

vaccine   a suspension of attenuated or dead microbes given to elicit an immune response and confer specific immunity.

vasodilator   a drug that produces vasodilatation by relaxing smooth muscle in the blood vessel walls by either a direct or indirect action.

vehicle   the formulation in which a drug is administered, e.g. the ointment base or injection solution; the drug needs to leave the vehicle to be available for absorption.

very-low-density lipoproteins (VLDL)   one of three primary classes of lipoproteins found in the blood of fasting individuals.

volatile liquid anaesthesia   controlled vaporisation of a volatile liquid into a flow of gas (oxygen with or without nitrous oxide), so that a known concentration of volatile agent in oxygen is administered via a mask.

volume of distribution   (V) the volume in which the amount of drug in the body would need to be uniformly distributed to produce the observed concentration in blood.

Some definitions adapted from Youngson RM. *Collins Dictionary: Medicine*. Glasgow: Harper Collins, 1999.

APPENDIX 5
AUSTRALIAN AND NEW ZEALAND SCHEDULES FOR DRUGS AND POISONS

The National Drugs and Poisons Schedule Committee recommends the classification of drugs and poisons into Schedules, in the Standard for the Uniform Scheduling of Drugs and Poisons (SUSDP) (see Chapter 4). The recommendations of this Committee are usually incorporated in legislation and regulations of the states and territories; confusingly, the names of the Schedules still vary among states. An agreement between Australia and New Zealand has led to Trans-Tasman Scheduling Harmonisation. The two countries now have compatible Schedules, labelling and packaging requirements (although minor discrepancies still exist). Scheduling is a means of classifying chemicals, including poisons and drugs, to identify the degree of control over their availability to the public. The criteria for classification include toxicity, abuse potential, safety and the actual need for the chemical.

There are very strict labelling requirements for scheduled substances, and this includes the use of **signal words**, e.g. PHARMACY ONLY MEDICINE. Drugs are now labelled with the name of the classification rather than the 'S' number. This change was made to counteract the false perception in the community that higher S numbers necessarily meant higher toxicity.

The Schedule can depend on the strength and form of a substance; for example, paracetamol 500 mg tablets in packets of 24 are unscheduled (and therefore available in supermarkets), whereas packets of 100 are S2, PHARMACY ONLY. Codeine can appear in various Schedules, depending on the strength of the formulation and whether other drugs are present.

Most drugs are in Schedule 2, 3, 4 or 8. There may be varying requirements within a Schedule, e.g. both clomiphene and isotretinoin are S4 PRESCRIPTION ONLY MEDICINES, but there are special provisions in state and territory laws regarding their prescription. (Clomiphene is an ovarian stimulant used by specialist physicians to treat anovulatory infertility, and isotretinoin is used to treat severe acne but is teratogenic, so great caution must be used in prescribing it for women of childbearing age.) A few medicines are included in Schedules 5 and 6 Poisons, such as head lice preparations and some essential oils.

It is important to note that drug scheduling is not 'set in stone', and drugs are moved around between Schedules as clinical experience and drug usage patterns change. Hence the most recent version of the SUSDP or *MIMS Bimonthly* data should always be consulted for the definitive answer to the question 'What schedule is this drug in?'.

CLASSIFICATION OF POISONS
Unscheduled substances

Unscheduled substances are those not requiring control by scheduling. They are not considered to be poisons. Many therapeutic preparations are unscheduled substances.
INCLUDES: antacids, laxatives, contact lens products, infant formulae, vitamins, sunscreens, many topical antiseptics and many herbal remedies.

Schedule 1 Poisons

This schedule is not currently used. It formerly included substances requiring proof of age, identity and the signature of the purchaser. It has been suggested that some complementary and alternative medicines be moved into this Schedule so that they can be subject to control.

Pharmaceutical substances
Schedule 2 Poisons (or Medicinal/ Therapeutic Substances/Poisons/ Products)
LABELLED: PHARMACY MEDICINE

Available to the public only from pharmacies, or, where a pharmacy service is unavailable, from persons licensed to sell Schedule 2 poisons. A pharmacist's advice is available if required.
INCLUDES: most cough and cold preparations; some antihistamines, mild analgesics, worm tablets, an antianginal spray, some anti-inflammatory agents, many topical antifungal preparations, some histamine H_2-receptor antagonists (in small packs, for relief of heartburn), and decongestant eye-drops.

Schedule 3 Poisons (or Medicinal/ Therapeutic/Potent Substances/ Poisons/Products)
LABELLED: PHARMACIST ONLY MEDICINE

Available to the public only from a pharmacist or from medical, dental or veterinary practitioners, but without need for a prescription. The safe use of these substances requires professional advice. The storage must not be accessible to the public.

INCLUDES: some metered-dose bronchodilator asthma aerosols, topical corticosteroids (some low-strength preparations in small packs) and adrenaline injections (high-strength, for anaphylaxis).

Schedule 4 Poisons (or Restricted/ Therapeutic Drugs/Substances/ Products/Poisons)
LABELLED: PRESCRIPTION ONLY MEDICINE or PRESCRIPTION ANIMAL REMEDY

May be used or supplied only under prescription from a medical, dental or veterinary practitioner. Must be stored in a dispensary. In some Australian states, specially qualified nurses, optometrists and podiatrists may prescribe a limited range of S4 PRESCRIPTION ONLY drugs.

INCLUDES: many drugs: all new drugs, antibiotics, antidepressants, hormones including insulins and hormonal contraceptives (except for emergency contraception, when they are S3 PHARMACIST ONLY), most cardiovascular and central nervous system drugs, antineoplastic agents, antiglaucoma eyedrops, vaccines and most injections.

Agricultural, domestic and industrial substances
Schedule 5 Poisons (Domestic/ Household Type Poisons or Hazardous Substances, or Industrial/Agricultural/Veterinary Products)
LABELLED: CAUTION

Substances with a low potential for causing harm, which can be minimised by the use of appropriate packaging with simple warnings and safety directions on the label. For sale by a pharmacist, Poisons licence holder or general dealer. Must not be stored or supplied in a drink or food container.

INCLUDES: some household poisons, ether, naphthalene, petrol and borax; some head lice lotions.

Schedule 6 Poisons (Domestic/ Industrial/Agricultural and Veterinary Poisons)
LABELLED: CAUTION or POISON (depending on whether for internal or external use)

More dangerous chemicals than those in Schedule 5, with

a moderate potential for causing harm. Extra storage and packaging controls and warning labels are required.

INCLUDES: household and garden pesticides and solvents; some iodine tinctures.

Schedule 7 Poisons (Dangerous Agricultural/Industrial Poisons)
LABELLED: DANGEROUS POISON

Substances with a high potential for causing harm at low exposure, and which require special precautions during manufacturing, handling, storage or use. A permit is required to buy these chemicals, and the purchaser must be over 18 years of age. These poisons should be available only to specialised or authorised users who have the skills necessary to handle them safely. Special regulations restricting their availability, possession, storage or use may apply.

INCLUDES: arsenic, strychnine, cyanide and commercial pesticides.

Controlled drugs and prohibited substances
Schedule 8 Poisons (or Drugs of Addiction/Dependence or Controlled Drugs or Narcotic Substances)
LABELLED: CONTROLLED DRUG

Substances that may produce addiction or dependence. Possession without authority is illegal. The tightest controls are used to reduce abuse, misuse and dependence. Prescriptions are valid for only 3 months. Drugs must stored in a locked cabinet and records kept for 3 years.

INCLUDES: opioids (such as morphine, methadone, buprenorphine, and high-dose codeine alone); CNS stimulants such as dexamphetamine and methylphenidate.

Schedule 9 Poisons
LABELLED: PROHIBITED SUBSTANCES

Substances of which the manufacture, possession, sale or use is prohibited except in special circumstances. Drugs that may be abused or misused and drugs possibly required for teaching, research or analytical purposes, but which are too toxic for therapeutic use.

INCLUDES: heroin and most recreational drugs (except alcohol and tobacco).

Adapted from: *Medicines Regulation and the TGA:* www.tga.gov.au/docs/html/medregs.htm, accessed 31 May 2006; Caswell A (ed.). *MIMS Annual 2005,* Sydney: CMPMedica Australia Pty Ltd, 2005; *MIMS Bimonthly* 2006; 2. Sydney: CMPMedica Australia, 2006.

APPENDIX 6

POISONS INFORMATION CENTRES

In Australia, call **13 11 26** in all states and territories (24-hour line) for connection to the nearest available Poisons Information Centre for information and advice on emergency treatment of poisoning, bites and stings.

In New Zealand, the standard telephone number is 0800 764 766 (= 0800 POISON).

ACT
ACT Poisons Service
The Canberra Hospital
Garran ACT 2605
Ph: 13 11 26

NSW
Poisons Information Centre
The Children's Hospital at Westmead
Hawkesbury Road
Westmead NSW 2145
Ph: 13 11 26

NT
Ph: 13 11 26

QLD
Poisons Information Centre
Royal Children's Hospital, Brisbane
Herston Road
Herston QLD 4029
Ph: 13 11 26

SA
Ph: 13 11 26

TAS
Ph: 13 11 26

VIC
Poisons Information Centre
Royal Children's Hospital
Flemington Road
Parkville VIC 3052
Ph: 13 11 26

WA
Poisons Information Centre
Sir Charles Gairdner Hospital
Hospital Avenue
Nedlands WA 6009
Ph: 13 11 26

NEW ZEALAND
NZ Poisons Information Centre
Ph: 0800 764 766 [0800 POISON]

DRUG (OR MEDICINES) INFORMATION CENTRES

ACT
Drug Information Pharmacist
ACT Drug Information Service
The Canberra Hospital
Garran ACT 2605
Ph: (02) 6244 3333
Fax: (02) 6244 3334

NSW
Drug Information Pharmacist
NSW Medicines Information Centre
PO Box 766
Darlinghurst NSW 2010
Ph: (02) 8382 2136
Fax: (02) 9360 1005
E-mail: nswmic@stvincents.com.au
Website:* www.ciap.health.nsw.gov.au/specialties/MIC/index.html

NT
Drug Information Pharmacist
Royal Darwin Hospital
PO Box 41326
Casuarina NT 0811
Ph: (08) 8922 8424
Fax: (08) 8922 8499
E-mail: andrew.crowhurst@nt.gov.au

QLD
Drug Information Pharmacist
Queensland Drug Information Centre
Royal Brisbane Hospital
Level 1, Ned Hanlon Building
Bowen Bridge Road
Herston QLD 4029
Ph: (07) 3636 7599
Fax: (07) 3636 1393

SA
Specialist Pharmacist
Drug Information Services
Flinders Medical Centre
Flinders Drive
Bedford Park SA 5042

* Note: this is an excellent website for drug information, the Clinical Information Access Program, with links to the *Australian Prescriber* journal and to many databases including Medline, CINAHL, PubMed, to online journals and books, the Cochrane Library, and MIMS publications.

Ph: (08) 8204 5301
Fax: (08) 8204 6245
E-mail: gaileasterbrook@fmc.sa.gov.au

TAS

Drug Information Pharmacist
Royal Hobart Hospital
GPO Box 1061L
Hobart TAS 7001
Ph: (03) 6222 8737
Fax: (03) 6222 8029

Victoria

Drug Information Pharmacist
Austin Health
Studley Rd
Heidelberg VIC 3084
Ph: (03) 9496 5668
Fax: (03) 9459 4546
E-mail: druginfo@austin.org.au

Drug Information Pharmacist
Drug Information Centre
Monash Medical Centre
246 Clayton Road
Clayton VIC 3168
Ph: (03) 9594 2361
Fax: (03) 9594 6595

Western Australia

Drug Information Pharmacist
Sir Charles Gairdner Hospital
Hospital Ave
Nedlands WA 6009
Ph: (08) 9346 2923
Fax: (08) 9346 4480

NEW ZEALAND

In New Zealand, as in Australia, the Poisons Information Centre is run separately from Drug Information (DI) Centres. The latter are considered to be mainly for professional queries from within the respective institutions. The specialist drug information pharmacists and pharmacologists can provide expert advice and answer questions from other health professionals and students on clinical placements, in the clinical context. As such, the contact numbers of Drug Information Centres are not usually made available to the public.

The emphasis in NZ is on encouraging members of the public to contact a health professional (doctor or pharmacist) for advice and information about their medicines, whereas the DI Centres are for professional queries.

Adapted from: Caswell A (ed.). *MIMS Annual 2005*, Sydney: CMPMedica Australia Pty Ltd, 2005; and information supplied by the Drug Information Pharmacists, with thanks.

APPENDIX 7
THE WORLD HEALTH ORGANIZATION LIST OF ESSENTIAL MEDICINES

The World Health Organization (WHO) 14th Expert Committee meeting on the selection and use of essential medicines has derived a model list of 312 individual medicines in some 27 categories, which can provide safe and effective treatment for most communicable and non-communicable diseases (see Chapter 1, under Drug Classifications).

The following table is adapted from the WHO model list of drugs. Categories of essential medicines are noted and, where possible, examples of therapeutic groups are given.

Section	Subsection	Examples*
1. Anaesthetics	1.1. General anaesthetics and oxygen 1.2. Local anaesthetics 1.3. Preoperative medication and sedation for short-term procedures	Thiopental (injection), oxygen (inhalation) *Lignocaine (injection, topical), *bupivacaine (injection) *Promethazine (elixir or syrup), atropine (injection)
2. Analgesics, antipyretics, non-steroidal anti-inflammatory medicines (NSAIMs), medicines used to treat gout, and disease-modifying agents used in rheumatoid disorders (DMARDs)	2.1. Non-opioids and non-steroidal anti-inflammatory medicines (NSAIMs) 2.2. Opioid analgesics 2.3. Medicines used to treat gout 2.4. Disease-modifying agents used in rheumatoid disorders (DMARDs)	*Ibuprofen (tablet), aspirin (tablet and suppository) *Codeine (tablet), *morphine (injection, oral solution and tablets) Allopurinol (tablet) Chloroquine (tablet)
3. Antiallergics and medicines used in anaphylaxis		*Chlorpheniramine (tablet or injection), adrenaline (injection), prednisolone (tablet)
4. Antidotes and other substances used in poisonings	4.1. Non-specific 4.2. Specific	*Charcoal (powder) activated Naloxone (injection), acetylcysteine (injection)
5. Anticonvulsants/ antiepileptics		*Diazepam (injection), sodium valproate (tablet)
6. Anti-infective medicines	6.1. Anthelmintics 6.2. Antibacterials 6.3. Antifungal medicines	6.1.1. Intestinal: *mebendazole (tablet), pyrantel (tablet and oral suspension) 6.1.2. Antifilarials: ivermectin (tablet) 6.1.3. Antischistosomals and antitrematode medicines: praziquantel (tablet) 6.2.1. β-lactam medicines: *amoxycillin (tablet, capsule or powder for oral suspension), ampicillin (injection) 6.2.2. Other antibacterials: *doxycycline (tablet or capsule), trimethoprim (tablet) 6.2.3. Antileprosy medicines: dapsone (tablet), clofazimine (capsule), rifampicin (capsule or tablet) 6.2.4. Antituberculosis medicines: ethambutol (tablet), rifampicin (capsule or tablet), isoniazid (tablet) *Fluconazole (injection, capsule and oral suspension), nystatin (tablet, lozenge or pessary)

(Continued)

Section	Subsection	Examples*
6. Anti-infective medicines—cont'd	6.4. Antiviral medicines	6.4.1. Antiherpes medicines: aciclovir (tablet or injection) 6.4.2. Antiretrovirals: zidovudine (capsule, oral solution or injection). Commence 3 or 4 drugs simultaneously 6.4.2.1 Nucleoside reverse transcriptase inhibitors: abacavir (tablet, oral solution) 6.4.2.2 Non-nucleoside reverse transcriptase inhibitors: nevirapine (tablet, oral suspension) 6.4.2.3 Protease inhibitors: indinavir (capsule), ritonavir (capsule, oral solution)
	6.5. Antiprotozoal medicines	6.5.1. Antiamoebic and antigiardiasis medicines: *metronidazole (tablet, injection or oral suspension) 6.5.2. Antileishmaniasis medicines: *meglumine (injection) 6.5.3. Antimalarial medicines 6.5.3.1 For curative treatment: *quinine (tablet or injection), 6.5.3.2 For prophylaxis: chloroquine (tablet or syrup) 6.5.4. Antipneumocystosis and antitoxoplasmosis medicines: pentamidine (tablet) 6.5.5. Antitrypanosomal medicines 6.5.5.1 African: suramin (injection) 6.5.5.2 American: nifurtimox (tablet)
7. Antimigraine medicines	7.1. For treatment of acute attack 7.2. For prophylaxis	Aspirin (tablet), paracetamol (tablet) *Propranolol (tablet)
8. Antineoplastic, immunosuppressives and medicines used in palliative care	8.1. Immunosuppressive medicines 8.2. Cytotoxic medicines 8.3. Hormones and antihormones 8.4. Medicines used in palliative care	*Cyclosporin (capsule and injection), *azathioprine (tablet) Doxorubicin (injection), cisplatin (injection) *Prednisolone (tablet), tamoxifen (tablet) Those listed in WHO publication *Cancer Pain Relief: With A Guide to Opioid Availability*. 2nd edn.
9. Antiparkinsonism medicines		*Biperiden (tablet and injection), levodopa and carbidopa (tablet)
10. Medicines affecting the blood	10.1. Antianaemia medicines 10.2. Medicines affecting coagulation	Ferrous salt (tablet and oral solution), folic acid (tablet), hydroxocobalamin (injection) *Warfarin (tablet), heparin sodium (injection), protamine sulfate (antidote: injection)
11. Blood products and plasma substitutes	11.1. Plasma substitutes 11.2. Plasma fractions for specific use	*Dextran 70 (injection), *polygeline (injection) *Factor VIII concentrate
12. Cardiovascular medicines	12.1. Antianginal medicines 12.2. Antiarrhythmic medicines 12.3. Antihypertensive medicines 12.4. Medicines used in heart failure 12.5. Antithrombotic medicines 12.6. Lipid-lowering agents	*Atenolol (tablet), glyceryl trinitrate (tablet, sublingual) *Atenolol (tablet), verapamil (tablet, injection) *Atenolol (tablet), enalapril (tablet) *Enalapril (tablet), digoxin (tablet, oral solution or injection) Aspirin (tablet) Statins: choice determined for those at highest risk of myocardial infarction

(Continued)

Section	Subsection	Examples*
13. Dermatological medicines (topical)	13.1. Antifungal medicines	*Miconazole (ointment or cream), benzoic and salicylic acids (ointment or cream)
	13.2. Anti-infective medicines	*Gentian violet (aqueous solution or tincture), silver sulfadiazine (cream)
	13.3. Anti-inflammatory and antipruritic medicines	*Betamethasone (ointment or cream), *calamine lotion
	13.4. Astringent medicines	Aluminium diacetate (solution)
	13.5. Medicines affecting skin differentiation and proliferation	*Podophyllum resin (solution), coal tar (solution)
	13.6. Scabicides and pediculicides	*Benzyl benzoate (lotion), permethrin (cream or lotion)
14. Diagnostic agents	14.1. Ophthalmic medicines	*Tropicamide (eye-drops), fluorescein (eye-drops)
	14.2. Radiocontrast media	*Iohexol (injection), barium sulfate (aqueous suspension)
15. Disinfectants and antiseptics	15.1. Antiseptics	*Chlorhexidine (solution), *ethanol (solution)
	15.2. Disinfectants	*Chloroxylenol (solution), glutaraldehyde (solution)
16. Diuretics		*Hydrochlorothiazide (tablet), spironolactone (tablet)
17. Gastrointestinal medicines	17.1. Antacids and other antiulcer medicines	*Ranitidine (tablet, injection or oral solution), aluminium hydroxide (tablet or oral suspension)
	17.2. Antiemetic medicines	*Promethazine (tablet, elixir or injection), metoclopramide (tablet or injection)
	17.3. Anti-inflammatory medicines	*Sulfasalazine (tablet or suppository),
	17.4. Laxatives	Senna (tablet)
	17.5. Medicines used in diarrhoea	17.5.1. Oral rehydration: Oral rehydration salts (for glucose electrolyte solution) 17.5.2. Medicines for diarrhoea in children: zinc sulfate (tablet or syrup) 17.5.3. Antidiarrhoeal (symptomatic) medicines in adults: *codeine (tablet)
18. Hormones, other endocrine medicines and contraceptives	18.1. Adrenal hormones and synthetic substitutes	*Prednisolone (tablet)
	18.2. Androgens	Testosterone (injection)
	18.3. Contraceptives	18.3.1. Oral hormonal contraceptives: *ethinyloestradiol + levonorgestrel (tablet) 18.3.2. Injectable hormonal contraceptives: medroxyprogesterone acetate (depot injection) 18.3.3. Intrauterine devices: copper-containing device 18.3.4. Barrier methods: condoms, diaphragms
	18.4. Oestrogens	*Ethinyloestradiol (tablet)
	18.5. Insulins and other antidiabetic agents	*Glibenclamide (tablet), insulin (injection)
	18.6. Ovulation inducers	*Clomifene (tablet)
	18.7. Progestogens	Norethisterone (tablet)
	18.8. Thyroid hormones and antithyroid medicines	*Propylthiouracil (tablet), thyroxine (tablet)

(Continued)

Section	Subsection	Examples*
19. Immunologicals	19.1. Diagnostic agents 19.2. Sera and immunoglobulins 19.3. Vaccines	Tuberculins (injection) *Antitetanus immunoglobulin (injection), antivenom serum (injection) 19.3.1. For universal immunisation: BCG, tetanus (injections) 19.3.2. For specific groups of individuals: influenza, meningococcal meningitis (injections)
20. Muscle relaxants (peripherally acting and cholinesterase inhibitors		*Neostigmine (tablet and injection), suxamethonium (injection)
21. Ophthalmological preparations	21.1. Anti-infective agents 21.2. Anti-inflammatory agents 21.3. Local anaesthetics 21.4. Miotics and antiglaucoma medicines 21.5. Mydriatics	*Gentamicin (eye-drops), tetracycline (eye ointment) *Prednisolone (eye-drops) *Tetracaine (eye-drops) *Pilocarpine (eye-drops), acetazolamide (tablet) Atropine (eye-drops)
22. Oxytocics and antioxytocics	22.1. Oxytocics 22.2. Antioxytocics	*Ergometrine (injection), oxytocin (injection) *Nifedipine (capsule)
23. Peritoneal dialysis solution		Parenteral solution of appropriate composition
24. Psychotherapeutic medicines	24.1. Medicines used in psychotic disorders 24.2. Medicines used in mood disorders 24.3. Medicines used in generalised anxiety and sleep disorders 24.4. Medicines used for obsessive–compulsive disorders and panic attacks 24.5. Medicines used in substance dependence programs	*Chlorpromazine (tablet, injection, syrup), *haloperidol (tablet, injection) 24.2.1. Medicines used in depressive disorders: *amitriptyline (tablet) 24.2.2. Medicines used in bipolar disorders: carbamazepine (tablet), lithium carbonate (capsule or tablet) *Diazepam (tablet) Clomipramine (capsules) Methadone (oral solution)
25. Medicines acting on the respiratory tract	Antiasthmatic and medicines for chronic obstructive pulmonary disease	*Beclomethasone (inhalation), salbutamol (tablet, inhalation, injection, syrup, respirator), adrenaline (injection)
26. Solutions correcting water, electrolyte and acid–base disturbances	26.1. Oral 26.2. Parenteral 26.3. Miscellaneous	Oral rehydration salts (for glucose electrolyte solution): see Section 17.5.1. *Sodium lactate (injection), glucose (injection) Water for injection
27. Vitamins and minerals		*Retinol (tablet, capsule, oral oily solution, water-miscible injection), ascorbic acid (tablet), iodine (oil, capsule, solution)

BCG = bacille Calmette–Guérin.
*Note: various other medicines may suffice as alternatives, depending on cost and availability.
Adapted from the WHO Model List, revised March 2005. For further information, see: www.who.int/medicines/services/essmedicines_def/en/index.html, accessed 23 October 2006.

FIGURE AND PICTURE CREDITS

Figure 2-2 designed and printed by Rolls Printing P/L; reproduced with permission.

Figure 4-1 from National Prescribing Service Newsletter 2001: 19; used with permission.

Figure 4-2 published by the Australian Adverse Drug Reactions Advisory Committee, Woden, ACT; reproduced with permission.

Figure 5-1 from Katzung BG (ed.). *Basic and Clinical Pharmacology*. 9th edn. 2004. New York: The McGraw-Hill Companies, Inc, 2004 [ch. 2]. Reproduced with permission of The McGraw-Hill Companies.

Figure 6-5 from Birkett DJ. Bioavailability and first-pass clearance. In: Birkett DJ. *Pharmacokinetics Made Easy*. Sydney: McGraw-Hill 2002 [ch. 5]. Reproduced with permission.

Figure 6-7 from Birkett DJ, Grygiel JJ, Meffin PJ, Wing LMH. Fundamentals of Clinical Pharmacology; 4. Drug biotransformation. *Current Therapeutics* 1979; 6: 129–38. Reproduced with permission.

Figure 7-4 from Brody TM, Larner J, Minneman KP. *Human Pharmacology: Molecular to Clinical*. 3rd edn. St Louis: Mosby, 1998. Reproduced with permission.

Figure 8-1 reprinted, by permission, from *Problems in Pediatric Drug Therapy*. 4th edn. p. 92. © 2002 by the American Pharmaceutical Association.

Clinical Interest Box 8-1 photo from Streissguth AP, Aase JM, Clarren SK et al. Fetal alcohol syndrome in adolescents and adults. *Journal of the American Medical Association* 1991; 265: 1961–7.

Table 8-1 reproduced from Australian Drug Evaluation Committee. *Prescribing Medicines in Pregnancy*. 4th edn. Canberra: Government Publishing Service, 1999. Copyright Commonwealth of Australia, reproduced by permission. Disclaimer: 'The Commonwealth does not warrant that the information is accurate, comprehensive or up-to-date and you should make independent inquiries, and obtain appropriate advice, before relying on the information in any important matter.'

Figure 8-2 from Barone MA. *The Harriet Lane Handbook*. 14th edn. St Louis: Mosby, 1996.

Figure 8-3 Goodman RM, Gorlin RJ. *Atlas of the Face in Genetic Disorders*. 2nd edn. St Louis: Mosby, 1977, courtesy Dr Charles Linder, Medical College of Georgia.

Figure 10-4 reproduced with permission of John W Stirling, Electron Microscope Unit, South Path, Flinders Medical Centre, Adelaide, Australia.

Figure 13-3 Bowman WC. Therapeutically useless drugs from unusual sources. *Pharmaceutical Journal* 1973; 211: 219–23. Published with permission from the *Pharmaceutical Journal*.

Figure 14-5 from Bowman WC, Rand MJ. *Textbook of Pharmacology*. 2nd edn. Oxford: Blackwell, 1980 [ch. 6], used with permission.

Figure 15-1 data from: Speight TM, Holford NHG (eds). *Avery's Drug Treatment*. 4th edn. Auckland: Adis International, 1997; Oberoi G, Phillips G. *Anaesthesia and Emergency Situations: A Management Guide*. Sydney: McGraw-Hill, 2000.

Figure 15-2 Bowman WC, Rand MJ. *Textbook of Pharmacology*. 2nd edn. Oxford: Blackwell, 1980; used with permission.

Figure 15-4 Bowman WC, Rand MJ. *Textbook of Pharmacology*. 2nd edn. Oxford: Blackwell, 1980; used with permission.

Figure 16-3B diagrams by Victor Iwanov, University of Melbourne; reproduced from *Therapeutic Guidelines: Analgesic, version 4*. Melbourne: Therapeutic Guidelines, 2002; with permission.

Figure 16-4 developed by McCaffery M, Pasero C. *Pain: Clinical Manual*. St Louis: Mosby, 1999; from Salerno E. *Pharmacology for Health Professionals*. St Louis: Mosby, 1999.

Figure 16-5 adapted from: Salerno E. *Pharmacology for Health Professionals*. St Louis: Mosby, 1999; Carr DB, Jacox AK, Chapman CR et al. *Acute Pain Management: Operative or Medical Procedures and Trauma. Clinical Practice Guideline*. AHCPR Pub. No 92-0032. Rockville, MD: Agency for Health Care Policy and Research, Public Health Service, US Department of Health and Human Services, 1992.

Figure 16-6 from Wong D, Hockenberry-Eaton M, Wilson D et al. *Wong's Essentials of Pediatric Nursing*. 6th edn. St Louis: Mosby, 2001. Reproduced with permission.

Figure 16-8 Courtesy of Baxter Healthcare Corporation, Deerfield, IL.

Figure 17-2 from Beare PB, Myers JL. *Adult Health Nursing*. 3rd edn. St Louis: Mosby, 1998.

Figure 18-1 adapted from: Tortora GJ, Grabowski SR. *Principles of Anatomy and Physiology*. 9th edn. HarperCollins, New York, 2000 [ch. 14]; Vander A, Sherman J, Luciano D. *Human Physiology: The Mechanisms of Body Function*. 7th edn. McGraw-Hill, Boston; 1998 [ch. 13]; Rang HP, Dale MM, Ritter JM, Moore PK. *Pharmacology*. 5th edn. Edinburgh: Churchill Livingstone, 2003.

Figure 18-2 adapted from: Rang HP, Dale MM, Ritter JM, Moore PK. *Pharmacology*. 5th edn. Edinburgh: Churchill Livingstone, 2003, with permission; data redrawn from Richens A, Dunlop A. Serum-phenytoin levels in management of epilepsy. *Lancet* 1975: 2: 247–8.

Figure 20-1 courtesy of Dr Andrew Herxheimer, in Laurence DR. *Clinical Pharmacology*. 4th edn. Edinburgh: Churchill Livingstone, 1973; used with permission.

Figure 22-1 reproduced from NASA. Using spider-web patterns to determine toxicity. *NASA Tech Briefs* 1995; 19(4): 82, with permission.

Figure 22-2 from data reviewed in Wallgren H, Berry M. *Actions of Alcohol*. Amsterdam: Elsevier, 1970; as shown in Bowman WC, Rand MJ. *Textbook of Pharmacology*. 2nd edn. Oxford: Blackwell, 1980 [ch. 42]; used with permission.

Figure 22-3 from Bowman WC, Rand MJ. *Textbook of Pharmacology*. 2nd edn. Oxford: Blackwell, 1980 [ch. 42], used with permission; data obtained by Dr M.P. Giles, Department of Pharmacology, University of Melbourne.

Figure 26-1 from Rang HP, Dale MM, Ritter JM, Moore PK. *Pharmacology*. 5th edn. Edinburgh: Churchill Livingstone, 2003 [ch. 19]. Reproduced with permission.

Figure 28-1 Data from Greger R. Physiology of sodium transport. *American Journal of Medical Science* 2000; 319: 51–62. Reproduced from Rang HP, Dale MM, Ritter JM, Moore PK. *Pharmacology*. 5th edn. Edinburgh: Churchill Livingstone, 2003 [Ch. 23], with permission.

Figure 30-1 after Rang HP, Dale MM, Ritter JM, Moore PK. *Pharmacology*. 5th edn. Edinburgh: Churchill Livingstone, 2003 [chs 20–21], with permission.

Figure 30-2 after Rang HP, Dale MM, Ritter JM, Moore PK. *Pharmacology*. 5th edn. Edinburgh: Churchill Livingstone, 2003 [chs 20–21], with permission.

Figure 31-2 A, C and D courtesy GlaxoSmithKline, Australia; used with permission.

Figure 32-1 C and F: photographs courtesy of BOC Gases Australia Ltd, reproduced with permission.

Figure 33-3 adapted from: Rang HP, Dale MM, Ritter JM, Moore PK. *Pharmacology*. 5th edn. Edinburgh: Churchill Livingstone, 2003. By permission of the publisher.

Figure 38-2 from Tanner JM. *Foetus into Man: Physical Growth from Conception to Maturity*. Ware: Castlemead, 1989. Reproduced with permission from Castlemead Publications.

Figure 39-1 adapted from: Rang HP, Dale MM, Ritter JM, Moore PK. *Pharmacology*. 5th edn. Edinburgh: Churchill Livingstone, 2003 [Figure 25-1], with permission.

Figure 39-3 from Tanner JM. *Foetus into Man: Physical Growth from Conception to Maturity*. 2nd edn. Ware: Castlemead, 1990. Reproduced with permission from Castlemead.

Figure 42-1 adapted from: Grills B. Osseous structure and function: study guide. Melbourne: La Trobe University, 2002 [unpublished].

Figure 43-1 modified from: Salerno E. *Pharmacology for Health Professionals*. St Louis: Mosby, 1999.

Figure 43-2 modified from: Salerno E. *Pharmacology for Health Professionals*. St Louis: Mosby, 1999.

Figure 43-4 modified from: Salerno E. *Pharmacology for Health Professionals*. St Louis: Mosby, 1999.

Figure 48-1 adapted from Beare PG, Myers JL. *Adult Health Nursing*. 3rd edn. St Louis: Mosby, 1998.

Figure 48-2 reproduced from Souhami R, Tobias J. *Cancer and its Management*, 5th edn. Malden, MA: Blackwell, 2005, with permission.

Figure 48-4 adapted from Beare PG, Myers JL. *Adult Health Nursing*. 3rd edn. St Louis: Mosby, 1998.

Figure 51-1 from Raper KB, Alexander DF. Penicillin. V. Mycological aspects of penicillin production. *Journal of the Elisha Mitchell Scientific Society* 1945; 61, 74–113.

Figure 53-2 with kind permission of John Rumpff and Ros Biebrick, Haematology, *SouthPath*, Flinders Medical Centre, Adelaide, Australia.

Figure 54-4 from Mudge-Grout CL. *Immunologic Disorders*. St Louis: Mosby, 1992.

Figure 55-3 reproduced with kind permission of Karen Lillywhite, Computer Assisted Learning Unit, School of Medicine, Flinders University, Adelaide, Australia.

Figure 56-2 from Beare PG, Myers JL. *Adult Health Nursing*. 3rd edn. St Louis: Mosby, 1998.

Chapter 59 Irukandji—Jack Barnes; Stonefish—Neville Coleman; Sea snake—Dr Peter Fenner; King Brown (Mulga), Death adder, Eastern brown snake, Taipan, Katipo—Lochman Transparencies; Tiger snake—Australian Picture Library; Sydney funnel-web spider—ANT Photo Library.

INDEX

Notes about the index

- This is a combined index to drugs, diseases and other topics.
- Drug Monographs are indicated by a bold entry (e.g. **234**).
- Material in Tables is indicated by the page number followed by the letter 't' (e.g. 655t).
- Material in Boxes is indicated by the page number followed by the letter 'b' (e.g. 42b).
- References to figures are in italics (e.g. *194*).
- Material in Clinical Interest Boxes is indicated by the page number followed by the letter 'c' (e.g. 217c).
- Drug names starting with a numeral are indexed ignoring the numeral (so *5-hydroxytriptamine* is found under 'H').
- Greek letters have been spelt out, so 'α-blockers' appears as 'alpha-blockers'.
- Many topics relating to drugs are indexed at the more specific word, e.g. 'drug interactions' at 'interactions between drugs'.

A

A-delta fibre pain 252
AAN 12–3
abacavir 836
  pregnancy safety 844
abbreviations and symbols, in prescriptions 39, 40–1t
ABC powders 275c
abciximab
  platelet effects 500, 509–10
  pregnancy safety 512
abducent nerve 215t
Aboriginals and Torres Strait Islanders, *see also* indigenous remedies
  diabetes in 669c
  gastric remedies 577c
  health workers among 33
  indigenous health workers 33
  psychiatric disorders 321c
  renal disorders 475c
  traditional medicine 65, 797c
absence seizures 297, 299c, 300t
absinthe, toxicity 67t
absorbers of UV radiation 913–4
absorption 112b, 113–5
  defined 114b
  drug interactions affecting 157–8
  gastrointestinal 553
  in the elderly 148b
  variables affecting 114–5
  via skin 905, 908
abuse of drugs 371, *see also* sport, drugs in
  ADHD treatments 342
  amphetamines 339
  fetal effects 729
  myths about 377c
  parkinsonism from 350c
  sexual function affected by 746
acamprosate **391**
  for treatment of alcohol abuse 390–1
  pregnancy safety 405
Acanthamoeba infection 595, 597
acarbose, *see* alpha-glucosidase inhibitor
accommodation of the eye 585, 588
ACE, *see* angiotensin-converting enzyme
ACE inhibitors 454–7
  Alzheimer's disease treatment 362
  combined with diuretics 486t
  cyclosporin interactions 892
  drug groups 13t
  incontinence caused by 489t

ACE inhibitors—cont'd
  loop diuretic interactions 482
  pharmacokinetics 455t
  potassium-sparing diuretic interactions 487
  psoriasis treatment 920
  sexual function affected by 750
  sleep pattern effects 284t
  stroke treatment 362
  taste and smell effects 617t
  teratogenic potential 142t, 726
  thiazide diuretic interactions 485
acetaminophen, *see* paracetamol
acetazolamide 307, 481
  CO_2 level effects 527
  glaucoma treatment 593t, 594
  membrane-stabilising actions 303
  pregnancy safety 309, 606
acetic acid
  ear treatment 611c, 613–614
  pregnancy safety 618
acetic acid NSAIDS 879t, 881t
acetylation, conjugation reaction 122t
acetylcholine (ACh)
  affects 5-HT receptors 314
  as neurotransmitter 221
  balance with dopamine *350*
  CNS effects of imbalance 223–4
  drugs affecting 178
  miotic effects 590
  muscarinic actions 178t
  nicotine effects on 394
  pregnancy safety 606
  release of *203*
  role in SNS 202
  transmitter in PNS 169–72
acetylcholinesterase
  inactivation by 172
  role in SNS 202
acetylcholinesterase inhibitors, *see* anticholinesterases
acetylcysteine **530**
  for paracetemol overdose 272
  mucolytic 529
  pregnancy safety 549
N-acetyltransferases 123
  conjugation reaction 122t
  genetic deficiency in 124
ACHT, skin conditions from 907t
aciclovir 831, **832**
  for mouth blistering 565
  mycophenolate mofetil interactions 895

aciclovir—cont'd
  ocular use 597
  pregnancy safety 597, 606, 844
  skin conditions from 907t
  topical administration 915
'acid', *see* lysergic acid diethylamide
acid–base balance, *see* pH
acid-fast bacilli 795t
acid-labile drugs, in neonates 145t
acidic drugs
  absorption of 115
  bind to albumin 119
acidity, *see* pH
acidosis 232, *see also* carbon dioxide
acitretin
  acne treatment 920–1
  pregnancy safety 928
  psoriasis treatment 920
acne vulgaris 920–2
  drugs causing 907t
  neomycin treatment 915
acoustic nerve 215t
acquired immunity 874–5
acrolein, tear gas 606
acromegaly 632
ACT, regulation in 76t
ACTH, *see* adrenocorticotrophic hormone
action plans for asthma 541
action potentials 167–9, *170*
  CNS 219–24
  generation and transmission 165–9
activated charcoal, toxic binding by 569c
activated partial thromboplastin time (APTT) 503c
Active Australia campaign 948
active constituents, plant drugs 7–11
active immunity 875t
active transport 114
active tubular secretion from kidneys 125
acupuncture for pain relief 276
acute lymphoblastic leukaemia, combination therapy 764
acute pain 255
adalimumab 886–7
  pregnancy safety 900
adapalene
  acne treatment 920
  pregnancy safety 928
addiction 372, *see* abuse of drugs; dependence; withdrawal from drugs
Addison's disease 656, 656c

ADE, *see* adverse drug events
ADEC 82, 138–9, 139t
adefovir 831, 834
  pregnancy safety 844
adenine 757
adenohypophysis, *see* anterior pituitary
    hormones
adenomas 633c, 634–5
adenosine diphosphate (ADP), in blood
    clotting 495
adenosine, dipyridamole interactions 509
adenosine triphosphate (ATP)
  caffeine interactions 345
  cardiac treatment with 437
  in cardiac action 417
  inhibitors, *see* proton pump inhibitors
  pregnancy safety 437
  sodium–potassium neural pump 220
ADH, *see* vasopressin
ADHD, *see* attention deficit hyperactivity
    disorder
Adie's tonic pupil syndrome 588c
adipose tissue, *see* body fat
adjustment disorder 284
adjuvant therapy
  analgesics 276
  cancer treatment 761
  for chronic pain 255t
administration of drugs
  aerosol therapy 519–21
  analgesics 259–61
  drug delivery systems 42b, 90t
  for the ear 613
  general anaesthetics 231
  legal issues 78–9
  liposome delivery 788
  oxygen delivery 526
  routes for 115–7
  topical 908–11
  transtympanic perfusion 612
adolescents, *see* age factors; paediatrics
ADP, *see* adenosine diphosphate
ADR (adverse drug reactions), *see* adverse
    drug events
ADRAC 91–2
adrenal cortex 627t, 650–62
  androgens produced by 734
  cancer treatment effects 781
  fetal 727
adrenal insufficiency 660c
adrenal medulla 653
  catecholamine synthesis 173
  fetal 727
  histamine effects 897t
adrenaline
  adjunct to local anaesthesia 243
  adverse drug events 190
  asthma treatment 534
  beta-blocker interaction 198t
  chlorpromazine interactions 323
  effects of 187–90
  glaucoma treatment 593
  hyperglycaemia linked to 672t
  in cardiac action 419
  in insulin release 666
  MAO inhibitor interactions 331
  methyldopa interactions 453
  pancuronium interactions 205
  pregnancy safety 199t
  shock, treatment for 192t
  snake bite treatment 959

adrenaline—cont'd
  stress induces release of 653
adrenergic agonists, *see* sympathomimetic
    drugs
adrenergic antagonists, *see* sympatholytic
    drugs
adrenergic receptors, *see* adrenoceptors
adrenergic transmission 169, 172–5, 174, *see*
    also adrenoceptors
adrenoceptor agonists, *see* sympathomimetic
    drugs
adrenoceptor antagonists, *see* sympatholytic
    drugs
adrenoceptors 174, 188t, *see also* alpha-
    adrenoceptors; beta-adrenoceptors
adrenocorticoids
  amphotericin B interactions 828
  phenytoin interactions 306
adrenocorticotrophic hormone 308, 626t,
    654, *see also* corticotrophin-releasing
    factor
  for infantile spasms 308
  membrane-stabilising actions 303
  regulation in sport 936
adsorbents, antidiarrhoeal agents 579–80
adverse drug events 153–6, *see also specific*
    drugs
  definition 3t
  drugs affecting the PNS 181t
  in the elderly 149–50, 149t
  information about 16
  monitoring for 45–7
  ocular effects 603c, 603–6
  reporting 91–2
  to over-the-counter drugs 51, 57
  with 'natural' products 7
Adverse Drug Reactions Advisory Committee,
    blue form 91–2
advertising, *see* marketing
AEDs, *see* antiepileptic drugs
aerosol therapy 519–21, *see also* inhaled
    drugs
aesculus, toxicity 67t
aetiology, *see* disease
affective disorders 325–7, *see also* anxiolytics;
    depression; mania
afferent pathways in CNS 213
afferent stimulation to relieve pain 253
African traditional medicine 66
age factors 147–8, 298–9, *see also* elderly;
    paediatrics
agonist analgesics 263, *see also* morphine
agonists, defined 107
AHF, *see* antihaemophilic factor (factor VIII)
AIDS, *see* HIV
akathisia 316t, 317c
Akhenaton 734c
akinesia, dopamine levels and 349–55
alafacept 919
albendazole 864
  pregnancy safety 866
albumin, binds acidic drugs 119
alcohol (ethanol) **388**
  abuse of 371, 386–92
  amantadine interactions 834
  anaesthesia and 234
  analgesic effects 276
  anticoagulant interactions 506
  antihistamine interactions 899
  Australian use of 378–9
  barbiturate interactions 290

alcohol (ethanol)—cont'd
  benzodiazepine interactions 288
  beverages containing 387t
  biguanide interactions 678
  caffeine interactions 346
  chloral hydrate interactions 291c
  chlorpromazine interactions 323
  cycloserine interactions 857
  deaths resulting from 376
  depression evoked by 326
  diabetic effects 673c
  diazepam interactions 287
  didanosine interactions 838
  diphenoxylate interactions 579
  drug interactions with 158
  efavirenz interactions 840
  fetal alcohol syndrome 141c
  gastrin stimulant 572
  glyceryl trinitrate interactions 442
  griseofulvin interactions 830
  headaches from 365
  hypoglycaemia linked to 672t
  isoniazid interactions 858
  lignocaine interactions 241
  methadone interactions 386
  methotrexate interactions 775
  metronidazole interactions 819
  morphine interactions 268
  mouth-washes and gargles 563, 563c
  neonatal withdrawal symptoms 143t
  ocular adverse effects 604t
  opioid interactions 543
  OTC pharmaceuticals 387t
  oxytocin inhibited by 635
  phentermine interactions 952
  phenytoin interactions 306
  plasma concentrations 390
  plasma lipid profile effects 464t, 470
  praziquantel interactions 865
  pregnancy safety 405
  psychotropic agent interactions 318
  regulation in sport 934, 939
  retinopathy induced by 604
  rifampicin interactions 859
  salbutamol compared with 2c
  sexual function impaired by 750–1
  skin treatment 911
  sleep effects 284t
  symptoms of abuse 374t
  teratogenic potential 142t
  tocolytic effects 728
  topical astringent 909
  valproate interactions 307
  zalcitabine interactions 840
aldesleukin (interleukin-2) 785
  as orphan drug 80t
  pregnancy safety 896t
  role in immunostimulation 896
aldosterone 659–63
  determines sodium uptake 477
  potency of 657
  stress induces release of 653
alefacept, pregnancy safety 928
alendronate **692**
  effect on bone 693
  osteoporosis treatment 692
  pregnancy safety 693
alendronic acid, in Australia's top 10 drugs
    17t
alertness, *see* attention deficit hyperactivity
    disorder; CNS stimulants; narcolepsy

alfentanil 267
    as anaesthetic 239
    pregnancy safety 278
alginic acid, in antacids 565
alkalinity, see acidic drugs; basic drugs; pH
alkaloids, see also belladonna alkaloid; ergot
        alkaloids
    chemical structure 10
    drugs from 8–11
alkylating agents 907t
    cancer treatment 761, 770, 784
    indications and toxicity 771t
    infertility related to 767
allatoxins, carcinogenesis induced by 759–60
allergic reactions 874, see also anaphylactic
        reactions
    asthma 531
    OTC drugs for 53t
    to drugs 155, 156t
allergic rhinitis 547–8, 898
allopurinol 888
    azathioprine interactions 158, 893
    gout treatment 887
    ocular adverse effects 604t
    penicillin interactions 806
    phenytoin interactions 306
    pregnancy safety 789, 900
    skin conditions from 907t
    tumour lysis syndrome 784
    warfarin interactions 505
aloe vera (aloes) 62t, 910, 927c
alopecia, drugs causing 765, 907t
alpha-adrenoceptor agonists
    CNS effects 222
    drug groups 13t
alpha-adrenoceptor antagonists, see
        alpha-blockers
alpha-adrenoceptors 174
    drugs acting on 441
    effects of 186–7, 187b
    food intake regulation 949
alpha-blockers 193–5
    adrenaline interactions 190t
    benign prostatic hyperplasia treatment 736
    glaucoma treatment 593t
    incontinence caused by 489t
    nicotine interactions 397
    sexual function affected by 749–50
    taste and smell effects 617t
5-alpha-dihydrotesterone, regulation in sport
        934
alpha-glucosidase inhibitor (acarbose) 679–80
    diabetes treatment 677
    pharmacokinetics 678t
    pregnancy safety 681
alpha-latrotoxin 962
alpha₁-adrenoceptor blockers, see
        alpha-blockers
alpha₁-glycoprotein, binds basic drugs 119
alpine cider plum 826c
alprazolam
    abuse of 392
    anxiolytic 287
    pharmacokinetics 286t
    recommended for elderly 285
    sexual function affected by 750
alprostadil
    erectile dysfunction treatment 749
    pregnancy safety 751
alteplase 506
    fibrinolysis effects 500

alteplase—cont'd
    heparin interactions 501
    pregnancy safety 512
alternative medicine, see complementary and
        alternative medicine
altretamine, cancer treatment 776
aluminium acetate
    ear treatment 614
    skin condition treatment 910
aluminium hydroxide
    adverse drug events 566t
    antacids containing 565, 565t
    antidiarrhoeal agents 579
    constipation treatment 574
    mycophenolate mofetil interactions 895
    tacrolimus interactions 891
    thyroxine interactions 645t
aluminium silicate, protectant effect 911
aluminium solutions, pregnancy safety 928
aluminium subacetate, antipruritic agent
        909
alveolar ventilation, in anaesthesia 230
Alzheimer's disease 361t
    nicotine reduces prevalence of 394–5
    treatment of 179c, 360–3
amantadine 353–4, 831, 834
    adjuvant analgesic 276
    antiparkinsonian 546
    decongestant 546
    pregnancy safety 366, 844
ambulance paramedics 31
amenorrhoea 704c
    progesterone treatment 711–2
American names (USAN) 14
amethocaine
    local anaesthetic 240, 243t
    ocular use 599
    pregnancy safety 606
    topical administration 247t
    toxicity of 244
amide-linked anaesthetics 240
amifostine
    hydration therapy 784
    pregnancy safety 789
amikacin 814
    ototoxicity 615
    pregnancy safety 821
amiloride 485–6
    blocks ion channels 105
    cyclosporin interactions 892
    pharmacokinetics 484t
amino acids
    as neurotransmitters 221–2
    taste of 616
aminobenzoic acid 907t, 913
aminobutyric acid 222, 358
aminoglutethimide 662
    cancer treatment 779t, 781
    glucocorticoid interactions 660t
    medroxyprogesterone acetate interactions
        713
    pregnancy safety 662
    warfarin interactions 505
aminoglycosides 814–5
    age-related adverse drug events 149t
    amoebiasis treatment 855
    botulinum toxin interactions 601
    capreomycin interactions 857
    cidofovir interactions 834
    combined with cephalosporins 809
    cyclosporin interactions 892

aminoglycosides—cont'd
    loop diuretic interactions 482
    neonatal dose 145t
    ocular use 596
    ototoxicity 615–6, 615t
    pancuronium interactions 205
    penicillin interactions 806
    plasma concentrations 815
    teicoplanin interactions 812
    vancomycin interactions 812
    zalcitabine interactions 840
aminopenicillins 806
aminophylline
    asthma treatment 344, 535
    pregnancy safety 549
    rifampicin interactions 859
aminoquinolines 359c
aminosalicylates, for inflammatory bowel
        disease 580–1
amiodarone 430, 436, 436t
    avoid during breastfeeding 144t
    cytochrome P450 isoform inhibition 158t
    digoxin interactions 426t
    fosamprenavir interactions 842t
    mefloquine interactions 850
    pharmacokinetics 430t
    phenytoin interactions 306
    photosensitising effects 907t
    pregnancy safety 437
    procainamide interactions 433t
    quinidine interactions 432t
    saquinavir interactions 843
    skin conditions from 907t
    thiourea interactions 649
    thyroid effects 643, 645–6
    warfarin interactions 505
amisulpride 325
    major effects 315t
    pregnancy safety 320
amitriptyline 366
    adverse events 319t
    age-related adverse drug events 149t, 150
    migraine treatment 364
    pregnancy safety 320
    sedative effects 328
    sexual function affected by 750
    skin conditions from 907t
amlodipine 446t
    angina treatment 445
    pharmacokinetics 446t
    pregnancy safety 457
ammonia, respiratory stimulation by 528
amnesia
    anterograde amnesic effect 288
    drug-induced 287
amoebiasis 854–5
amoebicidal agents 855
    metronidazole 819
amorolfine 917, 918t
    pregnancy safety 928
    topical antifungal 916
amoxycillin
    adverse drug events 807
    clavanulic acid with 806
    ear treatment 612
    effect of food on absorption 808t
    peptic ulcer treatment 570–1
    pharmacokinetics 807t
    pneumonia treatment 546
    pregnancy safety 821
    sinusitis treatment 544, 549

amoxycillin—cont'd
  sugar-free medications 673c
  urinary tract infection treatment 820
amphetamines 193, 339–40
  abuse of 374t, 380, 393–4
  addiction to 340
  bicarbonate interactions 567
  hospitalisations due to abuse 376
  intoxication with 377t
  RAS affected by 217
  regulation in sport 938
  sexual function affected by 747
  spider's webs affected by 373
  sport stimulant 933
  taste and smell effects 617t
amphotericin B 826, **828**
  capreomycin interactions 857
  cidofovir interactions 834
  digoxin interactions 426t
  glucocorticoid interactions 660t
  imidazole antifungal interactions 829t
  liposome delivery 788
  loop diuretic interactions 482
  pregnancy safety 844
  sugar-free medications 673c
  zalcitabine interactions 840
ampicillin
  food affects absorption of 808t
  oestradiol valerate interactions 711
  pharmacokinetics 807t
  pregnancy safety 821
  resistance to 798t
  taste and smell effects 617t
  urinary tract infection treatment 820
amprenavir 836, 841
  drug interactions 842t
  pregnancy safety 844
amyl nitrate
  abuse of 375t
  sexual function affected by 747
amyotrophic lateral sclerosis 360
anabolic steroids 735–6, 935c
  adverse drug events 936
  hypoglycaemia linked to 672t
  regulation in sport 933, 934–5
  sexual function affected by 751
  warfarin interactions 505
anaemia 493–4, 512–3, see also iron
anaerobes, infections caused by 796t
  drug resistance 805t, 809t
anaesthesiology 32, 228c
anaesthetics 227–48
  adjuncts to 209, 235, 527
  adrenaline as adjunct to 190
  benzodiazepine interactions 288
  CNS effects 214c
  diazepam interactions 287
  dosage measurement 23
  drug groups 13t
  effect on CNS 220
  effect on reticular activating system 217
  history of 5–6
  neuromuscular blocking drugs in 203
  palliative care with 787
  pancuronium interactions 205
  perinatal use 729
  potency 230
  psychotropic agent interactions 318
  sodium nitroprusside interactions 449
  tocolytic effects 728
  valproate interactions 307

anagrelide
  cancer treatment 782
  pregnancy safety 789
anakinra 887
anal canal 559–60
analeptics (restorative drugs) 339, 528
analgesics 252–78, see also local anaesthetics
  age-related adverse drug events 149t, 150
  burn treatment 924
  caffeine an adjunct to 344
  during childbirth 234
  ear treatment 612
  headache treatment 366
  history of 5–6
  liniments and rubs 910
  migraine treatment 364
  nephrotoxicity 488c
  non-pharmacological 276–7
  OTC drugs 53t
  ototoxicity 615t
  Paget's disease 691
  palliative care with 787–8
  perinatal use 729
  postoperative 235
  regulation in sport 938
  respiratory depression from 528
  stage 1 of anaesthesia 227
anandamide (endogenous cannabinoid) 401
anaphylactic reactions 874
  adrenaline treatment 189–90
  histamine effects 897, 898
  to bivalirudin 505
  to neuromuscular blocking drugs 205
  to penicillin 808c
  to snake bites 960
  to spider bites 962
anastrozole
  cancer treatment 779t, 781
  pregnancy safety 789
  use in sport 935
ancestim, during cancer chemotherapy 784
Ancylostoma duodenale 864
androgens 653, 698, see also anabolic
    steroids; sex hormones
  breast cancer treatment 779
  contraceptive use 742
  in male reproductive system 734–5
  pregnancy safety 737
  sexual function affected by 746–7
  skin conditions from 907t
  teratogenic potential 142t, 726
androstenedione
  for athletes 940
  in male reproductive system 734
  regulation in sport 934
angel dust, see phencyclidine
angina pectoris 197, 441
angiogenesis-inhibiting agents, cancer
    treatment 762
angioneurotic oedema 898
angiotensin-converting enzyme 453, see also
    ACE inhibitors
angiotensin II 453, 661
angiotensin II agonists 13t
angiotensin-II-receptor antagonists 457
  potassium-sparing diuretic interactions 487
  teratogenic potential 142t
animals
  animal rights 97
  drugs from 7
ankylosing spondylitis 886

Anopheles mosquito 848
anorectic agents 339, 342–3
  noradrenergic drugs 950–1
  taste and smell effects 617t
anorexigenic neurotransmitters 949
anosmia 618
anovulation 740
ANS, see autonomic nervous system
antacids 565–7
  adverse drug events 566t
  alendronate interactions 692
  amprenavir interactions 842t
  chloroquine interactions 851
  digoxin interactions 426t
  drug interactions 566t
  flucytosine interactions 830
  glucocorticoid interactions 660t
  imidazole antifungal interactions 829t
  mycophenolate mofetil interactions 895
  nitrofurantoin interactions 822
  OTC drugs 55
  peptic ulcer treatment 570
  phenytoin interactions 306
  pregnancy safety 566, 581
  quinidine interactions 432t
  quinolone interactions 818
  sucralfate interactions 573
  tetracycline interactions 816
antagonists, defined 107–8
antazoline
  ocular use 598
  pregnancy safety 606
anterior pituitary hormones 626, 626t,
    630–5, 656
anterograde amnesic effect 288
anthelmintic drugs 864–6
anthracyclines 778c
  adverse drug events 783
  cancer treatment 762, 773–6
  mechanism of action 776
anthranilates, in sunscreens 913
anti-inflammatory agents, see also
    inflammation
  ginseng 64
  glucocorticoids 656
  ocular use 585
  ototoxicity 616
  retinopathy induced by 604
  taste and smell effects 617t
  topical administration 917–20
antiallergens, ocular use 585, 598
antianaemic drugs, DUB treatment 720
antiandrogens 737
  acne treatment 922
  cancer treatment 779, 779t
  contraceptive use 742
  drug groups 13t
  sexual function affected by 751
antianginal agents 196, 728
antianxiety drugs, see anxiolytics
antiarrhythmics 196–7, 428–37
  adjuvant analgesics 276
  amiodarone interactions 436t
  anaesthetic interactions 233
  disopyramide interactions 432t
  flecainide interactions 435
  ginseng 64
  lignocaine interactions 241
  mexiletine interactions 435
  pharmacokinetics 430t
  procainamide interactions 433t

antiarrhythmics—cont'd
    quinidine interactions 432t
    ritonavir interactions 843
    taste and smell effects 617t
antiatherosclerotic agents 466
antibacterials 804–22
    asthma treatment 541
    topical 915
antibiotics, see also antifungals; antimalarials;
        antimicrobials; antivirals; resistance to
        antibiotics
    acne treatment 922
    adverse systemic effects of ocular treatment
        605t
    anaesthetic interactions 233
    antitumour activity 778c
    cancer treatment 772t, 773–6
    COPD treatment 542
    ear-drops **614**
    ear treatment 612, 613
    in food sources/animals 800c
    introduction of 794
    lactulose interactions 577
    ocular use 592, 596
    oestradiol valerate interactions 711
    ototoxicity 615t
    pancuronium interactions 205
    sildenafil interactions 748
    simvastatin interactions 467
    skin condition treatment 920
    skin treatment 912c
    statin interactions 466
    suxamethonium interactions 207
    taste and smell effects 617t
    upper respiratory tract infection treatment
        544
antibodies 871, 873–4, see also monoclonal
        antibodies
antibody-dependent cytotoxic drug allergies
        156t, 874
anticholinergic effects, psychotropic agents
        316
anticholinergics
    adverse systemic effects of ocular treatment
        605t
    age-related adverse drug events 149, 149t
    alcohol interactions 391
    amantadine interactions 834
    antihistamine interactions 899
    antihistamines as 899
    chlorpromazine interactions 323
    constipation treatment 574
    diphenoxylate interactions 579
    diuretic use 488–9
    drug interactions with 157
    erectile dysfunction due to 745
    incontinence caused by 489t
    nasal condition treatment 549
    ocular adverse effects 604t
    ocular use 588–9, 589t
    parkinsonism treatment 349, 355
    peptic ulcer treatment 570
    perceptual states altered by 373
    premedication with 235t
    psychotropic agent interactions 318
    quinidine 431
    vertigo treatment 612
anticholinesterases 207
    Alzheimer's disease treatment 362
    anaesthetic interactions 233
    bethanechol interactions 179

anticholinesterases—cont'd
    miotic effects 590
    muscle relaxants 355–6
    myasthenia gravis treatment 603
    ocular adverse effects 604t
    pancuronium interactions 205
    procainamide interactions 433t
    sites of action 208
anticoagulants 500–6, see also oral
        anticoagulants
    adverse drug events 154
    age-related adverse drug events 149t
    alopecia from 907t
    carbamazepine interactions 307
    griseofulvin interactions 830
    metronidazole interactions 819
    oestradiol valerate interactions 711
    penicillin interactions 806
    phenytoin interactions 306
    rifampicin interactions 859
    skin conditions from 907t
    thiourea interactions 649
    thyroxine interactions 645t
    valproate interactions 307
anticonvulsants 299, see also seizures
    adjuvant analgesics 276
    adverse drug events 300
    carbamazepine interactions 307
    cephalosporin interactions 810
    drug interactions with 158
    hormonal factors 124
    ideal properties 303
    levodopa–carbidopa interactions 352
    mefloquine interactions 850
    migraine treatment 364
    multiple sclerosis treatment 360
    oestradiol valerate interactions 711
    seizure treatment 287
    sildenafil interactions 748
    tamoxifen interactions 780
antidepressants 328–34
    ADHD treatment 342
    adrenaline interactions 190
    adverse drug events 329
    age-related adverse drug events 150
    alcohol interactions 391
    Alzheimer's disease treatment 362
    antiepileptic interactions 302
    balancing levels of 223–4
    benzodiazepine interactions 288
    choosing between 316
    CNS effects 214c
    diazepam interactions 287
    drug dependence treatment 382
    mechanism of action 326
    migraine treatment 364
    mood disorder treatment 312
    multiple sclerosis treatment 360
    ocular effects 589, 604t
    palliative care in cancer treatment 787
    peptic ulcer treatment 570
    pregnancy safety 329
    ritonavir interactions 843
    safer varieties for elderly 285
    salbutamol interactions 536
    sexual function affected by 750
    taste and smell effects 617t
    TCA interactions 329
    terbutaline interactions 536
antidiabetic drugs
    alcohol interactions 391

antidiabetic drugs—cont'd
    beta-blocker interaction 198t
    diethylpropion interactions 952
    glucocorticoid interactions 660t
    phentermine interactions 952
    rifampicin interactions 859
    testosterone interactions 735
antidiarrhoeal agents 578–80
    clindamycin interactions 814
    digoxin interactions 426t
    OTC drugs 55
antidiuretic hormone 222, 477, 635
    inhaled use 677
    oxytocic effects 727
    pregnancy safety 636
antiemetics 567–70, see also nausea; vomiting
    during cancer treatment 778, 783, 787
    during pregnancy 725
    haloperidol 325
    migraine treatment 364
    postoperative 235
    prochlorperazine 324
    psychotropic agent interactions 318
    sedative effects 292
antiepileptic drugs 297–309
    diazepam interactions 287
    ethosuximide interactions 307
    oestradiol valerate interactions 711
    palliative care in cancer treatment 787
    psychotropic agent interactions 318
    teratogenic potential 726
    topiramate interactions 304
    valproate interactions 307
antiestrogens, see antioestrogens
antifever agents, see antipyretics; NSAIDs
antifungals 826–31
    glucocorticoid interactions 660t
    oral candidiasis treatment 564
    orphan drugs 80t
    sildenafil interactions 748
    simvastatin interactions 467
    sites of action 827
    statin interactions 466
    tamoxifen interactions 780
    topical administration 916, 918t
antiglaucoma agents 592–5, 593t
antihaemophilic factor (factor VIII) 495t
    haemostatic effects 510–1
    pregnancy safety 512
antihistamines, see also histamine
    age-related adverse drug events 149t
    alcohol interactions 391
    antiemetic effects 567t
    antiepileptic interactions 302
    antipruritic agents 909
    atropine interactions 180
    benzodiazepine interactions 288
    conjunctivitis treatment 598
    cough suppressants 542
    diazepam interactions 287
    immunostimulation by 896–901
    Ménière's disease treatment 613c
    methadone interactions 386
    migraine treatment 364
    nasal condition treatments 548
    neonatal withdrawal symptoms 143t
    ocular effects 589
    ocular use 592, 598
    opioid interactions 543
    OTC drugs 55
    paradoxical reactions 285

antihistamines—cont'd
  photosensitising effects 907t
  pregnancy safety 899
  psychotropic agent interactions 318
  sedative effects 284t, 292
  sexual function affected by 751
  skin condition treatment 920
  skin conditions from 907t
  urticaria treatments 920
antihyperlipidaemic agents 462–71, 603
antihypertensives
  age-related adverse drug events 149t, 150
  anaesthetic interactions 233
  aspirin interactions 274
  chlorpromazine interactions 323
  depression evoked by 326
  dexamphetamine interactions 341
  glyceryl trinitrate interactions 442
  levodopa–carbidopa interactions 352
  NSAID interactions 157, 883
  olanzapine interactions 325
  procainamide interactions 433t
  risperidone interactions 325
  sexual function affected by 749, 750
  sodium nitroprusside interactions 449
antimalarials 849–54
  photosensitising effects 907t
  retinopathy induced by 604
antimanic agents 214c, 334–5
antimetabolites 104, 773
  alopecia from 907t
  cancer treatment 761
  indications and toxicity 771t
  taste and smell effects 617t
antimicrobials 794–7
  adverse systemic effects of ocular treatment 605t
  ear treatments 613
  ocular use 585, 595–7
  pressure sore treatment 927
  sites of action 805
  sugar free medications 673c
  taste and smell effects 617t
  topical 914–7
antimigraine drugs 276, 617t
antimuscarinics, see muscarinic receptor antagonists
antimycobacterials, see also antituberculous agents
  atazanavir interactions 842t
antineoplastic agents 761–3
  atazanavir interactions 842t
  cancer treatment 770–89
  chemical structures 773
  monoclonal antibodies 781–2
  orphan drugs 80t
  ototoxicity 615t
  taste and smell effects 617t
  teratogenic potential 726
antinicotinics, see non-depolarising blocking drugs
antioestrogens 710
  cancer treatment 779t, 780–1
  infertility related to 767
  regulation in sport 933, 935
antioxidants, for athletes 940
antiparkinsonian agents 349–55, see also Parkinson's disease
  age-related adverse drug events 149t
  CNS effects 214c
  ocular effects 589

antiparkinsonian agents—cont'd
  taste and smell effects 617t
antiplatelet drugs 507–10
  dipyridamole interactions 509
  glycoprotein IIb/IIIa receptor inhibitor interactions 510
  oxpentifylline interactions 452
  stroke treatments 362
  thrombolytic interactions 506
antiporters 476
antipruritic agents 909
antipseudomonal penicillins 806
antipsychotics 312, 322–5, see also neuroleptics; psychotropic agents
  alcohol interactions 391
  Alzheimer's disease treatment 362
  antiepileptic interactions 302
  CNS effects 214c
  depression evoked by 326
  extrapyramidal system effects 218
  falls and fractures associated with 286c
  sedative effects 284t
  TCA interactions 329
antipyretics, see also fever
  for coughs 542
  sinusitis treatment 549
antiretroviral agents
  foscarnet interactions 835
  St John's wort interactions 327c
antirheumatics 617t, 884–7, 886
antisense oligonucleotides 762
antiseptics 915
  acne treatment 921
  for pressure sores 927
  history of 6
  ocular use 597
  OTC drugs 53t
  skin condition treatment 910
antiserotonin agents, migraine treatment 364
antispasmodic agents, see also muscle spasms
  adjuvant to analgesics 276
  age-related adverse drug events 149t
  alcohol interactions 391
  irritable bowel syndrome treatment 581
antithrombin III 501
  pregnancy safety 512
antithrombin III-dependent and independent coagulants 504–5
antithrombotic drugs 236, see also aspirin
antithymocyte globulins 893
antithyroid agents 640–9
  lithium interactions 333
  taste and smell effects 617t
  teratogenic potential 726
antituberculous agents 856–61
antitumour antibiotic agents, see also antibiotics
  alopecia from 907t
  cancer treatment 761
antitussives, see cough preparations
antivenoms 957–64
antivirals 831–44
  benzodiazepine interactions 288
  drug groups 13t
  ergometrine interactions 728
  ocular use 597
  orphan drugs 80t
  sildenafil interactions 748
  tamoxifen interactions 780
  taste and smell effects 617t
  topical administration 915

anxiety disorders 284
anxiolytics 282–93, see also benzodiazepines; sedatives
  alcohol interactions 391
  Alzheimer's disease treatment 362
  CNS effects 214c
  for children 292
  palliative care with 787
  peptic ulcer treatment 570
  sexual function affected by 750
ANZCCART 97
APF 16, 84
'aphrodisiacs' 746–8
apnoea, see sleep disorders
apocrine glands 904
apolipoproteins 463–4
apomorphine
  emetic agent 353
  parkinsonism treatment 353
  pregnancy safety 366
apoptosis 758, 762
apothecary system 19, 31
appetite-suppressant drugs, see anorectic agents
approved (generic) names 12–4
apraclonidine 590
  glaucoma treatment 590t, 593, 593t
  pregnancy safety 606
aprepitant 570
  antiemetic use 567t
  cancer treatment 783
  pregnancy safety 581
  warfarin interactions 505
aprotinin
  haemostatic effects 511
  pregnancy safety 512
aqueous humour 585
arachidonic acid, role in pain 254–5
area under the plasma concentration versus time curve 130–1, 131
aripiprazole 315t, 325
  pregnancy safety 320
arnica, toxicity 67t
aromatase inhibitors
  cancer treatment 779t, 781
  use in sport 935
aromatherapy 63
aromatic amino acid decarboxylase, see dopa decarboxylase
arrhythmia
  drug-induced 245, 318c, 432
  treatment of 422
arsenic trioxide, cancer treatment 782
artemether 852–3
  pregnancy safety 866
arterial thrombi 496
arteries 419
arterioles 419
  adrenoceptors 188t
  histamine effects 897t
  innervation of 166t
arteriopathic dementia 362
arthrus reaction 874
articaine
  local anaesthetic 243t
  nerve block anaesthesia 247t
  pregnancy safety 248
artificial sweeteners 616
artificial tear solutions 602
artificially acquired immunity 874–5
Ascaris lumbricoides 864, 866

ASCEPT 29
Asclepias 5
ascorbic acid, *see* vitamin C
asparaginase, *see* colaspase
aspartame, taste of 616
aspartate 222
Aspergillus infections 796t
aspirin 271-2, **274**, 879t
    abuse of 405
    age-related adverse drug events 149t, 262
    angina treatment 442c
    antiplatelet action 500, 507, 509
    as NSAID 270
    asthma induced by 533c
    avoid during breastfeeding 144t
    combination analgesics 273
    cyclophosphamide interactions 774
    dipyridamole interactions 509
    headache treatment 366
    heparin interactions 501
    hypoglycaemia linked to 672t
    in Australia's top 10 drugs 17t
    mechanism of action 29, 879
    methotrexate interactions 775
    migraine treatment 364
    mouth blister treatment 564
    ocular adverse effects 604t
    ototoxicity 615t
    overdose 275b
    pregnancy safety 278, 512
    probenecid interactions 890
    stroke treatment 362
    taste and smell effects 617t
    teratogenic potential 726
    ulcer risk 879
    valproate interactions 307
    vs paracetamol 275b
    warfarin interactions 157, 505
assays, standards established by 84-5
asthma 531-41
    airways in 529
    aminophylline treatment 344
    drugs used by athletes with 935, 942c
    histamine effects 898
    mediators of 532
    therapeutic tips 548c
asthma weed 67t
astringents 909
    diarrhoea treatments 577c
    tretinoin interactions 922
atazanavir 836, 841
    drug interactions 842t
    pregnancy safety 844
atelectasis 527
atenolol 197t, 436
    avoid during breastfeeding 144t
    insulin interactions 675
    pharmacokinetics and dosages 198t
    pregnancy safety 199t
atheroma, ocular effect of 603
atherosclerosis, high lipid levels associated
        with 462
athletes, *see* sport, drugs in
atomoxetine, ADHD treatments 342
atopy 898
atorvastatin
    dosage 467
    hyperlipidaemia treatment 466
    in Australia's top 10 drugs 17t
    pregnancy safety 470
    saquinavir interactions 843

atosiban, tocolytic effects 728
atovaquone
    malaria treatment 853
    pregnancy safety 866
atracurium 204, 206t
    pregnancy safety 248
    premedication with 235t
atria (heart) 411
atrial fibrillation 435b
    digoxin treatment 425, 427
    warfarin for 29c
atrioventricular node, *see* AV node
atropine 179, **180**, *see also* anticholinergics
    adverse drug events 181t, 605t
    age-related adverse drug events 149t
    antidiarrhoeal agents 579
    cancer treatment 776
    clinical use and administration 182t
    diphenoxylate adjunct 579, 580
    erectile dysfunction due to 745
    nerve toxin antidote 209c
    ocular effects 589, 589t
    parkinsonism treatment 355
    pregnancy safety 182, 606
    premedication with 230, 235t
    respiratory disorder treatment 530
    skin conditions from 907t
    substitute drugs 181-2
attapulgite
    antidiarrhoeal agent 579
    clindamycin interactions 814
attention deficit hyperactivity disorder
        (ADHD) 328, 340-2
atypical antipsychotics 324-5, 672t
AUC 130-1, *131*
auditory ossicles 611
augmented (Type A) ADRs 154-5
auranofin
    antirheumatic effects 884
    pregnancy safety 900
aurothiomalate
    antirheumatic effects 884-5
    pregnancy safety 900
Australasian Society of Clinical and
        Experimental Pharmacologists and
        Toxicologists 29
Australia, *see also* Aboriginals and Torres
        Strait Islanders; indigenous remedies;
        regulation
    adverse drug reaction incidence 153-4
    alcohol abuse in 389
    anabolic steroid use in 935
    antidepressant use in 332c
    asthma in 531, 531c
    Australian Sports Anti-Doping Authority
        934
    cancers in 755c
    CMI handouts 18
    complementary and alternative medicine
        use 59c
    controlled substances 372
    coronary heart disease, deaths from 500
    criminal offences in 82-3
    deaths from heart failure 423c
    dementia in 179c, 360
    depression in 328
    diabetes in 668-9
    diet treatment for dyslipidaemia 465
    diuretic use in 486
    drug abuse in 376, 378
    drug availability in 27-8

Australia—cont'd
    drug development in 93
    drugs developed or trialled in 90t, 94
    drugs from plants 11
    ethical marketing code 98
    fluoridated water 563c
    helminthiasis in 864c
    herbal remedies in 63
    HIV infections 831c
    leprosy in 861
    malaria in 848
    musculoskeletal disorders in 879
    obesity in 947, 948
    orphan drugs in 80
    plant drugs 797c
    psychiatric disorders in 314
    skin cancers in 912c
    snake bites 957
    strokes due to clotting or haemorrhage 496
    thalidomide use in 785-6
    top 10 drugs 15, 17t
    tuberculosis in 856
Australia New Zealand Therapeutic Products
        Authority 77
Australian and New Zealand Council for
        the Care of Animals in Research and
        Teaching 97
Australian Approved Names 12-3
Australian Capital Territory, regulation in 76t
Australian Drug Evaluation Committee 82
    pregnancy categories 138-9, 139t
Australian National Prescribing Service 28
Australian Pharmaceutical Benefits Scheme 31
Australian Pharmaceutical Formulary 16, 84
Australian Pharmaceutical Handbook 16
Australian Sports Anti-Doping Authority 82
autoimmune disorders 643
autoinduction of metabolism 305
automaticity (cardiac conduction system)
        414-5
    digoxin effects 425
    treatment of 429
autonomic drugs
    multiple sclerosis treatment 360
    nicotine interactions 397
autonomic nervous system 163-75, *164*
    cardiac action 419
    drugs affecting 178-83
    gastrointestinal tract nerves 553
    hypothalamus in 216
    ocular effects 588-92, 589t
    responses to 166t
    sexual function role 745, 749
autonomic reflexes 163
autumn crocus 778c
AV node (cardiac conduction system) 414
    calcium-channel blocker effects 443
axons 165
Ayurvedic medicine 4
azatadine, pregnancy safety 899
azathioprine
    allopurinol interactions 158, 888
    cyclophosphamide interactions 774
    didanosine interactions 838
    immunosuppressant 892-3
    inflammatory bowel disease 580
    muromonab-CD3 combination 894
    mycophenolate mofetil interactions 895
    pregnancy safety 900
    warfarin interactions 505
    zalcitabine interactions 840

azelaic acid
  acne treatment 921
  pregnancy safety 928
azithromycin 812
  for trachoma 595
  pharmacokinetics 813t
  pregnancy safety 606, 821
  warfarin interactions 505
azole antifungals 826–7
  benzodiazepine interactions 288
  cyclosporin interactions 892
  disopyramide interactions 432t
  drug groups 13t
  drug interactions 829t
  pharmacokinetics 829t
  phenytoin interactions 306
  rifampicin interactions 859
AZT, see zidovudine
aztreonam 804, 812
  pregnancy safety 821

B

B lymphocytes 872–4
babies, see neonates; paediatrics
bacille Calmette–Guérin (BCG)
  cancer treatment 785
  pregnancy safety 789
bacitracin
  ear treatment 613–4
  ocular use 596
  pregnancy safety 606
  topical administration 915
  triple antibiotic ointment 915
baclofen 358
  multiple sclerosis treatment 360
  muscle relaxant 356–7
  pregnancy safety 366
bacteraemia 794
bacteria, classification of 794
bacterial protein synthesis inhibitors 812–9
bactericidal agents 796 see also microbial
    infections
bacteriostatic agents 796
Bacteroides infections 795t, 796t
balanced anaesthesia 230
barbitone 290
barbiturates 290
  abuse of 374t, 380
  anaesthetics 238–9
  anticonvulsant effects 303
  antiepileptic interactions 301, 302
  calcium-channel blocker interactions 447t
  chloramphenicol interactions 817
  CNS effects 300t
  depression evoked by 326
  disuse of 282
  GABA receptor agonists 303, 305
  intoxication with 377t
  metronidazole interactions 819
  mode of action 287
  neonatal withdrawal symptoms 143t
  ocular adverse effects 604t
  oestradiol valerate interactions 711
  paradoxical reactions 285
  photosensitising effects 907t
  pregnancy safety 293
  sexual function affected by 750
  simvastatin interactions 467
  skin conditions from 907t
  valproate interactions 307
  warfarin interactions 505

barbiturates—cont'd
  withdrawal affects sleep patterns 284t
barriers to drug distribution 120
Bartholin's glands 705
Basal–bolus regimen for insulin administration
    676
basal cell carcinomas, see skin cancers
basal ganglia 202, 217, 218
basedoxifene 710
basic drugs
  absorption of 115
  bind to alpha₁-glycoprotein 119
basiliximab
  for rejection control 894
  pregnancy safety 900
basophils 494, 896
baths for skin disorders 909
beclomethasone 538
  asthma treatment 536, 538, 548c
  inhaled corticosteroid 658
  nasal condition treatment 548
  OTC vs prescription variants 52t
  pregnancy safety 549
bedsores, see pressure sores
belladonna alkaloids
  antidiarrhoeal agents 579
  hallucinogens 403
  toxicity 67t
benign prostatic hyperplasia 193–4, 736–7
benoxaprofen, adverse drug events 154t
benserazide
  parkinsonism treatment 350
  pregnancy safety 366
bentonite, in calamine lotion 910
benzalkonium chloride
  antiseptic effects 915
  contact lens solutions 602
  ear treatment 614
  skin condition treatment 910
benzathine benzylpenicillin 804
benzhexol
  clinical use and administration 182t
  parkinsonism treatment 355
  pregnancy safety 182, 366
benzimidazoles 864–5
benzocaine
  antipruritic agent 909
  liniments and rubs 910
  local anaesthetic 240, 243t
  metabolism of 242
  mouth-washes and gargles 563
  pregnancy safety 618
  topical administration 247t
benzodiazepines
  abuse of 380, 392
  adjuvant analgesics 276
  adverse drug events 288–9
  anaesthetics 239
  angina treatment 445
  anticonvulsant effects 303
  atazanavir interactions 842t
  depression evoked by 326
  drug groups 13t
  drug interactions 288
  drugs related to 289–90
  falls and fractures linked to 286c
  GABA receptor agonists 303, 304
  limbic effects 218
  macrolide antibiotic interactions 812
  Ménière's disease treatment 613c
  overdose 289, 289b

benzodiazepines—cont'd
  paediatric risks 292
  parental administration 302
  perinatal use 729
  pharmacokinetics 286t, 288
  photosensitising effects 907t
  pregnancy safety 293
  premedication with 235t
  replace barbiturates 282
  safer for elderly 285
  sedative effects 285–9
  sexual function affected by 750
  vertigo treatment 612
  withdrawal affects sleep patterns 284t
benzoic acid esters, local anaesthetics 240
benzophenones, in sunscreens 913
benzopyrene, carcinogenesis induced by 759
benzoyl peroxide
  acne treatment 921
  pregnancy safety 928
  tretinoin interactions 922
benzphetamine 951
benztropine
  adjunct to psychotropic agents 316
  clinical use and administration 182t
  parkinsonism treatment 355
  pregnancy safety 182, 366
benzydamine, in mouth-washes and gargles
    563
benzyl benzoate 917
benzylpenicillin 804
  bile acid-binding resin interactions 468
  pharmacokinetics 807t
  pregnancy safety 821
  resistance to 805t
bergamot, photosensitising effects 907t
Bernard, Claude 204, 228c
beta-adrenoceptor agonists 191
beta-adrenoceptors 174, 186–7, 187b
  food intake regulation 949
beta-blockers 195–8, 430
  adrenaline interactions 190t
  adverse drug events 197, 605t
  angina treatment 442c
  asthma exacerbated by 535
  asthma treatment 532, 548c
  biguanide interactions 678
  calcium-channel blocker interactions 447t
  cardiac action 424
  clonidine interactions 452
  depression evoked by 326
  dexamphetamine interactions 341
  disopyramide interactions 432t
  drug groups 13t
  drug interactions 198t
  effects compared 448t
  glaucoma treatment 592, 593t
  hyperthyroidism treatment 647
  hypoglycaemia linked to 672t
  insulin interactions 675
  isoprenaline interactions 191
  latanoprost interactions 594
  lignocaine interactions 241, 434
  mefloquine interactions 850
  migraine treatment 364
  minoxidil interactions 448
  noradrenaline interactions 191
  pharmacokinetics 198t, 430t
  plasma lipid profile effects 464t, 470
  prazosin interactions 195
  psoriasis treatment 920

beta-blockers—cont'd
  quinidine interactions 432t
  regulation in sport 934, 935, 938, 939
  salbutamol interactions 536
  sexual function affected by 750
  sleep pattern effects 284t
  suxamethonium interactions 207
  taste and smell effects 617t
  terbutaline interactions 536
  theophylline interactions 537
  vertigo treatment 612
beta-endorphin
  delta-receptor antagonist 264t
  kappa-receptor agonist 264t
  mu-receptor agonist 264t
beta-hydroxy-beta-methylbutyrate, for athletes
    940
beta-interferon, multiple sclerosis treatment
    360
beta-lactamase 797, 804
betahistine, vertigo treatment 612
betamethasone
  pharmacokinetics 657t
  potency 657
  pregnancy safety 662
  topical administration 919
betaxolol 197t
  glaucoma treatment 592, 593t
  pharmacokinetics and dosages 198t
  pregnancy safety 199t, 606
betel nut and leaf 67t, 403
bethanechol 178, **179**
  adverse drug events 181t
  pregnancy safety 182
bevacizumab, cancer treatment 782
beverages, see alcohol (ethanol); caffeine; tea
bicalutamide
  antiandrogens 737
  cancer treatment 779, 779t
bicarbonate
  adverse drug events 566t
  for athletes 940
  gastric effects 559
  hexamine interactions 820
bicuspid valve 388
Bier's block 245–6, 247
bifonazole, topical antifungal 916, 918t
biguanides
  diabetes treatment 677–9
  pharmacokinetics 678t
bile acid-binding resins 467–8
  digoxin interactions 426t
  hypercholesterolaemia treatment 467t
  statin interactions 466
  teicoplanin interactions 812
  tetracycline interactions 816
  vancomycin interactions 812
bilharziasis, see Schistosoma spp.
biliary system 126, 574
bilirubin 220c
bimatoprost
  glaucoma treatment 593t, 594
  pregnancy safety 606
binding proteins (hormones) 621
bioassays, standards established by 85
bioavailability 114b, 117, 118
bioequivalence 14, 117–8
bioethics 96–7, see also ethical issues
biological membranes, see cell membranes
biological response modifiers, see
    immunomodulating drugs

biological variability 85
biosurgery (maggots), for pressure sores 926
biotechnology, see genetic engineering
biotransformation, see metabolism of drugs
biperiden
  clinical use and administration 182t
  parkinsonism treatment 355
  pregnancy safety 182, 366
bipolar affective disorder 312, 327, 332c,
    334–5
birthwort, toxicity 67t
bisacodyl 576t
  pregnancy safety 581
  stimulant laxative 575–6
bishydroxycoumarin 505
bismuth
  peptic ulcer treatment 570–1
  protectant effect 911
  skin conditions from 907t
bisoprolol 197t
  pharmacokinetics and dosages 198t
  pregnancy safety 199t
bisphosphonates
  adjuvant analgesics 276
  bony metastasis treatment 786
  drug groups 13t
  effect on bone 693
  osteoporosis treatment 692
  Paget's disease treatment 691
bitumen 911
bivalirudin 500, 504–5
  pregnancy safety 512
bizarre (Type B) ADRs 155
blackwood 884c
bladder 474, 487–8, 736
bleomycins 778c
  cancer treatment 772t, 773–6
  emetic potential 766c
  mechanism of action 776
  pregnancy safety 789
  taste and smell effects 617t
blepharitis 595
blepharospasm 359, 600c, 601
blinking 585, 600c
blistering of the mouth 564–5
blockers, see antagonists
blood, see also factors in blood coagulation;
      names of blood components, e.g. red blood
      cells
  absorption from 114–5
  blood products developed in Australia 90t
  cells 492
  coagulation of 274, 494–7, 500
  composition of 492
  drug distribution to 118t
  pH of 476
  skin reservoir of 905
  types and groups 497
blood–brain barrier 120, 219, 220c
blood doping 934, 938–9
blood glucose levels, see also hyperglycaemia;
      hypoglycaemia
  control of 667, 668
  monitoring 670, 671–2
  obesity and 948
blood pressure, see also hypertension;
      vasodilators
  control of 451, 455
  glucocorticoids in 654
blood sugar, see blood glucose levels
blood vessels, see also cardiovascular system

blood vessels—cont'd
  adrenoceptors 188t
  constrict when injured 494
blue form 91–2, 92
body chart for pain assessment 256–7, 257
body compartments, drug distribution to
    118t
body fat
  adrenoceptors 188t
  distribution of 947–8
  drug binding 119
  drug distribution to 118t
  in neonates 145t
  in the elderly 147
body image 905
body mass index 140, 947, 947c
body surface area as basis for dosage 21–2,
    145
body temperature, regulation via skin 905
body weight, see also obesity
  dosage based on 21
boils 611, 915
boldenone, regulation in sport 934
bone
  drug binding 119–20
  drug distribution to 118t
  effect of drugs on 692–3
  metastases of 786
  methylxanthine effects on 345
  mobilisation of calcium 686
bone marrow suppressants, see also
    haemopoietic system
  amphotericin B interactions 828
  cancer treatment 765, 784
  cyclophosphamide interactions 774
  flucytosine interactions 830
  ganciclovir interactions 833t
  methotrexate interactions 775
  valganciclovir interactions 833t
  zidovudine interactions 837
bone mineral density
  corticosteroid effects 538
  homeostasis 690–2
boric acid
  antipruritic agent 909
  ear treatment 614
botulinum toxin 204c, **601**
  as muscle relaxant 359
  for blepharospasm 600c
  ocular use 599–600
  pregnancy safety 366, 606
bowel cancer, aspirin decreases risk 272
Bowman's capsule 474
box jellyfish 962–3
BP 14, 16, 84
bracken fern 884c
Bradford Hill, Austin 89c
bradycardia 207, 429
bradykinesia 349
bradykinin, involved in coughs 456c, 457
brain 214–8, see also central nervous system
  dopamine levels 349–55
brainstem 214–6
bran, laxative effects 574–5
brand names 14
breakthrough pain, palliative care for 788
breast cancer
  antioestrogen treatment 780
  combination therapy 764t
  hormone treatments 751
  oestrogen treatment 780

breastfeeding 730
  analgesics during 262
  antidepressants during 329
  drug excretion via breast milk 126
  drug use during 142–4, 144c, 730
  drugs to avoid during 144t, 353
  during cancer treatment 767
breathing, *see* respiratory system
brimonidine
  glaucoma treatment 593, 593t
  ophthalmic use 590t
  pregnancy safety 606
brinzolamide
  glaucoma treatment 593t, 594
  pregnancy safety 606
British National Formulary 16
British Pharmacopoeia 16
  drug standards in 84
  for approved names 14
bromazepam
  anxiolytic 287
  pharmacokinetics 286t
bromhexine, mucolytic 529–30
bromides 290–1
  strychnine interactions 291c
bromoacetone, tear gas 606
bromocriptine
  avoid during breastfeeding 144t
  erectile dysfunction treatment 749
  hyperprolactinaemia treatment 635
  infertility treatment 740
  lactation inhibited by 730
  macrolide antibiotic interactions 812
  neuroleptic malignant syndrome treatment 316
  on–off syndrome treatment 352
  parkinsonism treatment 353
  pregnancy safety 366, 636, 751
Brompton cocktail 264c
bronchial glands 517
bronchial smooth muscle *516*, 517–8
  histamine effects 897t
  mechanism of action on *534*
bronchioles, in asthma *529*
bronchoconstriction 518, 531
bronchodilators
  asthma treatment 532, 532–6
  caffeine as 344
  for COPD 542
buccal cavity, *see* mouth
buckeyes, toxicity of 67t
budesonide
  asthma treatment 536, 538
  eformoterol combined with 539
  inhaled corticosteroid 658
  nasal condition treatment 548
  pregnancy safety 549, 662
buffering function of blood 492
bufotenine 403
bulbocavernosus 746
bulbourethral glands 697
bulk-forming laxatives 574–5
bullas *906*
bumetanide 482
  ototoxicity 615t
  pharmacokinetics 484t
bupivacaine
  local anaesthetic 240–2, 243t
  nerve block anaesthesia 247t
  perinatal use 729
  pregnancy safety 248

bupivacaine—cont'd
  spinal block anaesthesia 247t
  toxicity of 244
buprenorphine
  as substitute drug 384
  dosage forms 266t
  morphine interactions 268
  mu-receptor agonist 264t
  pregnancy safety 278
  regulation in sport 937
bupropion
  drug dependence treatment 382
  nicotine dependence treatment 396
  pregnancy safety 405
  regulation in sport 938
Burkitt's lymphoma 763
burn treatment 922–5, *923*
Burrow's solution 614, 910
buspirone 290
  macrolide antibiotic interactions 812
  pregnancy safety 293
  sexual function affected by 750
  unsafe for children 292
busulfan
  cancer treatment 770
  emetic potential 766t
  indications and toxicity 771t
  ocular adverse effects 604t
butyl methoxydibenzoylmethane 913t
butyl nitrate, symptoms of abuse 375t
butyrophenone 325
butyrylcholinesterase 207

C

C-fibre pain 252
cabergoline
  inhibits lactation 730
  parkinsonism treatment 353
  pregnancy safety 366, 636
Cade, John 334c
caecum 559–60
caffeine **343**
  abuse of 371
  affects sleep patterns 284t
  alcohol interactions *346*
  antiemetic use 569
  avoid during breastfeeding 144t
  beverages containing 400t
  combination analgesics 273
  effect on spider's webs *373*
  gastrin stimulant 572
  MAO inhibitor interactions 331
  metabolism during pregnancy 124
  migraine treatment 364
  nicotine interactions 397
  pregnancy safety 346, 405
  regulation in sport 938, 939
  social use of 398–9
  sport stimulant 933
calamine lotion 910
  antipruritic agent 909
  pregnancy safety 928
calcineurin inhibitors
  immunosuppressants 890–2
  topical administration 919
calcipotriol
  pregnancy safety 928
  psoriasis treatment 920
calcitonin 627t, 640, 687–9
  osteoporosis treatment 692
  Paget's disease treatment 691

calcitriol 689, **691**
  hypocalcaemia treatment 689t
  kidneys synthesise 474
  pregnancy safety 693
  psoriasis treatment 920
  sodium uptake determined by 477
calcium 687, *see also* calcium-channel
    blockers; hypercalcaemia; hypocalcaemia
  balancing 654, *685*
  dietary supplements 688c
  in blood coagulation 495t
  in cardiac action 417
  messenger system 105
  osteoporosis treatment 691–2
  phenytoin interactions 306
  tetracycline interactions 816
calcium alginate, for pressure sores 927
calcium carbonate
  adverse drug events 566t
  antacids containing 565, 565t
  thyroxine interactions 645t
calcium-channel blockers 430
  angina treatment 443–5
  atazanavir interactions 842t
  beta-blocker interaction 198t
  biguanide interactions 678
  cardiac action 417, 424
  compared 446t, 448t
  cyclosporin interactions 892
  digoxin interactions 426t
  drug groups 13t
  drug interactions 447t
  headache treatment 366
  in the elderly 445b
  incontinence caused by 489t
  interactions between drugs 447t
  mefloquine interactions 850
  migraine treatment 364
  mode of action 105
  pancuronium interactions 205
  pharmacokinetics 430t
  prazosin interactions 195
  quinupristin interactions 818
  saquinavir interactions 843
  sexual function affected by 750
  smooth muscle effects 441
  taste and smell effects 617t
  vertigo treatment 612
calcium chloride, pancuronium interactions 205
calcium folinate
  cancer chemotherapy **783**
  in combination therapy 764t
  methotrexate interactions 775
  pregnancy safety 789
  rescues myelosuppression 784
  toxoplasmosis treatment 855
calcium gluconate, hypocalcaemia treatment 689t
calcium hydroxide astringent 909
calcium salts, pregnancy safety 693
calculation of dosage, *see* dosage
CAM, *see* complementary and alternative medicine
cAMP 105
camphor 528, 910
camptothecins 776, 778c
canals of Schlemm *591*
cancer (neoplasia), *see also* carcinogens; skin cancers; teratogens
  carcinogenesis 759–60

cancer (neoplasia)—cont'd
  tumour cell burdens 760
cancer treatment 755–67
  adverse drug events 764–6, 776, 779, 783–5
  cell response to 758
  chemotherapy 761
  combinations of drugs 764
  pain management 256
  research into 788–9
  sex hormones in 751
  suxamethonium interactions 207
  vomiting induced by 567–8
candesartan 457
  pregnancy safety 457
Candida infections 796t, 797, 826
cane toads 11
cannabinoids 399–402
  analgesic effects 276
  decrease intraocular pressure 595
  diabetic effects 673c
  ocular adverse effects 604t
  regulation in sport 934, 938
  sexual function affected by 746
cannabis
  abuse in Australia 380
  abuse in New Zealand 379c
  hospitalisations due to 376
  intoxication with 377t
  pregnancy safety 405
  sedative effects 284t
  teratogenic potential 726
cannulae 525
cantharidin, sexual function affected by 747
capacitance vessels, *see* systemic vascular
    resistance
capecitabine
  cancer treatment 773
  indications and toxicity 771t
  pregnancy safety 789
  warfarin interactions 505
capillaries 419, 897t
capreomycin 857
  pregnancy safety 866
capsaicin 275
captopril
  ACE inhibitor 456
  antacid interactions 566t
  pharmacokinetics 455t
  pregnancy safety 457
  sexual function affected by 750
  taste and smell effects 617t
carbachol
  glaucoma treatment 178, 593t, 594
  miotic effects 590
  pregnancy safety 606
carbamazepine
  anticonvulsant effects 300t, 303
  antiepileptic interactions 302
  calcium-channel blocker interactions 447t
  caspofungin interactions 830
  CNS effects 300t
  delavirdine interactions 840
  diabetes treatment 636c
  drug interactions with 158, 306–7
  H_2-receptor antagonist interactions 572t
  hormonal factors 124
  isoniazid interactions 858
  low hepatic clearance 132t
  macrolide antibiotic interactions 812
  medroxyprogesterone acetate interactions
    713

carbamazepine—cont'd
  pain treatment 303
  phenytoin interactions 306
  photosensitising effects 907t
  praziquantel interactions 865
  pregnancy safety 309
  saquinavir interactions 843
  simvastatin interactions 467
  skin conditions from 907t
  sodium channel inhibitor 303, 305
  teratogenic potential 142t, 726
  tiagabine interactions 305
  topiramate interactions 304
  triazole antifungal interactions 829t
  warfarin interactions 505
carbamide peroxide 614
  for pressure sores 927
  pregnancy safety 618
carbapenems 804, 810
carbidopa
  levodopa combination **351–2**
  parkinsonism treatment 350
  pregnancy safety 366
carbimazole 603, 646, 648–9, **649**
  pregnancy safety 650
  taste and smell effects 617t
carbogen 525c, 527
carbohydrates
  chemical structure *10*
  drugs from 11
  for athletes 940
  glucocorticoids in metabolism of 654
carbomers, artificial tear solutions 602
carbon dioxide
  as medical gas 525c, 526–8
  blood levels of 518
carbon monoxide poisoning 527
carbonic anhydrase 519
carbonic anhydrase inhibitors 481
  drug groups 13t
  glaucoma treatment 592–4, 593t
carboplatin
  cancer treatment 762c, 776
  emetic potential 766t
  indications and toxicity 772t
  pregnancy safety 789
carbuncles 915
carcinogens 139b, 759
  ganciclovir 832
cardiac conduction system, *see* cardiovascular
    system
cardiac myocytes *424*
cardioactive glycosides, *see* digitalis glycosides;
    glycosides
cardiomyopathy 435b
cardiovascular system, *see also* heart
  action potentials *432*
  adrenaline effects 187–8, 190
  alcohol effects 387
  anaesthetic effects 234
  atropine effects 180
  beta-blocker effects 196–8
  caffeine effects 344
  cannabinoid effects 401
  cardiac conduction system 443
  cardiac function control 418–9
  cardiac muscle 411, *413*
  cardiogenic shock 435b
  drugs affecting 318, 422–37, 617t
  drugs toxic to 765
  histamine effects 896–7

cardiovascular system—cont'd
  innervation of 166t
  muscarinic actions 178t
  ocular effect of disorders 602–3
  over-the-counter drugs for 53t
  rofecoxib adverse effects 882c
carmellose, pregnancy safety 606
carmustine
  cancer treatment 770
  hepatotoxicity 765
  indications and toxicity 771t
  pregnancy safety 789
carotenes, *see* vitamin A
carrier transport 104, 114
  in kidneys 476
Carukia barnesi 963c
carvedilol 197t
  pharmacokinetics and dosages 198t
  pregnancy safety 199t
caspase enzymes 762
caspofungin 828–30
  pregnancy safety 844
castanospermine, plant production of 11
castor oil, components of 11
cataplexy 342
cataracts 585
  antioxidants for 601c
  drugs causing 605
catechol-*O*-methyltransferase 174
catecholamines 172–5, 186–91, *see also*
    adrenaline; dopamine; monoamines;
    noradrenaline
  CNS effects 222
  entacapone interactions 355
  involvement in psychiatric disorders 313
  nicotine interactions 397
  role in labour 727
caudal anaesthesia 248
caustic bush 797c
cef. . ., *see also* ceph. . .
cefaclor
  ear treatment 612
  pharmacokinetics and dosages 811t
  pregnancy safety 821
  sinusitis treatment 549
cefepime 808
  pharmacokinetics and dosages 811t
  pregnancy safety 821
cefotaxime
  pharmacokinetics and dosages 811t
  pregnancy safety 606, 821
cefoxitin
  pharmacokinetics and dosages 811t
  pregnancy safety 821
cefpirome
  pharmacokinetics and dosages 811t
  pregnancy safety 821
ceftazidime 808
  pharmacokinetics and dosages 811t
  pregnancy safety 821
  probenecid interactions 810
ceftriaxone
  anticoagulant interactions 810
  pharmacokinetics and dosages 811t
  pregnancy safety 821
  probenecid interactions 810
  warfarin interactions 505
cefuroxine
  ear treatment 612
  pharmacokinetics and dosages 811t
  pregnancy safety 821

celecoxib 879t
    as NSAID 270
    peptic ulcer risk 879
    pharmacokinetics 881t
    regulation in NZ 883c
    TGA recommendations 882
    warfarin interactions 505
celery 60t, 650c
cell bodies, neurons 165
cell-kill fraction 758–9
cell-mediated immune reactions 156t, 871–3, 874
cell membranes
    absorption across 113–4
    antimicrobials affecting 796
    cancer cells 760
    synthesis inhibitors 804–12
cells 756
    life cycle of 755–8, 761–2
    respiration 516
cellulitis 915
Celsus 5
central nervous system 163, 213–24, see also brain; CNS depressants; CNS stimulants; neurotransmitters; spinal cord
    adrenaline effects 189
    anticonvulsant effects 300t
    atropine effects 180
    caffeine effects 343–4
    cannabinoid effects 401
    drugs affecting 214c
    glucocorticoids in 654
    histamine effects 897
    muscle relaxant effects 356–7
    opioid effects 263
    OTC drugs for 53t
    pain pathways 254
    pituitary gland regulation 630
    psychiatric disorders 313–4
    sexual function role 745
centrally acting adrenergic inhibitors, for hypertension 450–3
Centre for Adverse Reactions Monitoring (NZ) 159c, 951c
ceph. . ., see also cef. . .
cephalexin
    pharmacokinetics and dosages 811t
    pregnancy safety 821
    urinary tract infection treatment 820
cephalosporins 808–10
    alcohol interactions 391
    aminoglycoside interactions 814–5
    drug groups 13t
    mechanism of action 804
    pharmacokinetics and dosages 811t
    probenecid interactions 890
    resistance to 798t
    skin conditions from 907t
    superinfection from 798
cephalothin
    pharmacokinetics and dosages 811t
    pregnancy safety 821
cephamandole 808
    anticoagulant interactions 810
    pharmacokinetics and dosages 811t
    pregnancy safety 821
    warfarin interactions 505
cephazolin
    anticoagulant interactions 810
    pharmacokinetics and dosages 811t
    pregnancy safety 821

cephazolin—cont'd
    warfarin interactions 505
cercariae 863
cerebellum 214, 216
    role in autonomic nervous system 163
    role in sympathetic nervous system 202
cerebral cortex 163, 214, 217
cerebral spasticity 356
cerumen, impacted 614
cestodes 863
cetirizine, pregnancy safety 899
cetrimide, antiseptic effects 915
cetrorelix 699, 740
cetuximab 782
cetylpyridinium chloride 563
chaparall, toxicity 68–9
checkpoints (cell life cycle) 757
chemical assay, standards established by 84–5
chemical burns 924
chemical messengers, see neurotransmitters
chemical warfare agents 209c
chemistry
    advances in 6
    chemical structures 10
    in drug discovery 87
    of anaesthetics 240–1
    of sedatives 291
    size of molecules 4
chemoprophylaxis of malaria 849
chemoreceptor trigger zone 556–8, 558
chemotherapy, see cancer treatment
Cheyne–Stokes respiration, caffeine treatment 344
childbirth, see also perinatal drug use; pregnancy
    analgesia during 234, 261–2
children, see paediatrics
Chinese medicine 4, 63, 65–6, see also complementary and alternative medicine
Chlamydia trachomatis 595
chloral hydrate 291
    effect on spider's webs 373
    ocular adverse effects 604t
    pregnancy safety 293
    skin conditions from 907t
    warfarin interactions 505
chlorambucil
    cancer treatment 770
    emetic potential 766t
    indications and toxicity 771t
    pregnancy safety 789
chloramphenicol 816–7
    bacteriocidal actions 796
    clindamycin interactions 814
    didanosine interactions 838
    ear treatment 613
    neonatal dose 145t
    ocular use 596
    phenytoin interactions 306
    pregnancy safety 606, 821
    rifampicin interactions 859
    skin conditions from 907t
    stavudine interactions 838
    topical, adverse drug events 915
    warfarin interactions 505
    zalcitabine interactions 840
chlorhexidine
    antiseptic effects 915
    in mouth-washes and gargles 563
    photosensitising effects 907t
    plaque inhibited by 563

chlorhexidine—cont'd
    pregnancy safety 928
    pressure sore treatment 927
    skin conditions from 907t
chloride, absorption in the nephron 481
chlorinated sugar, contraceptive effects 742
chlorocresol 910
chloroform 6, 237
chlorophyll, photosensitising effects 907t
chloroquine 359c, 849, 851–2
    antirheumatic effects 884, 885
    mefloquine interactions 850
    ocular adverse effects 604t
    praziquantel interactions 865
    pregnancy safety 866, 900
    retinopathy induced by 604
    skin conditions from 907t
    teratogenic potential 726
chlorotrianisene, inhibits lactation 730
chloroxylenol, in liniments and rubs 910
chlorpheniramine, sexual function affected by 751
chlorpromazine 322, 323
    apomorphine interactions 353
    development of 312c
    major effects 315t
    pregnancy safety 320
    sedative effects 316
    sexual function affected by 750
chlorpropamide, diabetes treatment 677
chlorthalidone 482, 484t
chocolate, social use of 399c
cholecalciferol, pregnancy safety 693
cholecystitis 559
cholecystokinin 949–50
cholestatic hepatitis 807
cholesterol, see also hypercholesterolaemia
    corticosteroids synthesised from 653
    lipoproteins containing 462
    tissue transport 463
cholestyramine 467–8
    calcitriol interactions 691
    digoxin interactions 426t
    drug interactions with 157
    effects compared 469t
    mycophenolate mofetil interactions 895
    pregnancy safety 470
    tetracycline interactions 816
    thiazide diuretic interactions 485
    thyroxine interactions 645t
    vancomycin interactions 812
choline esters 178
choline salicylate, in mouth-washes and gargles 563
choline theophyllinate, asthma treatment 535
cholinergic transmission 169–72, 173, 178–83, see also acetylcholine; anticholinergics; muscarinic receptor agonists
cholinergics, glaucoma treatment 592, 594
cholinesterase inhibitors, see anticholinesterases
cholinomimetic alkaloids, see muscarinic receptor agonists
CHOP regimen, cancer treatment 782
choriocarcinoma 763
Christianity, in history of medicine 5–6
Christie, Agatha 291c
Christmas disease 510–1
chromosomes
    abnormal 760

chromosomes—cont'd
  duplication of 758
chronic obstructive pulmonary disease
    (COPD) 524, 541–2
chronic pain 255
chronotropic effects 187, 422–5, *see also* heart
    rate
chylomicrons 462
chyme 554–5
ciclesonide, asthma prophylaxis 536
cidofovir 831, 834
  pregnancy safety 844
cimetidine
  benzodiazepine interactions 288
  biguanide interactions 678
  cyclosporin interactions 892
  diazepam interactions 287
  drug interactions with 158
  lignocaine interactions 241, 434
  peptic ulcer treatment 572, 572t
  phenytoin interactions 306
  praziquantel interactions 865
  pregnancy safety 581
  procainamide interactions 433t
  sexual function affected by 751
  tamoxifen interactions 780
  taste and smell effects 617t
  theophylline interactions 537
  warfarin interactions 505
cinacalcet, pregnancy safety 693
cinchocaine, toxicity of 244
cinchona bark 6, 359c, 853c
cineoles, for respiratory disorders 543c
cinnamates, in sunscreens 913
ciprofloxacin 818
  ear treatment 613
  foscarnet interactions 835
  Legionnaire's disease treatment 546
  ocular use 596
  pregnancy safety 606
  resistance to 798t
  sucralfate interactions 573
  tamoxifen interactions 780
  theophylline interactions 537
  urinary tract infection treatment 820
  warfarin interactions 505
circadian rhythms 216, 653–4
circulatory system, *see* blood; cardiovascular
    system; shock
cisapride
  amprenavir interactions 842t
  efavirenz interactions 840
  indinavir interactions 842
  macrolide antibiotic interactions 812
cisplatin
  cancer treatment 776
  capreomycin interactions 857
  chemical structure 773
  didanosine interactions 838
  emetic potential 766t
  hydration therapy 784
  indications and toxicity 772t
  liposome delivery 788
  loop diuretic interactions 482
  ototoxicity 765
  pregnancy safety 789
  renal toxicity 765
  stavudine interactions 838
  vomiting induced by 567–8
  zalcitabine interactions 840
cistracurium 204, 206t

cistracurium—cont'd
  pregnancy safety 248
citalopram 329
  adverse effects 319t
  pregnancy safety 320
cladribine
  cancer treatment 773
  indications and toxicity 771t
  pregnancy safety 789
clarithromycin 812–3
  cytochrome P450 isoform inhibition 158t
  ergometrine interactions 728
  ototoxicity 615t
  peptic ulcer treatment 570–1
  pharmacokinetics 813t
  pregnancy safety 821
  simvastatin interactions 467
class Ia antiarrhythmics 430–4, 430t
class Ib antiarrhythmics 430, 430t, 433–4
class Ic antiarrhythmics 435–6
class II antiarrhythmics 436
class III antiarrhythmics 430, 430t, 436–7
class IV antiarryhthmics 430, 430t, 437
classification
  of adverse drug events 154–5
  of drug interactions 156–7
  of drugs 13t, 14–6, *see also* regulation;
    scheduling
Claviceps purpurea 352
clavulanate
  adverse drug events 807
  effect of food on absorption 808t
  penicillins combined with 804, 806
  pharmacokinetics 807t
  pregnancy safety 821
  urinary tract infection treatment 820
cleansers 909, 927
clearance 131–2, *see also* excretion
  drug interactions affecting 158
  effect on half-life *135*
clematis 271c
clenbuterol 942c
climacteric, *see* male climacteric; menopause
clindamycin 814
  acne treatment 922
  pregnancy safety 821, 928
  saquinavir interactions 843
  toxoplasmosis treatment 596
clinical depression, *see* depression
clinical pharmacology 3t
clinical trials 89–92
  Australia and New Zealand 93–4
  cancer treatment 788
  ethical issues 98–9
  legal issues 79
clobazam 287
  pharmacokinetics 286t
clodronate
  bony metastasis treatment 786
  effect on bone 693
  pregnancy safety 693
clofazimine
  leprosy treatment 861–2
  pregnancy safety 866
clomiphene 710, **741**
  infertility treatment 740
  ocular adverse effects 604t
  pregnancy safety 721, 751
clomipramine 329
  adverse drug events 319t
  lumefantrine interactions 853

clomipramine—cont'd
  pregnancy safety 320
clonazepam
  age-related adverse drug events 292
  anticonvulsant effects 300t, 303
  antiepileptic interactions 301
  CNS effects 300t
  conjugation reaction 122t
  GABA receptor agonist 304
  pregnancy safety 309
  seizure treatment 287
clonidine
  adjuvant analgesic 276
  beta-blocker interaction 198t
  hypertension treatment 450–3
  ocular adverse effects 604t
  phentermine interactions 952
  pregnancy safety 457
  sedative effects 284t
  sexual function affected by 750
  withdrawal treatment 384
clopamide 942c
clopidrogel
  antiplatelet action 500, 509
  in Australia's top 10 drugs 17t
  pregnancy safety 512
clostebol 942c
Clostridium infections 795t, 796t, *see also*
    botulinum toxin
  cephalosporin-resistant 809t
  drug resistance 805t
clotrimazole 916, 918t
clotting of blood, *see* coagulation (clotting of
    blood)
cloves, for pain relief 277c
clozapine 325
  major effects 315t
  pregnancy safety 320
  schizophrenia treatment 322c
  sexual function affected by 750
cluster headache 366
CMI 18, 58, 97
CMV, *see* cytomegalovirus treatment
CNS, *see* central nervous system
CNS depressants 282–93, *see also* hypnotics;
    sedatives
  abuse of 374t, 386–92
  adverse drug events 234
  alcohol effects 750–1
  alcohol interactions 388
  anaesthetic interactions 233
  antihistamine interactions 899
  baclofen interactions 358
  barbiturate interactions 290
  benzodiazepine interactions 288
  chlorpromazine interactions 323
  dantrolene interactions 360
  diazepam interactions 287
  general anaesthetics 227
  interactions between 157
  intoxication with 377t
  methadone interactions 386
  metoclopramide interactions 568
  morphine interactions 268
  muscle relaxants 356–7
  ocular adverse effects 604t
  olanzapine interactions 325
  opioid interactions 543
  phenytoin interactions 306
  propofol interactions 239
  risperidone interactions 325

CNS depressants—cont'd
  sedative effects 284t, 316
  sevoflurane interactions 238
  sexual function affected by 745, 746, 749
  TCA interactions 329
  topiramate interactions 304
  valproate interactions 307
CNS stimulants 339–46
  abuse of 392–9
  caffeine interactions 345
  CNS effects 214c
  dexamphetamine interactions 341
  diabetic effects 673c
  psychotropic agent interactions 318
  regulation in sport 933, 938
  sleep pattern effects 284t
co-trimoxazole 819–20
coagulation (clotting of blood) 494–7, 500, see also anticoagulants
  after snake bite 957
  sites of drug action 500
  tests of function 503c
coal tar 907t, 910, 920
Coca-Cola, history of 398
cocaine
  abuse of 374t, 380, 396–8
  adrenaline interactions 190
  carrier transport 104
  during breastfeeding 144t
  during pregnancy 140
  for nasal conditions 245
  high toxicity 244
  history of 6, 228c, 240c, 398
  intoxication with 377t
  local anaesthetic 240
  methyldopa interactions 453
  neonatal withdrawal symptoms 143t
  noradrenaline interactions 191
  pregnancy safety 405
  regulation in sport 933, 938
  teratogenic potential 142t
  topical administration 247t
  vasoconstrictive action 244
cochlea 611
Cochrane Collaboration 18
cocky apple 797c
cocoa, social use of 399c
Code of Good Clinical Practice, in clinical trials 94
codeine 267, 543
  abuse of 375t, 380
  antidiarrhoeal 579
  antitussive 544
  combination analgesic 273
  conjugation reaction 122t
  dosage forms 266t
  genetic failure to metabolise 264
  migraine treatment 364
  neonatal withdrawal symptoms 143t
  OTC vs prescription variants 52t
  pregnancy safety 278
  regulation in sport 938
coffee, see also caffeine
  for respiratory disorders 543c
cognitive decline (dementia) 179c, 360–3
coitus interruptus 745
colaspase
  cancer treatment 776
  methotrexate interactions 775
  pregnancy safety 789

colchicine
  asthma treatment 540
  discovery of 6, 778c
  gout treatment 887–8
  NZ guidelines 889
  pregnancy safety 900
cold sores 915
colds, see also cough preparations
  treatment of 55, 544–5, 934
colestipol 467–8
  digoxin interactions 426t
  lipid-lowering effects 469c
  mycophenolate mofetil interactions 895
  pregnancy safety 470
  tetracycline interactions 816
  thiazide diuretic interactions 485
  thyroxine interactions 645t
  vancomycin interactions 812
  warfarin interactions 505
collagen, in blood clotting 494–5
collagen diseases, ocular effects 603
collecting duct 477
Collodion 910
Colman, Peter 93c
colon 559–60
colon cancer, combination therapy 764t
colonisation by microorganisms 794
colony-stimulating factors, see granulocyte colony-stimulating factors
combinations of drugs, see also formulations
  antimalarials 852–4
  cancer chemotherapy 764
  diuretics 485, 486t
  interactions among 156
  OTC products 58
  problems with 30
comfort drops 602
comfrey, toxicity 67t
Commonwealth of Australia, see Australia
Community Quality Use of Medicines program 18
competition for protein binding sites 119, 124, 157
competitive antagonists, see depolarising blocking drugs; non-depolarising blocking drugs
complement system 871, 872
complementary and alternative medicine 59–70
  adverse drug events 154
  cancer treatment 763, 786c, 788–9
  diabetes treatments 679c
  drug dependence treatment 381c
  drug use in 32
  for athletes 940
  gynaecological treatments 720c
  home and folk remedies 30, 60t
  interactions between drugs 789
  neurological treatments 363c
  NSAIDS in 884c
  ocular medicine 601c
  pain treatment 277
  respiratory treatments 543c
  safety of 7
  sedatives 292, 292c
complex-mediated drug allergies 874
complex partial epilepsy, see partial complex (psychomotor) seizures
compliance
  among children and teenagers 320
  anticonvulsant regimes 300

compliance—cont'd
  antidepressant treatment 328
  drug regimes 44–5
  psychiatric treatment 318
compound A 238
compound analgesics 272–4, 275c
Compound Tincture of Benzoin 911
compressed air, as medical gas 525c
computer-aided design, drugs developed from 87
COMT 174
concentration–response relationship 107, 107, 108, 109
conception rates 741
condoms 743
conduction block anaesthesia, see nerve block anaesthesia
conductivity (cardiac) 414–5
  digoxin effects 425
  treatment of 429
conflicts of interest 98
confusional states, see dementia
conium, toxicity 67t
conjugated equine oestrogens 709
  hormone replacement therapy 719
  pregnancy safety 721
conjugation reactions 121, 122t
conjunctiva 585
conjunctivitis 595
Conn's syndrome 660c
consent 97, 315
constipation 560, 574
consumer medical information 16–9, 36, 58, 97
contact lens solutions 600–2
contaminants in medications, herbal remedies 69
continuous (Type C) ADRs 155
contraceptives 740–5, see also oral contraceptives
  anticonvulsant interactions 300
  failure rates 742t
  griseofulvin interactions 830
  methods used 744t
  sites of action 744
  St John's wort interactions 159
contractile mechanism (cardiac) 417
contraindications, information about 16
controlled-release preparations 43
controlled substances, see drug abuse; illicit drugs; regulation
COPD 524, 541–2
copper, contraceptive use 743
corneas 585
coronary arteries 412, 414, 462
coronary heart disease, deaths resulting from 412c, 500
corpus luteum 627t
corpus striatum 218
cortex of the kidney 474
cortex of the lymph node 871
cortical nephrons 474
corticosteroids 627t, 653–9, see also mineralocorticoids
  adjuvant analgesics 276
  adverse drug events 659
  aminoglutethimide interactions 662
  amphotericin B interactions 828
  anaesthetic interactions 233
  antiemetic use 570
  antimicrobials with 915

corticosteroids—cont'd
  aspirin interactions 274
  asthma treatment 532, 536–9, 548c
  azathioprine interactions 893
  bone effects 692–3
  cancer treatment 778, 781, 784
  carbamazepine interactions 307
  cataracts caused by 605
  COPD treatment 542
  cyclophosphamide interactions 774
  depression evoked by 326
  digoxin interactions 426t
  ear treatment 613–4, **614**
  gout treatment 887
  headache treatment 366
  hyperglycaemia linked to 672t
  immunosuppressants 890
  inflammatory bowel disease treatment 580
  insulin interactions 675
  interactions between 659
  maternal administration enhances fetal lung maturation 531
  multiple sclerosis treatment 360
  muromonab-CD3 with 894
  mycophenolate mofetil interactions 895
  nasal condition treatment 548
  neostigmine interactions 209
  nicotine interactions 397
  ocular adverse effects 597c, 604t
  ocular use 592, 597–8, 598t
  palliative care in cancer treatment 787
  pancuronium interactions 205
  perceptual states altered by 373
  pharmacokinetics 657–8
  photosensitising effects 907t
  plasma lipid profile effects 464t
  pregnancy safety 928
  regulation in sport 933, 936, 938–9
  rifampicin interactions 859
  sildenafil interactions 748
  skin condition treatment 906, 920
  skin conditions from 907t
  sleep pattern effects 284t
  suxamethonium interactions 207
  tamoxifen interactions 780
  taste and smell effects 617t
  teratogenic potential 726
  topical administration 917–9
  toxoplasmosis treatment 596
  urticaria treatments 920
corticotrophin, *see* adrenocorticotrophic hormone
corticotrophin-releasing factor 630, 654
  food intake regulation 949
  levels during pregnancy 725
cortisol, *see* hydrocortisone
cortisone
  discovery of 653
  pharmacokinetics 657t
  pregnancy safety 662
  warfarin interactions 505
Corynebacterium diphtheriae 795t
coryza, *see* colds
cost of drug development 31, 88, *see also* pharmacoeconomics
cough preparations 542–4
  OTC drugs 55
  regulation in sport 934
coughs, bradykinin involved in 456c
coumarins, testosterone interactions 735

counterirritants
  in liniments and rubs 910
  pain management 276
COX-2 (cyclo-oxygenase-2) inhibitors (coxibs) 879t, 880
  ACE inhibitor interactions 454
  as NSAIDs 270
  availability of 882
  pharmacokinetics 881t
  regulation in NZ 883c
'crack', *see* cocaine
cramps, *see* muscle spasms
cranberry, as folk remedy 60t
cranial nerves 214–5, 215t
cranium, raised pressure 216c
creams, skin treatment 909
creatine, for athletes 940
cretinism 612–5, 640, 644, *see also* hypothyroidism
Creutzfelt–Jakob disease 632c
criminal offences, in Australia 82–3
Crohn's disease 560c, 580–1, 886
cromoglycate **539**
  asthma treatment 539
  nasal condition treatment 549
  ocular use 598
  pregnancy safety 549, 606
cromolyns, *see* cromoglycate; mast-cell stabilisers
crotamiton 917
  pregnancy safety 928
croup 547
Cryptococcus infections 796t
crystal hydrate theory of anaesthesia 229
crystal methamphetamine, *see* methamphetamines
crystalline carbohydrates, developed in Australia 90t
CSF (cerebrospinal fluid) 614
CSFs, *see* granulocyte colony-stimulating factors
CTZ 556–8, *558*
curare 204, 357
cure of cancers 763
Cushing's syndrome 656, 656c
cyanocobalamin, skin conditions from 907t
cyclamates, taste of 616
cyclic AMP 105
cyclin-dependent kinases, cancer treatment 762
cyclins, in cell cycle 756–7
cyclo-oxygenase inhibition 13t, 271, 879
cyclopentolate
  adverse systemic effects of ocular treatment 605t
  clinical use and administration 182t
  glaucoma treatment 590
  ocular use 589, 589t
  pregnancy safety 606
cyclophosphamide **774**
  avoid during breastfeeding 144t
  azathioprine interactions 893
  Burkitt's lymphoma treatment 763
  cancer treatment 770
  chemical structure 773
  CHOP regimen 782
  combination therapy 764t
  emetic potential 766t
  hydration therapy 784
  immunosuppressant 892
  indications and toxicity 771t

cyclophosphamide—cont'd
  mycophenolate mofetil interactions 895
  pregnancy safety 789
  renal toxicity 765
  resistance to 766
  teratogenic potential 142t, 726
cycloplegics 180, 585
cyclopropane 237
cycloserine, tuberculosis treatment 857
cyclosporin **892**
  avoid during breastfeeding 144t
  azathioprine interactions 893
  calcium-channel blocker interactions 447t
  capreomycin interactions 857
  caspofungin interactions 830
  cyclophosphamide interactions 774
  epoetin alfa interactions 937
  everolimus interactions 895
  imidazole antifungal interactions 829t
  immunosuppressant 891
  inflammatory bowel disease treatment 580
  macrolide antibiotic interactions 812
  metoclopramide interactions 568
  muromonab-CD3 with 894
  mycophenolate mofetil interactions 895
  NSAID interactions 883
  plasma lipid profile effects 464t
  potassium-sparing diuretic interactions 487
  pregnancy safety 900
  psoriasis treatment 920
  quinupristin interactions 818
  simvastatin interactions 467
  sirolimus interactions 895
  St John's wort interactions 327c
  statin interactions 466
  sulfonamides/trimethoprim interactions 820
  topical administration 917
CYP, *see* cytochrome P450 isoforms
CYP2C19, *see* proguanil
CYP2D6: 853
CYP3A4 enzyme inducers
  cyclophosphamide interactions 774
  tamoxifen interactions 780
CYP3A4 inhibitors 827
cyproheptadine, pregnancy safety 899
cyproterone 712, 714, 737
  acne treatment 922
  cancer treatment 779, 779t
  contraceptive use 715t
  'male pill' 743
  pregnancy safety 721, 737
cysteic acid 222
cystic fibrosis 517c, 530
cysts *906*
cytarabine
  cancer treatment 773
  indications and toxicity 771t
  pregnancy safety 789
cytochrome P450 isoforms 122
  drug interactions inhibiting 158t
  genetic deficiency in 124
  Maori polymorphism in 123c
cytokines 492
  cancer treatment 762
  cytokine release syndrome 894
  from immune response 873
  role in inflammation 871
cytomegalovirus treatment 832, 834
cytoprotective agents, peptic ulcer treatment 570, 572–3

cytosine 737
cytotoxic agents 761–2
  adverse drug events 154
  cancer treatment 770–7
  handling of 765c
  immunosuppressants 890, 892–4
  infertility related to 767
  skin cancer treatment 912c
cytotoxic cells 873

D

DA, see dopamine
dacarbazine
  cancer treatment 770
  emetic potential 766t
  hepatotoxicity 765
  indications and toxicity 771t
  pregnancy safety 789
daclizumab
  for rejection control 894
  pregnancy safety 900
dactinomycin 778c
  cancer treatment 763, 772t
  emetic potential 766t
  mechanism of action 776
  pregnancy safety 789
Dale, Sir Henry 171
dalfopristin 817–8
  pregnancy safety 821
dalteparin 502–3
  pregnancy safety 512
damania, as herbal remedy 62t
danaparoid 502–3
  pregnancy safety 512
danazol 699
  cyclosporin interactions 892
  for DUB 720
  in male reproductive system 737
  pregnancy safety 721
  teratogenic potential 726
  warfarin interactions 505
dandelion, as herbal remedy 62t
dandruff treatment 910
dantrolene 360
  malignant hyperthermia treatment 232
  multiple sclerosis treatment 360
  muscle relaxant 359
  neuroleptic malignant syndrome treatment 316
  pregnancy safety 366
dapsone
  didanosine interactions 838
  leprosy treatment 861, 862
  pregnancy safety 866
  saquinavir interactions 843
  stavudine interactions 838
darbopoietin 512, 936–7
Dark Ages medicine 5–6
daunorubicin 778c
  cancer treatment 772t, 773–6
  cardiac toxicity 765
  emetic potential 766t
  mechanism of action 776
  pregnancy safety 789
day surgery procedures 231–2
DDC, see dopa decarboxylase (DDC)
de Sade, Marquis 747
deadly nightshade 179
  toxicity 67t
deaths
  from asthma 531c

deaths—cont'd
  from cancer 755c
  from digitalis glycosides 622c
  from drug abuse 376
  from heart failure 423c
debriding agents 926–7
debrisoquine, see cytochrome P450 isoforms
decisions before prescribing 35–6
Declaration of Ethical Intention 96c
decongestants 544–5
  ocular use 591–2, 597
  sinusitis treatment 549
decubitus ulcer (pressure sores), see pressure sores
defecation 560
deglution 553–4
dehydroepiandrosterone (DHEA), regulation in sport 934
delavirdine 836, 840
  pregnancy safety 844
delayed hypersensitivity to drugs 156t
delayed (Type D) ADRs 155
delta-opioid-receptor agonists 264t
delta^9-tetrahydrocannabinol, see cannabinoids
dementia 179c, 360–3
demulcents, for coughs 542
dendrites 165
dental disorders 554
dentifrices 564
dentists, drugs administered by 32
deoxyribonucleic acid (DNA)
  synthesis and replication 757–8
  synthesis inhibitors 818–9
Department of Essential Drugs and Medicines (WHO) 15
dependence 371–405, see also tolerance; withdrawal from drugs
  in New Zealand 84
  on amphetamines 340
  on benzodiazepines 289
  on nicotine 395–6
  pharmacological factors 375–6
  treatment of 380–3
depolarisation 220
  cardiac system 415–6
depolarising blocking drugs 108, 204–5
  adjuncts to anaesthesia 235
  irreversible antagonists 108
  muscle relaxants 357–8
depressants, see CNS depressants
depression 312, 327–8, see also antidepressants; bipolar affective disorders
  not treated with CNS stimulants 339
  sexual function affected by 750
dermatitis, otic 611, see also eczema
dermatophytosis 916
dermatoses, tar treatments 911
dermis 904, 908, see also skin
DES, see diethylstilboestrol
desacetyldiltiazem 445
desensitisation 106
desflurane 237, 237t
  optimal anaesthetic 232
  pregnancy safety 248
designer drugs (amphetamine-like agents) 350c, 393–4
desipramine, photosensitising effects 907t
desloratadine, pregnancy safety 899
desmopressin 636
  pregnancy safety 636
desogestrel 712

desonide, topical administration 919
destruction of drugs, legal issues 79
detoxification, from opioids 384, see also withdrawal from drugs
detrusor muscle 478
development of drugs 88–95
dexamethasone
  adjuvant analgesic 276
  antiemetic use 568, 570
  aprepitant interactions 570
  balance disorder treatment 612
  cancer treatment 778, 783
  caspofungin interactions 830
  ear treatment 613, 614
  infertility treatment 740
  ocular use 597, 598t
  pharmacokinetics 657t
  potency of 657
  praziquantel interactions 865
  pregnancy safety 606, 618, 662
  saquinavir interactions 843
  suppression test 625
dexamphetamine 341
  abuse of 393
  controlled substance 340
  for ADHD 342
  pregnancy safety 346, 405
dexchlorpheniramine, pregnancy safety 899
dexfenfluramine
  adverse drug events 154t
  anorectic agent 343, 951, 951c
dexmedetomidine
  pregnancy safety 293
  sedative effects 292
dextranomers, for pressure sores 927
dextrans
  artificial tear solutions 602
  glycoprotein IIb/IIIa receptor inhibitor interactions 510
  heparin interactions 501
  warfarin interactions 505
dextroamphetamines
  abuse of 374t, 393
  obesity treatment 950–1
dextromethorphan 543
  adjuvant analgesics 276
  antitussives 544
  pregnancy safety 278
  sugar-free medications 673c
dextropropoxyphene 267
  age-related adverse drug events 150, 262
  dosage forms 266t
  migraine treatment 364
  neonatal withdrawal symptoms 143t
  not controlled drug 265
  pregnancy safety 278
  regulation in sport 938
dextrothyroxine, warfarin interactions 505
DHEA 934
diabetes insipidus 477, 636c
diabetes mellitus 665–81, see also antidiabetic drugs
  diabetic nephropathy 669c
  history of 667c
  ocular effects 603
diacetylmorphine, see heroin
diacylglycerol, messenger system 105
diagnostic aids
  endocrine tests 625
  hypothyroidism 643c
  OTC drugs 53t

diagnostic aids—cont'd
  stains 599
diamorphine, *see* heroin
diaphragms (contraceptives) 741–3
diarrhoea 560, 578b, *see also* antidiarrhoeal
  agents
diastole 414, 418–9
diazepam **287**, 366
  abuse of 392
  adjunct to psychotropic agents 316
  age-related adverse drug events 149, 149t,
    150
  amphetamine overdose treated with 340b
  anaesthetic 239
  anxiolytic 287
  avoid during breastfeeding 144t
  GABA receptor agonist 304
  generic equivalents 118c
  low hepatic clearance 132t
  multiple sclerosis treatment 360
  muscle relaxant 357
  muscle spasm treatment 288, 356
  neonatal withdrawal symptoms 143t
  omeprazole interactions 571
  pancuronium interactions 205
  pharmacokinetics 286t
  pregnancy safety 309, 366
  preoperative 288
  sedative effects 285–9
  seizure treatment 287
  sexual function affected by 750
  withdrawal symptoms treated with 288
diazoxide
  angina treatment 445, 447
  ocular adverse effects 604t
  pregnancy safety 457
dibromopropamidine, ocular use 597
diclofenac 879t
  as NSAID 270
  ocular use 598
  pharmacokinetics 881t
  pregnancy safety 606
  risk of GIT effects 882
dicloxacillin 806
  adverse drug events 807
  pharmacokinetics 807t
  pregnancy safety 821
  warfarin interactions 505
dicyclomine, teratogenic potential 726
didanosine 836–7
  dapsone interactions 862
  indinavir interactions 842
  pregnancy safety 844
  stavudine interactions 838
  zalcitabine interactions 840
diencephalon 214
diet, *see also* obesity
  antibiotics in food animals 800c
  calcium sources 688c
  cancer linked with 759–60
  cancer treatment 786c
  constipation treatments 574
  effect of food on penicillin absorption 808t
  energy balance 948–50
  food allergies 898
  food intake regulation *949*
  lipid management 465
  manipulation for athletes 940
  nephrotoxicity 488c
  nutritional supplements 55, 158–9
  tetracycline interactions 816

diethylpropion **952**
  anorectic agent 339, 343, 951
  pregnancy safety 346, 952
  sibutramine interactions 951
diethylstilboestrol 710
  cancer treatment 780
  linked to abnormalities 138
dietitians, drugs administered by 32
diffusion of drugs 114
digestion 553, *see also* gastrointestinal tract
digitalis glycosides 11, 422
  adrenaline interactions 190
  amphotericin B interactions 828
  CNS effects 220
  death from 622c
  dexamphetamine interactions 341
  discovery of 6
  fludrocortisone interactions 661
  glucocorticoid interactions 660t
  loop diuretic interactions 482
  noradrenaline interactions 191
  ocular adverse effects 603, 604t
  rifampicin interactions 859
  thiazide diuretic interactions 485
  thiourea interactions 649
digoxin 423–8
  age-related adverse drug events 149t
  amiodarone interactions 436t
  beta-blocker interactions 198t
  biguanide interactions 678
  bile acid-binding resin interactions 468
  calcitriol interactions 691
  calcium-channel blocker interactions 447t
  diuretics interactions 157
  dose for neonates 145t
  ginseng interactions 64
  hydrocortisone interactions 659
  intraocular pressure reduced by 595
  loop diuretic interactions 482
  macrolide antibiotic interactions 812
  mechanism of action 424
  metoclopramide interactions 568
  pharmacokinetics 425–6
  plasma concentrations 428b
  pregnancy safety 437
  quinidine interactions 432t
  quinine interactions 852
  skin conditions from 907t
  sources of 11
  St John's wort interactions 327c
  sucralfate interactions 573
  thyroid-mediated sensitivity 643
  thyroxine interactions 645t
digoxin-specific antigen-binding fragment
  427
  dosage 429b
  pregnancy safety 437
dihydrocodeine, pregnancy safety 278
dihydroergotamine 353, 729c
  migraine treatment 364
  pregnancy safety 366
dihydrogen sodium versenate 587
dihydropyridine calcium-channel blockers,
  angina treatment 445
dihydrotestosterone 698, 705, 734
dihydroxyphenylalanine 172–3
diltiazem 430, 446t
  angina treatment 442c, 445
  beta-blocker interaction 198t
  cyclosporin interactions 892
  cytochrome P450 isoform inhibition 158t

diltiazem—cont'd
  digoxin interactions 426t
  disopyramide interactions 432t
  in Australia's top 10 drugs 17t
  pharmacokinetics 446t
  pregnancy safety 457
diluents of respiratory secretions 529
dimenhydrinate
  antiemetic use 567t
  pregnancy safety 899
dimethoxymethamphetamine 403c
dimethyltryptamine, perceptual states altered
  by 402
dinoprost
  oxytocic effects 728
  pregnancy safety 730
dinoprostone
  oxytocic effects 728
  pregnancy safety 730
Dioscorides 5
dipevefrine, glaucoma treatment 593
diphenhydramine
  migraine treatment 364
  nasal condition treatment 548
  neonatal withdrawal symptoms 143t
  pregnancy safety 726, 899
  sedative effects 292
  sexual function affected by 751
diphenoxylate **579**
  antidiarrhoeal agent 579–80
  pregnancy safety 581
diphenylhydantoin, *see* phenytoin
Diphyllobothrium latium 863
dipivefrine
  ocular use 590
  ophthalmic use 590t
  pregnancy safety 606
diplopia 356c
dipyridamole
  glycoprotein IIb/IIIa receptor inhibitor
    interactions 510
  heparin interactions 501
  penicillin interactions 806
  platelet effects 500, 509
  pregnancy safety 512
  warfarin interactions 505
direct-acting sympathomimetics 186–93
direct-acting vasodilators 441–8
direct pharmacodynamic interactions 157
direct-to-consumer marketing 98
Directly Observed Treatment – Short Course
  856
discovery of drugs 86–8
disease
  affects drug metabolism 124
  anaesthesia and 234
  neurotransmitter imbalances 223–4
  understanding of 4, 29–30
disease-modifying antirheumatic drugs
  (DMARDs) 884–7, *886*
disodium cromoglycate, *see* cromoglycate
disopyramide 430, 432
  hypoglycaemia linked to 672t
  pharmacokinetics 430t
  photosensitising effects 907t
  pregnancy safety 437
  rifampicin interactions 859
dispensing, legal issues 78
displacement interactions 157
disseminated intravascular coagulation 501
dissociative anaesthetics 239

dissolution 112
distal convoluted tubule 477
distribution through the body 119–21
  defined 114b
  drug interactions affecting 157
  in the elderly 148b
disulfiram
  alcohol abuse treatment 390
  alcohol interactions 391
  isoniazid interactions 858
  metronidazole interactions 819
  phenytoin interactions 306
  pregnancy safety 405
  skin conditions from 907t
  warfarin interactions 505
dithranol, pregnancy safety 928
diuretics 481–9
  ACE inhibitor interactions 454
  age-related adverse drug events 149t
  combinations of drugs 486t
  cyclosporin interactions 892
  digoxin interactions 157, 426t
  fludrocortisone interactions 661
  glucocorticoid interactions 660t
  hydrocortisone interactions 659
  incontinence caused by 489t
  lithium interactions 318, 333
  losartan interactions 456
  NSAID interactions 883
  pharmacokinetics 484t
  plasma lipid profile effects 464t
  prazosin interactions 195
  quinidine interactions 432t
  regulation in sport 933, 937
  salbutamol interactions 536
  sexual function affected by 751
  stroke treatment 362
  terbutaline interactions 536
  theophylline 345
diverticular disease 560
DMT, perceptual states altered by 402
DNA, see deoxyribonucleic acid (DNA)
DNA polymerase inhibitors 831
dobutamine
  pregnancy safety 199t
  shock, treatment for 192–3, 192t
docetaxel 778c
  cancer treatment 776
  indications and toxicity 772t
  pregnancy safety 789
doctors
  drugs administered by 32
  electronic prescribing 39
docusate
  laxative effects 575
  pregnancy safety 581
dolasetron
  antiemetic use 567t, 569
  cancer treatment 783
  pregnancy safety 581, 789
DOM 403c
Domagk, Gerhard 794
domperidone
  antiemetic use 567t
  apomorphine interactions 353
  migraine treatment 364
donepezil
  Alzheimer's disease treatment 362
  pregnancy safety 366
dong quai
  gynaecological treatments 720c

dong quai—cont'd
  warfarin interactions 504
DOPA 172–3
dopa decarboxylase (DDC) 350
dopa (dihydroxyphenylalanine), see carbidopa;
    levodopa
dopamine 186, 630, 634, see also neuroleptics
  age-related decline in receptors 149
  brain levels 353–5
  drug dependence involves 375
  lactation involves 730
  love involves 221
  parkinsonism involves 349–55
  pregnancy safety 199t
  presynaptic receptors 223
  psychiatric disorders involve 313, 324
  shock, treatment for 192, 192t
dopamine agonists
  drug dependence treatment 382
  olanzapine interactions 325
  risperidone interactions 325
dopamine antagonists
  amantadine interactions 834
  antiemetic use 567t, 568
  parkinsonism from 350c
dopaminergic pathways 221, 745
doping of athletes 405, 933, 933c
dornase alfa, mucolytic 530
dorzolamide
  carbon dioxide levels affected by 527
  glaucoma treatment 592, 593t, 594
  pregnancy safety 606
dosage, see also administration of drugs;
    clearance
  antimicrobials 800
  decisions about 36
  dose forms 3t
  hormones 625–6
  intravenous vs. oral 124
  local anaesthetics 243, 244c
  measurement and calculation 19–23
  neonates 145t
  non-linear pharmacokinetic parameters 305
  OTC drugs 59
  pain management 258–9
  paracetamol 54
  parkinsonism treatment 349
  pharmacokinetics 129–35
dothiepin, pregnancy safety 320
Down syndrome, thyroid effects 643
downregulation 106
doxepin
  adverse drug events 319t
  age-related adverse drug events 149t
  pregnancy safety 320
doxorubicin 778c
  avoid during breastfeeding 144t
  cancer treatment 772t, 773–6
  cardiac toxicity 765
  combination therapy 764t
  emetic potential 766t
  hepatotoxicity 765
  liposome delivery 788
  mechanism of action 776
  pregnancy safety 789
  sedative effects 328
doxycycline 815–6
  dosage 815t
  malaria treatment 849
  pneumonia treatment 546
  pregnancy safety 821

doxycycline—cont'd
  sinusitis treatment 544, 549
doxylamine
  pregnancy safety 726
  teratogenic potential 726
dreaming 283
dressings 911, 927
drip rate, dosage measurement 22
dromotropic effects 189, 422, 424–5
dronabinol 402
droperidol 325
  antiemetic use 567t
  pregnancy safety 320
  sexual function affected by 750
dropsy, see oedema
drospinerone 712, 714
drowsiness, see sleep disorders
drug abuse, see abuse of drugs
drug administration, see administration of
    drugs
drug allergies, see adverse drug events
drug courts 83
drug delivery systems, see administration of
    drugs
Drug Houses of Australia 9–10
drug information centres 18
drug interactions, see interactions between
    drugs
drug metabolism, see metabolism of drugs
drug regulation, see regulation
drug resistance, see resistance
drug transporters, see active transport
drugs 2
  allergic reactions 898
  Australia's top 10: 17t
  availability in Australia 27–8
  bone effects 692–3
  classification of 13t, 14–6
  criminal offences involving 82–3
  developed in Australia 94
  discovery and development 86–95
  dosage measurement 19–23
  ethical issues 96–9
  formulations 39–45, 42b
  history of 8c
  in sports 933–44
  individual and lifespan aspects 137–50
  information sources 16–9
  legal issues 73–84
  names of 12c, 12–4
  ototoxicicity 615t
  responses to 44
  sources of 7–12
  standardisation of 84–6
  taste and smell effects 617t
  testing in sports 941–2
  usage evaluation 28–9
  used by anaesthetists 231c
dry powder devices 519
DUB 720
ductless glands, see endocrine system
ducts, innervation of 166t
DUE 28–9
duodenal ulcers 555–6
dwarfism 633c
dydrogesterone, pregnancy safety 721
dyflos 905c
dymenhydrinate, antiemetic use 569
dynorphin 254, 264t
dysbetalipoproteinaemia 464t
dysfunctional uterine bleeding 720

dysgeusia 616–7
dyslipidaemia 462–71
dysmenorrhoea 704c, 742
dyspepsia 565
dysphagia 554
dyspnoea, in COPD 541
dysrhythmia, *see* arrhythmia
dystonia (impaired muscle tone) 316t, 317c, 359
dystrophia adiposogenitalis 734c

E

EAN, *see* approved (generic) names
ear-drops **614**
ears 611–6, *see also* otic. . .; ototoxicosis
    administration to 117
    OTC drugs for 53t
East Timor, malaria in 850
eastern medicine 65
Ebers Papyrus 4, 153
eccrine glands 126, 904
echinacea 62t, 543c
echiocandins 828–30
eclampsia 301c, 726
econazole, topical administration 918t
economics, *see* pharmacoeconomics
ecothiopate 208, 590
'ecstasy' 393–4, 403c
    abuse in Australia 380
    affects 5-HT receptors 314
    perceptual states altered by 402
    symptoms of abuse 374t
ectoparasiticidal drugs 916
ectopic beats 429
eczema 909, 920, *see also* dermatitis
ED 740, 748–9
edrophonium 207
EDTA contact lens solutions 602
EE, *see* ethinyloestradiol
efalizumab 919
    pregnancy safety 928
efavirenz 836, 840
    pregnancy safety 844
efferent pathways 214
efficacy (effectiveness)
    measuring 107
    of over-the-counter drugs 51, 57–8
efflux pumps 797
eformoterol
    asthma treatment 534
    budesonide combined with 539
    pregnancy safety 549
    regulation in sport 935
Ehrlich, Paul 104c
ejaculation 746
elapid snakes 958t
elderly, *see also* dementia
    adverse drug events 154
    anaesthesia 233–4
    analgesics 262
    anticoagulants 506
    anticonvulsants 308
    antidepressant treatment 328–9
    calcium-channel blockers 445b
    cancer rates 755c
    cancer treatment 767
    CNS depressant use 285
    constipation treatment 574
    digoxin treatment 428
    diuretic use 486
    drug use 147–50

elderly—cont'd
    epilepsy in 299
    falls and fractures 286c
    female predominance 321
    gastric ulcers 570
    hypothyroidism 644
    incontinence 487–8
    lipid-lowering drugs 470
    pharmacokinetics in 147, *148*
    psychotropic agents 318, 320
    sedatives 293
    sleeping patterns *283*
electrical burns 924
electrical excitation (cardiac) 415–7
electrocardiography 417–8, *418*, 425
electroconvulsive therapy 312c, 322, 334
electroencephalography
    diagnosing epilepsy 289, 298
    during sleep 282
electronic prescribing 39
elimination 114b, 125, 130b, *see also* clearance
emboli 497, 500
embryo development, *see* fetus
emergency contraception 714–6
emetics, *see also* antiemetics; vomiting
    apomorphine 353
    emetic centre in brain 556–8
    emetic weed 67t
    in cancer chemotherapy 766t
EMLA cream (lignocaine with prilocaine) 240, 245
    pregnancy safety 248
emollients 909
emotional disorders, *see* mood disorders
empirical therapy 800
emtricitabine 836–8
    pregnancy safety 844
enalapril
    ACE inhibitor 456
    pharmacokinetics 455t
    pregnancy safety 457
end-stage renal disease 475c
endocrine drugs
    psychotropic agent interactions 318
    taste and smell effects 617t
    teratogenic potential 726
endocrine system 621–8
    cannabinoid effects 401
    disorders of, and anaesthesiology 234
    effect of alcohol 388
    glands *621*
    hypothalamus 216
    infertility related to 740
    mechanism of action 623
    ocular involvement 603
    reproductive systems 697–8
endogenous depression 327
endogenous opioids 253–4, *see also* opioids
endometriosis 720–1
endometrium 701
endopeptidases 758
endorphins 253–4, *see also* beta-endorphin
endothelial cells, drug administration across 908
endotracheal intubation 230
energy balance and obesity 948–50, *948*
enflurane 237, 237t
    pregnancy safety 248
enfuvirtide 836, 843
    pregnancy safety 844

enkephalins 253–4, 264t, 265c
enoxaparin 502–3
    pregnancy safety 512
entacapone
    isoprenaline interactions 191
    on–off syndrome treatment 352
    parkinsonism treatment 354–5
    pregnancy safety 366
Entamoeba histolytica 854
enteral administration, *see* oral administration
enteric coatings 43, 115
enteric nervous system 164–5, 553
Enterobacter infections 795t
Enterobius vermicularis 864, 866
Enterococcus infections, drug-resistant 797, 798t, 805t, 809t
enterohepatic cycling, excretion by 126
enteroviral infections 796t
entonox, as medical gas 525c
enuresis, antidepressant treatment 328
environmental factors
    drug metabolism 124
    nephrotoxicity 488c
enzyme inducers
    medroxyprogesterone acetate interactions 713
    methadone interactions 386
    oestradiol valerate interactions 711
enzyme inhibitors, cancer treatment 762
enzymes
    drug-metabolising 122–3
    orphan drugs 80t
    skin conditions from 907t
    targeting 104
eosinophils 494
ephedra, toxicity 67t
ephedrine 193, **194**, *see also* noradrenaline
    asthma treatment 532
    avoid during breastfeeding 144t
    bicarbonate interactions 567
    drugs developed from 87
    pregnancy safety 199t
    regulation in sport 938, 939
epidermal growth factor 781
epidermis 904, 908, *see also* skin
Epidermophyton infections 916
epidural anaesthesia 117, 247–8, 247t
    perinatal use 234, 729
epilepsy 289–99, *see also* antiepileptic drugs; seizures
Epilepsy Foundation of Victoria 301c
epimetendiole 942c
epinephric glands, *see* adrenal cortex
epinephrine, *see* adrenaline
epirubicin 772t, 776
episcleritis 597
epitestosterone 935, 937
epitopes 872
epoetin alfa **937**
eprosartan 457
Epstein–Barr virus infections 796t
eptacog alfa 511t
    pregnancy safety 512
eptifibatide
    platelet effects 500, 509–10
    pregnancy safety 512
erectile dysfunction 740, 748–9
ergocalciferol
    hypocalcaemia treatment 689t
    pregnancy safety 693
ergogenic aids for competitive athletes 940

ergometrine (ergonovine) **728**, 729c
  oxytocic effects 727
  parkinsonism treatment 353
ergot alkaloids 352–3, 729c
  analgesic effects 276
  macrolide antibiotic interactions 812
  oxytocic effects 727
  pregnancy safety 730
  ritonavir interactions 843
  saquinavir interactions 843
  skin conditions from 907t
ergotamine 729c
  avoid during breastfeeding 144t
  caffeine an adjunct to 344
  headache treatment 366
  migraine treatment 364
  pregnancy safety 366
ergotoxine 729c
ertapenem 810
  pregnancy safety 821
eruptions of the skin, drugs causing 907t
erythema
  following infection 871
  from UV radiation 912
erythrocytes, see red blood cells
erythromycins 812–4
  acne treatment 922
  benzodiazepine interactions 288
  clindamycin interactions 814
  cyclosporin interactions 892
  cytochrome P450 isoform inhibition 158t
  delavirdine interactions 840
  disopyramide interactions 432t
  drug interactions with 158
  ergometrine interactions 728
  everolimus interactions 895
  Legionnaire's disease treatment 546
  ototoxicity 615t
  pharmacokinetics 813t
  pregnancy safety 821, 928
  simvastatin interactions 467
  sirolimus interactions 895
  skin conditions from 907t
  tamoxifen interactions 780
  theophylline interactions 537
  warfarin interactions 505
erythropoietin 492
  drug testing for 942c
  kidneys synthesise 474
  regulation in sport 936–7
eschar 927
Escherichia coli infections 795t
  cephalosporin-resistant 809t
  drug-resistant 798t, 805t
escitalopram 329
  pregnancy safety 320
eserine 591c
esmolol 197t, 436
  pharmacokinetics and dosages 198t
  pregnancy safety 199t
esomeprazole 17t, 571
essential drugs list (WHO) 15–6
essential oils 63
  photosensitising effects 907t
  skin condition treatment 911
ester-linked anaesthetics 240, 242
  pregnancy safety 737
estrogens, see oestrogens
etanercept 886
  antirheumatic effects 884
  pregnancy safety 900

etanercept—cont d
  topical administration 917
ethacrynic acid 482
  capreomycin interactions 857
  ototoxicity 615t
  pharmacokinetics 484t
ethambutol 860
  ocular adverse effects 604t
  pregnancy safety 866
  tuberculosis treatment 546, 856–7
ethanol, see alcohol
ether 6, 237
ethical issues 96–9, see also bioethics
  drugs in sport 942–3
  institutional ethics committees 89
ethinyloestradiol 709
  cancer treatment 780
  contraceptive use 712, 714, 715t
  dosage 710, 713c
ethosuximide 307
  anticonvulsant effects 300t
  antiepileptic interactions 301
  pregnancy safety 309
ethyl alcohol, see alcohol
ethyl chloride for pain relief 240
ethynodiol, contraceptive use 712
etidocaine, toxicity of 244
etidronate
  effect on bone 693
  pregnancy safety 693
etonogestrel
  contraceptive use 715t, 742
  depot preparations 716–7
etoposide
  cancer treatment 776
  combination therapy 764t
  emetic potential 766t
  indications and toxicity 772t
  pregnancy safety 789
etoricoxib, regulation in NZ 883c
eucalyptus oil 797c, 907t
eugenol, in liniments and rubs 910
euglycaemia, see blood glucose levels
eunuchoidism 734
euphoria 339, 372
European Approved Names 12–4
European Pharmacopoeia 16
eustachian tubes 611
euthyroid state 644
evening primrose, as herbal remedy 62t
everolimus 894
  pregnancy safety 900
evidence-based medicine 27, 66–8
  complementary and alternative methods
      evaluated by 61
evidence–relevance gap 27
excitatory amino acids 222–3
excitement, stage 2 of anaesthesia 227–8
excitotoxins 222
excretion 114b, 125–6, 125, see also clearance
  drug interactions affecting 158
  in children 144
  in infants 143
  in the elderly 148b
  in the fetus 141
  in urine 125
  via skin 905
exemestane
  cancer treatment 779t, 781
  pregnancy safety 789
  use in sport 935

exfoliative dermatitis 907t
exocrine cells 897, 904
exocytosis 170
exoerythrocytic phase in malaria 848
exogenous depression 327
exophthalmic goitre 647c
expectorant drugs 528–9, 542
Expert Committee on Complementary
      Medicines in the Health System 60, 68c
expiration 516
expired air drug excretion 126
external ear 611
extracellular water, drug distribution to 118t
extradural anaesthesia, see epidural anaesthesia
extrapyramidal system 218, 349
  antipsychotic effects on 313, 316, 317c,
      355
extrinsic pathway (coagulation) 495, 496
eye drops 586–7
eye gels 587
eye lotions 587
eye ointments 587
eyes, see also ocular . . .
  administration to 117
  adrenoceptors 188t
  atropine effects 180
  drugs affecting 585–606
  innervation of 166t
  muscarinic actions 178t
  OTC drugs for 53t
ezetimibe
  effects compared 469t
  lipid-lowering effects 467t, 470
  pregnancy safety 470
  simvastatin combined with 471

F

F, see bioavailability
Fab, see digoxin-specific antigen-binding
      fragment
Faces pain scale 258
facial nerve 215t
factor VIII, see antihaemophilic factor
factor IX complex 511
  pregnancy safety 512
factors in blood coagulation 495t
faecal softening agents 575, 575b
failure of therapy (Type F) ADRs 155
fallopian tubes 697, 745
Fallot's tetralogy 197
falls and fractures in the elderly 286c
famciclovir 831
  emtricitabine interactions 838
  pregnancy safety 844
families of drugs 13t
family planning 745c, see also contraceptives
famotidine
  peptic ulcer treatment 572, 572t
  pregnancy safety 581
'fantasy', see gamma-hydroxybutyric acid
farnesyl molecules 760
farnesyltransferase, cancer treatment 762
fasciculations 205
fast-acting polypeptides, see tachykinins
fat, see body fat; lipid metabolism
fatigue, see sleep disorders
febrile convulsions 299
feedback mechanism, autonomic nervous
      system 163
felodipine
  angina treatment 445

felodipine—cont'd
  pharmacokinetics 446t
  pregnancy safety 457
female reproductive system 697, 700–5
  contraception 741–2
  drugs affecting 709–21
  hypothalamic factors 702
  sexual response 704–5
fenemates 879t, 881t
fenfluramine, anorectic agent 342–3, 951, 951c
fenofibrate 468–9, 469t
  pregnancy safety 470
fenoterol, deaths attributed to 533, 533c
fentanyl 267
  adjunct to anaesthetic 230
  anaesthetic 239
  dosage forms 266t
  during childbirth 234
  for day procedures 232
  mu-receptor agonist 264t
  pregnancy safety 278
  premedication with 235t
  topical administration 908
  transdermal administration 267c
ferrous sulfate
  quinolone interactions 818
  thyroxine interactions 645t
fertilisation 697
fertility, drugs affecting 740–5
fetal alcohol syndrome 141c
fetal distress syndrome 261
fetal screening 95
fetus, see also placenta; pregnancy; teratogens
  alcohol effects 388–9
  development of 139–42
  drug distribution to 120
  drugs affecting 138–42
  lung prophylaxis 531
  pharmacokinetics 141
fever 531, see also antipyretics
feverfew
  herbal remedy 62t
  migraine treatment 365
  neurological treatments 363c
  pain treatment 277c
fexofenadine 901
  nasal condition treatment 548
  pregnancy safety 899
fibrates, for hyperlipidaemia 467t, 468–9
fibrin-stabilising factor 495t
fibrinogen 492, 495t
fibrinolysis, drugs affecting 13t, 500
fight-or-flight system, see sympathetic nervous system
filgrastim, pregnancy safety 789
financial costs of drug development, see pharmacoeconomics
finasteride 736–7, **736**
first aid
  for burns 924
  for snake bite 957c
first-generation antipsychotics, see antipsychotics
first-pass effect 124
fish oil
  folk remedy 60t
  hypertriglyceridaemia treatment 467t
  neurological treatment 363c
five rights 33, 36
flashback phenomena 403

flecainide 430, 435–6
  disopyramide interactions 432t
  lumefantrine interactions 853
  pharmacokinetics 430t
  pregnancy safety 437
Flockhart, D. 159
floxacins, glycaemic levels linked to 672t
flucloxacillin 806
  adverse drug events 807
  pharmacokinetics 807t
  pregnancy safety 821
fluconazole 827
  cyclosporin interactions 892
  cytochrome P450 isoform inhibition 158t
  oral candidiasis treatment 564
  pharmacokinetics 829t
  pregnancy safety 844
  rifampicin interactions 859
  simvastatin interactions 467
  warfarin interactions 505
flucytosine 830
  amphotericin B interactions 828
  pregnancy safety 844
fludarabine
  cancer treatment 773
  indications and toxicity 771t
fludrocortisone **661**
  pharmacokinetics 657t
  potency 657
  pregnancy safety 662
fluid distribution, changes during pregnancy 140
fluid imbalances 39
flumazenil 287
  benzodiazepine overdose treatment 289, 392
  pregnancy safety 293
flumethasone, ear treatment 613
flunitrazepam
  pharmacokinetics 286t
  premedication with 235t
  rapid absorption 288
  sleep disorder treatment 287
fluorescein 599, **600**
  pregnancy safety 606
fluoridated mouth-washes 564
fluoridated water 563c
fluorometholone
  ocular use 597, 598t
  pregnancy safety 606, 662
fluoroquinolones 818–9
  indications and toxicity 772t
  sleep pattern effects 284t
5-fluorouracil, see fluorouracil
fluorouracil
  calcium folinate interactions 783
  cancer treatment 773
  chemical structure 773
  combination therapy 764t
  emetic potential 766t
  indications and toxicity 771t
  photosensitising effects 907t
  pregnancy safety 789
  taste and smell effects 617t
fluoxetine 329, **330**
  adverse drug events 319t
  cytochrome P450 isoform inhibition 158t
  drug dependence treatment 382
  drug interactions with 158
  fast-tracking of development 749c
  lithium interactions 333

fluoxetine—cont'd
  no hypertensive effects 318c
  pharmacokinetics 330
  pregnancy safety 320, 330
  selegiline interactions 354
  sexual function affected by 750
  use in Australia 332c
  warfarin interactions 505
fluoxymesterone
  breast cancer treatment 779
  regulation in sport 934
  skin conditions from 907t
flupenthixol 324
  major effects 315t
  pregnancy safety 320
  sexual function affected by 750
fluphenazine
  avoids anticholinergic effects 316
  extrapyramidal effects 324
  major effects 315t
  piperazine compound 324
  pregnancy safety 320
  sexual function affected by 750
flurbiprofen
  ocular use 598
  pregnancy safety 606
flutamide
  antiandrogens 737
  cancer treatment 779, 779t
  pregnancy safety 789
fluticasone
  asthma prophylaxis 536
  in Australia's top 10 drugs 17t
  inhaled corticosteroid 658
  pregnancy safety 549
  salmeterol with 539
fluvastatin
  hyperlipidaemia treatment 466
  pregnancy safety 470
fluvoxamine 329
  cytochrome P450 isoform inhibition 158t
  pregnancy safety 320
  theophylline interactions 537
foetal alcohol syndrome, see fetal alcohol syndrome
foetus, see fetus
folic acid 513
  during pregnancy 725
  in metabolism 773
folinic acid, see calcium folinate
foliotropins 700
folk remedies, see complementary and alternative medicine
follicle-stimulating hormone 626t, 698, 700, 709, see also gonadotrophin-releasing hormone
  in male reproductive system 734
  infertility treatment 740
follicle-stimulating hormone inhibitors 742
follicular hormones, see oestrogens
folliculitis 915
follitropins, pregnancy safety 751
fondaparinux 500, 504
  pregnancy safety 512
food, see diet
fool's parsley, toxicity 67t
formalin 389
formularies, information in 16
formulations 39–45, 42b, see also combinations of drugs
  absorption affected by 115

formulations—cont'd
 definition 3t
 local anaesthetics 244
 topical administration 908–9
fosamprenavir 836, 841
 drug interactions 842t
 pregnancy safety 844
foscarnet 831, 834–5
 cidofovir interactions 834
 ganciclovir interactions 833t
 pregnancy safety 844
 valganciclovir interactions 833t
 zalcitabine interactions 840
fosinopril
 ACE inhibitor 456
 pharmacokinetics 455t
 pregnancy safety 457
fosphenytoin 305
fotemustine 770, 771t
foxglove 67t, 423
framycetin
 ear treatment 613–4
 for pressure sores 927
 ocular use 596
 pregnancy safety 606, 618
 topical administration 915
Frank–Starling relation (cardiac function) 419
free radicals 526
Friar's Balsam 911
Frohlich's syndrome 734c
frusemide **483**
 age-related adverse drug events 149t
 bile acid-binding resin interactions 468
 capreomycin interactions 857
 didanosine interactions 838
 diuretic use 482
 drug testing for 942c
 hydration therapy 784
 in Australia's top 10 drugs 17t
 ototoxicity 615t
 pharmacokinetics 484t
 skin conditions from 907t
 zalcitabine interactions 840
FSH, see follicle-stimulating hormone
FSH-releasing hormone, see gonadotrophin-
  releasing hormone
Fuchs, Leonhard 423
functionalisation reactions 121
fungal infections 796t, 797, see also
  antifungals
funnel-web spiders 961
furuncles 611, 915
Fusobacterium infections 796t

G

γ-aminobutyric acid 222, 358
G-protein-coupled receptors 104–5, *105,
  106,* see also adrenoceptors; muscarinic
  receptors
GABA 222, 358
GABA receptors
 agonists 275, 303–5
 benzodiazepines act on 286
gabapentin 275, 307
 anticonvulsant effects 303
 neuropathy and neuralgia treatment 303
 pregnancy safety 309
galactorrhoea 634c, 730
galantamine
 neurological treatment 363c
 pregnancy safety 366

Galen of Pergamon 5, 933
galenicals, *see* combinations of drugs
gallbladder 166t, 559, *see also* biliary
  system
gallium-67 cancer treatment 761
gallstones 559c
gamete intrafollicular transfer 740
gametes 697
gamma-aminobutyric acid 222, 358
gamma-hydroxybutyric acid 357, 358c, 403
gamma interferon, from immune response
  873
ganciclovir 831–3
 mycophenolate mofetil interactions 895
 pregnancy safety 844
 stavudine interactions 838
 zidovudine interactions 837
ganglia 169
ganglion-blocking drugs 182
 adverse drug events 181t
 bethanechol interactions 179
 sexual function affected by 746, 749
ganirelix 699, 740
gargles 563–4
garlic
 as folk remedy 60t
 for respiratory disorders 543c
 warfarin interactions 504
gas transport 516
gases, *see also* inhaled drugs
 in respiratory disorders 524–8
 medical 525c
gastrin 555
gastritis 555, 565
gastro-oesophageal reflux disease 554c, 565
gastrointestinal tract 553–60
 adrenaline effects 189
 adrenoceptors 188t
 alcohol effects 387
 amoebiasis 854–5
 atropine effects 180
 caffeine effects 343
 cannabinoid effects 401
 drugs affecting 563–81
 gastric acid 147, 555
 gastric emptying time 157, 555
 gastric secretions 556, 557
 histamine effects 897t
 in neonates 145t
 innervation of 166t
 muscarinic actions 178t
 NSAID adverse drug events 879, 882
 OTC drugs for 53t
gate control theory of pain 253
gatifloxacin 818
gefitinib 782
 pregnancy safety 789
gelatin, for pressure sores 927
gels, skin treatment 909
gemcitabine
 cancer treatment 762c, 773
 emetic potential 766t
 indications and toxicity 771t
 pregnancy safety 789
 warfarin interactions 505
gemeprost
 oxytocic effects 728
 pregnancy safety 730
gemfibrozil 468–9, **469**
 cytochrome P450 isoform inhibition 158t
 effects compared 469t

gemfibrozil—cont'd
 pregnancy safety 470
 warfarin interactions 505
gender differences
 cluster headache 366
 complementary and alternative medicine
  use 154
 duodenal ulcers 556
 fetal development 745
 haemoglobin 493
 heart disease treatment 412c
 migraine 363
 pelvis cross-section 475
 psychiatric disorders 320
 urinary tract 474
gene doping 934, 938–9
gene therapy 95, 762
general anaesthetics 227–39
 ACE inhibitor interactions 454
 interactions between drugs 233–4
 pharmacokinetics 229
 vancomycin interactions 812
general practitioners, *see* doctors
generalised absence seizures, *see* absence
  seizures
generalised tonic–clonic seizures, *see*
  tonic–clonic generalised epilepsy
generic names 12–4
genetic engineering 94
genetic factors, *see also* chromosomes
 adverse drug events 156
 carcinogenesis 759
 codeine metabolism 264
 polymorphism 123–4
 prolactin effects 634
 role in obesity 950
 screening for 95
genitourinary system, OTC drugs for 53t
gentamicin 814
 balance disorder treatment 612
 Legionnaire's disease treatment 546
 ocular use 596
 pregnancy safety 606, 821
 resistance to 798t
 topical administration 915
 urinary tract infection treatment 820
geranyl molecules 760
geriatrics, *see* elderly
gestodene 712, 714, 715t
gestrinone 699
 pregnancy safety 721
GG167, *see* zanamivir
GH, *see* growth hormone
GHB, *see* gamma-hydroxybutyric acid
GHRF, *see* growth hormone-releasing factor
GHRIF, *see* growth hormone release-inhibiting
  factor
gigantism 633c
ginger 62t, 720c
gingival hyperplasia 445
gingko
 glaucoma treatment 601c
 neurological treatments 363c
 tinnitus treatment 614
ginseng **64**
 adverse drug events 64
 herbal remedy 62t
 toxicity 67t
 warfarin interactions 504
GIT, *see* gastrointestinal tract
glatiramer, multiple sclerosis treatment 360

glaucoma 197, 585, *591*, 592–5
  adrenergic treatments 590
  complementary and alternative medicine 601c
glial cells 219–20
glibenclamide **679**
  diabetes treatment 677
  pharmacokinetics 678t
  pregnancy safety 681
gliclazide
  diabetes treatment 677
  pharmacokinetics 678t
  pregnancy safety 681
glimepiride, pregnancy safety 681
glipizide
  diabetes treatment 677
  pharmacokinetics 678t
  pregnancy safety 681
glitazones, *see* thiazolidinediones (glitazones)
Global Alliance for Elimination of Leprosy 862
globulins 492
globus pallidus 218
glomerular filtration 125, 145t, 475
glomerulus 474
glossopharyngeal nerve 215t
glucagon 627t, 667, **680**, 681
  hyperglycaemia linked to 672t
  octreotide interactions 634
  pregnancy safety 681
glucocorticoids, *see* corticosteroids
glucocorticosteroids, *see* corticosteroids
glucosamine 884c
glucose 681, *see also* blood glucose levels
glucosidase inhibitor, *see* alpha-glucosidase inhibitor
glucuronidation, conjugation reaction 122t
glue ear 612
glutamate 222
  Alzheimer's disease linked to 362
  amyotrophic lateral sclerosis associated with 360
  anticonvulsant effects 303
  receptors 223, 339
glutaraldehyde, wart treatment 916
glutathione transferases, conjugation reaction 122t
glycerin
  ear treatment 614
  Magnoplasm 910
  suppositories 577
glycerol
  calamine lotion 910
  glaucoma treatment 595
  laxative effects 577
glyceryl trinitrate **442**
  alcohol interactions 391
  ocular adverse effects 604t
  oral administration 116
  OTC vs prescription variants 52t
  pharmacokinetics 444t
  pregnancy safety 457
  sexual function affected by 747
  sildenafil interactions 749
  topical administration 908
  transdermal administration 910
  vasodilators 441–3
glycocalyx 797
glycopeptide antibiotics 810–2
glycoprotein IIb/IIIa receptor inhibitors, antiplatelet action 509–10

glycoproteins 114, 119
glycopyrrolate 181–2
  adverse drug events 181t
  clinical use and administration 182t
  pregnancy safety 182
  premedication with 235t
glycosides *10*, 11, *see also* cardiac glycosides
GnRH analogues
  cancer treatment 779–80, 779t
  contraceptive use 742
goblet cells 517
goitre 640c, 643–5
goitrogens 647–9, 650c
gold salts
  antirheumatic effects 884–5
  avoid during breastfeeding 144t
  photosensitising effects 907t
  skin conditions from 907t
Golden Eye Ointment 597
Gompertzian growth kinetics in tumours 760
gonadorelin 699
gonadotrophin-releasing hormone 630, 630t, 698, 698–9, 709
  agonists 720
  cancer treatment 779–80
  contraceptive use 742
  in male reproductive system 734, 737
  infertility treatment 740
  inhibitors 699, 700t
  prostate cancer treatment 778
gonadotrophins 698, 700, 709, 740, 936
gonads 697
Good Manufacturing Practice principles 57
GORD 554c, 565
goserelin
  cancer treatment 779–80, 779t
  GnRH analogue 700t
  pregnancy safety 789
gossypol, contraceptive use 742
gout 6, 887–90, *see also* hyperuricaemia
GP Asthma Initiative 541
GPCRs, *see* G-protein-coupled receptors
gram-negative anaerobic infections 796t
gram-negative bacilli 795t
  drug resistance 805t
  superinfection with 798
gram-negative cocci 795t
gram-negative fungi, superinfection with 798
gram-positive bacilli 795t
  drug resistance 805t
gram-positive cocci 795t
Gram staining 794
gramicidin
  ear treatment 613–4
  ocular use 596
  topical administration 915
grand mal, *see* tonic–clonic generalised epilepsy
granisetron
  antiemetic use 567t, 569
  cancer treatment 783
  pregnancy safety 581
granulation tissue 926
granules 170
granulocyte colony-stimulating factors 492
  cancer treatment 785
  drug groups 13t
  epoetin alfa 937
  immunostimulation by 895–6
  myelosuppression rescued by 784

granulocytes 494
grapefruit juice
  cyclosporin interactions 892
  drug interactions 123c, 158–9
  everolimus interactions 894
  sildenafil interactions 748
  simvastatin interactions 467
  sirolimus interactions 894
  statin interactions 466
  tamoxifen interactions 780
Graves' disease 603, 643, 645, 647c
Greek medicine 5
green-lipped mussels 884c
green plum 797c, 826c
green tea, as folk remedy 60t
grey baby syndrome 816–7
grey matter (brain) 214
griseofulvin 830–1
  alcohol interactions 391
  amorolfine interactions 917
  photosensitising effects 907t
  pregnancy safety 844
  simvastatin interactions 467
  skin conditions from 907t
  topical antifungal 916
growth factors, in cell cycle 756, 757
growth hormone 626t, 631–4
  effect of *633*
  hyperglycaemia linked to 672t
  regulation in sport 936
  secretion of *631*
growth hormone release-inhibiting factor, *see* somatostatins
growth hormone-releasing factor 630
growth phase of cells 756
growth, thyroxine effects *646*
guanethidine 604t, 672t
guanine 757
guanine nucleotide protein-coupled receptors, *see* G-protein-coupled receptors
guarana (*Paullinia cupana*), social use of 398
Guedel, Arthur 227
guinea-pig ileum smooth muscle preparation 85
gums and mucilages, sources of 11
gustation, drugs affecting 616–7
gynaecological disorders 720–1
gynaecomastia 730, 735, 747
gyrase, *see* topoisomerases

H

H$_1$-receptor antagonists, *see* antihistamines
H$_2$-receptor antagonists
  age-related adverse drug events 149t
  drug interactions 572t
  imidazole antifungal interactions 829t
  peptic ulcer treatment 570–2, 572t
  taste and smell effects 617t
haematinics 512–3
  epoetin alfa interactions 937
haematocrit 492, *see also* platelets
haemoconcentration 232
haemodyalisis, Aboriginals treated with 475c
haemoglobins 493–4, 512–3, 939
Haemophilus influenzae infections 795t
  cephalosporin-resistant 809t
  drug-resistant 798t, 805t
haemopoietic system 492–7, 512–3, *see also* bone marrow suppressants
haemorrhagic anaemia 494

haemorrhagic cystitis 765
haemorrhoids 560
haemostatic drugs 510–2
haemostatics 494–6
Hageman factor 495t
Hahnemann, Samuel 64
hair loss 765, 907t
half-life 130b, 133–5
halitosis, mouth-washes for 563
hallucinogens 402–4
    5-HT receptors affected by 314
    abuse of 375t, 380
    chemical structure 404
    depression evoked by 326
    intoxication with 377t
    pregnancy safety 405
    reticular activating system effects 218
halogenated anaesthetics
    adrenaline interactions 190t
    noradrenaline interactions 191
haloperidol 325
    amphetamine overdose treatment 340b
    antiemetic use 567t
    avoids anticholinergic effects 316
    avoids sedative effects 316
    lithium interactions 333
    major effects 315t
    photosensitising effects 907t
    pregnancy safety 320
    sexual function affected by 750
    warfarin interactions 505
halothane 237, 237t
    pregnancy safety 248
hamamelis 909
hangovers 390
Hansen's disease (leprosy) 861–2
Hashimoto's disease 643, 647c
hashish 399–402, see also cannabinoids
    regulation in sport 938
    symptoms of abuse 374t
hawthorn, as herbal remedy 62t
hay fever, see allergic rhinitis; vernal
    conjunctivitis
HCG, see human chorionic gonadotrophin
HDLs 462, 464
head, respiratory structures 547
headaches 344, 363–6, see also migraine
    treatment
health information managers, drugs
    administered by 32–3
health professionals, see also doctors;
    prescribing
    drug abuse among 378
    relation to pharmaceutical industry 98
    roles of 31–5
hearing loss, see ototoxicosis
heart 411–9, see also cardiovascular system
    adrenoceptors 188t
    innervation of 166t
    muscle fibres 413
heart block 435b
heart failure 422
    deaths resulting from 423c
    digoxin treatment 425
    dopamine treatment 192
    ocular effects of treatment 603
    spironolactone treatment 486c
    treatment of 197, 422
heart rate 418
heartburn 554, 725
heavy metals, nephrotoxicity 488c

Helicobacter pylori 555c, 570–1, see also
    peptic ulcer disease
helium, as medical gas 525c
helminthiasis 797, 862–4
helper T cells 873
hemlock, toxicity 67t
hemp, see cannabinoids
henbane 179, 403
heparin antagonists 503–4
heparins 500–3, see also thrombocytopenia
    age-related adverse drug events 149t
    comparison with other drugs 501–2
    dipyridamole interactions 509
    overdose treatment 503–4
    pregnancy safety 512
    standard heparin 501
    thrombolytic interactions 506
hepatic . . ., see also liver
hepatic clearance 132
hepatic encephalopathy, lactulose treatment
    577
hepatic enzyme-inducing drugs, see also
    barbiturates; phenytoin
    calcium-channel blocker interactions 447t
    fludrocortisone interactions 661
    glucocorticoid interactions 660t
    hydrocortisone interactions 659
hepatic first-pass effect 124
hepatitis C, in New Zealand 835c
hepatocytes 559
hepatoma 763
hepatotoxicity
    cancer chemotherapy 765
    dantrolene 360
    isoniazid 858
    methotrexate 775
    paracetamol 54
    rifampicin 859
herbal remedies 62t, 63, see also
    complementary and alternative medicine;
    indigenous remedies; names of plants;
    plant drugs
    adverse drug events 68–9
    drugs developed from 86
    interactions between drugs 69, 158–9
    pain treatment 277c
    polypharmacy 66c
    psychiatric treatments 327c
    respiratory treatments 543c
    toxicity 67t
    traditional medicine 65–6
    warfarin interactions 504
hereditary factors, see genetic factors
heroin 267, see also abuse of drugs
    abuse of 375t, 380, 383–6
    during breastfeeding 144t
    neonatal withdrawal symptoms 143t
    sexual function affected by 746
herpes 564–5, 796t, 915
hexamethonium, sexual function affected by
    749
hexamine hippurate 820–1
    pregnancy safety 821
hiatal hernia 554
hiccups, carbon dioxide treatment 527
high-density lipoproteins 462, 464
high-throughput screening 87c, 88
Hildegard of Bingen 5, 927c
Hippocrates 5, 35
Hippocratic oath 96
hirsutism 720

histamine receptor antagonists 13t, see also
    antihistamines; H₁-receptor antagonists;
    H₂-receptor antagonists
histamines
    5-HT receptors affected by 314
    drugs developed from 87
    gastric acid secretion and 555, 571
    immunostimulation by 896–901
    neuromuscular blocking drugs release 205
    opiods release 264
    role in inflammation 871
histone deacetylase, cancer treatment 762
HIV
    antivirals 836–40
    from immune response 873
    in Australia 831c
    inhibition sites 839
    resistance to treatment 797
    vaccine 836c
HIV-protease inhibitors, statin interactions 466
HMB 940
HMG-CoA reductase inhibitors, see statins
Hodgkin's disease, combination therapy 764
holistic medicine 61, see also complementary
    and alternative medicine
homatropine
    clinical use and administration 182t
    ocular use 589t
    pregnancy safety 606
home remedies, see complementary and
    alternative medicine
homeopathy 63–4
homeostasis 163, 905
homocysteic acid 222
homosalate 913t
honey 60t, 927
hopwood 797c
hordeolum 595
hormonal effects, on drug metabolism 124
hormone replacement therapy 709–10, 718c
    osteoporosis treatment 692
hormones 621–8, see also sex hormones
    acne treatment 922
    cancer treatment 762, 777–8, 779t
    depression evoked by 326
    mechanism of action 622
    regulation in sport 933
    role in inflammation 871
    use in sport 936–7
Horner's syndrome 588c
horse chestnut, toxicity 67t
horseradish 60t, 543c
hospital admissions due to adverse drug
    events 154, 159
hospitals
    drug charts 38–9, 38
    invention of 5
    palliative care in 787
5-HT, see 5-hydroxytryptamine
5-HT₃ receptor antagonists, antiemetic use
    567t, 569
human chorionic gonadotrophin 698, 700,
    701, see also luteinising hormone
    choriogonadotrophin alfa 700
    infertility treatment 740
    levels during pregnancy 725
    pregnancy safety 751
    regulation in sport 936
human growth hormone, see growth hormone;
    recombinant growth hormone

human insulin **675**, *see also* insulin
human papilloma virus 916
human rights 90–1, 96–7
humans, drugs from 7
humoral immunity 871, 873–4, *see also* antibodies
hunger, *see* anorectic agents
hydantoins, skin conditions from 907t
hydralazine 448–9
    didanosine interactions 838
    ocular adverse effects 604t
    pregnancy safety 457
    skin conditions from 907t
    stavudine interactions 838
    zalcitabine interactions 840
hydration therapy 784
hydrocarbons
    abuse of 392
    chemical structure 10
    drugs from 11
hydrochloric acid, gastric 147, 555
hydrochlorothiazide 482, **483**
    diuretic combinations 485
    pharmacokinetics 484t
    sexual function affected by 751
hydrocortisone 654, 656–7, **659**
    antipruritic agent 909
    ear treatment 613
    ocular use 597, 598t
    OTC vs prescription variants 52t
    pharmacokinetics 657t
    pregnancy safety 606, 662
    stress induces release of 653
    topical administration 919
hydromorphone 263, 267, 383
    dosage forms 266t
    mu-receptor agonist 264t
    pregnancy safety 278
3-hydroxy-3-methylglutaryl coenzyme
        inhibitors, *see* statins
hydroxy-beta-methylbutyrate, for athletes 940
hydroxybenzoates, dermatitis from 910
hydroxychloroquine
    antirheumatic effects 884–5
    pregnancy safety 866, 900
hydroxydaunomycin, CHOP regimen 782
hydroxyethylrutosides
    peripheral vascular treatments 450
    pregnancy safety 457
hydroxyprogesterone 698, 710
5-hydroxytryptamine, *see also* selective
        serotonin reuptake inhibitors
    associated with depression 326
    CNS pathways 222
    food intake regulation 949
    in sexual response 705
    involved in migraine 363–4
    involvement in psychiatric disorders 313–4
    receptors for 223
5-hydroxytryptamine agonists
    analgesic effects 276
    anorectic agents 951
    drug groups 13t
5-hydroxytryptamine antagonists
    Alzheimer's disease treatment 362
    drug groups 13t
    during cancer chemotherapy 783
hydroxyureas, cancer treatment 776
Hymenoleptis nana 863
hyoscine 179, 181
    adverse drug events 181t

hyoscine—cont'd
    antidiarrhoeal agents 579
    antiemetic use 567t, 568–9
    clinical use and administration 182t
    early use of 9–10
    irritable bowel syndrome treatment 581
    parkinsonism treatment 355
    pregnancy safety 182
    topical administration 908
hyoscyamine, antidiarrhoeal agents 579
hyoscyamus, discovery of 6
hyperactivity, *see* attention deficit hyperactivity
        disorder
hyperalgesia 253, 269–70
hyperbaric oxygen 525
hypercalcaemia 427b, 687, 689t
hypercapnia 518, 524, *see also* carbon dioxide
hypercholesterolaemia 462–71, 464t, 467t, 603
hyperglycaemia, *see also* blood glucose levels
    in indigenous populations 669c
    lowers glucagon production 667
    results of 672
    symptoms of 672c
    thiazide diuretic involvement 484
hyperglycaemic agents 680–1
hyperkalaemia 486c, 488b, 766
hyperlipidaemia 464t, 467t
hyperlipoproteinaemias 464–5
hyperparathyroidism 686–7
hyperphosphataemia 766
hyperpituitarism 634–5
hyperprolactinaemia 324, 634c, 740, 749
hyperpyrexia, *see* malignant hyperthermia/
        hyperpyrexia
hypersensitivity 874, *see also* adverse drug
        events; allergic reactions; anaphylactic
        reactions
    to drugs 155, 156t
    to penicillin 808c
hypertension, *see also* antihypertensives
    adrenoceptor antagonists for 193–5
    management of 450–7
    moclobemide-induced 318c
    ocular effect of disorders 602
    treatment of 197
hyperthermia, *see* malignant hyperthermia/
        hyperpyrexia
hyperthyroidism 603, 645–9, 647c
hypertriglyceridaemia 464t, 467t
hyperuricaemia 784, 887–90, 889
hypnotics, *see also* sleep disorders
    age-related adverse drug events 149t, 150,
        285, 293
    alcohol interactions 391
    anaesthetics 239
    CNS effects 214c
    diazepam interactions 287
    risk of dependence 283
    withdrawal affects sleep patterns 284t
hypoalbuminaemia 119
hypocalcaemia 488b, 687, 689t, 766
hypochloraemia 488b
hypochlorite, antiseptic effects 915
hypodermis 904
hypoglossal nerve 215t
hypoglycaemia, *see also* blood glucose levels
    glucagon production stimulated by 667
    results of 672
    symptoms of 672c
hypoglycaemic agents
    aminoglutethimide interactions 662

hypoglycaemic agents—cont'd
    antacid interactions 566–7
    retinal oedema relieved by 603
    sildenafil interactions 748
    taste and smell effects 617t
hypogonadism 734
hypokalaemia 427b, 484, 488b
hypolipidaemics, *see* lipid-lowering drugs
hypomagnesaemia 427b, 488b
hyponatraemia 307, 488b
hypoparathyroidism 686
hypopituitarism 635
hypoprothrombinaemia 506
hyposmia 618
hypothalamic factors 621
    anterior pituitary regulation 630–1
    food intake regulation 949
    mechanism of action 622
    reproductive systems 698–700, 702
hypothalamic–pituitary–adrenal axis
    endocrine system 623
    suppression of 654
hypothalamic–pituitary–gonadal axis 699
hypothalamus 216–7
    adrenal cortex controlled by 654
    negative feedback to 656
    reproductive system disorders 734–5
    role in ANS 163
hypothyroidism
    clinical features 647c
    congenital 640c
    treatment of 643–5
hypovolaemia 232, 488b
hypoxaemia 518–9, 524
hypoxia 524
hypromellose (artificial tears) 602

I

ibuprofen 879t
    as NSAID 270
    combination analgesics 273
    ear treatment 612
    migraine treatment 364
    ocular adverse effects 604t
    pharmacokinetics 881t
    risk of GIT effects 879, 882
ichthammol 911
    pregnancy safety 928
    skin condition treatment 920
ICP 216c
ICSH, *see* luteinising hormone
idarubicin 772t, 776
IDDM, *see* diabetes mellitus
ideal drugs 3–4
idiopathic epilepsy 298c
idoxuridine, topical administration 915
IECs 89, 97
ifosfamide
    cancer treatment 770
    emetic potential 766t
    hydration therapy 784
    indications and toxicity 771t
    pregnancy safety 789
illicit drugs 267, 372, *see also* abuse of drugs;
        regulation
imatinib 782
imidazole antifungals 826, 916
    dandruff treatment 910
    drug interactions 829t
    pregnancy safety 928
    topical 918t

imipenem 804, 810
  ganciclovir interactions 833t
  pregnancy safety 821
  valganciclovir interactions 833t
imipramine 329, see also tricyclic
      antidepressants
  adverse drug events 319t
  development of 312c
  phenytoin interactions 306
  pregnancy safety 320
  sexual function affected by 750
  taste and smell effects 617t
imiquimod
  cancer treatment 785
  pregnancy safety 789
  wart treatment 916
immune responses 874
immune system 870–1, 870, 874–5
immunisation, see vaccinations
immunocompetent cells 872
immunodeficiency, see immunosuppressants
immunoglobulins 873–4
immunomodulating drugs
  cancer chemotherapy 784
  immunostimulatory agents 895–6
  topical administration 917–20
immunosuppressants 890–5
  azathioprine interactions 893
  cancer treatment 761, 784
  cyclophosphamide interactions 774
  glucocorticoids 656, 658
  inflammatory bowel disease treatment 580
  multiple sclerosis treatment 360
  mycophenolate mofetil interactions 895
  psoriasis treatment 920
  sites of action 891
impetigo 915
implants 42b
impotence 746, 748–9, see also erectile
      dysfunction
in-vitro fertilisation 740
inactivation 172, 174
incontinence, urinary 328, 478c, 487–8
indanedione, testosterone interactions 735
indapamide 482
Indian medicine 4
Indian tobacco, toxicity 67t
indigenous people, see Aboriginals and Torres
      Strait Islanders; Maoris
indigenous remedies 65c, see also herbal
      remedies
  antifungals 826c
  gastric disorders 577c
  NSAIDS in 884c
  pain relief 271c
  phyto-oestrogens 719
  respiratory disorders 543c
indinavir 836, 841, 842
  atazanavir interactions 842t
  cytochrome P450 isoform inhibition 158t
  didanosine interactions 838
  emtricitabine interactions 838
  imidazole antifungal interactions 829t
  nevirapine interactions 841
  pregnancy safety 844
  quinupristin interactions 818
indirect-acting sympathomimetics 186, 193
indirect pharmacodynamic interactions 157
indomethacin 879t
  age-related adverse drug events 150
  as NSAID 270

indomethacin—cont'd
  mechanism of action 879
  ocular adverse effects 604t
  pharmacokinetics 881t
  probenecid interactions 890
  warfarin interactions 505
induction of metabolism 124, 158
infant respiratory distress syndrome 530–1
infantile spasms 299c, 308
infants, see also breastfeeding; neonates;
      paediatrics
  anticonvulsants for 300
  breastfeeding 142–4
  drug metabolism in 144–7
  epilepsy in 298
  sleep patterns 282, 283
infections, see antibiotics; microbial infections
infertility, see also reproductive systems
  drug-induced 740–5
  following cancer treatment 767
  treatments for 740
infestations, OTC drugs for 53t
infiltration anaesthesia 245, 247t
inflammation, see also anti-inflammatory
      agents
  histamine effects 897
  NSAID treatment for 271
  ocular 597–8
  response to infection 794, 871
  role in pain 254–5
inflammatory bowel disease 560, 580–1
infliximab 886–7, 917
  antirheumatic effects 884
  Crohn's disease treatment 581
  pregnancy safety 900
influenza
  Olympic Games precautions 541c
  treatment of 544–5
  vaccines for 542, 545, 549
information sources 16–9, 36, 58, 97
informed consent 97, 315
infusion pumps 261, see also parenteral
      administration
  dosage measurement 22–3
  total intravenous anaesthesia 238
ingestion, see oral administration
inhaled drugs 117, see also aerosol therapy
  abuse of 375t, 392
  anaesthetic–oxytocin interactions 637
  anaesthetics 236
  analgesics 261
  diabetes treatment 676–7
  glucocorticoids 658
  medical gases 525c
  sevoflurane interactions 238
inhibin 698, 700
inhibition of enzyme activity 124
injections, see parenteral administration
INN 14
inner ear 611–2
inositol triphosphate, messenger system
      105
inotropic effects 187, 422
insecticides, anaesthetic interactions 233
insomnia, see sleep disorders
inspiration 516
institutional ethics committees 89, 97
insulin analogues 673
insulin-dependent diabetes mellitus, see
      diabetes mellitus
insulin-like growth factors, see somatomedins

insulins 627t, 666–81
  beta-blocker interaction 198t
  formulations 674t
  glucocorticoid interactions 660t
  human 675
  hypoglycaemia linked to 672t
  nicotine interactions 397
  pharmacokinetics 674
  pregnancy safety 681
  retinal oedema relieved by 603
  skin conditions from 907t
  taste and smell effects 617t
Intensive Medicines Monitoring Programme
      (NZ) 92c
interactions between drugs 45, 156–9, see
      also names of drugs
intercalated disc 412
interferons 784–5
  immunostimulation by 895–6
  multiple sclerosis treatment 360
  pregnancy safety 789, 896t
interindividual variability 123–4, 137–50
interleukins 492
  anakinra based on 887
  cancer treatment 762
  from immune response 873
  immunosuppression by 890
  role in immunostimulation 896
International Narcotics Control Board 74
International Non-Proprietary Names 14
international normalised ratio test 503c
International Olympic Committee 933,
      941–2
international regulation of drugs 74–5
International System of Units 19–20
International Units of activity 85–6
Internet (websites)
  adverse reactions reported on 92
  information from 18–9
  pharmacies on 74
interstitial-cell-stimulating hormone, see
      luteinising hormone
intestinal tract 574–81, see also
      gastrointestinal tract; large intestine;
      small intestine
intoxication, see abuse of drugs; alcohol
      (ethanol)
intra-articular administration 117b
intracytoplasmic sperm injection 740
intradermal implants, formulations for 42b
intradural anaesthesia, see spinal block
      anaesthesia
intralesional administration of glucocorticoids
      658
intramuscular injections 116
intraocular pressure 585, 592
intraosseous administration 117b
intraperitoneal administration 117b
intrapleural administration 117b
intrathecal anaesthesia 116–7, see also spinal
      block anaesthesia
intrauterine devices 742, 743
intravenous infusions 116, see also parenteral
      administration
  anaesthetics 237–8, 238c
  dosage measurement 22–3
  formulations of 42b
  opioids 260
  regional anaesthesia 245–6, 247t
intrinsic factor, as gastric secretion 555
intrinsic pathway (coagulation) 495, 496

intrinsic sympathomimetic activity 195
iodides, skin conditions from 907t
iodinated glycerol, thiourea interactions 649
iodine **648**, 783
    cancer treatment 761
    deficiency 640c
    goitrogenic effects 647–8
    hypothyroidism treatment 643
iodophors, for pressure sores 927
ion channels (membrane pores) 114
    anaesthetic effects on 229
    in CNS 220
    targeting 104–5
ionisation, effect on absorption 115
iontophoresis 587
ipecacuanha, vomiting induced by 569c
ipratropium
    asthma treatment 532, 535, 548c
    clinical use and administration 182t
    nasal condition treatment 549
    pregnancy safety 549
    respiratory treatments 530
iproniazide 328
irbesartan 457
    in Australia's top 10 drugs 17t
    pregnancy safety 457
irinotecan
    cancer treatment 776
    emetic potential 766t
    indications and toxicity 772t
iris 585
iron, *see also* haemoglobin
    during pregnancy 725
    epoetin alfa interactions 937
    iron-deficiency anaemia 494
    methyldopa interactions 453
    tetracycline interactions 816
irreversible antagonists, *see* depolarising
        blocking drugs
irreversible anticholinesterase agents 208–9
irrigating solutions 602, *see also* saline
        solutions
irritable bowel syndrome 560, 581
irritant expectorants 529
Irukandji syndrome 963c
ischaemia, *see* heart failure; stroke
ischiocavernosus 746
Islamic medicine 5
islets of Langerhans 666, *see also* pancreas
isoflurane 237, 237t
    pregnancy safety 248
isoniazid **858**
    antacid interactions 566t
    conjugation reaction 122t
    cycloserine interactions 857
    didanosine interactions 838
    imidazole antifungal interactions 829t
    ocular adverse effects 604t
    phenytoin interactions 306
    pregnancy safety 866
    skin conditions from 907t
    stavudine interactions 838
    tuberculosis treatment 546, 856–7
    zalcitabine interactions 840
isophane insulin 674t
isoprenaline 191
    asthma treatment 533
    pregnancy safety 199t
    selectivity of 104, 186
    shock, treatment for 192t
isoprenoids, chemical structure *10*

isopropyl alcohol
    ear treatment 611c, 614
    pregnancy safety 618
isosorbides 441
    pharmacokinetics 444t
    pregnancy safety 457
    sexual function affected by 747
isotretinoin
    acne treatment 920
    pregnancy safety 789, 928
    teratogenic potential 142t, 726
itraconazole 826, 827
    benzodiazepine interactions 288
    cytochrome P450 isoform inhibition
        158t
    didanosine interactions 838
    everolimus interactions 895
    glucocorticoid interactions 660t
    pharmacokinetics 829t
    pregnancy safety 844
    rifampicin interactions 859
    simvastatin interactions 467
    sirolimus interactions 895
IV, *see* intravenous infusions
ivermectin **865**
    pregnancy safety 866

J

jacksonian seizures, *see* epilepsy
jimson weed 179
juvenile-onset diabetes, *see* type 1 diabetes
juxtamedullary nephrons 475

K

kainate, receptors for 223
kaolins
    antidiarrhoeal agents 579, 580
    clindamycin interactions 814
    digoxin interactions 426t
kappa-opioid receptors, agonists 264t
katipo spider 961c
kava kava 392
    for pain relief 277c
    sedative effects 292c
Keppra, *see* levetiracetam
keratin 908
keratitis 595
kerato-conjunctivitis sicca 602
keratolytics 910
    acne treatment 921
    wart treatment 916
keratoplastics 910
ketamine 237, 403
    adjuvant analgesics 276
    anaesthetic 239
    pregnancy safety 248
ketoconazole 826–7
    antacid interactions 566t
    aprepitant interactions 570
    benzodiazepine interactions 288
    cyclosporin interactions 892
    cytochrome P450 isoform inhibition 158t
    delavirdine interactions 840
    didanosine interactions 838
    everolimus interactions 895
    glucocorticoid interactions 660t
    H_2-receptor antagonist interactions 572t
    indinavir interactions 842
    isoniazid interactions 858
    oral candidiasis treatment 564
    pharmacokinetics 829t

ketoconazole—cont'd
    pregnancy safety 844
    rifampicin interactions 859
    sexual function affected by 751
    simvastatin interactions 467
    sirolimus interactions 895
    topical antifungal 916, 918t
ketoprofen 879t
    pharmacokinetics 881t
    probenecid interactions 890
    risk of GIT effects 882
    warfarin interactions 505
ketorolac 879t
    ocular use 598
    pharmacokinetics 881t
    pregnancy safety 606
    warfarin interactions 505
ketotifen
    ocular use 598
    pregnancy safety 606
key (prototype) drugs 15
kidneys 474–7, *474*, *see also* nephrotoxicity;
        renal . . .; renin–angiotensin–aldosterone
        system
    adrenoceptors 188t
    drug excretion from 125
    innervation of 166t
    transplants 894
kinase-linked receptors 104
kinins, role in inflammation 871
Klebsiella infections 795t
    cephalosporin-resistant 809t
    drug resistance 805t
'knockout drops' 291c
kombucha mushroom 69

L

L-aromatic amino acid decarboxylase, *see* dopa
        decarboxylase
L-tryptophan, sedative effects 292c
labelling, *see* regulation
labetalol 195, 197t
    pharmacokinetics and dosages 198t
    pregnancy safety 199t
labour, *see* childbirth
lacrimal glands 167t, 585
lacrimators 606
lactamases 797, 804
lactation, *see* breastfeeding
lactulose **577**
lamivudine 836, 838
    pregnancy safety 844
lamotrigine 307
    anticonvulsant effects 300t, 303
    bipolar affective disorder treatment 334
    pregnancy safety 309
    sodium channel inhibitor 303
Langley, John N. 104c
lanolin
    emollient effects 909
    skin conditions from 907t
lanreotide 630t
    pregnancy safety 636
lansoprazole
    peptic ulcer treatment 571
    pregnancy safety 581
large intestine 559–60, 854–5
lasofoxifene 710
latanoprost **594**
    glaucoma treatment 592, 593t, 594
    pregnancy safety 606

latrodectism 962
Latrodectus katipo 961
latrotoxin, *see* alpha-latrotoxin
laxatives 574–8
  irritable bowel syndrome treatment 581
  OTC drugs 55
  palliative care in cancer treatment 787
  sites of action 576
LDLs 462, 464
leeches 504
leflunomide 885
  antirheumatic effects 884
  pregnancy safety 900
  warfarin interactions 505
legal issues, *see* illicit drugs; regulation;
    scheduling
Legionnaire's disease 546
lemon balm, sedative effects 292c
lemon-scented gum 797c
lenograstim, pregnancy safety 789
lens of the eye 585
lepirudin 500, 504–5
  pregnancy safety 512
leprosy 861–2
leptin analogues 953
leptin, role in obesity 949
lercanidipine 445, 446t
letrozole 779t, 781
leucocytes, *see* white blood cells
leucocytosis 494
leucopenia 494
Leucovorin, *see* calcium folinate
leukaemia, combination therapy 764
leukotriene-receptor antagonists, asthma
    treatment 532, 539
leukotrienes, role in inflammation 871
leuprorelin
  cancer treatment 779–80, 779t
  GnRH analogue 700t
  pregnancy safety 789
levamisole 785
  pregnancy safety 789
levetiracetam 307
  anticonvulsant effects 303
  pregnancy safety 309
levo-thyroxine, *see* thyroxine
levobunolol 197t
  glaucoma treatment 592, 593t
  pharmacokinetics and dosages 198t
  pregnancy safety 199t, 606
levobupivacaine
  local anaesthesia 243t
  nerve block anaesthesia 247t
  pregnancy safety 248
  spinal block anaesthesia 247t
levocabastine
  ocular use 598
  pregnancy safety 606
levodopa
  antihistamine interactions 899
  baclofen interactions 358
  carbidopa with **351–2**
  chlorpromazine interactions 323
  parkinsonism treatment 350–1, *351*
  perceptual states altered by 373
  pregnancy safety 366
  selegiline interactions 354
  sexual function affected by 747
  sleep pattern effects 284t
  taste and smell effects 617t
levonorgestrel 712, 714

levonorgestrel—cont'd
  contraceptive use 715t, 716
  depot preparations 716
  phased dosage 713c
  pregnancy safety 721
LH, *see* luteinising hormone
LH-releasing hormone (LHRH), *see*
    gonadotrophin-releasing hormone
libido, drugs affecting 746–8, *see also* sexual
    response
lice infestations 916–7
lichenification of the skin *906*, 907t
licorice
  as folk remedy 60t
  irritant expectorant 529
  mineralocorticoid activity 660c
  toxicity 67t
lidocaine, *see* lignocaine
lifestyle diseases 7
lifestyle drugs 92
ligand-gated ion channels 104, 220
lignocaine **241**, 430, 433–4, *see also* EMLA
    cream
  childbirth analgesia 234
  cimetidine interactions 572
  disopyramide interactions 432t
  erectile dysfunction treated with 749
  high hepatic clearance 132t
  infiltration anaesthesia 247t
  lipid solubility 242
  local anaesthetic 240–1, 243t
  mouth-washes and gargles containing 563
  nerve block anaesthesia 247t
  perinatal use 729
  pharmacokinetics 430t
  pregnancy safety 248, 437
  premature ejaculation treated with 751
  spinal block anaesthesia 247t
  suxamethonium interactions 207
  topical administration 244, 247t
  toxicity of 244
limbic system 217–8, *218*
  benzodiazepines act on 286
  role in ANS 163
  surgery to 322
lincomycin, pregnancy safety 821
lincosamides 814
linezolid 817
  pregnancy safety 821
liniments 910
liothyronine, *see* tri-iodothyronine
lipase, in pancreatic enzyme supplements
    573–4
lipid-lowering drugs 462–71, 603
lipid metabolism, *see also* hyperlipidaemia
  alcohol effects 388
  glucocorticoids in 654
lipid solubility of anaesthetics 229, *230*, 242
lipid theory of anaesthesia 229
lipodystrophy 675
lipolytic growth hormone fragments 953
lipoprotein lipase 462, 464t
lipoproteins 462
liposome delivery, cancer treatment 788
5-lipoxygenase inhibitors, asthma treatment
    539
liquid paraffin
  laxative effects 575
  pregnancy safety 581
liquids
  anaesthetics 237–9

liquids—cont'd
  dose calculation 21
  formulations of 42b
liquorice, *see* licorice
lisinopril
  ACE inhibitor 456
  pharmacokinetics 455t
  pregnancy safety 457
listed products, *see* regulation
lithium 290–1, **333**
  ACE inhibitor interactions 454
  age-related adverse drug events 319–20
  alopecia from 907t
  avoid during breastfeeding 144t
  bipolar affective disorder treatment 333–4
  chlorpromazine interactions 323
  didanosine interactions 838
  discovery of 312c
  headache treatment 366
  history of 334c
  loop diuretic interactions 482
  NSAID interactions 883
  ocular adverse effects 604t
  pancuronium interactions 205
  plasma concentration 332b
  potassium-sparing diuretic interactions 487
  pregnancy safety 320
  psoriasis treatment 920
  stavudine interactions 838
  suxamethonium interactions 207
  teratogenic potential 142t, 726
  thiazide diuretic interactions 485
  thiourea interactions 649
  thyroid effects 643
  zalcitabine interactions 840
live viruses, azathioprine interactions 893
livedo reticularis 354
liver 559
  adrenoceptors 188t
  anaesthesia and 234
  drugs extracted by 117
  function of 115t, 148
  innervation of 166t
  opioid sensitivity and 264
LMWHs 502–3, 510
loading doses 121, 133
lobelia, toxicity 67t
local anaesthetics 239–48, 243t
  adverse drug events 244–5
  for children 262
  interactions between 245
  ocular use 585, 598–9
  pharmacokinetics 241–2, *242*
  routes of administration *246*
  skin conditions from 907t
locomotor stimulation 339
lodoxamide 598
  pregnancy safety 606
lomustine
  cancer treatment 770
  hepatotoxicity 765
  indications and toxicity 771t
loop diuretics 481–2
  aminoglycoside interactions 815
  digoxin interactions 426t
  ototoxicity 615t
  pharmacokinetics 484t
  phenytoin interactions 306
  plasma lipid profile effects 464t
  pregnancy safety 482
  regulation in sport 937

loop of Henle 476–7
loperamide
  antidiarrhoeal agent 579–80
  cancer treatment 776
  for irritable bowel syndrome 581
  pregnancy safety 581
lopinavir 836, 841
  pregnancy safety 844
loratadine 900
  nasal condition treatment 548
  pregnancy safety 899
lorazepam
  abuse of 392
  anaesthetic 239
  antiemetic use 568
  anxiolytic 287
  pharmacokinetics 286t
  preoperative 288
  recommended for elderly 285
losartan **456**, 457
  pregnancy safety 457
lotions 910
low-density lipoproteins 462, 464
low-molecular-weight heparins 502–3, 510
LSD, see lysergic acid diethylamide
Lugol's solution 648c
lumefantrine 852–3
  pregnancy safety 866
luminal amoebicides 855
lumiracoxib, regulation in NZ 883c
lung cancer
  combination therapy 764t
  statistical studies 89c
  treatment regimen 762c
lungs 166t, 188t, 516–7
lupus erythematosus
  drug-induced 433, 449, 907t
  ocular effects 603
luteal hormones, see progestogens
luteinising hormone 626t, 698, 700, 709, see
    also human chorionic gonadotrophin
  in male reproductive system 734
  infertility treatment 740
luteinising-hormone-releasing hormone, see
    gonadotrophin-releasing hormone
luteolytic agents, contraceptive effects 742
lutropin alfa 700
  pregnancy safety 751
lymph nodes 870–1, 870
lymphocytes 494, 870–1, see also immune
    system
lymphokines, immunostimulation by 896
lypressin 636
lyprinol 884c
lysergic acid diethylamide 353, 402–3, 729c
  sexual function affected by 747
  symptoms of abuse 375t

M

ma huang 67t, 543c
macrolide antibiotics 812–4
  benzodiazepine interactions 288
  cyclosporin interactions 892
  drug groups 13t
  theophylline interactions 537
macromolecules 757, 758
macrophages 494, 871
macules 906
madderwort, toxicity 67t
maggots, debridation with 926
magic bullet drugs 6

'magic mushrooms', see psilocybin
magnesium, see also hypomagnesaemia
  cardiac system requires 417
  tetracycline interactions 816
magnesium hydroxide
  antacids 565, 565t
  mycophenolate mofetil interactions 895
magnesium salts
  adverse drug events 566t
  laxative effects 577
  pancuronium interactions 205
magnesium sulfate 308
  magnoplasm 910
  pre-eclampsia treatment 725
  tocolytic effects 728
magnoplasm 910
maidenhair tree 62t
maintenance dose rates 132b
  anticonvulsants 301–2
  phenytoin 302
major depression, see depression
malaria 6, 359c, 848–9, see also antimalarials
maldison (malathion) 916–7
  pregnancy safety 928
  topical poisoning by 905c
male climacteric 698, 736
male pill **743**
male reproductive system 698, 705–6, see also
    reproductive systems; sex hormones
  contraception 742
  drugs affecting 734–7
  infertility 740
malignant hyperthermia/hyperpyrexia 207
  anaesthesia-related 232
  neuroleptic malignant syndrome 316, 316t
  ryanodine receptor mutation 344
malignant tumours, see cancer treatment;
    neoplasia
mammotrophin, see prolactin
Manderson, Desmond 82
mania 312, 334–5, see also bipolar affective
    disorders
manna gum 884c
mannitol 487
  glaucoma treatment 595
  laxative effects 577c
manufacture of drugs 78–9, 82–3
MAO, see monoamine oxidase
MAO inhibitors, see monoamine oxidase
    inhibitors
Maoris, see also New Zealand
  diabetes in 669c
  dietary calcium 688c
  psychiatric disorders 321c
  renal disorders 475c
marijuana 399–402, see also cannabinoids
  abuse of 374t
  avoid during breastfeeding 144t
  regulation in sport 938
  sexual function affected by 746
  spider's webs affected by 373
  theophylline interactions 537
marine creatures, stinging 962–4
marketing
  ethical issues 98
  legal issues 79
  of OTC drugs 57
mast-cell stabilisers 548c
  asthma treatment 532, 534, 539–40
  conjunctivitis treatment 598
  nasal condition treatment 549

mast-cell stabilisers—cont'd
  ocular use 598
mast cells
  effect of blockers on 205
  role in immunostimulation 896
maternal pharmacokinetics 140–1
matrix metalloproteinases, cancer treatment
    762
maturity-onset diabetes, see type 2 diabetes
Mawson, Sir Douglas 921c
maximal efficacy 107
MDA 403c
MDIs 519, 520
MDMA, see 'ecstasy'
MDR1 114
mebendazole 864–5
  pregnancy safety 866
mebeverine, clinical use and administration
    182t
mecamylamine, sexual function affected by
    749
medical gases 525c
medical practitioners, see doctors; health
    professionals
medication
  definition 2, 3t
  for the elderly 149t
  hospital drug charts 38–9, 38
medicinal leeches 504
medicine cabinets 46c
Medicines Act 1981 (NZ) 83
medieval period, medicine in 5–6
Medimate booklets 18
medroxyprogesterone acetate 712, **713**
  cancer treatment 779t, 781
  contraceptive use 715c
  pregnancy safety 789
medulla oblongata 215
  anaesthetic paralysis 229
  emetic trigger zone 783
  respiratory involvement 518
  role in ANS 163
medulla of the kidney 474, see also adrenal
    cortex
medulla of the lymph node 871
mefenamic acid 879t
  pharmacokinetics 881t
  warfarin interactions 505
mefloquine 849–51
  pregnancy safety 866
  quinine interactions 852
megestrol 712
  cancer treatment 779t, 781
  pregnancy safety 789
Melaleuca 271c, 543c, 797c
melanin, synthesis of 904
melanocyte-stimulating hormone 626t
melanocytes 904
melanoma 755c, see also skin cancers
melatonin 56c, 292c
meloxicam 879t
  COX-2 inhibitor 880
  pharmacokinetics 881t
  regulation 882, 883c
melphalan 770, 771t
memantine
  Alzheimer's disease treatment 362
  pregnancy safety 366
membrane pores, see ion channels (membrane
    pores)
membrane potentials 169, 220

membranes, *see* cell membranes
memory, *see also* amnesia
  drugs enhancing 344c
  impaired by ECT 322
memory T cells 873
men, *see* gender differences; male reproductive
    system
menarche 701
Ménière's disease 613c
meningococcal disease 876c
menopause 321, 698, 717–8
menorrhagia 704c
menstrual cycle 701–4, *703*
  anticonvulsants and 300
  contractions during 726
  disorders of 704c
  role in contraception 741
mental illness, *see* psychiatric disorders;
    psychotropic agents
menthol 528, 580, 909
mepacrine 359c
meperidine, *see* pethidine
mepivacaine
  infiltration anaesthesia 247t
  local anaesthetic 243t
  pregnancy safety 248
  toxicity of 244
merbaphen 481c
6-mercaptopurine, *see* mercaptopurine
mercaptopurine 158, 770c
  allopurinol interactions 888
  cancer treatment 773
  chemical structure 773
  emetic potential 766t
  hepatotoxicity 765
  immunosuppressant 892
  indications and toxicity 771t
  inflammatory bowel disease treatment 580
  photosensitising effects 907t
  pregnancy safety 789
mercurous chloride 481c
meropenem, pregnancy safety 821
merozoites 848
mesalazine **580**
  in sulfasalazine 885
  inflammatory bowel disease treatment 580
  pregnancy safety 581
mescaline 403
  abuse of 375t
  perceptual states altered by 402
mesna
  hydration therapy 784
  pregnancy safety 789
mesolimbic pathway, involved in dependence
    375
mesterolone 734, 737
mestranol 709, 714
  contraceptive use 712, 715t
mesylate, *see* phentolamine
meta-analyses 27, 91
metabolic tolerance, *see* tolerance
metabolism of drugs 121–6, *see also*
    excretion
  defined 114b
  drug interactions affecting 157–8
  enzymes in 122–3
  fetal 141
  in children 144–7
  in the elderly 148b
  paracetamol 273
metabolites 87, 121

metaraminol 193
  pregnancy safety 199t
metastasis of cancers 755
metered-dose inhalers 519, *520*
metformin 669c, 677–9
  infertility treatment 740
  pharmacokinetics 678t
  pregnancy safety 681
methadone 267, **385–6**
  abuse of 374t
  as substitute drug 384
  dosage forms 266t
  drug dependence treatment 382
  mu-receptor agonist 264t
  neonatal withdrawal symptoms 143t
  nevirapine interactions 841
  phenytoin interactions 306
  pregnancy safety 278, 405
  regulation in sport 937
  rifampicin interactions 859
methamphetamines
  abuse of 374t, 379c, 393
  anorectic agents 951
methanol 386c, 604, 604t
methdilazine, pregnancy safety 899
methicillin, resistance to 798t
methohexitone, pregnancy safety 248
methotrexate 104, **775–6**
  antirheumatic effects 884
  avoid during breastfeeding 144t
  cancer treatment 762–3, 773
  chemical structure 773
  combination therapy 764t
  emetic potential 766t
  hepatotoxicity 765
  immunosuppressant 892
  indications and toxicity 771t
  inflammatory bowel disease treatment 580
  liposome delivery 788
  myelosuppression from 784
  neurotoxicity 765
  NSAID interactions 883
  pregnancy safety 789
  probenecid interactions 158, 890
  psoriasis treatment 920
  renal toxicity 765
  resistance to 766
  sulfonamides/trimethoprim interactions 820
  taste and smell effects 617t
  teratogenic potential 142t, 726
  topical administration 917
methoxsalen
  photosensitising effects 907t, 911
  pregnancy safety 928
methoxyflurane 237
  pregnancy safety 248
methoxypsoralen, photosensitising effects
    907t
1-methyl-4-phenyl-1,2,3,6-tetrahydropyridine
    350c
methyl aminolevulinate, cancer treatment 782
methyl anthranilate 913t
4-methyl-benzylidene camphor 913t
N-methyl-d-aspartate receptors 223, 362
methyl salicylate (Oil of Wintergreen) 616, 910
methylated spirits 386c, 604, 604t
methylcellulose 574–5, 602
methyldopa
  age-related adverse drug events 150
  hypertension treatment 450–3
  MAO inhibitor interactions 331

methyldopa—cont'd
  phentermine interactions 952
  pregnancy safety 457
  sexual function affected by 750
  sleep pattern effects 284t
  zalcitabine interactions 840
methylenedioxyamphetamine 403c
3,4-methylenedioxymethamphetamine, *see*
    'ecstasy'
methylphenethylamine, *see* amphetamine
methylphenidate
  for ADHD 342
  potential for abuse 340, 340c
  pregnancy safety 346
methylprednisolone
  antiemetic use 570
  pharmacokinetics 657t
  pregnancy safety 662
  topical administration 919
methylxanthines 339, 343–6
  asthma treatment 535
  perceptual states altered by 373
methysergide 353, 729c
  analgesic effects 276
  headache treatment 366
  migraine treatment 364
  pregnancy safety 366
metoclopramide **568**
  alcohol interactions 391
  antiemetic use 567t, 568
  cancer treatment 783
  levodopa–carbidopa interactions 352
  migraine treatment 364
  morning sickness treatment 569c
  postoperative 230
  pregnancy safety 581, 726, 789
  sleep pattern effects 284t
  stimulates lactation 730
metoprolol 197t, 436
  insulin interactions 675
  lumefantrine interactions 853
  pharmacokinetics and dosages 198t
  pregnancy safety 199t
  sexual function affected by 750
metric system 19–20, 20t
metronidazole 819
  alcohol interactions 391
  amoebicidal agent 855
  didanosine interactions 838
  peptic ulcer treatment 570
  pregnancy safety 821
  pressure sore treatment 927
  stavudine interactions 838
  topical administration 915
  trichomoniasis treatment 855
  warfarin interactions 505
  zalcitabine interactions 840
metrorrhagia 704c
mexiletine 430, 435
  pharmacokinetics 430t
  pregnancy safety 437
  rifampicin interactions 859
mianserin 333
  adverse drug events 319t
  pregnancy safety 320, 329
  recommended treatment 328
  sedative effects 328
MICA paramedics 31
'Mickey Finns' 291c
miconazole 826, 827
  isoniazid interactions 858

miconazole—cont'd
    oral candidiasis treatment 564
    pharmacokinetics 829t
    pregnancy safety 844
    skin conditions from 907t
    topical antifungal 916, 918t
    warfarin interactions 505
microbial infections 794
    following burns 924
    links with cancer 760
    ocular, treatment 595–7
    OTC drugs for 53t
    pressure sores 925
microorganisms, drugs from 7
micropump systems 42b
Microsporum infections 916
micturition, *see* urinary tract
midazolam
    adjunct to anaesthesia 237
    adverse drug events 234
    amprenavir interactions 842t
    anaesthetic 239
    efavirenz interactions 840
    for day procedures 232
    indinavir interactions 842
    macrolide antibiotic interactions 812
    parenteral administration 288
    pharmacokinetics 286t
    premedication with 230, 235t, 288
    quinupristin interactions 818
    ritonavir interactions 843
    saquinavir interactions 843
midbrain 163, 214–5
middle ear 611–2
midwives, drugs administered by 33
migraine treatment 363–5
    antidepressants 328
    CNS effects 214c
milk–alkali syndrome 567c
milkwood tree 797c
milrinone
    cardiac treatment 428
    dobutamine interactions 193
    mechanism of action 424
mind and emotions 313–4, *see also*
        antidepressants; anxiolytics; psychotropic
        agents
mineral oil, ear treatment 614
mineralocorticoids 627t, 653, 659–63, *see*
        also corticosteroids
    amphotericin B interactions 828
    rifampicin interactions 859
minerals, *see also names of individual minerals*
    drugs from 7
    nutritional supplements 55–6, 692
minimum pricing policy 28
minipill (oral contraceptive) 714–5
minocycline 815–6
    dosage 815t
    leprosy treatment 862
    pregnancy safety 821
minor tranquillisers, *see* anxiolytics
minoxidil
    angina treatment 445, 447–8
    fast-tracking of 749c
    pregnancy safety 457, 928
miosis of the eye 588
miotic agents 590
    glaucoma treatment 592, 593t, 594
mirtazapine 334
    pregnancy safety 320

miscarriage 533, 725
misoprostol
    combination analgesics 274
    for drug-induced GIT effects 882
    peptic ulcer treatment 570, 573
    pregnancy safety 581, 730
missed doses 133c
misuse of drugs 371, *see also* abuse of drugs
mitochondria, in heart muscle 412
mitomycin
    cancer treatment 772t
    emetic potential 766t
    mechanism of action 776
mitosis 756
mitotic inhibitors
    cancer treatment 761, 776
    indications and toxicity 772t
mitozantrone
    cancer treatment 772t
    mechanism of action 776
mivacurium 204, 206t
    pregnancy safety 248
mixed infections 800
mixed seizures 289
Mobile Intensive Care Ambulance service 31
mobilisation of calcium 690
moclobemide 332–3
    adverse drug events 319t
    cytochrome P450 isoform inhibition 158t
    hypertension due to 318c
    mechanism of action 328
    morphine interactions 268
    pregnancy safety 320, 329
    sexual function affected by 750
    sumatriptan interactions 365
modafinil, for narcolepsy 342
mole (number) 19
molecular biology 7
molecular targets 104–7, *see also*
        neurotransmitters; receptors
mometasone
    nasal condition treatment 548
    pregnancy safety 662
    topical administration 919
monitoring therapy
    anticonvulsants 301
    decisions about 35–6
    plasma digoxin 428b
monkshood, toxicity 67t
monoamine neurotransmitters *404*
monoamine oxidase 174
monoamine oxidase inhibitors
    acetylcholine balance 224
    adrenaline interactions 190
    adverse drug events 319t
    antidepressants 330–3
    baclofen interactions 358
    beta-blocker interactions 198t
    dexamphetamine interactions 341
    diethylpropion interactions 952
    diphenoxylate interactions 579
    entacapone interactions 355
    hydralazine interactions 449
    levodopa–carbidopa interactions 352
    mechanism of action *326*, 327–8
    methyldopa interactions 453
    migraine treatment 364
    morphine interactions 268
    noradrenaline interactions 191
    phentermine interactions 952
    pseudoephedrine interactions 544

monoamine oxidase inhibitors—cont'd
    selegiline interactions 354
    sexual function affected by 750
    sleep pattern effects 284t
    sumatriptan interactions 365
    sympathomimetic drugs interact with 157
monoamine pathways 222
monoamine theory 326
monoamines 221–4, *see also* 5-
        hydroxytryptamine; neurotransmitters
monobactam antibiotics, mechanism of action
        804
monoclonal antibodies, *see also names of*
        specific agents
    cancer treatment 762, 781–2
    drug groups 13t
    monitoring 760
monocytes 494, 871
monophasic oral contraceptives 714–5
monosodium glutamate 222, 365
monotherapy for epilepsy 299
monovalent antivenoms 959, 960t
montelukast
    asthma treatment 539
    pregnancy safety 549
mood disorders 312, *see also* bipolar affective
        disorder; depression
MOPP combination, for Hodgkin's disease 764
morning after pill 714–6, 741
morning sickness 569c, 725
morphine 265, **268–9**
    abuse of 374t
    adjunct to anaesthetic 230
    analgesic use 262–3
    biguanide interactions 678
    conjugation reaction 122t
    dosage forms 266t
    during childbirth 262
    high hepatic clearance 132t
    kappa-receptor agonist 264t
    limbic effects 218
    mu-receptor agonist 264t
    neonatal withdrawal symptoms 143t
    pregnancy safety 278
    premedication with 230, 235t
    regulation in sport 937
    sexual function affected by 746
mosquitoes 848, *see also* malaria
motility of gastrointestinal tract 553
motor cortex *202*, 217, *see also* muscles
    output 163
    role in SNS 202
motor end-plate nicotinic receptors, role in
        SNS 202–5
motor pathways *202*
mountain pepper 826c
mountain tobacco, toxicity 67t
mouth 553–4, *see also* oral administration
    absorption from 116
    drugs affecting 563–5
mouth-washes 563–4
moxifloxacin 818
MPA, *see* medroxyprogesterone acetate
MPPP 403c
MPTP, parkinsonism from 350c
MSH 626t
MTX, *see* methotrexate
mu-opioid receptors, agonists 264t
mucilages 11
mucociliary blanket 517, 528–31
mucolytic drugs 529–30, 542

mucous membranes
    administration via 42b
    effect of atropine 180
    gastrointestinal tract 554
    respiratory system 517
mugwort, toxicity 67t
multi-infarct dementia 362
multiple drug use, *see* polypharmacy
multiple sclerosis 172c, 359–60
mumps 554, 796t
mupirocin
    pregnancy safety 928
    pressure sore treatment 927
    topical antimicrobial 915
muromonab-CD3:
    for rejection control 894
    pregnancy safety 900
muscarinic receptor agonists 178, 181t, *see also* miotic agents
    adverse drug events 178
    in sexual response 705
    interactions among 179
muscarinic receptor antagonists 178–9, 181t, 182t, *see also* anticholinergics; parasympatholytics
    antiemetic use 567t, 568–9
    asthma treatments 535–6
    cough treatments 542
    drug interactions with 157
    miotic effects 590
    respiratory treatments 530
muscarinic receptors 171–2
    density decreases with age 149
    drugs acting on 178, 178t
    pesticides and nerve gas effects 209
muscle relaxants 355–9
    adjuncts to anaesthesia 235
    age-related adverse drug events 150
    aminoglycoside interactions 815
    botulinum toxin interactions 601
    palliative care in cancer treatment 787
    premedication with 235t
    psychotropic agent interactions 318
    vancomycin interactions 812
muscle spasms, *see also* antispasmodic agents; epilepsy
    benzodiazepines for 288
    nociceptive pain 256
    treatment of 356–7
muscles, *see* motor cortex; musculoskeletal system; smooth muscle
muscularis 554
musculoskeletal system
    caffeine effects 344
    cardiac muscle 411
    effect of blockers on 204–5
    ocular effect of disorders 603
    over-the-counter drugs for 53t
mushrooms
    psilocybin 375t, 402–3
    toxicity 67t
mussels
    anti-inflammatory effects 884c
    as folk remedy 60t
    respiratory treatment 543c
mustine, for Hodgkin's disease 764
mutagens 139b, *see also* teratogens
    cancer treatment 767
    carcinogenesis induced by 759
myasthenia gravis 356c, 357
    ocular effect of 603

myasthenia gravis—cont'd
    treatment of 209, 355–6
mycobacterial infections 785, 795t, *see also* leprosy; tuberculosis
mycophenolate mofetil 895
    pregnancy safety 900
Mycoplasma infections 795t
mycoses 826
mydriatic agents 585, 588–90
    atropine 180
    ocular use 597
myelin sheaths 167, *168*
myelosuppression, *see* bone marrow suppressants
myocardial infarction, treatment of 197
myocardial ischaemia, *see* stroke
myocardium 411–2
    action potentials *416*
    calcium-channel blocker effects 443
    contraction 415
myoclonic seizures 297, 300t
myofibrils 412
myolysis from snake bite 959
myosin 412, 417
Mytacea 797c
myxoedema 640, 643–4

N

NA, *see* noradrenaline
nafarelin, GnRH analogue 700t
nalorphine, mu-receptor antagonist 264t
naloxone 269–70
    conjugation reaction 122t
    during childbirth 262
    kappa-receptor antagonist 264t
    morphine interactions 268
    mu-receptor antagonist 264t
    overdose treatment with 383
    perinatal use 729
    postoperative 235
    pregnancy safety 278, 405
naltrexone 269–70, **382**
    morphine interactions 268
    pregnancy safety 278, 405
names of drugs 12c, 12–4
nandrolone
    anabolic steroid 735
    as orphan drug 80t
    drug testing for 942c
    regulation in sport 934
    synthetic androgen 734
naphazoline
    ocular use 590, 590t, 591–2
    pregnancy safety 606
naphthalene, photosensitising effects 907t
naphtholophenol, contraceptive effects 742
naproxen 879t
    age-related adverse drug events 262
    dosage 880
    migraine treatment 364
    pharmacokinetics 881t
    probenecid interactions 890
    ulcer risk 879
naratriptan
    migraine treatment 364
    pregnancy safety 366
narcolepsy 342, *see also* sleep disorders
narcotic drugs 265c
    legislation against 378
    regulation in sport 933, 937–8
Narcotic Goods Act (Cth) 83

narrow-spectrum penicillins 804
nasal administration 117
nasal conditions
    antihistamine treatment 898
    drugs for 53t, 547–9
nasolacrimal ducts 585
nasopharyngeal glands, innervation of 167t
National Competition Review of Drugs, Poisons and Controlled Substances 77
National Drugs and Poisons Schedule Committee 77
National Medicines Policy (NMP) 28
native cabbage 826c
native senna 577c
natriuresis 481
NATs, *see* acetyltransferases
natural killer cells 871
'natural products', *see* complementary and alternative medicine; herbal remedies
naturally acquired immunity 874–5
naturopathy 63, *see also* complementary and alternative medicine; herbal remedies
nausea, *see also* antiemetics; vomiting
    cancer treatment 765, 783
    ear disorders 612
    morning sickness 725
nebulisers 519
Necator americanus 864
neck, respiratory structures 547
nedocromil **539**
    asthma treatment 539
    pregnancy safety 549
nefazodone
    adverse drug events 319t
    pregnancy safety 320
    recommended treatment 328
negative feedback, endocrine system 623
negative inotropic effects 422, 449
Neisseria infections 795t
    cephalosporin-resistant 809t
    drug-resistant 798t, 805t
nelfinavir 836, 841–3
    cytochrome P450 isoform inhibition 158t
    pregnancy safety 844
    saquinavir interactions 843
nematodes 863–4
neomycin
    ear treatment 613–4
    lactulose interactions 577
    ocular use 595–6
    ototoxicity 615
    pregnancy safety 606, 618, 821, 915
    skin conditions from 907t
    topical administration 915
neonates, *see also* babies; infants; paediatrics
    anaesthesia 233
    analgesia 262
    dosage 145t
    drug metabolism in 144
    epilepsy in 298
    fetal alcohol syndrome 141c
    fetal distress syndrome 261
    neonatal withdrawal symptoms 143t
    oxygen-induced blindness 605
    retrolental fibroplasia 527c
neoplasia, *see* cancer treatment
neostigmine 104, 207, **209**
    myasthenia gravis treatment 603
    pancuronium interactions 205
    pregnancy safety 366
nephrons 477, *481*

nephrotoxicity
ABC powders 275c
amphotericin B 828
cyclosporin 892
foscarnet 835
NSAIDs 883
snake bite 959
nerve block anaesthesia 246–7, 247t
nerve cells, *see* neurons
nerve fibres, *see* axons
nerve gases (anticholinesterases) 208–9
nervous system *168, see also* autonomic
nervous system; central nervous system;
parasympathetic nervous system;
peripheral nervous system; sympathetic
nervous system
cardiac innervation *414*
drugs toxic to 765
gastrointestinal tract nerves 553
OTC drugs for 53t
respiratory involvement 518–9
response to high sympathetic drive *189*
susceptibility to anaesthesia 241
neuraminidase inhibitors 831, 833
neuroactive peptides, *see* neuropeptides
neurochemical transmission 169, 221, *see also*
neurotransmitters
neurodegenerative disorders 349–63
neuroeffector junctions 169, *173, 174*
neurogenic pain 256
neurohypophysis 626, 626t, 630–5, 656
neurokinins A and B, respiratory involvement
518
neuroleptanalgesia 231–2
neuroleptic malignant syndrome, *see*
malignant hyperthermia/hyperpyrexia
neuroleptics, *see also* antipsychotics;
psychotropic agents
age-related adverse drug events 149t
discovery of 312c
levodopa–carbidopa interactions 352
sexual function affected by 750
neurological disorders 349–63
neuromuscular blocking drugs 178, 204–5,
357–8, *see also* depolarising blocking
drugs; non-depolarising blocking drugs
adjuncts to anaesthesia 235
capreomycin interactions 857
clindamycin interactions 814
pesticides and nerve gases 209
procainamide interactions 433t
sites of action *208*
neuromuscular junctions 202–4, *203*
neurons 165–7, *167*
action potentials 219–24
in efferent pathways 165
neuropathic pain 256, 276
analgesics for 258
anticonvulsant treatment 303
antidepressant treatment 328
neuropeptides 221–2, 518
hypothalamic factors 630–1
neuropeptide Y 949, 953
neuroses 284, 312, 328
neurotransmitters 169, 172c, *see also*
acetylcholine; monoamines
anaesthetic effects on 229
autonomic nervous system *171*
food intake regulation 948–9
imbalances in *223*
in CNS 220–4

neurotransmitters—cont'd
in migraine 363–4
in psychiatric disorders 313
in sexual response 705
in vomiting 567
pain pathways *254*
regulate anterior pituitary 630
neutrophils 494
nevirapine 836, 840–1
pregnancy safety 844
new drugs 30–1
new genetics 94–5
New South Wales, regulation 76t
New Zealand, *see also* Maoris
antibiotic resistance control 806c
asthma incidence 531, 533c
Centre for Adverse Reactions Monitoring
159c
clinical trials in 93–4
complementary and alternative medicine
in 59
coronary heart disease 412c
diabetes 669c
dietary calcium 688c
drug abuse and misuse 340c, 379c
drug information 18
drug regulation 83–4
Fantasy abuse 358c
fluoridated water 563c
health surveys 453c
hepatitis C 835c
Intensive Medicines Monitoring Programme
92c
meningococcal disease 876c
methadone maintenance program 385c
obesity 947, 947c
Preferred Medicines List 28
Primary Health Care Strategy 32c
selenium use 56c
Trans-Tasman Scheduling Harmonisation 77
venomous spiders 961c
newborns, *see* neonates
niacin, *see* nicotinic acid
nicorandil
angina treatment 445–7
pregnancy safety 457
nicotine **397–8**, *see also* nicotinic receptors;
tobacco use
abuse of 371, 374t, 394–6
avoid during breastfeeding 144t
diabetic effects 673c
oestradiol valerate interactions 711
oxytocin released by 635
pregnancy safety 405
replacement therapy 396
sexual function affected by 747
sleep pattern effects 284t
taste and smell effects 617t
theophylline interactions 537
topical administration 908
transdermal administration 910
nicotinic acid
hyperlipidaemia treatment 467t, 469t, 470
pregnancy safety 470
nicotinic receptor agonists, *see* depolarising
blocking drugs
nicotinic receptors 171–2
nifedipine 446t
angina treatment 445
cimetidine interactions 572
pharmacokinetics 446t

nifedipine—cont'd
pregnancy safety 457, 730
quinupristin interactions 818
sexual function affected by 750
skin conditions from 907t
taste and smell effects 617t
tocolytic effects 728
nigrostriatal tracts, involved in parkinsonism
349
nikethamide 942c
nilutamide
antiandrogens 737
cancer treatment 779, 779t
nimodipine
Alzheimer's disease treatment 362
angina treatment 445
pregnancy safety 457
nitrates
alcohol interactions 391
effects compared 448t
migraine triggered by 363
pharmacokinetics 444t
sildenafil interactions 748
vasodilators 441–3
nitrazepam
pharmacokinetics 286t
sleep disorder treatment 287
nitric oxide
blood transport of 493
in angina 442
in childbirth 727
in penile erection 745
in sexual function 748
respiratory involvement 518
nitrites, symptoms of abuse 375t
nitroferricyanide, *see* sodium nitroprusside
nitrofurantoin
didanosine interactions 838
drug interactions 822
probenecid interactions 890
quinolone interactions 818
skin conditions from 907t
stavudine interactions 838
urinary tract infection treatment 820
zalcitabine interactions 840
nitrogen mustards
cancer treatment 770
emetic potential 766t
indications and toxicity 771t
nitroglycerine, *see* glyceryl trinitrate
nitroprusside, *see* sodium nitroprusside
nitrosamines, links with cancer 760
nitrosoureas
cancer treatment 762, 770
emetic potential 766t
indications and toxicity 771t
nitrous oxide **236**
anaesthesia 230
analgesia 261
didanosine interactions 838
medical gas 525c
perinatal use 261, 729
pregnancy safety 248
waste gases a hazard 233c
zalcitabine interactions 840
nizatidine
peptic ulcer treatment 572, 572t
pregnancy safety 581
NK cells 871
NK$_1$ receptor antagonists, antiemetic use 567t
NMDA 223, 362

NMDA channel modulators, adjuvant analgesics 276
NMJs 202–4, *203*
NMP (National Medicines Policy) 28
NNRTIs 836, 840–1
nociceptin, discovery of 95
nociceptive pain 252, 256, 258, *see also* pain
nodes of Ranvier 167
nodules of the skin *906*
nomograms 145, *146*
non-barbiturate anaesthetic agents 239
non-competitive antagonists 109
non-depolarising blocking drugs 204–5, 206t
   adjuncts to anaesthesia 235
   cancer treatment 763
   muscle relaxants 357
   reversible antagonists 108
non-drug contraception 742–5
non-drug therapy, psychiatric disorders 321–2
non-linear pharmacokinetic parameters 305
non-nucleoside reverse transcriptase inhibitors 836, 840–1
non-rapid eye movement (non-REM) sleep 282
non-selective alpha-adrenoceptor antagonists 194–5
non-selective beta-adrenoceptor antagonists 197t
non-specific resistance to disease 870–1
non-steroidal anti-inflammatory drugs 270–5, 879–84, *see also* aspirin
   abuse of 405
   ACE inhibitor interactions 454
   adverse drug events 234, 882
   age-related adverse drug events 149t, 150
   Alzheimer's disease treatment 362
   aminoglycoside interactions 815
   anticoagulant interactions 506
   antihypertensives interactions 157
   aspirin interactions 274
   avoid during pregnancy 261
   beta-blocker interaction 198t
   cephalosporin interactions 810
   cidofovir interactions 834
   cyclophosphamide interactions 774
   cyclosporin interactions 892
   dysfunctional uterine bleeding treatment 720
   glycoprotein IIb/IIIa receptor inhibitor interactions 510
   gout treatment 887
   heparin interactions 501
   lithium interactions 318, 333
   loop diuretic interactions 482
   methotrexate interactions 775
   ocular use 597, 598
   ototoxicity 615t
   pain treatment 255t
   palliative care in cancer treatment 787
   paracetamol combined with 273
   penicillin interactions 806
   pharmacokinetics 880, 881t
   postoperative 235
   potassium-sparing diuretic interactions 487
   probenecid interactions 890
   prostaglandins inhibited by 255
   psoriasis treatment 920
   sites of action *880*
   taste and smell effects 617t
   thiazide diuretic interactions 485
   tocolytic effects 728
   urticaria treatment 920
   zidovudine interactions 837

noradrenaline 172–3, 190–1
   adverse drug events 191
   cardiac action linked to 419
   in peripheral nervous system 169
   mania associated with 326
   mechanism of action *326*
   pregnancy safety 199t
   psychiatric disorders linked to 313
   reuptake 174
   selectivity of 186
   shock, treatment for 192t
   stress induces release of 653
noradrenergic transmission *197*
   drugs affecting 186–99, 950–1
norepinephrine, *see* noradrenaline
norethisterone 712, 714
   alopecia from 907t
   contraceptive use 712, 715t
   hormone replacement therapy 719
   pregnancy safety 721
norethynodrel, contraceptive use 712
norfloxacin 818
   sucralfate interactions 573
   urinary tract infection treatment 820
norfluoxetine 330
Northern Territory, drug legislation 76t
nortriptyline
   adverse drug events 319t
   age-related adverse drug events 328
   pregnancy safety 320
norverapamil 445
nose, *see* nasal administration; olfaction, drugs affecting
NRTIs 836–40
NSAIDs, *see* non-steroidal anti-inflammatory drugs
nuclear receptors 104
nucleic acids, synthesis of 757
nucleoside reverse transcriptase inhibitors (NRTIs) 836–40
null hypotheses 86
nurses, drugs administered by 33
nutritional supplements, *see also* diet
   drug interactions with 158–9
   OTC drugs 55
nystatin **564**, 826
   ear treatment 613–4
   griseofulvin interactions 830
   oral candidiasis treatment 564
   OTC vs prescription variants 52t
   pregnancy safety 581, 618, 844, 928
   topical administration 918t
   topical antifungals 916

O

oats, as folk remedy 60t
obesity
   anaesthesia and 234
   drugs in 947–54
   sites of treatment action *950*
occlusive dressings 908, 919
occupational therapists, drugs administered by 34
octocrylene 913t
octreotide 630t, **634**
   cancer treatment 779t
   hypoglycaemia linked to 672t
   pregnancy safety 636, 789
octyl methoxycinnamate 913t
octyl salicylate 913t
ocular . . ., *see also* eyes

ocular effects, cannabinoids 401
ocular hypertension, *see* glaucoma
ocular inserts 587
oculomotor nerve 215t
oedema 6, 482
   digitalis treatment 423
   diuretic therapy 481
   following infection 871
oesophagus 554, 816
oestradiol 627t, 698, 709
   hormone replacement therapy 718–9
   transdermal administration 910
oestradiol valerate **711**
   pregnancy safety 721
oestriol 698, 709
   hormone replacement therapy 719
   pregnancy safety 721
oestrogen receptors 709
oestrogens 698, 709–10, *see also* antioestrogens
   acne treatment 922
   affects sexual function 745
   Alzheimer's disease treatment 362
   bone effects 692
   cancer treatment 780
   contraceptive use 715t
   contraceptives containing 741
   dantrolene interactions 360
   didanosine interactions 838
   griseofulvin interactions 830
   in male reproductive system 734
   lactation inhibited by 730
   levels during pregnancy 725
   migraine triggered by 363
   nevirapine interactions 841
   ocular adverse effects 604t
   phenytoin interactions 306
   prostate cancer treatment 778
   ritonavir interactions 843
   sexual function affected by 746–7
   tetracycline interactions 816
   topical administration 908
oestrone 698, 709
ofloxacin 818
   leprosy treatment 862
   ocular use 596
   pregnancy safety 606
   sucralfate interactions 573
   taste and smell effects 617t
oil-in-water creams 909
oil of cloves 910
oils, drugs from 12
ointments 909
OITP 114
olanzapine 325
   bipolar affective disorder treatment 334
   in Australia's top 10 drugs 17t
   major effects 315t
   pregnancy safety 320
   sexual function affected by 750
old man weed 884c
older people, *see* elderly
olfaction, drugs affecting 617t, 618
olfactory nerve 215t
oligospermia treatment 740
olive oil, as ear treatment 614
olopatadine
   ocular use 598
   pregnancy safety 606
olsalazine 580–1
   pregnancy safety 581

Olympic Games
  drug testing at 941–2, 941t
  influenza precautions 541c
omalizumab 539
omeprazole **571**
  diazepam interactions 287
  in Australia's top 10 drugs 17t
  peptic ulcer treatment 571
  phenytoin interactions 306
on–off syndrome 351, 352c
Onchocerca volvulus 865
oncogenes 760
oncology, *see* cancer treatment
ondansetron **569**
  antiemetic use 567t, 569
  postoperative 230
  pregnancy safety 581, 789
onychomycoses 916
ophthalmic administration, *see* eyes
opiates, *see* opioids
opioid agonists 263, 264t, 265–9
opioid antagonists 269–70
opioid peptides 222
opioids, *see also* abuse of drugs; narcotic drugs
  abuse of 374t, 376, 383–6
  adverse drug events 259
  age-related adverse drug events 149t
  alcohol interactions 390, 391
  anaesthetics 239
  analgesics 262–3
  antidiarrhoeal agents 579–80
  antitussives 543–4
  benzodiazepine interactions 288
  cancer treatment 755c
  CNS effects 214c
  constipation treatment 574
  depression evoked by 326
  dosage forms 266t
  during childbirth 234
  during pregnancy 261, 727
  endogenous 253–4
  from Tasmania 11
  incontinence caused by 489t
  intoxication with 377t
  naltrexone interactions 382
  neonatal withdrawal symptoms 143t
  ocular adverse effects 605t
  overdose 270b
  pain management with 255t
  palliative care in cancer treatment 787
  pharmacokinetics 264–5
  pregnancy safety 405
  premedication with 235t
  psychotropic agent interactions 318
  respiratory depression by 528
  sevoflurane interactions 238
  sexual function affected by 746
  skin conditions from 907t
  undertreatment with 258
  withdrawal from 276, 284t
opium 265c, 378
opposed hormone replacement therapy 718
optic nerve 215t
optometrists, drugs administered by 34
oral administration 116
  dose calculation 20–1
  formulations for 39–43
  of analgesics 259–60
oral anticoagulants 505
  aminoglutethimide interactions 662
  cimetidine interactions 572

oral anticoagulants—cont'd
  dipyridamole interactions 509
  glycoprotein IIb/IIIa receptor inhibitor
    interactions 510
  testosterone interactions 735
  thrombolytic interactions 506
oral candidiasis 564
oral cavity, *see* mouth
oral contraceptives 710, 712–7, 741, *see also*
    contraceptives
  carbamazepine interactions 307
  depression evoked by 326
  during breastfeeding 144t
  hyperglycaemia linked to 672t
  infertility treatment 740
  modafinil interactions 342
  nevirapine interactions 841
  orlistat interactions 953
  penicillin interactions 806
  phenytoin interactions 306
  photosensitising effects 907t
  plasma lipid profile effects 464t
  recommended treatment 716t
  rifampicin interactions 859
  ritonavir interactions 843
  skin conditions from 907t
  St John's wort interactions 327c
  tetracycline interactions 816
  'The Pill' 718c
  theophylline interactions 537
oral hygiene 563
oral hypoglycaemic agents 676, 677–80, *see
    also* hypoglycaemic agents
  beta-blocker interaction 198t
  teratogenic potential 726
orchidectomy 737
orexigenic neurotransmitters 949
organic ion transporting polypeptides 114
organic molecules, drugs as 4
organic nitrates
  mechanism of action *443*
  sexual function affected by *747–8*
  vasodilators 441–8
organic sulfides, tears induced by 606
organophosphate anticholinesterases 605,
    905c
orgasm 746
orlistat
  anorectic agent 951–3
  pregnancy safety 953
  sibutramine interactions 951
orphan drugs 79–80, 80t
orphenadrine
  age-related adverse drug events 150
  clinical use and administration 182t
  parkinsonism treatment 355
  pregnancy safety 182, 366
orthoptists, drugs administered by 34
orthotists, drugs administered by 34
oseltamivir 546, 831, 833
  pregnancy safety 844
Osler, William 750
osmotic agents, glaucoma treatment 594
osmotic diuretics 487
osmotic laxatives 575b, 577
osteomalacia 689, 690
osteonectin 95
osteoporosis 691–2
  after menopause 718
  corticosteroid effects 538
  methylxanthine implicated in 345

OTC drugs, *see* over-the-counter drugs
otic administration of drops, *see* ears
otitis media 611c, 612
ototoxicosis 612
  drug-induced 614–6, 615t, 765
ovaries 627t, 697, 740
over-the-counter drugs 15, 28, 51–8, *see also*
    regulation
  alcohol content 387t
  examples of 53t
  for weight loss 953c
  with prescription variants 52t
overdose
  amphetamines 340
  aspirin 275b
  benzodiazepines 289, 289b
  carbon dioxide 528
  digoxin 427
  heroin 383
  illicit drugs 381–2
  NSAIDs 405
  opioids 270b
  paracetamol 272, 272b
  tricyclic antidepressants 331b
overmedication, *see* polypharmacy
overweight, *see* obesity
oviducts 697, 745
ovulation 701–4
oxaliplatin
  cancer treatment 776
  indications and toxicity 771t
oxandrolone 734–5, 737
oxazepam
  anxiolytic 287
  nicotine interactions 397
  pharmacokinetics 286t
  recommended for elderly 285
  withdrawal symptom treatment 288
oxazolidones 817
oxcarbazepine 307
  pregnancy safety 309
oxicams 879t, 881t
oxidative stress 526
oxpentifylline
  hypertension treatment **452**
  pregnancy safety 457
  vascular disorder treatment 450
oxprenolol 197t
  pharmacokinetics and dosages 198t
  pregnancy safety 199t
oxybenzone 913t
oxybuprocaine, ocular use 599
oxybutynin
  clinical use and administration 182t
  diuretic use 488
  pregnancy safety 182
oxycodone 269
  dosage forms 266t
  pregnancy safety 278
oxygen
  as medical gas 525c
  blood levels of 518–9, 939
  headache treatment 366
  ocular adverse effects 605, 605t
  ototoxicity 615
  respiratory treatments 524–6, 542
  toxicity of 232
  transport of 493–4, 516
oxymetazoline, topical decongestant 340
oxytocics 727
  adrenaline interactions 190

oxytocics 727—cont'd
noradrenaline interactions 191
oxytocin 222, 635–6, **637**, 698, 727
love involves 221
pregnancy safety 730
sexual function affected by 705, 747

P

p-aminobenzoic acid (PABA) 907t, 913
P-glycoprotein, in active transport 114
p34 protein, in cell cycle 756
p53 protein 757–8
P450 enzyme system 826
packaging 58, 78
paclitaxel 778c
cancer treatment 762c, 776
indications and toxicity 772t
pregnancy safety 789
padimate-O 913t
Paediatric Pharmacopoeia 16
paediatrics, *see also* infants; neonates
adverse reactions 154
anaesthesia 233
analgesia 262
antibiotics 821
anticonvulsants 308
antidepressant treatments 329
body chart for pain assessment 256–7
cancer treatment 766
CNS depressants 285
digoxin treatment 428
drug metabolism 144–7
epilepsy 298
faces pain scale 258
migraine 363
paracetamol 272
population studies 97
psychotropic agents 319–20
sedatives 292
Paget's disease of bone 691
pain, *see also* anaesthetics; analgesics;
nociceptive pain
assessing 258
myths about 259c
physiology of 252–6
tolerance 252
palivizumab 831, 835
palliative care in cancer treatment 786–7, 787c
pamidronate
bony metastasis treatment 786
effect on bone 693
hypercalcaemia treatment 689t
pregnancy safety 693
Pan Pharmaceuticals 68c
Panadol, *see* paracetamol
pancreas 188t, 558–9, 627t, 666–7
pancreatic enzyme supplements 573–4
pancreatic lipase inhibitors 951–3
pancuronium 204–5, **205**, 206t
as muscle relaxant 357
pregnancy safety 248
panic disorder 288c
pantoprazole
in Australia's top 10 drugs 17t
peptic ulcer treatment 571
pregnancy safety 581
papaverine 749
pregnancy safety 751
papaya, warfarin interactions 504
Papua New Guinea, malaria in 850
papules *906*

paraben preservatives, skin conditions from 907t
Paracelsus 6, 481c
paracetamol **54**, 272
abuse of 405
adverse drug events 54
alcohol interactions 391
as NSAID 270
aspirin compared to 275c
conjugation reaction 122t
ear infection treatment 612
headache treatment 366
in Australia's top 10 drugs 17t
interactions 54
metabolism of 273
migraine treatment 364
mouth blistering treatment 564
nicotine interactions 397
overdose 272b, 530
pain management 255t
palliative care in cancer treatment 787
pharmacokinetics 54, 272
pregnancy safety 54, 278
skin conditions from 907t
sugar-free medications 673c
paracrines 339
paradoxical reactions, *see also* adverse drug
events
anticonvulsants 300
CNS depressants 285
paraffins, emollient effects 909
paraldehyde 291–2
pregnancy safety 293
paraoxonase-1, discovery of 95
parasympathetic nervous system 164–5,
168t, *see also* acetylcholine; muscarinic
receptors
cardiac involvement 419
drugs affecting 181t
gastrointestinal tract nerves 553
respiratory involvement 518
sexual function 745–6
parasympatholytics, *see* anticholinergics;
muscarinic receptor antagonists
parasympathomimetics 590, 605t, *see also*
cholinergic transmission; muscarinic
receptor agonists
parathyroid glands 627t, 640, 685–7
parathyroid hormone 627t, 685–6
determines sodium uptake 477
osteoporosis treatment 692
parecoxib 879t
pharmacokinetics 881t
regulation in NZ 883c
parenteral administration 116–7
antiepileptic drugs 302
dosage measurement 22
formulations for 43–4
of analgesics 260–1
parietal cells 555
Parker, Gordon 12c
parkinsonian effects of psychotropic agents
316t, 317c
Parkinson's disease 349–55, *see also*
antiparkinsonian agents
nicotine reduces prevalence of 394–5
treatment of 224, 747
paromomycin
amoebicidal agent 855
capreomycin interactions 857
pregnancy safety 821, 866

parotid glands 553
paroxetine 329
adverse drug events 319t
cytochrome P450 isoform inhibition 158t
pregnancy safety 320
pars intermedia 630
partial agonists 263, 269
partial complex (psychomotor) seizures 156t,
297, 299c
anticonvulsants 300t
treatment of 303
partial simple motor epilepsy 297
parturition, *see* childbirth
passionflower, sedative effects 292c
passive immunity 874–5, 875t
passive reabsorption 125
passive smoking 395
passive transport (diffusion) 114
pastes, skin treatment 910
patches, *see* transdermal administration
pathogens, *see* microbial infections
patient-controlled analgesia (PCA) infusions
260
patients, *see also* consumer medical
information; humans
drug responses 44, 123–4
information needs 763c
interindividual variability 123–4, 137–50
pain management plans 259
special requirements of 36
testing on 90
Paullinia cupana, *see* guarana
PBS 28, 80–1, 465t
PCA pumps 260
PCP, *see* phencyclidine
pectins 579–80
digoxin interactions 426t
pediculicides 916–7
Pediculus humanus (lice) 916–7
peginterferon alfa 835–6
pelvic inflammatory disease, from
contraceptives 742
pelvis cross-section 475
pelvis of the kidney 474
penicillamine
antirheumatic effects 884
gold salt interactions 884
heavy-metal poisoning treatment 885
pregnancy safety 900
taste and smell effects 617t
penicillins
aminoglycoside interactions 815
aminoglycosides used with 814
bacteriostatic agents 796
drug groups 13t
drug interactions 806
introduction of 794
mechanism of action 804–8
neonatal dose 145t
probenecid interactions 890
resistance to 798t
skin conditions from 907t
taste and smell effects 617t
penis 697, 745
pentamidine
didanosine interactions 838
foscarnet interactions 835
lamivudine interactions 838
stavudine interactions 838
zalcitabine interactions 840
pentazocine, pregnancy safety 278

pep pills, *see* amphetamines
peppermint oil **580**, 581
pepsin 555
pepsinogen 571
peptic ulcer disease 29–30, 555–6, 565, 570–3
peptides, *see* neuropeptides
Peptococcus infections 796t
Peptostreptococcus infections 796t
perfluorocarbons, blood doping with 939
pergolide
    parkinsonism treatment 353
    pregnancy safety 366, 636
pericardium 411
pericyazine 324
    pregnancy safety 320
peridural administration, *see* epidural
    anaesthesia
perimenopause 717
perinatal drug use 729
perindopril
    ACE inhibitor 456
    pharmacokinetics 455t
    pregnancy safety 457
perinephric glands, *see* adrenal cortex
peripheral nervous system 163
    muscle relaxant effects 357
    opioid effects 263–4
    pain factors 253
    psychotropic agent effects 314
    respiratory involvement 518–9
peripheral neuropathy, drug interactions 838
peripheral vascular system 419, *see also* blood
    vessels
    disorders of 449–50
    nicotinic acid treatment 470
peristalsis 554
peritoneal dialysis solutions, orphan drugs 80t
periwinkle, toxicity 67t
permethrin 916–7
    pregnancy safety 928
permetrexed
    cancer treatment 773
    indications and toxicity 771t
permissive effects of thyroid hormones 622
pernicious anaemia 494
perphenazine
    cytochrome P450 isoform inhibition 158t
    piperazine compound 324
personality factors in drug abuse 372
peru balsam, skin conditions from 907t
pesticides (anticholinesterases) 208–9, 488c
pethidine 269
    age-related adverse drug events 262
    dosage forms 266t
    high hepatic clearance 132t
    MAO inhibitor interactions 331
    mu-receptor agonist 264t
    neonatal withdrawal symptoms 143t
    perinatal use 729
    phenytoin interactions 306
    pregnancy safety 278
    regulation in sport 937
    RIMA interactions 333
    selegiline interactions 354
    sexual function affected by 746
    symptoms of abuse 374t
petit mal epilepsy, *see* epilepsy
petroleum jelly, emollient effects 909
Peyer's patches 870
peyote, *see* mescaline
PGE, PGF, *see* prostaglandins

pH, *see also* antacids
    of blood 476, 492
    of skin 904
    of the body 115, *115*, 519
    urinary 125
phaeochromocytoma 172, 193c, 194–5, 197
phagocytosis 494, 871
PHARM 28
PHARMAC (NZ) 84, 806c
Pharmaceutical Benefits Scheme 28, 80–1,
    465t
Pharmaceutical Health and Rational Use of
    Medicines Committee 28
pharmaceutical industry 92–3, 98, *see also*
    pharmacoeconomics
pharmaceutical phase 112
pharmaceutics, *see* formulations
pharmacists
    drugs administered by 34, 52
    information from 18
    legal issues 81–2
pharmacodynamics 2, 106–10
    definition 3t
    drug interactions 157
    ginseng 64
    responses to drugs 44
pharmacoeconomics 3t, 31, 97–8
pharmacogenetics, interindividual variability
    123–4, 137–50
pharmacogenomics 95
pharmacokinetics 2, 3t, 113–26, *see also*
    names of drugs
    autoinduction of metabolism 305
    dosing schedules 129–35
    drug interactions 157–8
    non-linear pharmacokinetic parameters 305
    responses to drugs 44
pharmacological factors, in drug abuse 372–6
pharmacology 2, 87
pharmacopoeias 3t, 6, 16
pharmacotherapy 27–49, 73–84
pharmacy, definition 3t
pharmacy-only drugs 52
pharynx 554
phase I and II trials 90, *see also* clinical trials
phase I reactions, *see* functionalisation reactions
phase II reactions, *see* conjugation reactions
phase IV trials 91, *see also* clinical trials
phased dosage of sex hormones 713c, 714
phases of activity 112–26, *113*
    cardiac system 415–6
phencyclidine 403
    as adjuvant analgesic 276
    perceptual states altered by 402
    symptoms of abuse 375t
phendimetrazine, anorectic agent 951
phenelzine 331
    adverse drug events 319t
    morphine interactions 268
    pregnancy safety 320
    sexual function affected by 750
phenformin 678
phenindione
    avoid during breastfeeding 144t
    bile acid-binding resin interactions 468
    gemfibrozil interactions 469
    orlistat interactions 953
    thiourea interactions 649
    thyroxine interactions 645t
pheniramine
    ocular use 598

pheniramine—cont'd
    pregnancy safety 899
phenobarbitone 290
    abuse of 374t
    amprenavir interactions 842t
    anticonvulsant effects 300t, 303
    bile acid-binding resin interactions 468
    CNS effects 300t
    drug interactions with 158
    griseofulvin interactions 830
    medroxyprogesterone acetate interactions
    713
    neonate dose 145t
    parenteral administration 302
    pregnancy safety 309
    saquinavir interactions 843
    sexual function affected by 750
    tiagabine interactions 305
phenol
    analgesic effects 276
    antipruritic agent 909
    calamine lotion 910
    skin conditions from 907t
phenolics, chemical structure *10*
phenols 11, 907t
phenothiazines 322, 324
    adjuvant analgesics 276
    atropine interactions 180
    cancer treatment 783
    cataracts caused by 605
    'dirty' drugs 316
    during breastfeeding 730
    levodopa–carbidopa interactions 352
    lithium interactions 333
    major effects 315t
    Ménière's disease treatment 613c
    ocular adverse effects 605t
    photosensitising effects 600, 605, 907t
    premedication with 235t
    retinopathy induced by 604
    sedative effects 284t
    sexual function affected by 750
    skin conditions from 907t
phenoxybenzamine 194
    pregnancy safety 199t
    sexual function affected by 750
phenoxymethylpenicillin 804
    pharmacokinetics 807t
    pregnancy safety 821
    strep throat treatment 544
phentermine **952**
    anorectic agent 339, 343, 951
    pregnancy safety 346, 952
    sibutramine interactions 951
phentolamine 194–5
    pregnancy safety 199t
phenylalanine, dopamine derived from 350
phenylalkylamine calcium-channel blockers,
    angina treatment 445
phenylephrine 193
    adjunct to local anaesthesia 243
    glaucoma treatment 593
    ocular use 590–2, 590t, 605t
    pregnancy safety 606
    taste and smell effects 617t
    topical decongestant 340
phenylethanolamine *N*-methyltransferase 173
phenylethylamines, *see also* amphetamines
    involved in love 221
phenylketonuria, cholestyramine
    contraindicated with 468

phenylpropanolamine, regulation in sport 938–9
phenytoin **306**
  alcohol interactions 391
  amiodarone interactions 436t
  amprenavir interactions 842t
  anticonvulsant effects 300t, 303
  antiepileptic interactions 301–2
  calcium-channel blocker interactions 447t
  caspofungin interactions 830
  chloramphenicol interactions 817
  cimetidine interactions 572
  CNS effects 300t
  delavirdine interactions 840
  didanosine interactions 838
  disopyramide interactions 432t
  drug interactions with 158
  H₂-receptor antagonist interactions 572t
  hormonal factors 124
  imidazole antifungal interactions 829t
  in pregnancy 308
  insulin interactions 675
  isoniazid interactions 858
  maintenance dose rates 302
  medroxyprogesterone acetate interactions 713
  migraine treatment 364
  neonate dose 145t
  ocular adverse effects 595, 605t
  omeprazole interactions 571
  parenteral administration 302
  photosensitising effects 907t
  praziquantel interactions 865
  pregnancy safety 309
  rifampicin interactions 859
  saquinavir interactions 843
  simvastatin interactions 467
  skin conditions from 907t
  sleep pattern effects 284t
  sodium channel inhibitor 303, 305
  stavudine interactions 838
  sucralfate interactions 573
  sulfonamides/trimethoprim interactions 820
  teratogenic potential 142t, 726
  theophylline interactions 537
  tiagabine interactions 305
  topiramate interactions 304
  warfarin interactions 505
  withdrawal from 302
  zalcitabine interactions 840
phlegm 528
phocomelia 140
pholcodine 269, **543**
  antitussive 544
  not a controlled drug 265
  pregnancy safety 278, 549
  regulation in sport 938
  respiratory depression by 528
phosphamide alkylating agents, hydration therapy 784
phosphate, levels in bone 690
phosphate supplements, pregnancy safety 693
phosphodiesterase inhibitors
  asthma treatment 535
  for cardiac disorders 428
phosphoinositides 105
phosphorus-32: 761, 783
photoallergy 911–2
photodynamic therapy 600
photophobia 364

photosensitivities 605
  drugs causing 907t, 911, 915
phototoxicity 911–2
Phthirus pubis (lice) 916–7
physical aspects of drugs 4
physical dependence 371–2
physiotherapy 34, 276
physostigmine 207, 591c
phyto-oestrogens 719, 720c
phytomenadione, *see* vitamin K₁
PI-88, developed in Australia 90t
Pick's disease 360
pilocarpine
  adverse drug events 605t
  glaucoma treatment 178, 593t, 594
  miotic effects 590
  pregnancy safety 606
pimecrolimus 917, 919–20
  pregnancy safety 928
pimozide 325
  amprenavir interactions 842t
  atazanavir interactions 842t
  macrolide antibiotic interactions 812
  major effects 315t
  pregnancy safety 320
  saquinavir interactions 843
  sexual function affected by 750
pindolol 197t
  pharmacokinetics and dosages 198t
  pregnancy safety 199t
pine tar, antipruritic agent 909
pioglitazone 680
  pharmacokinetics 678t
  pregnancy safety 681
  tamoxifen interactions 780
Piper methysticum, see kava kava
piperacillin 806–7
  pharmacokinetics 807t
  pregnancy safety 821
  warfarin interactions 505
piperazine compounds 324
piperidine compounds 324
pirenzipine 181
piroxicam 879t
  age-related adverse drug events 262
  pharmacokinetics 881t
  risk of GIT effects 879, 882
  warfarin interactions 505
PIs, *see* protease inhibitors
pituitary gland 626, 630–7
  cancers of 781
  gonadotrophins 700, 709
  hormones influenced by *626*, 698–700, *702*
  reproductive system disorders 734–5
pizotifen
  migraine treatment 364
  pregnancy safety 366
placebo effects, may affect responses 45
placenta 627
  drug transfer across 120, 141
  IgG can cross 874
  role in pregnancy 725
placental lactogen 698
plant drugs 7–8, 9c, *see also* herbal remedies
  antifungals 826c
  antineoplastic agents 778c
  antithyroid agents 650c
  Australian 90t, 797c
  cancer treatment 786c
  laxatives 574–5
  nephrotoxicity 488c

plant drugs—cont'd
  NSAIDS in 884c
  phyto-oestrogens 719
  skin condition treatment 911
  sterols 466c
plaque on skin *906*
plasma 492
  drug distribution to 118t
  role in immunity 872
plasma cholinesterase, *see* butyrylcholinesterase
plasma concentrations 129–31, *129*, *130*
  antidepressants 328
  drug interactions affecting 157–8
  monitoring 47
plasma expanders, blood doping with 937, 939
plasma lipid profile, *see* hyperlipidaemia; lipid-lowering drugs
plasma proteins 492
  binding of 119
  role in inflammation 871
plasma thromboplastin 495t
plasma uric acid, thiazide diuretic interactions 484
plasmablasts 873
plasmin 507
Plasmodium spp. 848, *849*, *see also* malaria
platelet aggregation inhibitors
  heparin interactions 501
  penicillin interactions 806
platelet plugs 494–5
platelets (thrombocytes) 492, 494, *see also* thrombocytopenia
  activation of *508*
  drugs affecting 500, 765
  suppressed by chemotherapy 784
platinum compounds
  cancer treatment 762, 777
  ototoxicity 615t
platyhelminths 863
plicamycin, for Paget's disease 691
pneumonia 546
PNMT 173
PNS, *see* peripheral nervous system
podiatrists, drugs administered by 34
podophyllotoxins 778c
  cancer treatment 761, 776
  wart treatment 916
poisons, *see also* scheduling; toxicology
  pesticides and nerve gases 209
  poisons information centres 18
  regulation of 77–8
polarisation of nerve cells, *see* depolarisation
poloxamer, laxative effects 575
polyacrylic acids, artificial tear solutions 602
polydrug abuse, *see* polypharmacy
polyethylene glycol electrolytes, laxative effects 577
polygodial 826c
polymorphonuclear leukocytes 872
polymyxins
  ocular use 596
  pregnancy safety 606
  topical administration 915
Polynesians 669c, *see also* Maoris
polypeptide hormones (endocrine system) 621
polypharmacy
  may affect responses 45
  herbal remedies 66c

polypharmacy—cont'd
  in the elderly 147
  monitoring for 46c
  over-the-counter drugs 58
  polydrug abuse 371
  with NSAIDS 274–5
polyphenols 399
polyvalent antivenoms 959, 960t
polyvinyl alcohol, eye lubrication with 602
pons 215
popularity of drugs 30
population studies 97
pores (ion channels), *see* ion channels
    (membrane pores)
porphyria 605
porphyrins, photosensitising effects 600, 907t
positive feedback (endocrine system) 624
positive inotropic effects 422–4
possession of drugs, legal issues 78
post-marketing studies 91
posterior pituitary hormones 626, 626t, 635–6
postganglionic neurons 165
postnatal depression 321
postoperative management 235–6
postpartum psychiatric disorders 321
postsynaptic receptors 186
postsynthesis phase of cells 756
potassium, *see also* hypokalaemia
  ACE inhibitor interactions 454
  cyclosporin interactions 892
  glucocorticoid interactions 660t
  hypertensive loss 484
  potassium-sparing diuretic interactions 487
  reabsorption in kidneys 477
potassium arsenite 770c
potassium bromide 290–1
potassium channel activators, angina
    treatment 445–8
potassium chloride, pancuronium interactions
    205
potassium citrate, hexamine interactions 820
potassium clavulanate, *see* clavulanate
potassium-depleting drugs, digoxin
    interactions 426t
potassium iodide 648
  thiourea interactions 649
potassium nitrate, in desensitising dentifrice
    564
potassium permanganate
  antipruritic agent 909
  for pressure sores 927
potassium-sparing diuretics 481, 485–7
  ACE inhibitor interactions 454
  amphotericin B interactions 828
  cyclosporin interactions 892
  pharmacokinetics 484t
  pregnancy safety 487
  regulation in sport 937
potency 2–3, 107
povidone, artificial tear solutions 602
povidone-iodine
  antiseptic effects 915
  burn treatment 925
  pressure sore treatment 927
  topical antifungal 916
powders for skin 910
PQRST approach to pain assessment 256
pramipexole, parkinsonism treatment 353
pravastatin
  developed in Australia 90t
  dosage 467

pravastatin—cont'd
  hyperlipidaemia treatment 466
  in Australia's top 10 drugs 17t
  pregnancy safety 470
praziquantel 865
  pregnancy safety 866
prazosin 193–4, **195**
  benign prostatic hyperplasia treatment 736
  pregnancy safety 737
pre-eclampsia 301c, 725
preclinical pharmacology 88
prednisolone
  asthma treatment 538
  cancer treatment 782
  combination therapy 764t
  conjunctivitis treatment 598
  infantile spasm treatment 308
  inflammatory bowel disease treatment 580
  ocular use 597–8, 598t
  pharmacokinetics 657t
  potency of 657
  pregnancy safety 606, 662
  taste and smell effects 617t
prednisone 658
  cancer treatment 778
  Hodgkin's disease treatment 764
  pharmacokinetics 657t
  pregnancy safety 662
Preferred Medicines List (NZ) 28
prefrontal lobotomies 322
pregabalin 275
  pregnancy safety 309
preganglionic neurons 165
pregnancy, *see also* childbirth; fetus; pregnancy
    safety
  anaesthesia during 234
  analgesia during 261–2
  drug use during 138–42, 144c, 725–9
  eclampsia 301c
  nausea and vomiting 569c
  urinary tract infections 820t
  uterine changes during 727
pregnancy safety 3t, *see also* names of drugs;
    teratogens
  Australian categories 726
  drugs affecting cholinergic transmission
    182
  fetal screening 95
  regulation of drugs 82
premature ejaculation 751
premature labour, adrenaline treatment 189
premenstrual syndrome 321, 328, 704c
prenylation of proteins 760
preoperative management 234–5, 235t
  benzodiazepines for 288
  for anaesthesia 234–5, 235t
prescribing 37
  decisions before 35–6
  regulation 28, 78, 92c
prescription-only drugs 15, 52
  characteristics of 51
  over-the-counter variants 52t
presenile dementia, *see* Alzheimer's disease
preservatives in skin treatments 910
pressure-immobilisation 957
pressure sores 925–7, 926
presynaptic receptors 186, 223
preventers (antiasthma drugs) 536–9
priapism 745, 747
prickly fanflower, cancer treatment 786c
PRIF, *see* dopamine

prilocaine 247t, *see also* EMLA cream
  local anaesthetic 240, 243t
  pregnancy safety 248
  toxicity of 244
primaquine 359c, 851
  malaria treatment 850
  pregnancy safety 866
primary active transport, in kidneys 476
primary epilepsy 289
Primary Health Care Strategy (NZ) 32c
primary tissue schizonts 848
primidone 305
  pregnancy safety 309
  tiagabine interactions 305
  warfarin interactions 505
Prinzmetal angina 441b
private prescriptions 28
proaccelerin 495t
proarrhythmogenic agents 437
probenecid
  aciclovir interactions 832
  aspirin interactions 274
  cephalosporin interactions 810
  drug interactions with 158
  ganciclovir interactions 833t
  gout treatment 888–90
  methotrexate interactions 158, 775
  nitrofurantoin interactions 822
  NSAID interactions 883
  penicillin interactions 806
  pregnancy safety 900
  regulation in sport 937
  valganciclovir interactions 833t
  zidovudine interactions 837
procainamide 430, 432–3
  bethanechol interactions 179
  biguanide interactions 678
  disopyramide interactions 432t
  pharmacokinetics 430t
  pregnancy safety 437
  skin conditions from 907t
  taste and smell effects 617t
procaine
  infiltration anaesthesia 247t
  local anaesthesia 240, 243t
  low toxicity of 244
  metabolism of 242
  nerve block anaesthesia 247t
  photosensitising effects 907t
  pregnancy safety 248
procaine penicillin 804
  pharmacokinetics 807t
  pregnancy safety 821
procarbazine
  alcohol interactions 391
  Hodgkin's disease treatment 764
  indications and toxicity 771t
  pregnancy safety 789
prochlorperazine
  antiemetic use 567t, 568
  cancer treatment 783
  extrapyramidal effects 324
  major effects 315t
  migraine treatment 364
  morning sickness treatment 569c
  piperazine compound 324
  pregnancy safety 320, 568, 581
  premedication with 235t
  sexual function affected by 750
proconvertin 495t
prodrugs, metabolism of 121

progesterones 627t, 698, 709–12
    in menstrual cycle 702
    infertility treatment 740
    levels during pregnancy 725
    pregnancy safety 721
progestogens 698, 709–12
    cancer treatment 779t, 781
    contraceptive use 715t, 741–2
    depot preparations 716–7
    dysfunctional uterine bleeding treatment
        720
    hyperglycaemia linked to 672t
    in 'male pill' 743
    sexual function affected by 746
    tocolytic effects 728
proguanil
    malaria treatment 853
    pregnancy safety 866
prohibited substances, see regulation
prokinetic drugs, alcohol interactions 391
prolactin 626t, 634, 698
    lactation maintained by 730
    levels during pregnancy 725
prolactin release-inhibiting factor, see
    dopamine
promethazine
    antiemetic use 567t
    morning sickness treatment 569c
    nasal condition treatment 548
    pregnancy safety 899
    premedication with 235t
    sedative effects 292
    sexual function affected by 751
promotion, see marketing
prontosil 794
propamidine
    ocular use 595, 597
    pregnancy safety 606
propanolol
    sexual function affected by 750
    taste and smell effects 617t
propantheline
    clinical use and administration 182t
    diuretic use 488
    pregnancy safety 182
proparacaine, see proxymetacaine
prophylactic antiasthma drugs 536–9
Propionibacterium acnes 920–2
propionic acid NSAIDs 879t
    pharmacokinetics 881t
    topical antifungals 916
propofol 237, 239
    anaesthetic 230, 238–9
    for day procedures 232
propranolol 197t
    adjunct to psychotropic agents 316
    age-related adverse drug events 150
    bile acid-binding resin interactions 468
    cytochrome P450 isoform inhibition 158t
    high hepatic clearance 132t
    hyperthyroidism treatment 647
    nicotine interactions 397
    pancuronium interactions 205
    pharmacokinetics and dosages 198t
    pregnancy safety 199t, 248, 650
    warfarin interactions 505
proprietary names 14
propylene glycol
    artificial tear solutions 602
    ear treatment 614
    pregnancy safety 618

propylthiouracil 646, 648–9, **649**
    pregnancy safety 650
    warfarin interactions 505
proscribed drugs, see regulation
prostaglandin agonists, glaucoma treatment
        593t, 594
prostaglandin analogues, drug groups 13t
prostaglandins
    as neurotransmitters 223
    contraceptive use 742
    emetic involvement 570
    glaucoma treatment 592
    inhibitors of 270–1, 879
    oxytocic effects 728
    oxytocin interactions 637
    role in inflammation 871
    role in labour 727
    role in pain 254–5
prostate cancer 777–8, 780
prostate gland 697
prostate specific antigen 760
prosthetists, drugs administered by 34
protamine 503–4
protease inhibitors 836, 841–3
    efavirenz interactions 840
    nevirapine interactions 841
proteasomes, cancer treatment 762
protectants, skin treatment 910
protein binding, in neonates 145t
protein hormones, endocrine system 621
protein metabolism 654, 757, 796
protein theory of anaesthesia 229
protein tyrosine kinases, cancer treatment
        762
Proteus infections 795t
prothrombin 495t, 511t
    pregnancy safety 512
proton pump inhibitors
    atazanavir interactions 842t
    drug groups 13t
    drug-induced GIT effect treatment 882
    imidazole antifungal interactions 829t
    peptic ulcer treatment 570–1
prototype drugs 15
protozoa 909
proximal convoluted tubule 476
proxymetacaine
    ocular anaesthetic 599
    pregnancy safety 606
Prozac, see fluoxetine
prunes for constipation 574
pruritus
    bile acid-binding resin treatment 468
    caused by laxatives 575
pseudoaddiction 259c
pseudocholinesterase, see
    butyrylcholinesterase
pseudoephedrine **544**
    abuse of 379c, 380
    bicarbonate interactions 567
    pregnancy safety 549
    priapism treatment 749
    regulation in sport 938–9
pseudomembranous colitis 810
Pseudomonas aeruginosa infections 795t
    cephalosporin-resistant 809t
    drug-resistant 805t
psilocybin 403
    perceptual states altered by 402
    symptoms of abuse 375t
psoralens 911, 920

psoriasis 905, 909, 920
psychiatric disorders, see also antipsychotics;
        depression; psychotropic agents
    ADHD 328, 340–2
    anxiety disorders 284
    bipolar affective disorder 312, 327, 332c,
        334–5
    mania 312, 334–5
    mood disorders 312
    neuroses 312, 328
    psychoses 312
    schizophrenia 312, 322c, 322–3
psychogenic pain 256
psychological dependence 371
psychomotor seizures, see epilepsy
psychostimulants, see CNS stimulants
psychotherapies 321c, 321–2
    bipolar affective disorder 334
    cancer treatment 786c
    pain management 277
psychotomimetics 399–404, see also
        cannabinoids; hallucinogens
psychotropic agents 312–35, see also
        antidepressants; antipsychotics
    adjuvant analgesics 276
    adverse drug events 315–20, 316t
    age-related adverse drug events 149t
    anabolic steroids 735
    antihistamine interactions 899
    benzodiazepine interactions 288
    lactation effects 730
    methadone interactions 386
    perceptual states altered by 373
    sexual function affected by 750
psyllium 574–5, **575**
PTA 495t
ptosis 356c
puffers 520c
pulmonary system 166t, 188t, 516–7, see also
        tuberculosis
purine antagonists, cancer treatment 773
purine antimetabolites, cancer chemotherapy
        784
purine nucleotides, as neurotransmitters 223
purines 757, 761
Purkinje fibres 187–8, 414
purpuras, drugs causing 907t
pustules 906
pygeum, for benign prostatic hyperplasia
        736
pyrantel 866
    pregnancy safety 866
pyrazinamide
    pregnancy safety 866
    tuberculosis treatment 856–7, 860–1
pyrethrins 11–2
    pregnancy safety 928
pyridostigmine 207, 355–6
    myasthenia gravis treatment 603
    pregnancy safety 366
pyridoxine
    morning sickness treatment 569c
    teratogenic potential 726
pyrimethamine
    malaria treatment 850, 854
    pregnancy safety 866
    toxoplasmosis treatment 596, 855
pyrimidine antagonists, cancer treatment 773
pyrimidines 757, 761
pyrithione zinc 910
    pregnancy safety 928

Q

quality use of medicines 27–31
quaternary ammonium compounds 179
Queensland, drug legislation 76t
quercetin, for cataracts 601c
quetiapine 325
    bipolar affective disorder treatment 334
    major effects 315t
    pregnancy safety 320
quinagolide, pregnancy safety 636
quinapril
    ACE inhibitor 456
    pharmacokinetics 455t
    pregnancy safety 457
quinidine 430–2
    bethanechol interactions 179
    bicarbonate interactions 567
    biguanide interactions 678
    chlorpromazine interactions 323
    cytochrome P450 isoform inhibition 158t
    digoxin interactions 426t
    disopyramide interactions 432t
    fosamprenavir interactions 842t
    pharmacokinetics 430t
    pregnancy safety 437
    rifampicin interactions 859
    saquinavir interactions 843
    skin conditions from 907t
    suxamethonium interactions 207
    warfarin interactions 505
quinines 851–2, 853c
    biguanide interactions 678
    cytochrome P450 isoform inhibition 158t
    drug groups 13t
    mefloquine interactions 850
    muscle relaxants 359c
    ocular adverse effects 605t
    photosensitising effects 907t
    pregnancy safety 866
    psoriasis treatment 920
    skin conditions from 907t
quinolones 818–9
    antacid interactions 566t
    didanosine interactions 838
    drug groups 13t
    glycaemic levels linked to 672t
    nitrofurantoin interactions 822
    ocular use 596
    pregnancy safety 821
    taste and smell effects 617t
    theophylline interactions 537
quinupristin 817–8
    pregnancy safety 821
QUM 179

R

rabeprazole, peptic ulcer treatment 571
rabies vaccine, as orphan drug 80t
radiation, carcinogenesis induced by 759
radiation therapy, cancer treatment 761,
        783
    amphotericin B interactions 828
    cyclophosphamide interactions 774
    flucytosine interactions 830
    infertility related to 767
    methotrexate interactions 775
    zidovudine interactions 837
radioactive iodine **648**
radioactive isotopes, for bony metastasis 786
radiopharmaceuticals 761
raised intracranial pressure 216c

raloxifene 710
    bone effects 692
    cancer treatment 781
    osteoporosis treatment 692
    pregnancy safety 693, 721, 789
raltitrexed
    cancer treatment 773
    indications and toxicity 771t
ramipril
    ACE inhibitor 456
    in Australia's top 10 drugs 17t
    pharmacokinetics 455t
    pregnancy safety 457
randomised controlled clinical trials (RCCT)
        27, 89c, 89–92
ranitidine
    age-related adverse drug events 149t
    biguanide interactions 678
    over-the-counter formulations 52t
    peptic ulcer treatment 572, 572t
    pregnancy safety 581
    sexual function affected by 751
rapid acetylators 124
rapid eye movement (REM) sleep 282
RAS 215, 217–8, 284
rasagiline, parkinsonism treatment 354
rasburicase
    hyperuricaemia treatment 784
    pregnancy safety 789
rational molecular design, drugs developed
        from 87
rationing of drugs 97–8
RBCs, see red blood cells
RCCT 27, 89c, 89–92
re-entry phenomena (cardiac) 429–30, 431
reactions, see adverse drug events
reboxetine 333–4
    pregnancy safety 320
receptor-site tolerance 375
receptors, see also names of neurotransmitters
    autonomic nervous system 171
    desensitisation and turnover 106
    for acetylcholine 171
    for neurotransmitters 223
    for opioids 263
    targeting 105
recombinant blood factors VIII and IX, orphan
        drugs 80t
recombinant growth hormone 631, **632**
    as orphan drug 80t
    pregnancy safety 636
    regulation in sport 936
    supplies restricted 633c
recombinant tissue plasminogen activator, see
        alteplase
record keeping, legal issues 79
rectal administration 261, 659, see also
        suppositories
rectum 116, 559–60
red blood cells 492–4, 848
red-neck syndrome 812
red nuclei 218
redback spiders 961
reflectors of UV radiation 913–4
reflex arcs 219, 219
reflex respiratory stimulants 528
reflux oesophagitis 554
refractoriness (cardiac) 415
    digoxin effects 425
    quinidine treatment 431
regional anaesthesia 245

registered products 61
regulation 51–9, see also abuse of drugs; illicit
        drugs; scheduling
    complementary and alternative medicine
        61–3
    controlled substances 77, 84
    criminal offences 82–3
    in Australia 75–83, 76t, 81, 378, 380
    in sport 933–44
    international 74–5
    labelling 57–8, 78
regulatory proteins 104
reinforcement (drug abuse) 373
relaxants, see muscle relaxants
relaxin, levels during pregnancy 725
Relenza, see zanamivir
REM sleep 282
remifentanil 232c, 267
    adjunct to anaesthetic 230
    postoperative 235
remission of cancers 763
remodelling of bone 690
Renaissance medicine 6
renal . . ., see also kidneys
renal cell carcinoma 763
renal clearance 132
renal excretion 122, see also excretion
renal function
    anaesthesia and 234
    caffeine effects on 345
    changes during pregnancy 140
    drug excretion and 125
    in the elderly 148
    paracetamol effects 54
    tubular network 474
renin 661
renin–angiotensin–aldosterone system 451,
        453–7, 454
repaglinide 679–80
    diabetes treatment 677
    pharmacokinetics 678t
    pregnancy safety 681
replacement therapy for hormones 625
repolarisation (heart ventricles) 415–6
reproductive systems 696–706, see also female
        reproductive system; male reproductive
        system
    effect of cancer treatment 766–7
    fertility 740–5
    sexual functioning 745–51
reserpine
    affects 5-HT receptors 314
    CNS effects 222
    depression evoked by 326
    sexual function affected by 749
resistance to antibiotics 797–8, 799
    cephalosporins 809t
    vancomycin 810–1
resistance to antituberculous agents 856
resistance to chemotherapy 766
resistance to disease 871–4
resistance vessels, peripheral vascular system
        419
resistin 950
resorcinol
    acne treatment 921
    keratolytic effects 910
    pregnancy safety 928
    tretinoin interactions 922
respiratory system 516–21
    adrenaline effects 189

respiratory system   cont'd
   anaesthesia effects 234
   antiemetic effects 558
   atropine effects 180
   caffeine effects 344
   cannabinoid effects 401
   depressants 528
   disorders of 523–49
   infections 542–7, 796t
   opioid effects 259
   OTC drugs for 53t
   structures in 547
responses to drugs, *see* adverse drug events
resting membrane potential, *see* membrane
    potential
resting phase of cells 756
restorative drugs 339, 528
retailing, legal issues 78
retention of urine 478
reteplase 506
   fibrinolysis effects 500
   heparin interactions 501
   pregnancy safety 512
reticular activating system 215, 217–8, 284
retinoblastoma gene 757, 759
retinoic acid 921c
retinoids (vitamin A analogues)
   acne treatment 920–2
   cancer treatment 763, 782
   psoriasis treatment 920
   skin cancer treatment 912c
   teratogenic potential 726
retinopathy, drug-induced 885
retrolental fibroplasia 527c
reuptake of noradrenaline 174
reversible antagonists, *see* competitive
    antagonists
reversible dementia 361
reversible inhibitors of MAO-A 341, *see also*
    moclobemide
reversible neutropenia 333
reward (drug abuse) 373
Rh antigen 497
rhabdomyolysis 467
Rhesus blood group 497
rheumatoid disorders 884, *see also* disease-
    modifying antirheumatic drugs
   ocular effects of treatment 603
   penicillamine treatment 885
rhinitis, allergic 547–8, 898
rhythm method 745c
rhythmicity (cardiac) 415
ribavirin 831, 835–6
   pregnancy safety 844
   zidovudine interactions 837
ribonucleotide reductase, cancer treatment
    762
rickets 689–90
rifabutin 861
   fosamprenavir interactions 842t
   indinavir interactions 842
   nevirapine interactions 841
   pregnancy safety 866
   saquinavir interactions 843
rifampicin 546, 856–7, **859**
   amprenavir interactions 842t
   benzodiazepine interactions 288
   caspofungin interactions 830
   drug interactions with 158
   everolimus interactions 895
   indinavir interactions 842

rifampicin—cont'd
   isoniazid interactions 858
   leprosy treatment 861–2
   nevirapine interactions 841
   pregnancy safety 866
   saquinavir interactions 843
   sirolimus interactions 895
   tamoxifen interactions 780
   warfarin interactions 505
rifamycins
   imidazole antifungal interactions 829t
   medroxyprogesterone acetate interactions
    713
riluzole 360
   pregnancy safety 366
RIMA 341, *see also* moclobemide
risedronate 692–3
   pregnancy safety 693
risk–benefit ratio, drugs during pregnancy
    138
risk factors, adverse drug events 155–6
risperidone 325
   major effects 315t
   pregnancy safety 320
   schizophrenia treatment 322c
ritonavir 836, 841, 843
   cytochrome P450 isoform inhibition 158t
   fosamprenavir interactions 842t
   nevirapine interactions 841
   pregnancy safety 844
rituximab 782
   pregnancy safety 789
rivastigmine 362
   pregnancy safety 366
river blindness 865
river red gum 797c
rocuronium 204–5, 206t
   pregnancy safety 248
rofecoxib
   adverse drug events 154t
   cardiovascular adverse drug events 882c
   introduction of 30–1
   ulcer risk 879
Roman medicine 5
ropinirole 353
   pregnancy safety 366
ropivacaine
   local anaesthia 243t
   nerve block anaesthesia 247t
   pregnancy safety 248
rose bengal 599
   pregnancy safety 606
rosiglitazone 680
   pharmacokinetics 678t
   pregnancy safety 681
rosy periwinkle 778c
roundworms 863–4
routes of administration, *see* administration
    of drugs
roxithromycin 812–4
   cytochrome P450 isoform inhibition 158t
   pharmacokinetics 813t
   pneumonia treatment 546
   pregnancy safety 821
   strep throat treatment 544
Royal Australian College of Physicians,
    position on doping athletes 942
rt-PA, *see* alteplase
rubs 910
rule of nines in burn treatment 923
ryanodine receptor family, caffeine effects 344

S
SA node, *see* sinoatrial node
saccharin, taste of 616
saddle block 248
safety, *see* adverse drug events; interactions
    between drugs; pregnancy safety
salbutamol
   asthma treatment 534, **536**, 548c
   conjugation reaction 122t
   ethanol compared to 2c
   hyperglycaemia linked to 672t
   in Australia's top 10 drugs 17t
   OTC vs prescription variants 52t
   pregnancy safety 549, 730
   selectivity of 104
   sugar-free medications 673c
   tocolytic effects 727, 728
   use in sport 935
salcatonin **690**
   hypercalcaemia treatment 689, 689t
   pregnancy safety 693
salicylates 271c, 271–2, 879t, *see also* aspirin
   alcohol interactions 391
   discovery of 6
   hypoglycaemia linked to 672t
   methotrexate interactions 158, 775
   ototoxicity 616
   penicillin interactions 806
   photosensitising effects 907t
   probenecid interactions 890
   prostaglandins inhibited by 270–1
   skin conditions from 907t
   sources of 11
   sunscreens 913
   warfarin interactions 505
salicylic acid
   keratolytic effects 910
   tretinoin interactions 922
   wart treatment 916
saline solutions 529
   antipruritic agents 909
   artificial tear solutions 602
   hypercalcaemia treatment 689t
   laxative effects 575b, 577
   mouth-washes and gargles 563
   nasal condition treatments 548
   sinusitis treatments 549
saliva
   drug excretion by 126
   substitutes for 564
salivary glands 553
salmeterol
   asthma treatment 534
   fluticasone combined with 539
   pregnancy safety 549
   regulation in sport 935
Salmonella infections 795t
salted fish, links with cancer 760
salvarsan, adverse drug events 154t
salvia, glaucoma treatment 601c
samarium-153:
   cancer treatment 761
   for bony metastases 786
   pregnancy safety 789
sample manipulation, banned in sports 939
sampling for regulation, legal issues 78
saquinavir 836, 841, 843–4
   nevirapine interactions 841
   pregnancy safety 844
sarcolemma 412
sarcomas, more common in children 766

sarin 208–9
saturable metabolism 134–5
saw palmetto 62t, 736
scabicides 916–7
scale (skin condition) 906
scheduling 51, 77–8, see also regulation
Schistosoma spp. 863
schizonticides, see antimalarials
schizophrenia 312, 322c, 322–3
schizophreniform psychosis 323
scientific medicine 6, 88
sclera 585
scleritis 597
scopolamine, see hyoscine
SCOTT (NZ) 94
scripts, see prescribing
scurvy, treatment of 6
second messengers 105
secondary epilepsy 289, 298c
secretins 222
secretions of the gastrointestinal tract 553,
    555
sedatives, see also antihistamines; anxiolytics;
    H₁-receptor antagonists; hypnotics
    age-related adverse drug events 149t, 150
    chemistry of 291
    CNS effects 214c, 222
    depression evoked by 326
    diazepam interactions 287
    incontinence caused by 489t
    methadone interactions 386
    palliative care in cancer treatment 787
    psychotropic agent interactions 318
    psychotropic agents as 316
seizures, see also anticonvulsants; antiepileptic
    drugs; epilepsy
    classification of 299c
    epilepsy diagnosis 298
    treatment for 287–8
selective androgen receptor modulators, in
    'male pill' 743
selective beta₁-adrenoceptor antagonists
    197t
selective oestrogen receptor modulators 710,
    719, 781
selective progesterone receptor modulators
    742
selective serotonin reuptake inhibitors (SSRIs)
    329–30, see also 5-hydroxytryptamine
    5-HT receptors affected by 314
    adverse drug events 319t
    anorectic agents 343
    balance with acetylcholine 224
    mechanism of action 326, 328
    selegiline interactions 354
    sexual function affected by 750
    sumatriptan interactions 365
    warfarin interactions 505
selectivity 2–3, 104
selegiline 354, 354
    Alzheimer's disease treatment 362
    morphine interactions 268
    pregnancy safety 366
selenium, risks of 56c
selenium sulfide
    for dandruff 910
    pregnancy safety 928
self-medication 51–2, 57, see also over-the-
    counter drugs; polypharmacy
semilunar valves 411
seminal vesicles 697

senna preparations 576t
    pregnancy safety 581
    stimulant laxative 575–6
sensitivity to OTC drugs 58
sensory areas of cortex 217
sensory input 163, 905
sepsis 794
septicaemia 794
serendipity in drug discovery 86
Serenoa repens 62t, 736
SERMs 710, 719, 781
serotonin, see hydroxytryptamine
serotonin and noradrenaline reuptake
    inhibitors 343
serotonin syndrome 329
serpentary, toxicity 67t
Serratia infections 795t
sertraline 329
    adverse drug events 319t
    in Australia's top 10 drugs 17t
    pregnancy safety 320, 321
    selegiline interactions 354
    taste and smell effects 617t
sevoflurane 237, 237t, 238
    anaesthesia 230, 232
    pregnancy safety 248
sex hormones 627t, 699
    female reproductive system 700–4
    role in sexual function 745, 747, 751
    teratogenic potential 726
sex organs
    adrenoceptors 188t
    male, innervation of 167t
sexual functioning, drugs affecting 745–51
sexual intercourse, conception rates 741
sexual reproduction, see reproductive systems
sexual response 704–6
Shakespeare, William 750
shampoos for dandruff 910
Shigella infections 795t, 798t
shock, see also anaphylactic reactions
    cardiogenic shock 435b
    from burns 922
    treatment of 191–3
SI units 19–20
sibutramine, anorectic agent 343, 951
sick sinus syndrome 435b
side effects 3t, 153, see also adverse drug
    events
signal transduction, cell life cycles 756
sildenafil 748
    fast-tracking of 749c
    glyceryl trinitrate interactions 442
    pregnancy safety 751
silicones, emollient effects 909
silver salts, photosensitising effects 907t
silver sulfadiazine
    burn treatment 924–5, 925
    pregnancy safety 925, 928
    pressure sore treatment 927
    topical administration 915
simethicone, in antacids 565, 565t
simple epilepsy, anticonvulsants 300t
simvastatin 467
    cyclosporin interactions 892
    ezetimibe combined with 471
    hyperlipidaemia treatment 466
    in Australia's top 10 drugs 17t
    lipid-lowering effects 469t
    pregnancy safety 470
    saquinavir interactions 843

Single Convention on Narcotic Drugs 74
single-dose packs 587
sinoatrial node 414, 416–7
    action potentials 417
    calcium-channel blocker effects 443
sinus bradycardia, see bradycardia
sinus tachycardia 429
sinusitis, antibiotics for 549
sinusoids of the liver 559
sirolimus 894
sitosterol 466c
Sjogren's syndrome, ocular effects 603
skeletal muscle, see muscles; musculoskeletal
    system
skin 903–29, see also transdermal
    administration
    adrenoceptors 188t
    atropine effects 180
    depth of burn damage 923, 924
    drugs applied to 117
    grafts, rapid growth of 924
    histamine effects 897t
    innervation of 167t
    over-the-counter treatments 53t
skin cancers 755c, 912, 912c
sleep 282–4
    sleep hygiene 283c
    sleeping patterns 283
    stages of 282
sleep disorders, see also barbiturates; hypnotics
    insomnia 283, 293
    narcolepsy 342
    sleep apnoea 207, 344
slippery elm 62t
slow acetylators 124, 448
small intestine 116, 559
smell, drugs affecting 617t, 618
smoking, see tobacco use
smooth muscle, see also muscles
    adrenaline effects 189
    histamine effects 897
    innervation of 166t
snake bite 957–60
sneezeweeds 797c
soaks for skin disorders 909
soaps 911
social pharmacology 371–405
sociocultural factors in drug abuse 372
sodium, see also hyponatraemia
    absorption in the nephron 481
    fludrocortisone interactions 661
    glucocorticoid interactions 660t
    reabsorption in kidneys 477
sodium aurothiolamate, see aurothiomalate
sodium bicarbonate, see bicarbonate
sodium bromide 290–1
sodium carbonate, hexamine interactions 820
sodium channel inhibitors 303, 305
sodium chloride, see also saline solutions
    oxytocin interactions 637
    pancuronium interactions 205
sodium chondroitin sulfate, ocular use 602
sodium clodronate, see clodronate
sodium cromoglycate, see cromoglycate
sodium fluoride, in mouth-washes and gargles
    563
sodium fusidate, topical administration 915
sodium hyaluronate
    ocular use 587, 602
    pregnancy safety 606
sodium iodide, thiourea interactions 649

sodium nitrite, for sodium nitroprusside overdose 449b
sodium nitroprusside 193, 449, 449b
sodium picosulfate 575–6, 576t
sodium propionate, topical administration 918t
sodium salts 577
    lithium interactions 318
sodium thiosulfate, for sodium nitroprusside overdose 449b
sodium valproate, see valproate
solids, formulations of 42b
solubility
    effect on absorption 115
    lipid solubility of anaesthetics 229, 230, 242
solutions, skin treatment with 910
solvents, abuse of 375t
soman 208–9
somatic nervous system 202–9, 206
somatomedins 632, 936, see also insulin-like growth factors
somatostatins 222, 630, 630t, 632, 666
    cancer treatment 781
somatotropin, see recombinant growth hormone
sorbitol, laxative effects 577
sotalol 197, 197t, 430, 436–7
    avoid during breastfeeding 144t
    pharmacokinetics 198t, 430t
    pregnancy safety 199t, 437
sources of drugs 7–12, see also plant drugs
South Australia, drug legislation 76t
Spanish fly 747
SPARC gene, discovery of 95
spasms, see muscle spasms
spasticity 356–7, 360
Special Access Scheme of TGA 28, 788, 855
specific resistance to disease 870–4
specificity 2–3, 104
specified substances, in sport 939
spectinomycin 818
    pregnancy safety 821
speech pathologists and therapists, drugs administered by 35
'speed', see amphetamines; methamphetamines
sperm 705, 740
spermicidal agents 741, 743
sphincter of the bladder 487–8
spider bites 960–2
spiders, web shapes 373
spinal accessory nerve 215t
spinal block anaesthesia 247t, 248
spinal cord 213, 218–9, 219, see also central nervous system
spinal spasticity 356
spirochaetal infections 795t
spironolactone 485–6
    acne treatment 922
    alopecia from 907t
    cyclosporin interactions 892
    digoxin interactions 426t
    heart failure treatment 486c
    pharmacokinetics 484t
    sexual function affected by 751
splanchnic nerves 553
spleen 188t, 870
split-mixed regimen for insulin administration 676
sport, drugs in 82, 405, 933–44
spotted cowbane, toxicity 67t
spotted hemlock, toxicity 67t

spotted parsley, toxicity 67t
sprays, skin treatment 911
sputum 528
SSRIs, see selective serotonin reuptake inhibitors
St Bennet's herb, toxicity 67t
St John's wort 62t
    amprenavir interactions 842t
    antidepressant 327c
    atazanavir interactions 842t
    benzodiazepine interactions 288
    cyclosporin interactions 892
    digoxin interactions 426t
    drug interactions with 159
    fosamprenavir interactions 842t
    pain management 277c
    tamoxifen interactions 780
    warfarin interactions 504
stages of anaesthesia 227–9
stains, ocular 599
standard heparin, see heparins
standardisation of drugs 84–6
Standards for the Uniform Scheduling of Drugs and Poisons (SUSDP) 51, 77–8
Standing Committee on Therapeutic Trials (NZ) 94
standing orders 36–7
stanozolol
    anabolic steroid 735
    drug testing for 942c
    regulation in sport 934
Staphylococcus infections 795t, 809t
    drug-resistant 797, 798t, 805t
    superinfection with 798
    topical 915
starch powders 910
State and territory legislation 83, see also names of states and territories
statins (HMG-CoA reductase inhibitors)
    amprenavir interactions 842t
    atazanavir interactions 842t
    cyclosporin interactions 892
    drug groups 13t
    fosamprenavir interactions 842t
    gemfibrozil interactions 469
    hypercholesterolaemia treatment 467t
    hyperlipidaemia treatment 465–7
    nicotinic acid interactions 470
statistical methods 86, 89c
status epilepticus 297
stavudine 836, 838–9
    didanosine interactions 838
    emtricitabine interactions 838
    pregnancy safety 844
    zidovudine interactions 837
steady state plasma drug concentration 129
    clearance and 132
    defined 130b
    phenytoin 302
stem cells 677, 872
stenosis 517
stepwise management of pain 259, 260
stereotyped behaviours 339
sterilisation (reproductive) 745
sterility of ocular formulations 586
steroid hormones 621
    abuse of 380
    anabolic steroids 735–6
    chemical structure 622
    mechanism of action 625
    salbutamol interactions 536

steroid hormones—cont'd
    sources of 11–2
    terbutaline interactions 536
Stevens–Johnson syndrome, drug-induced 907t
stilboestrol, teratogenic potential 726
stimulant laxatives 575–6, 575b
stimulants, see CNS stimulants
stinkwood 271c
Stokes–Adams syndrome 191, 435b
stomach 554–5, 556, see also gastrointestinal tract
    absorption from 116
    drugs affecting 565–70
stomach cancer, combination therapy 764t
stonefish stings 963–4
storage of drugs 58, 79
strabismus 600–1
stratum corneum 904, 908
stratum germinativum 904
stratum granulosum 904
stratum lucidum 904
Streptococcus infections 795t
    drug-resistant 798t, 805t
    topical 915
streptogramins 817–8
streptokinase 506
    fibrinolysis effects 500
    heparin interactions 501
    pregnancy safety 512
    warfarin interactions 505
Streptomyces avermitilis 865
streptomycin
    capreomycin interactions 857
    pregnancy safety 821
    resistance to 798t
    skin conditions from 907t
    statistical studies 89c
    tuberculosis treatment 856–7, 861
streptozocin (streptozotocin), emetic potential 766t
stress
    glucocorticoids in reaction to 654
    hormonal responses 625c, 630
stroke
    ischaemic brain damage 362
    myocardial ischaemia 412
stroke volume (cardiac function) 418
strontium 783
    cancer treatment 761
    for bony metastases 786
    osteoporosis treatment 692–3
    pregnancy safety 693
Strongyloides stercoralis 865
structural specificity 104
structure–activity studies 6
strychnine
    bromide interactions 291c
    sport stimulant 933
subarachnoid anaesthesia, see spinal block anaesthesia
subcutaneous fat 904
subcutaneous injections 116
sublingual administration 116, 442
substance P 263
    emetic involvement 570
    respiratory involvement 518
substantia nigra 218
substitute drugs 80–1
    drug dependence treatment 382
    withdrawal symptom treatment 384

succinylcholine, *see* suxamethonium
sucralfate
    digoxin interactions 426t
    loop diuretic interactions 482
    peptic ulcer treatment 570, 573
    phenytoin interactions 306
    pregnancy safety 581
    quinolone interactions 818
    thyroxine interactions 645t
    warfarin interactions 505
sufentanil 239, 267
suffering 252–5, 252, *see also* pain
sugar content of medications 672, 673c
sulfacetamide
    adverse systemic effects of ocular treatment
      605t
    pregnancy safety 606
sulfadiazine, for toxoplasmosis 855
sulfadoxine
    malaria treatment 850, 854
    pregnancy safety 866
sulfamethoxazole
    dapsone interactions 862
    pregnancy safety 821
    sugar-free medications 673c
    trimethoprim combined with 819–20
sulfanilamide, adverse drug events 154t
sulfapyridine 885
sulfasalazine 885
    antirheumatic effects 884
    inflammatory bowel disease treatment 580,
      581
    photosensitising effects 907t
    pregnancy safety 581, 900
sulfation, conjugation reaction 122t
sulfinpyrazone
    nitrofurantoin interactions 822
    warfarin interactions 505
sulfite sensitivity 191b
sulfonamides
    bacteriostatic agents 796
    cytochrome P450 isoform inhibition 158t
    didanosine interactions 838
    hexamine interactions 820
    methotrexate interactions 775
    ocular use 596
    phenytoin interactions 306
    photosensitising effects 600, 605, 907t
    skin conditions from 907t
    success of 794
    warfarin interactions 505
    zalcitabine interactions 840
sulfonylureas
    diabetes treatment 677–8
    drug groups 13t
    pharmacokinetics 678t
    photosensitising effects 907t
    taste and smell effects 617t
sulfotransferases 122t, 123
sulfur mustard gas 209c
sulfur preparations 910
    acne treatment 921
    pregnancy safety 928
    tretinoin interactions 922
sulindac 879t
    didanosine interactions 838
    pharmacokinetics 881t
    warfarin interactions 505
    zalcitabine interactions 840
sulthiame 307–8
    membrane-stabilising actions 303

sulthiame—cont'd
    pregnancy safety 309
sumatriptan **365**
    analgesic effects 276
    headache treatment 366
    migraine treatment 364
    pregnancy safety 366
    selegiline interactions 354
sun protection factors 914t
sunscreens 911–4, 912c
    photosensitising effects 907t
superinfection 798, 806c
supply of drugs, legal issues 79
supportive cancer therapy 783–8
suppositories 659, *see also* rectal
    administration
supraventricular tachycardia 435b
surface anaesthesia 245
surface area dosage 21–2, 145
surgery, *see also* anaesthetics
    cancer treatment 760
    pain management 277
    psychiatric disorders 322
SUSDP 51, 77–8
sustained-release preparations 43
suxamethonium 204–5, **207**
    adjunct to anaesthesia 230, 235
    cyclophosphamide interactions 774
    digoxin interactions 426t
    metoclopramide interactions 568
    muscle relaxant 357–8
    pancuronium interactions 205
    pregnancy safety 248
    premedication with 235t
SVR 419
swallowing 553–4
sweat glands 126, 904
swimmer's ear 611c
Sydney 2000 Olympic Games 736
    drug testing at 941–2, 942c
symbols in prescriptions 39, 40–1t
sympathetic nervous system 164–5, 168t
    in cardiac action 419
    respiratory involvement 518
sympatholytic drugs 178, 193–8
    sexual function affected by 749
sympathomimetic drugs 178, 186–93
    amphetamines related to 339
    anorectic agents 342–3
    as decongestants 542
    dexamphetamine interactions 341
    glaucoma treatment 592, 593
    hyperglycaemia linked to 672t
    isoprenaline interactions 191
    MAO inhibitor interactions 157, 331
    methyldopa interactions 453
    nasal condition treatment 548
    nicotine interactions 397
    ocular effects 589
    ophthalmic use 590t
    oxpentifylline interactions 452
    phenoxybenzamine interactions 194
    psychotropic agent interactions 318
    regulation in sport 938, 939
    RIMA interactions 333
    salbutamol interactions 536
    terbutaline interactions 536
    theophylline interactions 537
    thyroxine interactions 645t
symporters, in kidneys 476
symptomatic epilepsy 298

synapses 169, 218, 221
synaptic vesicles 170
synthesis phase of cells 756
synthesised drugs 7
syphilis 795t
systemic anaphylaxis, *see* anaphylactic
    reactions
systemic clearance, defined 130b
systemic vascular resistance 419
systole 414, 419

T
T lymphocytes 872–3
T₃, *see* tri-iodothyronine
T₄, *see* thyroxine
tablets 39–43
tabun 208–9
tachycardia 197, 425, 429
tachykinins 222, 255
tachyphylaxis 106
tacrolimus
    caspofungin interactions 830
    chloramphenicol interactions 817
    imidazole antifungal interactions 829t
    immunosuppressant 891
    macrolide antibiotic interactions 812
    pregnancy safety 900
    sulfonamides/trimethoprim interactions
      820
tadalafil
    glyceryl trinitrate interactions 442
    pregnancy safety 751
    role in sexual function 748
Taenia spp. 863
talcum powder 910–1
tamoxifen 710, **780**
    aminoglutethimide interactions 662
    bone effects 692
    cancer treatment 779t, 780
    combination therapy 764t
    pregnancy safety 721, 789
    use in sport 935
    warfarin interactions 505
tamsulosin 193–4, 736
Tanacetum parthenium, *see* feverfew
tannins, sources of 11
tapeworms 863
tardive dyskinesia 313, 316t, 317c
target glands in endocrine system 622
tars
    coal tar 907t, 910, 920
    pine tar 909
    pregnancy safety 928
    skin condition treatment 911
Tasmania, drug legislation 76t
taste, drugs affecting 615c, 616–7
taxanes 778c
    cancer treatment 776
    emetic potential 766t
tazobactam 806
    penicillins combined with 804
    pharmacokinetics 807t
    pregnancy safety 821
TB, *see* tuberculosis
TCAs, *see* tricyclic antidepressants
TDM 45–7
tea 399, *see also* caffeine
    for respiratory disorders 543c
    social use of 399c
tea-tree oil 63, 797c
tear gases 606

tears (from the eye) 585, 608
technetium-99 cancer treatment 761
technological change 29, 97, *see also*
    computer-aided design
teenagers, *see* age factors; paediatrics
teicoplanin 810–2
    pregnancy safety 821
telemedicine 97
telephone orders 36–7
telmisartan 457
    pregnancy safety 457
telomerase 758, 762
temafloxacin, adverse drug events 154t
temazepam 392
    perinatal use 729
    pharmacokinetics 286t
    recommended for elderly 285
    sleep disorder treatment 287
temozolomide 770, 771t
temporal arteritis, ocular effects 603
tenecteplase 506
    fibrinolysis effects 500
    pregnancy safety 512
teniposide
    cancer treatment 776
    emetic potential 766t
    indications and toxicity 772t
    pregnancy safety 789
tenofovir 836, 843
    pregnancy safety 844
tenoxicam, age-related adverse drug events
    262
TENS 276
tension headache 366
teratogens 138–42, 139b, 726, *see also*
    cancer; fetus; pregnancy safety
    antiandrogens 737
    cancer treatment 767
    LSD 747
    retinoids (vitamin A analogues) 782
terazosin 193–4, 736
    pregnancy safety 737
terbinafine 917, 918t
    topical antifungal 916
terbutaline
    asthma treatment 534, **536**, 548c
    pregnancy safety 549
    regulation in sport 935
    sugar-free medications 673c
terfenadine, adverse drug events 154t
teriparatide 686, **686**
    osteoporosis treatment 692
    pregnancy safety 693
terpenes, sources of 11–2
tertiary amines 179
testes 627t, 736–7
testosterone 627t, 698, 705, 734–5
    depot preparations **735**
    derivatives from 712
    erectile dysfunction treated with 749
    'male pill' 743
    marijuana lowers levels of 746
    pregnancy safety 737
    regulation in sport 934, 935
    sexual function affected by 745
tetanus, following burns 924
tetrabenazine, as muscle relaxant 357
tetracaine, *see* amethocaine
tetracosactrin
    pregnancy safety 636, 662
    regulation in sport 936

tetracyclines 815–6
    acne treatment 922
    adverse drug events 319t
    antacid interactions 566t
    avoid during breastfeeding 144t
    bacteriostatic actions 796
    bile acid-binding resin interactions 468
    bone binding 119–20
    didanosine interactions 838
    disopyramide interactions 432t
    dosage 815t
    drug groups 13t
    ocular use 596
    peptic ulcer treatment 570–1
    photosensitising effects 605, 907t
    pregnancy safety 606, 821, 928
    skin conditions from 907t
    sucralfate interactions 573
    superinfection from 798
    teratogenic potential 142t, 726
    zalcitabine interactions 840
tetrahydrocannabinol, *see* cannabinoids
tetrahydrozoline
    ocular use 590–2, 590t
    pregnancy safety 606
thalidomide 75c
    adverse drug events 154t
    as orphan drug 80c
    cancer treatment 785–6
    effects of 139–40
    pregnancy safety 789
    regulation prompted by 75
    teratogenic potential 726
thallium-201 cancer treatment 761
THC, *see* cannabinoids
thebaine, developed in Australia 90t
theobromine, social use of 398
theophylline
    aciclovir interactions 832
    asthma treatment 532, **537**, 548c
    avoid during breastfeeding 144t
    cimetidine interactions 572
    H_2-receptor antagonist interactions 572t
    low hepatic clearance 132t
    macrolide antibiotic interactions 812
    mexiletine interactions 435
    neonatal dose 145t
    nicotine interactions 397
    pregnancy safety 549
    quinolone interactions 818
    rifampicin interactions 859
    ritonavir interactions 843
    sleep pattern effects 284t
    social use of 398
    St John's wort interactions 327c
    sucralfate interactions 573
    vasoconstrictor 344
    zafirlukast interactions 538
therapeutic drug monitoring 45–7
Therapeutic Goods Act 1989 (Cth) 76, 79–80
Therapeutic Goods Administration 27
    NSAID recommendations 882
    regulatory role 51
    reviews alternative medicines 60
therapeutic interventions, decisions before 35
therapeutic ranges 47, 129
thiazide diuretics 481–5
    adverse drug events 485
    age-related adverse drug events 149t
    bile acid-binding resin interactions 468
    calcitriol interactions 691

thiazide diuretics—cont'd
    didanosine interactions 838
    digoxin interactions 426t
    drug interactions 485
    hyperglycaemia linked to 672t
    insulin interactions 675
    ocular adverse drug events 605t
    pharmacokinetics 484t
    photosensitising effects 605, 907t
    plasma lipid profile effects 464t, 470
    regulation in sport 937
    skin conditions from 907t
    zalcitabine interactions 840
thiazolidinediones (glitazones) 679–80
    diabetes treatment 677
    drug groups 13t
    imidazole antifungal interactions 829t
thioguanine
    cancer treatment 773
    indications and toxicity 771t
    pregnancy safety 789
thionamides 646, 648–9
thiopentone 230, 237–9
    lipid reservoir for 119
    pregnancy safety 248
    sexual function affected by 750
thioridazine 324
    cytochrome P450 isoform inhibition 158t
    major effects 315t
    pregnancy safety 320
    risk of arrhythmia 318c
    sedative effects 316
    sexual function affected by 750
thiotepa 770, 771t
thiothixene, avoids anticholinergic effects 316
thiourea drugs 646, 648–9
thioxanthines 315t, 324, 750
thornapple, toxicity 67t
throat, over-the-counter drugs for 53t
thrombi 500
thrombocytes, *see* platelets (thrombocytes)
thrombocytopenia 494
    from chemotherapy 765, 784
    heparin-induced 502
thrombokinase 495t
thrombolytics 506–7
    aprotinin interactions 511
    dipyridamole interactions 509
    glycoprotein IIb/IIIa receptor inhibitor
        interactions 510
    heparin interactions 501
    oxpentifylline interactions 452
    stroke treatment 362
thrombopoietin 492
thromboxane A_2 495t, *880*
thrush, *see Candida* infections
thujone, respiratory stimulation by 528
thymidylate synthetase, cancer treatment 762
thymine 757
thymol, in liniments and rubs 910
thymus gland 870
thyroglobulin, production of 641
thyroid 627t
thyroid hormones 621, 640–9, *see also*
    hyperthyroidism; hypothyroidism
    control of 642
    dexamphetamine interactions 341
    hyperglycaemia linked to 672t
    sleep pattern effects 284t
    synthesis of *641*
    warfarin interactions 505

thyroid-stimulating hormone 626t, 641–2
thyroid storm 646
thyrotoxicosis, *see* hyperthyroidism
thyrotrophin-releasing hormone 630
thyroxine 627t, 640, 644, **645**
 bile acid-binding resin interactions 468
 dosage 644t
 pregnancy safety 650
tiagabine
 anticonvulsant effects 303
 GABA receptor agonist 303, 305
 pregnancy safety 309
tiaprofenic acid 879t, 881t
tibolone 719–20
 pregnancy safety 721
ticarcillin 804, 806
 adverse drug events 807
 pharmacokinetics 807t
 pregnancy safety 821
 warfarin interactions 505
ticlopidine
 glycoprotein IIb/IIIa receptor inhibitor
  interactions 510
 platelet effects 500, 509–10
 pregnancy safety 512
tiludronate, pregnancy safety 693
timolol 197t
 adverse systemic effects of ocular treatment
  605t
 asthma induced by 603c
 glaucoma treatment 592, 593t
 latanoprost interactions 594
 pharmacokinetics and dosages 198t
 pregnancy safety 199t, 606
tinctures, skin treatment 911
tinidazole
 alcohol interactions 391
 amoebicidal agent 855
tinnitus 612, 614–6
tiotropium
 asthma treatment 535
 pregnancy safety 549
tirofiban 500, 509–10
 pregnancy safety 512
tissue amoebicides 855
tissue binding, and drug distribution
 119–20
tissue thromboplastin 495t
titanium dioxide, in sunscreens 913
TIVA 238
TNM method of tumour monitoring 760
tobacco use 394–6
 anaesthesia and 234
 cancer linked to 760
 COPD due to 542, 542c
 deaths resulting from 376
 in Australia 378–9
 in New Zealand 379c
 oestradiol valerate interactions 711
 pregnancy safety 405
 statistical studies 89c
 symptoms of abuse 374t
 theophylline interactions 537
tobramycin 814
 as orphan drug 80t
 ocular use 596
 ototoxicity 615
 pregnancy safety 606, 821
tocolytics 727–9
tocopherols, *see* vitamin E
tolbutamide, diabetes treatment 677

tolerance 372
 pharmacological factors 375–6
 to alcohol 390
 to analgesics 255–6
 to opioids 263
tolnaftate 916, 918t
tolterodine 182t, 488
toluene, photosensitising effects 907t
tonic–clonic generalised epilepsy 297
 anticonvulsants 300t
 treatment of 303
tonic water 853c
tonsils 870
toothpaste 564
topical administration 117, *see also*
  transdermal administration
 formulations for 42b
 glucocorticoids 658
 in children 145–7
 local anaesthetics 244, 245, 247t
topical antimicrobials 914–7, 918t
topiramate **304**
 anticonvulsant effects 303
 GABA receptor agonist 303, 305
 migraine treatment 364
 pregnancy safety 309
topoisomerase I inhibitors
 cancer treatment 761, 776
 indications and toxicity 772t
topoisomerase II inhibitors, *see*
  fluoroquinolones
topoisomerases, in DNA synthesis 757–8
topotecan
 cancer treatment 776
 emetic potential 766t
 indications and toxicity 772t
 pregnancy safety 789
toremifene
 cancer treatment 779t, 781
 pregnancy safety 789
 use in sport 935
torsade de pointes 435b
total body clearance *131*
total body water
 drug distribution to 118t
 in neonates 145t
total intravenous anaesthesia 238
total peripheral resistance 419
Tourette's syndrome, haloperidol treatment 325
toxaemia of pregnancy (eclampsia) 301c
toxicology 3t, *see also* adverse drug events
 anaesthesia 229
 anticholinesterases 207
 antineoplastic agents 772t
 digoxin 427b
 envenomation 957–64
 excitotoxins 222
 herbal remedies 67t
 kombucha mushroom 69
 neuromuscular blocking 204c, *206*, 241
 nicotine 395
 oxygen 525
 studies of 88
 thyroid glands 640c
 topical poisons 905c
toxoplasmosis 596, 855
tracheobronchial tree *516*
trachoma 595
trade names 14
traditional medicine 65–6, *see also*
  complementary and alternative medicine

traffic accidents, alcohol and *389*
tramadol 269
 dosage forms 266t
 not a controlled drug 265
 pregnancy safety 278
trandolapril 456
 pregnancy safety 457
tranexamic acid
 dysfunctional uterine bleeding treatment
  720
 haemostatic effects 511
 pregnancy safety 512
tranquillisers 322, 595, *see also*
  antipsychotics; anxiolytics
Trans-Tasman Scheduling Harmonisation 77
transcutaneous absorption of drugs, *see*
  transdermal administration
transcutaneous electrical nerve stimulation
 276
transdermal administration 910, *see also* skin;
  topical administration
 analgesics 261
 fentanyl 267c
 glyceryl trinitrate 443, *444*
 skin conditions from 907t
transferase enzymes 123
transplants
 pancreatic tissue 677
 rejection control 893–5
transtympanic perfusion 612
tranylcypromine
 adverse drug events 319t
 morphine interactions 268
 pregnancy safety 320
 tyramine reaction 331, 331c
trastuzumab 781–2
 pregnancy safety 789
travellers' diarrhoea 579c
travoprost
 glaucoma treatment 593t, 594
 pregnancy safety 606
trematodes 863
Treponema pallidum infections 795t
tretinoin
 acne treatment **922**
 cancer treatment 782
 pregnancy safety 928
 wrinkle treatment 921c
tri-iodothyronine 627t, 640, 642, 644
 dosage 644t
 pregnancy safety 650
trials, *see* clinical trials
triamcinolone
 ear treatment 613–4
 pharmacokinetics 657t
 pregnancy safety 618, 662
 topical administration 919
triamterene 485–6
 biguanide interactions 678
 cyclosporin interactions 892
triazolam
 adverse drug events 289
 amprenavir interactions 842t
 efavirenz interactions 840
 imidazole antifungal interactions 829t
 indinavir interactions 842
 macrolide antibiotic interactions 812
 pharmacokinetics 286t
 recommended for elderly 285
 ritonavir interactions 843
 saquinavir interactions 843

triazolam—cont'd
sleep disorder treatment 287
triazole antifungals 826, 829t
Trichinella spiralis 864
trichloracetic acid, wart treatment 916
trichloro-ethane-diol, *see* chloral hydrate
trichomoniasis 855
Trichophyton infections 916
triclosan 915, 927
tricuspid valve 411
tricyclic antidepressants 329
acetylcholine balance 224
adjuvant analgesics 276
adrenaline interactions 190
adverse drug events 319t
age-related adverse drug events 149t, 319–20
atropine interactions 180
baclofen interactions 358
carrier transport 104
chlorpromazine interactions 323
cimetidine interactions 572
clonidine interactions 452
constipation treatment 574
dexamphetamine interactions 341
diphenoxylate interactions 579
disopyramide interactions 432t
entacapone interactions 355
fosamprenavir interactions 842t
H₂-receptor antagonist interactions 572t
mechanism of action 326, *326*, 328
noradrenaline interactions 191
overdose 331b
photosensitising effects 907t
sexual function affected by 750
thyroxine interactions 645t
urticaria treatment 920
vertigo treatment 612
withdrawal affects sleep patterns 284t
trifluoperazine
extrapyramidal effects 324
major effects 315t
piperazine compound 324
pregnancy safety 320
trigeminal nerve 215t
triglycerides 462, 470
trigone area 478
trimeprazine, pregnancy safety 899
trimetaphan, adverse drug events 181t
trimethoprim
biguanide interactions 678
cytochrome P450 isoform inhibition 158t
dapsone interactions 862
lamivudine interactions 838
pregnancy safety 821
procainamide interactions 433t
sugar-free medications 673c
sulfonamides combined with 819–20
urinary tract infection treatment 820
trimipramine 329
pregnancy safety 320
triphasic oral contraceptives 715
triptan drugs
migraine treatment 364
taste and smell effects 617t
trochlear nerve 215t
troglitazone 680
adverse drug events 154t
diabetes treatment 677
trophic hormones 622, 630
tropicamide
clinical use and administration 182t

tropicamide—cont'd
glaucoma treatment 590
ocular use 589, 589t
pregnancy safety 606
tropisetron
antiemetic use 567t, 569
cancer treatment 783
pregnancy safety 581
tropomyosin 417
tryptophan, sedative effects 292c
tuberculosis 546, 856
dissemination of *860*
drug-resistant 797
statistical studies 89c
treatment of 264c
tubular reabsorption 476
tubular secretion 145t, 476
tumour lysis syndrome 765–6, 784
tumour necrosis factor
as orphan drug 80t
cancer treatment 762
etanercept 886
tumours, *see also* cancer treatment; skin
cancers
in the skin *906*
turbocurarine 204–5
Turning the Tide program 381
turnover of receptors 106
twin studies, interindividual variability 124
twitching 205
tympanic membrane 612
type 1 diabetes 670
type 2 diabetes 670–1
obesity linked to 948, 950
Type A to F adverse drug events 154–5
tyramine
MAO inhibitor interactions 157, 331,
331c
selegiline interactions 354
tyrosine
dopamine derived from 350
in nerve transmission 172
tyrosine kinase inhibitors 13t, 782

U

UDP-glucoronosyltransferases 123
conjugation reaction 122t
drug-related inhibition 158
UK 60, 63
ulcerative colitis 580–1, 855
ulcers, *see* peptic ulcer disease
ultrashort-acting barbiturates 238–9
ultraviolet radiation
carcinogenesis induced by 759
photosensitisation to 911
skin damage from 912–3
un-ionised drugs (or states), effect on
absorption 115
undecenoic acid 918t
undecylenic acid, topical antifungal 916
under-treatment of pain 257
unfractionated heparin, *see* heparins
United Kingdom 60, 63
United Nations drug regulations 74–5, 84
United States
alcohol-related incidents 376
alternative medicine in 60
herbal remedies 159
orphan drugs in 80
unscheduled drugs 51–2
upregulation 106

urea hydrogen peroxide, *see* carbamide
peroxide
ureters 474
urethra 474, 478
uric acid production *889*, *see also*
hyperuricaemia
urinary alkalisers
hexamine interactions 820
quinidine interactions 432t
urinary bladder, *see* bladder
urinary excretion of drugs, *see* excretion
urinary tract 474, 478, *see also* kidneys
adrenaline effects 189
adrenoceptors 188t
antimicrobial treatments 820–1
atropine effects 180
innervation of 166t
urofollitrophin, infertility treatment 740
urokinase 506
fibrinolysis effects 500
heparin interactions 501
pregnancy safety 512
warfarin interactions 505
ursodeoxycholic acid 574
pregnancy safety 581
urticaria (hives) 897–8, 920
drugs causing 907t
USA, *see* United States
USAN (US approved names) 14
uterus
adrenoceptors 188t
drugs affecting 726–9
perforation by contraceptives 742
uveitis 597
UVR, *see* ultraviolet radiation

V

vaccinations
azathioprine interactions 893
cancer treatment 762
cyclophosphamide interactions 774
etanercept interactions 886
HIV 836c
immunostimulation by 895–6
meningococcal disease 876c
methotrexate interactions 775
skin conditions from 907t
spacing of 874
vagina 742, 855
vagus nerve 215t, 419
valaciclovir 831, 833
pregnancy safety 844
valerian 62t, 292c
Valerius Cordus 6
valganciclovir 831–3
pregnancy safety 844
Valium, *see* diazepam
valproate 307
age-related adverse drug events 308
anticonvulsant effects 300t, 303
antiepileptic interactions 301–2
aspirin interactions 274
bipolar affective disorder treatment 334
carbamazepine interactions 307
CNS effects 300t
migraine treatment 303, 364
pregnancy safety 309
sodium channel inhibitor 303
sugar-free medications 673c
warfarin interactions 505
withdrawal from 302

valproic acid
  didanosine interactions 838
  low hepatic clearance 132t
  mefloquine interactions 850
  penicillin interactions 806
  teratogenic potential 142t, 726
  zalcitabine interactions 840
van Gogh, Vincent 332c
vancomycin 810–2
  aminoglycosides used with 814
  biguanide interactions 678
  capreomycin interactions 857
  cidofovir interactions 834
  ototoxicity 615t
  pregnancy safety 821
  resistance to 798t
Vane, Sir John 879
vardenafil
  glyceryl trinitrate interactions 442
  pregnancy safety 751
  sexual function affected by 748
varicella 564–5, 796t, 833
vas deferens 705, 746
vasa recta 475
vascular dementia, treatment of 360–3
vascular headaches, treatment of 197
vascular system 419, 441–57, see also
    blood vessels; cardiovascular system;
    vasoconstrictors; vasodilators
  adrenaline effects 189
  calcium-channel blocker effects 444
  smooth muscle 166t, 189, 417, 897
vasectomy 745
vasoconstrictors
  adjuncts to local anaesthesia 243–4
  analgesics 276
  ergometrine interactions 728
  local anaesthetic interactions 245
  nicotine interactions 397
  ocular decongestants 591–2
  oxytocic effects 728
vasodilators 441–57
  benign prostatic hyperplasia treatment 736
  glyceryl trinitrate interactions 442
  hypertension treatment 450–7
  loop diuretics 482
  migraine triggered by 363
  oxytocic effects 728
  sexual function affected by 747
  tocolytic effects 728
vasomotor reversal effect 323
vasopressin, see antidiuretic hormone
vecuronium 204–5, 206t
  adjunct to anaesthetic 230
  pregnancy safety 248
veins 419
  adrenoceptors 188t
  innervation of 166t
venlafaxine 333–4
  adverse drug events 319t
  pregnancy safety 320, 329
  recommended treatment 328
venous thrombi 496
ventolin, see salbutamol
ventricles of the heart 411, 415–6
ventricular escape 429
venules 419
verapamil 430
  angina treatment 442c, 445
  beta-blocker interaction 198t
  constipation treatment 574

verapamil—cont'd
  cytochrome P450 isoform inhibition 158t
  digoxin interactions 426t
  disopyramide interactions 432t
  effects compared 446t
  pharmacokinetics 446t
  pregnancy safety 457
  quinidine interactions 432t
  rifampicin interactions 859
  sexual function affected by 750
  simvastatin interactions 467
vernal conjunctivitis 598, see also allergic
    rhinitis
vertebrae, see spinal cord
verteporfin 600, 782
  pregnancy safety 606
vertigo, from ear disorders 612
very-low-density lipoproteins 462
vesicles in skin 906
vestibulocochlear nerve 215t
Viagra, see sildenafil
Victoria, drug legislation 76t
vigabatrin
  anticonvulsant effects 303
  GABA receptor agonist 303–4
  pregnancy safety 309
VIGOR study 882c
vinblastine 778c
  cancer treatment 761, 776
  emetic potential 766t
  indications and toxicity 772t
  pregnancy safety 789
vinca alkaloids
  cancer treatment 761, 776
  toxicity 67t, 615t, 765
vincristine 778c
  cancer treatment 761, 776
  CHOP regimen 782
  didanosine interactions 838
  emetic potential 766t
  Hodgkin's disease treatment 764
  indications and toxicity 772t
  neurotoxicity 765
  ocular adverse effects 605t
  pregnancy safety 789
  stavudine interactions 838
  zalcitabine interactions 840
vinorelbine 762c, 772t
Vioxx Gastrointestinal Outcomes Research
    882c
viral infections 796t
virilisation, from anabolic steroids 735
visceral fat 947–8
visceral nociceptive pain 256
visceral reflexes, see autonomic reflexes
viscosity of the blood 492
vitamin A
  dietary requirements 921c
  emollient effects 909
  for athletes 940
  ocular adverse effects 605t
  teratogenic potential 142t
vitamin A analogues, see retinoids
vitamin B$_{12}$ 513
vitamin C 544, 940
vitamin D 689
  calcitriol 691
  calcium regulation by 687
  emollient effects 909
  hypocalcaemia treatment 689t
  ocular adverse effects 605t

vitamin D—cont'd
  osteoporosis treatment 692
  skin synthesises 905, 912
vitamin D analogues, psoriasis treatment
    920
vitamin E (tocopherols) 747, 940
vitamin K, intestinal production 560
vitamin K$_1$
  for anticoagulant overdose 505–6
  pregnancy safety 512
  warfarin interactions 505
vitamins 55c, 55–6
vitiligo 911
vitreous humour 585
VLDLs 462
Vogl, Alfred 481c
volatile hydrocarbons, see inhaled drugs
volatile liquid anaesthetics 237–9, see also
    inhaled drugs
volatile oils 549, 563
voltage-gated ion channels 220
volume of distribution 120–1, 120, 133
  defined 114b, 130b
  effect on half-life 135
voluntary nervous system, see somatic nervous
    system
vomiting 556–8, see also antiemetics
  cancer treatment causing 765, 783
  drugs for 567–70
voriconazole 826–7
  pharmacokinetics 829t
  pregnancy safety 844

W

waist:hip ratio 948
warfarin **504**
  age-related adverse drug events 149t
  alcohol interactions 391
  allopurinol interactions 888
  amiodarone interactions 436t
  aspirin interactions 157
  atrial fibrillation treatment 29c
  bile acid-binding resin interactions 468
  carbamazepine interactions 307
  chloramphenicol interactions 817
  comparison with other drugs 501
  efavirenz interactions 840
  fosamprenavir interactions 842t
  gemfibrozil interactions 469
  ginseng interactions 64
  griseofulvin interactions 830
  H$_2$-receptor antagonist interactions 572t
  imidazole antifungal interactions 829t
  loop diuretic interactions 482
  low hepatic clearance 132t
  macrolide antibiotic interactions 812
  metronidazole interactions 819
  miconazole interactions 826c
  NSAID interactions 883
  omeprazole interactions 571
  orlistat interactions 953
  paracetamol interactions 54
  phenytoin interactions 306
  pregnancy safety 512
  quinidine interactions 432t
  quinine interactions 852
  quinolone interactions 818
  rifampicin interactions 859
  sildenafil interactions 748
  St John's wort interactions 327c
  stroke treatment 362

warfarin—cont'd
  sulfonamides/trimethoprim interactions
    820
  teratogenic potential 142t, 726
  thiourea interactions 649
  thyroxine interactions 645t
warnings, see regulation; safety
warts 916
waste gases hazards 233c
water, see also saline solutions
  as respiratory diluent 529
water-in-oil creams 909
water resistance of sunscreens 914
WBCs, see white blood cells
weight, see dosage
Western Australia, regulation in 76t
wet dressings 911
wheals in skin 906
white blood cells 492, 494, 765
  suppressed by chemotherapy 784
white matter (brain) 214
WHO, see World Health Organization
wholesaling, legal issues 78–9
wild chervil 778c
wild tobacco, toxicity 67t
willow bark 271c
Wilson's disease 885
Wise Use of Antibiotics campaign (NZ)
    806c
withdrawal from drugs
  adverse drug events related to 155
  alcohol (ethanol) 390
  anticonvulsants 302
  benzodiazepine treatment for 288
  beta-blockers 197c
  heroin 384
  illicit drugs 376
  insomnia induced by 284t
  opioids 263
  symptom relief 269–70
  treatment of 276
  withdrawal syndrome 372
withdrawal of drugs from market 30
Withering, William 153, 423
Wolff–Parkinson–White syndrome 435b

wolfsbane, toxicity 67t
women, see also childbirth; female
    reproductive system; gender differences;
    pregnancy
  anticonvulsants for 300
  infertility in 740
  psychiatric disorders 320–1
wood alcohol 386c, 604, 604t
Wood, Fiona 924c
World Anti-Doping Agency 933
World Health Organization
  analgesic guidelines 261c
  essential drugs list 15–6
  ethical marketing code 98
  hyperlipoproteinaemia classification 464t
  Stop TB Strategy 856
worms 797, 862–4
wormwood, toxicity 67t
wound management 926

X

xanthines, see also caffeine
  asthma treatment 534–5
  oxpentifylline interactions 452
  quinolone interactions 818
  rifampicin interactions 859
  salbutamol interactions 536
  sleep pattern effects 284t
  social use of 398–9
  terbutaline interactions 536
xylene, photosensitising effects 907t

Y

yellow box 797c
yohimbine 746
young adults, see also age factors
  epilepsy 299

Z

zafirlukast 538
  asthma treatment 539
  pregnancy safety 549
  warfarin interactions 505
zalcitabine 836, 839–40
  didanosine interactions 838

zalcitabine—cont'd
  pregnancy safety 844
  stavudine interactions 838
zanamivir 93c, 546, 831, 833
  developed in Australia 90t
  pregnancy safety 549, 844
zidovudine 836, 837
  cidofovir interactions 834
  combinations of drugs 838
  emtricitabine interactions 838
  ganciclovir interactions 833t
  high hepatic clearance 132t
  NSAID interactions 883
  pregnancy safety 844
  probenecid interactions 890
  rifabutin interactions 861
  stavudine interactions 838
  taste and smell effects 617t
  triazole antifungal interactions 829t
  valganciclovir interactions 833t
zileuton, asthma treatment 539
zinc oxide
  calamine lotion 910
  powder for skin 910
  pregnancy safety 928
  protectant effect 911
  sunscreens 913
zinc stearate 911
zinc sulfate, in ocular decongestants 592
zinc supplements, for olfactory dysfunction
    618
zinc undecenoate 918t
zoledronic acid
  bone effects 693
  bony metastasis treatment 786
  pregnancy safety 693, 789
zolmitriptan, pregnancy safety 366
zolpidem 290
  pregnancy safety 293
  ritonavir interactions 843
zomepirac, adverse drug events 154t
zopiclone 289–90
  pregnancy safety 293
zuclopenthixol 324
  pregnancy safety 320